O9-BHL-982

MRI
of the
Musculoskeletal System

Second Edition

MRI of the Musculoskeletal System

Second Edition

Editor

Thomas H. Berquist, M.D., F.A.C.R.
Professor of Radiology
Mayo Medical School
Chair, Department of Diagnostic Radiology
Mayo Clinic Jacksonville
Jacksonville, Florida

Raven Press New York

Raven Press, 1185 Avenue of the Americas, New York, New York 10036

Made in the United States of America

Library of Congress Cataloging-in-Publication Data

MRI of the musculoskeletal system/editor, Thomas H. Berquist.—2nd ed.
p. cm.
Rev. ed. of: Magnetic resonance of the musculoskeletal system. c1987.
Includes bibliographical references.
Includes index.
ISBN 0-88167-667-5
1. Musculoskeletal system—Magnetic resonance imaging.
I. Berquist, Thomas H. (Thomas Henry), 1945–. . II. Magnetic resonance of the musculoskeletal system.
[DNLM: 1. Bone Diseases—diagnosis. 2. Magnetic Resonance Imaging. 3. Muscular Diseases—diagnosis. WE 141 M939]
RC925.7.M34. 1990
616.7'07548—dc20
DNLM/DLC
for Library of Congress 90-38462
CIP

The material contained in this volume was submitted as previously unpublished material, except in the instances in which some of the illustrative material was derived.

Great care has been taken to maintain the accuracy of the information contained in the volume. However, neither Raven Press nor the editors can be held responsible for errors or for any consequences arising from the use of the information contained herein.

9 8 7 6 5 4 3 2

To my patient family:
my wife, Kay,
and sons, Aric, Matthew, and Andrew

Preface

The first edition of this book was prepared and published in 1987. Magnetic resonance imaging (MRI) has expanded rapidly since that time. Improvements in hardware and new software technology have permitted examinations to be performed more rapidly and with greater sensitivity, and have even improved specificity compared with early experience. Musculoskeletal magnetic resonance imaging is the second most common application for MRI. Since the first edition, the significance of these applications and the need for an understanding of anatomy in all image planes used with MRI has become readily apparent.

The purpose of this second edition is to update the principles and applications of magnetic resonance as they apply to musculoskeletal diseases. Chapter 1 reviews the basic principles for MRI, especially as they apply to the musculoskeletal system. Chapter 2 provides essentials for interpretation of MR images based on tissue characteristics with various pulse sequences. Chapter 3 describes the general technical principles used in MRI. This includes patient positioning, coil selection, and pulse sequences for the various types of MR examinations. Safety factors and artifacts are also discussed in this section.

Chapters 4 through 12 are anatomically oriented. Important musculoskeletal anatomy principles, particularly in the commonly used MR image planes, are thoroughly discussed. Emphasis is placed on soft tissue anatomy, especially muscular and neurovascular structures that are important in assessing mass lesions and other traumatic and nontraumatic conditions involving the musculoskeletal system.

Discussion of specific pathology, except trauma, in each anatomic chapter would result in redundancy. Brief discussions of conditions such as infection, neoplasms, arthritis, and osteonecrosis are included in each chapter, especially as they apply to a given anatomic region. More in-depth discussions of neoplasms, infection, diffuse bone-marrow disorders, and miscellaneous conditions such as arthropathies, pediatric imaging, myopathies, metabolic disease, and spectroscopy are discussed in Chapters 12–15.

Technical advances are continuing in magnetic resonance and this will result in continued expansion of the clinical applications. This revised edition will update clinicians and radiologists involved in musculoskeletal imaging on the current techniques and applications for MRI.

Preface to the First Edition

The number of clinical magnetic resonance (MR) units is growing rapidly. Software, coil technology, and many hardware developments are evolving. MR imaging has become an accepted clinical tool for evaluating neurological diseases. In general, body imaging has progressed more slowly for a variety of reasons, but musculoskeletal MR is the exception. Musculoskeletal applications of MR are expanding rapidly. Motion artifact is generally not encountered in the extremities. Superior soft tissue contrast and direct coronal and sagittal imaging make MR superior to computed tomography (CT) in many situations. In addition, there is no bone artifact with MR, and nonferromagnetic metal causes less artifact on MR than CT images. Therefore, it is essential for practicing radiologists and clinicians to become aware of the clinical applications of MR in the musculoskeletal system.

The purpose of this volume is to review the principles and applications of MR as they apply to musculoskeletal diseases. The first two chapters, by Nixon and Ehman, provide information on basic principles and how these principles can be applied to provide optimal tissue contrast and characterization. The third chapter, by Berquist, is devoted to patient selection, positioning, and coil techniques. Because MR procedural aspects differ from CT and conventional imaging techniques, it is important to be aware of these factors so that information can be obtained effectively. Factors that affect image quality (coils, number of averages, matrix size, repetition time, etc.), the most commonly used pulse sequences, and patient throughput are thoroughly discussed.

The remaining chapters discuss the applications of MR in specific musculoskeletal diseases. Chapters are pathologically oriented to avoid redundancy. The chapter by Richardson is an exception in that it is devoted to spinal disorders. The final chapter, by Berquist et al., discusses future potential and miscellaneous conditions (areas where MR experience is less extensive). Comparisons of MR with CT, ultrasound, isotopes, and other conventional techniques are emphasized.

Many questions remain unanswered, including optimal field strength and clinical utilization of spectroscopy. Images in this volume demonstrate the use of a variety of radio frequency coils (surface and volume) and field strengths (0.15 to 1.5 tesla).

This volume will be of interest to physicians involved in MR imaging and to clinicians dealing with musculoskeletal diseases who may not be familiar with the principles and applications of MR.

THOMAS R. BERQUIST
RICHARD L. EHMAN
MICHAEL L. RICHARDSON

Acknowledgments

Preparation of this book would not have been possible without the able assistance of our magnetic resonance imaging technologists. Many technologists were involved; however, our supervisor, Kristie Nelson, and our technical and training supervisor, John Rasmusson, were particularly helpful.

I am particularly indebted to my secretary, Cindy Franke, for her diligent support in not only preparing the manuscript, but in hand labeling each of the anatomic images for this text. James Martin, Tom Flood, and John Hagen were invaluable in the preparation of images and illustrations.

Finally, I wish to thank the production staff at Raven Press, specifically Nicholas Radhuber, and our editor, Mary Rogers, for assistance in the preparation and editing of this text.

Contents

Chapter 1	Basic Principles and Terminology of Magnetic Resonance Imaging *Richard L. Morin and Joel E. Gray*	1
Chapter 2	Interpretation of Magnetic Resonance Images *Richard L. Ehman*	27
Chapter 3	General Technical Considerations in Musculoskeletal MRI *Thomas H. Berquist and Richard L. Morin*	53
Chapter 4	Temporomandibular Joint *Clyde A. Helms*	75
Chapter 5	The Spine *Gary M. Miller*	87
Chapter 6	Pelvis, Hips, and Thighs *Thomas H. Berquist*	149
Chapter 7	The Knee *Thomas H. Berquist and Richard L. Ehman*	195
Chapter 8	Foot, Ankle, and Calf *Thomas H. Berquist*	253
Chapter 9	Shoulder and Arm *Thomas H. Berquist*	313
Chapter 10	Elbow and Forearm *Thomas H. Berquist*	357
Chapter 11	Hand and Wrist *Thomas H. Berquist*	395
Chapter 12	Musculoskeletal Neoplasms *Thomas H. Berquist*	435
Chapter 13	Musculoskeletal Infection *Thomas H. Berquist*	475
Chapter 14	Diffuse Marrow Diseases *James B. Vogler III and William A. Murphy, Jr.*	491
Chapter 15	Miscellaneous Conditions *Thomas H. Berquist*	517
	Subject Index	529

Contributors

Thomas H. Berquist, M.D. *Professor of Radiology, Mayo Medical School; Consultant in Diagnostic Radiology, Department of Diagnostic Radiology, Mayo Clinic, Rochester, Minnesota 55905*

Richard L. Ehman, M.D. *Associate Professor of Radiology, Mayo Medical School; Consultant in Diagnostic Radiology, Department of Diagnostic Radiology, Mayo Clinic, Rochester, Minnesota 55905*

Joel E. Gray, Ph.D. *Professor of Radiologic Physics, Mayo Medical School; Consultant in Diagnostic Radiology, Department of Diagnostic Radiology, Mayo Clinic, Rochester, Minnesota 55905*

Clyde A. Helms, M.D. *Associate Professor of Radiology, University of California School of Medicine, San Francisco, California 94143*

Gary M. Miller, M.D. *Assistant Professor of Radiology, Mayo Medical School; Consultant in Neuroradiology, Mayo Clinic, Rochester, Minnesota 55905*

Richard L. Morin, Ph.D. *Associate Professor of Radiology, Mayo Medical School; Senior Associate Consultant in Diagnostic Radiology, Department of Diagnostic Radiology, Mayo Clinic, Rochester, Minnesota 55905*

William A. Murphy, Jr., M.D. *Professor of Radiology, Mallinckrodt Institute of Radiology, Washington University School of Medicine, St. Louis, Missouri 63110*

James B. Vogler III, M.D. *Senior Associate Consultant, Department of Radiology, Mayo Clinic, Jacksonville, Florida 32224*

MRI of the Musculoskeletal System, 2nd Edition, edited by T. H. Berquist.
Raven Press, Ltd., New York © 1990.

CHAPTER 1

Basic Principles and Terminology of Magnetic Resonance Imaging

Richard L. Morin and Joel E. Gray

The Nuclear Magnetic Resonance Experiment, 2
The Nuclear Magnetic Resonance Signal, 3
Magnetic Resonance Imaging, 4
Magnetic Resonance Imaging Pulse Sequences, 7
Flow and Motion Compensation Techniques, 13
Fast Scanning Techniques, 14
Chemical Shift Imaging Techniques, 15
Magnetic Resonance Imaging Artifacts, 15
Practical Aspects of Magnetic Resonance Imaging, 16
Biological Effects, 16
Siting Requirements, 18
Operational Aspects, 21
Summary, 22
Appendix, 22
References, 25

This chapter is presented to acquaint those new to magnetic resonance imaging (MRI) with the fundamental concepts and basic principles responsible for the nuclear magnetic resonance (NMR) phenomenon and MRI. At the outset, it is important to understand that this chapter is intended to be tutorial in nature. In addition to fundamental concepts of the physical phenomenon of NMR itself, clinically relevant techniques are discussed in the context of a tutorial presentation of fundamentals for those new to MRI. It is important to appreciate that the physics principles often take awhile to assimulate. There are many approaches to the discussion and presentation of the fundamental physics of MRI. Technical details and in-depth coverage can be found in MRI texts and review articles (1–5) and the educational materials provided by MRI vendors. The appendix lists terms that have been selected from the ACR glossary of MR terms (6) and are provided for the sake of completeness and reference.

A chronology of the historical development of MRI is listed in Table 1-1. The principle of NMR was first elucidated in the late 1940s by Professor Bloch at Stanford and Professor Purcell at Harvard. They shared the Nobel Prize in physics for their work in 1952. The importance of this technique lies in the ability to define and study the molecular structure of the sample under investigation. In the 1970s, the principle of NMR was utilized to generate cross-sectional images similar in format to x-ray computed tomography (CT). By 1981, clinical research was underway.

The intense enthusiasm and the rapid introduction of MRI stem from the abundance of diagnostic information present in MR images and the possibility of physiologic images in the future. Although the image format is similar to CT, the fundamental principles are quite different; in fact, an entirely different part of the atom is responsible for the image formation. In MRI it is the *nucleus* that provides the signal used in generating an

TABLE 1-1. *Historical development of MRI*

1946	Elucidation of NMR phenomena and technique—Bloch and Purcell
1951	Single dimension spatial localization—Gabillard
1952	Nobel Prize to Bloch and Purcell
1959	Blood flow by NMR—Singer
1971	*In vitro* cancer detection by NMR—Damadian
1972	*In vivo* cancer detection by NMR—Weisman
1972	NMR imaging—Damadian
1973	NMR Zeugmatography—Lauterbur
1975	Commercial development
1981	Clinical trials with prototypes

R. L. Morin and J. E. Gray: Mayo Medical School and Mayo Clinic, Rochester, Minnesota 55905.

image. We note that this differs from conventional diagnostic radiology in which the *electrons* are responsible for the imaging signal. Furthermore, it is not only the nucleus of the atom but also its structural and biochemical environment that influence and provide the signal.

Throughout this discussion we illustrate the underlying physics principles with analogies and discuss the nature of the physics from a "classical" rather than a "quantum mechanical" point of view. Both approaches result in accurate explanations of the NMR phenomenon; however, they differ in their mathematical constructs and visualization of the underlying physical principles.

THE NUCLEAR MAGNETIC RESONANCE EXPERIMENT

When certain nuclei (those with an odd number of protons, an odd number of neutrons, or an odd number of both) are placed in a strong magnetic field, they align themselves with the magnetic field and begin to rotate at a precise rate or frequency (Larmor frequency). If a radio transmission is made at this precise frequency, the nuclei will absorb the radiofrequency (RF) energy and become excited. After termination of the radio transmission, the nuclei will calm down (or relax) with the emission of radio waves. The emission of RF as the nuclei relax is the source of the NMR signal. The ability of a system to absorb energy that is "packaged" in a particular kind of way is termed *resonance.* This condition is analogous to the pushing of a child on a swing. If the child is pushed at the highest point of return, then the maximum amount of energy is transmitted to the swing. Attempting to push the child at the midpoint of return results in a suboptimal transfer of energy, and in this sense would be *off-resonance.* Hence, the resonance condition in this case is the timing of pushes with the exact frequency of the pendulum movement of the swing.

The precession of nuclei about a magnetic field is similar in concept to the precession of a spinning top in the presence of a gravitational field as illustrated in Fig. 1-1. This type of rotation occurs whenever a spinning motion interacts with another force. Nuclei with an odd number of protons or neutrons or both possess a property of "spin," which in this case interacts with the magnetic field, thereby inducing precession of the nuclei about the magnetic field. The precessional or Larmor frequency is determined by a property of the individual nuclei and the magnetic field strength [given in the SI unit tesla (T) or the cgs unit gauss (G), 1 T = 10,000 G] (Table 1-2). The mathematical definition of the Larmor frequency is given by

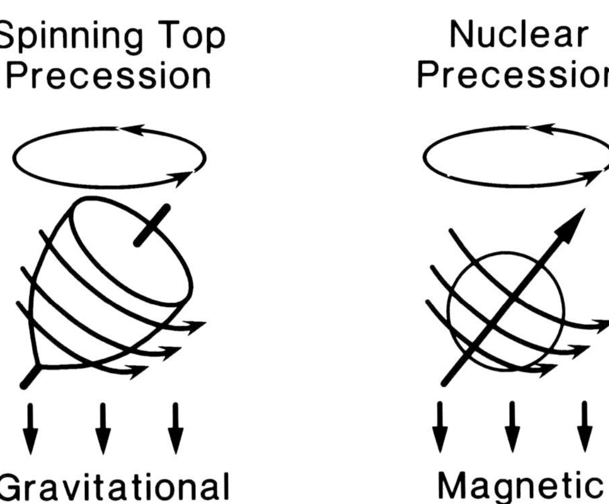

FIG. 1-1. Illustration of precession. (Adapted from ref. 1.)

TABLE 1-2. *Larmor (resonance) frequencies for hydrogen*

Field strength (tesla)	Resonance frequency (MHz)
0.15	6.4
0.35	14.9
0.50	21.3
1.00	42.6
1.50	63.9
2.00	85.2
4.00	170.3

$$\omega = \gamma \mathbf{B}_0$$

where γ is the Larmor frequency, $\mathbf{B}_0$ is the static magnetic field strength, and α is the gyromagnetic ratio (a constant that is different for each nucleus). Larmor frequencies for various nuclei and field strengths are given in Tables 1-2 and 1-3. At a field strength of 1.5 T, the Larmor frequency is 64 megahertz (MHz), which is the same frequency used for transmitting the television signal of channel 3.

In summary, the fundamentals of the NMR experiment are illustrated in Fig. 1-2 and consist of three steps: (a) placing a sample in a magnetic field, thereby inducing nuclear precession, (b) transmitting a RF pulse at the Larmor frequency, and (c) listening for the NMR signal.

TABLE 1-3. *Larmor (resonance) frequencies at 1.0 tesla*

Nucleus	Larmor frequency
^{1}H	42.6
^{13}C	11.0
^{14}N	3.0
^{31}P	17.1

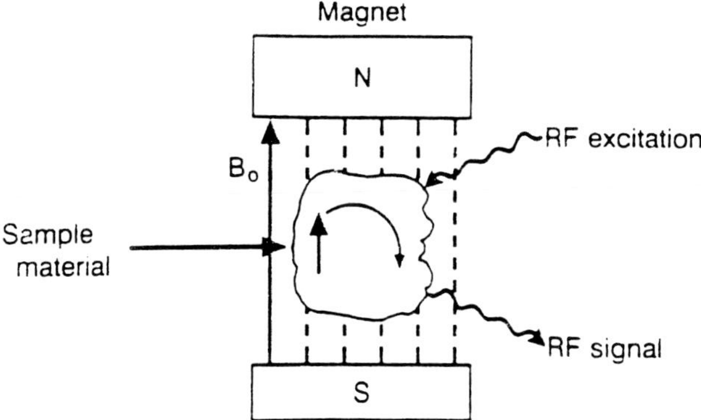

FIG. 1-2. Basics of NMR measurements. (Adapted from ref. 1).

THE NUCLEAR MAGNETIC RESONANCE SIGNAL

The form of the RF signal produced by the NMR experiment depends on the number of nuclei present (spin density) and the time it takes for the nuclei to relax (T1 and T2). The parameter T1 (spin–lattice relaxation time) measures the longitudinal return of the nuclei to alignment with the static magnetic field and reflects the chemical environment of the proton. T2 (spin–spin relaxation time) measures the transverse dephasing of the nuclei and reflects the relationship of the proton to the surrounding nuclei. These processes are shown diagrammatically in Fig. 1-3. The degree to which the NMR signal depends on spin density, T1 or T2, is strongly affected by the pulse sequence, which we discuss later. The nature of this signal and its decay due to relaxation are of fundamental importance and we discuss this process in detail.

The form of the basic NMR signal (free induction decay, FID) is shown in Fig. 1-4. The signal is a time oscillating waveform that is detected in the *xy* or transverse plane defined by the coordinate system for the experiment as shown in Fig. 1-5. The oscillating nature of the signal is due to the fact that we measure the signal in the transverse plane as it rotates about the longitudinal axis. Hence, a rotating signal is translated into a sinusoidal time-varying voltage.

It is important to understand that we can only measure the macroscopic magnetization vector, that is, the algebraic summation of all nuclear spins under investigation (Fig. 1-6). In reality, not all nuclear spins in a sample precess at the same frequency. Each individual nuclei "sees" a slightly different magnetic field due to the interactions of electrons that surround individual nuclei. The first process that occurs upon RF transmission is the phasing of individual nuclear spins to create the macroscopic magnetic vector (similar to the military command "fall in" given to a group of soldiers). This ensemble of phased nuclear spins then change their orientation with regard to the *z* axis. The rotation of this phased macroscopic magnetic vector is the property that we detect in an oscillatory sense over time.

The decay of the signal as shown in Fig. 1-4 occurs because following cessation of the radio transmission, the nuclear spins dephase and since magnetization is a vector quantity, the macroscopic magnetic vector decreases in magnitude. Since this activity takes place in the *xy* or transverse plane, this process is also called *transverse* relaxation. In a chemical sense, this relaxation is due to interactions that occur between adjacent nuclei and is therefore termed *spin–spin relaxation.* The overall behavior of substances with different T2 is illustrated in Fig. 1-7.

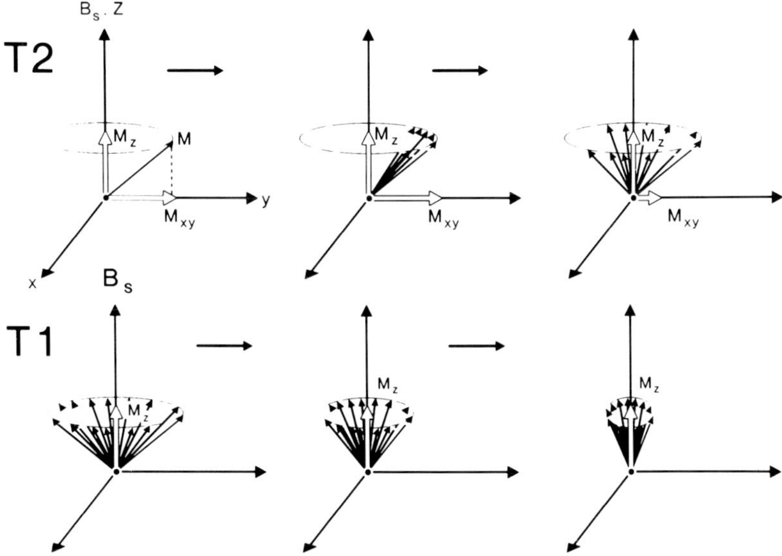

FIG. 1-3. Diagrammatic representation of T2 (spin–spin, transverse) relaxation and T1 (spin–lattice, longitudinal) relaxation.

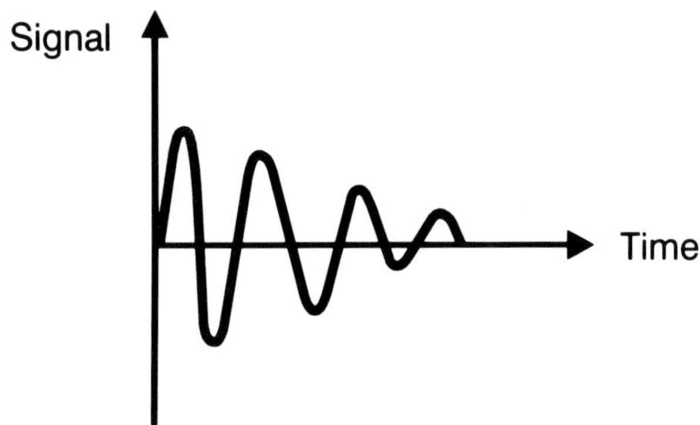

FIG. 1-4. Plot of free induction decay (FID), the basic NMR signal.

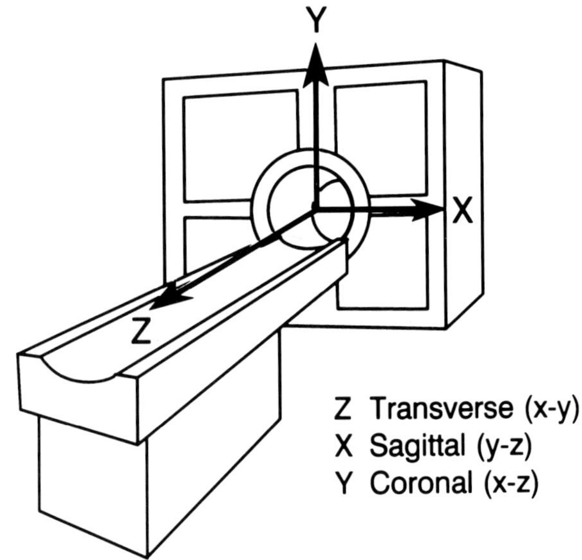

FIG. 1-5. MRI coordinate system.

As the above mentioned dephasing or T2 relaxation is occurring, the entire ensemble of nuclei are returning to alignment with the main magnetic field, which is oriented along the *z* axis. Hence, the longitudinal or *z* component of the macroscopic magnetic vector "grows" or increases with time, returning to an equilibrium value. Since this T1 recovery occurs along the longitudinal direction, it is termed *longitudinal* relaxation. In a chemical sense, this process is governed by the strength with which an individual nucleus is bound to its chemical backbone (water, lipid, protein, etc.) and hence this process is often termed *spin–lattice relaxation.* This process is diagrammatically represented in Fig. 1-8 for substances of different T1 values.

MAGNETIC RESONANCE IMAGING

A diagrammatic representation of a MRI system is shown in Fig. 1-9. To conduct the NMR experiment, a strong magnet, radiotransmitter, and radio receiver are necessary. To produce MR images, additional magnetic coils (gradient coils) are necessary to encode the signal and thus allow us to determine its origin. In addition, a computer system is necessary to control the sequencing of these operations and perform image reconstruction.

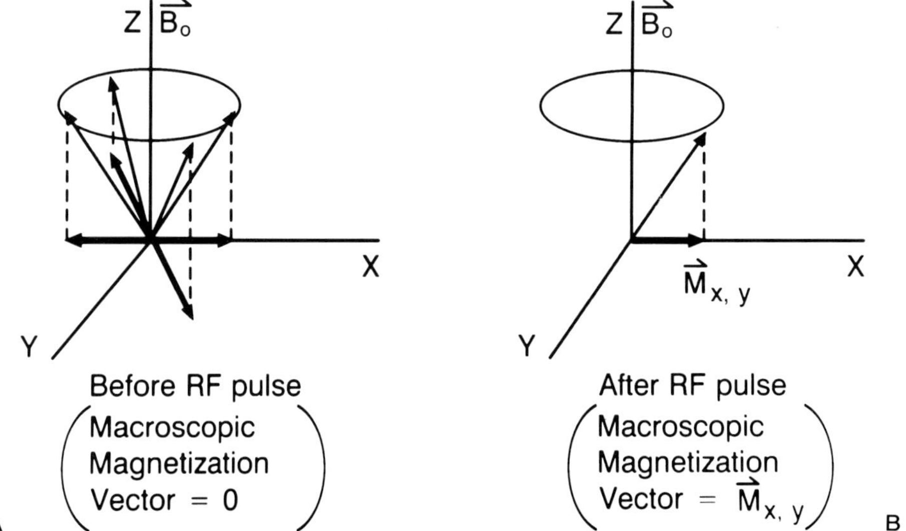

FIG. 1-6. Illustration of the macroscopic magnetic vector formed by individual nuclei. **A:** Individual nuclei 1, 2, 3, and 4 precessing about the magnetic field $\vec{\mathbf{B}}_0$. Measured macroscopic magnetization vector is zero due to algebraic summation of *x*,*y* components of dephased or randomly oriented nuclei. **B:** Macroscopic magnetization vector formed by the phasing of individual nuclei 1, 2, 3, and 4. Macroscopic magnetization vector measured is $\vec{M}_{x,y}$.

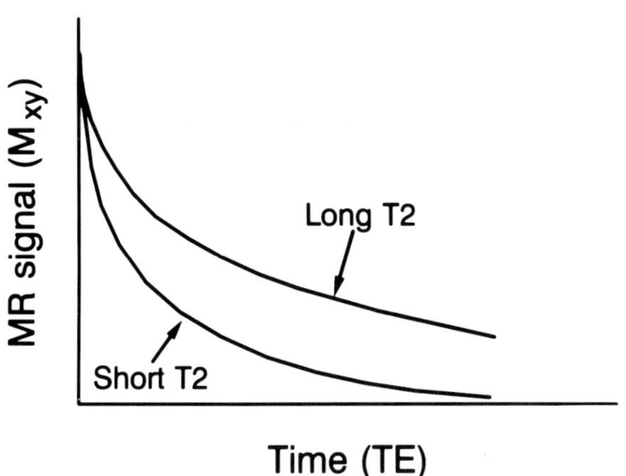

FIG. 1-7. Plot of the loss of magnetization in the transverse (*xy*) plane following cessation of RF transmission.

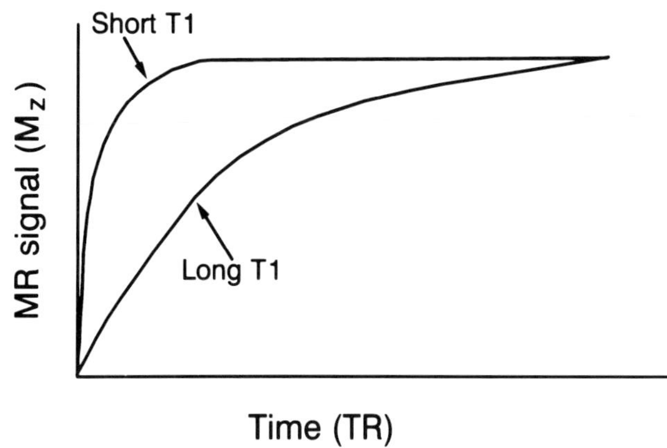

FIG. 1-8. Plot of recovery of magnetization in the longitudinal (*z*) direction.

In the most common type of MRI, spatial localization is obtained through the use of additional magnetic fields superimposed on the main magnetic field. The key to understanding this phenomenon lies in the Larmor equation. Recall that the precessional frequency is directly related to magnetic field strength. If a spatially varying magnetic field is superimposed on the main magnetic field, then precessional frequencies will be related to a location in space, analogous to the frequency obtained by the specific location of keys on a piano. This translation between frequency and spatial location is shown in Fig. 1-10.

The most common imaging technique (two-dimensional Fourier transform or 2DFT) (7–9) involves the use of three such gradient fields to localize a point in space. It is important to understand that all three gradients will be turned on and off at different times. The particular application and relative timing of the *x*, *y*, and *z* gradients determines which axis (*x*, *y*, or *z*) is being localized. In general, signals will be localized by selective application of slice selection, phase encoding, and frequency encoding gradients. A schematic diagram of the timing of these gradients is given in Fig. 1-11. We describe each in detail for the acquisition of a transverse slice.

The slice is first selected by applying a gradient along the *z* axis while applying a RF pulse with a narrow frequency range. This excites the nuclei only in the slice of interest so that they are all precessing at the same frequency and phase (Fig. 1-10). However, the signal we detect is from the entire slice, so it is not possible to form an image.

Next, the relative phase of spin precession is modified by applying a gradient in the *y* direction. This gradient

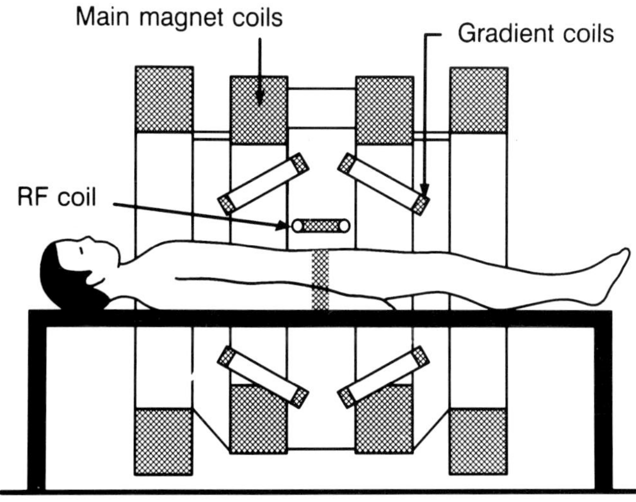

FIG. 1-9. Diagrammatic representation of MRI system. (Adapted from ref. 1.)

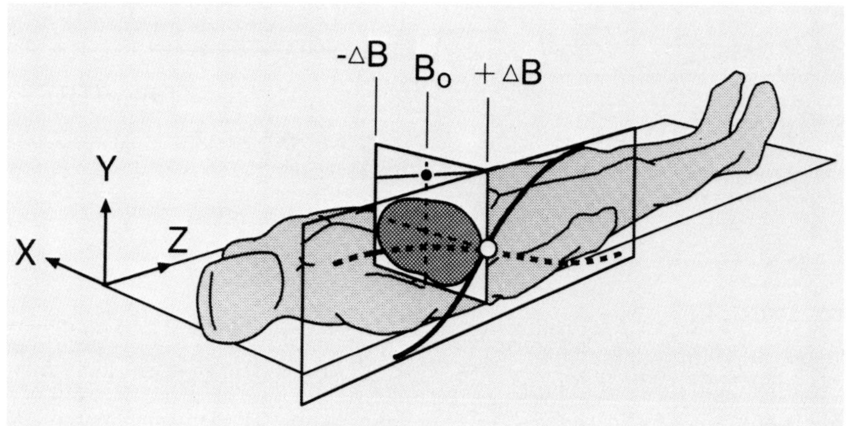

FIG. 1-10. Diagram of spatial encoding of MR signal by superposition of magnetic field gradients (different resonance frequencies correspond to different positions in the cephalocaudad direction).

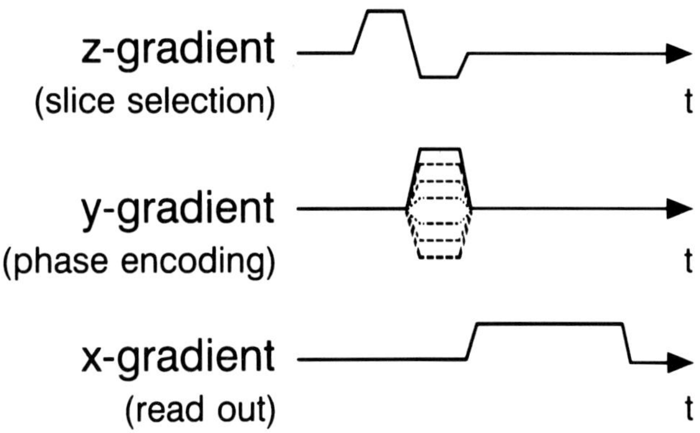

FIG. 1-11. Diagram of gradient activation versus time for MRI acquisition of a single transverse slice. For this case, slice selection is in the C-C direction, phase encoding in the A-P direction, and frequency in the R-L direction.

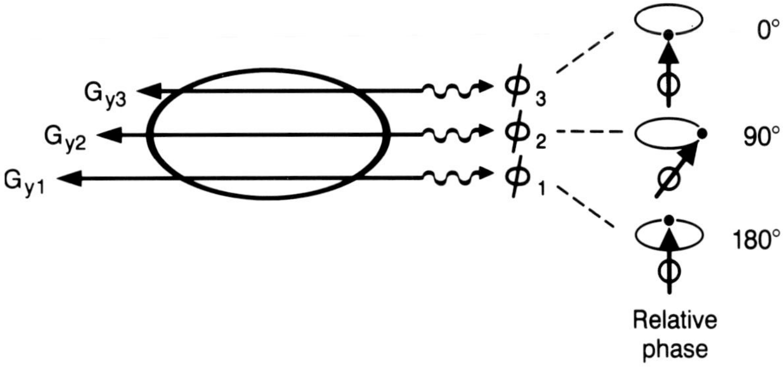

FIG. 1-12. Illustration of phase encoding in the *y* direction. Gradient increases from top to bottom.

causes the atoms to precess at different frequencies *while it is applied* (a schematic representation of phase encoding is given in Fig. 1-12). If no gradient is present, the nuclei precess at the Larmor frequency corresponding to the main magnetic field strength. If a slightly higher magnetic field is superimposed with a gradient, the nuclei in row 1 precess at a slightly higher frequency than those in row 2. Likewise for rows 2 and 3. When the gradient is turned off, all the rows will once again precess at the same frequency. However, since row 2 was previously precessing at a slightly higher frequency than row 1, all the nuclei in row 2 will be slightly ahead of those in row 1; that is, they will be precessing at the same frequency but at different phase. Likewise, each successive row will process at the same frequency but at a slightly different phase. In order to obtain discrimination in the phase encoding direction, this process must be repeated many (often 256) times. This principle of phase encoding is shown pictorially in Fig. 1-13 for a sagittal image with phase encoding in the A-P direction (10).

Last, the precessing nuclei are frequency encoded by the application of a magnetic gradient in the *x* direction. This gradient causes the atoms to precess at different frequencies (Fig. 1-14) and is usually applied while the signal is being collected (hence, it is sometimes called the readout gradient).

MAGNETIC RESONANCE IMAGING PULSE SEQUENCES

MRI pulse sequences are basically the recipe for the application of RF pulses, the sequencing of gradient pulses in the *x*, *y*, and *z* direction, and the acquisition of the resultant MR signal.

The most basic component of a pulse sequence is the specification of the RF excitation and subsequent signal detection. Timing diagrams for three pulse sequences (partial saturation, inversion recovery, and spin echo) are given in Figs. 1-15 to 1-17. We discuss each sequence in detail.

The most basic of pulse sequences is the *partial saturation* sequence. This sequence is composed of a RF pulse with sufficient power (due to the width or the amplitude of the pulse) to cause the nuclei to rotate through 90°. Following cessation of the RF pulse, the FID is measured. After a delay period, termed the repetition time (TR), the pulse sequence is repeated. Thus, the partial saturation sequence consists of a 90° RF pulse separated by a constant time, TR. By varying the parameter TR, the recovery of the magnetization along the longitudinal direction can be measured. With a short TR, only those substances with a short T1 will have fully recovered before the next RF pulse is delivered. Hence, this sequence is useful in demonstrating differences due to variation in spin–lattice relaxation times within the sample. Examples using this pulse sequence are given in Fig. 1-18.

The schematic diagram for the *inversion recovery* (IR) pulse sequence is shown in Fig. 1-16. This sequence is characterized by the application of a RF pulse of sufficient power to tip the nuclei through 180°, an inversion time (TI), and the subsequent application of a 90° pulse (to rotate the magnetization into the readout plane), followed by signal detection. This pulse sequence can also be used to measure the longitudinal recovery of magnetization (Fig. 1-19). Since the range of measured magnetization for this pulse sequence varies from $-m_z$ to $+m_z$, the magnitude of measured differences for a sample due to T1 relaxation may be larger with the IR sequence than those with the partial saturation tech-

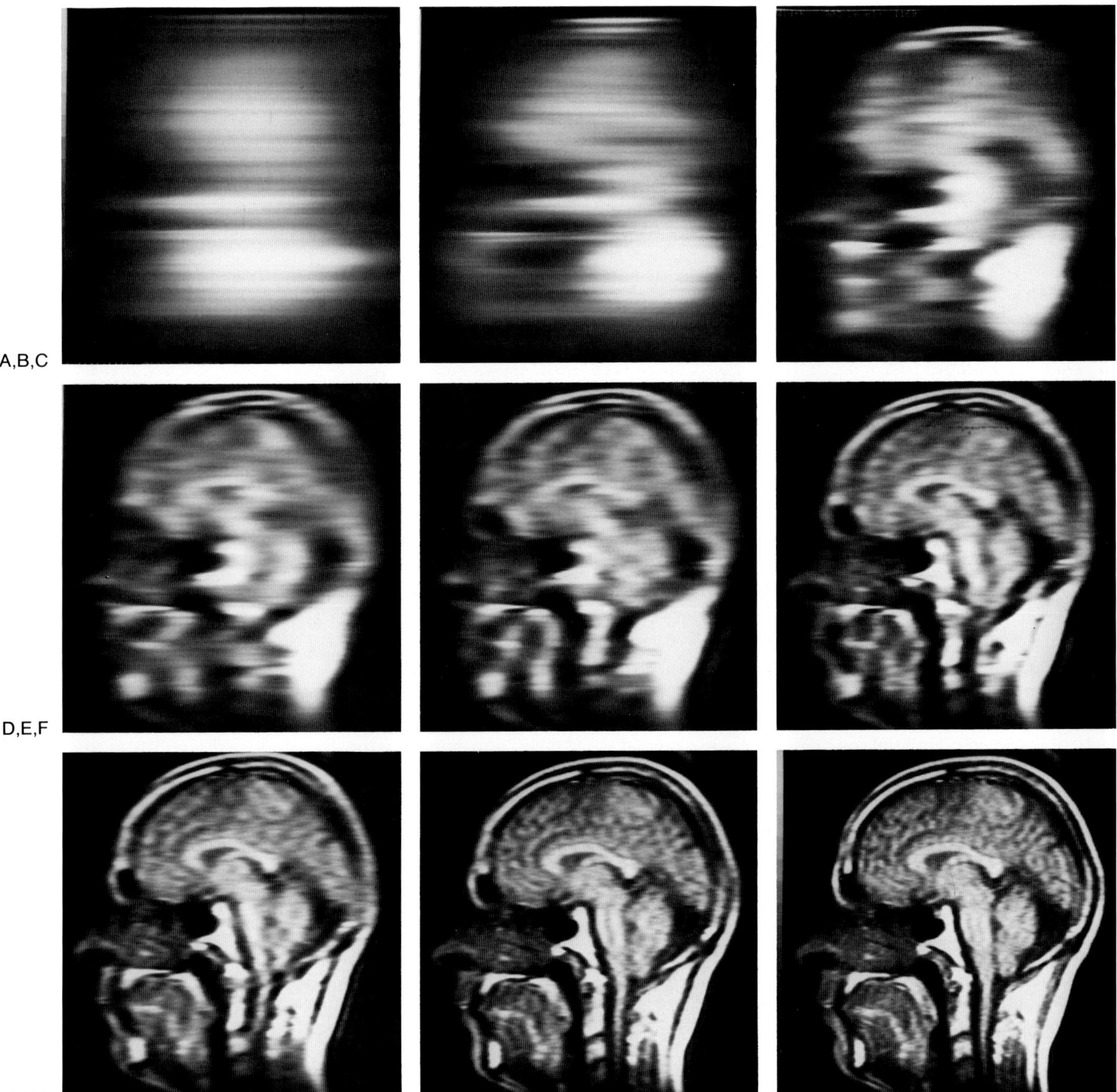

FIG. 1-13. Pictorial demonstration of MRI phase encoding (10). All images are from the same acquisition (TR = 500, TE = 25, 2 excitations, 10 mm slice, 256 phase encoding steps). The original raw data were truncated to demonstrate the effect of phase encoding. **A:** 2 steps. **B:** 4 steps. **C:** 8 steps. **D:** 12 steps. **E:** 16 steps. **F:** 24 steps. **G:** 32 steps. **H:** 48 steps. **I:** 64 steps. **J:** 128 steps. **K:** 192 steps. **L:** 256 steps.

J,K,L

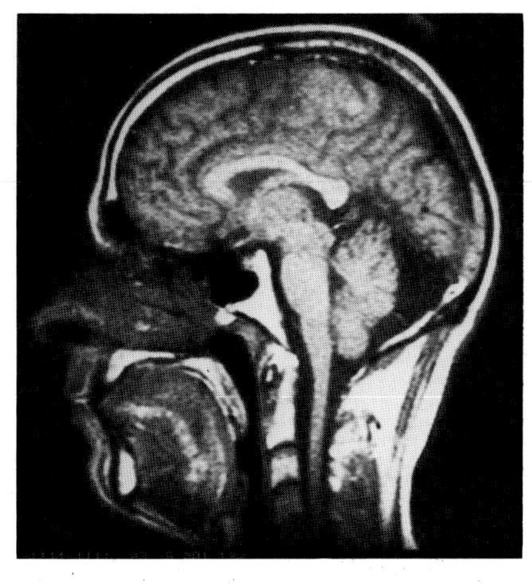

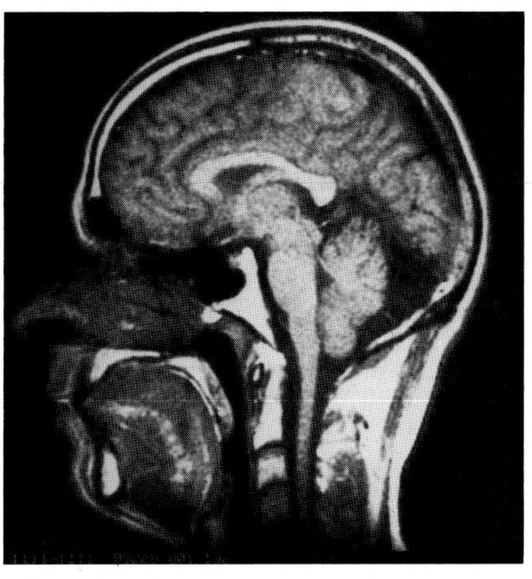

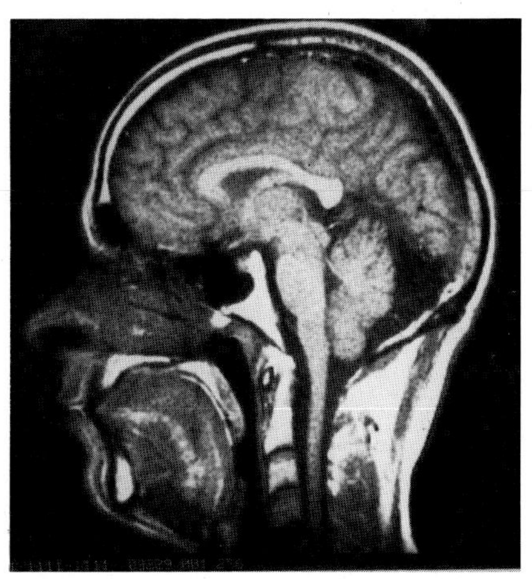

FIG. 1-13. *Continued.*

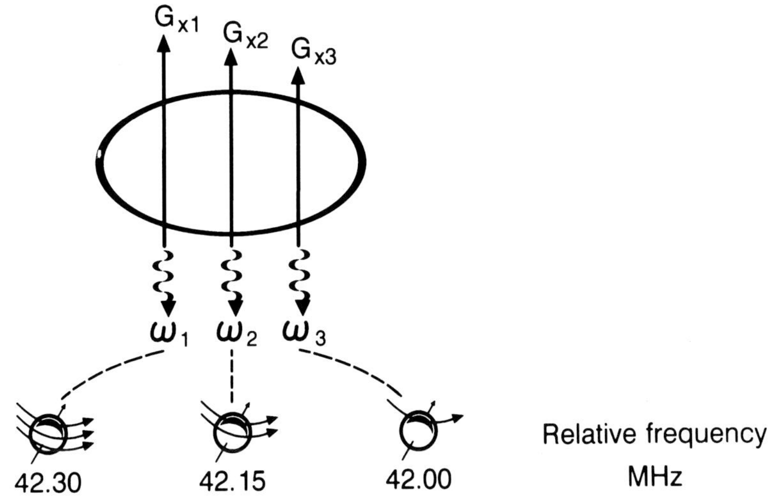

FIG. 1-14. Schematic illustration of frequency encoding in the *x* direction. Gradient decreases from left to right.

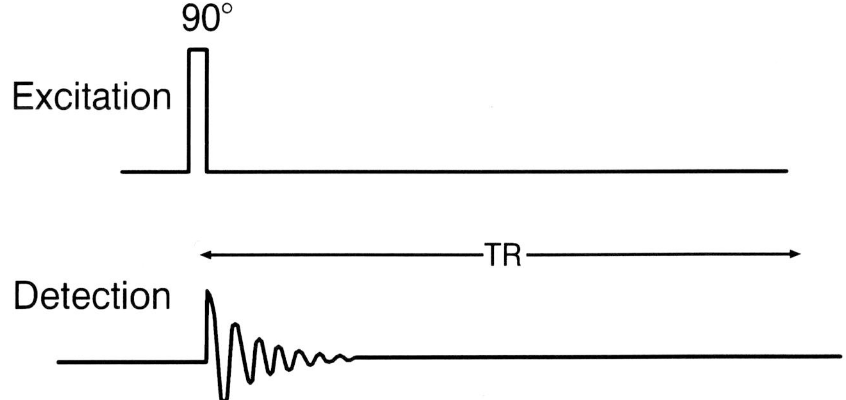

FIG. 1-15. Pulse diagram for partial saturation pulse sequence.

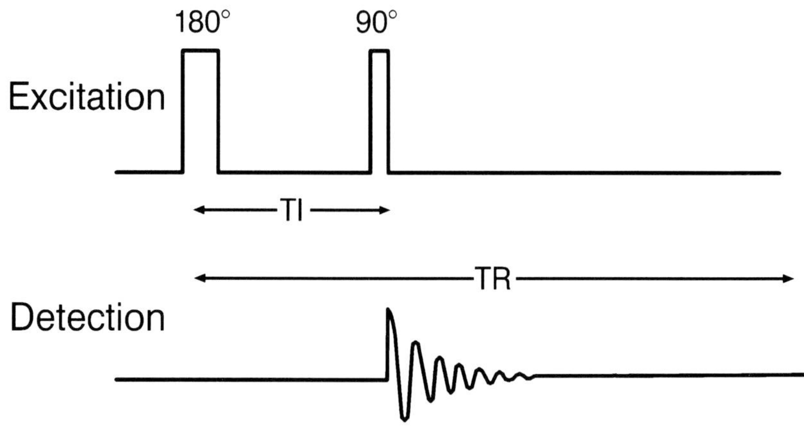

FIG. 1-16. Pulse diagram for inversion recovery pulse sequence.

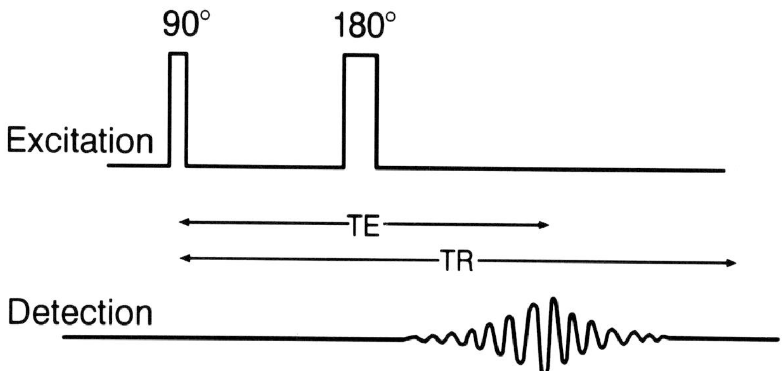

FIG. 1-17. Pulse diagram for spin-echo pulse sequence.

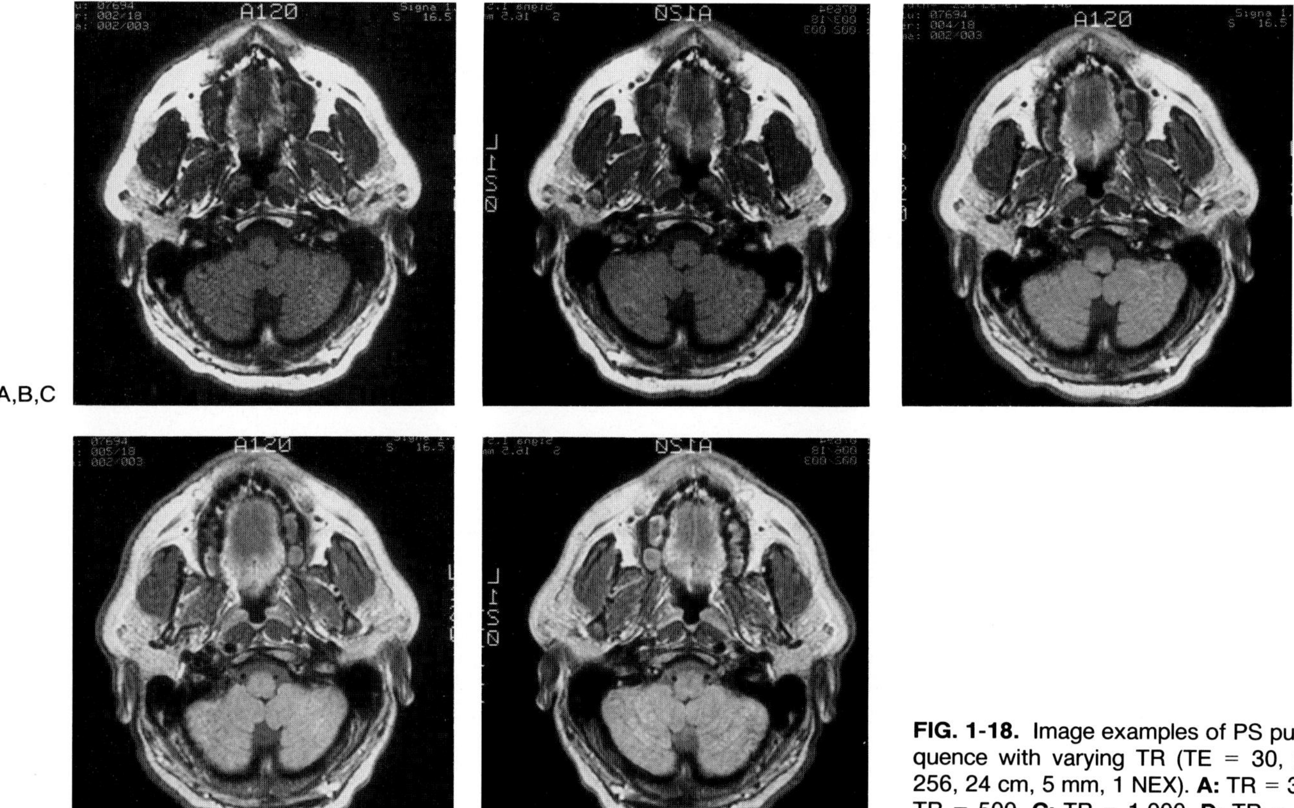

FIG. 1-18. Image examples of PS pulse sequence with varying TR (TE = 30, 256 × 256, 24 cm, 5 mm, 1 NEX). **A:** TR = 300. **B:** TR = 500. **C:** TR = 1,000. **D:** TR = 1,500. **E:** TR = 2,000.

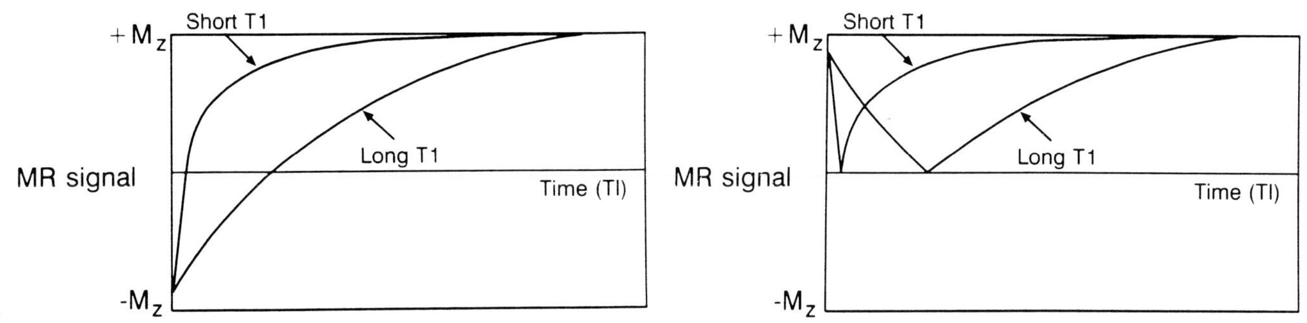

FIG. 1-19. Recovery of magnetization for inversion recovery pulse sequence. **A:** Phase sensitive image reconstruction and **B:** magnitude reconstruction.

nique (in which the longitudinal magnetization varies from 0 to $+m_z$) if phase-sensitive image reconstruction is employed. These differences may not be as pronounced with magnitude reconstruction (Fig. 1-19). Hence, image contrast due to T1 differences can be greater with IR. Examples using this pulse sequence and magnitude reconstructions are given in Fig. 1-20.

The pulse diagram for the *spin-echo* (SE) pulse sequence is shown in Fig. 1-17. The spin-echo pulse sequence is characterized by the application of a 90° pulse which therefore tips the nuclei into the measurement or *xy* plane, followed by successive 180° pulses, separated by the delay period TE, which cause the formation of successive signals for detection, which are termed spin echoes. The entire pulse sequence is repeated following the delay interval TR. The formation of spin echoes is demonstrated in Fig. 1-21. The fundamental characteristic of this sequence lies in the fact that the nuclei are

A,B,C

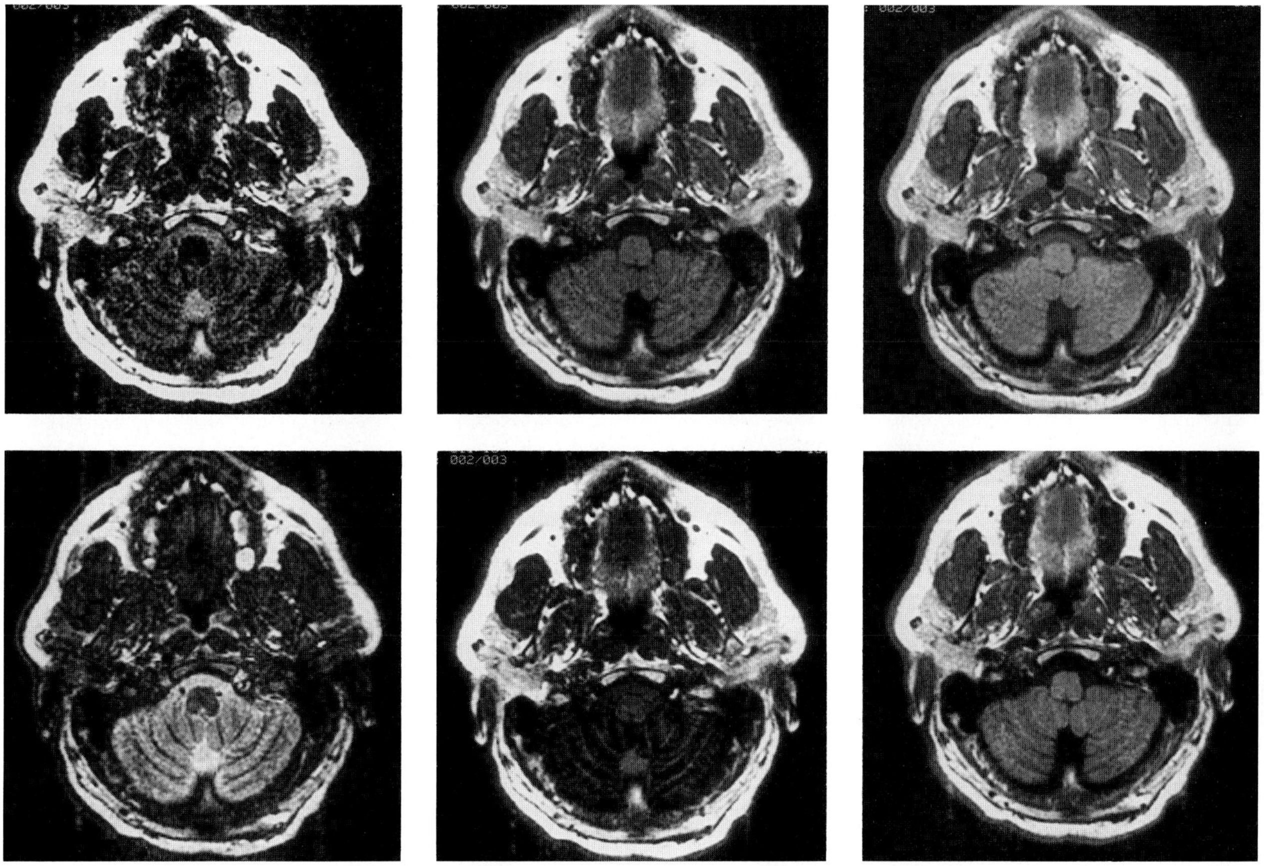

D,E,F

FIG. 1-20. Image examples using the IR pulse sequence (magnitude reconstructions) with varying TI and TR (TE = 30, 256 × 256, 24 cm, 5 mm, 1 NEX). **A:** TR = 1,000, TI = 300. **B:** TR = 1,000, TI 500. **C:** TR = 1,000, TI = 700. **D:** TR = 1,500, TI = 300. **E:** TR = 1,500, TI = 500. **F:** TR = 1,500, TI = 700.

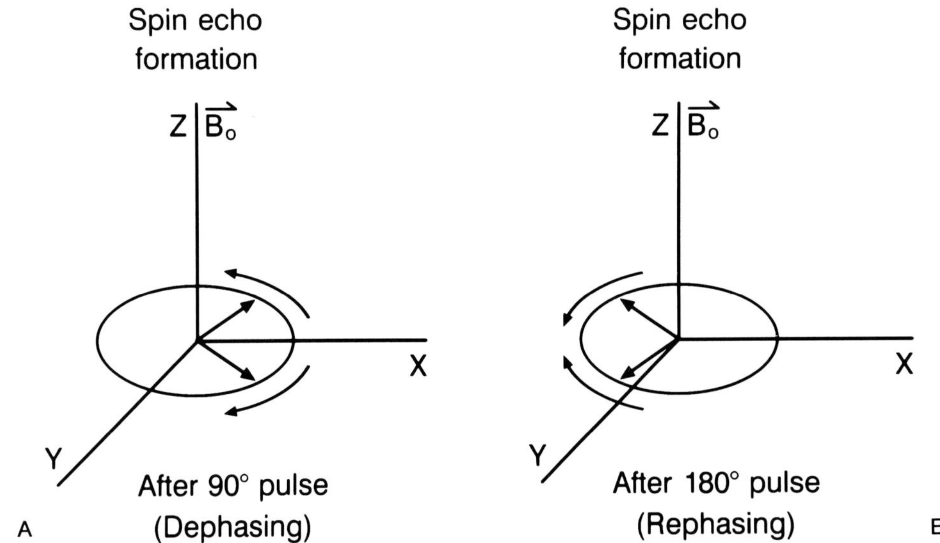

FIG. 1-21. Spin-echo formation. **A:** Individual nuclei are precessing away from one another following 90° RF pulse. **B:** Individual nuclei are precessing toward one another following 180° (rephasing) RF pulse.

dephasing following the 90° pulse. If this dephasing spin system is rotated through 180°, individual spins will now be traveling toward one another instead of away from one another. When all spins meet one another, a spin echo is produced. Following that moment in time, the spin system once again will be dephasing and can be refocused or rephased with another 180° pulse. This sequence can be useful in demonstrating differences due to either differences in spin–lattice relaxation time or differences due to spin–spin relaxation time as shown in Fig. 1-22. Examples of the use of this pulse sequence are given in Fig. 1-23.

The previous discussion dealt with pulse sequences that were concerned only with RF excitation and signal detection. Hence, this discussion would be germane to spectroscopy as well as imaging. For MRI, the pulse sequence must also identify the timing information associated with the gradients necessary to prepare or localize the signal for image reconstruction.

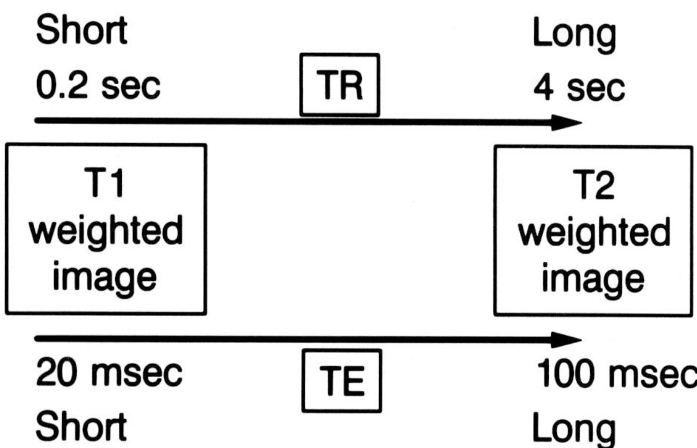

FIG. 1-22. Nomogram for contrast dependence using the spin-echo sequence.

An example of a MRI pulse sequence is shown in Fig. 1-24. We note that the gradients are labeled as slice selection, phase encoding, and readout (or frequency encoding). The reason for this specification is that slice selection can be along the transverse, coronal, or sagittal planes with phase and readout gradients along the other two orthogonal planes. The dotted lines indicating progression of phase encoding implies that this pulse sequence will be repeated many times with a differing amount of phase encoding at each repetition. The rest of the sequence will remain the same with each repetition.

It is the variation in timing and relative temporal placements of the three magnetic gradient sequences that are largely responsible for the plethora of the imaging sequences currently available. We use such diagrams in later sections to understand the differences and consequences of employing various pulse sequences. An understanding of the effects of frequency shifts and dephasing effects are of central importance to understanding image characteristics and artifacts in MRI. Because this is a currently active area of development, similar techniques have been developed by different sources, resulting in different acronyms for essentially the same procedure. It is important to note that although essentially similar results have been accomplished by various investigational groups and vendors, due to differences in hardware the exact realization may result in subtle but sometimes important differences. Table 1-4 presents a compilation of the acronyms for similar procedures (11). These acronyms represent in some cases broad classifications provided by various manufacturers, yet they are routinely used in the literature. For more information about any of these techniques, the reader is referred to the technical representatives of the particular vendor of interest.

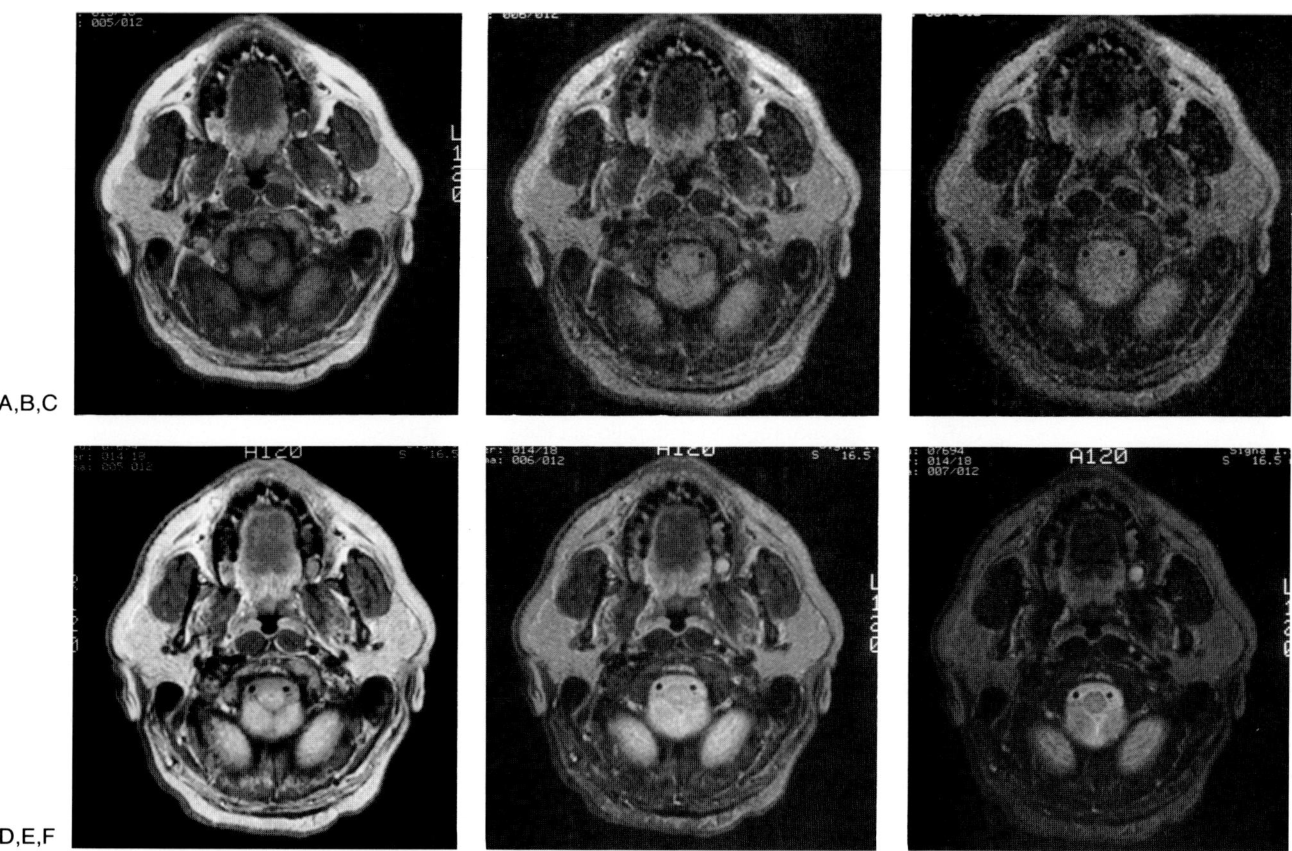

FIG. 1-23. Image examples using the SE pulse sequence with varying TE and TR (256 × 256, 24 cm, 5 mm, 1 NEX). **A:** TR = 500, TE = 30. **B:** TR = 500, TE = 60. **C:** TR = 1,000, TE = 90. **D:** TR = 1,500, TE = 30. **E:** TR = 1,500, TE = 60. **F:** TR = 1,500, TE = 90.

FLOW AND MOTION COMPENSATION TECHNIQUES

Any movement of structures during MRI data acquisition can cause artifacts ranging from image "unsharpness" (as experienced in other modalities) to intense streaks that totally obscure the image. Such movements in patients can be caused by fluid flow or physiologic motion. Since the total sampling time in the phase encoding direction is substantially greater than the sampling time in the frequency encoding direction, the amount of movement is much greater in the phase encoding direction and artifacts generally appear as linear bands in the phase encoding direction. Although the fundamental principles of physical movement during data acquisition are the same for both sources of motion, the nature of the movement produces different artifacts and, therefore, different strategies are needed for artifact elimination or compensation.

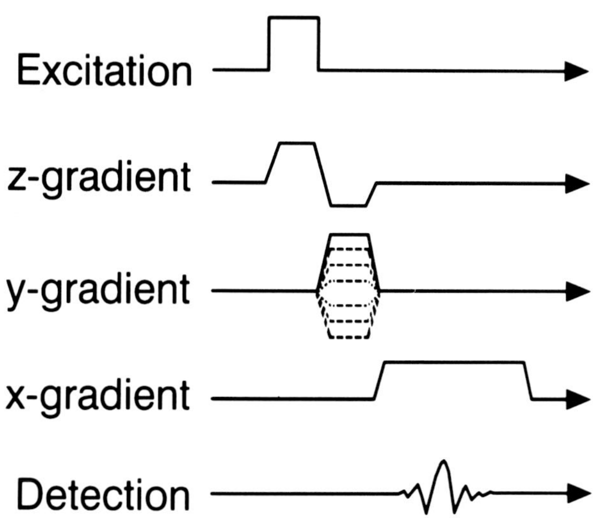

FIG. 1-24. Schematic diagram of a MRI pulse sequence.

Flow artifacts such as those shown in Fig. 1-25 occur because the spins in the flowing blood are not in phase due to their movement in the presence of the gradient (12). In 2DFT, this phase dispersal is translated to a distribution of intensities in the phase encoding direction. Two approaches are often used to eliminate flow artifacts: gradient moment nulling (GMN) and spatial presaturation (SAT). Both techniques involve changes in the basic pulse sequence yet provide different corrections. GMN (13) essentially rephases the spin systems, thereby decreasing the artifact and producing an image in which the vessel is of high intensity, while SAT (14)

TABLE 1-4. *Cross-reference of acronyms for MRI imaging sequences (11)*

Imaging sequence description	General Electric	Philips	Picker	Siemens
Flow artifact suppression				
Spatial presaturation	SAT	Rest	BOSS	Saturation
Gradient moment nulling	Flow compensation	Flow compensated gradient	MAST	GMR
Respiratory motion compensation	EXORCIST		ROPE	
Gradient recalled echo imaging				
Steady-state	GRASS/GRIL	FFE/FAME	FAST	FISP
Non-steady-state				FLASH

BOSS	Bimodal out of slice saturation
FAST	Flow artifact suppression technique
FFE	Fast field echo
FISP	Fast imaging with steady-state precession
FLASH	Fast low angle shot
GRASS	Gradient recalled acquisition in the steady state
GMR	Gradient moment refocusing
GRIL	GRASS interleaved
MAST	Motion artifact suppression technique
ROPE	Respiratory ordered phase encoding
SAT	Saturation

eliminates signal and produces a vessel of low intensity. The pulse sequences for each technique are given in Figs. 1-26 and 1-27. As demonstrated, GMN is accomplished by variation in the slice selection and frequency encoding gradients while SAT is accomplished by the addition of a 90° pulse and a localization gradient. The effects of GMN and SAT are shown in Figs. 1-28 and 1-29, respectively.

FAST SCANNING TECHNIQUES

In general, the fundamental limit on image resolution in MRI is motion unsharpness due to physiologic movement within the patient. Techniques have been developed (15–17) to acquire MRI data in very short time periods. The most popular of these use an approach to limit the flip angle of RF stimulation (less than the usual 90°) and thereby decrease the time necessary to wait for recovery. Hence, the repetition time can be decreased, allowing faster acquisitions. The concept of limited flip angle is illustrated in Fig. 1-30. The signal that is acquired is most often an echo as described earlier, except that the echo is produced not by successive 180° RF pulses but by reversal of the gradient field. The pulse sequence for this technique of gradient recalled echo (GRE) or field echo (FE) imaging is shown in Fig. 1-31. The principle of GRE imaging lies in the fact that the application of a gradient actually dephases the spins due to a difference in field strength which is dependent upon position. By reversing the direction of the gradients ($-G$ to $+G$), the effect is to rephase the spins that were ini-

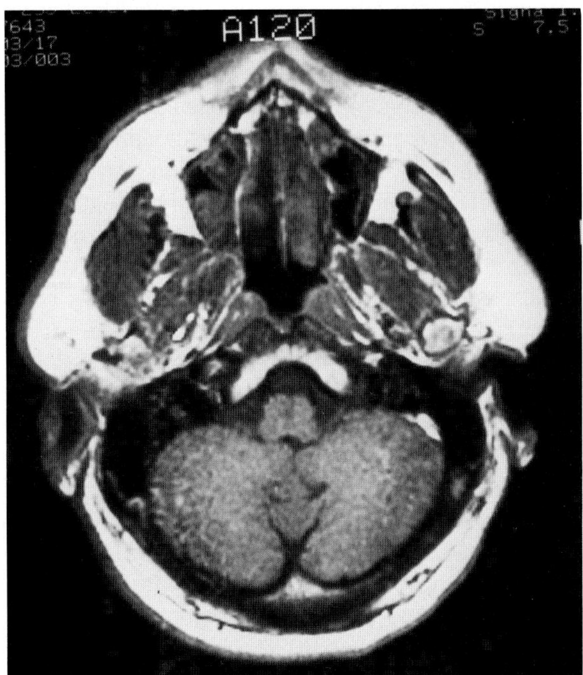

FIG. 1-25. Demonstration of flow artifacts in MRI.

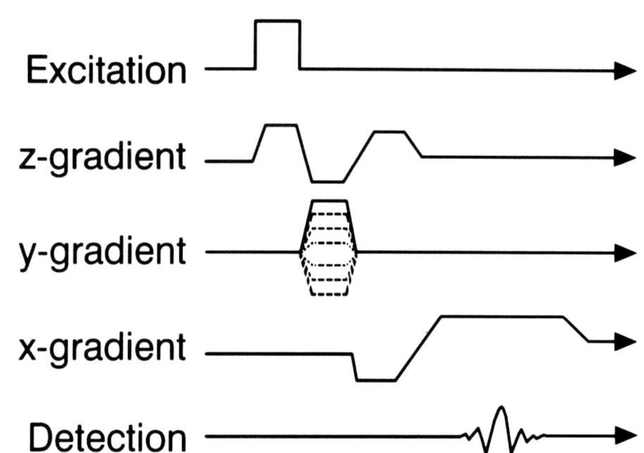

FIG. 1-26. Pulse sequence that illustrates gradient moment nulling. Extra applications of the slice selection (*z*) and frequency encoding (*x*) gradients are utilized to compensate for flow.

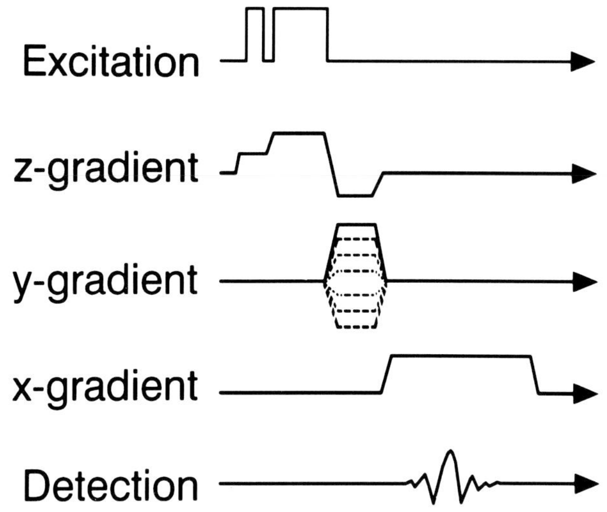

FIG. 1-27. Pulse sequence that illustrates spatial presaturation. An extra RF pulse and application of the *z* gradient is used for presaturation in the superior-inferior direction.

tially dephasing (Fig. 1-32). Alternative fast scanning techniques such as echo planar imaging can acquire data in a time as short as 40 msec. A compilation of various fast scanning techniques is presented in Table 1-5 (15).

CHEMICAL SHIFT IMAGING TECHNIQUES

The principle involved in the phenomenon described as "chemical shift" relates to the difference in Larmor frequencies for spins at different field strengths. The

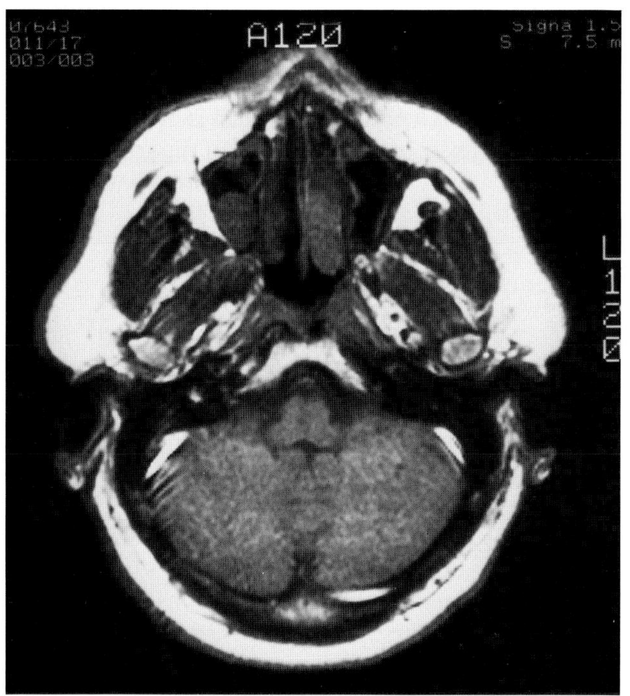

FIG. 1-28. Demonstration of flow compensation using gradient moment nulling (other parameters same as Figure 1-25).

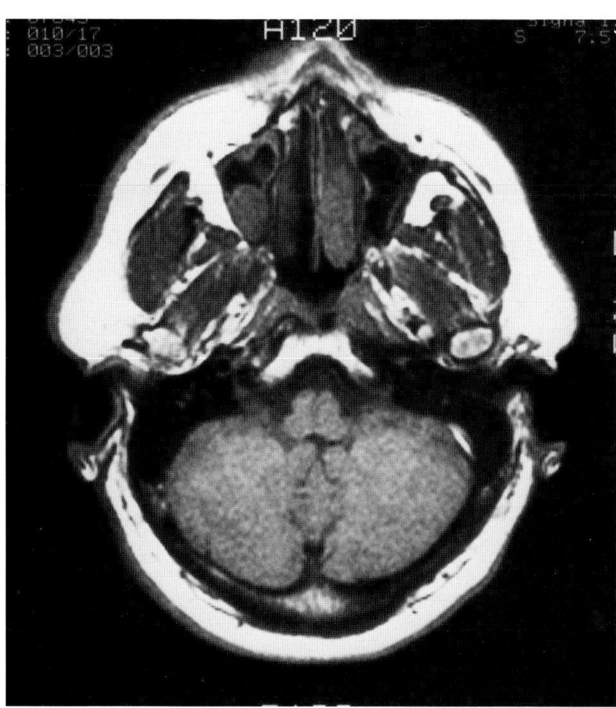

FIG. 1-29. Demonstration of flow compensation using spatial presaturation (other parameters same as Figure 1-25).

magnetic field actually experienced by a nucleus will depend on the molecular configuration of the chemical backbone to which the nucleus is attached. This depends on the configuration of electrons about the atom, which results in slight changes of the magnetic field due to the shielding effects of the electrons. Hence, at a constant field strength, the precessional frequency of fat is different from the precessional frequency of water (e.g., by about 220 Hz at 1.5 T). Therefore, the "shift" refers to the precessional frequency that results because of the "chemical" environment of the nuclei.

This phenomenon can be exploited in imaging to obtain images that suppress either the fat or water signals. The technique, first reported by Dixon (18), uses the pulse sequence shown in Fig. 1-33. As demonstrated in Fig. 1-34, due to differences in precessional frequencies, the fat and water signals can be obtained when the two are either together (in phase) or opposite (opposed). Algebraic combination of these images results in the suppression of one or the other signal, as demonstrated in Fig. 1-35. Other techniques are also useful to suppress "unwanted" signal intensities. Fat suppression can also be accomplished using the STIR (19) pulse sequence as illustrated in Fig. 1-36. The use of this sequence is shown in Fig. 1-37.

MAGNETIC RESONANCE IMAGING ARTIFACTS

Artifacts in MRI can come from many sources (20–22). In general, the primary sources of artifacts are

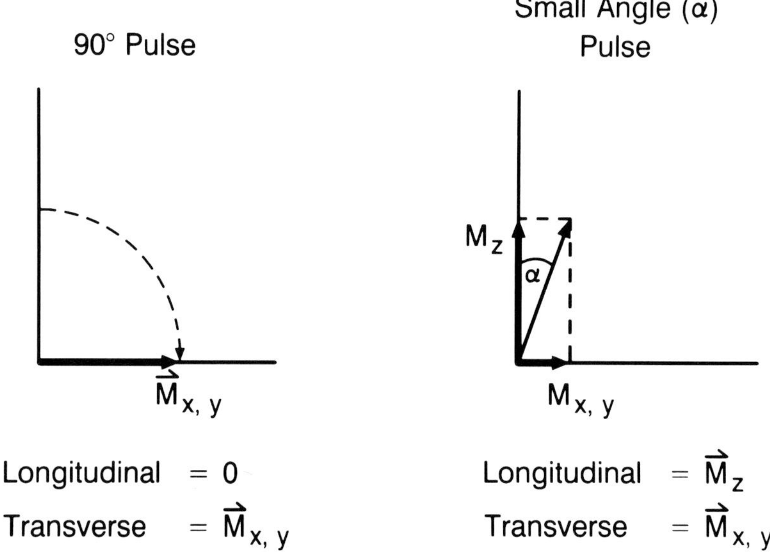

FIG. 1-30. Illustration of limited flip angle RF stimulation showing presence of longitudinal magnetization following stimulation.

those that affect the frequency or phase dispersion of the spin system. Recall that, fundamentally, the signal strength at a particular frequency is interpreted to reside at a particular point in space. Hence, anything that changes the frequency or adds signal at a particular frequency will result in a displacement or addition of intensity in the direction of the frequency encoding gradient. In an analogous fashion, something that changes the relative order of the phase of the spin precessions (either during or between views) will produce artifacts in the phase encoding direction. The sources of such artifacts are wide ranging, such as data sampling techniques, electromagnetic noise, patient motion, magnetic field inhomogeneities, magnetic susceptibility, computer malfunctions, and chemical shift. A listing of some of the common artifacts and their effects is given in Table 1-6. Detailed explanations of the source of these artifacts are given in refs. 20–22. Examples of several of these artifacts are demonstrated in Fig. 1-38. It is also important to understand that particular types of artifact may be associated with specific types of imaging procedure (e.g., spin-echo imaging versus gradient recalled echo imaging).

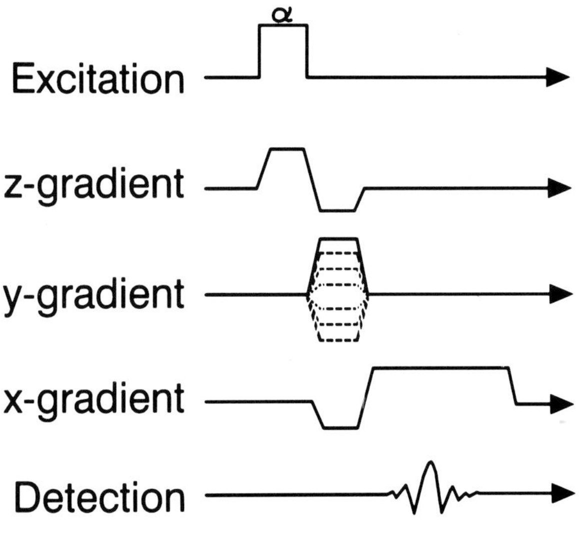

FIG. 1-31. Pulse sequence that illustrates gradient recalled echo production. Extra application of the frequency encoding gradient (*x*) causes rephasing and hence echo production.

PRACTICAL ASPECTS OF MAGNETIC RESONANCE IMAGING

Biological Effects

Three areas have received attention in terms of the biological effects of MRI: high static magnetic fields, time-varying magnetic fields (gradients), or radiofrequency irradiation (23–25).

The first area concerned the use of strong static magnetic fields. The primary theoretical concerns had to do with the effects of the magnetic fields on the protons and electrons within molecules which could affect chemical bonding or biochemical reactions. Experiments have been conducted both *in vitro* as well as *in vivo* for cellular preparations, tissues, and organisms (26–28). The conclusion from these data is that no deleterious biological effects have been demonstrated for magnetic field strengths commonly found in MRI.

The second area of concern centered on the use of time-varying magnetic fields (gradient fields). Changing

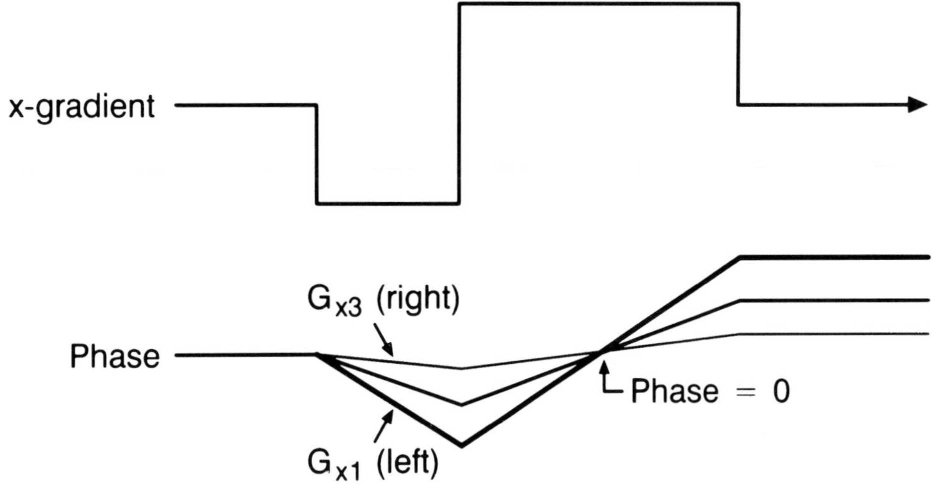

FIG. 1-32. Illustration of the production of echoes by gradient reversal. G_{x1} and G_{x3} refer to Figure 1-11.

TABLE 1-5. *Acronyms for FAST MRI*[a]

Acronym	Definition
CE-FAST	An SFP sequence that refocuses in the phase encoding direction but reads out the data just before the RF pulse. Also called PSIF.
CORE	Constrained reconstruction: a method to reconstruct artifact-free images from a finite amount of data.
EPI	Echo planar imaging. Includes (a) BLIP-EPI when gradient pulses between read intervals are applied and (b) SEPI when spiral EPI is used.
FAST	Also called FISP or GRASS. An SFP sequence that refocuses only in the phase encoding direction (enhances T1/T2 effects).
FATE	A FAST-TE sequence (i.e., a spin echo form of FLASH), essentially a double-echo spin echo with the 90° pulse replaced by a variable flip angle pulse to remove gradient-echo sensitivity to field inhomogeneities and allow for T2 weighted fast imaging. Also known as FADE.
FFI	Fast Fourier imaging—a subset of HYBRID.
FISP	Fast imaging with steady-state free precession—see FAST.
FLASH	Fast low-angle single-shot imaging. Dephases transverse magnetization prior to next RF pulse. Signal depends on T1 and T2*.
GRASS	Gradient recalled steady state—see FAST.
GFE	Gradient field echo imaging. Fast GFE is also known as FGFE or FFE.
HALF FOURIER	Any technique that uses only one-half of the usual number of phase encoding steps to obtain the same resolution as if all steps had been used.
HYBRID	A hybrid technique between spin-echo and EPI. Used to cover a fraction of *k*-space with oscillating gradients. Can be used with EPI to improve resolution.
LASE	Low-angle spin echo. Similar to FATE but the 90° pulse is replaced by a RF pulse greater than 90° and only one 180° pulse is used.
PSIF	Time reversed FISP—see CE-FAST.
RARE	Rapid acquisition with relaxation enhancement. Phase encodes between multiple 180° pulses to reduce acquisition time (rather than collecting multiple echoes).
SFP	Steady-state free precession.
SSFP	Another widely used short form for SFP.
STEAM	Stimulated echo acquisition mode. A method using three 90° pulses to generate up to five echoes. The stimulated echo and SE are generally used.
TRUE FISP	An SFP experiment that rephases in both read and phase encoding. Signal varies with T1/T2 and T2*.

[a] Adapted from ref. 15.

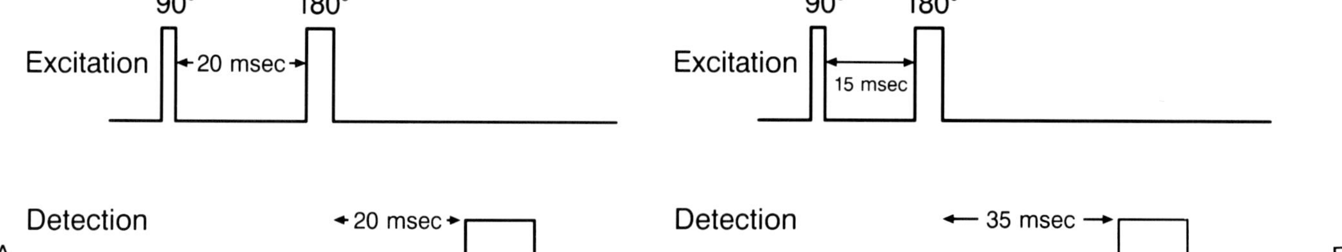

FIG. 1-33. Pulse sequences for chemical shift imaging. **A:** Equal timing to acquire in-phase image. **B:** Unequal timing to acquire opposed image.

magnetic fields can induce electric currents in biological tissues. The two tissues of primary concern are the heart and the nervous system. In addition, it is possible to stimulate the retina with an appropriate gradient. These effects are related to the gradient (rate of change of the magnetic field) and the duty cycle (the relationship of pulse width and the interpulse delay). In the systems studied, the thresholds for these biological effects are sufficiently high that a biological stimulation does not occur for the gradient field strengths typically found in MRI.

The third area of concern centered on the biological effects with the use of radiofrequency radiation. This field of investigation has been the subject of scientific inquiry (apart from MRI) for quite a long time. The primary biological effect of interest is that of heating due to the oscillation of the atoms and molecules stimulated by the radiofrequency radiation. Several factors are important in understanding this biological phenomenon in humans. The amount of heating is dependent on several factors, including the RF frequency, the absorption of the RF energy, and the thermoregulatory mechanisms within humans. The quantity used to characterize the absorption is the specific absorption rate (SAR), which is a measure of power deposition in watts per unit mass. This absorption is essentially dependent on the conductivity and density of the medium and the electric field strength of the RF radiation. The SAR is related to the RF pulse height, the RF pulse width, the interpulse delay, and the absorption properties of the patient. Most current MRI systems require an input of patient weight and calculate the SAR for a given pulse sequence. This calculation in general is an overestimate of the RF heating due to the fact that most current models do not account for the astoundingly efficient thermoregulatory mechanism of healthy humans (29). Although a rise in body temperature is possible, it is usually not a problem in patients whose cardiovascular or thermoregulatory systems are not compromised. Hence, RF heating is not deemed to be a contraindication for the use of routine clinical MRI.

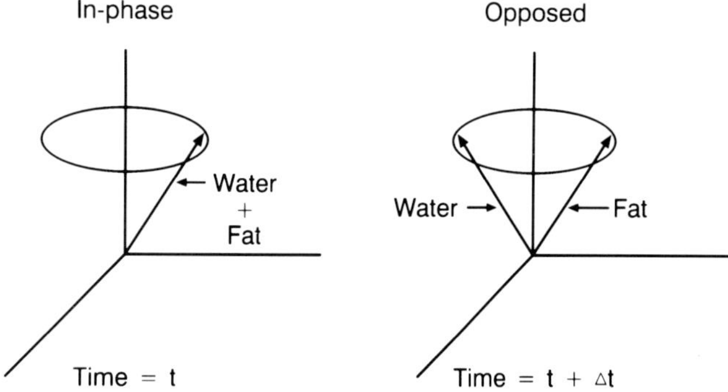

FIG. 1-34. Precessional behavior for water and fat. Water precesses faster than fat.

Although not a formal regulation, the FDA has promulgated guidelines (30) regarding the strength of static, time-varying, and radiofrequency fields for MRI. The current guidelines are listed in Table 1-7. At the present time, clinical MRI systems operate within (often well within) these guidelines.

Siting Requirements

The placement of MRI systems within a hospital is significantly different from other imaging modalities. In general, most systems use superconducting magnets and operative field strengths between 1 and 2 T. These systems will in general require radiofrequency as well as magnetic shielding for clinical operation. The radiofrequency shield is used primarily to attenuate environmental radiofrequency radiation transmission so that the very weak MR signal may be detected above the usually intense background.

The purpose of the magnetic shielding is actually twofold. The primary purpose is to shield the environment from the rather extensive stray magnetic fields which may have deleterious effects on all types of electronic equipment. In addition, it is necessary to maintain a high degree of magnetic field homogeneity. Recall that precessional frequencies are related to magnetic field strengths and, therefore, uniform stimulation requires a uniform magnetic field. Large masses of ferrous metal adjacent to the magnet will deform the magnetic field. However, the effects of environmental metal can

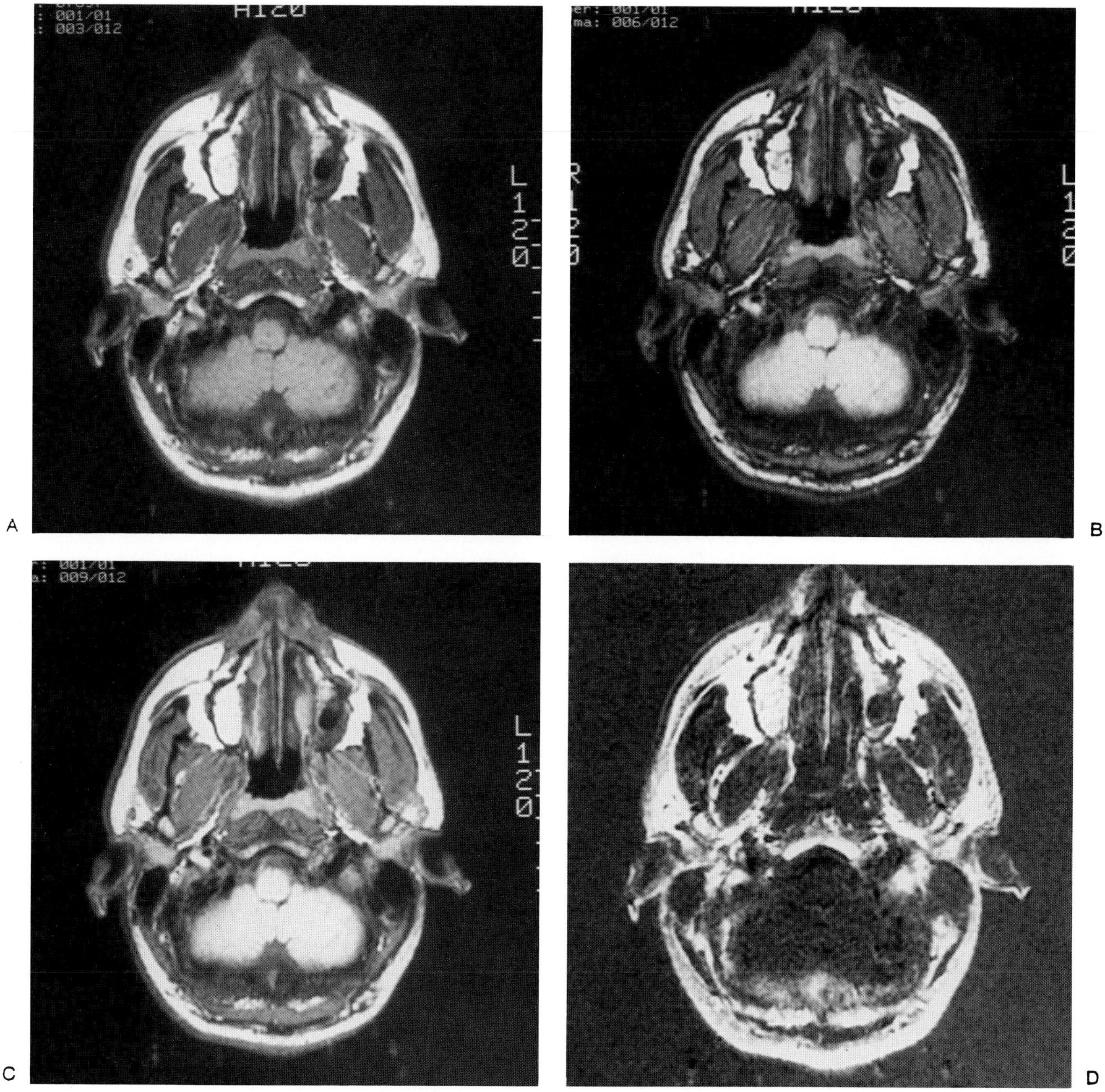

A B C D

FIG. 1-35. Chemical shift images. **A:** In-phase image. **B:** Opposed image. **C:** Water image. **D:** Fat image.

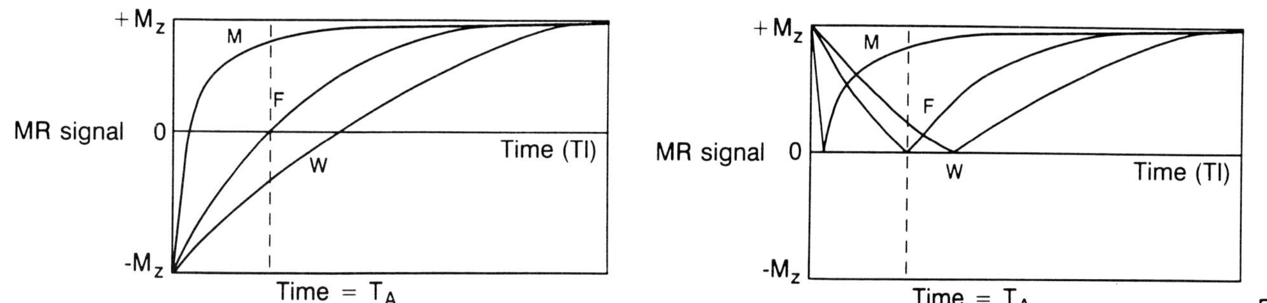

FIG. 1-36. Diagram of the effect obtained with short TI inversion recovery. By gathering data at time T_A, signal from tissue F will be zero whereas both other tissues of shorter and longer T_1 will be enhanced. **A:** Phase sensitive reconstruction. **B:** Magnitude reconstruction.

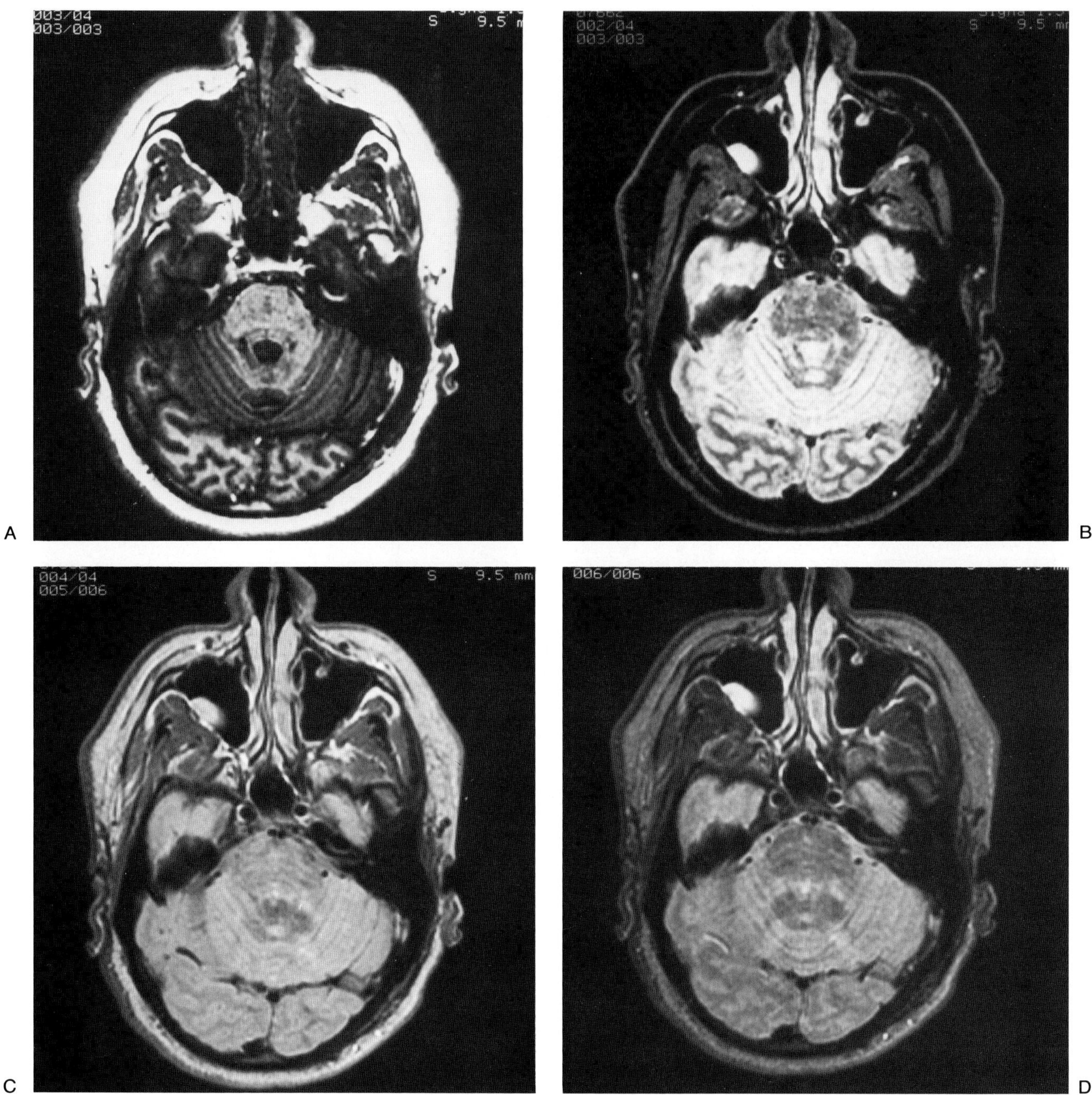

FIG. 1-37. Images using STIR sequence (with magnitude reconstruction). For all images: 256 × 192, 2 NEX, 24 cm FOV, 3 mm, 1.5 mm skip, frequency encoding along *x*-axis, no frequency wrap, TR = 2,000. **A:** Conventional IR, TI = 700, TE = 25. **B:** STIR, TI = 170. **C:** SE, TE = 30. **D:** SE, TE = 60.

TABLE 1-6. *MRI artifacts*

Frequency effects	Phase effects
Wrap-around	Wrap-around
Chemical shift	Gibbs
Susceptibility	Motion
Zipper	Zipper
Magnetic field inhomogeneity	

be counteracted with a process of "shimming." This is performed by placing pieces of metal within the magnet (passive shimming) and by the use of additional magnetic coils (shim coils) to produce small magnetic fields that increase or decrease the observed field to produce a uniform field (active shimming). Therefore, the primary concern is not large stationary metallic objects but

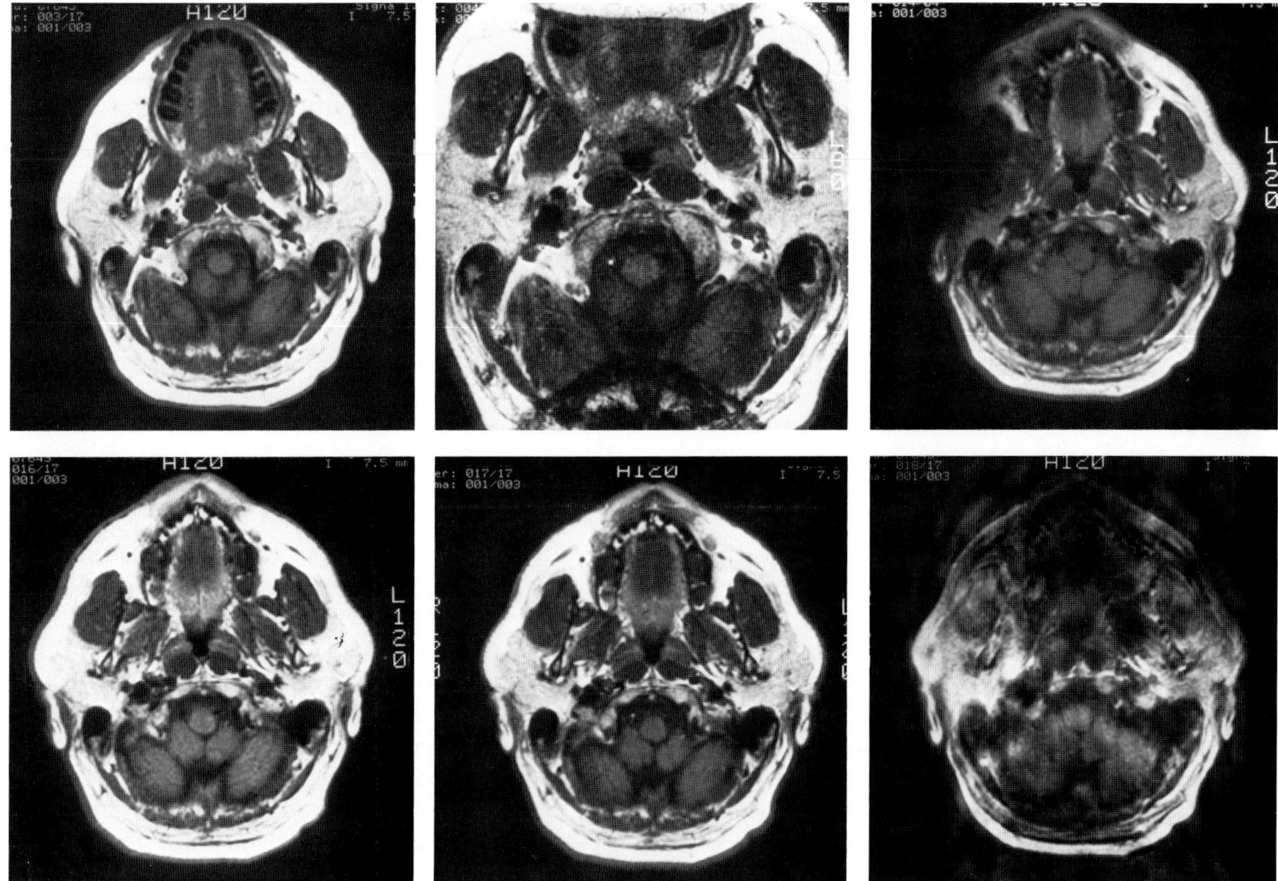

FIG. 1-38. Image artifacts in MRI. **A:** Basic sequence: TR = 300, TE = 30, 256 × 256, 2 NEX, 24 cm FOV, 5.0 mm, skip 2.5 mm. **B:** Image fold over with 16 cm FOV. **C:** Metallic artifact (wire-reinforced endotracheal tube, held on skin surface). **D:** RF artifacts (door open-frequency encoding along *x*-axis). **E:** RF artifacts (door open-frequency encoding along *y*-axis. **F:** patient motion (head rocking left to right) during acquisition.

moving metallic structures such as elevators or heavy traffic.

There are several different approaches to both radiofrequency and magnetic shielding, and this aspect does not provide a serious obstacle to the current siting of MRI systems. Equipment suppliers often will provide all the planning details necessary to design and construct the appropriate shielding.

For superconducting magnet systems, a structure must be provided to allow for the escape of large quantities of helium gas in the event the magnet were to lose its superconductive state (quench). Also, appropriate accessibility must be provided for the replenishment of cryogenic coolants. Additional site considerations are listed in Table 1-8.

TABLE 1-7. *FDA guidelines for MRI* (30)

Static magnetic field of ≤2 T.
Time-varying magnetic field of ≤3 T.
Radiofrequency power such that the body core temperature will rise no more than 1°C or localized heating no greater than 38°C in the head, 39°C in the trunk, or 40°C in the extremities.

Operational Aspects

As with other imaging systems, the detailed operational procedures for any MRI system are dependent to a large extent on factors related to the operation of the

TABLE 1-8. *Site considerations for MRI*

Space (horizontal and vertical)
Equipment accessibility—magnet and cryogens
Structural integrity
Mechanical and electrical services
Venting of gases
Magnetic and RF field interference
Nonferrous building materials
No fluorescent lights or SCR dimmers
Moving masses of metal
Effect of magnet on the environment
Isolated (filtered) power supplies
Power cables and transformers
Adjacencies
Expansion capabilities
Patient accessibility
Rapid direct patient exit from exam room
Installation and service access
Security (24 hours per day)

department and institution. However, some general observations regarding operational parameters unique to MRI can be made.

Security issues are more important for MRI than most other imaging systems. Magnetic field strengths of 1 to 2 T (Tesla) have sufficient power to lift a wheelchair off the ground and pull it to the magnet. Hence, it is important that entrance to the magnet room be limited and under the control of appropriate personnel. Many facilities also restrict access such that maintenance personnel, emergency teams, and even firefighters are denied access to the magnet room. Since pacemakers may change pacing modes in fields of 5 G (gauss) or greater, general access should be restricted in those areas where the field is greater than 5 G. Metallic objects should be tested with a strong, small magnet to determine if they contain any ferromagnetic material prior to placing them in the magnetic room. This is particularly true for equipment that may leave the room for servicing or modification.

There are many patient as well as personnel safety issues that must be discussed and decided during the design and installation of the MRI system. MRI is contraindicated for some patients due to the presence of certain biomedical implants. A determination must be made by the facility as to which devices, if present, would constitute a contraindication for a MRI exam (31).

The emergency procedures must be explicit. Significant harm can come to both personnel and patient if the emergency resuscitation team were to enter the magnet room. It is important that both visual and audio contact be provided for both patient comfort and assurance of patient safety. Both respiratory and cardiac monitoring must be available if any critically ill patients are to be scanned.

With regard to personnel, it is useful to bring all alarm systems (scan room oxygen, patient oxygen, computer room temperature, cryogen storage, smoke detectors, halon release, etc.) to one annunciator panel so that the technologist may locate the source of an alarm quickly and easily. Many facilities also utilize a lock for the magnet room door with only authorized personnel (normally MRI technologists) having access to the key. It is also useful to install a warning device, such as a photooptical or infrared chime system, to alert the MRI technologist that someone is approaching the magnet room door.

It is important that emergency air packs be available in the unlikely event of a quench with the release of helium into the magnet room. This is a situation with a low probability of occurrence yet catastrophic consequences. A technologist rushing into the magnet room during such an event in order to assist the patient may quite likely die of asphyxia before the patient is withdrawn from the room. In the presence of halon, nonferrous fire extinguishers are necessary.

In facilities experiencing their initial encounter with MRI, it is essential that the radiology staff as well as support staff, engineers, security personnel, custodial personnel, and fire department personnel receive adequate safety training prior to routine operation of the MRI system.

Perhaps of greatest importance from an operational sense is the design and implementation of acquisition protocols to optimize the diagnostic capability of MRI. With the vast armament of scan sequences and scan parameters available, a balance must be made between the number and type of scans that are performed and the amount of time available to scan an individual patient.

SUMMARY

Magnetic resonance imaging is a technique that makes use of both magnetic and radiofrequency fields to produce images of the internal structures of the body. The fundamentals of the technique involve placing the patient in a strong magnetic field, stimulation of the atomic nuclei with a radio transmission, and the detection of a radio transmission from the nuclei as they return to their prestimulation state. The technique uses nonionizing electromagnetic radiation for stimulation and detection. The available tissue contrast (due primarily to differences in relaxation times) is currently the highest among all medical imaging modalities. The technique is noninvasive and at present demonstrates no untoward biological effect. The placement and operation of MRI systems are markedly different from conventional imaging systems and demand a greater level of attention and forethought.

ACKNOWLEDGMENTS

The authors thank Joel P. Felmlee for his consultation and assistance.

APPENDIX (ADAPTED FROM REF. 6)

Aliasing Consequence of sampling in which any components of the signal that are at a higher frequency than the Nyquist limit will be "folded" in the spectrum so that they appear to be at a lower frequency. In Fourier transform imaging, this can produce an apparent wrapping around to the opposite side of the image of a portion of the object that extends beyond the edge of the reconstructed region.

Artifacts False features in the image produced by the imaging process. The random fluctuation of intensity due to noise can be considered separately from artifacts.

Attenuation Reduction of power, for example, due to passage through a medium or electrical component. Attenuation in electrical systems is commonly expressed in decibels (dB).

B_0 A conventional symbol for the constant magnetic field in a NMR system (units of tesla).

B_1 A conventional symbol for the radiofrequency magnetic field used in a MR system. It is useful to consider it as composed of two oppositely rotating vectors, usually in a plane transverse to $\mathbf{B}_0$. At the Larmor frequency, the vector rotating in the same direction as the precessing spins will interact strongly with the spins.

Bandwidth A general term referring to a range of frequencies (e.g., contained in a signal or passed by a signal processing system).

Carr–Purcell (CP) sequence Sequence of a 90° RF pulse followed by repeated 180° RF pulses to produce a train of spin echoes; useful for measuring T2.

Carr–Purcell–Meiboom–Gill (CPMG) sequence Modification of Carr–Purcell RF pulse sequence with 90° phase shift in the rotating frame of reference between the 90° pulse and the subsequent 180° pulses in order to reduce accumulating effects of imperfections in the 180° pulses. Suppression of effects of pulse error accumulation can alternatively be achieved by switching phases of the 180° pulses by 180°.

Chemical shift The change in the Larmor frequency of a given nucleus when bound in different sites in a molecule, due to the magnetic shielding effects of the electron orbitals. Chemical shifts make possible the differentiation of different molecular compounds and different sites within the molecules in high-resolution NMR spectra. The amount of the shift is proportional to magnetic field strength and is usually specified in parts per million (ppm) of the resonance frequency relative to a standard. The actual frequency measured for a given spectral line may depend on environmental factors such as effects on the local magnetic field strength due to variations of magnetic susceptibility.

Chemical shift imaging A magnetic resonance imaging technique that provides mapping of the regional distribution of intensity (images) of a restricted range of chemical shifts, corresponding to individual spectral lines or groups of lines.

Chemical shift spatial offset Image artifact of apparent spatial offset of regions with different chemical shifts along the direction of the frequency encoding gradient.

Coherence Maintenance of a constant phase relationship between rotating or oscillating waves or objects. Loss of phase coherence of the spins results in a decrease in the transverse magnetization and hence a decrease in the MR signal.

Echo planar imaging A technique of planar imaging in which a complete planar image is obtained from one selective excitation pulse. The FID is observed while periodically switching the y-magnetic field gradient field in the presence of a static x-magnetic field gradient field. The Fourier transform of the resulting spin-echo train can be used to produce an image of the excited plane.

Filter Filtering is any process that alters the relative frequency content. This can be done with an analog (conventional electrical) filter, for example, to remove higher frequency components so as to avoid aliasing in digitizing. Filtering can be carried out numerically on the digitized data.

Flip angle Amount of rotation of the macroscopic magnetization vector produced by a RF pulse, with respect to the direction of the static magnetic field.

Flow-related enhancement The increase in intensity that may be seen for flowing blood or other liquids with some MRI techniques, due to the washout of saturated spins from the imaging region.

Fourier transform imaging MRI techniques in which at least one dimension is phase encoded by applying variable gradient pulses along that dimension before "reading out" the MR signal with a magnetic field gradient perpendicular to the variable gradient. The Fourier transform is then used to reconstruct an image from the set of encoded MR signals. An imaging technique of this type is spin warp imaging. A commonly used technique is two-dimensional Fourier transform (2DFT) imaging.

Free induction decay (FID) If transverse magnetization of the spins is produced, for example, by a 90° pulse, a transient MR signal results which decays toward zero with a characteristic time constant T2 (or T2*); this decaying signal is the FID. In practice, the first part of the FID is not observable due to residual effects of the powerful exciting RF on the electronics of the receiver and the receiver dead time.

Frequency encoding Encoding the distribution of sources of MR signals along a direction by detecting the signal in the presence of a magnetic field gradient along that direction so that there is a corresponding gradient of resonance frequencies along that direction. In the absence of other position encoding, the Fourier transform of the resulting signal is a projection profile of the object.

Gauss (G) A unit of magnetic flux density in the older (cgs) system. The Earth's magnetic field is approximately 0.5 to 1 G, depending on location. The currently preferred (SI) unit is the tesla (T) (1 T = 10,000 G).

Gradient echo Spin echo produced by reversing the direction of a magnetic field gradient or by applying balanced pulses of magnetic field gradient before and after a refocusing RF pulse so as to cancel out the position-dependent phase shifts that have accumulated due to the gradient. In the latter case, the gradient echo is generally adjusted to be coincident with the RF spin echo.

Gradient magnetic field A magnetic field that changes in strength in a certain given direction. Such fields are used in MRI with selective excitation to select a region for imaging and also to encode the location of MR signals received from the object being imaged. Measured in tesla per meter (T/m).

Gyromagnetic ratio The ratio of the magnetic moment to the angular momentum of a particle. This is a constant for a given nucleus.

Image acquisition time Time required to carry out a MRI procedure comprising only the data acquisition time. The total image acquisition time will be equal to the product of the repetition time, TR, the number of excitations, and the number of different signals (encoded for position) to be acquired for use in image reconstruction. The additional image reconstruction time will also be important to determine how quickly the image can be viewed. In comparing sequential plane imaging and volume imaging techniques, the equivalent image acquisition time per slice must be considered, as well as the actual image acquisition time.

Interpulse time Times between successive RF pulses used in pulse sequences. Particularly important are the inversion time (TI) in inversion recovery, and the time between 90° pulse and the subsequent 180° pulse to produce a spin echo, which will be approximately one-half the spin-echo time (TE). The time between repetitions of pulse sequences is the repetition time (TR).

Inversion recovery A pulse NMR technique that can be incorporated into MRI, wherein the nuclear magnetization is inverted at a time on the order of T1 before the regular imaging pulse-gradient sequences. The resulting partial relaxation of the spins in different structures being imaged can be used to produce an image that depends strongly on T1. This may bring out differences in the appearance of structures with different T1 relaxation times. Note that this does not directly produce an image of T1. T1 in a given region can be calculated from the change in the NMR signal from the region due to the inversion pulse compared to the signal with no inversion pulse or an inversion pulse with a different inversion time (TI).

Longitudinal magnetization (M_z) Component of the macroscopic magnetization vector along the static magnetic field. Following excitation by a RF pulse, M_z will approach its equilibrium value M_0, with a characteristic time constant T1.

Longitudinal relaxation Return of longitudinal magnetization to its equilibrium value after excitation; requires exchange of energy between the nuclear spins and the lattice.

Macroscopic magnetization vector Net magnetic moment per unit volume (a vector quantity) of a sample in a given region, considered as the integrated effect of all the individual microscopic nuclear magnetic moments. Most MR experiments actually deal with this.

Magnetic field gradient A magnetic field that changes in strength in a certain given direction. Such fields are used in NMR imaging with selective excitation to select a region for imaging and also to encode the location of NMR signals received from the object being imaged. This is measured in millitesles (mT/m) or gauss per centimeter (G/cm).

Magnetic resonance (MR) Resonance phenomenon resulting in the absorption and/or emission of electromagnetic energy by nuclei or electrons in a static magnetic field, after excitation by a suitable RF magnetic field. The peak resonance frequency is proportional to the magnetic field and is given by the Larmor equation. Only unpaired electrons or nuclei with a nonzero spin exhibit magnetic resonance.

Magnetic susceptibility Measure of the ability of a substance to become magnetized. A difference in susceptibility between tissues can therefore lead to a difference in stimulation and the resultant signal.

Partial saturation (PS) An excitation technique applying repeated RF pulses in times on the order of or shorter than T1. In MRI systems, although it results in decreased signal amplitude, there is the possibility of generating images with increased contrast between regions with different relaxation times. It does not directly produce images of T1. The change in NMR signal from a region resulting from a change in the interpulse time, TR, can be used to calculate T1 for the region. Although partial saturation is also commonly referred to as saturation recovery, that term should properly be reserved for the particular case of partial saturation in which recovery after each excitation effectively takes place from true saturation.

Phase In a periodic function (such as rotational or sinusoidal motion), the position relative to a particular part of the cycle.

Phase encoding Encoding the distribution of sources of MR signals along a direction in space with different phases by applying a pulsed magnetic field gradient along that direction prior to detection of the signal. In general, it is necessary to acquire a set of signals with a suitable set of different phase encoding gradient pulses in order to reconstruct the distribution of the sources along the encoded direction.

Precession Comparatively slow gyration of the axis of a spinning body so as to trace out a cone; caused by the application of a torque tending to change the direction of the rotation axis, and continuously directed at right angles to the plane of the torque. The magnetic moment of a nucleus with spin will experience such a torque when inclined at an angle to the magnetic field, resulting in precession at the Larmor frequency. A familiar example is the effect of gravity on the motion of a spinning top or gyroscope.

Pulse sequences Set of RF (and/or gradient) magnetic field pulses and time spacings between these pulses; used in conjunction with magnetic field gradients and NMR signal reception to produce NMR images. A recommended shorthand designation of interpulse times used to generate a particular image is to list the repetition time (TR), the echo time (TE), and, if using inversion recovery, the inversion time, TI, with all times given in milliseconds (msec). For example, 2,500/30/1,000 would indicate an inversion recovery pulse sequence with TR of 2,500 msec, TE of 30 msec, and TI of 1,000 msec. If using multiple spin echoes, as in CPMG, the number of the spin echo used should be stated.

Rephasing gradient Magnetic field gradient applied for a brief period after a selective excitation pulse, in the opposite direction to the gradient used for the selective excitation. The result of the gradient reversal is a rephasing of the spins (which will have gotten out of phase with each other along the direction of the selection gradient), forming a gradient echo and improving the sensitivity of imaging after the selective excitation process.

Resonance A large amplitude vibration in a mechanical or electrical system caused by a relatively small periodic stimulus with a frequency at or close to a natural frequency of the system; in NMR apparatus, resonance can refer to the NMR itself or to the tuning of the RF circuitry.

Saturation recovery (SR) A particular type of partial saturation pulse sequence in which the preceding pulses leave the spins in a state of saturation, so that recovery at the time of the next pulse has taken place from an initial condition of no magnetization.

Spin The intrinsic angular momentum of an elementary particle, or system of particles, such as a nucleus, that is also responsible for the magnetic moment; or, a particle or nucleus possessing such a spin. The spins of nuclei have characteristic fixed values. Pairs of neutrons and protons align to cancel out each others, spins, so that nuclei with an odd number of neutrons and/or protons will have a net nonzero rotational component characterized by an integer or half integer quantum "nuclear spin number."

Spin echo Reappearance of a NMR signal after the FID has apparently died away, as a result of the effective reversal of the dephasing of the spins (refocusing) by techniques such as specific RF pulse sequences, for example, Carr–Purcell sequence (RF spin echo), or pairs of magnetic field gradient pulses (gradient echo), applied in times shorter than or on the order of T2. Unlike RF spin echos, gradient echos will not refocus phase differences due to chemical shifts or inhomogeneities of the magnetic field.

Spin-echo imaging (SE) Any of many MRI techniques in which the spin echo is used rather than the FID. Can be used to create images that depend strongly on T2 if TE has a value on the order of or greater than T2 of the relevant image details. Note that spin-echo imaging does not directly produce an image of T2 distribution. The spin echoes can be produced as a train of multiple echoes, for example, using the CPMG pulse sequence.

T1 ("T-one") Spin–lattice or longitudinal relaxation time; the characteristic time constant for spins to tend to align themselves with the external magnetic field. Starting from zero magnetization in the z direction, the z magnetization will grow to 63% of its final maximum value in a time T1.

T2 ("T-two") Spin–spin or transverse relaxation time; the characteristic time constant for loss of phase coherence among spins oriented at an angle to the static magnetic field, due to interactions between the spins, with resulting loss of transverse magnetization and NMR signal. Starting from a nonzero value of magnetization in the xy plane, the xy magnetization will decay so that it loses 63% of its initial value in a time T2.

T2* ("T-two-star") The observed time constant of the FID due to loss of phase coherence among spins oriented at an angle to the static magnetic field, commonly due to a combination of magnetic field inhomogeneities and spin–spin transverse relaxation with more rapid loss in transverse magnetization and NMR signal. NMR signals can usually still be recovered as a spin echo in times less than or on the order of T2.

TE Echo time. Time between middle of 90° pulse and middle of spin echo production. For multiple echos, use TE1, TE2, . . .

Tesla (T) The preferred (SI) unit of magnetic flux density. One tesla is equal to 10,000 gauss.

TI Inversion time. In inversion recovery, time between middle of inverting (180°) RF pulse and middle of the subsequent exciting (90°) pulse to detect amount of longitudinal magnetization.

TR Repetition time. The period of time between the beginning of a pulse sequence and the beginning of the succeeding (essentially identical) pulse sequence.

REFERENCES

1. Fullerton GD. Basic concepts for nuclear magnetic resonance imaging. *Magn Reson Imaging* 1982;1:39–55.
2. *RadioGraphics,* Volume 4, Special Edition, January 1984.
3. Young SW. *Nuclear magnetic resonance imaging: basic principles.* New York: Raven Press, 1984.
4. Balter S. An introduction to the physics of magnetic resonance imaging. *Radiographics* 1987;7:371–383.
5. Fullerton GD. Magnetic resonance imaging signal concepts. *Radiographics* 1987;7:579–596.

6. American College of Radiology. *Glossary of MR terms*, 2nd ed. Reston, Virginia: American College of Radiology, 1986.
7. Kumar A, Welti D, Ernst RR. NMR Fourier zeugmatography. *J Magn Reson* 1975;18:69–83.
8. Edelstein WA, Hutchison JMS, Johnson G, Redpath T. Spin warp NMR imaging. *Phys Med Biol* 1980;25:751–756.
9. Hutchison J. NMR scanning: the spin-warp method. In: *NMR imaging*. Winston-Salem, NC: Bowman-Gray School of Medicine, 1982.
10. Felmlee JP, Morin RL, Salutz JR, Lund GB. Magnetic resonance imaging phase encoding: a pictorial essay. *Radiographics* 1989;9:717–722.
11. Felmlee JP. Personal communication.
12. Hinks RS, Quencer RM. Motion artifacts in brain and spine MR. *Radiol Clin North Am* 1988;26:737–753.
13. Glover GH, Pelc MJ. A rapid gated cine MRI technique. In: Kressel HY, ed. *Magnetic resonance annual*. New York: Raven Press, 1988.
14. Felmlee JP, Ehman RL. Spatial presaturation: a method for suppressing flow artifacts and improving depiction of vascular anatomy in MR imaging. *Radiology* 1987;164:559–564.
15. Haacke EM. Editorial. *Magn Reson Imaging* 1988;6:353–354.
16. Haase A, Frahm J, Matthaei D, et al. FLASH imaging: rapid NMR imaging using low flip angle pulses. *J Magn Reson* 1986;67:258–266.
17. Mansfield P. Multi-planar image formation by NMR. *J Phys (E)* 1977;10:L55.
18. Dixon WT. Simple proton spectroscopic imaging. *Radiology* 1984;153:189–194.
19. Dwyer AJ, Frank JA, Sank VJ, et al. Short-TI inversion-recovery pulse sequence: analysis and initial experience in cancer imaging. *Radiology* 1988;168:827–836.
20. Bellon ER, Haacke EM, Coleman PE, et al. MR artifacts: a review. *Am J Roentg* 1986;147:1271.
21. Pusey E, Lufkin RB, Brown RKJ, et al. MRI artifacts: mechanism and clinical significance. *Radiographics* 1986;6:891.
22. Hahn FJ, Chu WK, Coleman PE, et al. Artifacts and diagnostic pitfalls on magnetic resonance imaging: a clinical review. *Radiol Clin North Am* 1988;26:717–735.
23. Persson BBR, Stahlberg F. *Health and safety of clinical NMR examination*. Boca Raton, FL: CRC Press, 1989.
24. NRPB advisory group on NMR clinical imaging. Revised guidance on acceptable limits of exposure during nuclear magnetic resonance clinical imaging. *Br J Radiol* 1983;56:974–977.
25. McRobbie D, Foster MA. Thresholds for biological effects of time-varying magnetic fields. *Clin Phys Physiol Meas* 1984;5:67–78.
26. Budinger TF. Thresholds for physiological effects due to RF and magnetic fields used in NMR imaging. *IEEE Trans Nucl Sci* 1979;NS-26:2812–2815.
27. Papatheofanis FJ. A review on the interaction of biological systems with magnetic fields. *Physiol Chem Phys Med NMR* 1984;16:251–255.
28. Jehenson P, Duboc D, Lavergne T, et al. Change in human cardiac rhythm induced by a 2T static magnetic field. *Radiology* 1988;166:227–230.
29. Pavlicek W, Salem D, Horton J. Comparative measurements of RF absorbed power using 0.15, 0.6, and 1.5 Tesla magnets. *Radiology* 1984;153(P):98.
30. Food and Drug Administration. Magnetic resonance diagnostic device: panel recommendation and report on petitions for MR reclassification. *Fed Reg* 1988;53:7575–7579.
31. Shellock FG, Crues JV. High-field-strength MR imaging and metallic biomedical implants: an *ex vivo* evaluation of deflection forces. *AJR* 1988;151:389–392.

MRI of the Musculoskeletal System, 2nd Edition, edited by T. H. Berquist.
Raven Press, Ltd., New York © 1990.

CHAPTER 2

Interpretation of Magnetic Resonance Images

Richard L. Ehman

Tissue Characterization, 27
Significance of Tissue Relaxation Times, 29
Relaxation Times of Musculoskeletal Tissues, 31
Effect of Pathology on Tissue Relaxation Times, 32
Inflammation, 32
Neoplasms, 32
Fibrosis, 33
Fatty Infiltration, 33
Hematoma, 33
Influence of Relaxation Times and Pulse Sequence Parameters on Contrast, 35
T1 and T2 Weighted Sequences, 36
Contrast in Gradient-Echo Sequences, 37
Approach for Selection of MRI Techniques, 39
Miscellaneous Techniques, 44
Appearance of Vascular Structures in MRI, 45
References, 50

The appearance of magnetic resonance images is determined by an entirely different set of physical principles than those that define other medical imaging techniques. This presents both a problem and an opportunity to physicians who interpret these images. It is a problem because there is less background knowledge to draw from in order to understand the pattern of black, white, and grey that is present in the images. It is an opportunity because, since magnetic resonance imaging (MRI) is based on a unique set of physical principles, it is inevitable that some features or disease processes will be displayed with higher clarity than with other imaging modalities. The challenge for any physician who would like to employ this powerful technique is therefore to gain a working understanding of the magnetic resonance properties of tissue and how they are portrayed in the images.

The purpose of this chapter is to describe the properties of tissue that are important in MRI of the musculoskeletal system. The dependence of these physical properties on tissue type and pathology has not yet been fully explained, but some of the general principles are useful in clinical practice. We outline methods for tailoring magnetic resonance examinations to make appropriate use of this information for common clinical problems. Approaches for interpreting image contrast are presented. The physical mechanisms that govern the appearance of flowing blood are also covered.

R. L. Ehman: Mayo Medical School and Mayo Clinic, Rochester, Minnesota 55905.

TISSUE CHARACTERIZATION

The process of extracting information about tissue type and pathology by magnetic resonance techniques has been called "tissue characterization." This often has been applied specifically to the use of quantitative measurements of relaxation times. Many studies of tissue characterization by *in vivo* measurement of relaxation times have appeared in the literature (14,38,44, 50,53,58,71). These generally have not demonstrated a strong clinical role for "tissue characterization" although it is fair to say that the hypothesis that accurate measurement of tissue relaxation times may be clinically useful has not yet been adequately tested.

It should be remembered at this point that "tissue characterization" is not something that is limited to MRI. It is performed in every branch of diagnostic imaging. Consider the case of a solitary pulmonary nodule that is observed in a chest radiograph. If a certain pattern of calcification is identified within the nodule, it can be judged benign. Other examples include assessing whether a mass is cystic or solid with ultrasonography and determining the presence or absence of fat within a renal mass with computed tomography. These processes

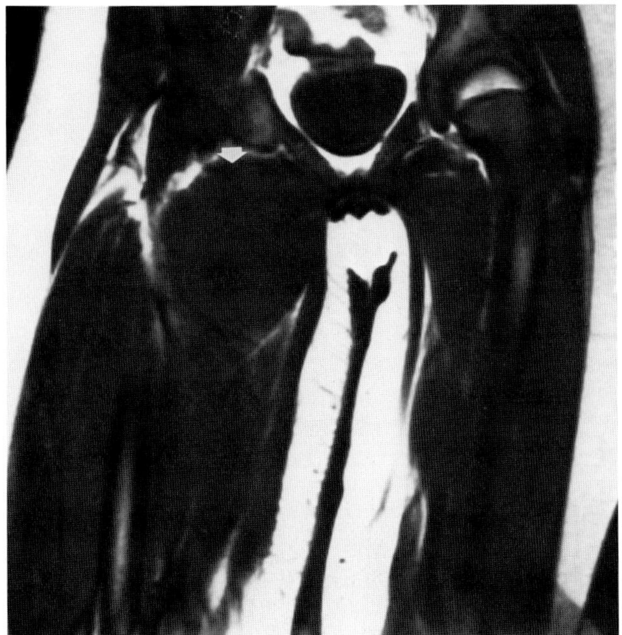

FIG. 2-1. Malignant soft tissue tumor (*arrow*) that is differentiated from muscle on the basis of its mass effect and homogeneity rather than a contrast difference.

are mostly qualitative, based on an understanding of the grey scale of the particular imaging modality. Some can be quantitative, as with CT. In any case, all these are examples of clinically useful tissue characterization. We believe that it is this type of tissue characterization, based on knowledge and manipulation of tissue contrast, that is most important in clinical MRI.

Given the expanded definition for tissue characterization described above, what are the properties that are important in clinical imaging? A key word in this question is "imaging." Some of the tissue properties that are important in this context are unique to the imaging process. This includes anatomic detail, which can demonstrate a lesion solely by its effect on morphology (Fig. 2-1). Another similar property is tissue texture: mass lesions in muscle are often characterized by their homogeneous texture, compared to the reticulated texture of normal muscle (Fig. 2-1). As we shall see, even some of the classical tissue characterization parameters have special meanings in the imaging context.

Magnetic resonance images basically reflect the distribution of mobile hydrogen nuclei. The brightness of each image pixel depends, among other things, on the density of mobile protons in the corresponding volume element and on the way that these protons respond to the externally superimposed static and fluctuating magnetic fields described in Chapter 1. This response depends on the chemical and biophysical environment of the protons and is described concisely by the relaxation times T1 and T2.

The spin–lattice relaxation time, T1, is an exponential time constant that describes the gradual increase in magnetization that takes place when a substance is placed in a strong magnetic field (Fig. 2-2). T1 predicts the time that it will take for nearly two-thirds (actually about 63%) of the longitudinal magnetization to be restored after it has been tipped 90° by a radiofrequency (RF) pulse. The spin–lattice relaxation time of water protons in tissue depends in a complex fashion on rotational, vibrational, and translational motions and on the way that these are modified by proximity to macromolecules.

The spin–spin relaxation time, T2, is a time constant that describes the rate of exponential decay of transverse magnetization that would occur if the field were perfectly homogeneous (Fig. 2-3). Thus, for a spin-echo sequence, the net transverse magnetization at an echo delay time of TE = T2 will be approximately two-thirds (actually 63%) less than what was present immediately after the 90° pulse. The transverse magnetization is the component that creates a signal in MRI. Like T1, the spin–spin relaxation time depends on the natural motions of molecules. It is also affected by other processes, which are described later in this chapter.

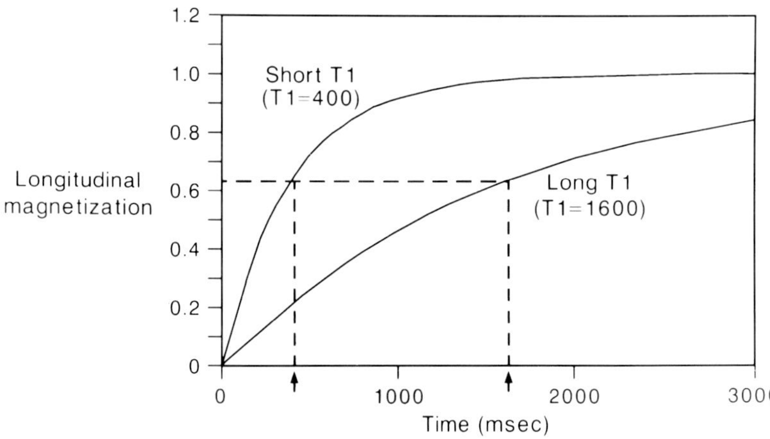

FIG. 2-2. The T1 relaxation time describes the regrowth of longitudinal magnetization after it is reduced to zero by a 90° radiofrequency pulse.

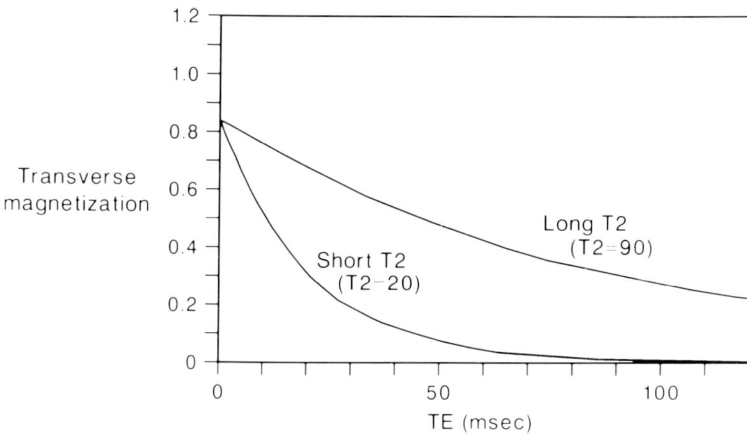

FIG. 2-3. The T2 relaxation time describes the exponential decay of magnetization in the transverse plane after it is placed there by a 90° radiofrequency pulse.

Accurate *in vivo* measurement of relaxation times is difficult with most MR imagers. These difficulties relate to the necessity of irradiating a large but well-defined volume with radiofrequency energy and performing the steps required to create an image. Slice-selective 90° and 180° RF pulses, for instance, tend to be inaccurate near the boundaries of the section (35). The signal obtained from tissue that is irradiated with inaccurate RF pulses will not be the same as what would be obtained with ideal pulses. Relaxation times calculated from such measurements will be correspondingly incorrect. Other problems include the effects of applied field gradients, motion, and the small number of data points that are typically acquired.

In spite of these problems, properly performed *in vivo* relaxation time measurements are surprisingly reproducible with the same imager when they are performed on tissues that are stationary (37,38). On the other hand, physiological motion can produce large random and systematic errors in relaxation times calculated from image data (17,19,20). Relaxation times obtained with one type of MR imager are usually not directly comparable to data obtained for the same tissue with another imager. This is because of the imager-specific systematic errors described above and the fact that relaxation times are field strength dependent. The T1 of muscle tissue, for instance, is nearly twice as long at 1.5T as it is at 0.15T (5,33).

Given these problems, it is not surprising that clinical applications requiring quantitative measurement of tissue relaxation times have been slow to emerge. In spite of this, it is essential to understand the relative relaxation time relationships of tissues and pathological processes because this is the key to understanding the highly variable grey scale of MRI.

Spin density (mobile proton density, hydrogen density) is another important property that determines the appearance of tissue in magnetic resonance images. Few *in vivo* measurements of tissue spin density have been reported. This is probably because absolute measurements are difficult to perform with imagers. The derived spin densities are relative values that can only be compared within the same image. Nevertheless, spin density differences are an important source of image contrast in some tissues. There are large differences between the spin density of adipose tissue and muscle, for instance (18).

Many other physical properties can potentially be measured or monitored by MR techniques in order to noninvasively characterize tissue. These include measuring the diffusion rate of water protons (67,68) and differentiating between groups of protons on the basis of the characteristic chemical shift in their resonant frequency (2,12,23,34,36,41,46,47,54,57,62).

SIGNIFICANCE OF TISSUE RELAXATION TIMES

A detailed discussion of the physical mechanisms that determine relaxation time in biological systems is beyond the scope of this chapter. Indeed, these processes are as yet poorly understood. Nevertheless, some of the concepts in the current view of this area are useful for understanding the appearance of normal and pathological tissue in clinical images.

Relaxation times are used to describe the time course of the bulk magnetization of resonating protons following the application of perturbing RF pulses. The bulk magnetization is a vector quantity (i.e., having a magnitude and direction), which is the sum of the minute magnetic contributions of each of the resonating protons in tissue. The magnetic behavior of individual protons is quantum mechanical in nature but the process of summing huge numbers of protons results in a bulk magnetization vector, which can assume a continuous range of magnitudes and orientations.

As already noted, the spin–lattice relaxation time (T1) describes the restoration of the longitudinal component of magnetization after it has been tipped by a RF pulse.

In order for this to happen, some of the protons that have been boosted into a higher energy level by the RF pulse must give up energy to the surrounding environment (sometimes called the "lattice"). This corresponds to reorienting individual proton magnetic moments from a direction that is roughly opposite to that of the main field to one that is, on average, in the same direction.

This process depends on interaction between the excited protons and neighboring nuclei in the lattice (21). The protons are subjected to a rapidly varying perturbation by the magnetic fields of adjacent nuclei. The frequency with which they vary is determined by the tumbling and translational motions of the protons and their neighbors. The perturbing motions are most effective for stimulating spin–lattice relaxation when they fluctuate at the Larmour frequency of the system.

The characteristic length of time during which the magnetic field of a proton interacts with that of an adjacent nucleus with a magnetic moment is called the correlation time, τ (tau) (21). Essentially, this quantity is proportional to the period (i.e., inversely proportional to the frequency) of the cyclic field fluctuations caused by motion. Each mode of molecular motion has a characteristic correlation time. For tumbling motion, the correlation time is proportional to the period of rotation (Fig. 2-4). For translational motion, the correlation time can be regarded as proportional to the average time between the Brownian "jumps." The combined correlation time is the parallel sum of the individual τ values associated with each of the perturbing motions:

$$\frac{1}{\tau_c} = \frac{1}{\tau_r} + \frac{1}{\tau_d} \qquad [1]$$

As shown in Fig. 2-5, the spin–lattice relaxation time decreases to a minimum as correlation time is lengthened and then increases again. The position of the minimum of this curve is dependent on the Larmour frequency and thus the strength of the B_0 field (4). Free

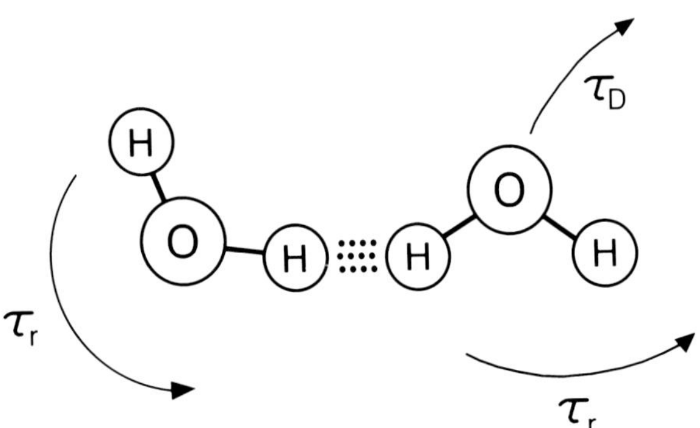

FIG. 2-4. As water molecules tumble and randomly jump in Brownian motion, the dipole moments of protons interact with a characteristic period called the correlation time.

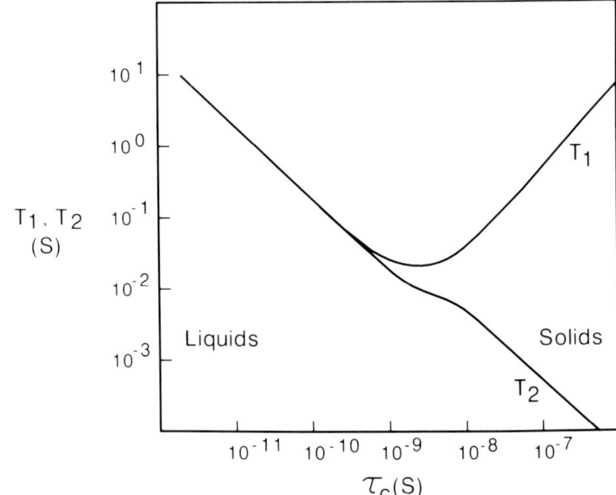

FIG. 2-5. Relationship between correlation time and the T1 and T2 relaxation times.

water has a short correlation time of about 10^{-12} sec and thus it has a long spin–lattice relaxation time.

The spin–spin or T2 relaxation time of protons is also dependent on correlation times. It is also strongly affected by slowly varying and static magnetic fields at the molecular level (21). Such fields form gradients, which cause moving protons to precess at rates that have a small random variation with time. Thus, they do not stay in phase with each other for as long as they would without the static field gradients and this is reflected as a reduction in the T2 relaxation time (see Chapter 1). Figure 2-5 shows that, in contrast to the T1 relaxation time, T2 continues to shorten as correlation times become longer and longer. Thus, the proton T1 and T2 relaxation times of solids, which have very slow molecular motion and longer correlation times, will be long and short, respectively.

Although pure water has long T1 and T2 relaxation times of over 2 sec, much shorter relaxation times are typically observed in tissue. This is a result of the hydrophilic properties of many macromolecules. These molecules, which include proteins and polynucleic acids, have electric dipole and ionic sites that allow hydrogen bonding with water molecules in solution (Fig. 2-6) (11,26,30). The water in this hydration layer is less mobile than free water and thus the correlation time is longer ($\tau_c = 10^{-9}$ sec). As a result, the T1 and T2 of hydration water is much shorter than that of free water.

The residence time of individual water molecules in the hydration layer of macromolecules is transient. Thus, individual water protons may alternately experience conditions that are favorable and unfavorable for relaxation as they exchange back and forth between bound and free states, respectively. Under these "fast-exchange" conditions, the observed relaxation time of water protons will be an average of the relaxation times

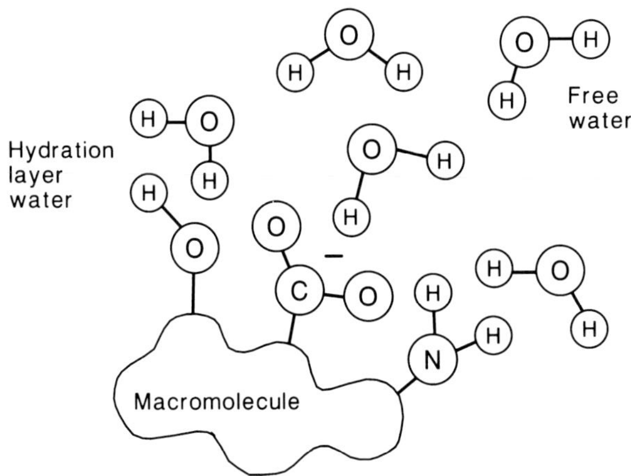

FIG. 2-6. Two-state model for organization of water in cytoplasm.

in the bound and free states, weighted by the fraction in each state (11):

$$\frac{1}{T1_o} = \frac{1 - F_b}{T1_f} + \frac{F_b}{T1_b} \qquad [2]$$

where $T1_o$ is the observed T1, $T1_f$ and $T1_b$ are the relaxation times in the free and bound states, respectively, and F_b is the fraction of bound protons. The equation for T2 is similar. More complex models have been created to explain tissue relaxation behavior (5), but this simple, two-state, fast-exchange model is very helpful for understanding clinical images. The T1 relaxation time of free water is approximately 2,500 msec, while that of hydration water is less than 100 msec. The model predicts that relaxation times of tissues with higher bound water fractions will be shorter than tissues that have a larger percentage of free water.

Tissue water proton relaxation times depend on many other factors. Field strength is one of the most important of these (5,10,25,33). The trough of the T1 relaxation time curve in Fig. 2-5 moves upward and to the left as field strength increases (4). This means that the relaxation times of protons with correlation times in this range (e.g., bound water protons) will be longer at higher field strengths. It follows that the T1 relaxation time of most tissues increases with field strength because of the influence on the bound water component. In contrast, the T2 relaxation times of most tissues are relatively independent of field strength, except for a clinically important exception described later.

Paramagnetic agents can strongly affect tissue relaxation times when they are present (8). These are substances with very strong magnetic moments, which can enhance the relaxation of neighboring protons by perturbing them in a manner analogous to the way that proton fields interact with other protons. Many of these agents are paramagnetic by virtue of the presence of an unpaired orbital electron. The magnetic dipole moment generated by the unopposed electron is about 700 times stronger than the magnetic moment of a proton. The proton relaxation enhancement effect of these molecules is correspondingly intense.

When a sufficient amount of paramagnetic agent is added to an aqueous solution, the T1 and T2 relaxation times are shortened. The effect can be represented by the following equations:

$$\frac{1}{T1_o} = \frac{1}{T1_d} + \frac{1}{T1_p} \qquad [3]$$

$$\frac{1}{T2_o} = \frac{1}{T1_d} + \frac{1}{T2_p} \qquad [4]$$

where $T1_o$ and $T2_o$ are the new observed relaxation times, $T1_d$ and $T2_d$ are the (diamagnetic) relaxation times of the solution or tissue without the paramagnetic agent, and $T1_p$ and $T2_p$ represent the extra relaxation process provided by the addition of the paramagnetic material. These latter quantities depend on the concentration of paramagnetic material:

$$\frac{1}{T1_p} = K1 \times (\text{concentration of paramagnetic material}) \qquad [5]$$

$$\frac{1}{T2_p} = K2 \times (\text{concentration of paramagnetic material}) \qquad [6]$$

where K1 and K2 are constants that depend on the type of paramagnetic agent and on the characteristics of the tissue or solution.

Paramagnetic material may be endogenous in origin or it may be exogenously administered as a contrast agent for MRI. Endogenous paramagnetic materials are not believed to be present in sufficient concentration to significantly affect the relaxation behavior of most normal human tissues, but they do have a substantial effect in some pathological states such as transfusional hemosiderosis (9).

RELAXATION TIMES OF MUSCULOSKELETAL TISSUES

Tables of quantitative *in vivo* relaxation time measurements (5) are of limited clinical usefulness because they are dependent on the field strength and on technical details of the imager and measurement method. Nevertheless, a general understanding of the relative relaxation characteristics of normal and pathological tissues is absolutely essential for competent interpretation

TABLE 2-1. *Relative relaxation times of musculoskeletal tissues*

Tissue	T1	T2
Muscle	Medium	Short
Adipose tissue	Short	Medium
Nerve	Medium	Medium
Other soft tissue	Medium to long	Medium to long
Tendon, bone	—	Very short

of clinical magnetic resonance imagery. This task is relatively easy for the musculoskeletal system because the number of different tissues is small.

At the field strengths that are commonly used for proton imaging (0.15–1.5T), the T1 relaxation times of most soft tissues range between 250 and 1,200 msec. The range of T2 values for most soft tissues is between approximately 25 and 120 msec. Fluids and fibrous tissue depart from this range. The relative relaxation times of musculoskeletal tissues are summarized in Table 2-1.

These relationships can be summarized in a relaxation time map (Fig. 2-7). This figure shows that most musculoskeletal soft tissues fall into three distinct classes. Adipose tissue is characterized by its short T1 relaxation time in comparison to most other tissues, which dominates its appearance with most common MRI techniques. Healthy skeletal muscle has a short T2 relaxation time that is characteristic. Most other soft tissues, including tumors, have T1 relaxation times that are longer than that of adipose tissue and T2 relaxation times that are longer than that of muscle. The mobile proton density of bone, tendon, and dense fibrous tissue is low so that these tissues have low intensity in most MR images. These relationships form the basis for understanding and manipulating contrast in clinical MRI of the musculoskeletal system.

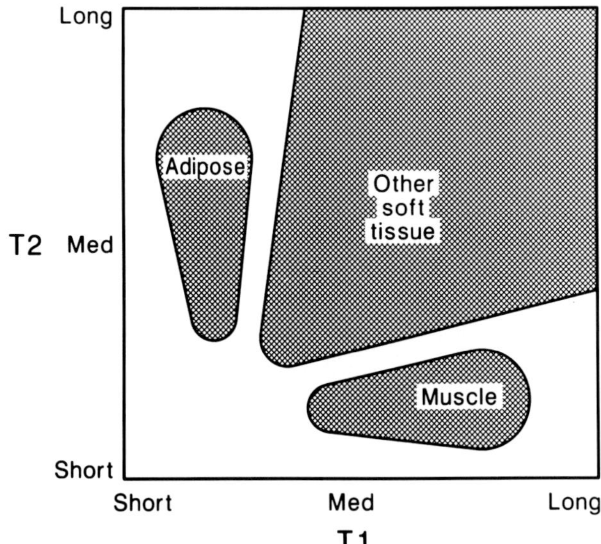

FIG. 2-7. Relaxation time map for musculoskeletal tissues.

EFFECT OF PATHOLOGY ON TISSUE RELAXATION TIMES

The relaxation times of many musculoskeletal tissues change in rather distinctive ways when they are affected by specific pathological processes (45). The significance and basic biophysical mechanisms for these changes are relatively poorly understood and few clinical applications have been demonstrated for their quantitative measurement. But they do cause diagnostically useful changes in the intensity and contrast of tissues in MR images. The general trend of the relaxation time changes for some important musculoskeletal disease processes is summarized in Table 2-2.

Inflammation

Inflammatory processes are generally characterized by prolongation of T1 and T2 relaxation times (32). The presence of edema seems to be the most likely mechanism to explain these changes. Accumulation of extracellular and possibly intracellular water causes an increase in the total water content of tissue. The previously described two-state, fast-exchange model is helpful for understanding how even a small change in water content can result in a large alteration in relaxation times. Since water protons freely diffuse between the intracellular and extracellular spaces and the number of macromolecular binding sites is relatively fixed, the increased water content represents an increase in the fraction of free water.

Figure 2-8 shows theoretically expected tissue T1 values for various free water fractions, calculated using Eq. 2. The relaxation times $T1_f$ and $T1_b$ were assigned values of 2,500 and 50 msec, respectively. Relaxation time rapidly increases as the fraction of free water increases above 85%. Note, for instance, that a 1% increase in free water from 91 to 92% causes a 10% increase in relaxation time.

Neoplasms

With certain exceptions, most solid neoplasms are characterized by relaxation times that are prolonged relative to their host tissues. Many studies of this phenomenon have appeared in the literature (3). Some studies

TABLE 2-2.

Disease process	T1	T2
Inflammation	Increased	Increased
Neoplasia	Increased	Increased
Fibrosis	—	Decreased
Fatty infiltration	Decreased	—
Interstitial hemorrhage	Increased	Increased

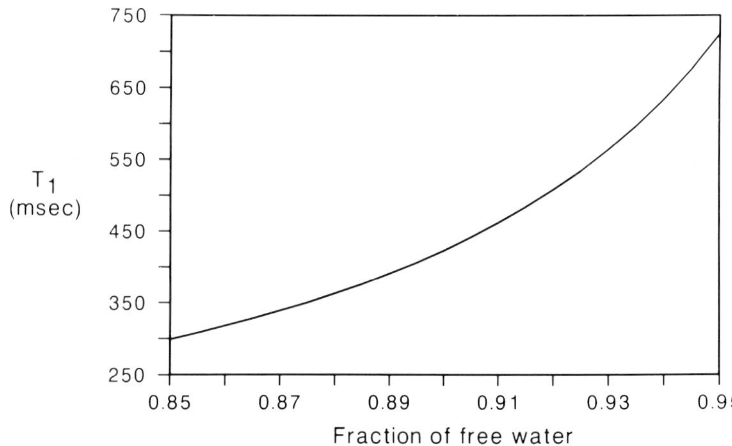

FIG. 2-8. Relationship between spin–lattice relaxation time and fraction of unbound or free water with a fast-exchange, two-state model for tissue relaxation times.

have demonstrated increases in tissue water content that correlate with the degree of relaxation time prolongation, while others have not (11). The changes probably reflect an alteration in the ratio of free to bound water in tumor tissue, possibly related to changes in the way that water is ordered within and adjacent to the hydration layer of macromolecules.

Although the elevation of T1 and T2 relaxation times in neoplastic tissue is usually less than that resulting from inflammation, there is considerable overlap, and distinction between these processes must usually be made on the basis of morphology and history.

Fibrosis

As noted above, the mobile spin density of predominantly fibrous tissue is low, thus providing little MR signal. Diffuse fibrosis of parenchymal tissues may be difficult to detect until it is well advanced and a substantial amount of the tissue has been replaced. The T2 relaxation time of mature fibrotic tissue is often reduced. In contrast, the T2 relaxation time of immature fibrosis in granulation tissue is usually long, causing high intensity in T2 weighted images.

Fatty Infiltration

Fatty infiltration of muscles and other musculoskeletal tissues causes a shortening of *in vivo* T1 relaxation times because of the very short T1 of fat. A distinguishing feature between this and most other spin–lattice relaxation time changes related to disease is that the relaxation curves are not uniexponential (24). This is because there is little exchange between the protons in fat and those in the host tissue. The relaxation is therefore biexponential, with a fast component due to fat protons and a slower component due to water protons in the host tissue. Most *in vivo* methods for measuring T1 are incapable of resolving the biexponential nature of the recovery curve and simply show that the relaxation time is short.

Hematoma

Interstitial hemorrhage in muscle and other tissues usually causes prolongation of both T1 and T2 relaxation times, probably due to the presence of inflammation and edema (13,61).

The relaxation time characteristics of hematomas (confluent collections of extravasated blood) are much more variable. They are strongly influenced by formation of paramagnetic substances (6,28,61). Oxygenated hemoglobin contains iron in a "low spin" ferrous state that is not paramagnetic. Thus, the proton relaxation times of stationary oxygenated blood are mainly determined by the concentration of protein (albumin and hemoglobin), which determines the fraction of water protons that are in the bound, fast relaxing state. The T1 and T2 relaxation times of fresh oxygenated blood are medium or long in comparison to most solid tissue. Deoxygenation of hemoglobin has little effect on the relaxation time of hematomas at imager fields of less than 1.0T. Deoxyhemoglobin contains iron in a "high spin" ferrous state that is paramagnetic, but the area of the unpaired electron is relatively inaccessible to water protons because of the conformation of the molecule. Thus, the net relaxation of water protons is not enhanced because they are unable to interact with the paramagnetic center.

As time passes, oxidative denaturation of deoxyhemoglobin causes formation of methemoglobin (44), which contains iron in a ferric form and is strongly paramagnetic. Water molecules have relatively free access to the paramagnetic site and thus the relaxation times are shortened. The T1 relaxation time of the hematoma is typically reduced more than T2 by the presence of methemoglobin. This can be rationalized by noting that the T2 of acute hematoma is short compared

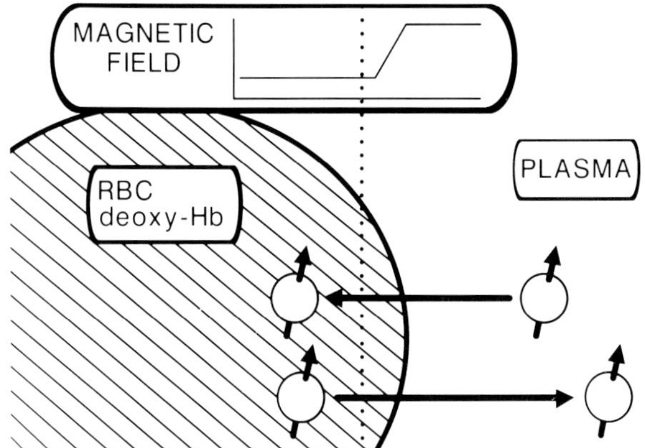

FIG. 2-9. Water protons diffusing through the cell membranes of erythrocytes containing deoxyhemoglobin experience a tiny shift in their resonant frequency due to the presence of a field gradient. This causes selective reduction of T2 relaxation time at high field strengths.

to its T1 relaxation time even though it is long in comparison to solid tissue. Even if $T1_p$ and $T2_p$ are relatively long, corresponding to a low concentration of methemoglobin, Eqs. 3 and 4 show that $T1_o$ will be affected more than $T2_o$. For instance, if the $T1_d$ and $T2_d$ values of an acute hematoma are 600 and 150 msec, respectively, and after a period of time a small amount of methemoglobin is formed to yield paramagnetic contributions ($T1_p$ and $T2_p$) on the order of 1,000 msec, then the observed $T1_o$ and $T2_o$ values of the hematoma will be 375 and 130 msec, respectively. In a T1 weighted image (see next section) this would result in a substantial increase in intensity.

At higher field strengths (>1.0T) an additional physical process begins to affect the relaxation times of hematogenous material. Empirical observations have shown that the T2 of hematomas can be extremely short at high field (1.5T) while it is long in comparison to soft tissue at low and medium field strengths (28). The explanation relates to the fact that while deoxyhemoglobin is not an effective proton relaxation enhancer, it does cause the magnetic susceptibility of the erythrocyte cytoplasm to differ significantly from that of plasma. When a substance is placed in a magnetic field, the strength of the local magnetization typically differs from the external field strength by a proportionality factor called the bulk magnetic susceptibility.

The difference in magnetic susceptibility between plasma and cytoplasm results in a small difference in the field strength between the interior and exterior of erythrocytes. This gradient across the cell membranes is only one or two ten-thousandths of 1 percent (1–2 ppm) of the main magnetic field, but that is enough to shorten the T2 relaxation at high field (63). The mechanism is due to diffusion of water protons through the field gradients at the erythrocyte membrane (Fig. 2-9). Protons moving in such a fashion accumulate phase differences that would not have been present if the field gradients were absent, resulting in more rapid decay of the transverse magnetization. The phase errors are proportional to the square of the gradient. Since the gradient is proportional to the field strength, this effect is much more pronounced at high field strength.

It is interesting to note that this T2 relaxation enhancement effect is operative only when erythrocyte membranes are intact. On lysis, the deoxyhemoglobin is distributed uniformly and the local field gradients abolished. Figure 2-10 shows a simple experiment in which two samples of diluted deoxygenated blood were imaged at 0.15 and 1.5T. The sample on the right in the images

A,B

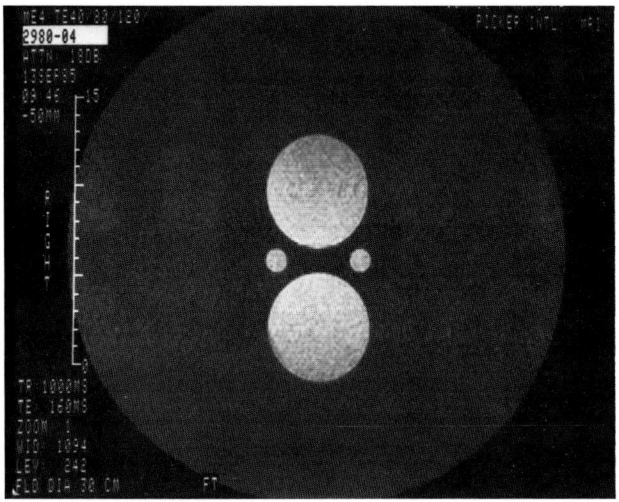

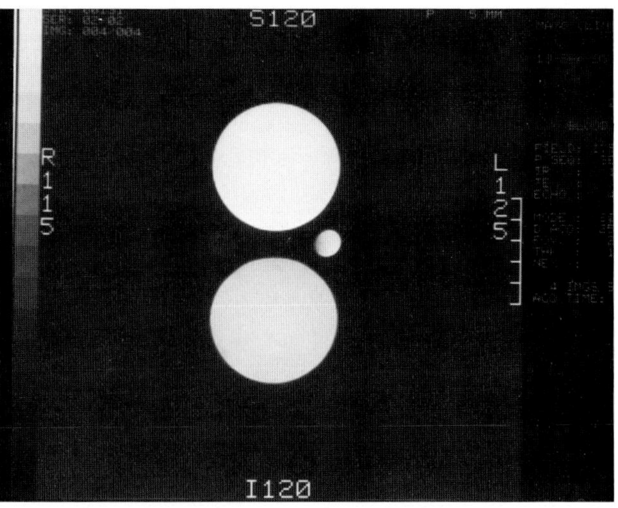

FIG. 2-10. A: Low-field T2 weighted image of two vials (small diameter disks) containing blood. The image demonstrates no intensity difference between lysed blood in the tube on the right of the picture and intact cells in the left. The two large disks are reference standards. **B:** High-field T2 weighted image of same vials as in (**A**) demonstrates striking reduction in the intensity of the nonlysed blood.

was osmotically lysed. Note that both samples have identical intensity in a T2 weighted image (see next section) at 0.15T, while the tube containing intact cells was dramatically reduced in intensity in a similar image at 1.5T. The measured T2 relaxation times of both tubes at 0.15T and the lysed tube at 1.5T were greater than 150 msec. The T2 of the intact cells at 1.5T was less than 45 msec.

Similar field-dependent T2 proton relaxation effect can also occur at the periphery of old hemorrhagic lesions due to susceptibility gradients in the vicinity of hemosiderin-laden macrophages (28).

In summary, the relaxation times of hematomas are affected by many factors, including protein concentration, formation of paramagnetic methemoglobin, and T2 proton relaxation enhancement by local heterogeneity in magnetic susceptibility at high field strength.

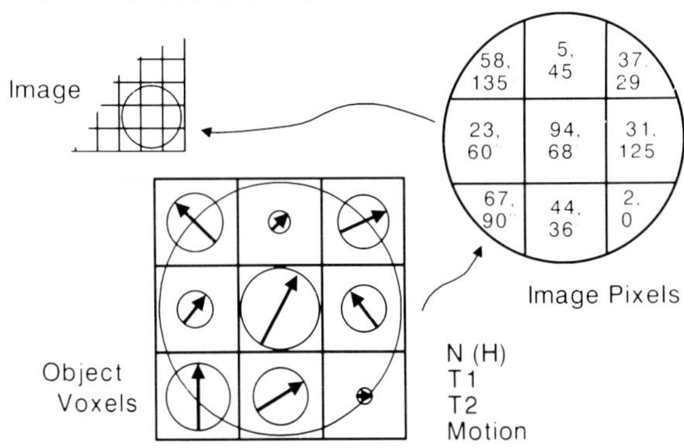

FIG. 2-11. Relationship between image pixels and object voxels.

INFLUENCE OF RELAXATION TIMES AND PULSE SEQUENCE PARAMETERS ON CONTRAST

The appearance of tissue in clinical MR images depends on tissue properties and on the parameters of the pulse sequence. As already noted, the most important tissue properties in this context are the relaxation times T1 and T2 and the spin density N(H). The most important pulse sequence parameters are the pulse repetition time TR and the echo delay time TE for the spin-echo sequence. The inversion recovery sequence has an additional important parameter: inversion time (TI). In the discussion that follows, we concentrate on spin-echo methods since these are the most frequently used techniques in current clinical MRI. A few unique features of gradient-echo imaging are outlined in a subsequent section.

The importance of understanding the influence of these tissue properties and pulse sequence parameters on the contrast between tissues cannot be overemphasized. It provides a basis for characterizing tissue in clinical images. It also provides guidance for selecting appropriate MRI techniques from the huge number of possible parameter combinations so that the examination can be tailored to individual diagnostic problems.

Typical MR images are displayed in such a way that the brightness of each pixel is dependent on the magnetic resonance signal that is obtained from each corresponding voxel (volume element) within the patient (Fig. 2-11). The precessing magnetization vector in each volume element has a certain magnitude and phase angle with respect to the magnetization vectors in neighboring voxels. These two quantities are dependent on the relaxation times, spin density, and motion of the protons within the volume element and on details of the magnetic resonance technique. The phase angle is usually used to determine the spatial location of the magnetic resonance signals. The magnitude of the magnetization vector in each volume element determines the brightness of each corresponding pixel in the final image.

It is useful to study a simplified model for the intensity of spin-echo signals from tissue:

$$\text{Intensity} = N(H)e^{-TE/T2}(1 - e^{-TR/T1}) \qquad [7]$$

where N(H) is the spin density, T1 and T2 are the spin–lattice and spin–spin relaxation times, respectively, TR is the pulse repetition time, and TE is the echo delay time. This model ignores many important factors that affect the spin-echo signal such as the presence of motion, flow, diffusion, and the technical details of the pulse sequence and imager. Nevertheless, it is helpful for understanding the basis for image contrast.

Note first that the intensity of the signal is proportional to the spin density and this is true for images with any combination of TR and TE. The dependence of intensity on T2 is governed by the first exponential in this equation and the dependence on T1 is modeled by the terms within the parentheses.

The behavior of the portion of the equation that is within the parentheses is shown in Fig. 2-2. A spin-echo sequence begins with a 90° RF pulse, which tips the magnetization that is parallel to the main magnetic field (longitudinal magnetization) into the transverse plane. The amount of longitudinal magnetization that is available is dependent on the time that has passed since the previous 90° pulse. Spin-echo sequences with long repetition times (TR) in comparison to the T1 of tissue will have large amounts of magnetization to tip into the transverse plane, while short TR values will cause the amount of available longitudinal magnetization to be reduced. When TR is at least three times as long as the T1 of the tissue, then the amount of longitudinal magnetization will be more than 95% of what would be present with an infinite waiting time. If TR is the same as T1, then the magnetization that is available will be about 63% of the maximum value. As TR is further reduced, the available magnetization becomes less and less. The latter condition is called a state of "partial saturation." Note that a particular repeated spin sequence may cause partial saturation of one tissue with a long T1 while some other tissue that has a short T1 may not be partially saturated.

Once the longitudinal magnetization is tipped into the transverse plane by the 90° RF pulse, a spin-echo signal is created at time TE by a 180° RF pulse applied at time TE/2. Equation 7 shows that the intensity or strength of the spin-echo signal depends on an exponential decay function that is governed by the ratio of TE/T2. Clearly, sequences with short echo delay times will produce stronger spin echos than those with long TE values in relation to the transverse relaxation time T2. As shown in Fig. 2-3, tissues with long T2 relaxation times will yield spin echos with higher intensity than those with short T2 values, all other factors being equal.

The significance of all this is that TR is a user selectable parameter that determines the maximum signal that a given tissue will yield (dependent on the rate of growth of longitudinal magnetization, i.e., T1). The selection of TE governs the exponential T2 decay of the potential signal before a spin echo is created. Given a pair of tissues with different relaxation times, it is possible to select TR and TE in such a way as to either minimize or maximize the intensity difference (contrast) between the two tissues.

Note that Eq. 7 indicates that if the T1 of a tissue is increased, its spin-echo intensity will be reduced. As shown in Fig. 2-2, this is because less longitudinal magnetization is available for tipping into the transverse plane and later creation of a spin echo. The reverse condition applies for T2. If the T2 relaxation time of a tissue is increased, its spin-echo intensity will increase because less transverse decay will occur before a spin echo is formed, as shown in Fig. 2-3.

T1 AND T2 WEIGHTED SEQUENCES

The concept of T1 and T2 weighted sequences is very useful for selecting sequences and understanding the gray scale of MR images. Consider a hypothetical case in which we wish to provide contrast between two tissues on the basis of their different T2 relaxation times. This means that it is desirable to select a sequence that is relatively insensitive to differences in T1 while yielding large intensity differences between tissues with different T2 values. The first goal can be achieved by selecting a TR time that is long in comparison to all the tissues. This will ensure that there is enough recovery time between 90° pulses so that full longitudinal magnetization develops in all tissues, regardless of the particular T1 relaxation time. The second goal is facilitated by selecting a TE that is relatively long so that there is a large difference in spin-echo intensity between tissues with slow and fast T2 decay.

A T2 weighted spin-echo sequence is therefore one in which the TR is long in relation to the T1 of the tissues of interest, and the TE is also relatively long. The freedom from T1 influence is dependent on the long TR, while the sensitivity to T2 differences is determined by TE. Although the relative intensity difference between tissues with differing T2 values increases with TE, there is a practical limit to the allowable maximum echo delay time. This is imposed by the fact that the absolute magnitudes of the signals decrease with echo delay time so that at some point the ratio of signal to noise in the image is degraded so much that further enhancement of relative contrast is useless.

Consider a second case in which we wish to differentiate between tissues on the basis of T1 differences. In order to minimize T2-dependent intensity differences, it is necessary to make TE as short as possible. By also selecting a short TR, tissues will be placed in a state of partial saturation, depending on their T1 relaxation time. Tissues with long T1 values will fail to remagnetize as much as those with shorter T1 times between 90° pulses and thus their spin-echo signals will be reduced.

A T1 weighted spin-echo sequence is therefore one with a relatively short TR and short TE. In practice, very short TE values are technically difficult to achieve in spin-echo sequences. The extent to which TR can be shortened in spin-echo sequences is also limited, because this progressively reduces the longitudinal magnetization resulting in lower signal-to-noise ratios.

T1 and T2 weighted sequences are very useful for a number of reasons. They allow qualitative recognition of the relaxation time characteristics of lesions in relation to adjacent tissues, which can be very helpful diagnostically. But the most important reason for employing such sequences is that they are most likely to provide lesion contrast. Many pathological processes, including inflammation, neoplasia, and parenchymal hemorrhage, are characterized by parallel increases in both T1 and T2 relaxation times. As already noted, these tend to produce opposite changes in spin-echo intensity, so that for certain combinations of TR and TE, the contrast between a lesion and adjacent normal tissue may be low. Isointensity between tumors and other soft tissue is particularly common with spin-echo sequences that are neither T1 or T2 weighted by the above criteria, especially spin-echo techniques with TR values of 500–1,500 and TE values in the range of 20–40 msec. Figure 2-12 shows such a situation. The frequency of such problems can be reduced by employing strongly T1 or T2 weighted sequences. In general, the best practice is to image the same area with at least two combinations of TR and TE.

The term "T1 weighted" is frequently misused when it is applied to describe partial saturation (short TR)

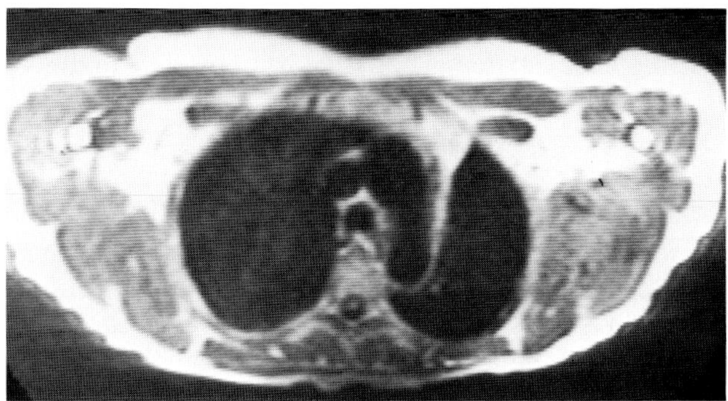
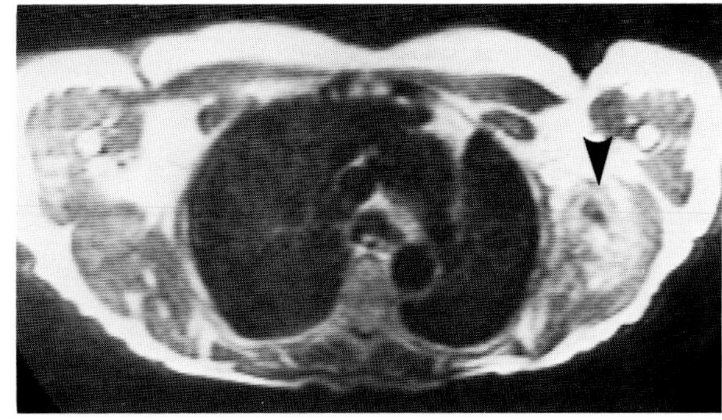

A,B

FIG. 2-12. **A:** Partial saturation spin-echo image fails to provide contrast between malignant soft tissue tumor and surrounding muscle. **B:** Tumor is apparent because of contrast provided by T2 weighted spin-echo image (*arrow*).

spin-echo sequences. Although these terms have not been formally defined, it seems clear that in order for a T1 weighted sequence to be useful as such, it must be substantially more sensitive to changes in T1 than to similar percentage changes in T2. Unless this condition is met, lesions that cause simultaneous elevation of T1 and T2 may be missed and few conclusions about relaxation time changes can be made. It is quite difficult to fulfill such a condition with partial saturation spin-echo sequences because the minimum echo delay time of most imagers still results in substantial T2 dependence.

One way to evaluate the weighting of particular MRI techniques is to determine the magnitude and direction of the change in image intensity that would result if the T1 and T2 of a particular tissue is changed by a small amount simultaneously. For example, if T1 and T2 were both increased, then a T1 weighted sequence would register a reduction of intensity and a T2 weighted sequence would show an increase. Mixed or unweighted techniques would yield small or no change of tissue intensity. By this standard, most long TR and long TE spin-echo sequences can be regarded as strongly T2 weighted. On the other hand, it is difficult to obtain strongly T1 weighted spin-echo images without using very short TE times (10–15 msec). Strongly T1 weighted techniques can easily be obtained using inversion recovery sequences (65).

Lesion conspicuity in MRI is not solely a function of contrast as measured by the relative or absolute intensity differences. Noise is an important additional factor that must be considered. This includes thermal noise and coherent noise (e.g., motion artifacts). It is tempting to try to find methods for "optimizing" the contrast-to-noise ratio for particular lesions (40,41,56). In practice, these approaches have limited value because the relaxation times of pathological and surrounding tissues are rarely known with sufficient precision to make such procedures worthwhile. In addition, the process of "optimizing" contrast may compromise the clarity of other tissue interfaces. Clearly, the important goal is simply to display the lesion with enough contrast so that it can be detected. This goal is best achieved by imaging with several different MRI techniques, at least some of which should be strongly T1 or T2 weighted.

CONTRAST IN GRADIENT-ECHO SEQUENCES

Gradient-echo techniques (Chapter 1) have seen increasing use for musculoskeletal imaging applications, especially for joint imaging (27,29,39,59,60). They provide interesting capabilities in terms of image contrast and acquisition speed. These sequences add an additional parameter to the list of settings that affect image contrast, namely, the tip angle α (alpha). Several features distinguish gradient-echo sequences from spin-echo sequences. One of the most important of these is that gradient-echo sequences can use very short pulse repetition times, thereby permitting rapid image acquisition. Such short TR times are possible because the low nutation angle RF pulses destroy only a fraction of the longitudinal magnetization in each pulse repetition cycle. This is in contrast to the spin-echo technique, in which longitudinal magnetization is reduced in each repetition cycle by the initial 90° RF pulse.

Gradient-echo techniques can be broadly divided into "steady-state" sequences, such as GRASS and FISP, and "spoiled" sequences, such as FLASH and SPGR (27,59). The concept of "residual transverse magnetization" is central to this classification. When short TR times are used with gradient-echo sequences, transverse magnetization created by each RF pulse may not have dephased appreciably before the next RF pulse is applied. This is especially likely to occur in tissues with long T2 relaxation times. If such transverse magnetization is present at the time of the next RF pulse, a portion of it will be rotated back into the longitudinal direction. The next RF pulse can then convert a portion of this same magnetization back into transverse magnetization. In this way, magnetization can be "recycled" back and

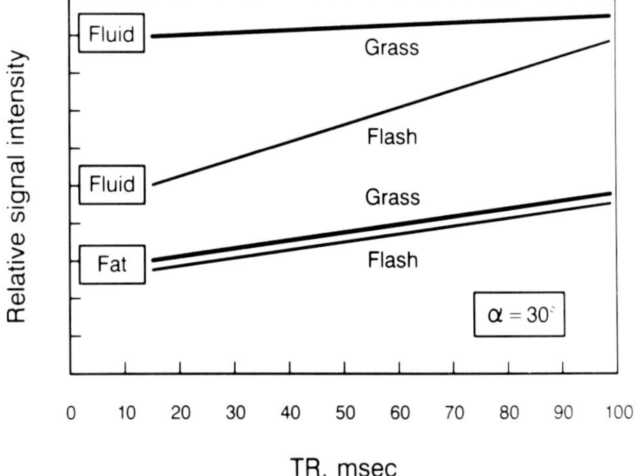

FIG. 2-13. Comparison of contrast characteristics of a "steady-state" type gradient-echo sequence (GRASS) with a "spoiled" type gradient-echo sequence (FLASH). The differences are most apparent for materials with long T2 relaxation times (i.e., fluid), and at short pulse repetitions times. The behavior illustrated here makes "steady-state" sequences suitable for providing T2 weighted contrast characteristics and "spoiled" sequences best for providing T1 weighted contrast.

forth between the longitudinal and transverse directions. This steady-state magnetization contributes to the signal generated in each gradient echo.

The sequences in the "steady-state" category employ measures to preserve and enhance the contribution of steady-state magnetization to the gradient-echo signal. The intensity of fluid and other materials with long T2 relaxation times is increased by this contribution in GRASS and FISP images. As a consequence, these images often have contrast characteristics reminiscent of T2 weighted spin-echo images.

The "spoiled" gradient-echo sequences, of which FLASH is the prototype, employ measures to eliminate the contribution of steady-state magnetization. This tends to reduce the intensity of structures with long T2 relaxation times. Spoiled gradient sequences are well suited for providing T1 weighted contrast characteristics.

The differences between "steady-state" and "spoiled" gradient-echo sequences tend to be reduced for sequences with long pulse repetition times because the longer time between successive RF pulses allows the transverse magnetization to die away (Fig. 2-13).

A,B

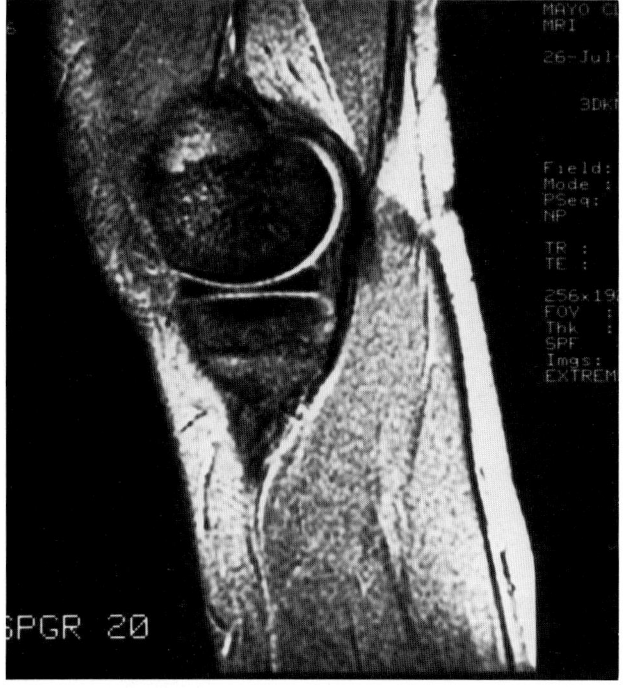

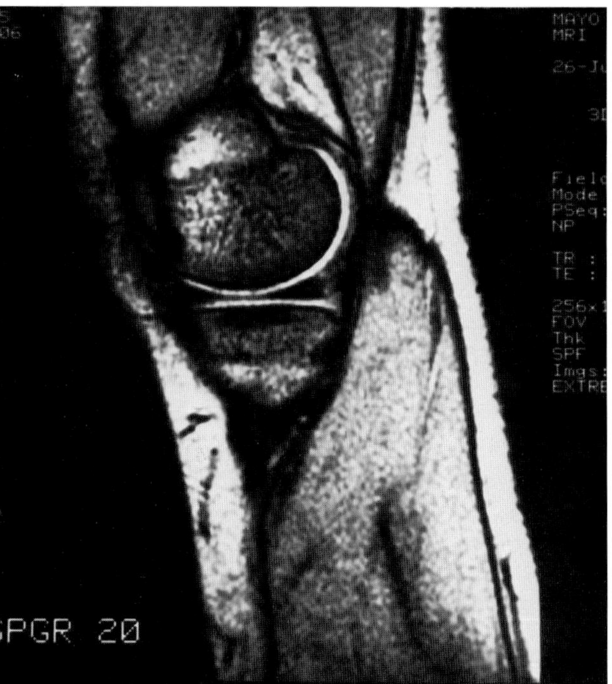

FIG. 2-14. Phase interference effects in gradient-echo images. **A:** Spoiled GRASS image of the knee, obtained with a TE time of 14 msec. **B:** A similar image obtained with a TE of 12 msec is markedly different in appearance. All interfaces between fat and water-containing tissues have markedly decreased signal intensity (*arrow*). This effect is a general property of all gradient-echo images and occurs at echo delay times in which the magnetization of water and fat is 180° out of phase, so that signal cancellation takes place in voxels containing mixtures of fat and water. The exact TE values in which such "phase opposition" effects are seen depend on the field strength of the imager. The phenomenon is completely independent from the "chemical shift" artifact. Please see cited reference for more information.

The contrast characteristics of gradient-echo sequences are more complex than spin-echo sequences. Gradient-echo images are strongly affected by a number of technical and tissue variables that tend to make the gray scale characteristics somewhat less predictable and consistent compared with spin-echo sequences. Gradient-echo sequences are more strongly affected by field inhomogeneity, magnetic susceptibility effects, and motion effects than spin-echo sequences. An important process that influences the appearance of gradient-echo images is a TE-dependent phase contrast phenomenon that affects the intensity of tissues containing a mixture of fat and water (66) (Fig. 2-14).

APPROACH FOR SELECTION OF MRI TECHNIQUES

Certain clinical problems in musculoskeletal MRI can serve as examples to clarify the rationale for selecting sequences and interpreting images. These problems include detection of primary soft tissue neoplasms, recurrent tumors after surgery, and identification of hematomas.

As shown in Chapter 12, one of the most successful applications of MRI is delineation of soft tissue tumors of the musculoskeletal system (16). Often these lesions are surrounded by muscle and it is this situation that is examined first. The ground rules are simple: most malignant lesions have T1 and T2 relaxation times that are longer than muscle. Healthy skeletal muscle tissue has a remarkably short T2 relaxation time in comparison to almost any other soft tissue, and certainly it is much shorter than most malignant soft tissue tumors. Given these facts, consider the expected time course of longitudinal magnetization that is shown in Fig. 2-15A. The longer T1 of tumor means that its longitudinal magnetization will be less than that of muscle, particularly with a short TR such as 500 msec.

Figure 2-15B shows the time course of the transverse magnetization that would occur after the 180° RF pulse in a sequence with a relatively short TR. The shorter T2 of muscle causes its transverse magnetization to decay more quickly than that of the tumor so that the curves cross. Thus, a partial saturation sequence (short TR) with a relatively short TE is unlikely to display a malignant soft tissue tumor with high contrast. Figure 2-16A demonstrates such an image in a patient with a malignant schwannoma. In Fig. 2-15C, the transverse magnetization is traced for the case in which a longer TR is used. Note that the starting transverse magnetization is stronger and that the initial difference between tumor and muscle is smaller. With a relatively long echo delay time, the relative intensity difference between tumor and muscle is much greater than in Fig. 2-15B. Figure

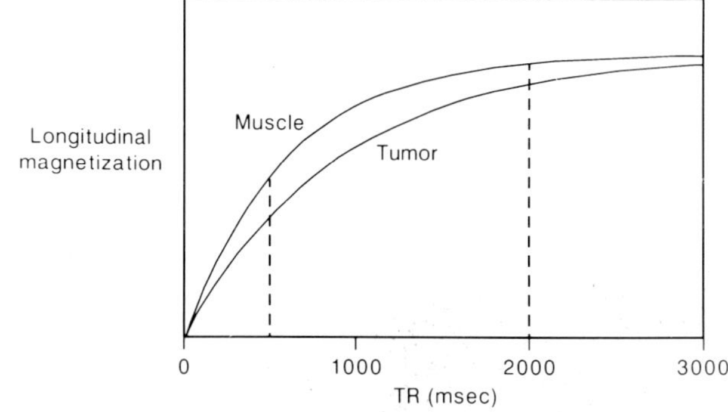

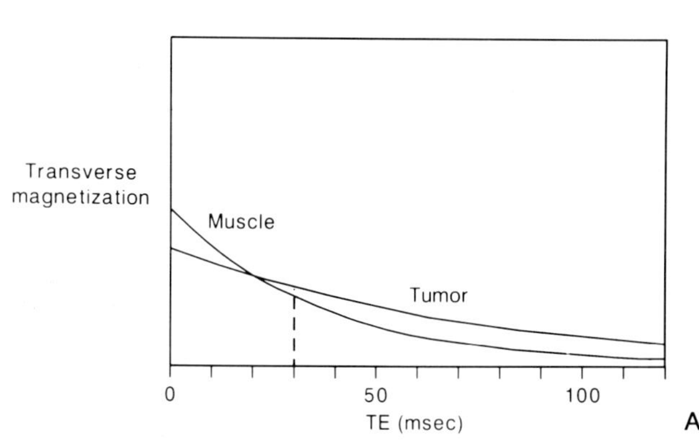

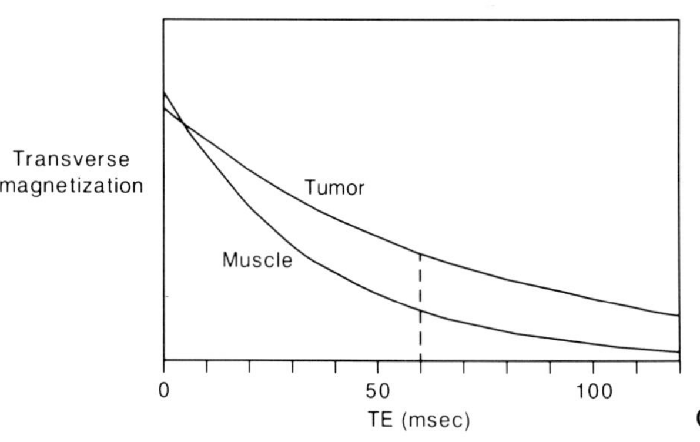

FIG. 2-15 A–C. Typical behavior of longitudinal and transverse magnetization of muscle and tumor in spin-echo sequences. T2 weighted sequence with long TR and TE provides best contrast.

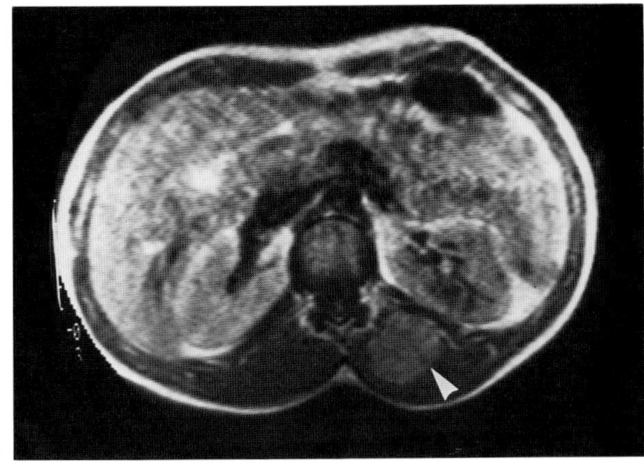

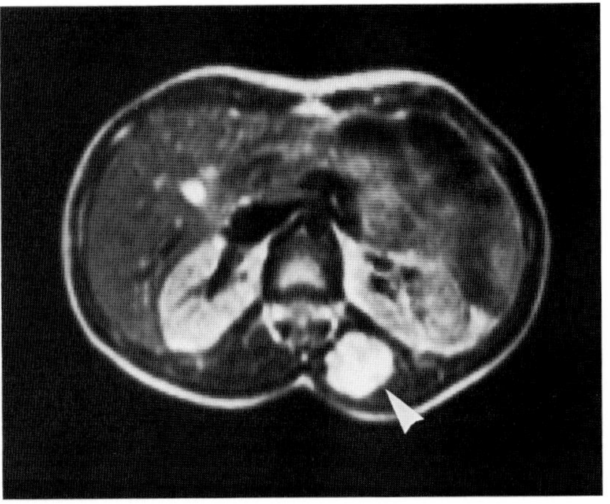

A,B

FIG. 2-16 A and **B.** Partial saturation and T2 weighted spin-echo images of patient with malignant schwannoma (*arrows*), analogous to the situation in Fig. 2-15.

16B shows a corresponding T2 weighted image of the same patient as in Fig. 2-16A.

The main lesson from this example is that since tumor and muscle differ markedly in their T2 relaxation times, a T2 weighted sequence is able to display the interface with a high degree of contrast. The partial saturation sequence provides a lower degree of contrast in this case because of its "mixed" response to both T1 and T2 differences.

Tumors are not always completely surrounded by a single tissue and in these situations several different MRI techniques may be necessary to completely delineate the borders of the lesion. A good example of this situation is a follow-up examination in a patient who has previously had a tumor resected from an extremity. Atrophy and fatty infiltration of surrounding muscles is frequently present. Figures 17A and 17B are partial saturation and T2 weighted images from such a patient. Does this patient have recurrent tumor? Figures 18A and 18B are partial saturation and T2 weighted images from a patient with a primary malignant soft tissue tumor in his left popliteal fossa. Can the complete boundaries of the lesion be identified in either image alone?

Adipose tissue has a T1 relaxation time that is dramatically shorter than almost any other soft tissue, as shown in Fig. 2-7. The T2 relaxation times of fat and tumor can overlap. Figure 2-19A demonstrates that the longitudinal magnetization that is available in fat is large even with a short TR. In Fig. 2-19B the transverse magnetization is traced in fat and tumor for a partial saturation sequence. Note that this sequence provides high contrast at short echo delay times. Although transverse magnetization is stronger when the TR is long, as shown

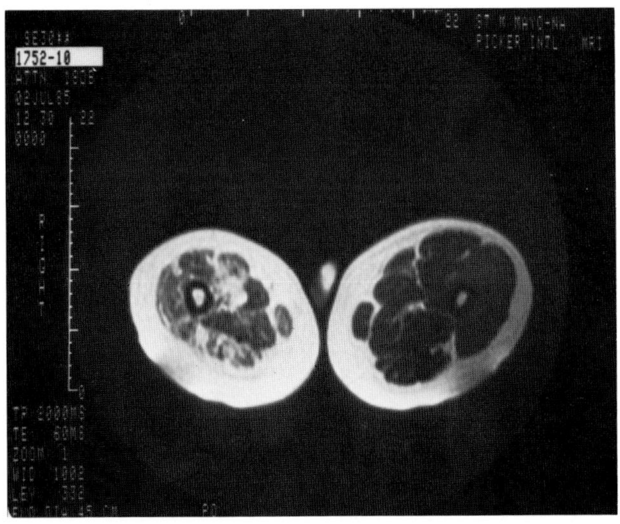

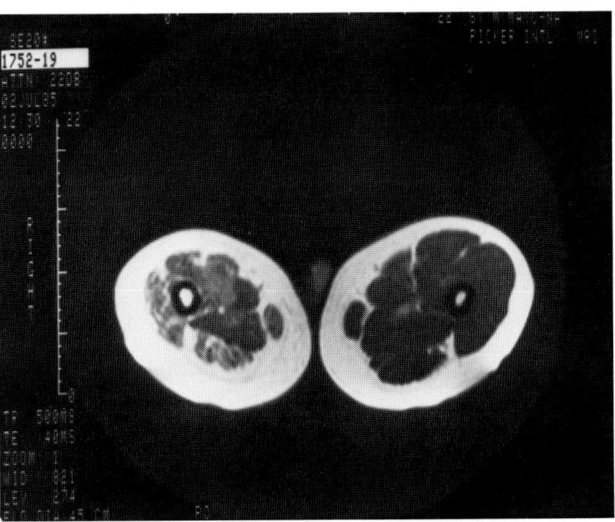

A,B

FIG. 2-17 A and **B.** Partial saturation and T2 weighted images of a patient with suspected recurrent malignant fibrous histiocytoma. See also Fig. 2-23.

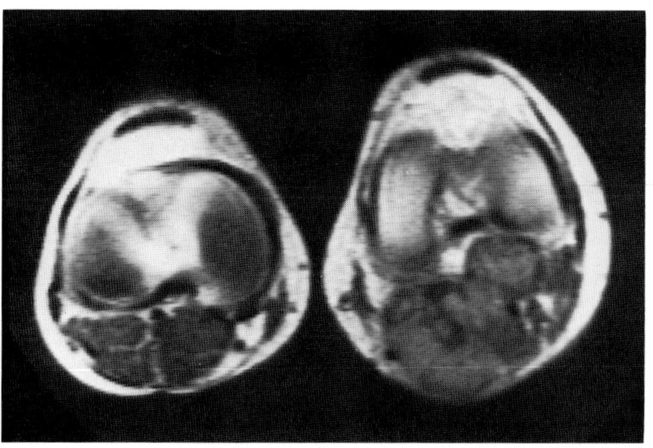

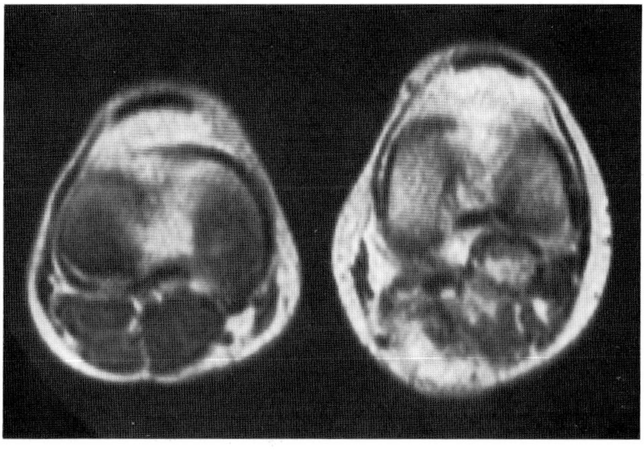

A,B

FIG. 2-18 A and B. Partial saturation and T2 weighted sequences are both needed to adequately trace the borders of the malignant tumor in the left popliteal region.

in Fig. 2-19C, the contrast between fat and tumor is poor.

Partial saturation sequences are therefore very helpful for differentiating fatty tissue from other tissues. Although they are not particularly T1 weighted, the very short T1 of fat provides sufficient T1-dependent contrast. Figure 2-17B (T2 weighted image) demonstrates an irregular area of high intensity which could be adipose tissue, but the partial saturation image (Fig. 2-17A) demonstrates that this is not fat and in fact this was recurrent tumor. The margins between tumor and adipose tissue are delineated in the partial saturation image in Fig. 2-18A, but those with muscle are difficult to identify. The T2 weighted image provides just the reverse.

As described in a previous section, hematomas can have a variety of different appearances because of the unique physical processes that can affect their relaxation

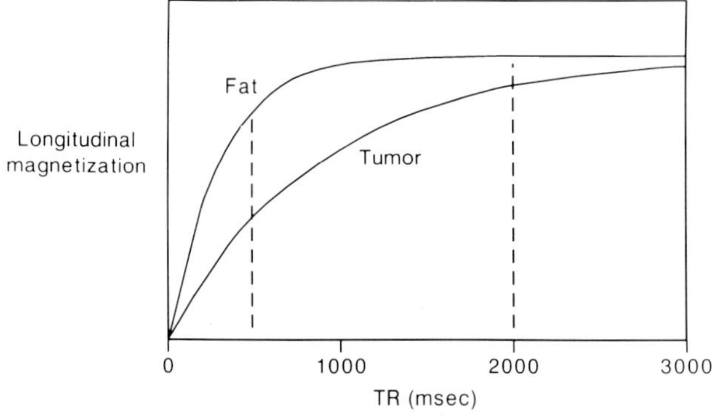

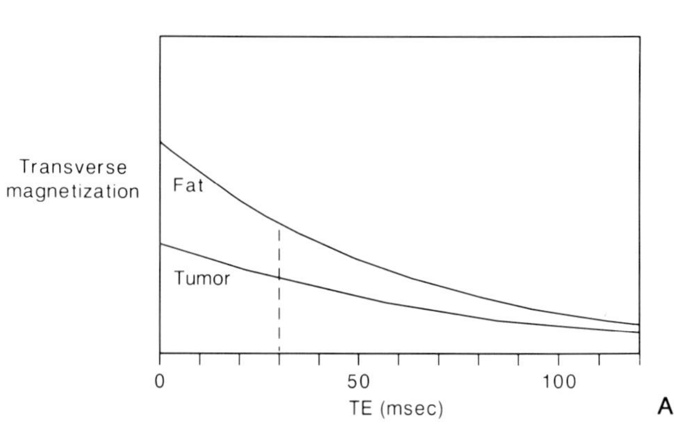

A,B

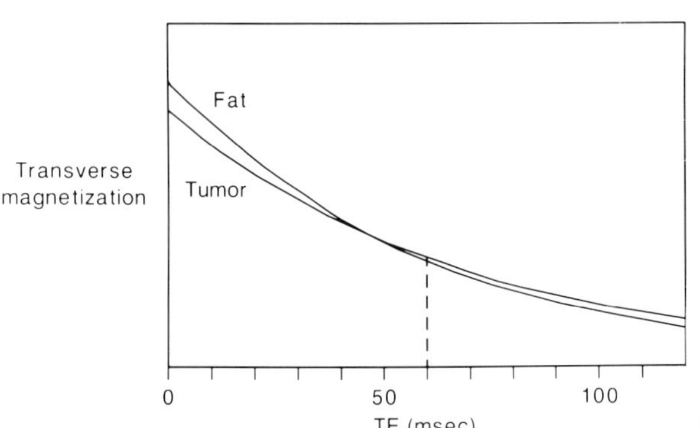

C

FIG. 2-19 A–C. Contrast between tumor and adipose tissue is clearly most easily achieved with a partial saturation spin-echo sequence with a relatively short TR and TE.

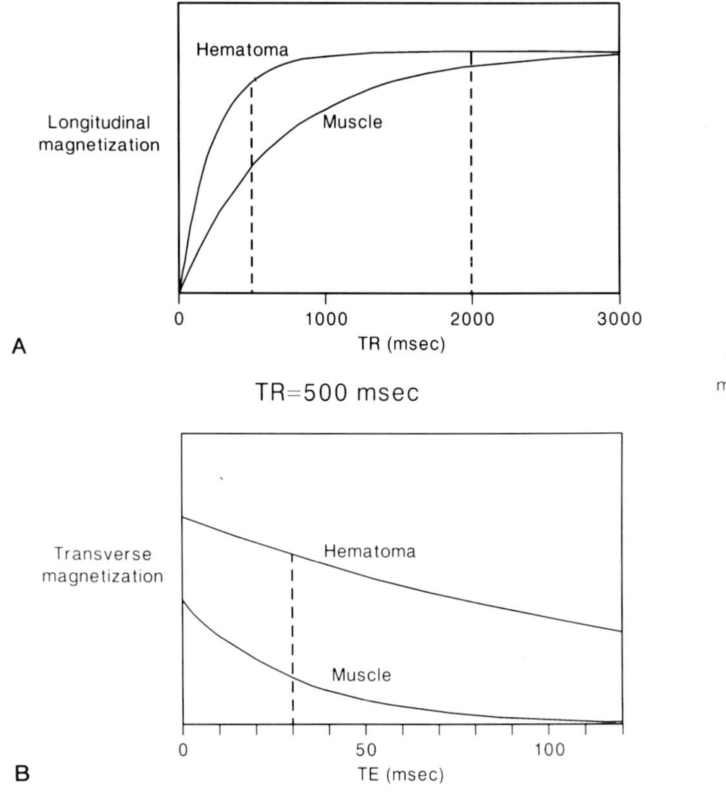

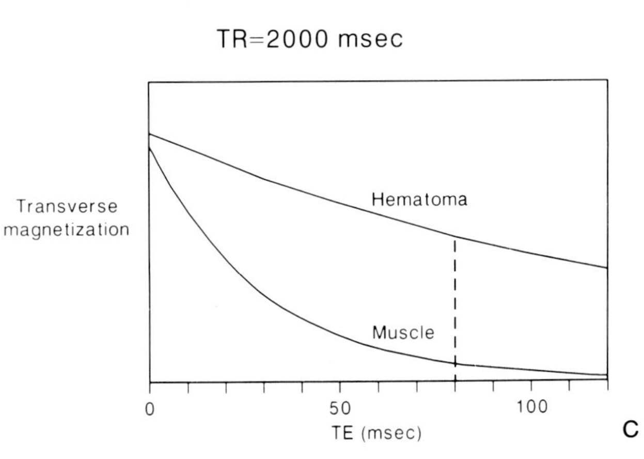

FIG. 2-20 A–C. Typical low and medium field behavior of magnetization in subacute hematoma.

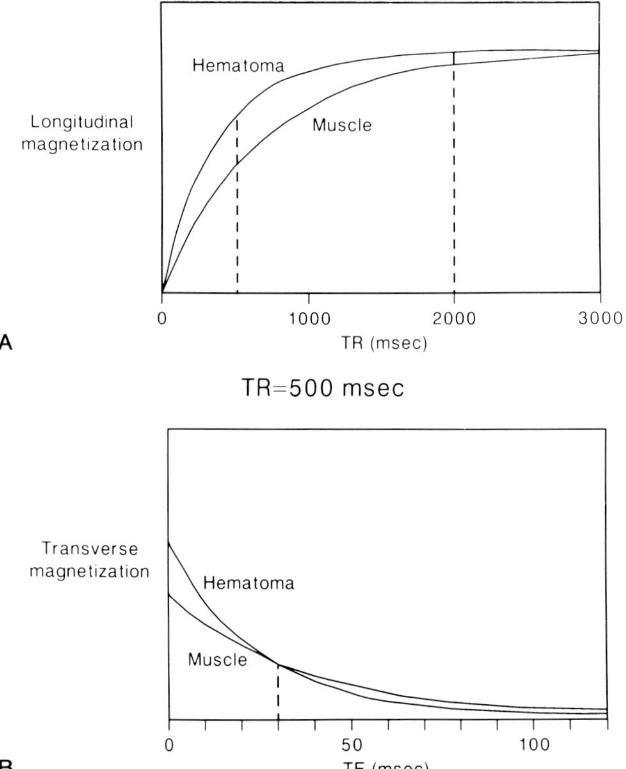

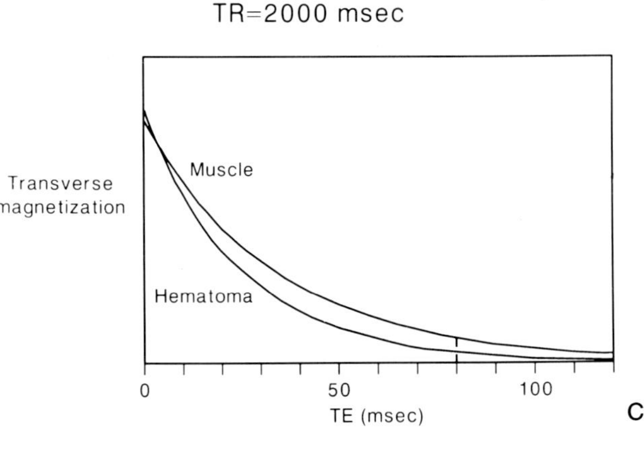

FIG. 2-21 A–C. Behavior of magnetization in subacute hematoma imaged at high field.

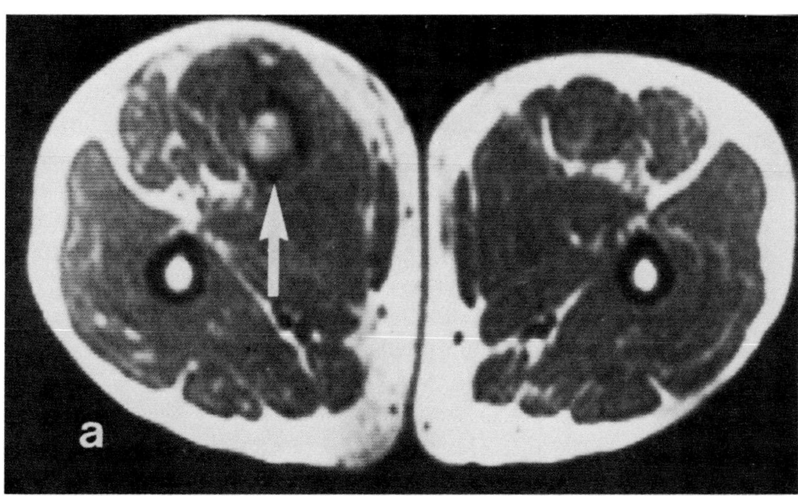

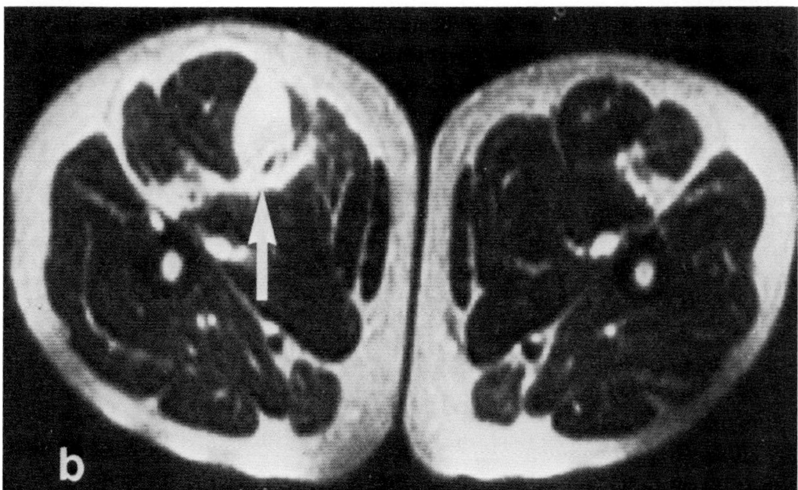

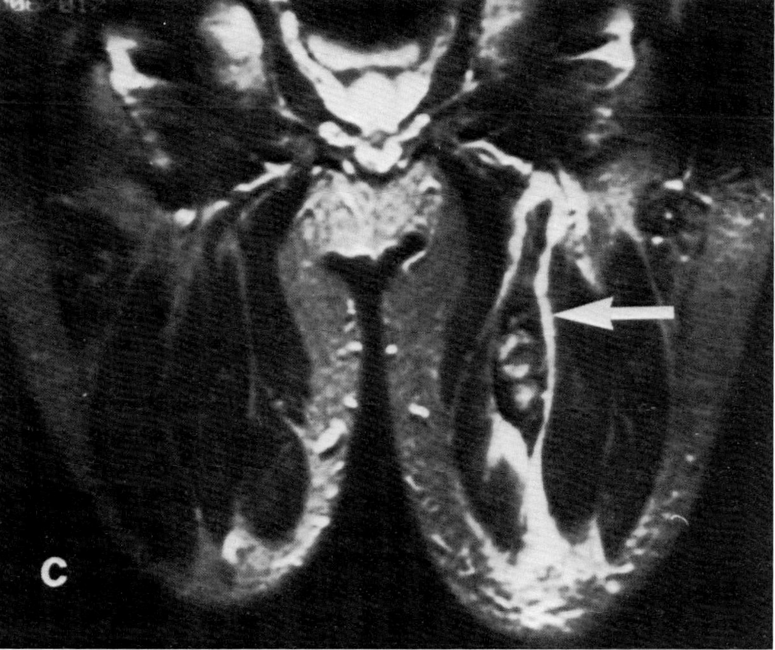

FIG. 2-22. A: Subacute hematoma imaged at low field (0.15T) with a strongly T1 weighted sequence. Image demonstrates a halo of low intensity (*arrow*), surrounding a central area of increased intensity. The low intensity is due to prolongation of T1. The area of high intensity is due to T1 shortening caused by a paramagnetic product of oxidative denaturation of hemoglobin. **B:** The hematoma has a high intensity in T2 weighted images at low field strength because of its long T2 relaxation time. **C:** This coronal T2 weighted image of the same hematoma was acquired on the same date but with a high field imager (1.5T). The peripheral areas that had the highest intensities with the same sequence in Fig. 2-22B are of low intensity here because of dramatic T2 shortening at high field.

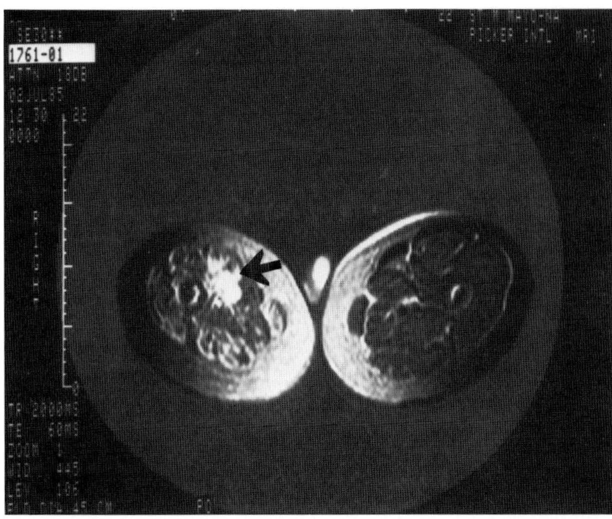

FIG. 2-23. Subtraction image clearly shows area of combined T1 and T2 prolongation at site of recurrent tumor (*arrow*).

times. Some of these are diagnostic. The T1 relaxation times of hematomas may be short at all field strengths due to the proton relaxation enhancement effect of methemoglobin. A second effect that may be characteristic is the selective T2 proton relaxation enhancement produced at high field by deoxyhemoglobin in intact erythrocytes. As demonstrated in Fig. 2-20, such lesions are of high intensity in both T1 and T2 weighted images at low and medium field strengths. At high field, the selective T2 shortening effect comes into play so that the hematoma may have a very low intensity in both T2 weighted and partial saturation sequences as shown diagrammatically in Fig. 2-21. A clinical example is shown in Fig. 2-22.

These examples have shown how it is possible to tailor the contrast of MRI sequences by choosing appropriate acquisition parameters. Coupled with a general knowledge of tissue relaxation behavior, this provides a useful qualitative tissue characterization capability, which goes one step beyond morphological imaging.

MISCELLANEOUS TECHNIQUES

A great deal of attention has been directed at the possibility of performing *in vivo* spectroscopy of proton and phosphorus resonances in order to characterize tissue at a biochemical level (2,23,34,42,46–50,54,55,70,72). These techniques offer potentially exciting prospects but they have not entered the realm of clinical practice.

Many additional techniques for tissue characterization are possible with MRI. Some of the simplest ones are most intriguing and seem to be particularly suitable for musculoskeletal problems.

A good example is computation of special-purpose images from standard MR images. Calculated maps of T1, T2, and spin density can be produced, and from them it is possible to generate supplementary images that can depend on any arbitrary function of T1, T2,

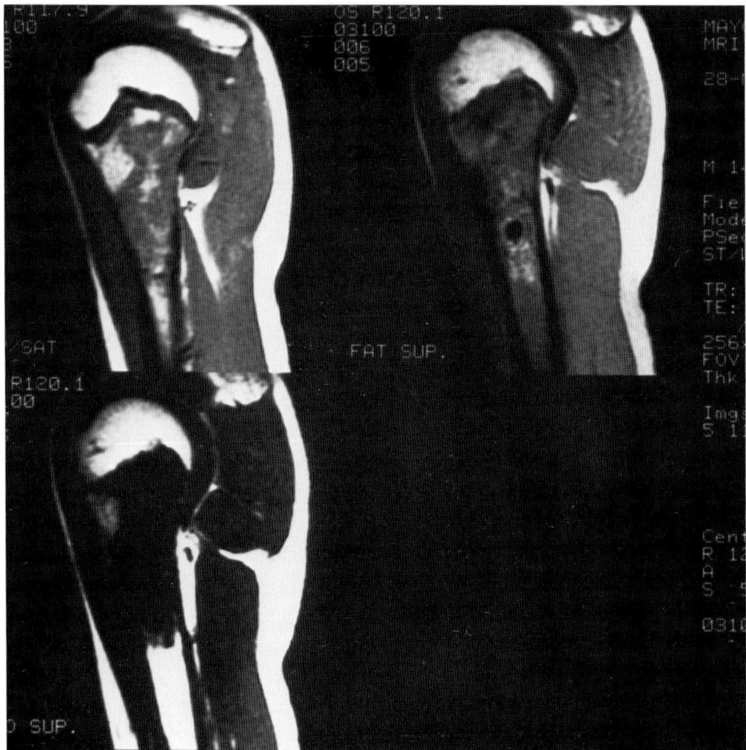

FIG. 2-24. Selective water and fat images, obtained using chemical shift presaturation. Patient has an osteogenic sarcoma in the proximal humerus. **A:** A conventional partial saturation image that clearly depicts the tumor (*arrow*). **B:** The signal from fat in the bone marrow has been suppressed by selective presaturation. (Fat signals remain high in the subcutaneous fat anteriorly, because field inhomogeneity has rendered the presaturation pulse ineffective in this region. The limited range over which spectral presaturation is effective is one of the primary limitations of the technique.) **C:** A fat image, generated by selective presaturation of water in the region.

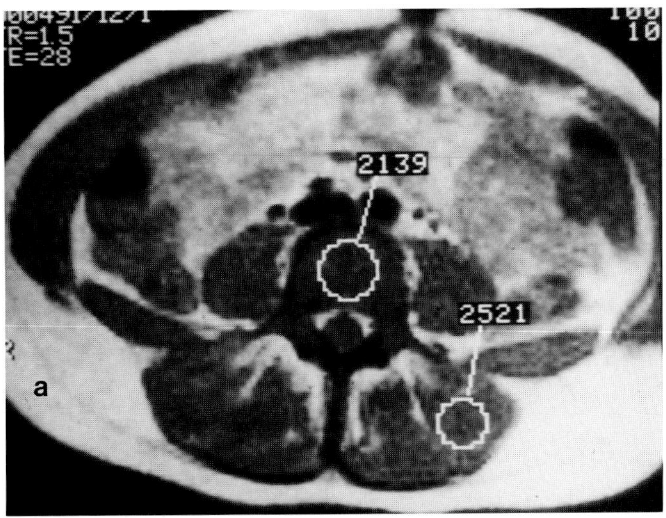

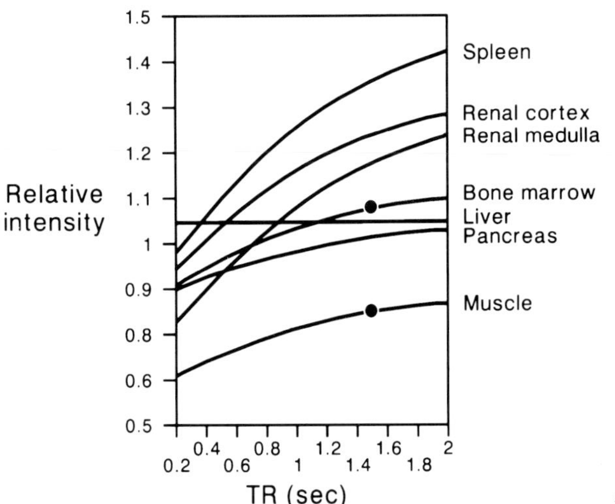

A,B

FIG. 2-25. No anatomic lesion is present in (**A**), yet a relatively gross abnormality is present. This can only be identified by understanding the gray scale relationships between tissues and how they depend on TR and TE. **B** is a quantitative representation of the normal relative intensities of tissues in spin-echo sequences at a field strength of 0.35T, based on average relaxation time and spin density measurements for a large group of patients. Clearly, the normal intensity of skeletal muscle is much less than that of medullary bone. As shown in (**A**), the intensity of bone marrow in the patient is actually lower than that of paraspinal muscle. This patient has hemosiderosis. Accumulation of hemoglobin breakdown products in bone marrow has shortened its T2 relaxation time.

and N(H) (51). A useful type of image would be one in which increased T1 and T2 relaxation times would both give increased intensity instead of having opposing effects as they do in ordinary images (43). A simple demonstration of the capability of this type of picture is provided by subtracting the image in Fig. 2-17A from image 2-17B. The resultant image has increased intensity in areas of prolonged T2 and prolonged T1 (Fig. 2-23). Inversion recovery sequences with short inversion times (T1) can provide a similar capability.

There are several approaches for generating MR images that selectively display only water or fat, as illustrated in Fig. 2-24 (36,62).

Finally, it should be noted that the quantitative measurements of relative intensity of tissue can be used as a basis for characterization. Figure 2-25 provides an example.

APPEARANCE OF VASCULAR STRUCTURES IN MRI

Arteries and veins of varying size can be identified in most musculoskeletal MR images. These vessels are of great intrinsic interest. It is important to define the relationship of major vessels to musculoskeletal tumors if surgery is planned. Many of the primary effects and complications of trauma can affect the vascular supply and drainage of an extremity. Atherosclerosis and deep venous thrombosis represent very important primary vascular diseases that affect extremities.

In most MR images, the appearance of normal arteries and veins is quite variable. The lumina of vessels may be of low intensity, high intensity, or mixed intensity. This is disturbing because it hinders reliable identification of such important lesions as venous thrombosis (Figs. 2-26 and 2-27).

In order to select examination techniques that facilitate diagnosis of vascular disease and to interpret the images, it is important to have a basic understanding of the physical processes that govern the appearance of moving blood in MRI (1,7,64). For simplicity, this discussion only considers vessels that are perpendicular to the plane of section.

The signal intensity of flowing blood is governed by three basic processes: saturation, spin phase, and washout effects. Saturation effects (Fig. 2-28) depend on the fact that the T1 relaxation time of fluid blood is longer than most soft tissues. Thus, the intensity of intravascular blood would be expected to be lower than adjacent tissue if the T1 weighting of a given pulse sequence is sufficient.

The saturation effect is often counteracted by a mechanism called "flow related enhancement" (Fig. 2-29). This results from flow of blood from outside the image volume in the interval between 90° RF pulses. These "fresh" spins carry full longitudinal magnetization because they have not been partially saturated by previous exposure to RF pulses. They can therefore provide more spin-echo signal. This is the main cause of the bright intraluminal signals that are often present in magnetic resonance images of blood vessels. Naturally, the effect

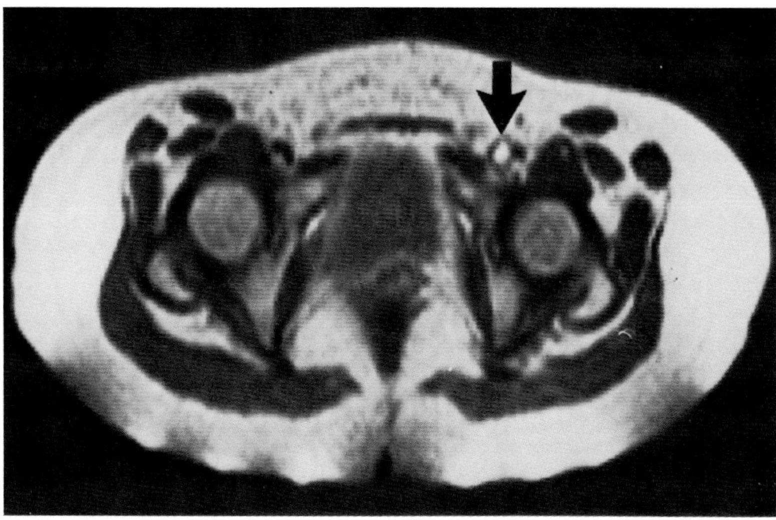

FIG. 2-26. Thrombosis of left common femoral vein (*arrow*). Note the normal flow void of the femoral artery lateral to the thrombosed vein, and the paired flow voids of the normal right femoral artery and vein.

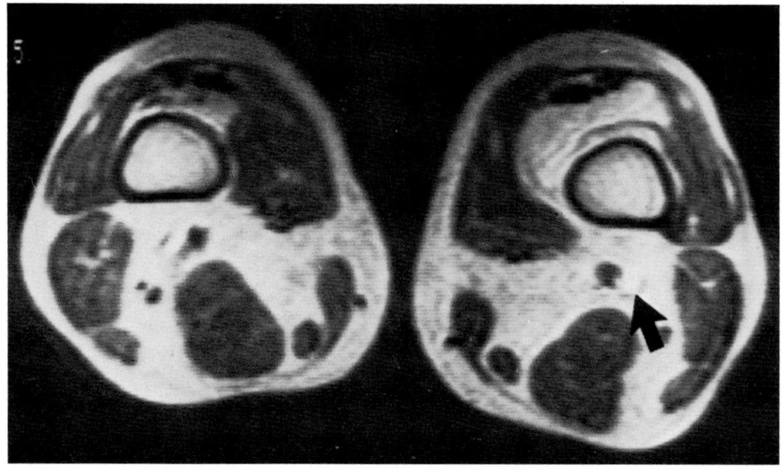

FIG. 2-27. The lumen of the normal popliteal vein in this image is high intensity due to flow related enhancement (*arrow*). Thrombosis is not present. Flow void of popliteal artery is located medial to vein. Dissimilar appearance of flowing vessels is due to differing balance of multiple mechanisms that increase and decrease intensity.

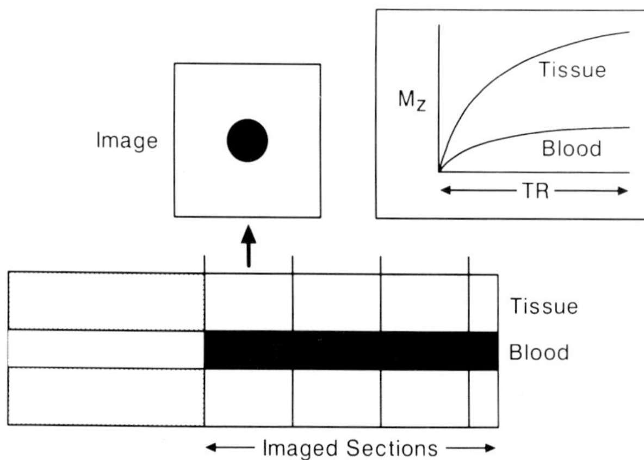

FIG. 2-28. Liquid blood has a longer T1 relaxation time than many tissues, especially perivascular fat. Disregarding the effect of flow, it tends to have a lower intensity than surrounding tissue in T1 weighted images because it is more saturated.

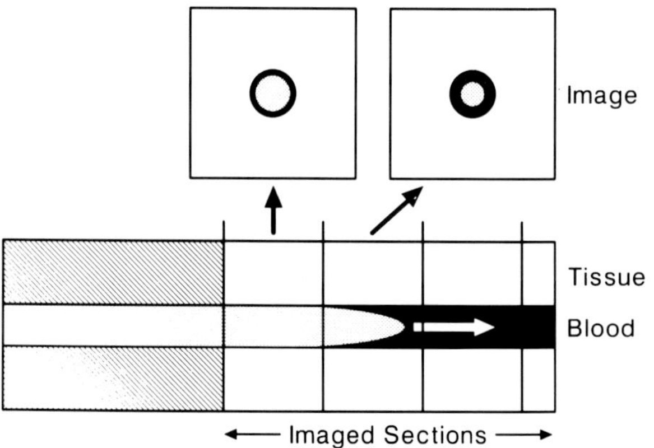

FIG. 2-29. Flow related enhancement counteracts the effect of saturation on blood in the vessel lumen. Spins that have not recently been irradiated with RF flow into the plane of section between repetitions. They yield more signal because they are unsaturated. The effect is more pronounced in sections close to the nonirradiated volume.

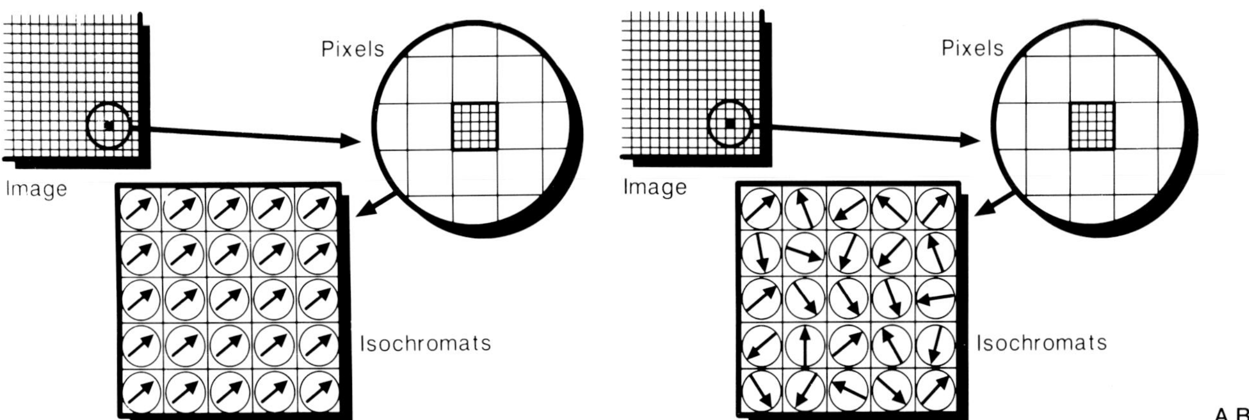

FIG. 2-30. The contents of a voxel can be conceptually divided into smaller elements called isochromats. The spin-echo signal from each isochromat is a vector quantity, having a magnitude and phase (direction). If the phase angles of most isochromats are similar (**A**), then the vectors add constructively. If the varied phase angles are present (**B**), then the net signal from the volume element will be reduced.

is most pronounced in the sections that are closest to the entry point of the vessel into the image volume. Flow related enhancement (and the flow artifacts that often accompany it) can be reduced by a technique called "spatial presaturation" (15,22).

Two other effects tend to decrease the intensity of flowing blood. One of these is known as the "spin dephasing" effect. Figure 2-30 demonstrates that the volume element corresponding to a single image pixel can conceptually be broken down into smaller volume elements called "isochromats." The net magnetization vector of the entire volume element is the vector sum of the individual magnetizations of the isochromats. If the phase angles of the isochromats are not identical, then the magnitude of their vector sum will be reduced. This is the basic principle for spin phase effects. The moving spins in flowing blood are subjected to magnetic field gradients in the course of imaging. These field gradients cause isochromats to accumulate phase differences with respect to stationary spins in tissue. The amount of phase shift depends on the velocity of the individual isochromats and the strength and duration of the field gradients. At the time of the spin echo, the magnetization isochromats with varying phase angles add together in an incoherent fashion so that signal intensity is reduced.

This situation is shown schematically for laminar flow on the right of Fig. 2-31. Figure 2-32B is a graph of the phase angle of three different isochromats flowing through the same field gradient. Note that the polarity of the phase errors is flipped by the 180° RF pulse. At the time of the first spin echo, the phase angles of the isochromats are different, so that these and the other elements of the voxel do not add coherently and the intensity of the spin-echo signal is reduced. This mechanism relies on the idea of velocity shear between isochromats to cause divergent phase angles, but shear is actually not required to cause intensity loss in an imaging situation, as described in the next paragraph.

The case of "plug flow," where all the isochromats move at the same velocity, is shown on the left in Fig. 2-31. The corresponding spin phase graph in Fig. 2-32A shows that although the phase angles of isochromats at the leading and trailing edges of the "plug" initially diverge, they reconverge at the time of the first spin echo. Although there is no phase divergence to reduce intensity in this case, there is a net phase error for the entire volume element. If flow is pulsatile, the process of imaging and averaging will result in a reduction of the intensity of the corresponding image pixel because individual phase encoding views and averages will obtain a random phase angle from the volume element. This plug flow mechanism may actually be a more important cause of first echo intensity loss in clinical images than the velocity shear mechanism described above.

The dephasing effects can reduce the intensity of blood in first echo (and other odd numbered echos in multiple spin-echo sequences) so that any flow related enhancement that may have been present is masked. "Even echo rephasing" is a striking phenomenon that can counteract the dephasing effects of gradients so that intensity is restored in even numbered echos (Fig. 2-33). This depends on a peculiar property of even numbered echos in multiple spin-echo sequences. Under certain circumstances, the even numbered 180° pulses may at least partially correct the phase errors that are induced by flow through gradients. This is schematically shown for the simulations of plug and laminar flow in Fig. 2-32. A technique called "gradient moment nulling" can be applied to most MR pulse sequences to reliably cause rephasing in any particular echo, thereby reducing motion artifacts and increasing luminal intensity (52).

The most important mechanism that reduces the MR image intensity of flowing blood has not yet been de-

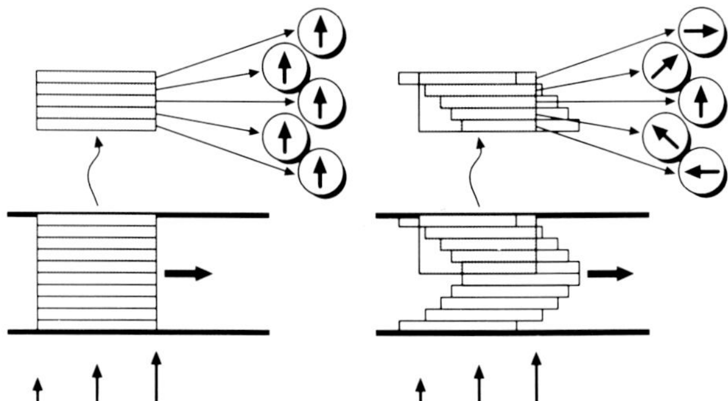

FIG. 2-31. Left: "Plug flow" is a model for flow that assumes that the velocity of fluid is the same near the center of the lumen as it is at the sides. Thus, each isochromat has the same velocity. The *vertical arrows* along the base of the vessel represent the strength of the local magnetic field at each point. This gradient causes the phase angle of each isochromat to change as it flows along the vessel, but since the velocities are identical the phase angles of all the isochromats in the volume element will be the same at the time of the spin echo. **Right:** "Laminar flow" is a situation in which the velocity has a parabolic profile across the lumen of the vessel. In this case, the phase errors accumulated by isochromats as they flow through the magnetic field gradient are variable because the velocities are different. Thus, the net signal intensity from a voxel is reduced at the time of spin-echo creation because the isochromats do not add constructively. This has been called the "dephasing effect."

scribed here. This is the "washout" effect, shown in Fig. 2-34. Protons must receive both 90° and 180° RF pulses in order to yield a spin-echo signal. In most imagers, these pulses are "slice selective" so that their effects are spatially limited to the confines of imaged sections. Flowing protons that escape the plane of section in the time interval between 90° and 180° RF pulses will not produce a signal. This establishes a "cutoff velocity" for blood flow, above which no intraluminal signal can be present. This velocity can be calculated by dividing the section thickness by the time interval between the 90° and 180° RF pulses. Note that the washout effect is not operative in gradient-echo imaging, since only a single RF pulse is employed.

In spin-echo imaging, it is often valuable to use techniques that will depict patent vessels with reliable flow voids. Such flow voids are promoted by avoiding flow related enhancement through the use of spatial presaturation, avoiding gradient moment nulling, and using a slightly longer echo delay if needed to permit more washout. An alternative approach is to depict patent vessels with high intensity. This method typically employs gradient-echo sequences (which are not subject to the washout effect) and gradient moment nulling to reduce dephasing.

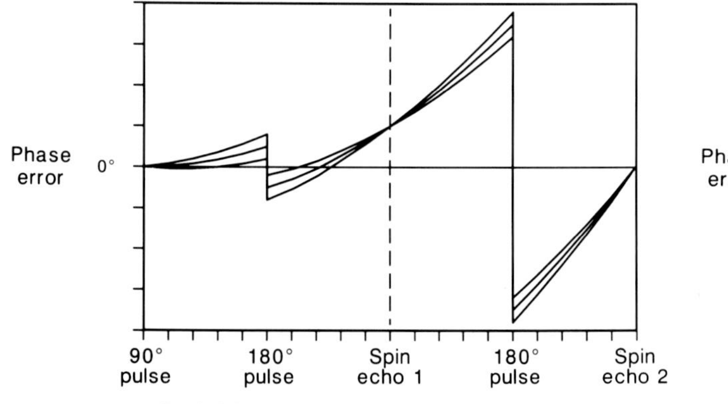

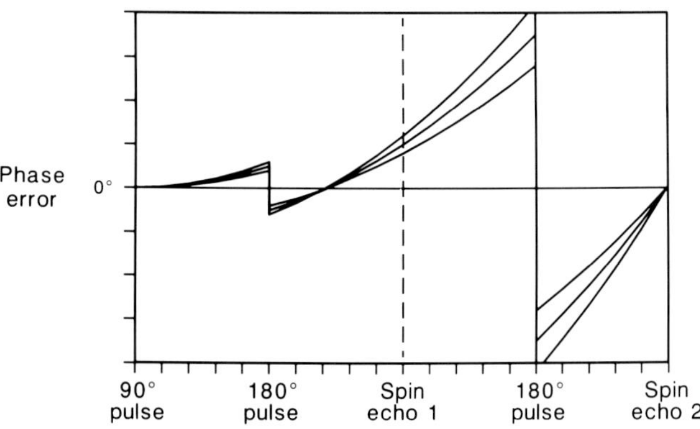

A,B

FIG. 2-32. In this mathematical simulation, the phase angles of three isochromats that are flowing through a magnetic field gradient are graphed versus time for a double spin-echo sequence. The phase angle of stationary tissue is zero throughout the sequence, so that the phase angles of the isochromats can be regarded as "phase errors" if they are not zero. **A:** The case of plug flow, in which each isochromat has the same velocity but a slightly different starting point along the vessel. Note that at the time of the first spin echo, the accumulated phase angles of each of the three isochromats are identical and nonzero. The intensity of the net spin-echo signal from a voxel in this case will be the same as if the fluid were stationary, but the phase angle will be different from that of stationary tissue. In practice, blood flow is variable and if the spin-echo experiment is repeated several times, the phase angle of each acquisition will be different. Thus, with averaging, the mean signal will be reduced. The simulation shows the surprising result that at the time of the second spin echo the phase angles of the isochromats are not only identical but the same as stationary tissue. This has been called the "rephasing phenomenon." **B:** The situation for laminar flow. Each of the three isochromats in the simulation is flowing at a slightly different rate. At the time of the first spin echo the phase angles are nonzero and different. This phase dispersion means that the signals from each isochromat will not add constructively and the net spin-echo signal will be reduced. Following the first echo, the phase angles of the isochromats continue to diverge, but the second 180° pulse has the effect of restoring phase coherence at the time of the second spin echo. The rephasing phenomenon can cause the signal intensity that was lost in the first echo due to phase dispersion to be restored in the second echo.

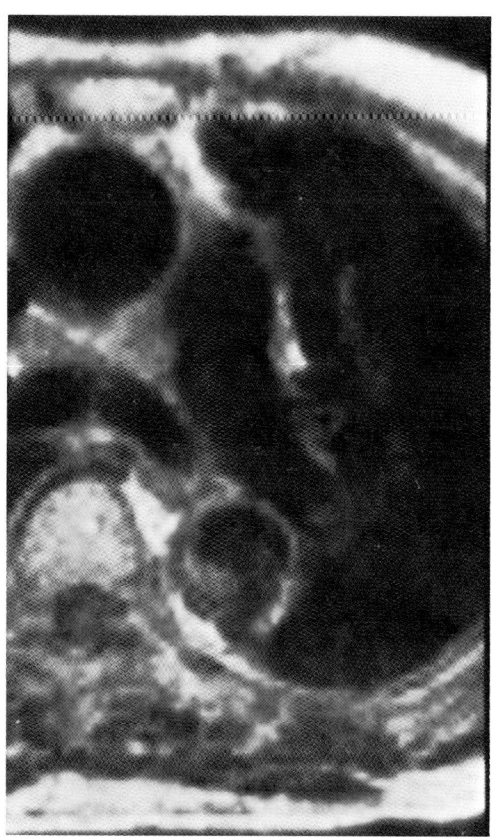

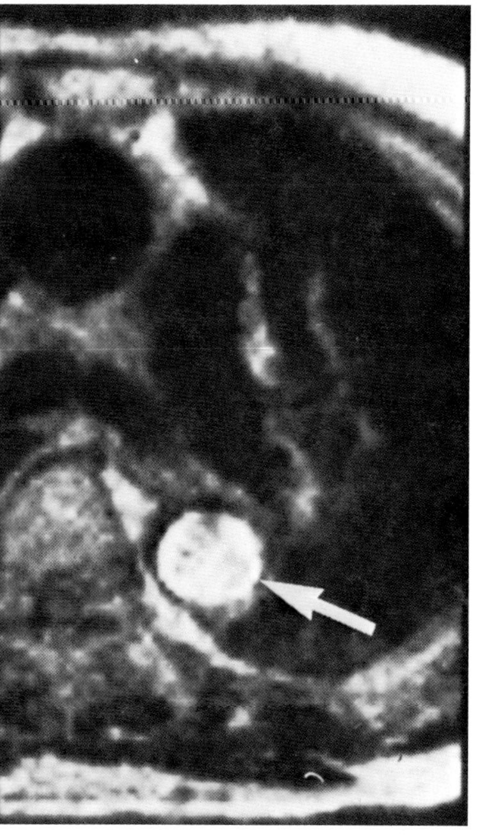

A,B

FIG. 2-33 A and **B.** An example of first echo dephasing and second echo rephasing in the descending aorta (*arrow*). The signal intensity observed in the lumen of a vessel is affected by the summation of flow effects. In the 28 msec first echo image, unsaturated spins from distant points outside the images volume are present within the lumen of the descending aorta, but flow related enhancement is not observed because the intensity is reduced by the dephasing phenomenon. This flow related enhancement is "uncovered" in the second echo image because of the rephasing effect, which corrects the phase dispersion that was present at the time of the first echo.

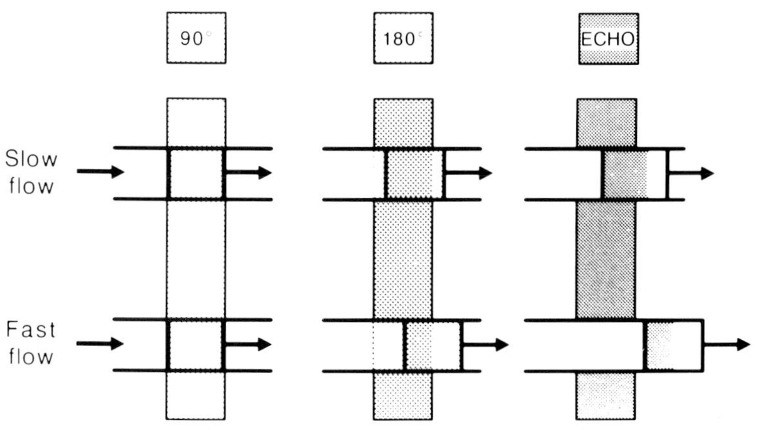

FIG. 2-34. Illustration of the "washout effect." Those flowing spins that move out of the section in the time between 90° and 180° pulses will not yield a spin-echo signal. The amount of signal loss due to washout increases with flow velocity. With very fast flow, all the blood in the segment of lumen may be replaced so that the spin-echo signal will be zero. The minimum velocity that replaces all spin in such a fashion is called the "cutoff velocity."

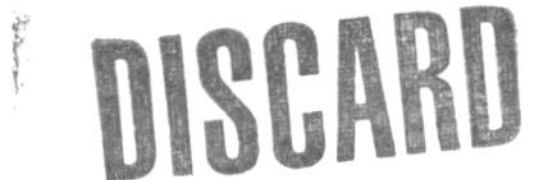

Many different flow effects can be observed in MRI, but the principles that have been described here can be used to explain the majority of them.

REFERENCES

1. Axel L. Blood flow effects in magnetic resonance imaging. *AJR* 1984;143:1157–1166.
2. Barany M, Lander BG, Glick RP, et al. *In vivo* H-1 spectroscopy in humans at 1.5 T. *Radiology* 1988;167:839–844.
3. Beall PT, Amtey SR, Kasturi SR. *NMR data handbook for biomedical applications.* New York: Pergamon, 1984: Table 9.10.
4. Bloemberger EM, Purcell EM, Pound RV. Relaxation effects in nuclear magnetic resonance absorption. *Phys Rev* 1948;73:679–712.
5. Bottomley PA, Foster TH, Argersinger RE, Pfeifer LM. A review of normal tissue hydrogen NMR relaxation times and relaxation mechanisms from 1–100 MHz: dependence on tissue type, NMR frequency. *Med Phys* 1984;11(4):425–448.
6. Bradley WG, Schmidt PG. Effect of methemoglobin formation on the appearance of subarachnoid hemorrhage. *Radiology* 1985;156:99–103.
7. Bradley WG, Waluch V. Blood flow: magnetic resonance imaging. *Radiology* 1985;154:443–450.
8. Brasch RC. Work in progress: methods of contrast enhancement for NMR imaging and potential applications. *Radiology* 1983;147:781–788.
9. Brasch RC, Wesbey GE, Gooding CA, Koerper MA. Magnetic resonance imaging of transfusional hemosiderosis complicating thalasemia major. *Radiology* 1984;150:767–771.
10. Crooks LE, Arakawa M, Hoenninger J, McCarten B, Watts J, Kaufman L. Magnetic resonance imaging: effects of magnetic field strength. *Radiology* 1984;151:127–133.
11. De Vre RM. Biomedical implications of the relaxation behavior of water related to NMR imaging. *Br J Radiol* 1984;57:955–976.
12. Dixon WT. Simple proton spectroscopic imaging. *Radiology* 1984;153:189–194.
13. Dooms GC, Fisher MR, Hricak H, Higgins CB. MR imaging of intramuscular hemorrhage. *J Comput Assist Tomogr* 1985;9:908–913.
14. Dooms GC, Hricak H, Moseley ME, Bottles K, Fisher M, Higgins CB. Characterization of lymphadenopathy by magnetic resonance relaxation times: preliminary results. *Radiology* 1985;155:691–697.
15. Edelman RR, Atkinson DJ, Silver MS, Loaiza FL, Warren WS. FRODO pulse sequences: a new means of eliminating motion, flow, and wraparound artifacts. *Radiology* 1988;166:231–236.
16. Ehman RL, Berquist TH, McLeod RA. MR imaging of the musculoskeletal system: a 5-year appraisal. *Radiology* 1988;166:313–320.
17. Ehman RL, Felmlee JP. Adaptive technique for high-definition MR imaging of moving structures. *Radiology* 1989;173:255–263.
18. Ehman RL, Kjos BO, Hricak H, Brasch RC, Higgins CB. Relative intensity of abdominal organs in magnetic resonance images. *J Comput Assist Tomogr* 1985;9:315–319.
19. Ehman RL, McNamara MT, Brasch RC, Felmlee JP, Gray JE, Higgins CB. Influence of physiological motion on the appearance of tissue in MRI. *Radiology* 1986;159:777–782.
20. Ehman RL, McNamara MT, Pallack M, Hricak H, Higgins CB. Magnetic resonance imaging with respiratory gating: techniques and advantages. *AJR* 1984;143:1175–1182.
21. Farrar TC, Becker ED. *Pulse and Fourier transform NMR: introduction to theory and methods.* New York: Academic Press, 1971.
22. Felmlee JP, Ehman RL. Spatial presaturation: a method for suppressing flow artifacts and improving depiction of vascular anatomy in MR imaging. *Radiology* 1987;164:559–564.
23. Frahm J, Haase A, Hanicke W, Matthaei D, Hartwin B, Helzel T. Chemical shift selective MR imaging using a whole body magnet. *Radiology* 1985;156:441–444.
24. Fullerton GD, Cameron IL, Hunter K, Fullerton H. Proton magnetic resonance relaxation behavior of whole muscle with fatty inclusions. *Radiology* 1985;155:727–730.
25. Fullerton GD, Cameron IL, Ord VA. Frequency dependence of magnetic resonance spin-lattice relaxation of protons in biological materials. *Radiology* 1984;151:135–138.
26. Fullerton GD, Potter JL, Dornbluth NC. NMR relaxation of protons in tissues and other macromolecular water solutions. *Magn Reson Imaging* 1982;1:209–228.
27. General Electric Medical Systems. *Introduction to fast scan magnetic resonance,* 1986:7299.
28. Gomori JM, Grossman RI, Goldberg HI, Zimmerman RA, Bilaniuk LT. Intracranial hematomas: imaging by high field MR. *Radiology* 1985;157:87–93.
29. Harms SE, Flamig DP, Fisher CF, Fulmer JM. New method for fast MR imaging of the knee. *Radiology* 1989;173:743–750.
30. Hazelwood CF. A view of the significance and understanding of the physical properties of cell-associated water. In: Drost-Hansen W, Clegg J, eds. *Cell associated water.* New York: Academic Press, 1979:165–260.
31. Hendrick RE, Nelson TR, Hendee WR. Optimizing tissue contrast in magnetic resonance imaging. *Magn Reson Imaging* 1984;2:193–204.
32. Herfkins R, Davis PL, Crooks LE, Kaufman L, Price D, Miller T, Marguus A. Nuclear magnetic resonance imaging of the abnormal live rat and correlations with tissue characteristics. *Radiology* 1981;141:211–218.
33. Johnson GA, Herfkins RJ, Brown MA. Tissue relaxation time: *in vivo* field dependence. *Radiology* 1985;156:805–810.
34. Joseph PM. A spin echo chemical shift MR imaging technique. *J Comput Assist Tomogr* 1985;9:651–658.
35. Joseph PM, Axel L. Potential problems with selective pulses in NMR imaging systems. *Med Phys* 1984;11:772–777.
36. Keller PJ, Hunter WW Jr, Schmalbrock P. Multisection fat–water imaging with chemical shift selective presaturation. *Radiology* 1987;164:539–541.
37. Kjos BO, Ehman RL, Brandt-Zawadzki M. Reproducibility of T1 and T2 relaxation times calculated from routine MR imaging sequences: phantom study. *AJNR* 1985;6:277–283.
38. Kjos BO, Ehman RL, Brant-Zawadzki M, Kelly WM, Norman D, Newton TH. Reproducibility of relaxation times and spin density calculated from routine MR imaging sequences: clinical study of the CNS. *AJNR* 1985;6:271–276.
39. Konig H, Sauter R, Deimling M, Vogt M. Cartilage disorders: comparison of spin-echo CHESS, and FLASH sequence MR images. *Radiology* 1987;164:753–758.
40. Kurtz D, Dwyer A. Isosignal contours and signal gradients as an aid to choosing MRI imaging techniques. *J Comput Assist Tomogr* 1984;8:819–828.
41. Lee JK, Dixon WT, Ling D, Levitt RG, Murphy WA. Fatty infiltration of the liver: demonstration by proton spectroscopic imaging. *Radiology* 1984;153:195–201.
42. Lenkinski RE, Holland GA, Allman T, et al. Integrated MR imaging and spectroscopy with chemical shift imaging of P-31 at 1.5 T: initial clinical experience. *Radiology* 1988;169:201–206.
43. Levin DN, Herrmann A, Spraggins TA, et al. Musculoskeletal tumors: improved depiction with linear combinations of MR images. *Radiology* 1987;163:545–549.
44. McSweeney MB, Small WC, Cerny V, et al. Magnetic resonance imaging in the diagnosis of breast disease: use of transverse relaxation times. *Radiology* 1984;153:741–744.
45. Mitchell DG, Burk DL Jr, Vinitski S, et al. Biophysical basis of tissue contrast in extracranial MR imaging. *AJR* 1987;149:831–837.
46. Narayana PA, Hazle JD, Jackson EF, et al. *In vivo* ^{1}H spectroscopic studies of human gastrocnemius muscle at 1.5 T. *Magn Reson Imaging* 1988;6:481–485.
47. Narayana PA, Jackson EF, Hazle JD, et al. *In vivo* localization proton spectroscopic studies in human gastrocnemius muscle. *Magn Reson Med* 1988;8:151–159.
48. Newman RJ, Bore PJ, Chan L, et al. Nuclear magnetic resonance studies of forearm muscle in Duchenne dystrophy. *Br Med J* 1982;284:1072–1074.
49. Nidecker AC, Muller S, Aue WP. Extremity bone tumors: evaluation by P-31 spectroscopy. *Radiology* 1985;157:167–174.

50. Ohtomo K, Itai Y, Furui S, et al. Hepatic tumors: differentiation by transverse relaxation time (T2) of MR resonance imaging. *Radiology* 1985;155:421–423.
51. Ortendahl DA, Hylton N, Kaufman L, Watts JC, Crooks LE, Mills CM. Star Analytical tools for magnetic resonance imaging. *Radiology* 1984;153:479–488.
52. Pattany PM, Phillips JJ, Chiu LC, et al. Motion artifact suppression technique (MAST) for MR imaging. *J Comput Assist Tomogr* 1987;11:369–377.
53. Pettersson H, Slone RM, Spanier S, et al. Musculoskeletal tumors: T1 and T2 relaxation times. *Radiology* 1988;167:783–785.
54. Pykett IL, Rosen BR. Nuclear magnetic resonance *in vivo* proton chemical shift imaging. *Radiology* 1983;149:197–201.
55. Redmond OM, Stack JP, Dervan PA, et al. Osteosarcoma: use of MR imaging and MR spectroscopy in clinical decision making. *Radiology* 1989;172:811–815.
56. Richardson ML, Amparo EG, Gillespy T, Helms CA, Demas BE, Genant HK. Theoretical considerations for optimizing intensity differences between primary musculoskeletal tumors and normal tissue with spin echo MRI. *Invest Radiol* 1985;20:492–497.
57. Rosen BR, Fleming DM, Kushner DC, et al. Hematologic bone marrow disorders: quantitative chemical shift MR imaging. *Radiology* 1988;169:799–804.
58. Schmidt HC, Tscholakoff D, Hricak H, Higgins CB. MR image contrast and relaxation times of solid tumors in the chest, abdomen, and pelvis. *J Comput Assist Tomogr* 1985;9:738–748.
59. Siemens Medical Systems. *FLASH and FISP gradient echo pulse sequences,* 1989.
60. Solomon SL, Totty WG, Lee JKT. MR imaging of the knee: comparison of three-dimensional FISP and two-dimensional spin-echo pulse sequences. *Radiology* 1989;173:739–742.
61. Swenson SJ, Keller PL, Berquist TH, Mcleod RA, Stephens DH. Magnetic resonance imaging of hemorrhage. *AJR* 1985;145:921–927.
62. Szumowski J, Plewes DB. Separation of lipid and water MR imaging signals by chopper averaging in the time domain. *Radiology* 1987;165:247–250.
63. Thulborn KR, Waterton JC, Matthews PM, Radda GK. Oxygenation dependence of the transverse relaxation time of water protons in whole blood at high field. *Biochim Biophys Acta* 1982:265–270.
64. Wehrli FW, MacFall JR, Axel L, Shutts D, Glover GH, Herfkins RJ. Approaches to in-plane and out-of-plane flow imaging. *Noninvasive Med Imaging* 1984;1:127–136.
65. Wehrli FW, MacFall JR, Shutts D, Breger R, Herfkens RJ. Mechanisms of contrast in NMR imaging. *J Comput Assist Tomogr* 1984;8(3):369–380.
66. Wehrli FW, Perkins TG, Shimakawa A, et al. Chemical shift-induced amplitude modulations in images obtained with gradient refocusing. *Magn Res Imaging* 1987;5:157–158.
67. Wesbey GE, Moseley M, Ehman RL. Translational molecular self-diffusion in magnetic resonance imaging: effects on observed spin–spin relaxation. *Invest Radiol* 1984;19:484–490.
68. Wesbey GE, Moseley M, Ehman RL. Translational molecular self-diffusion in magnetic resonance imaging: measurement of the self-diffusion coefficient. *Invest Radiol* 1984;19:491–498.
69. Wismer GL, Rosen BR, Buxton R, Stark DD, Brady TJ. Chemical shift imaging of bone marrow: preliminary experience. *AJR* 1985;145:1031–1037.
70. Vock P, Hoppeler H, Hartl W, Fritschy P. Combined use of MRI and MRS by whole body magnets in studying skeletal muscle morphology and metabolism. *Invest Radiol* 1985;20:486–491.
71. Zimmer WD, Berquist TH, Mcleod RA, et al. Bone tumors: magnetic resonance imaging versus computed tomography. *Radiology* 1985;155:709–718.
72. Zochodne DW, Thompson RT, Driedger AA, et al. Metabolic changes in human muscle denervation: topical ^{31}P NMR spectroscopy studies. *Magn Reson Med* 1988;7:373–383.

MRI of the Musculoskeletal System,
2nd Edition, edited by T. H. Berquist.
Raven Press, Ltd., New York © 1990.

CHAPTER 3

General Technical Considerations in Musculoskeletal MRI

Thomas H. Berquist and Richard L. Morin

Patient Selection, 53
Patient Positioning and Coil Selection, 63
Pulse Sequences and Slice Selection, 65
References, 72

Magnetic resonance imaging is an excellent technique for evaluation of the musculoskeletal system (8,20,24, 37,51,53). Respiratory motion, a significant problem in the chest and upper abdomen, is generally not a problem in the pelvis and extremities (7,8). Images can be obtained in the coronal, sagittal, transaxial, and oblique planes. Also, soft tissue contrast is superior to CT and conventional imaging techniques.

MRI examinations must be conducted differently than conventional radiographic or CT examinations. Patient selection, positioning, coil selection, and pulse sequences must all be considered to optimize image quality and properly characterize pathologic lesions. This chapter discusses general concepts in imaging techniques. More specific applications are discussed in the anatomic chapters that follow.

PATIENT SELECTION

MR images are produced using a static magnetic field, magnetic gradients, and radiofrequency (RF) pulses (57,73) (see Chapter 1). No ionizing radiation is used. To date, no untoward biological effects have been identified at the currently used field strengths (≤2 tesla) (69,72).

Most high-field MRI gantries are more confining than a conventional fluoroscopic unit or CT scanner. New mid- and low-field units (0.02–0.5 tesla) have shorter, more open gantries that allow easier patient access. Patients are positioned in the center of the cylindrical magnet chamber during the examination (Fig. 3-1). The dimensions of the gantry can be difficult for some patients to tolerate during lengthy examinations (17,61). Despite the confined feeling patients experience, we note problems with claustrophobia in only 3–4% of patients. Patients with claustrophobic tendencies seem to tolerate MR examinations more readily if they are in the prone position (Fig. 3-1B). If necessary, mild sedation with oral valium may be helpful. Patient size can also be a limiting factor. Body coils are usually only about 53 × 35 cm, which may make imaging of large patients difficult or impossible. In addition, many automatic imaging consoles do not function properly if patient weight exceeds 285 pounds.

The patient's clinical status must be considered. Patients with significant pain or inability to maintain the necessary positions may not be able to tolerate the potentially lengthy examinations. Premedication with valium or demerol may be useful in these cases. Young children (<6 years) may not be able to cooperate sufficiently to obtain an optimal examination. A parent or friend can be in the exam room adjacent to the gantry and talk with patients during the examination. When this technique is not possible, sedation may be indicated. Oral sedation is generally sufficient for children, but occasionally general or iv anesthetic agents may be required for pediatric patients and certain adults. Initially, there was concern that severely ill patients requiring cardiac monitoring and respiratory support could not be examined. Ferromagnetic anesthesia equipment cannot be moved into the magnet room or near the gantry without creating potential safety hazards or af-

T. H. Berquist and R. L. Morin: Mayo Medical School and Mayo Clinic, Rochester, Minnesota 55905.

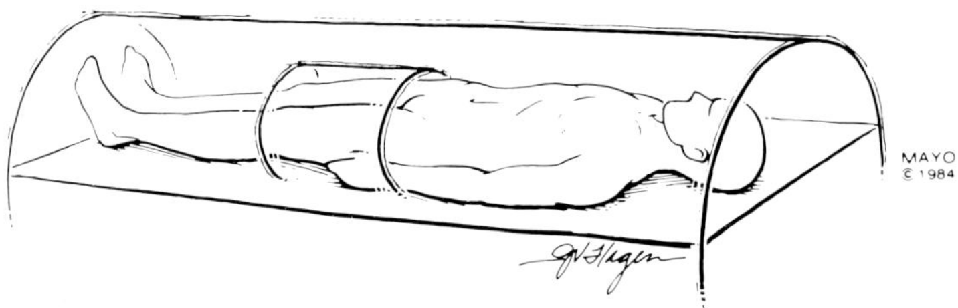

A

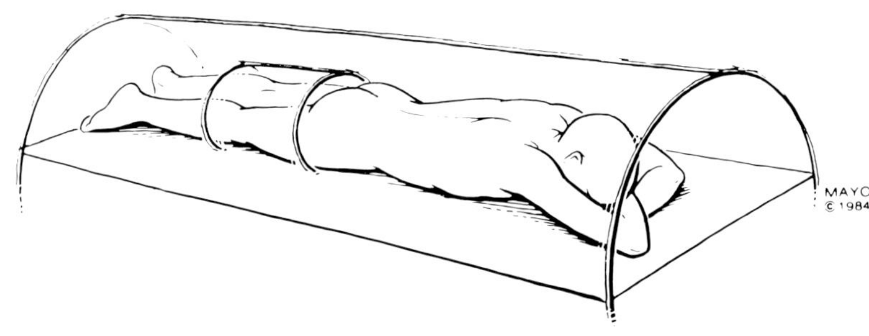

B

FIG. 3-1. Illustrations of patients positioned supine (**A**) and prone (**B**) in the gantry of an MR imager.

fecting the image quality. Our experience shows that critically ill patients or patients requiring general anesthesia can be monitored successfully without interfering with image quality. Initially, we studied 20 patients requiring cardiac and respiratory support. Patients were monitored with a blood pressure cuff with plastic connectors, an Aneuroid Chest Bellows for respiratory rate, and a Hewlett-Packard ECG telemetry system. The respiratory rate and ECG were monitored on a Saturn monitor. Certain problems were encountered during the study. Radiofrequency (RF) pulses caused ECG artifacts, especially if short repetition times were used. This problem was overcome by using a Doppler system to monitor the pulse during the imaging sequences. Satisfactory monitoring was achieved in all patients and equipment used did not affect image quality (65).

Magnetic fields may affect certain metal implants and electrical devices (8,59,60). In many situations the exact chemical structure of the implant cannot be determined (42). Although evaluations are still in progress, early reports have defined a number of implants that may be potentially dangerous to the patient or affect image quality (8,19,30,34,36,42,55,58,76). Synchronous pacemakers convert to the asynchronous mode when placed in magnetic resonance imagers. The pacemaker powerpack may change its orientation in the magnetic field. In addition, significant image degradation may occur if the powerpack is in the region being examined (58). Numerous heart valves have been studied at field strengths of 0.35–1.5 tesla (T). The artifacts created by most valves are negligible and it has been concluded that patients with these prosthetic valves can be imaged safely (74,76). However, pulling or torque was demonstrated with certain valves (Table 3-1). In spite of this response to the static magnetic field, the deflection is minimal and not considered a contraindication (58,74).

Most surgical clips at our institution are nonferromagnetic. However, a significant number of aneurysm clips (19 of 32) (Table 3-2) are ferromagnetic and will twist or turn in a magnetic environment (55,74). Brown

TABLE 3-1. *Heart valves: torque or deflection with static magnetic field* (19,55,74)

Beall (Coratomic, Indiana, PA)
Bjork–Shiley (universal/spherical) (Shiley)
Bjork–Shiley, model MBC (Shiley)
Bjork–Shiley, model 25 MBRC 11030 (Shiley)
Carpentier–Edwards, model 2650 (American Edwards, Santa Ana, CA)
Carpentier–Edwards (porcine) (American Edwards)
Hall–Kaster, model A7700 (Medtronic, Minneapolis, MN)
Hancock I (porcine) (Johnson & Johnson, Anaheim, CA)
Hancock II (porcine) (Johnson & Johnson)
Hancock extracorporeal, model 242R (Johnson & Johnson)
Hancock extracorporeal, model M 4365-33 (Johnson & Johnson)
Ionescu–Shiley (Universal ISM)
Lillehi–Kaster, model 300S (Medical, Inver Grove Heights, MN)
Lillehi–Kaster, model 5009 (Medical)
Medtronic–Hall (Medtronic)
Medtronic–Hall, model A7700-D-16 (Medtronic)
Omnicarbon, model 3523T029 (Medical)
Omniscience, model 6522 (Medical)
Smeloff–Cutter (Cutter Laboratories, Berkeley, CA)
Starr–Edwards, model 1260 (American Edwards)
Starr–Edwards, model 2320 (American Edwards)
Starr–Edwards, model Pre 6000 (American Edwards)
Starr–Edwards, model 6520 (American Edwards)
St. Jude, model A 101 (St. Jude Medical)
St. Jude, model M 101 (St. Jude Medical)

TABLE 3-2. *Aneurysm and hemostasis clips exhibiting torque in magnetic field* (16,21,55,74)

Drake (DR14, DR24) (Edward Weck, Triangle Park, NJ)
Drake (DR16) (Edward Weck)
Drake (301 SS) (Edward Weck)
Downs multipositional (17-7PH)
Heifetz (17-7PH) (Edward Weck)
Housepian
Kapp (405 SS) (V. Mueller)
Kapp curved (404 SS) (V. Mueller)
Kapp straight (404 SS) (V. Mueller)
Mayfield (301 SS) (Codman & Shurtleff, Randolph, MA)
Mayfield (304 SS) (Codman & Shurtleff)
McFadden (301 SS) (Codman & Shurtleff)
Pivot (17-7PH) (V. Mueller)
Scoville (EN58J) (Downs Surgical, Decatur, GA)
Sundt–Kees (301 SS) (Downs Surgical)
Sundt–Kees Multi-Angle (17-7PH) (Downs Surgical)
Vari-Angle (17-7PH) (Codman & Shurtleff)
Vari-Angle Micro (17-7PM SS) (Codman & Shurtleff)
Vari-Angle Spring (17-7PM SS) (Codman & Shurtleff)

et al. (16) demonstrated that the strongest torque and most significant image artifacts were present with clips made of 17-7HP stainless steel. Titanium and tantalum clips showed the least attractive force and minimal image distortion. We do not examine patients with cerebral aneurysm clips or pacemakers. However, hemostasis clips are usually not a significant problem in musculoskeletal imaging (Fig. 3-2).

Other nonorthopedic metallic devices, including dental materials, ear implants, vascular filters and coils, genitourinary prostheses, ocular implants, and intrauterine devices, have also been investigated (18,34,51,74,77,78). Some removable dental plates are ferromagnetic and cause significant local artifact (18,74) (Table 3-3). These materials should be removed prior to MR imaging (18). Permanent appliances such as braces may contain ferromagnetic material but patients can be studied safely (74). The facial region is not included on most musculo-

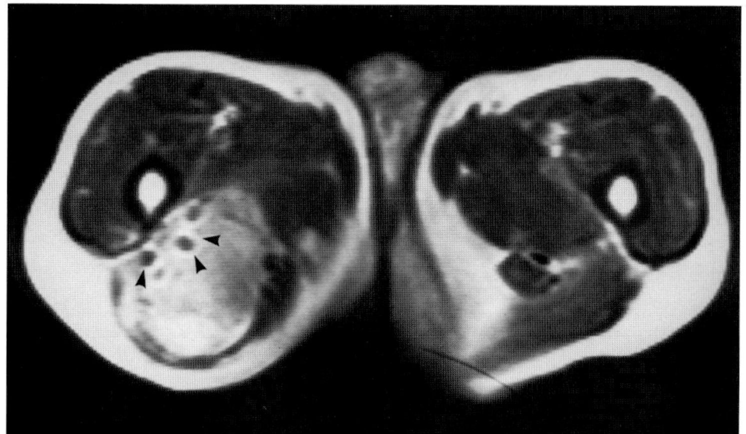

A

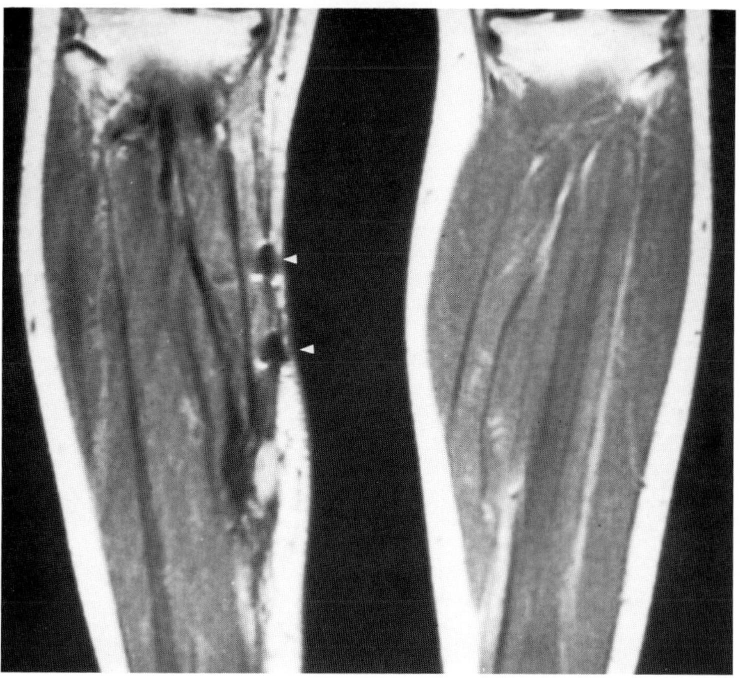

B

FIG. 3-2. MR artifacts created by hemostasis clips. **A:** 0.15 T SE 500/30 image in a patient with a partially resected liposarcoma. Note the focal areas of no signal with small bright halo (*arrows*) caused by the surgical clip artifacts. **B:** 1.5 T SE 500/20 coronal images of the calves. Note the surgical clip artifacts (*arrows*) in the right calf medially.

TABLE 3-3. *Dental appliances: MR image artifacts* (18,74)

Material or prosthesis	Artifact
Dental amalgam	No
Soft tissue conditioning material	No
Orthodontic wire	Yes
Type III gold	Yes
Type IV gold	Yes
Porcelain fixed to gold	No
Crown-and-bridge acrylic resin	No
Titanium implants	Yes
Polyurethane	No
Fixed partial denture, type III gold	Yes
Metal ceramic crown	Yes
Maxillary removable partial obturator	Yes

skeletal MR images. Therefore, artifacts from dental appliances are not usually a problem. We do not examine patients with permanent dental prostheses held in with magnetic posts because it is not yet clear what effect the magnetic field will have on these components.

To date, the only ear implants that may be contraindicated are cochlear implants (3M/House and 3M/ Vienna), which do deflect *in vitro* when placed in MR imagers. Patients with intraocular lens implants and copper intrauterine devices can be examined safely with MRI (74).

Genitourinary prostheses and vascular filters and coils, because of their location, are more likely to create artifacts and need to be considered carefully. Most penile implants and GU sphincter prostheses do not contain significant ferromagnetic material. An exception is the Omni Phase (Dacomed), which contains significant amounts of metal (74). Shellock (74) and Teitelbaum et al. (78) studied vascular coils, stents, and filters *in vitro* and *in vivo* (78) (Table 3-4). Their data indicate that artifact and torque are most significant with vascular appliances constructed with 304 and 316 stainless steel. Although the latter is not ferromagnetic in its original form, it does appear to undergo some change during configuration of appliances (i.e., Palmaz endo stent). Materials creating minimal artifact include the appliances made with Beta-3 titanium, Elgiloy, nitinol, and mP32-N alloys (78). Despite their magnetic susceptibility and the degree of artifact created (Table 3-4), patients with these devices generally can be imaged safely. The ferromagnetic devices (Greenfield filter—316L stainless steel) did not displace or perforate the inferior vena cava (78). The position of devices containing ferromagnetic material (Gianturco embolization coil, Gianturco bird nest filter, Gianturco zig-zag stent, Greenfield filter—316L stainless steel retrievable IVC filter, and Palmaz stent) should be confirmed radiographically prior to examination. If the device is perpendicular to the magnet or immediately adjacent to the area of interest, the examination may be inadequate and patient risk (due to change in position) is more significant (46,78).

A potentially more difficult problem exists in patients with nonmedical foreign bodies or ferromagnetic material. Patients with shrapnel or other metal foreign bodies may not be aware that this material is present (Fig. 3-3). In this setting there is little that can be done until an artifact is detected during the examination. If the patient expresses concern over a potential foreign body, one should consider a radiograph of the area or, if clinically indicated, cancel the examination. If an object is detected in the extremity and it is not near a nerve or in a region where its motion could cause damage, the examination can be performed with close monitoring (technologist in the room, questioning patient during and between pulse sequences). If the object has been present for 6 months or more it will likely be fixed by scar tissue, which reduces the risk of motion. Pigments in facial makeup (eyeliner, mascara, eye shadow) and certain tattoos may also contain ferromagnetic material (brown—ferric sulfate, flesh color—iron oxide, blue—cobalt chloride) and cause local heating and cutaneous inflam-

TABLE 3-4. *Vascular appliances: construction material and artifacts* (74,77,78)

Device	Material	Company	Artifact
Greenfield filter	(a) 316L stainless steel	Meditech, Watertown, MA	Significant
	(b) Beta-3 titanium	Ormco, Glendora, CA	Minimal–none
Mobin-Uddin IVC umbrella	Elginoy & silicone rubber	American Edwards, Santa Ana, CA	Mild
Amplatz retrievable IVC filter	MP 32N alloy	Cook, Bloomington, IN	Mild
Gunther retrievable IVC filter	304 stainless steel	William Cook, Europe	Severe
Gianturco bird nest IVC filter	304 stainless steel	William Cook, Europe	Severe
Retrievable filter	304 stainless steel	Thomas Jefferson University, Philadelphia, PA	Severe
Cragg nitinol spiral IVC filter			Mild
Maass helical IVC filter	Mediloy stainless steel	Medinvent, Lawanne, Switzerland	Moderate
Maass endovascular stent	Mediloy stainless steel	Medinvent, Lawanne, Switzerland	Moderate
Palmaz endo stent	316 stainless steel	Ethicon, Summerville, NJ	Severe
GEC coil	304 stainless steel	Cook, Bloomington, IN	Severe

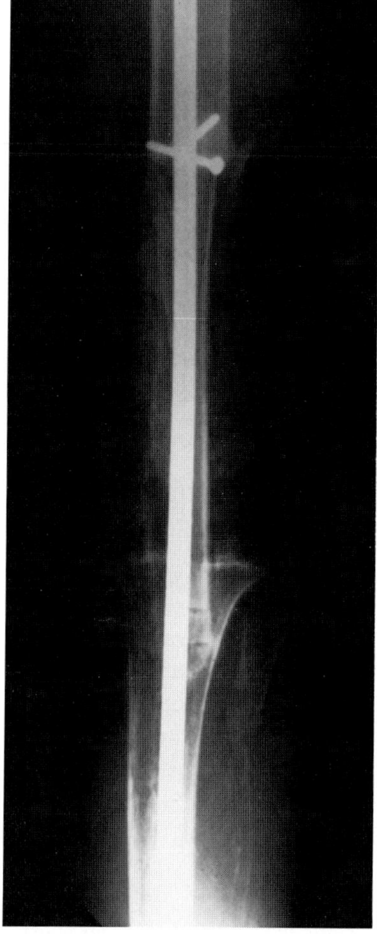

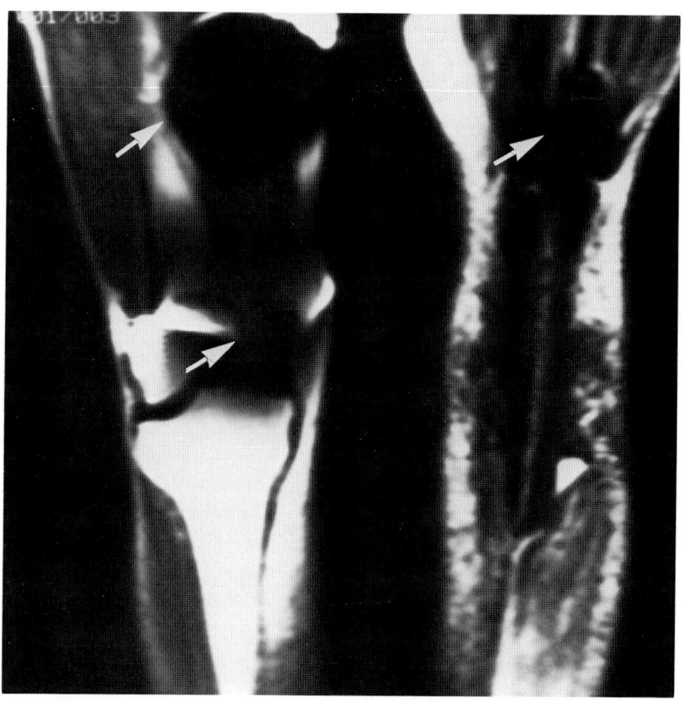

A,B

FIG. 3-3. Patient with a limb salvage procedure for a femoral sarcoma. **A:** AP radiograph shows rod and bone graft fusion with two screws superiorly. **B:** Coronal MR image (SE 500/20) shows artifact from the screws (*right arrow*) but little artifact from the medullary rod. Note the extensive artifact in the right thigh (*arrows*) due to iron shrapnel. The patient was not aware that these foreign bodies were present. The patient did not note any changes in this leg during the examination.

mation (36,68). Patients with tattooed eye liner are particularly susceptible. These factors should be considered; canceling these examinations may be indicated.

Manufacturers of orthopedic appliances (plates, screws, joint prostheses, etc.) generally use high-grade stainless steel, cobalt–chromium, titanium, or multiphase alloys (2). These materials are usually not ferromagnetic but may contain minimal ferromagnetic impurities. All orthopedic appliances at our institution have been tested for magnetic properties (torque or twisting in the magnet) and heating. No heating or magnetic response could be detected (8,31). Davis et al. (19) also studied the effects of RF pulses and changing magnetic fields on metal clips and prostheses. No heating could be detected with small amounts of metal. Heating was demonstrated with two adjacent hip prostheses in a saline medium. However, it was concluded that metal heating in patients should not be a problem even with large prostheses (31,42).

Metal materials typically cause significant artifact on CT images (8,19,50). Recently, reconstruction methods have been introduced to reduce metal artifacts on CT images (63). Nonferromagnetic metal materials cause less significant artifacts on MR images and, if small enough, the insignificant area of signal void may be overlooked. The extent of artifact created depends on the size, shape, magnetic susceptibility, and field strength of the imager. On low-field imagers one will note some local distortion (Fig. 3-4). The extent of artifact is usually more obvious on high-field (>1.0 T) images (Fig. 3-5). The artifacts noted on MR images are due to local magnetic field distortions caused by both ferromagnetic and nonferromagnetic appliances. The degree of artifact is greater with the former. These distortions result in signal amplitude reduction near the metal surface (78). The artifact generally is oriented in the direction of the frequency readout gradient (2,30,48,78).

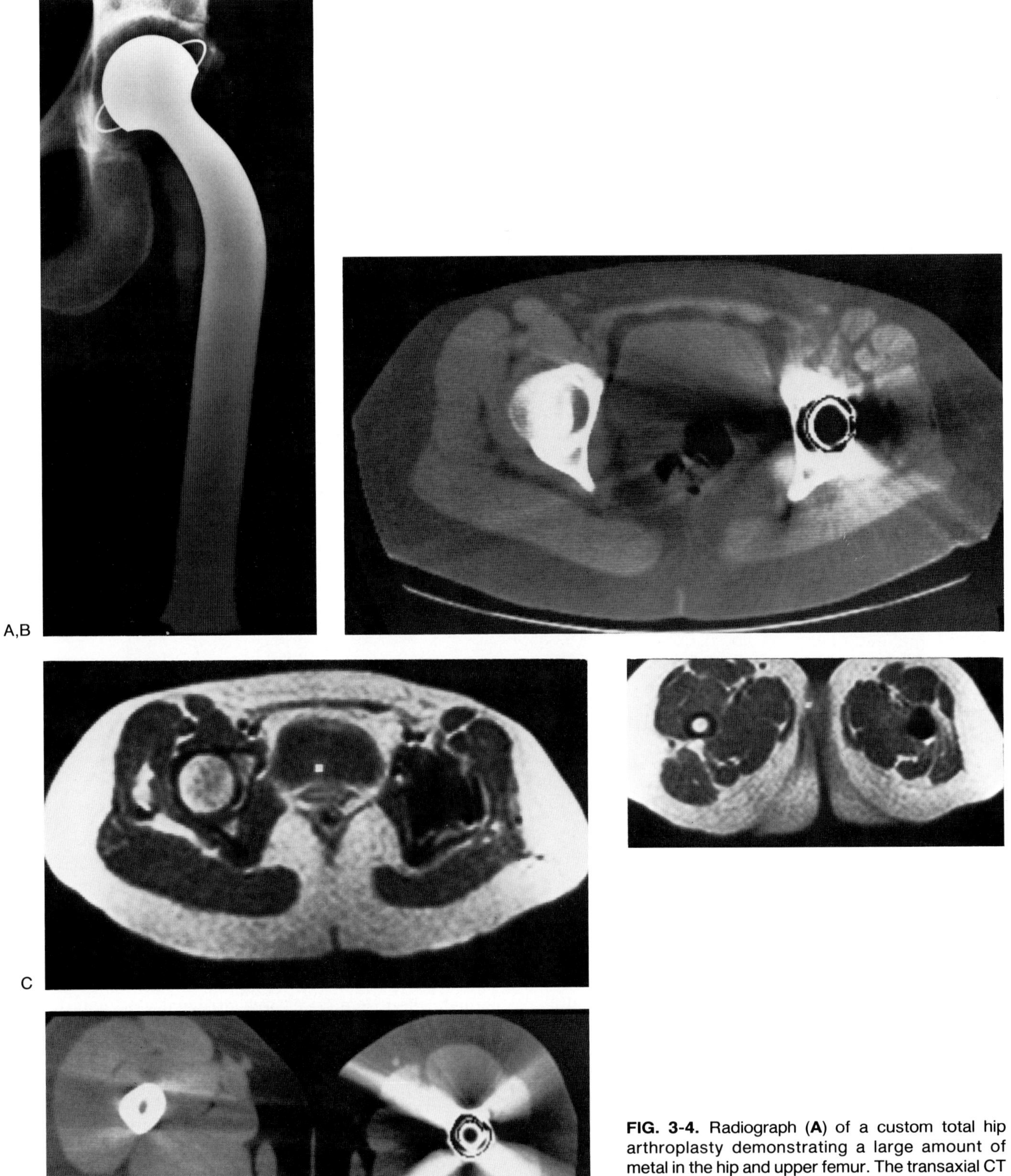

FIG. 3-4. Radiograph (**A**) of a custom total hip arthroplasty demonstrating a large amount of metal in the hip and upper femur. The transaxial CT image (**B**) through the femoral heads is degraded by artifact. Low-field (0.15 T) MR image (**C**) at the same level shows local distortion due to the size and configuration of the metal. In the region of the smaller, smoother femoral stem there is still significant artifact on the CT image (**D**) but no artifact on the low-field MR image (**E**).

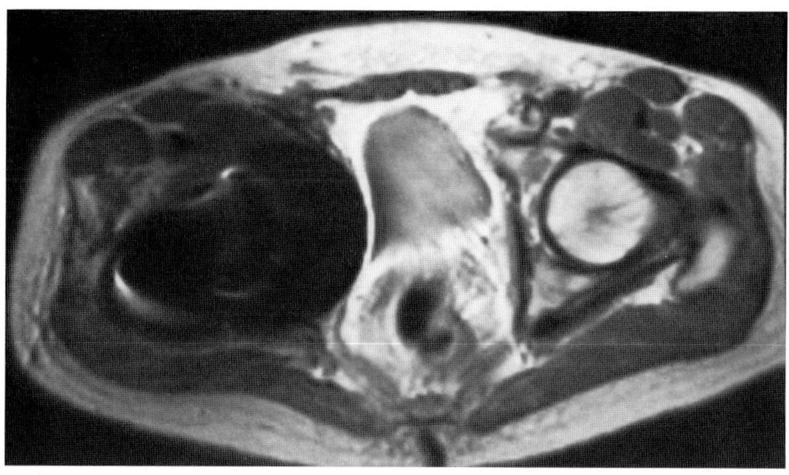

FIG. 3-5. Axial SE 2,000/30, 1.5 T image through the hips in a patient with a total hip arthroplasty. Note the increase in artifact compared to the lower field strength image in Fig. 3-4C.

The artifact created by orthopedic devices varies significantly. When imaging a hip prosthesis, more artifact is created by the large irregular head and neck region than the more regular and smaller femoral stem (Fig. 3-4). There is also more artifact from metal screws and Harrington rods (8,42) (see Fig. 3-3B). This may be due to the irregular contour (threads and ridges), screw position, or increased amounts of ferromagnetic impurities. The latter problem is demonstrated in Figs. 3-6 and 3-7. There are only two screws, yet there is a significant amount of artifact. There are also artifacts in the region of the old pin tracts. The radiograph (Fig. 3-6A) does not demonstrate metal in these old pin tracts. Even small amounts of ferromagnetic materials can cause significant artifact (55). This fact, coupled with histologic evidence of metal debris in histiocytes around screw tracts, suggests that small amounts of ferromagnetic material are present in screws used for internal fixation. A fibrohistiocytic response normally occurs around these screws if they are left in place for a significant length of time (>3 months). This phenomenon may allow artifact to occur even though no significant metal can be detected on routine radiographs (Fig. 3-7). When imaging patients with metal implants, it is important to select the sequences that are least susceptible to artifact. In our experience, there is less metal artifact when using spin echo sequences with short TR/TE (500/20) or short TR (<40 msec) and long TR (2,000 msec) (Fig. 3-8).

Methyl methacrylate is used to fill medullary cavities as well as to cement components. In the former situation there is no artifact created on MR images. Methacrylate is seen as a dark area of no signal but there is no image distortion (Fig. 3-9).

External fixation devices may be bulky, but most are not ferromagnetic (Fig. 3-10) as the materials are similar to those used in internal fixateurs (4,8). Magnetic properties can easily be checked with a hand-held magnet prior to the MR examination. The extent of image degradation will vary with the magnetic susceptibility. Re-

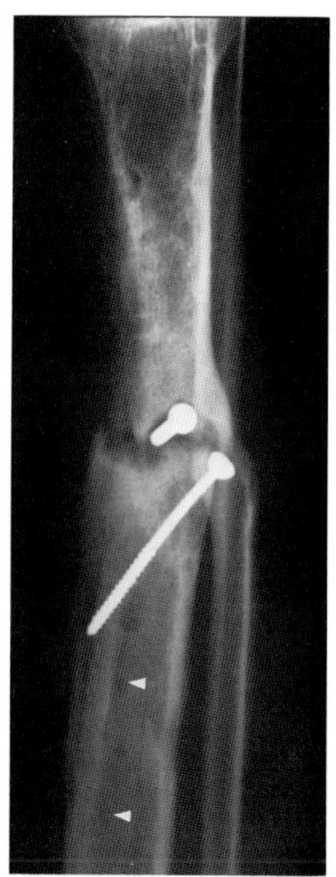

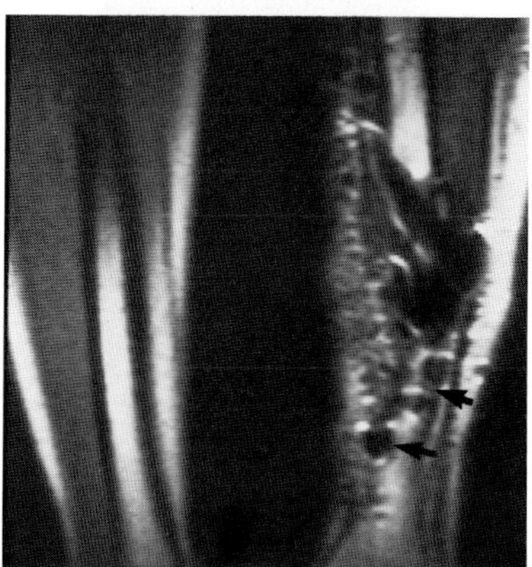

FIG. 3-6. A: Lateral radiograph of the tibia and fibula, demonstrating an old ununited fracture with two metal screws in place. Note the pin tracts in the distal tibia (*small arrows*). There is no metal evident in the tracts. **B:** Coronal 0.15 T image (SE 500/30) shows significant artifact from the screws and small artifacts in the pin tracts (*arrows*).

A,B

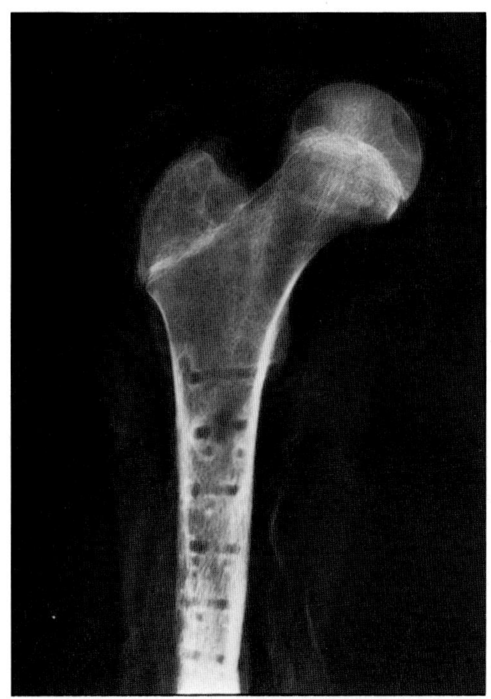

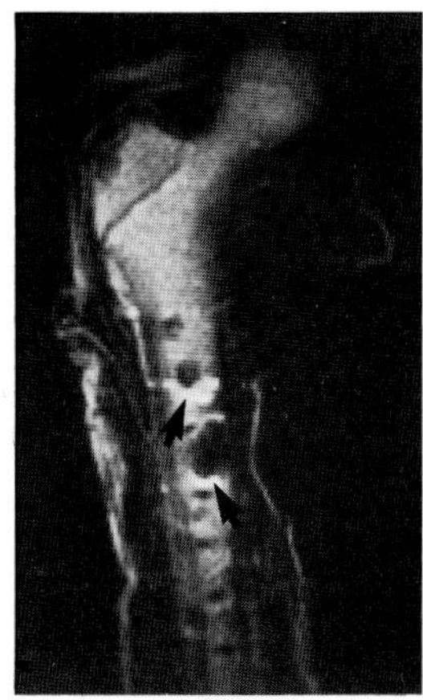

C

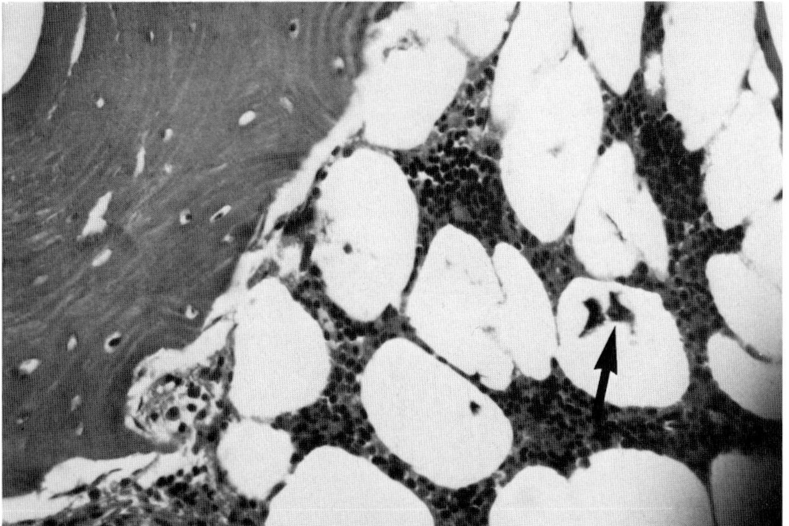

FIG. 3-7. A: Industrial film of a resected femur. The screws have been removed from the shaft and there is no evidence of residual metal. **B:** MR image of the femur (0.15 T, SE 500/30) shows multiple artifacts in the pin tracts (*arrows*). **C:** Histologic specimen of the pin tract with metal debris (*arrow*). (Courtesy of Les Wold, M.D., Department of Surgical Pathology, Mayo Clinic, Rochester, Minnesota.)

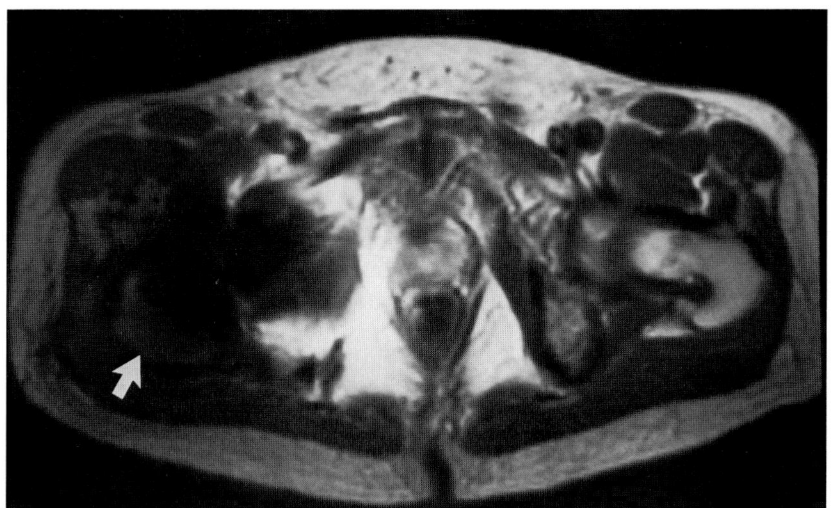

A

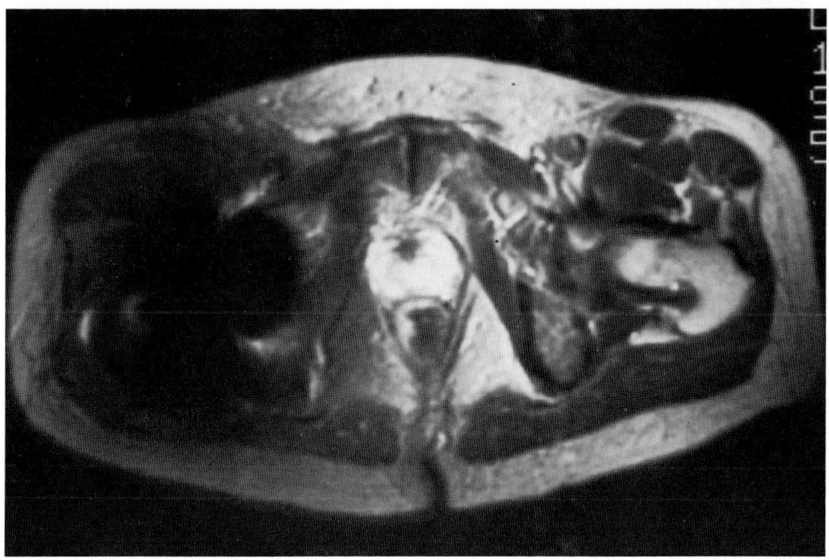

B

FIG. 3-8. Axial images of the hips in a patient with a total hip arthroplasty. The artifact created at 1.5 T using SE 2,000/30 (**A**) is significant but you can still identify the fluid collection around the hip (*arrow*). The artifact on the second echo SE 2,000/60 (**B**) is significantly greater, obscuring the pathology.

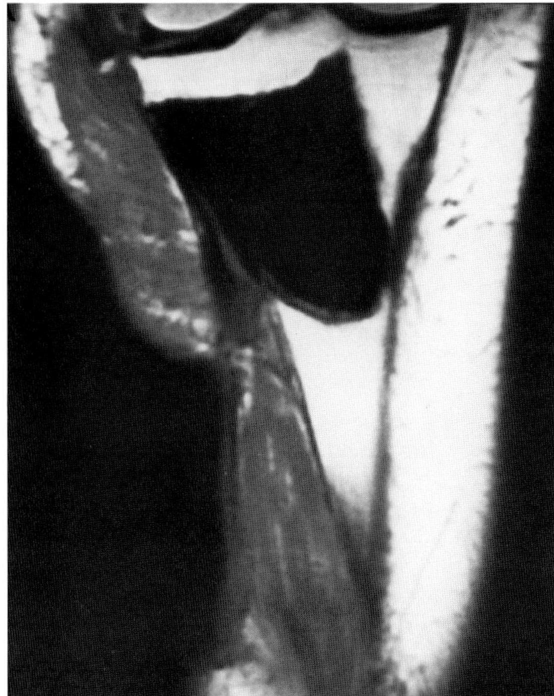

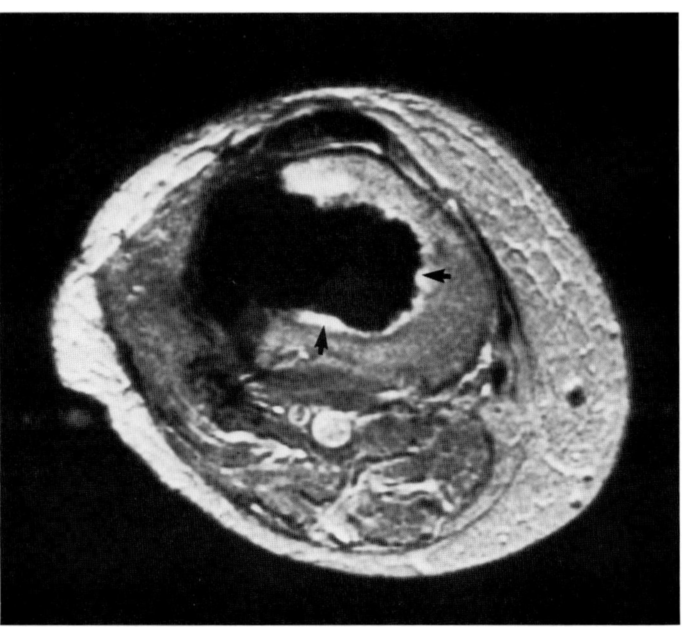

A,B

FIG. 3-9. MR images of the upper tibia in a patient who had curettage of a giant cell tumor with insertion of methyl methacrylate. **A:** Coronal SE 500/20 image shows no signal in the region of the methyl methacrylate but there is no artifact or image distortion. **B:** The axial T2WI (SE 2,000/60) shows a similar area of no signal with reactive edema (*arrows*) in the adjacent marrow.

cently, manufacturers of fixateurs have begun to use nonferromagnetic materials. Table 3-5 lists the materials used for external fixation devices in order of increasing artifact production on MR images (4). In addition to the artifact potential, coil selection may also be restricted due to the size of these fixation systems. This can result in a decreased signal-to-noise ratio (SNR) and reduced image quality. However, most patients can be examined using the head or body coils.

Evaluation of patients with casts and bulky dressings

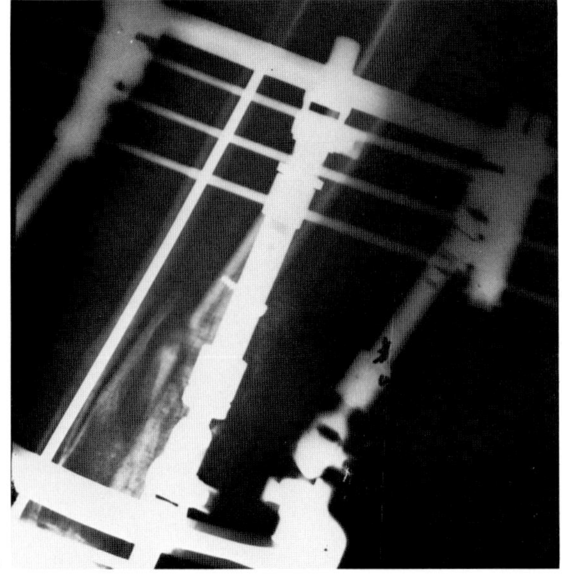

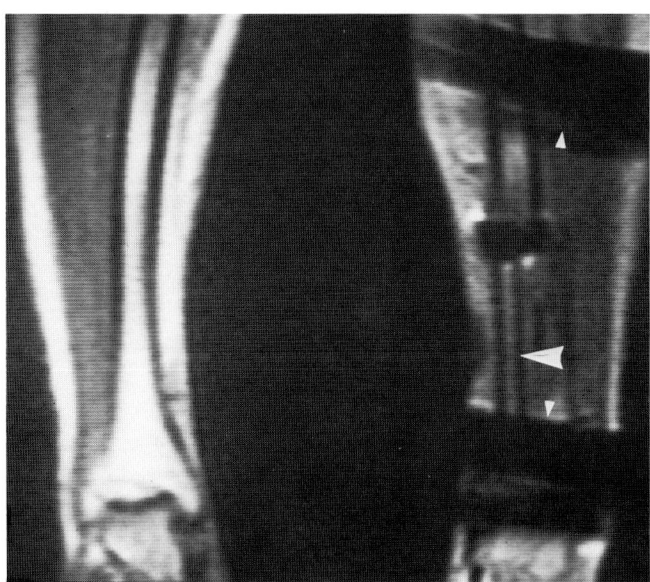

A,B

FIG. 3-10. Radiograph (**A**) taken in an Ace–Fischer external fixation device following placement of a fibular graft. The fixation device causes an area of no signal (*arrows*) on the coronal MR image (**B**), but the fibular graft (*large arrow*) is well demonstrated.

TABLE 3-5. *Artifacts on MR images due to external fixation devices* (4)

Composition	Artifact
Graphite	None–minimal
Titanium	Minimal
Aluminum	Mild–moderate
Stainless steel	Moderate–severe

(Robert–Jones, etc.) is also possible with MRI. Although coil selection is more restrictive, we have not detected any reduction in image quality because of these materials (8).

PATIENT POSITIONING AND COIL SELECTION

Patient positioning considerations include size, body part, and expected examination time. The patient should be studied with the most closely coupled (smallest possible that covers the anatomy) coil possible to achieve the maximum signal-to-noise ratio and best spatial resolution (1,8,9,26). The body coil is used to evaluate the trunk and thigh region (see Fig. 3-1). Patients can be positioned either supine or prone. The prone position should be used when pathology is suspected in the posterior soft tissues. This will prevent compression of soft tissues and anatomic distortion. The body coil may also be used for tumors in the lower extremity. Although the image quality is superior with surface coils, the body coil facilitates examination of the entire structure. In this way, one can perform the examination quickly and avoid overlooking skip lesions (Fig. 3-11).

The head coil, if open at both ends, can be used for children and when comparison of the calves is required. Again, in this setting the patient should be positioned prone to avoid compressing the posterior soft tissues (Fig. 3-12).

Many musculoskeletal examinations in the extremities are performed using surface coils. Surface coils can improve signal-to-noise ratios four to six times compared to head and body coils (1,26,35,70). The type of coil used depends on the anatomic site (Fig. 3-13). As a rule, one should match the sensitivity of the coil to the needed field of view (FOV) to maximize image quality (38,39). Surface coils (flat coils) are usually receive-only coils and minimally contoured. The depth of view is limited or equal to approximately one-half the radius of the coil. This results in exaggeration of fat signal adjacent to the coil and signal drop-off as the distance from the coil increases (Fig. 3-14). Although this has been a problem, new software programs are now available to create more uniform signal intensity throughout the image volume (54). Despite problems with uniformity

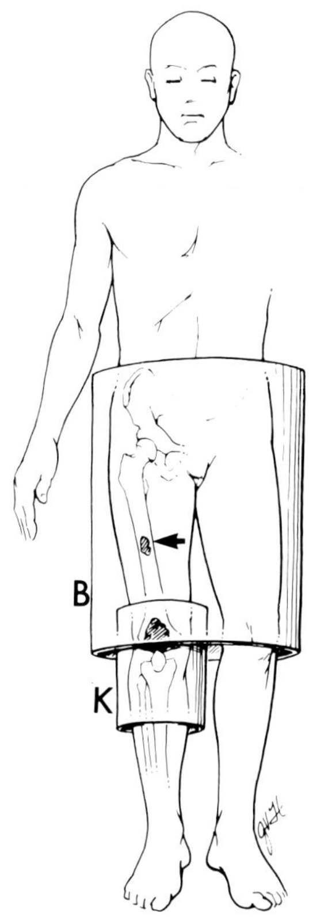

FIG. 3-11. Illustration of patient with a neoplasm in the distal femur. Use of the knee coil (K) would provide superior image quality. However, the skip lesion (*arrow*) would be missed if the body coil (B) were not used.

of signal, flat coils offer advantages in positioning and allow more motion for cine studies (Fig. 3-15).

The lack of uniformity with surface coils (flat coils) can be corrected with whole or partial volume coils. Partial volume coils include Helmholtz pairs or contoured coils. These coils partially surround the part to be examined (38,62). Whole volume coils are circumferential and provide uniform signal (Fig. 3-15) but restrict positioning to some degree.

Newer coil developments, including dual switchable coils for examining both extremities simultaneously and multiple coil arrays, will facilitate examinations and patient throughput (29,39,87). Multiple coil arrays allow use of multiple coils simultaneously to increase the signal-to-noise ratio and examination time can be halved (38).

Positioning of patients for lower extremity examinations is not difficult. Structures can be positioned near the midline, which allows optimal use of surface coils with small or reduced fields of view. Positioning of the upper extremity is more difficult. This is especially true with large patients and when software does not allow the selection of an off-center small field of view (some require the desired anatomy to be centered in the magnet base). The latter problem can partially be overcome by

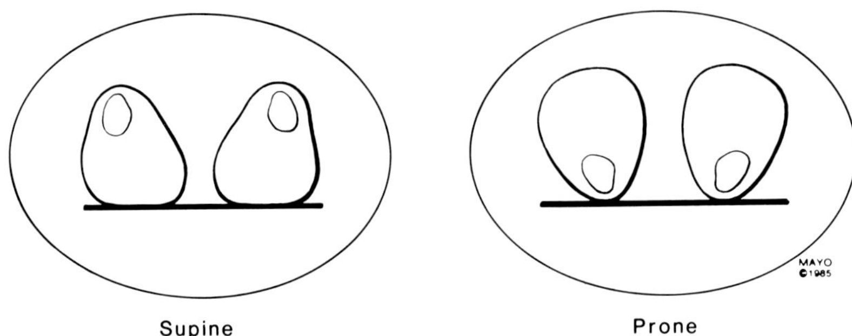

FIG. 3-12. Illustration of supine and prone positioning and the compression effect created on the calves when the patient is supine. The head or body coil is useful when comparison is needed.

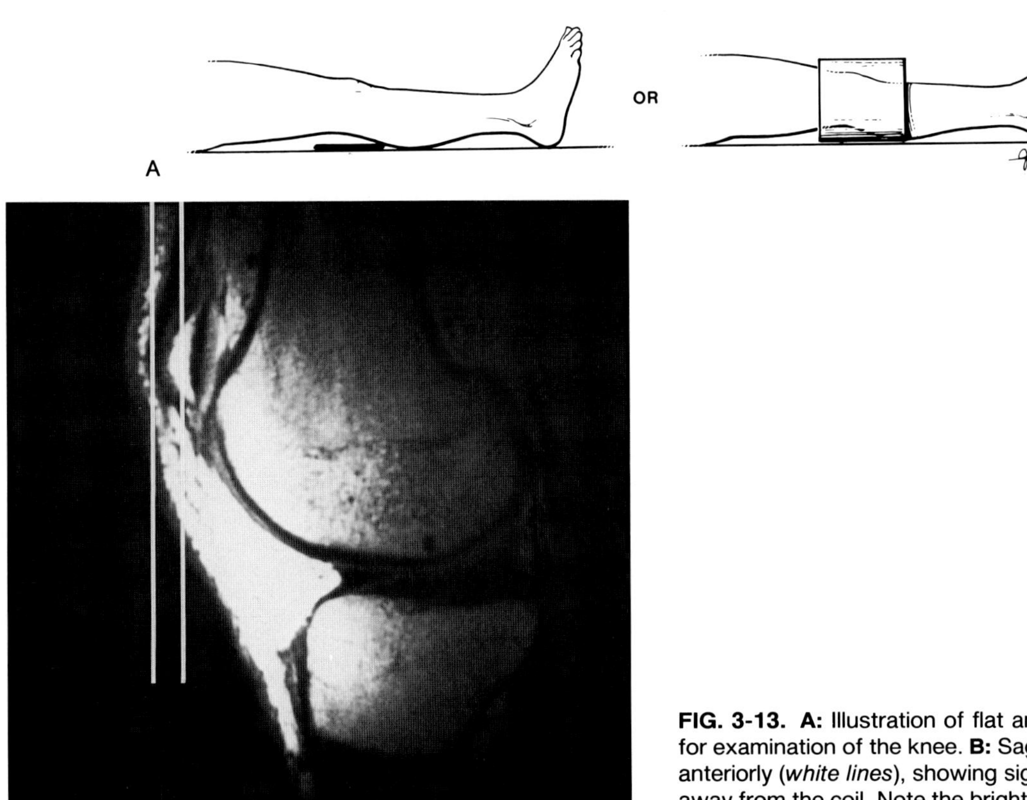

FIG. 3-13. A: Illustration of flat and volume coils positioned for examination of the knee. **B:** Sagittal image using a flat coil anteriorly (*white lines*), showing signal drop-off as one moves away from the coil. Note the bright signal from fat adjacent to the coil.

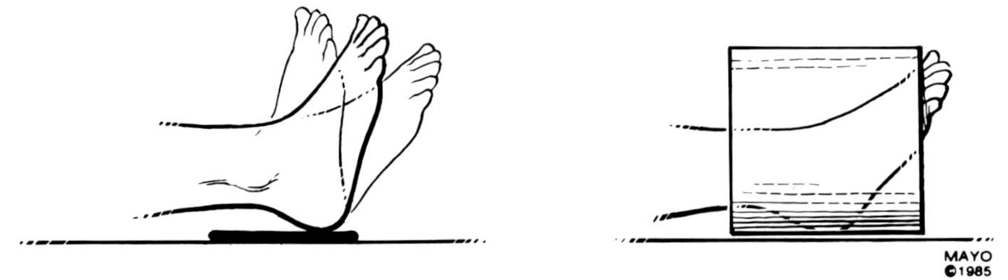

FIG. 3-14. Illustration of flat and volume coils for examination of the ankle. The flat coil permits more flexibility in positioning. The foot must be plantar flexed when the volume coil is employed.

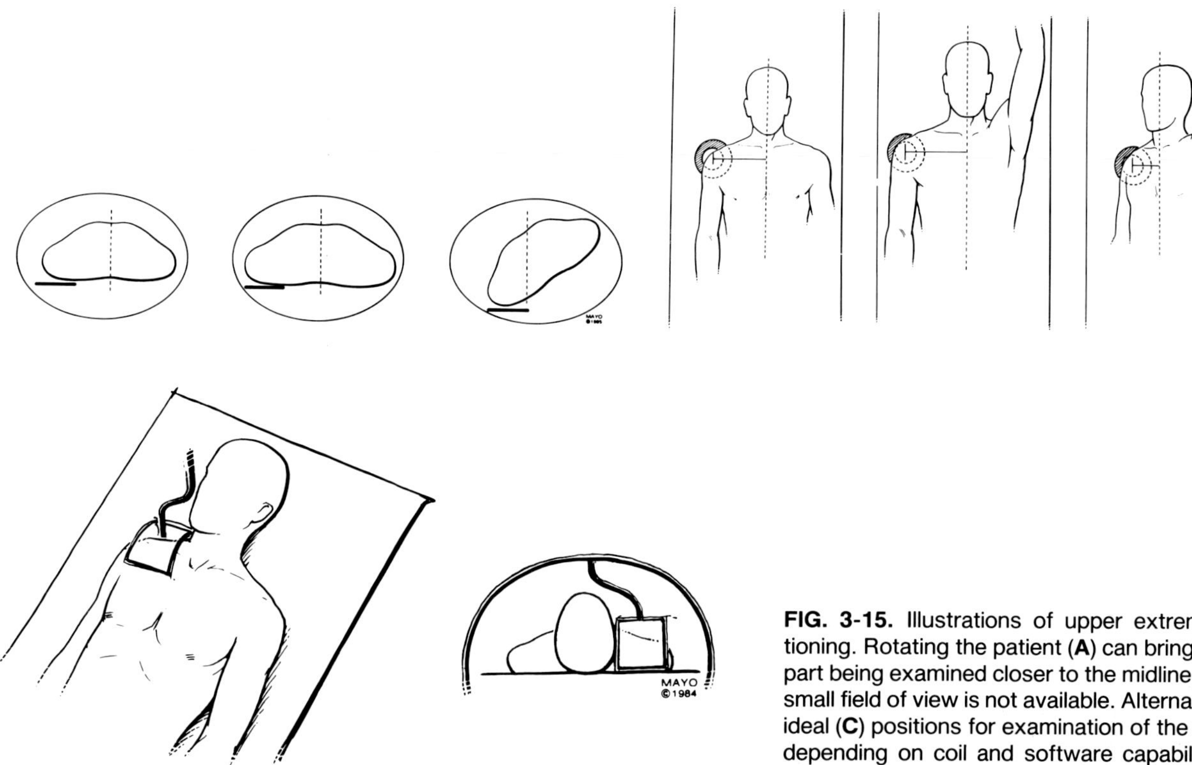

FIG. 3-15. Illustrations of upper extremity positioning. Rotating the patient (**A**) can bring the body part being examined closer to the midline if off-axis small field of view is not available. Alternate (**B**) and ideal (**C**) positions for examination of the shoulder, depending on coil and software capabilities. Off-axis field of view available in (**C**).

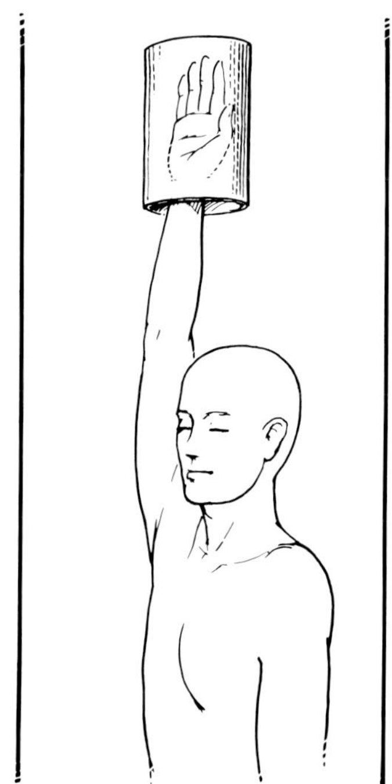

FIG. 3-16. Illustration of patient positioned for wrist examination with the arm above the head and using a volume coil.

rotating the patient to bring the elbow, wrist, or shoulder close to the midline (Fig. 3-15). If this is not possible, the extremity must be placed above the head during the examination (Fig. 3-16). This position is uncomfortable and cannot be maintained for significant time periods. Motion artifact degrades images in patients positioned with the arm above the head in up to 25% of cases. More specific information on coil selection and positioning will be provided in later chapters as they apply to specific clinical problems.

PULSE SEQUENCES AND SLICE SELECTION

Chapters 1 and 2 have discussed basic principles of MR pulse sequences and tissue characterization. Use of different pulse sequences [spin-echo, inversion recovery, short TI inversion recovery (STIR), gradient-echo sequences, etc.] and the many available TE and TR selections would, at first, seem very confusing (51,64, 75,79,81,82,85). However, current experience indicates that in most situations selection of a T1 and T2 weighted sequence will provide the necessary diagnostic information (20,51,82).

Spin-echo (SE) sequences with short TE and TR (TE ≤ 20, TR ≤ 500) and inversion recovery sequences are T1 weighted (contrast due primarily to T1 recovery). Short TE/TR spin-echo sequences provide excellent image quality and can be performed quickly due to the short TR [scan time = repetition time (TR) × number of acquisitions × number of phase-encoding steps (128–512)]. The TR (150–500 msec) allows these sequences to be performed more than four times as fast as most T2 weighted (TR 2,000–2,500) and inversion recovery sequences. Repetition times commonly used with inversion recovery are in the 1,500–2,100 msec range. Abnormal tissues and fluid collections (long T1 relaxation time) have low signal intensity (dark) using T1 weighted sequences. Therefore, T1 weighted sequences provide excellent contrast differentiation between normal marrow and fat (Fig. 3-17). However, lesions may be nearly the same signal intensity as muscle using short TE/TR (SE 500/20) sequences. Thus, T2 weighted sequences (contrast primarily due to T2 relaxation) are also required. Spin-echo sequences with long TE and TR (TE ≥ 60, TR ≥ 2,000) are T2 weighted. Abnormal tissues (long T2 relaxation time) have increased signal intensity, allowing differentiation from muscle, cortical bone, and fibrous structures (ligaments, tendon, scar tissue). We typically use a double-echo sequence (TE 30/60, TR 2,000), which provides an excellent anatomic display with the first echo (SE 2,000/30) and on the second echo (SE 2,000/60) T2 weighting causing increased intensity in tissues with long T2 relaxation times and suppresses the signal intensity of fat (Fig. 3-18).

Using conventional spin-echo and inversion recovery sequences, we find that normal tissues have a characteristic MR appearance. With short spin-echo sequences (SE 500/20), fat and marrow have high signal intensity and appear bright on MR images (Table 3-6). Muscle has intermediate signal intensity, neural tissue has slightly lower signal intensity than muscle, and cortical bone, ligaments, tendons, and fibrocartilage have low signal intensity (black). Hyaline cartilage appears gray or exhibits a signal intensity between that of muscle and fat. It has been suggested that the difference in appearance of hyaline and fibrocartilage may be due to variation in the type of collagen fibers and water content of these structures (37). The water content of hyaline cartilage (articular cartilage) is 75–80% higher than fibrocartilage (menisci). Fibrocartilage, ligaments, and tendons are composed of predominantly type I collagen (articular cartilage is type II) and contain less water (37).

The signal intensity of normal tissue is similar, with the exception of fat, on spin-echo and inversion recovery sequences (Table 3-6). Signal intensity of fat is suppressed on the second echo of long TE (≥60) spin-echo sequences.

Typically, flowing blood does not result in a signal so

A,B

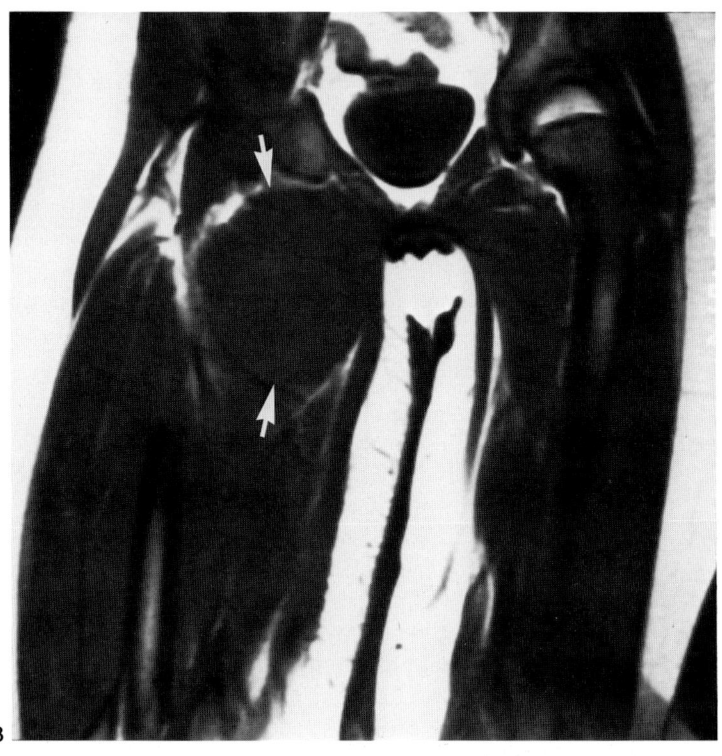

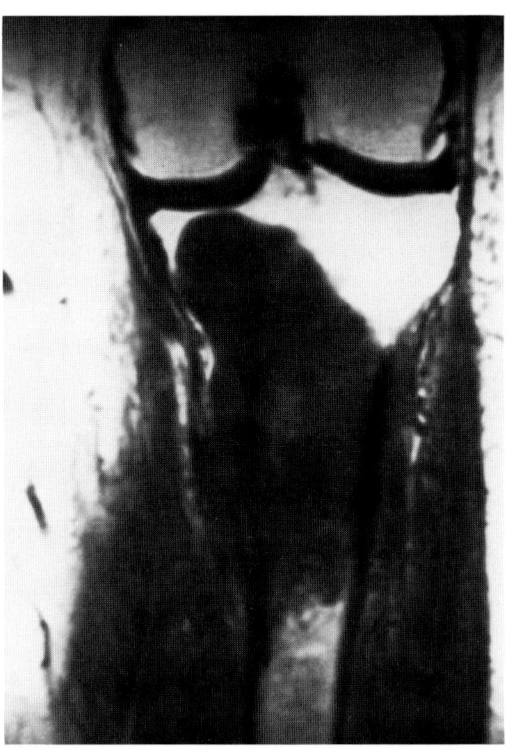

FIG. 3-17. T1 weighted sequences. **A:** There is excellent contrast between marrow and tumor in the upper tibia on this coronal MR image. **B:** Coronal image of the thighs. The mass (*arrows*) is isointense with muscle.

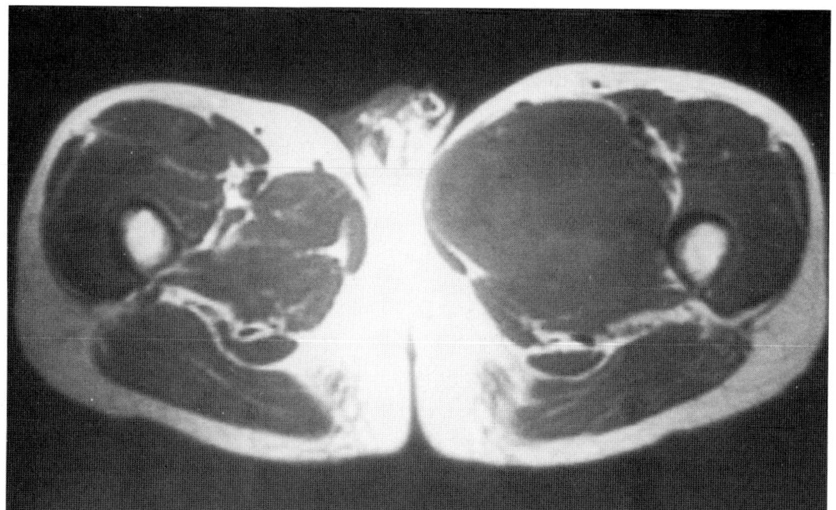
A

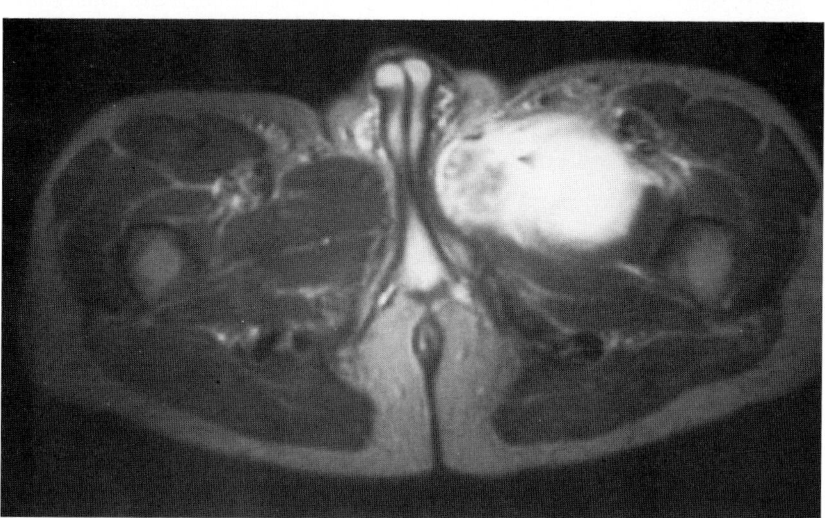
B

FIG. 3-18. Axial images of the thighs in a patient with a soft tissue sarcoma. **A:** SE 2,000/30 image shows excellent soft tissue anatomy with prominent soft tissue in the anteromedial left thigh. **B:** SE 2,000/60 image clearly demonstrates the high signal intensity tumor. Note the decreased signal intensity of fat and marrow.

vessels appear dark or black on MR images. This phenomenon is due to the fact that the moving protons are not stimulated along with stationary tissue or leave prior to signal collection (3,11,13,14,84). However, flow factors and pulse sequences can cause significant problems related to both interpretation and artifact creation. The signal intensity in blood vessels (Table 3-6) depends on the flow velocity, orientation of the vessel in the image plane (perpendicular or oblique), the presence of turbulence, pulse sequence selection, and single or multislice formats (3,25). Phenomena have clearly been described that explain certain signal changes noted in blood vessels (see Chapters 2 and 3). In large arteries the flow is more rapid, with most flow occurring in systole. Velocity is

TABLE 3-6. *Signal intensity of musculoskeletal tissues*

	SE 500/20[a]	SE 2,000/30	SE 2,000/60	IR 1,500/700/30[b]
Fat	High (white)	High (white)	Low intensity	High (white)
Marrow	High (white)	High (white)	Low intensity	High (white)
Hyaline cartilage	Gray	Gray	Bright	Gray
Muscle	Intermediate	Intermediate	Intermediate	Intermediate
Nerves	Intermediate (slightly < muscle)	Intermediate (slightly < muscle)	Intermediate (slightly < muscle)	Intermediate (slightly < muscle)
Fibrocartilage	Low (black)	Low (black)	Low (black)	Low (black)
Ligaments, tendons	Low (black)	Low (black)	Low (black)	Low (black)
Blood vessels	Low (black)[a]	Low (black)[a]	Low or high[a]	Low (black)[a]

[a] TR/TE.
[b] TR/TI/TE.

decreased in branch vessels. Flow is also faster in the lumen than along vessel walls. Venous flow is slower than arterial flow, but inconsistent velocity is present due to respiratory changes, transmitted pulsations, and muscle pressure (3). As noted previously, flowing blood produces a signal void because flow is rapid enough or there are areas of turbulence. Increased signal in vessels is seen with thrombosis (23,84). In this setting, especially venous thrombosis, the vessel lumen is often dilated (Fig. 3-19). Increased signal in vessels can also be noted with "flow-related enhancement" when unsaturated spins (those not stimulated) enter the image plane. This usually occurs with slow flow and is common in veins. Increased signal may also be noted with even echo rephasing set so the signal in the SE 2,000/60 may be higher than the first echo (SE 2,000/30). This should not be confused with thrombosis (11,13,14). Similarly, signal may increase in vessels during diastole due to the reduced flow rates. This is termed diastolic pseudogating (3,11,13,14).

An additional flow-related problem is the linear artifact created, usually by arteries when using 2DFT formats. The artifact occurs in the phase-encoding axis. Two methods can be used to solve this problem. First, if the site of suspected pathology is known, one can change the phase-encoding direction to prevent the artifact from obscuring the region of interest. Second, presaturation may be used to saturate spins entering the slice. This is also effective in reducing flow artifact (25) (see Chapter 2). Even though flow artifact can be a problem, it is occasionally useful. Figure 3-20 is a wrist imaged without presaturation.

Newer pulse sequences have improved patient throughput, increased image plane selection, and, in some cases, increased contrast of pathologic versus normal tissues. Short TI inversion recovery sequences are particularly useful in musculoskeletal imaging. Instead of the usual TI of 600–700 msec, a 100–150 msec TI is used with an echo time of 30 msec and a repetition time (TR) of 1,500 msec (22,75). The latter reduces the imaging time by 25–40% compared with a typical T2 weighted study which uses a TR of 2,000–2,500 msec. STIR sequences produce additive effects of T1 and T2 while nulling fat signal, so contrast or signal difference to noise ratios approach 18:1 in marrow between tumor and fat and 12:1 in muscle between tumor and muscle (22). STIR sequences allow easy detection of pathology, especially when subtle changes in marrow occur (Fig. 3-21) (75).

Gradient-echo sequences use reduced flip angles and short repetition times (12,27). The mechanisms and terms used by the vendors vary (FISP—fast imaging steady precession, FLASH—fast low-angle shot, GRASS—gradient reduced acquisition in steady state, and GRIL-GRASS interleaved) but the image appearances are similar. We typically use these sequences for examination of the knee and other joints where motion studies or complex anatomy may present a problem (Fig. 3-22) (32). Cine video studies can easily be performed using these fast sequences.

More recent developments include chemical shift imaging (44), MR angiography (Fig. 3-23), and volume reconstruction. These techniques will be discussed in detail as they apply to specific clinical problems (12,33,40,45,47,66,67,85).

Specificity of MR data such as T1 and T2 relaxation

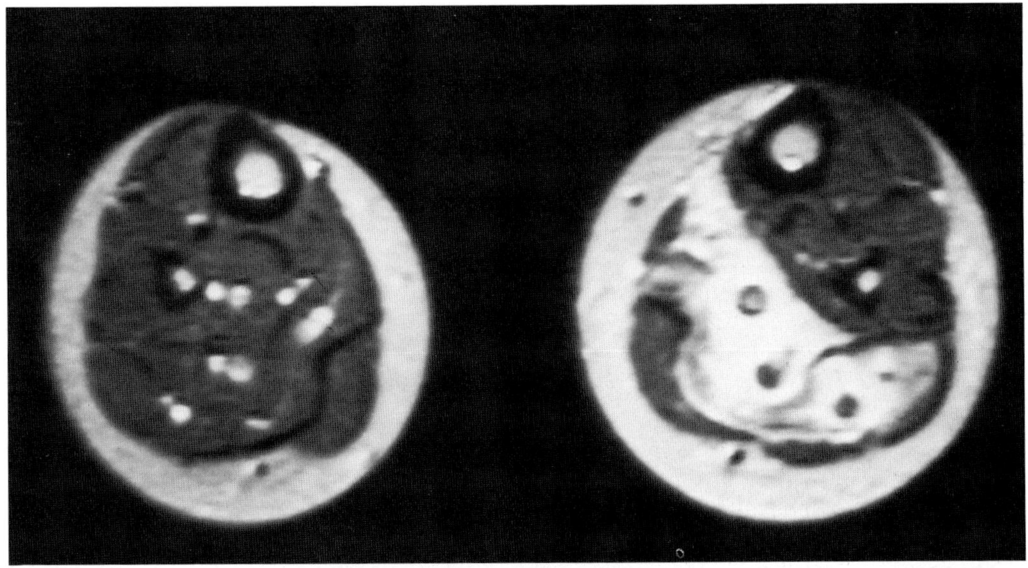

FIG. 3-19. Axial T2 WI (SE 2,000/60) of the calves showing a normal left calf. There is edema in the soleus and three of the right soleal veins are dilated and filled with thrombis. Note the size and high signal intensity in the normal left calf due to slow flow.

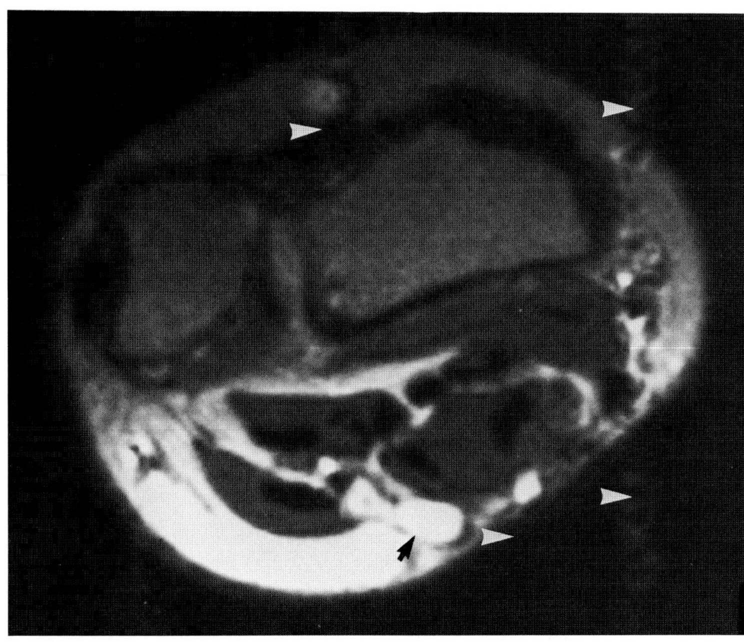

FIG. 3-20. Axial SE 2,000/60 image of the wrist. The signal intensity from the ganglion (*black arrow*) is similar to the vessels. The flow artifact (*arrows*) clearly differentiates the two different structures.

times has been disappointing thus far. However, recent data do indicate that 1.5 T imagers can measure T1 and T2 with reproducibilities of around 5% (15,41,43). Spectroscopy has not yet achieved widespread clinical use. However, muscle diseases, tumor therapy response, and transplant rejection appear to lead early applications (5,6,10,52,56).

The role of MR contrast agents (49), particularly in evaluating neoplasms and joint disorders, continues to evolve (28,83,86). These applications will be fully discussed in the subsequent chapters.

Slice selection will vary depending on the volume of tissue to be studied, size of the suspected pathology, and type of coil (body versus closely coupled or surface coil). It is usually best to image small areas, requiring fine anatomic detail, with thin (<5 mm) slices. Larger areas can be studied with 1 cm thick slices. This slice thickness is especially useful for screening examinations with double-echo T2 weighted sequences (TE 20,60; TR 2,000). When using T2 weighted sequences, an interslice gap is important. This is because slice profiles are not perfectly square and hence adjacent slices can be undesirably affected. This phenomenon can affect contrast and signal of adjacent slices (71). We typically use a gap equal to

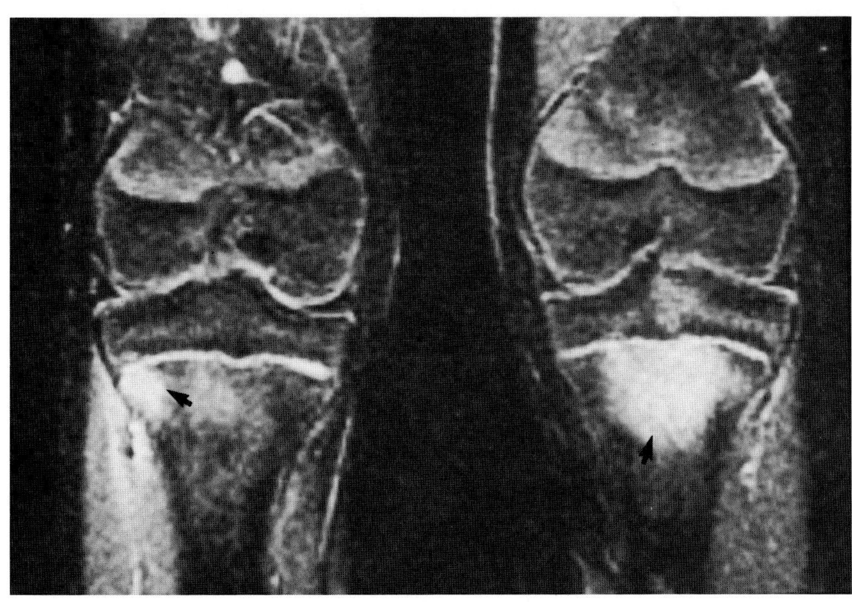

FIG. 3-21. STIR images (TR 1,500, TE 30, TI 150) of the knees, demonstrating suppression of marrow fat signal with marked increased signal in the metaphysis (*arrows*) due to osteomyelitis.

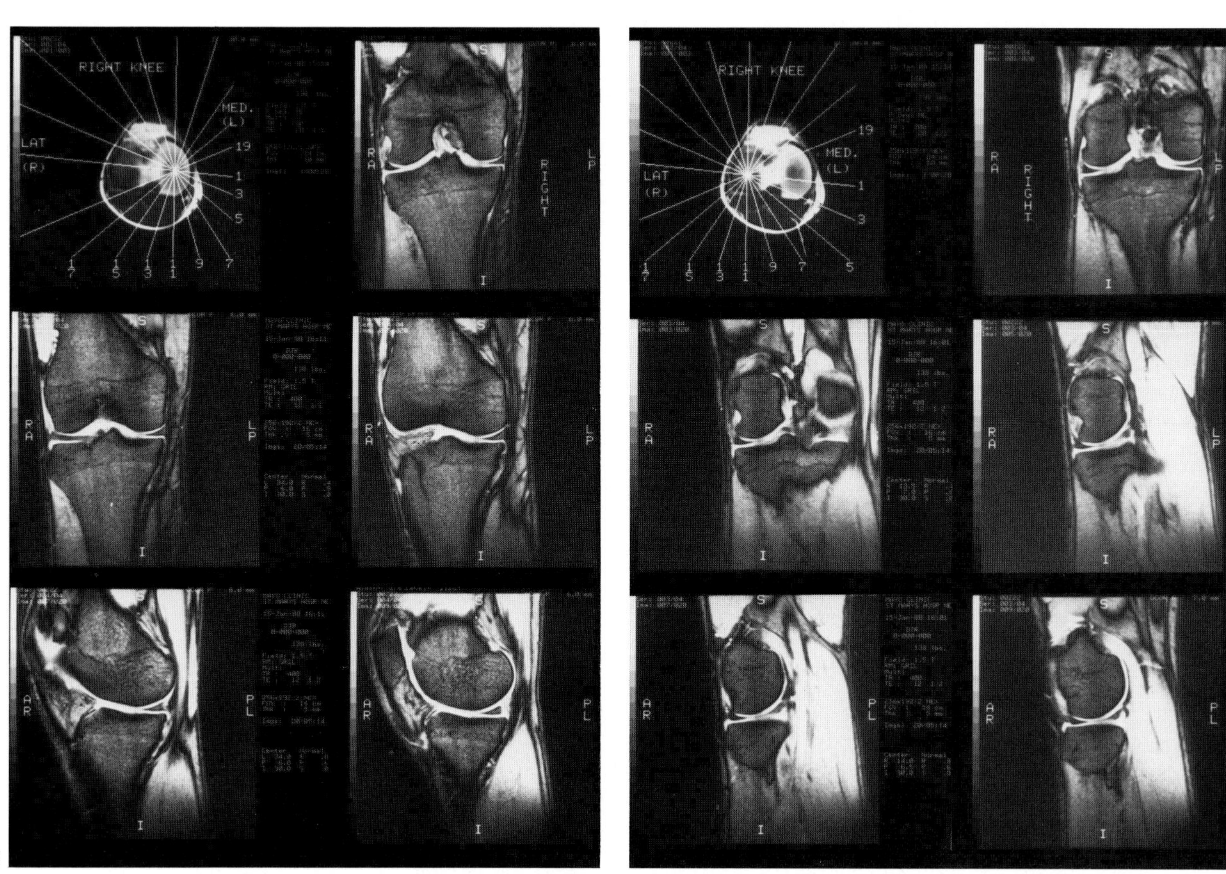

A,B

FIG. 3-22. Radial GRIL images of the right knee set up to evaluate the medial (**A**) and lateral (**B**) menisci. This technique provides tangential views of the menisci.

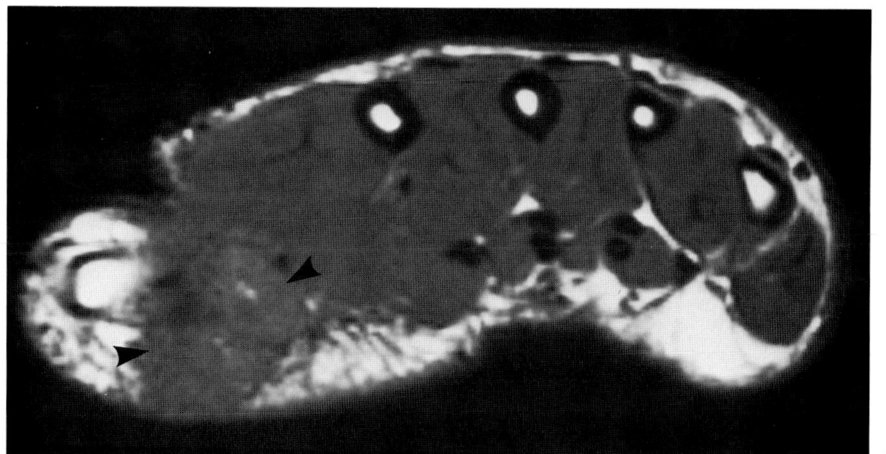

A

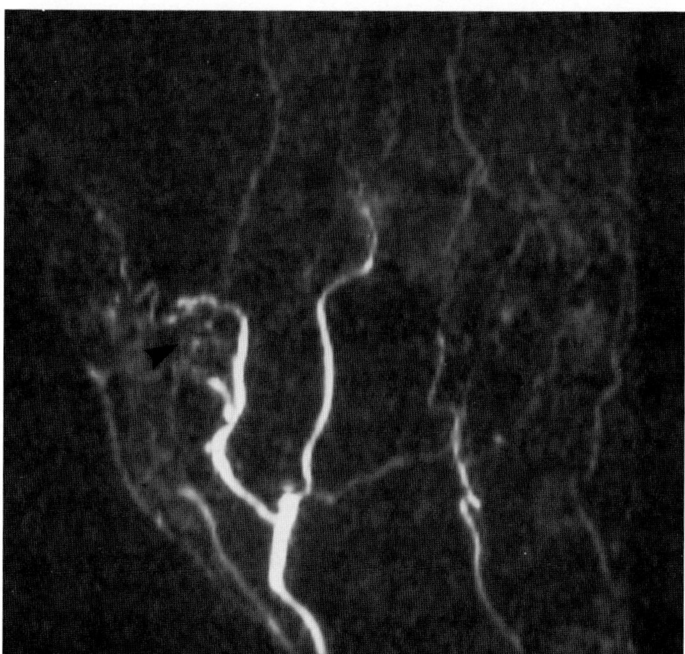

B

FIG. 3-23. Axial SE 500/20 (**A**) and coronal GRASS (**B**) images of the hand in a patient with a hypervascular renal cell metastasis (*arrows*).

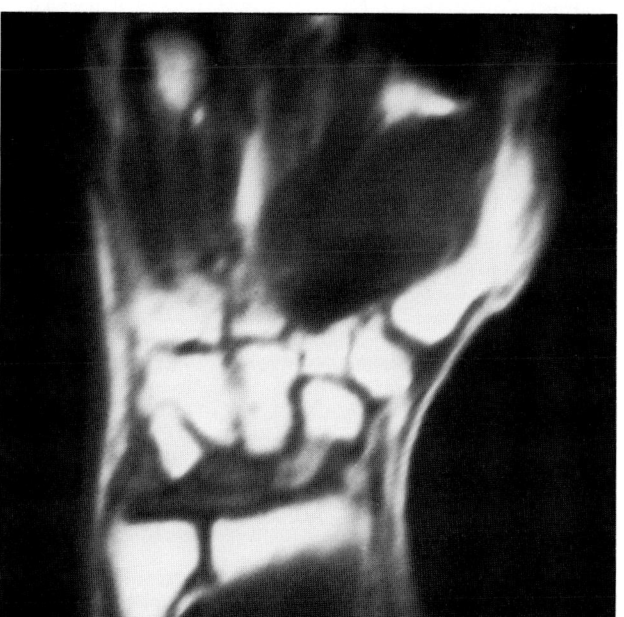

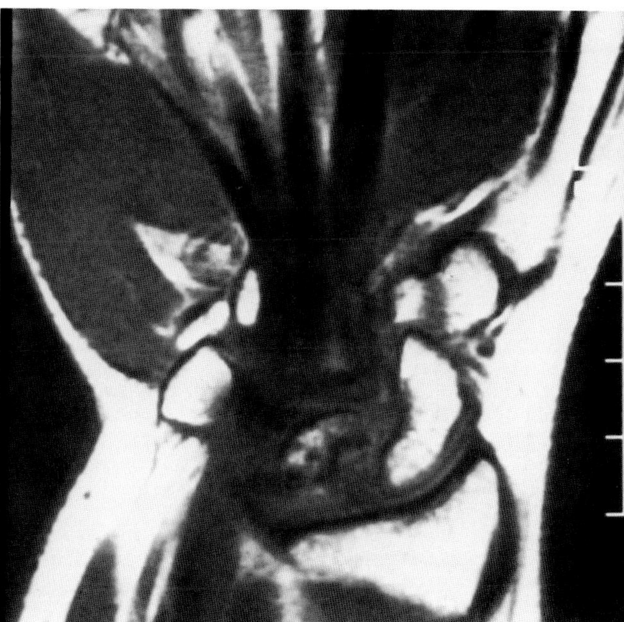

A,B

FIG. 3-24. Coronal SE 500/20 images of the wrist at 24 cm (**A**) and 12 cm (**B**) fields of view. The detail is much improved with the smaller field of view.

50% of the slice width with T2 weighted sequences. Contrast is less critical with typically anatomic T1 weighted sequences, so using interslice gaps is less critical.

It is also important to select the optimal field of view (FOV). This is especially important when using surface coils on the peripheral extremities. A smaller FOV improves spatial resolution significantly (Fig. 3-24). However, signal-to-noise ratios decrease with smaller FOV (73).

Additional parameters that not only affect image quality but also affect image time are the matrix and number of excitations or acquisitions. Spatial resolution or pixel size reduction is accomplished with matrices of 256 or 512, but this results in increased image time. The number of acquisitions used is also a factor. Increasing the acquisitions improves the signal-to-noise ratio and image quality but also increases image time. Image time is dependent on repetition time, the number of acquisitions, and the matrix chosen. For example, a T2 weighted sequence with a 2,000 TR, one acquisition, and a 256 × 256 matrix (2,000 × 1 × 256) takes 8.53 min.

One must consider the image quality, examination time, and use of other parameters such as flow compensation techniques, respiratory compensation (pelvis and trunk), presaturation, and compensation for phase or frequency wrap when setting up an MR examination. These factors will be discussed more completely in later chapters as they apply to specific anatomic and pathologic situations.

REFERENCES

1. Arakawa M, Crooks LE, McCarten B, Hoenninger JC, Watts JC, Kaufman L. A comparison of saddle shaped and solenoidal coils for magnetic resonance imaging. *Radiology* 1985;154:227–228.
2. Augustiny N, Gustav K, von Schulthess DM, Bösiger, P. MR imaging of large nonferromagnetic metallic implants at 1.5 T. *J Comput Assist Tomogr* 1987;11:678–683.
3. Axel L. Blood flow effects in magnetic resonance imaging. *AJR* 1984;143:1157–1166.
4. Ballock RT, Hajek PC, Byrne TP, Gartin SK. The quality of magnetic resonance imaging as affected by the composition of halo orthosis. *J Bone Joint Surg* [*Am*] 1989;71A:431–434.
5. Bárány M, Langer BG, Glick RP, Venkatasubramanian PN, Wilbur AC, Spigos D. *In vivo* H-1 spectroscopy in humans at 1.5 T. *Radiology* 1988;167:839–844.
6. Barfuss H, Fischer H, Hentschel D, Ladebeck R, Vetter J. Whole-body MR imaging and spectroscopy with a 4-T system. *Radiology* 1988;169:811–816.
7. Bellon EM, Haacke EM, Coleman PE, Sacco DC, Steiger DA, Gangarosa RE. MR artifacts: a review. *AJR* 1986;147:1271–1281.
8. Berquist TH. Magnetic resonance imaging: preliminary experience in orthopedic radiology. *Magn Reson Imaging* 1984;2:41–52.
9. Bodne D, Quinn SF, Cochran CF. Imaging foreign glass and wooden bodies of the extremities with CT and MR. *J Comput Assist Tomogr* 1988;12:608–611.
10. Bottomley PA. Human *in vivo* NMR spectroscopy in diagnostic medicine: clinical tool or research probe? *Radiology* 1989;170:1–15.
11. Bradley WG Jr. Flow phenomena in MR imaging. *AJR* 1988;150:983–994.
12. Bradley WG. When should GRASS be used? *Radiology* 1988;169:574–575.
13. Bradley WG Jr, Waluch V. Blood flow: magnetic resonance imaging. *Radiology* 1985;154:443–450.
14. Bradley WG Jr, Waluch V, Lai KS, Fernandes EJ, Spalter C. The appearance of rapidly flowing blood on magnetic resonance images. *AJR* 1984;143:1167–1174.
15. Breger RK, Rimm AA, Fischer ME, Papke RA, Haughton VM. T1 and T2 measurements on a 1.5-T commercial MR imager. *Radiology* 1989;171:273–276.
16. Brown MA, Carden JA, Coleman RE, McKinney R Jr, Spicer LD. Magnetic field effects on surgical ligation clips. *Magn Reson Imaging* 1987;5:443–453.
17. Brummett RE, Talbot JM, Charuhas P. Potential hearing loss resulting from MRI imaging. *Radiology* 1988;169:539–540.
18. Carr AB, Gibilisco JA, Berquist TH. Magnetic resonance imaging of the temporomandibular joint: preliminary work. *J Craniomand Disorders* 1987;1(2):89–96.
19. Davis PL, Crooks L, Arakawa M, McRee R, Kaufman L, Margulis AR. Potential hazards of MR imaging: heating and effects of changing magnetic fields and RF fields on small metallic implants. *AJR* 1981;137:857–860.
20. des Plantes BGZ, Falke THM, den Boer JA. Pulse sequences and contrast in magnetic resonance imaging. *RadioGraphics* 1984;4:869–883.
21. Dujovny M, Kossovsky N, Kossowsky R, et al. Aneurysm clip motion during magnetic resonance imaging: *in vivo* experimental study with metallurgical factor analysis. *Neurosurgery* 1985; 17:543–548.
22. Dwyer AJ, Frank JA, Sank VJ, Reinig JW, Hickey AM, Doppman JL. Short-T1 inversion-recovery pulse sequence: analysis and initial experience in cancer imaging. *Radiology* 1988;168:827–836.
23. Erdman WA, Weinreb JC, Cohen JM, Buja LM, Chaney C, Peshock RM. Venous thrombosis: clinical and experimental MR imaging. *Radiology* 1986;161:233–238.
24. Evens RG, Evens RG Jr. Economic and utilization analysis of MR imaging units in the United States in 1987. *Radiology* 1988;166:27–30.
25. Felmlee JP, Ehman RL. Spatial presaturation: a method for suppressing flow artifacts and improving depiction of vascular anatomy in MR imaging. *Radiology* 1987;164:559–564.
26. Fisher MR, Barker B, Amparo EG, Brandt G, Brant-Zawadzki M, Hricak H, Higgens CB. MR imaging using specialized coils. *Radiology* 1985;157:443–447.
27. Gullberg GT, Wehril FW, Shimakawa A, Simons MA. MR vascular imaging with a fast gradient refocusing pulse sequence and reformatted images for transaxial sections. *Radiology* 1987;165:241–246.
28. Hajek PC, Sartoris DJ, Neumann CH, Resnick D. Potential contrast agents for MR arthrography: *in vitro* evaluation and practical observations. *AJR* 1987;149:97–104.
29. Hardy CJ, Katzberg RW, Frey RL, Szumowski J, Totterman S, Mueller OM. Switched surface coil system for bilateral MR imaging. *Radiology* 1988;167:835–838.
30. Harris R, Wesbey G. Artifacts in magnetic resonance imaging. *Magn Reson Ann* 1988:71–112.
31. Hazel WA, Nestor BJ, Gray JE, Stauffer RN. Heating effects of magnetic resonance imaging on orthopedic metallic implants. *J Bone Joint Surg* [*Am*] (To be published).
32. Herman LJ, Beltran J. Pitfalls in MR imaging of the knee. *Radiology* 1988;167:775–781.
33. Heuck AF, Steiger P, Stoller DW, Glüer CC, Genant HK. Quantification of knee fluid volume by MR imaging and CT using 3-D data processing. *J Comput Assist Tomogr* 1989;13:287–293.
34. Hovsepain DM, Amis ES. Penile prosthetic implants. A radiographic atlas. *RadioGraphics* 1989;9:707–716.
35. Hyde JS, Kneeland JB. High resolution methods using surface coils. In: Wehrlie FW, Shaw D, Kneeland JB, eds. *Biomedical magnetic resonance imaging.* Weinheim, Germany: VCH, 1988:189–222.
36. Jackson JG, Acker JD. Permanent eyeliner and MR imaging (Letter). *AJR* 1987;149:1080.
37. King CL, Henkelman RM, Poon PY, Rubenstein J. MR imaging of the normal knee. *J Comput Assist Tomogr* 1984;8:1147–1154.
38. Kneeland JB, Knowles RJR, Cahill PT. Magnetic resonance imaging systems: optimization in clinical use. *Radiology* 1984;153:473–478.

39. Kneeland JB, Hyde JS. High-resolution MR imaging with local coils. *Radiology* 1989;171:1–7.
40. König H, Sauter R, Deimling M, Vogt M. Cartilage disorders: comparison of spin-echo, CHESS, and FLASH sequence MR images. *Radiology* 1987;164:753–758.
41. Kuno S, Katsuta S, Inouye T, Anno I, Matsumoto K, Akisada M. Relationship between MR relaxation time and muscle fiber composition. *Radiology* 1988;169:567–568.
42. Lackman RW, Kaufman B, Han JS, et al. MR imaging in patients with metallic implants. *Radiology* 1985;157:711–714.
43. LeBlanc A, Evans H, Schonfeld E, Ford J, Marsh C, Schneider V, Johnson P. Relaxation times of normal and atrophied muscle. *Med Phys* 1986;13:514–517.
44. Lenkinski RE, Holland GA, Allman T, et al. Integrated MR imaging and spectroscopy with chemical shift imaging of P-31 at 1.5 T: initial clinical experience. *Radiology* 1988;169:201–206.
45. Lenz GW, Haacke EM, Masaryk TJ, Laub G. In-plane vascular imaging: pulse sequence design and strategy. *Radiology* 1988;166:875–882.
46. Liebman CE, Messersmith RN, Levin DN, Lu CT. MR imaging of inferior vena caval filters: safety and artifacts. *AJR* 1988; 150:1174–1176.
47. Lufkin RB, Pusey E, Stark DD, Brown R, Leikind B, Hanafee WN. Boundary artifact due to truncation errors in MR imaging. *AJR* 1986;147:1283–1287.
48. Malko JA, Hoffman JC, Jarrett PJ. Eddy-current-induced artifacts caused by an "MRI-compatible" halo device. *Radiology* 1989;173:563–564.
49. Mattery RF. Perfluorooctylbromide: a new contrast agent for CT, sonography and MR imaging. *AJR* 1989;152:247–252.
50. Mechlin M, Thickman D, Kressel HY, Gefter W, Joseph P. Magnetic resonance imaging of postoperative patients with metallic implants. *AJR* 1984;143:1281–1284.
51. Merritt CRB. Magnetic resonance imaging—a clinical perspective: image quality, safety and risk management. *RadioGraphics* 1987;7:1001–1016.
52. Miller RG, Carlson PJ, Moussavi RS, Boska MD, Weiner MW. The use of magnetic resonance spectroscopy to evaluate muscle fatigue and human muscle disease. *Appl Radiol* 1989;18(3):33–38.
53. Moon KL, Genant HK, Helms CA, Chafetz NI, Crooks LE, Kaufman L. Musculoskeletal applications of nuclear magnetic resonance. *Radiology* 1983;147:161–171.
54. Narayana PA, Brey WW, Kulkarni MV, Sievenpiper CL. Compensation for surface coil sensitivity variation in magnetic resonance imaging. *Magn Reson Imaging* 1988;6:271–274.
55. New PF, Rosen BR, Brady TJ, et al. Potential hazards and artifacts of ferromagnetic and nonferromagnetic surgical and dental materials and devices in nuclear magnetic resonance imaging. *Radiology* 1983;147:137–148.
56. Ng TC, Majors AW, Vijayakumar S, et al. Human neoplasm pH and response to radiation therapy: P-31 MR spectroscopy studies *in situ*. *Radiology* 1989;170:875–878.
57. Pavlicek W. MR instrumentation and image formation. *RadioGraphics* 1987;7:809–814.
58. Pavlicek W, Geisinger M, Castle L, Barkowski GP, Meaney TF, Brean BL, Gallagher JH. The effects of nuclear magnetic resonance on patients with cardiac pacemakers. *Radiology* 1983;147:149–153.
59. Porter BA, Hastrup W, Richardson ML, Wesbey GE, Olson DO, Cromwell LD, Moss AA. Classification and investigation of artifacts in magnetic resonance imaging. *RadioGraphics* 1987;7:271–287.
60. Pusey E, Lufkin RB, Brown RKJ, Solomon MA, Stark DD, Tarr RW, Hanafee WN. Magnetic resonance imaging artifacts: mechanism and clinical significance. *RadioGraphics* 1986;6:891–911.
61. Quirk ME, Letendre AJ, Ciottone RA, Langley JF. Anxiety in patients undergoing MR imaging. *Radiology* 1989;170:463–466.
62. Reiman TH, Heiken JP, Totty WG, Lee JKT. Clinical MR imaging with a Helmholtz-type surface coil. *Radiology* 1988;169:564–566.
63. Robertson DD, Magid D, Poss R, Fishman EK, Brookes AF, Sledge CB. Enhanced computed tomographic techniques for the evaluation of total hip arthroplasty. *J Arthroplasty* 1989;4:271–276.
64. Rosen BR, Fleming DM, Kushner DC, et al. Hematologic bone marrow disorders: quantitative chemical shift MR imaging. *Radiology* 1988;169:799–804.
65. Roth JL, Nugent M, Gray JE, et al. Patient monitoring during magnetic resonance imaging. *Anesthesiology* 1985;62:80–83.
66. Rubin JB, Enzmann DR. Optimizing conventional MR imaging of the spine. *Radiology* 1987;163:777–783.
67. Rusenik H, Mourino MR, Firooznia H, Weinreb JC, Chase NE. Volumetric rendering of MR images. *Radiology* 1989;171:269–272.
68. Sacco DC, Steiger DA, Bellon EM, Coleman PE, Haacke EM. Artifacts caused by cosmetics in MR imaging of the head. *AJR* 1987;148:1001–1004.
69. Saunders RD. Biological effects of NMR clinical imaging. *Appl Radiol* 1982;11:43–46.
70. Schenck JR, Hart HR, Foster TH, et al. High field surface coil magnetic resonance imaging of localized anatomy. *Am J Neuroradiol* 1985;6:193–196.
71. Schwaighofer BS, Yu KK, Mattery RF. Diagnostic significance of interslice gap and imaging volume in body MR imaging. *AJR* 1989;153:629–632.
72. Schwartz JL, Crooks LE. NMR imaging produces no observable mutations or cytotoxicity in mammalian cells. *AJR* 1982; 139:583–585.
73. Shaw D. The fundamental principles of nuclear magnetic resonance. In: Wehrli FF, Shaw D, Kneeland JB, eds. *Biomedical magnetic resonance imaging*. Weinheim, Germany: VCH, 1988:1–45.
74. Shellock FG. MR imaging of metallic implants and materials: a compilation of the literature. *AJR* 1988;151:811–814.
75. Shuman WP, Baron RL, Peters MJ, Tazioli PK. Comparison of STIR and spin echo MR imaging at 1.5 T in 90 lesions of the chest, liver, and pelvis. *AJR* 1989;152:853–859.
76. Soulen RL, Budinger TF, Higgins CB. Magnetic resonance imaging of prosthetic heart valves. *Radiology* 1985;154:705–707.
77. Teitelbaum GP, Ortega HV, Vinitski S, et al. Low-artifact intravascular devices: MR imaging evaluation. *Radiology* 1988;168:713–719.
78. Teitelbaum GP, Bradley WG Jr, Klein BD. MR imaging artifacts, ferromagnetism and magnetic torque of intravascular filters, stents and coils. *Radiology* 1988;166:657–664.
79. Tkach JA, Haacke EM. A comparison of fast spin echo and gradient field echo sequences. *Magn Reson Imaging* 1988;6:373–389.
80. Tyrrell RL, Gluckert K, Pathria M, Modic MT. Fast three-dimensional MR imaging of the knee: comparison with arthroscopy. *Radiology* 1988;166:865–872.
81. van der Meulen P, Groen JP, Tinus AMC, Bruntink G. Fast field echo imaging: an overview and contrast calculations. *Magn Reson Imaging* 1988;6:355–368.
82. Wehrli FW, McFall JR, Glover GH, Grigsby N, Haughton V, Johanson J. The dependency of nuclear magnetic resonance image contrast on intrinsic and pulse sequence timing parameters. *Magn Reson Imaging* 1984;2:3–16.
83. Wesbey GE. Magnetopharmaceuticals. In: Wehrlie FW, Shaw D, Kneeland JB, eds. *Biomedical magnetic resonance imaging*. Weinheim, Germany: VCH, 1988:157–183.
84. White EM, Edelman RR, Wedeen VJ, Brady TJ. Intravascular signal in MR imaging: use of phase display for differentiation of blood-flow signal from intraluminal disease. *Radiology* 1986;161:245–249.
85. Wismer GL, Rosen BR, Buxton R, Stark DB, Brady TJ. Chemical shift imaging of bone marrow: preliminary experience. *AJR* 1985;145:1031–1037.
86. Wolf GL. Current status of MR imaging contrast agents. A special report. *Radiology* 1989;172:709–710.
87. Wright SM, Wright RM. Bilateral MR imaging with switched mutally coupled receiver coils. *Radiology* 1989;170:249–255.

MRI of the Musculoskeletal System, 2nd Edition, edited by T. H. Berquist.
Raven Press, Ltd., New York © 1990.

CHAPTER 4

Temporomandibular Joint

Clyde A. Helms

Anatomy, 75
Technique, 77
Internal Derangements, 80
Postoperative Joints, 84
Summary, 84
References, 84

Magnetic resonance imaging (MRI) of the temporomandibular joint (TMJ) has rapidly replaced arthrography and computed tomography (CT) in most imaging centers as the imaging modality of choice for suspected internal derangements (6,8,10,11,18–22,32,39,40). Its ability to directly visualize the disc and accurately determine the disc position in a noninvasive manner makes MRI an attractive alternative to the painful, invasive arthrogram. Although it will not rival the resolution of CT in examining bony detail, MRI will give an adequate picture of most bony abnormalities. In addition, MRI will image intra-articular abnormalities other than disc disease and give information on the state of hydration and morphology of the disc, which may be helpful in staging the degree of severity of an internal derangement (12,14).

An imaging protocol that will allow a rapid, complete exam should be sought in order to diminish the cost of a TMJ MRI study and therefore be competitive with the less expensive arthrogram and CT. If this is achieved, the only drawbacks to replacing arthrography or CT with MRI is the inability of MRI to demonstrate joint dynamics or disc perforations. These "shortcomings" of MRI are addressed later in this chapter.

ANATOMY

The normal TMJ has a fibrous disc that sits on the apex of the condyle in the closed-mouth position (Fig. 4-1). The disc has a saddle shape with a slightly thicker posterior portion called the posterior band. A less thick anterior band is connected by the thin intermediate zone, which is a very important structure to recognize when determining disc position with MRI. The disc is attached posteriorly to the bilaminar zone, which consists of loose, vascular connective tissue that is posteriorly joined to the temporal bone just anterior to the internal auditory canal. It is the bilaminar zone tissue that contains a rich vascular bed and neural elements that innervate the disc.

The disc is separated from the head of the condyle by a synovial-lined joint space called the lower joint. A separate upper joint lies just superior to the disc underneath the bony glenoid fossa and the articular eminence of the temporal bone. The upper and lower joints are not contiguous: they are separated by the disc; hence, a contrast agent placed into one of the joints should not fill both joint spaces. If both joints do fill simultaneously, a disc perforation is present. MRI is currently incapable of accuracy demonstrating disc perforations (1).

The disc attaches to the superior belly of the lateral pterygoid muscle anteriorly. The pterygoids coarse medially to attach to the pterygoid plates; hence, an anteriorly displaced disc has a tendency to lie somewhat anteromedially. It is unusual for a disc to displace laterally or solely medially, but this has been reported (23). Posterior disc displacements have not been reported.

As the mouth opens, the mandibular condyle initially rotates minimally and the jaw opens in a hinge fashion, with the condylar head remaining in the glenoid fossa. With further mouth opening, the condyle translates anteriorly to a variable degree. During translation the disc maintains a constant relationship between the condylar head and the eminence of the temporal bone. In all

C. A. Helms: University of California School of Medicine, San Francisco, California 94143.

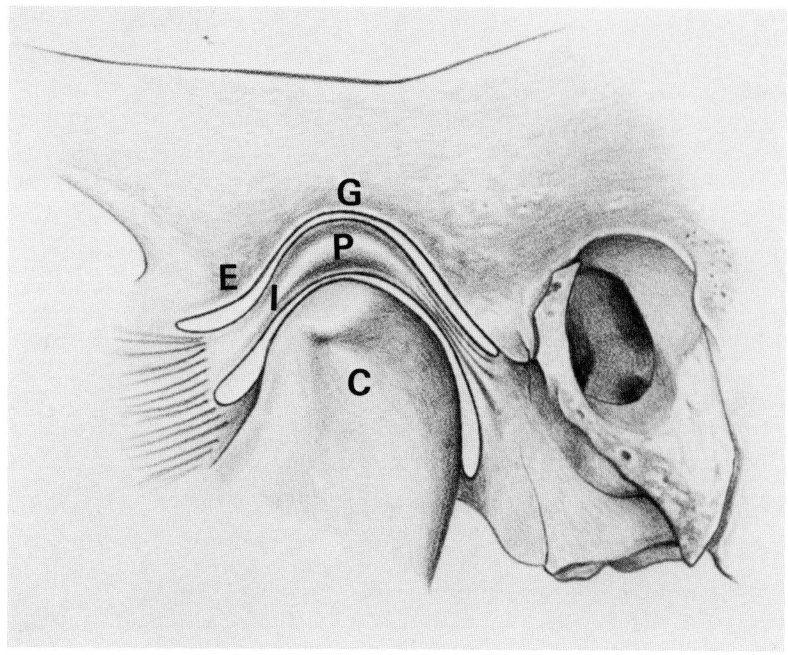

FIG. 4-1. Drawing of normal TMJ. This drawing illustrates the pertinent TMJ anatomy, including the condylar head (C) in the glenoid fossa (G). The posterior band (P) of the disc is on top of the apex of the condyle in this closed-mouth drawing, and the thin intermediate zone (I) is between the two most closely apposed bony surfaces of the condyle and the eminence of the temporal bone (E).

degrees of opening, the thin intermediate zone of the disc should be between the two most closely apposed cortical surfaces of the condyle and the eminence. This relationship holds even in the extremes of condylar translation (Fig. 4-2), during which the disc is at some risk for injury (9). Close attention to the position of the thin intermediate zone is very useful in determining normal versus abnormal disc position.

An "internal derangement" of the TMJ refers predominantly to an anteriorly displaced disc (also termed a "meniscus"). A typical anteriorly displaced disc is easily identified in the sagittal plane by its location just anterior to the condyle (Fig. 4-3). The posterior band causes a mass impression on the anterior recess of the lower joint space and the thin intermediate zone is no longer between the closely apposed cortical surfaces of the condyle and the eminence. If, with further mouth opening, the disc returns to its normal position (with a palpable, often painful and audible click), it is termed an anteriorly displaced disc *with* reduction. If the disc does not return to a normal position with mouth opening, it is termed an anteriorly displaced disc *without* reduction. These patients are said to have a "closed lock" presentation, although they are not really completely locked in a closed-mouth position.

Patients often alternate between having a reducing disc (with a click easily felt on clinical exam) and a nonreducing disc (with decreased mouth opening and no click). It is generally a very easy clinical determination as to when or if disc reduction occurs; therefore, many imaging centers do not make an effort to diagnose with imaging whether or not the disc reduces. Although one report found up to 15% of patients with clicks did not have reducing discs at arthrography (27), this is contrary to most investigators' experience and has not been

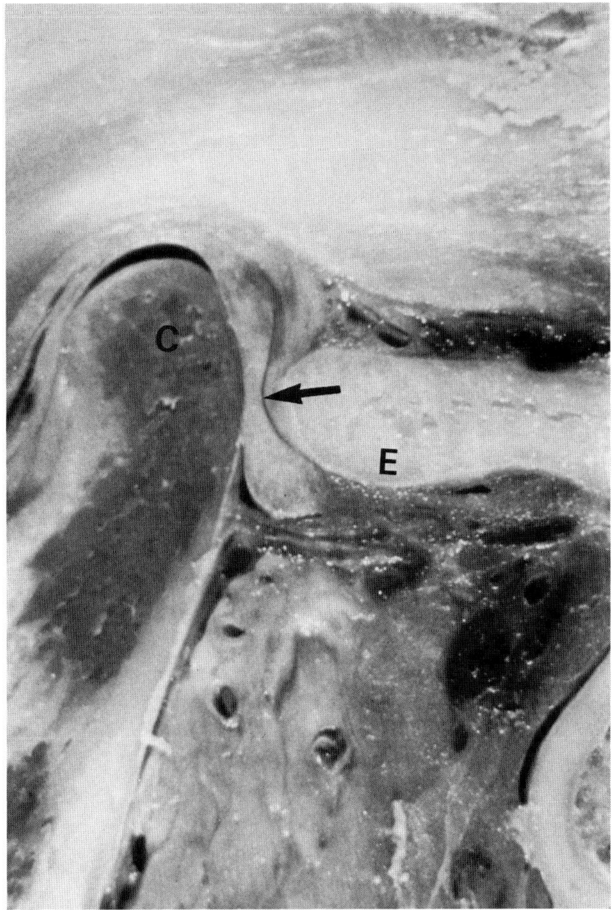

FIG. 4-2. Cadaver with extreme open-mouth position. The condyle (C) is far anterior to the glenoid fossa in this hyper-open-mouth position, yet the disc continues to have its thin intermediate portion (*arrow*) between the two most closely apposed bony surfaces. The disc is flexible and pliable and bends around the curved portion of the eminence (E) during mouth opening.

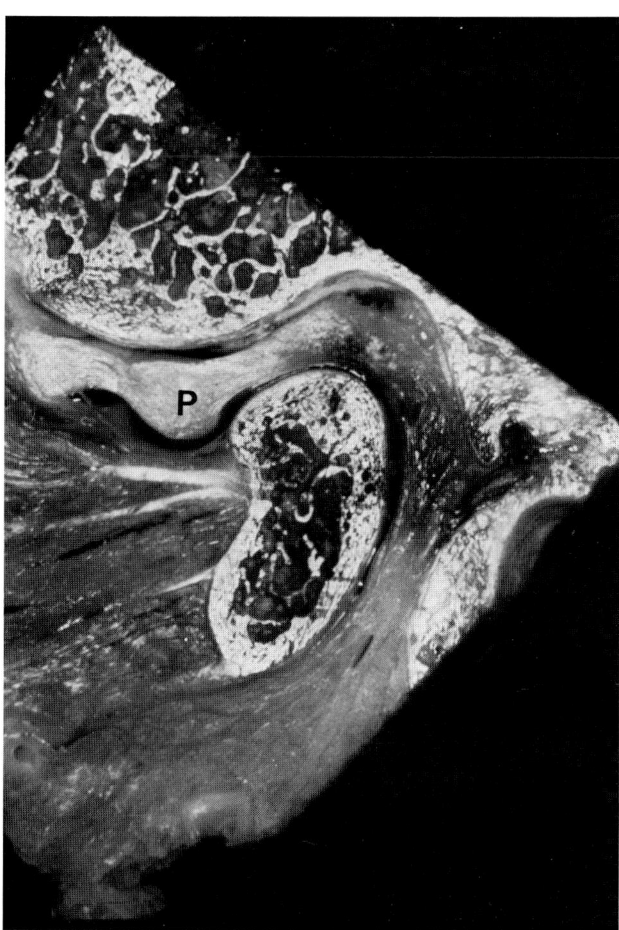

FIG. 4-3. Cadaver section with anteriorly displaced disc. The disc in this cadaver is far anteriorly displaced with the posterior band (P) distorting the anterior recess of the lower joint space. (Case courtesy of Dr. William Solberg.)

reproduced by others. Documenting disc reduction requires a full open-mouth image, which can be a very painful position for the patient to maintain. Patients with TMJ internal derangements often have painful muscle spasms when in the open-mouth position even for a short period of time. When attempting a full open-mouth MRI study, this often results in patient motion with degradation of the image and a nondiagnostic study. For these reasons, many prefer not to image patients in a full open-mouth position unless this is requested by the referring clinician.

TECHNIQUE

There are many different imaging protocols espoused by different investigators. Most agree, however, that only sagittal plane T1 weighted images are necessary for an adequate exam. Although a far medially or laterally displaced disc may be seen to better advantage with coronal images, these are such rare occurrences that routine coronal imaging is not practical. T2 weighted images will demonstrate joint fluid (13,34), but since this is rarely information that is useful to the clinician, T2 weighted images are not routinely performed in the TMJ. More recently, some institutions have began to use fast scan techniques (gradient echo sequences with reduced flip angles) to image the TMJ.

A small (3–5 inch) surface coil is mandatory to allow sufficient signal-to-noise and obtain a high-quality image. If bilateral coupled coils (Fig. 4-4) are available, a bilateral study can be performed in the same time frame as a unilateral study. Although this sounds attractive, it is not mandatory to have a bilateral study in the majority of cases. It is true that up to 80% of patients with a displaced disc on one side will have bilateral displaced disc (15); however, treatment applied to the most symptomatic joint invariably affects both joints with a satisfactory result. Hence, it is not necessary to routinely image both joints unless bilateral surgery is being entertained. Very few people advocated routine bilateral arthrograms; MR should be treated similarly.

Thin section slices (3–5 mm) are obtained through the TMJ in a straight sagittal plane. The condylar heads angle inwardly approximately 30° in most patients on the axial view, prompting some to recommend an oblique sagittal plane with the slices perpendicular to the condylar head (Fig. 4-5). Comparisons of straight sagittal versus oblique sagittal images have convinced most examiners that it is not necessary to perform oblique sagittal images. It simply adds another factor for the technician to worry about and does not improve the diagnostic yield or the image quality.

Two sequences of sagittal T1 weighted images should be obtained—one in the closed-mouth position and a second one in a partial open-mouth position (29). No attempt is made to obtain a full open-mouth image, unless specifically requested by the clinician, for the reasons stated previously. In the closed-mouth images, the condyle is seated in the glenoid fossa with the disc interposed between the condylar head and the glenoid (Fig. 4-6). Because the disc is predominantly low in signal and is tightly placed between two low-signal areas of cortex, it can be very difficult to adequately visualize in many instances. If the patient assumes a partial open-mouth position, the condylar head moves slightly out of the glenoid fossa, allowing the disc to be separated from the bony surfaces, and is more easily seen in its entirety (Fig. 4-7).

In the partial open-mouth position, the disc often is in a normal position, having reduced from an anteriorly displaced position. Hence, many false-negative studies could result if the partial open-mouth images are relied on for diagnosing disc position. It is mandatory to judge the disc position on the closed-mouth images and rely on the partial open-mouth images to note the size, shape, and signal characteristics. The information obtained on the partial open-mouth images concerning the disc size and shape can then be applied to the closed-mouth images to more confidently locate the disc posi-

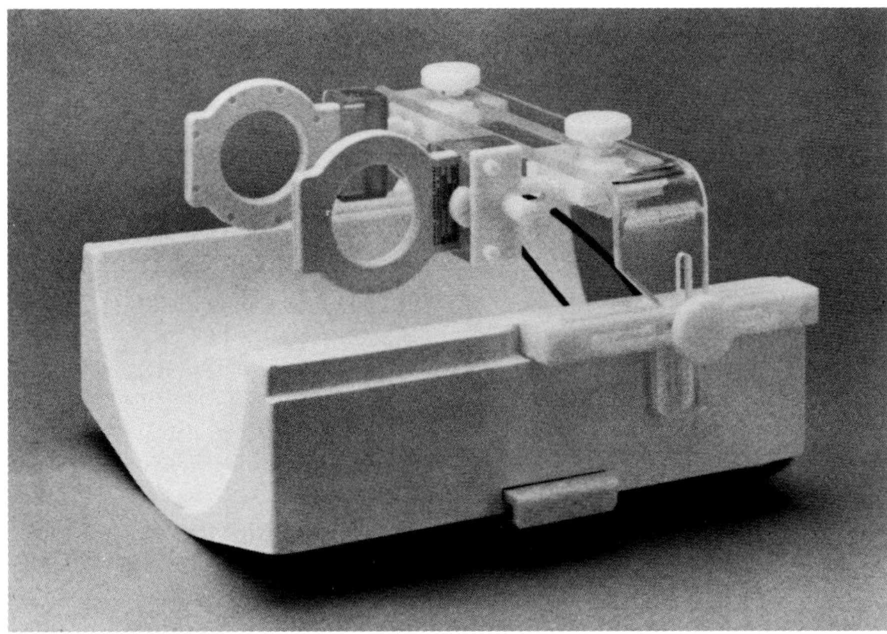

FIG. 4-4. Surface coil. This is a bilateral coupled surface coil for use in a 1.5 T magnet. Both joints can be imaged simultaneously with this coil.

tion (Fig. 4-8). If the closed-mouth images alone are used, a small but significant number of cases will be almost nondiagnostic.

A technique employing fast gradient-echo images has been used in conjunction with a device that will incrementally open the mouth in 1–3 mm steps for each image (2,5,7,35). A dozen or more images are obtained, each one in a different jaw position from fully closed to maximal opening. Each image takes 26 sec to obtain (GRIL, 67/12, 192 × 256 matrix, 2 NEX, flip angle 20°). When played as a video "loop," this shows condylar translation and disc movement, including disc re-

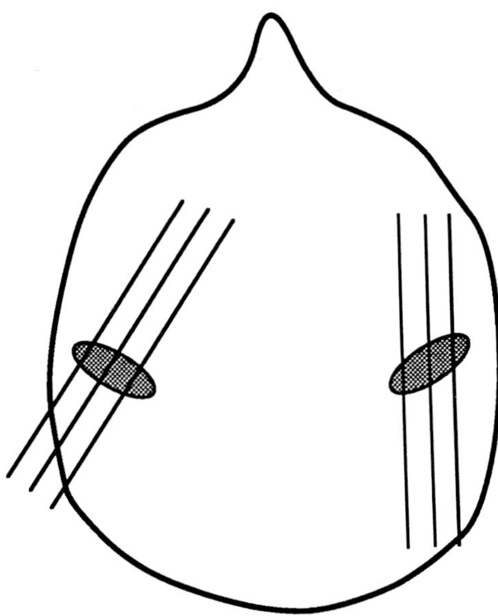

FIG. 4-5. Drawing of oblique sagittal versus straight sagittal cuts. The condylar heads angle medially 20–30° in most patients; therefore, some feel that the plane of the MR images should be angled accordingly. Straight sagittal images appear almost identical to angled images if the slice thickness is 3 mm or less.

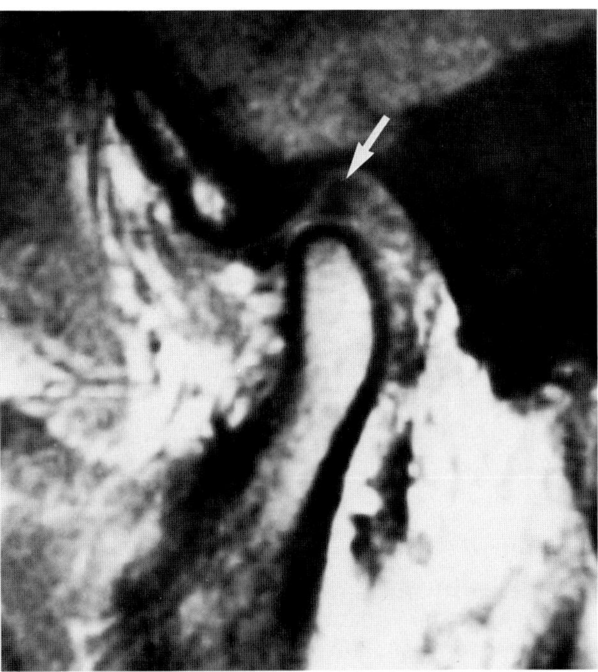

FIG. 4-6. Normal closed mouth. The disc is visualized with the posterior band (*arrow*) just above the condylar head in the closed-mouth position, but the disc can be difficult to fully evaluate because it is compressed between the dark cortical surfaces of the condyle and the eminence.

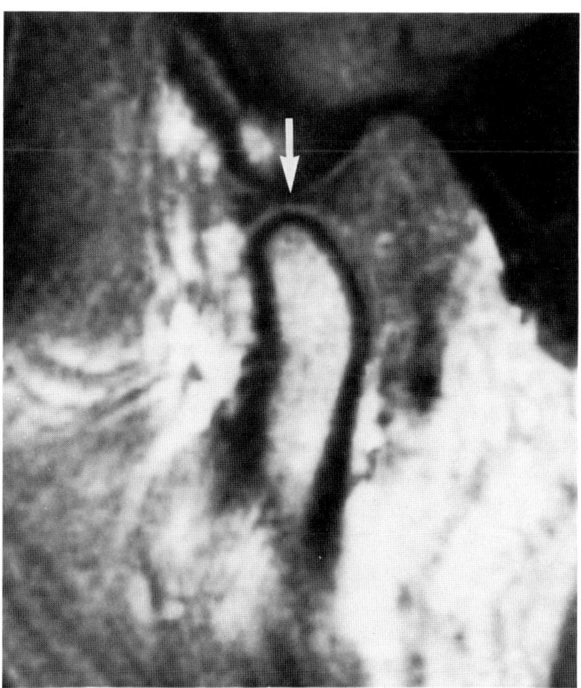

FIG. 4-7. Normal open mouth. The condyle has translated anteriorly beneath the eminence, allowing the disc to be removed off the dark cortical surfaces of the surrounding bone. The disc can be noted to have some signal in the posterior band, and the thin intermediate zone (*arrow*) is easily separated from the cortex of the eminence. This is the same patient as in Fig. 4-6.

duction, if it occurs. Although this is impressive to many clinicians, it gives a distorted picture of the true jaw mechanics because it relies on an external device to force mouth opening rather than the patient's intrinsic musculature. Also, since the dynamics of the TMJ can and do change quite frequently, any motion study—whether an arthrogram, CT, or MRI—must be viewed as a temporary set of events. Very few clinicians treat their patients based on the results of any motion study; therefore, few have adopted this technique. In addition, the resolution of the gradient-recalled echo images used in this technique is not nearly as good as that seen in standard spin-echo images.

A technique that has been used with some success is called three-dimensional (3-D) volume acquisition (31,44). This allows a volume of tissue to be rapidly imaged, rather than a slice, which can then be viewed as thin slices in the desired plane. In the TMJ the images would be sagittally oriented and could be as thin as 1 mm through each condylar head. This technique requires GRASS imaging, which employs a partial flip angle of varying degrees. It has been shown that smaller flip angles (around 20°) result in better disc visualization than do longer flip angles (31). Experience with 3-D volume techniques in the TMJ is somewhat limited but appears promising. Not all imaging centers have this capability, but it will be available in a more widespread manner in the future

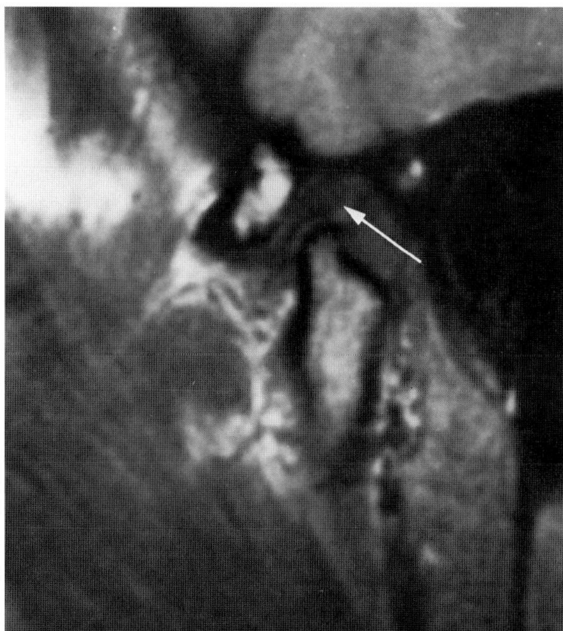

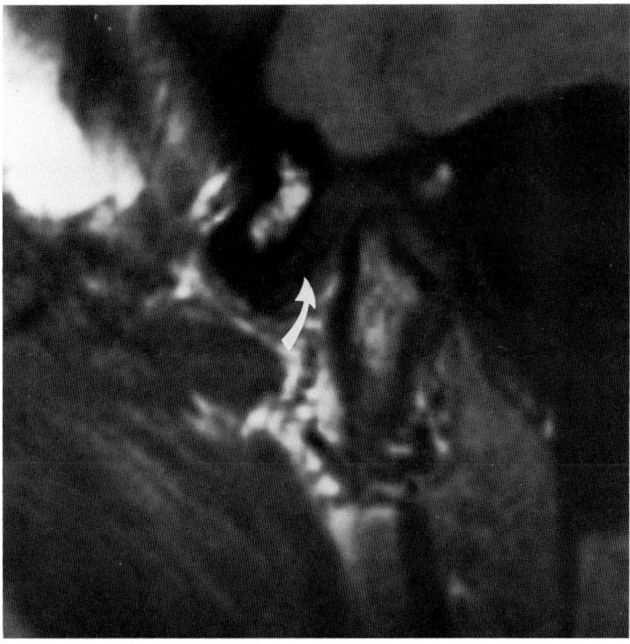

A,B

FIG. 4-8. Closed-mouth and partial open-mouth images with anteriorly displaced disc. **A:** The disc in this partial open-mouth image is normal in position with the thin intermediate zone between the two most closely apposed bony surfaces of the condyle and the eminence. Some intermediate signal can be identified in the posterior band (*arrow*), indicative of normal hydration. **B:** In the closed-mouth position, the thin intermediate zone (*arrow*) is anterior to the normal position and the posterior band is compressed between the condyle and the eminence. Disc signal in the posterior band is difficult to appreciate.

INTERNAL DERANGEMENTS

As mentioned previously, an internal derangement of the TMJ is basically an anteriorly displaced disc. This is seen most consistently and reliably in the closed-mouth position. The posterior band is normally over the apex of the condyle in a closed-mouth position, and the thin intermediate zone should be between the two most closely apposed bony surfaces of the condyle and the temporal eminence. It is often somewhat easier to judge the correct position of the thin intermediate zone than it is the posterior band in cases where the displacement is subtle (Fig. 4-9).

The normal disc has a bow-tie or drumstick appearance with the posterior band somewhat larger than the anterior band. On T1 weighted images a small amount of signal should be present in the disc, primarily in the posterior band, with the overall appearance of the disc being low signal. The disc is made up of proteoglycans somewhat like the nucleus pulposus in the spine (4,33); therefore, it should be expected to have some degree of hydration. This is seen best in the posterior band as intermediate signal on T1 weighted images and high signal on T2 or T2 images (Fig. 4-10). Some investigators have likened the TMJ disc to the menisci of the knee and stated that high signal in the disc indicates myxoid degeneration (22,36). The TMJ disc is not made up of fibrocartilage as are the menisci in the knee, and there is no evidence to show that it undergoes myxoid degeneration. Several reports show that with high-field-strength imaging the normal TMJ disc has some high signal in every instance (14,30). As an internal derangement progresses, the disc loses its normal hydration and the normal signal seen on T1 weighted images is no longer apparent. This is felt to be due to disc dessication and correlates with the duration of the patient's symptoms and the presence of degenerative joint disease (DJD) (12,14).

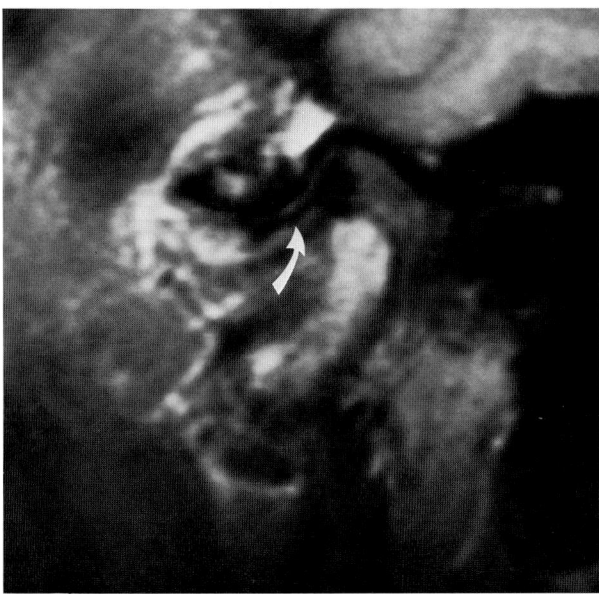

FIG. 4-9. Subtle anteriorly displaced disc. This closed-mouth image shows the thin intermediate zone (*arrow*) to be very minimally anteriorly displaced. If the posterior band were used to judge the proper position, this would probably be called normal. This patient has pain and clicking in this joint with clinically suspected internal derangement.

Surgeons and anatomists have reported that the normal disc is flexible and pliable and proceeds to a more stiff, inflexible state following internal derangement (16,17,28,41). The end result of a long-term or severe internal derangement is disc derangement and maceration with secondary bony changes of DJD (3,24,42,43). A grading system for internal derangements has been proposed which grades the severity of the internal derangement according to the morphology of the disc (14). An anteriorly displaced disc that maintains its normal bow-tie or drumstick configuration is a grade 1 joint (Figs. 4-11 and 4-12). An anteriorly displaced disc that does not have a normal morphology is a grade 2 joint (Figs. 4-11 and 4-13).

In a recent study (14) of over 200 joints, 17% of the grade 1 joints had DJD, while 95% of the grade 2 joints had DJD. The duration of symptoms and the presence of increased joint noise for the grade 2 joints were significantly greater than that of the grade 1 or normal joints (Fig. 4-14). Since the long-term sequela of an internal derangement is known to be DJD, it would appear that this grading system correlates with the severity of the disease process. Most of the grade 2 joints had discs that were irreparable at surgery, while virtually all the grade 1 joints had a disc repair attempted. The decreased signal seen with disc dessication was not incorporated into the grading scale because it was felt to be too subjective and dependent on too many variables—such as photography, window and level setting, and even the temperature of the film processor—to be reliable. Nevertheless, decreased disc signal was found to be statistically significant in its association with DJD and duration of symptoms (Fig. 4-15).

In addition to showing the disc position, therefore, MRI can grade the severity of the internal derangement by showing disc morphology and hydration. MRI is also useful in determining if bony abnormalities are present. DJD typically begins with cortical erosions and progresses to condylar head flattening with anterior osteophytosis (Fig. 4-16). As mentioned, DJD occurs with long-standing or severe internal derangements. Although the MRI appearance of condylar head avascular necrosis has been reported (37), this is not widely agreed on and remains controversial.

Disc perforations cannot currently be demonstrated with MRI unless they are extremely large (1). This is not a serious drawback for most clinicians, however, as very few surgeons use disc perforation as a criteria to operate,

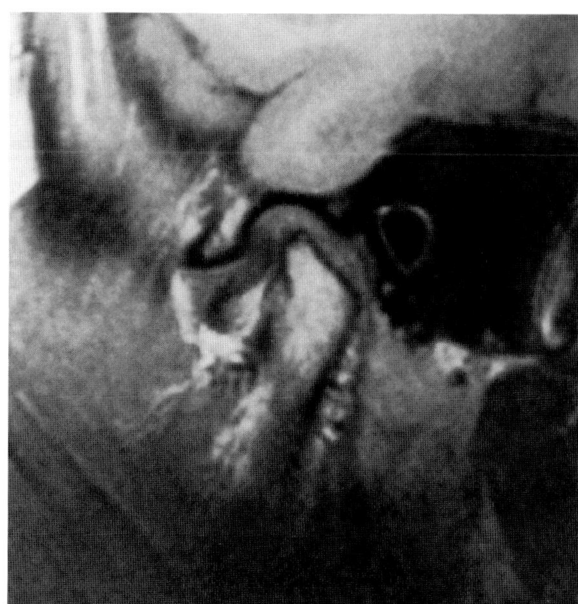

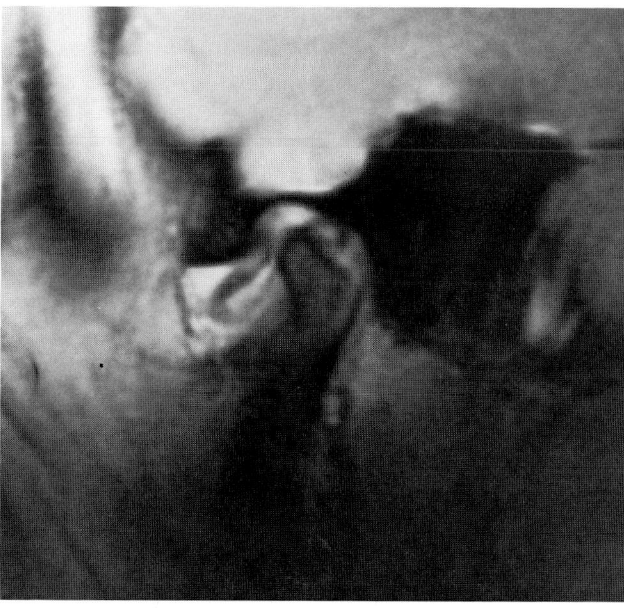

A,B

FIG. 4-10. T1 and GRASS images. **A:** This T1 weighted image shows the disc anteriorly displaced. Some intermediate signal is noted in the posterior band. **B:** With a GRASS image the signal in the posterior band is considerably higher, consistent with hydration. Note the joint fluid in the upper and lower spaces.

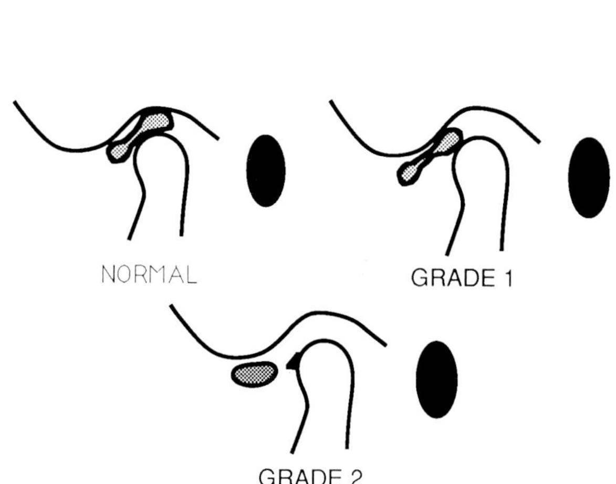

FIG. 4-11. Grading system (drawing). This schematic drawing illustrates the morphologic grading system for determining the severity of an internal derangement. The normal joint has a "drumstick"-shaped disc in normal position. A grade 1 joint has a "drumstick"-shaped disc that is anteriorly displaced. A grade 2 joint has a disc that is anteriorly displaced and deformed.

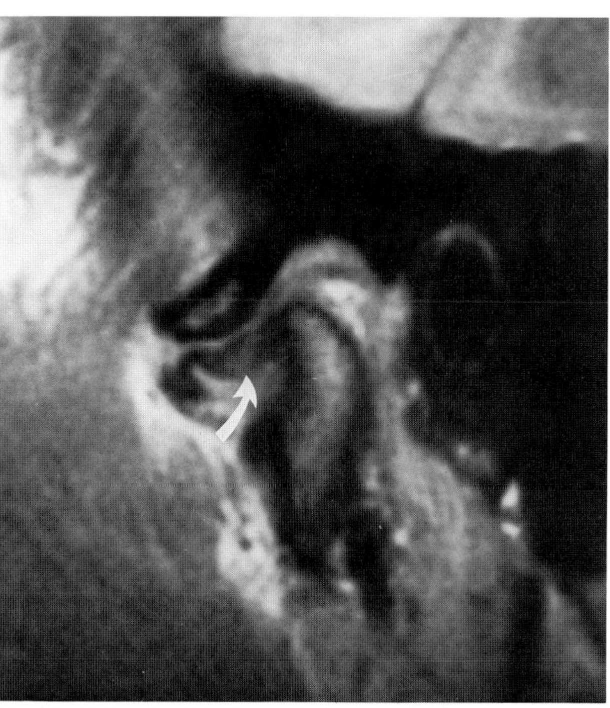

FIG. 4-12. Grade 1 joint. This patient suffered jaw trauma 6–8 weeks prior to this exam. The MRI shows an anteriorly displaced disc with normal morphology. Note the normal intermediate signal in the posterior band (*arrow*).

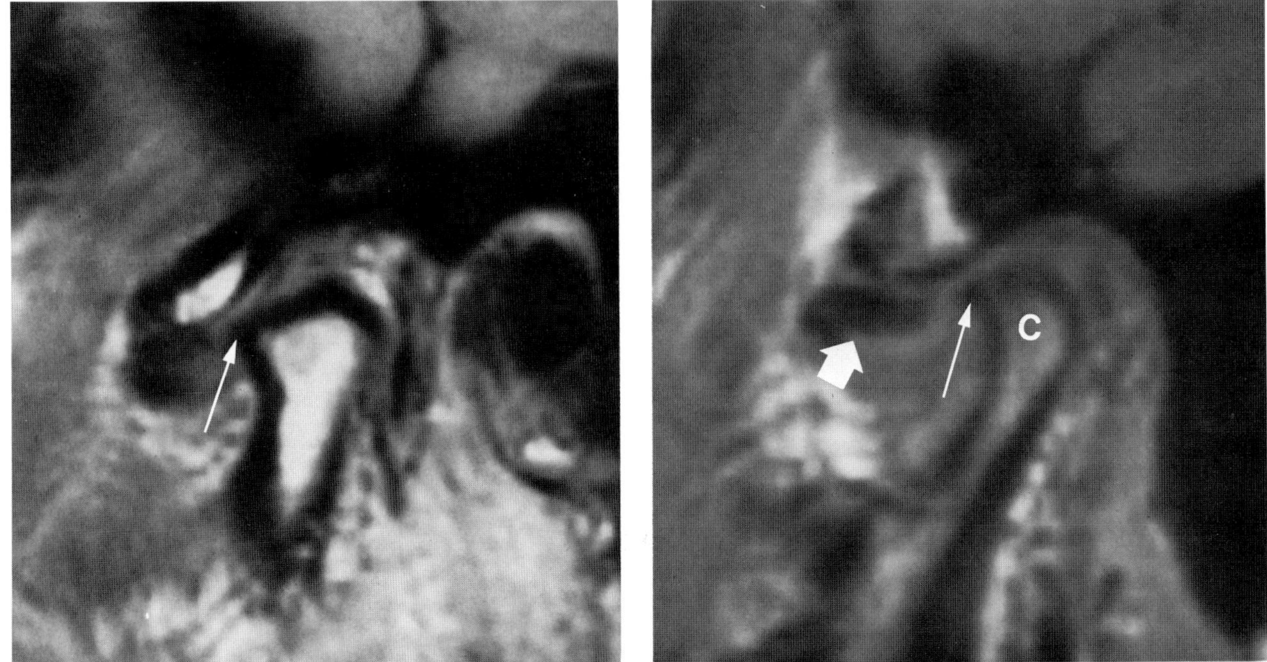

A,B

FIG. 4-13. Grade 2 joint. **A:** This patient has long-standing TMJ dysfunction. The MRI shows an anteriorly displaced disc that is abnormally shaped. Note the anterior osteophyte off the condyle (*arrow*). **B:** A similar appearance is noted in another patient with a long-standing history of TMJ dysfunction. The disc is deformed anteriorly (*arrow*) and an osteophyte (*thin arrow*) is present on the condyle (C).

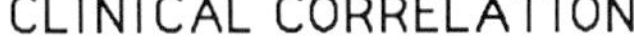

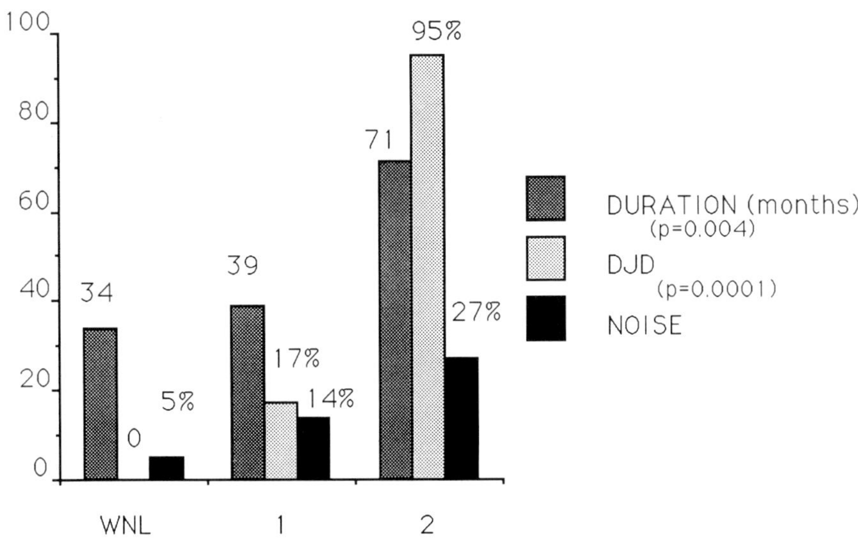

FIG. 4-14. Graph of DJD, duration, and joint noise (p values). Comparing the presence of DJD, duration of the patient's symptoms in months, and the patient's complaint of severe joint noise with the morphology grades in 216 joints shows a definite association between these parameters and the grading system.

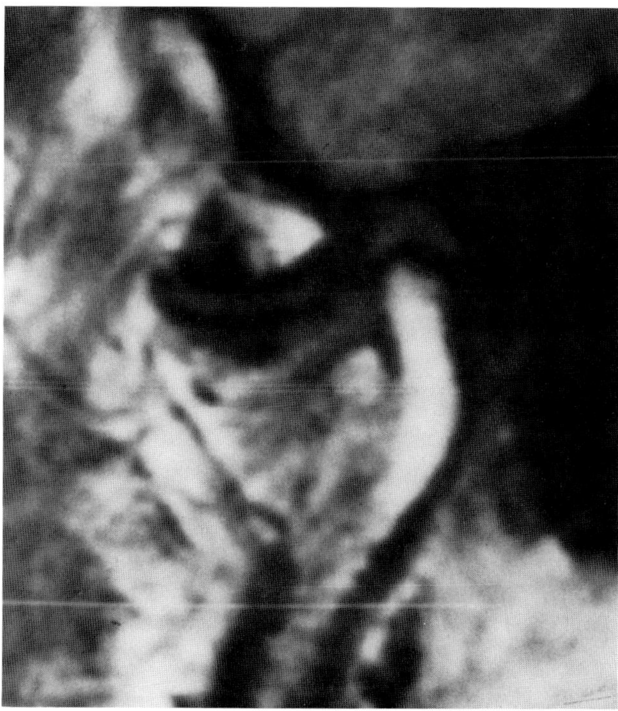

FIG. 4-15. Disc dessication. This patient has a normally shaped disc with decreased signal in the posterior band. This is felt to be due to disc dessication and indicates a more advanced internal derangement than the usual grade 1 joint. This is felt to precede disc deformity seen in grade 2 joints but is a very subjective finding and difficult to reproduce.

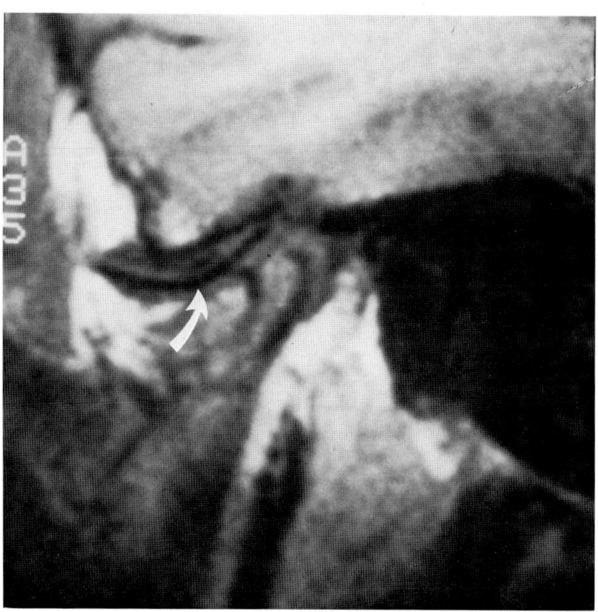

FIG. 4-17. Normal silastic implant. This patient has had placement of a silastic implant (*arrow*), which is of uniform, linear low signal. It is sutured into the glenoid fossa and covers the condyle during condylar translation. Note the irregularity of the condylar head, which may be secondary to surgical shaving or to DJD and remodeling.

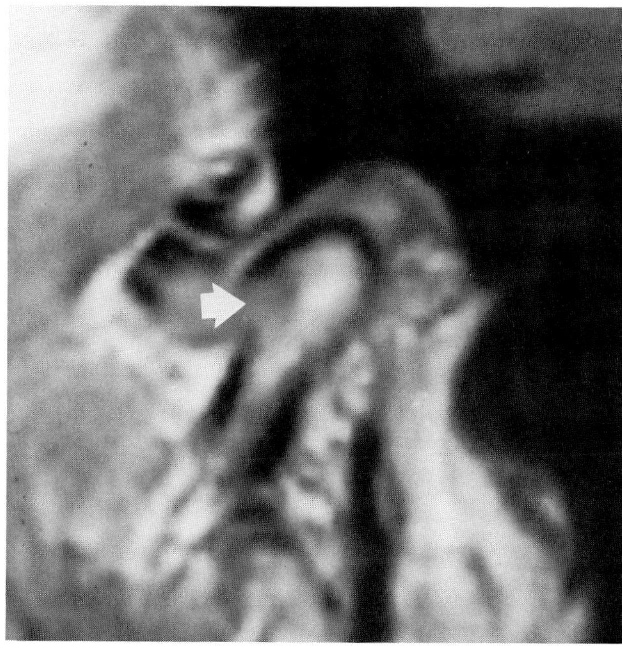

FIG. 4-16. DJD. This grade 2 joint has an anteriorly displaced disc that is deformed and an erosion of the cortical bone on the condyle (*arrow*), which is a finding of DJD in the TMJ. The most common finding of TMJ DJD is an anterior osteophyte off the condyle.

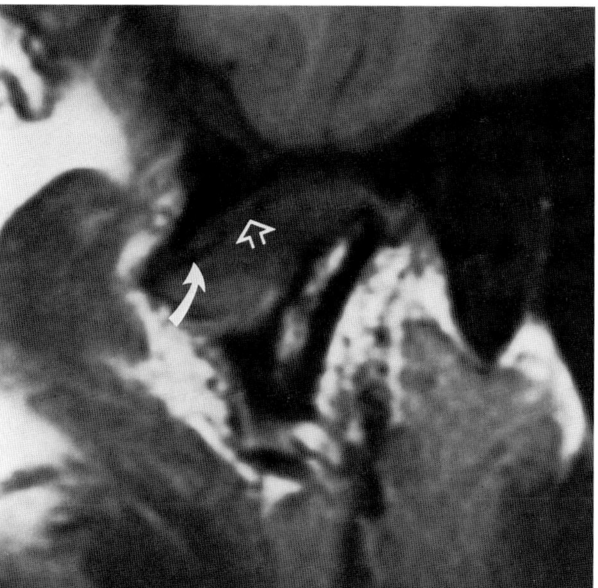

FIG. 4-18. Fractured implant with exuberant granulation tissue. This patient had placement of a proplast/Teflon graft (*arrow*), which is faintly identified as a linear low-signal structure beneath the eminence. Although it is in the normal position, it appears to have a disruption or fracture (*small arrow*). The joint has a large amount of granulation tissue, which makes normal function of the condylar head impossible. The condylar head is severely deformed, either from the surgery or from erosion by the mass of granulation tissue.

and no definitive treatment regimen is currently advocated for patients with disc perforations. Currently, arthrography must be performed to diagnose a disc perforation, because CT and MRI will not reliably give this information.

POSTOPERATIVE JOINTS

MRI is very useful in evaluating joints that have had silastic and proplast/Teflon implants (25,26,38). These implants have a signal void with a linear appearance on sagittal T1 weighted images (Fig. 4-17). MRI can show the position of the prosthesis and whether or not it is fractured. It can also demonstrate the amount of giant-cell tissue reaction and scar surrounding the prosthesis, which can interfere with function and result in having to remove the prosthesis (Fig. 4-18).

SUMMARY

MRI of the TMJ can rival arthrography and CT for accuracy in diagnosing internal derangements. In addition to showing the position of the disc, there is evidence that MRI can show the condition of the disc. Bony abnormalities and postoperative changes can readily be identified. MRI is clearly the imaging modality of choice for internal derangements of the TMJ.

REFERENCES

1. Abbott M, Carvlin MJ, Nowell M, Sherman J, Wu C, Schellinger D. Determination of the sensitivity of MR imaging in the identification of known perforationlike defects of the temporomandibular joint meniscus. *Radiology* 1989;173:100.
2. Bell KA, Miller KD, Jones JP. Cine MR imaging of the temporomandibular joint: Ochsner experience. *Radiology* 1989;173:101.
3. Blackwood HJ. Arthritis of the mandibular joint. *Br Dent J* 1963;115:317–324.
4. Blaustein DI, Scapino RP. Remodeling of the temporomandibular joint disk and posterior attachment in disk displacement specimens in relation to glycosaminoglycan content. *Plast Reconstr Surg* 1986;78:756–764.
5. Burnett K, Davis CL, Read J. Dynamic display of the TMJ meniscus by using "fast-scan" MRI. *AJR* 1987;149:959–962.
6. Carr AB, Gibilisco JA, Berquist TH. MRI of the temporomandibular joint: preliminary work. *J Craniomand Disorders Fac Oral Pain* 1987;1:89–96.
7. Conway WF, Hayes CW, Campbell RL, Laskin DM. Temporomandibular joint motion: efficacy of fast low-angle shot MR imaging. *Radiology* 1989;172:821–826.
8. Donlon WC, Moon KL. Comparison of magnetic resonance imaging, arthrotomography and clinical and surgical findings in temporomandibular joint internal derangements. *Oral Surg Oral Med Oral Pathol* 1987;64:2–5.
9. Griffin CJ, Sharpe CJ. Distribution of elastic tissue in the human temporomandibular meniscus especially in respect to "compression" areas. *Aust Dent* 1962;7:72.
10. Harms SE, Wilk RM, Wolford LM, Chiles DG, Milam SB. The temporomandibular joint: magnetic resonance imaging using surface coils. *Radiology* 1985;157:133–136.
11. Helms CA, Gillespy T III, Sims RE, Richardson ML. Magnetic resonance imaging of internal derangements of the temporomandibular joint. *Radiol Clin North Am* 1986;24:189–192.
12. Helms CA, Doyle GW, Orwig D, McNeill C, Kaban L. Staging of internal derangements of the TMJ with magnetic resonance imaging: preliminary observations. *J Craniomand Disorders* 1989;3:93–99.
13. Helms CA, Gillespy T III, Sims RE, Richardson ML. Magnetic resonance imaging of internal derangement of the temporomandibular joint. *Radiol Clin North Am* 1986;24:189–192.
14. Helms CA, Kaban L, McNeill C, Dodson T. Temporomandibular joint MR: morphology and signal characteristics of the disc. *Radiology* 1989;172:817–820.
15. Helms CA, Vogler JB, Morrish RB, Goldman SM, Capra RE, Proctor E. Diagnosis of TMJ internal derangements with computed tomography: review of 200 cases. *Radiology* 1984;152:459–462.
16. Isacsson G, Isberg A, Johansson AS, Larson O. Internal derangement of the temporomandibular joint: radiographic and histologic changes associated with severe pain. *J Oral Maxillofac Surg* 1986;44:771–778.
17. Isberg A, Isacsson G. Tissue reactions of the temporomandibular joint following retrusive guidance of the mandible. *J Craniomand Practice* 1986;4:143–148.
18. Kaplan PA, Helms CA. Current status of temporomandibular joint imaging of internal derangements. *AJR* 1989;152:697–706.
19. Kaplan PA, Tu HK, Williams SM, Lydiatt DD. The normal temporomandibular joint: MR and arthrographic correlation. *Radiology* 1987;165:177–178.
20. Katzberg RW, Schenck J, Roberts D, et al. Magnetic resonance imaging of the temporomandibular joint meniscus. *Oral Surg Oral Med Oral Pathol* 1985;59:332–335.
21. Katzberg RW, Bessette RW, Tallents RH. Normal and abnormal temporomandibular joint: MR imaging with surface coil. *Radiology* 1986;158:183–189.
22. Katzberg RW. Temporomandibular joint imaging. *Radiology* 1989;170:297–307.
23. Katzberg RW, Westesson P, Tallents RH, et al. Temporomandibular joint assessment of rotational and sideways disk displacements. *Radiology* 1988;169:741–748.
24. Katzberg RW, Keith DA, Guralnick WC, Manzione JV, Ten Eick WR. Internal derangements and arthritis of the temporomandibular joint. *Radiology* 1983;146:107–112.
25. Katzberg RW, Kaskin DM. Commentary. Radiographic and clinical significance of temporomandibular joint alloplastic disk implants. *AJR* 1988;151:736–738.
26. Kneeland JB, Ryan DE, Carrera GF, Jesmanowicz A, Froncisz W, Hyde JS. Failed temporomandibular joint prostheses: MR imaging. *Radiology* 1987;165:179–181.
27. Miller TL, Katzberg RW, Tallents RH, Bessette RW, Hayakawa K. Temporomandibular joint clicking with nonreducing anterior displacement of the meniscus. *Radiology* 1985;154:121–124.
28. Moffett BC Jr, Johnson LC, McCabe JB, Askew HC. Articular remodeling in adult human temporomandibular joint. *Am J Anat* 1964;115:119–141.
29. Orwig DS, Helms CA, Doyle GW. Optimal mouth position for magnetic resonance imaging of the temporomandibular joint disc. *J Craniomand Disorders Fac Oral Pain* 1989;3:138–142.
30. Port RB, Mikhael MA, Canzona JE. MR imaging of the temporomandibular joint: correlation with operative findings. Scientific Exhibit, presented at the 74th Scientific Assembly of the RSNA, Chicago, IL, Nov 27–Dec 2, 1988.
31. Rao VM, Vinitski S, Babaria A. Comparison of SE and short TE three-dimensional gradient-echo imaging of the temporomandibular region. *Radiology* 1989;173:99.
32. Roberts D, Schenk J, Joseph P, et al. Temporomandibular joint: magnetic resonance imaging. *Radiology* 1985;154:829–830.
33. Scapino RP. Histopathology associated with malposition of the human temporomandibular joint disc. *Oral Surg* 1983;55:382.
34. Schellhas KP, Wilkes CH. Temporomandibular joint inflammation: comparison of MR fast scanning with T1- and T2-weighted imaging techniques. *AJR* 1989;153:93–98.
35. Schellhas KP, Fritts HM, Heithoff KB, Jahn JA, Wilkes CH, Omlie MR. Temporomandibular joint: MR fast scanning. *J Craniomand Practice* 1988;6:209–216.

36. Schellhas KP, Wilkes CH, Omlie MR, et al. The diagnosis of temporomandibular joint disease: two compartment arthrography and MR. *AJR* 1988;151:341–350.

37. Schellhas KP, Wilkes CH, Fritts HM, Omlie MR, Lagrotteria LB. MR of osteochondritis and avascular necrosis of the mandibular condyle. *AJR* 1989;152:551–560.

38. Schellhas KP, Wilkes CH, El Deeb M, Lagrotteria LB, Omlie MR. Permanent proplast temporomandibular joint implants: MR imaging of destructive complications. *AJR* 1988;151:731–735.

39. Westesson P, Katzberg RW, Tallents RH, Sanchez-Woodworth RE, Svensson SA. CT and MR of the temporomandibular joint: comparison with autopsy specimens. *AJR* 1987;148:1165–1171.

40. Westesson PL, Katzberg RW, Tallents RH, Sanchez-Woodworth RE, Svensson SA, Espeland MA. Temporomandibular joint: comparison of MR images with cryosectional anatomy. *Radiology* 1987;164:59–64.

41. Westesson PL, Bronstein SL, Liedberg JL. Internal derangement of the temporomandibular joint: morphologic description with correlation to function. *Oral Surg Oral Med Oral Pathol* 1985;59:323–331.

42. Westesson PL. Structural hard-tissue changes in temporomandibular joints with internal derangement. *Oral Surg Oral Med Oral Pathol* 1985;59:220–224.

43. Westesson PL, Rohlin M. Internal derangement related to osteoarthrosis in temporomandibular joint autopsy specimens. *Oral Surg* 1984;57:17–22.

44. Wilk RM, Harms SE. Temporomandibular joint: multislab, three-dimensional Fourier transformation MR imaging. *Radiology* 1988;167:861–863.

MRI of the Musculoskeletal System, 2nd Edition, edited by T. H. Berquist.
Raven Press, Ltd., New York © 1990.

CHAPTER 5

The Spine

Gary M. Miller

Technical Considerations, 87
Normal Anatomy, 90
Spinal Column, 90
Intervertebral Discs, 95
Spinal Ligaments, 95
Spinal Cord and Nerves, 101
Dural Coverings, 102
Vascular, 102
Examination Technique, 102
MR Contrast Agents, 105
Pathologic Conditions, 105
Disc Diseases, 105
Postoperative Evaluation, 111
Neoplasms, 111
Inflammatory Conditions, 126
Demyelinating Disease, 133
Congenital Spinal Abnormalities, 134
Trauma, 138
Vascular, 139
Infarct, 145
References, 145

When multimodality imaging is available, the clinical uses of each modality tend to spread from a single niche. Magnetic resonance imaging (MRI), the only modality that directly images the spinal cord, is unique since no other invasive or noninvasive technique possesses this capability. Perhaps this explains why spinal imaging accounted for 27% of our first 26,000 exams. Whether MR's capacity to image other intraspinal and spinal column disorders will match the sensitivity and specificity of CT and myelography, as some authors claim, is less obvious. If technical developments such as contrast agents, increased spatial resolution, and artifact control continue, MRI should be at least somewhat competitive, providing the exams are tailored to match the clinical disorder.

A variety of considerations, including clinical, technical, and anatomical factors, influence MRI. Unlike the head, where a survey exam may be adequate to delineate many clinical disorders, a survey exam of the spine is apt to be less rewarding. Instead, spinal imaging requires clinical expertise, special equipment, specific imaging sequences, and perhaps imager interaction to obtain adequate exams.

G. M. Miller: Mayo Medical School and Mayo Clinic, Rochester, Minnesota 55905.

The application of multispecialty expertise seems essential to exploit MR's versatility. Translation of the clinical characterization and localization of neurologic disorders potentiates MR's effectiveness. The same thorough neurologic and neurosurgical evaluation that is key to an accurate clinical diagnosis is equally crucial in optimizing MR scanning sequences, since confirmation of the diagnosis is often possible with MRI. Additional consultation between radiologists and their clinical colleagues is sometimes important in handling those patients who have painful disorders or convoluted clinical problems.

TECHNICAL CONSIDERATIONS

Imaging of the spine is complex. In contrast to the head, where the volume and composition of its tissues are almost constant, the spine is less predictable. The length of the spinal column, its dorsal location, and the small size of the intraspinal content preclude effective imaging by a volume coil such as a body coil. To improve image quality, both a high-field-strength (1.5 T) magnet and surface coils must be used to increase the signal-to-noise ratio while smaller fields of view (16–24 cm) are often needed to improve spatial resolution. As a result, multiple coil placements are necessary for a complete study of the entire spine. When coupled with the desirability of obtaining more than one imaging sequence to detect or characterize pathology, the examination is prolonged to such an extent that the patient may be unable to cooperate.

As expected, motion—both patient and physiologic—obscures anatomic and pathologic detail. Sedatives may be necessary in children (chloral hydrate 50–75 mg/kg), while analgesics are sometimes needed in patients who are evaluated for a painful condition. If patient motion can be obviated, physiologic motion due to the proximity of the spine to the heart, great vessels, diaphragm, and aerodigestive system becomes a problem. Motion from the beating heart, flowing blood, diaphragmatic excursion, normal swallowing, and cerebral spinal fluid (CSF) pulsation create artifacts that simulate or obscure significant pathology (8). This is particularly true on T2W and gradient-echo sequences, where internal motion results in artifacts from the spatial mismapping of the signal intensities present (92,93). This lowers the contrast resolution between the CSF and spinal cord and causes areas of decreased signal in the CSF and corresponding areas of increased signal in the spinal cord parenchyma (Fig. 5-1). On T1W sequences, these artifacts are less apparent but can result in areas of increased signal in the CSF (Fig. 5-2). Because of this, a variety of motion compensation mechanisms have been and are being developed to reduce the effect of physiologic internal motion, to maximize the contrast between CSF and spinal cord, and to minimize misregistration artifacts. These include the use of flow compensation gradients, presaturation pulse sequences, phase and frequency gradient direction reversal, and cardiac/respiratory gating (36,94–96) (Fig. 5-3). Most vendors have many of these options available, and one or several must be used to reduce artifacts and enhance visualization of either pathology or normal anatomy.

Another artifact that can obscure pathology or simulate intramedullary lesions is the truncation artifact or Gibb's phenomenon (12,19,58). This is a sampling-related effect that occurs at high-contrast boundaries such as the CSF–cord interface. It is most apparent when the object imaged is small relative to the pixel size used, resulting in alternating bands of high and low signal that parallel the high-contrast interface. It is best seen on sagittal sequences where it can simulate a syrinx cavity.

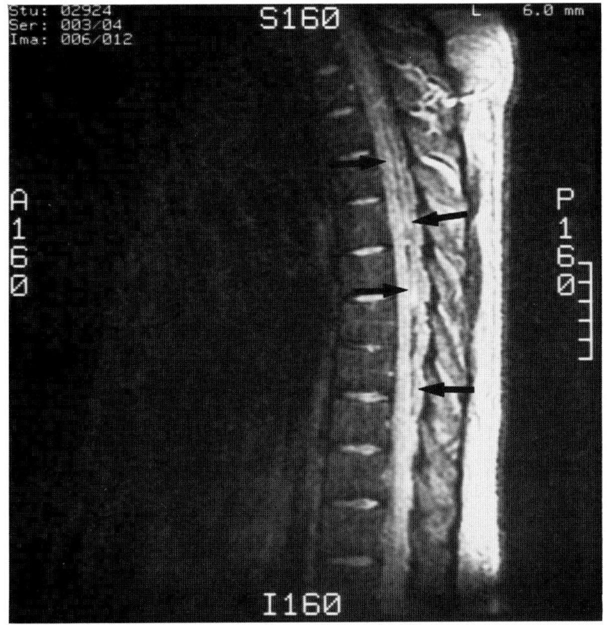

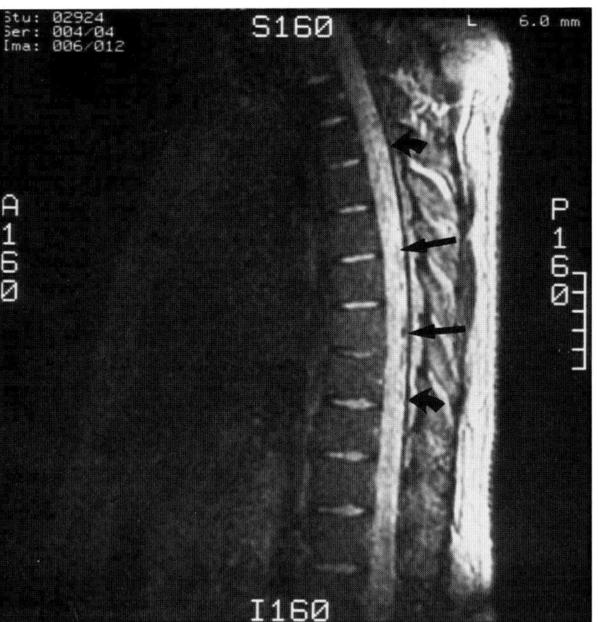

A,B

FIG. 5-1. A: Sagittal thoracic spine demonstrates the effect of cardiac motion on the image. The phase-encoding direction is anterior–posterior (AP), resulting in linear areas of increased and decreased signal in the spinal cord parenchyma and CSF from the phase misregistration of the beating heart and flowing blood (*arrows*). The CSF–cord and extradural interfaces are not identified. (TR 1,500 msec, TE 80 msec.) **B:** The phase-encoding direction has now been switched from AP in (**A**) to superior–inferior (SI). Note that the phase misregistration artifact now extends above and below the heart anterior to the spinal canal. While this improves the resolution of the cord–CSF interface, some artifacts persist within the CSF posterior to the spinal cord from CSF pulsations (*arrows*). The signal intensity of the spinal cord parenchyma is still inhomogeneous. Note the improved resolution of the extradural interface as the posterior longitudinal ligament and posterior dura are now visualized (*curved arrow*), as well as the posterior epidural fat. (TR 1,500 msec, TE 80 msec.)

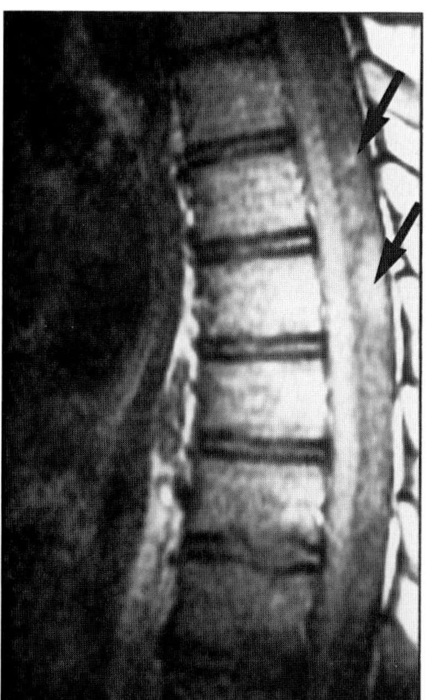

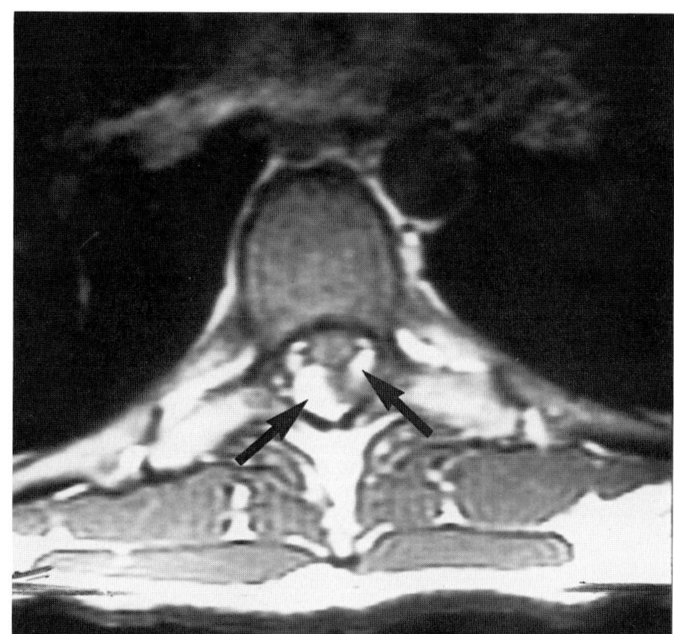

A,B

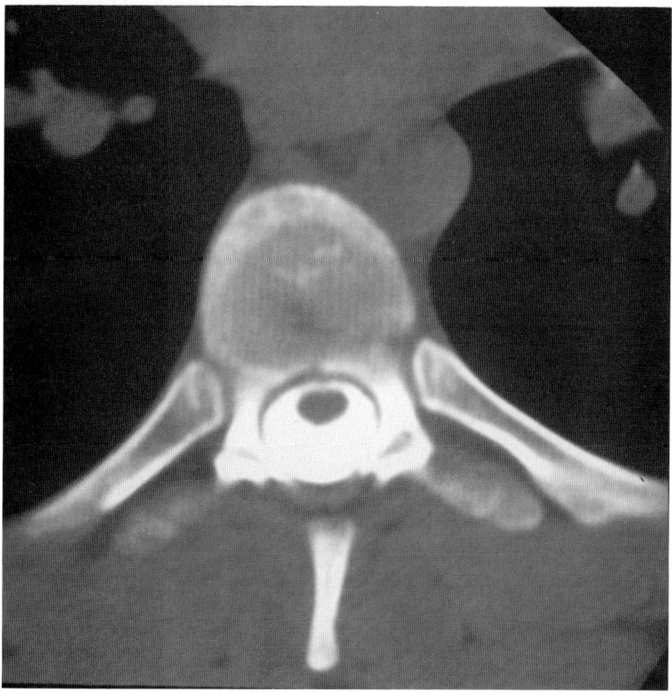

C

FIG. 5-2. A: Unusual ill-defined high signal intensity structures are seen posterior to the thoracic spinal cord on this sagittal image (*arrows*). (TR 500 msec, TE 20 msec.) **B:** These "lesions" can also be identified in the axial plane (*arrows*). (TR 450 msec, TE 30 msec.) **C:** A postmyelogram CT section obtained at the same location as (**B**) shows no intradural abnormalities, confirming that they are artifacts from CSF pulsations.

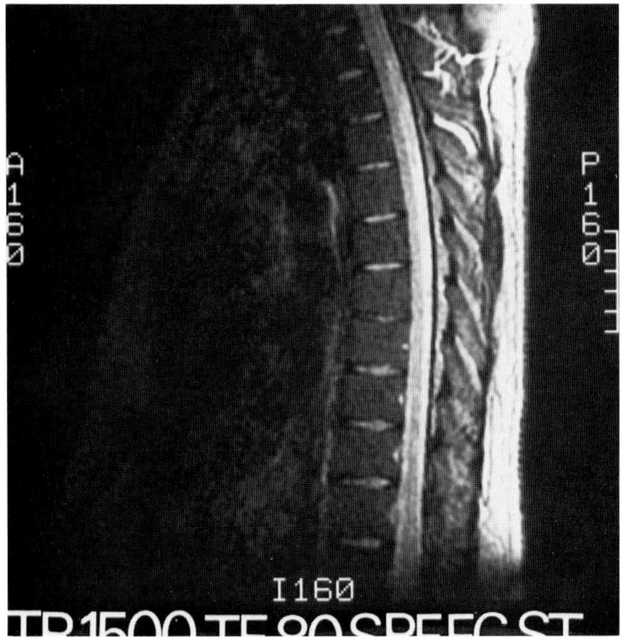

FIG. 5-3. A combination of presaturation pulses and flow compensation gradients were added to this pulse sequence to counteract the effects of CSF pulsations. Phase and frequency gradient directions were also switched so that the phase-encoding direction is SI. This is the same patient illustrated in Fig. 5-1. Note the improved spinal cord–CSF interface and the more homogeneous appearance of the spinal cord and CSF. On our imager, this combination provides the best images, which were equal to those obtained using cardiac gating alone. Cardiac gating, in combination with the above, did not result in additional improvement of image quality. (TR 1,500 msec, TE 80 msec.)

This artifact can be reduced by using small fields of view (FOV), small slice thicknesses, and a 192 or 256 matrix.

Body habitus, spinal curvature, and the size of the intraspinal components play a significant role and compound the technical difficulty of obtaining an adequate exam. Some patients exceed the weight limitations of the table, while others will not fit within the coil. Scoliosis precludes the possibility of visualizing the intraspinal structures on a single or few adjacent scans. The sizes of the spinal cord, which measures about 1 cm in diameter, of parenchymal pathology, which is no more than a few millimeters, and of nerve roots, which are 1 mm or less, demand excellent contrast and spatial resolution. As a result, even the most powerful commercially available magnets are taxed if the duration of the exam is compatible with reasonable patient comfort.

NORMAL ANATOMY

The anatomy of the spine is complex, being composed of multiple tissue types. The vertebral bodies provide mechanical support, and interposed intervertebral discs cushion motion. A variety of ligaments link these structures together. The spinal cord, which is bathed in the cerebral spinal fluid, lies within the protective environment of the bony spinal canal. At each segment, a pair of spinal nerves exit through the neural foramen. An extensive vascular network is also present with arteries segmentally supplying the bones, muscles, leptomeninges, cord, and a network of draining veins that extend both within the spinal canal and surround the vertebral bodies. Each of these structures has different signal characteristics, depending on pulse sequences selected. Figures 5-4 to 5-13 illustrate the normal MRI appearance of the spine in a variety of commonly used imaging planes and pulse sequences.

Spinal Column

There are 33 vertebrae with the usual distribution being seven cervical, twelve thoracic, five lumbar, five sacral, and four coccygeal segments. The sacral and coccygeal segments are usually fused. Some variability to this numbering pattern can occur within the lower segments (i.e., eleven thoracic and six lumbar). The morphology of each vertebra is similar with individual variations in each region (74). The first two cervical vertebrae are an exception, because they are highly specialized structures. In general, each vertebra is composed of a body, which is located anteriorly, and a posterior arch. The posterior arch is formed by two pedicles that extend from the body to an articular mass or pars interarticularis. Two bony projections extend above and below each articular mass, forming the superior and inferior facets that articulate with the corresponding facet of the adjacent vertebral bodies at a synovial joint. Two laminae extend posteriorly where they fuse to form the spinous process, thus completing a ring and forming the spinal canal. Laterally, transverse processes extend from the posterior arches, which together with the spinous processes act as levers for the attachment of many skeletal muscles. In addition to the synovial facet joints, an additional articulation is found in the cervical region. A lateral ridge of bone, the uncinate process, extends from the superior surface of each cervical vertebral body, which articulates with a notch in the inferior aspect of the vertebral body above, forming the uncovertebral joints of Luschka (74). This is not a true joint but rather is thought to represent the lateral extension of the intervertebral disc, which has partially degenerated by adulthood.

The spinal nerves course through the neural foramina at each vertebral body level. In the cervical region, the neural foramina can be elongated, forming a canal that is bordered by the pedicles of adjacent vertebrae above

Text continues on p. 95

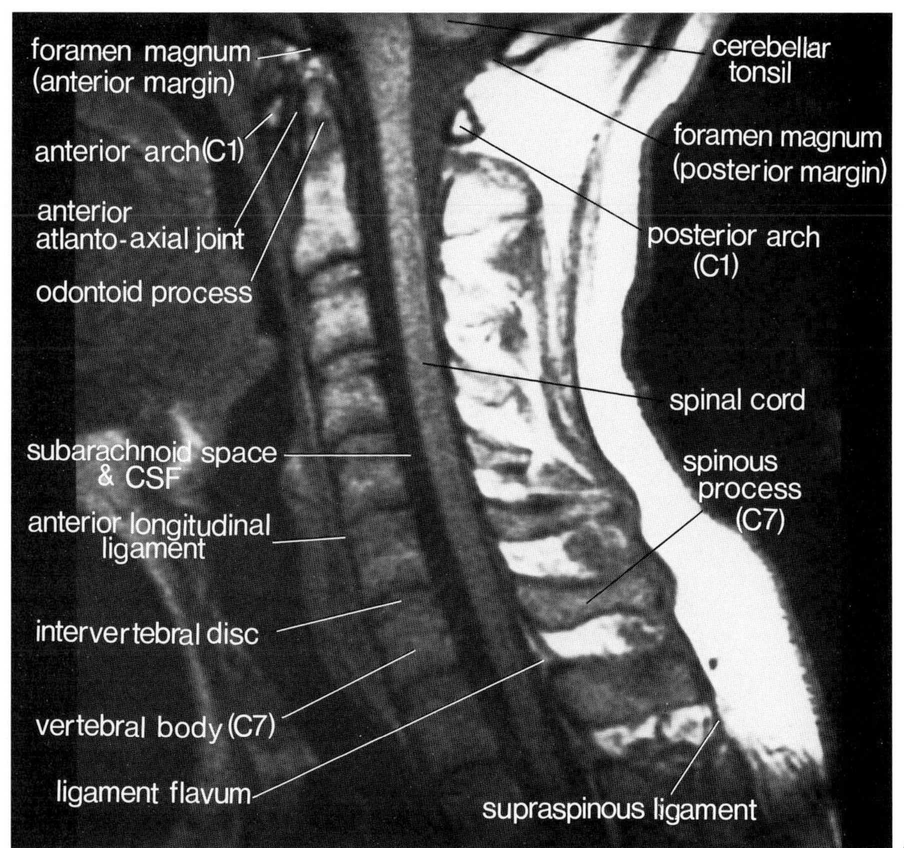

A

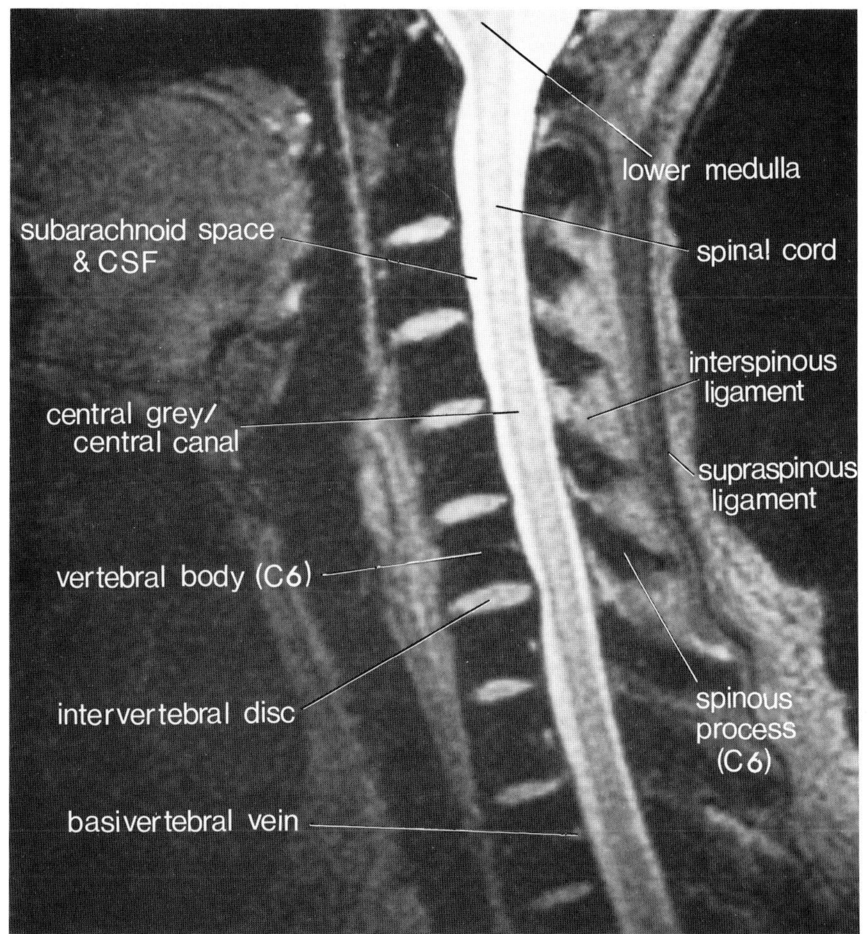

B

FIG. 5-4. Midline sagittal T1W (**A**) (TR 500 msec, TE 20 msec) and gradient-echo (**B**) (TR 250 msec, TE 20 msec, 12° flip angle) images through the cervical spinal canal using a 20 FOV.

A,B

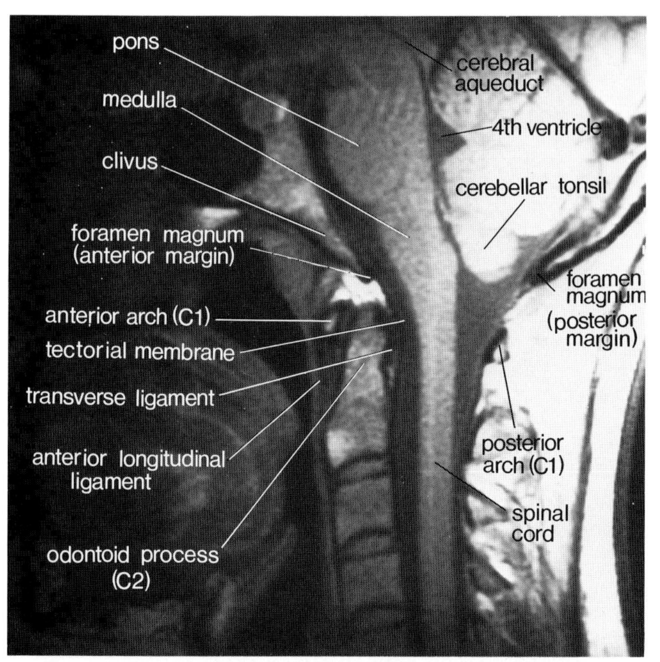

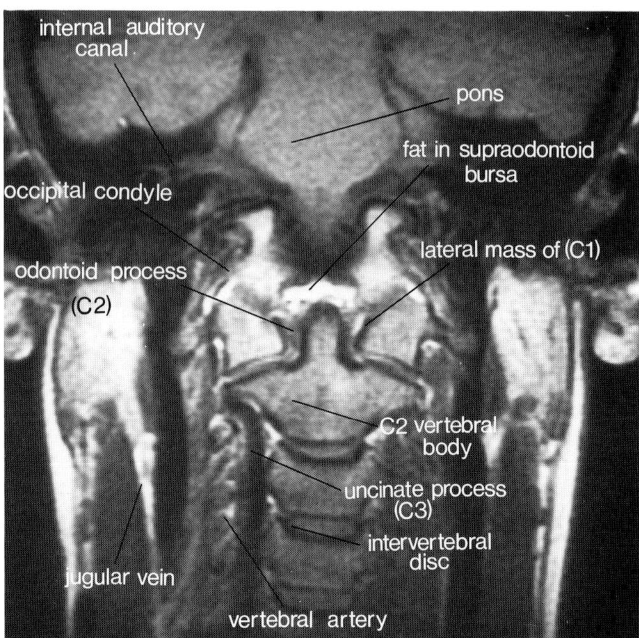

C

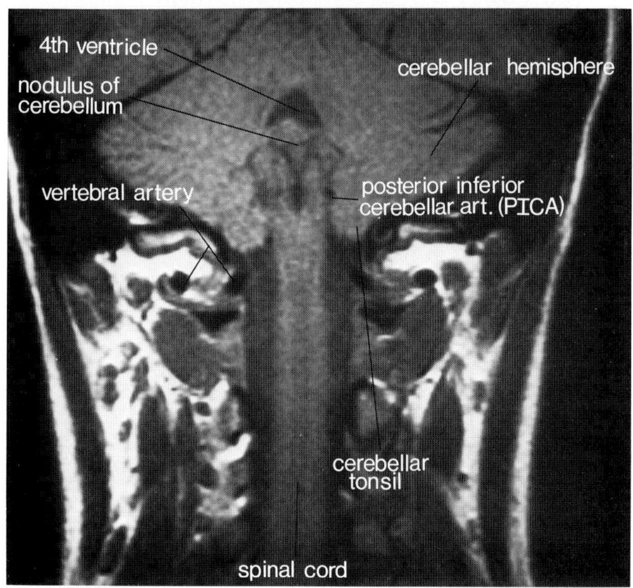

FIG. 5-5. High-resolution T1W (TR 500 msec, TE 20 msec) 16 FOV images through the cranial vertebral junction demonstrate the anatomy to better advantage. **A:** Midline sagittal. **B:** Coronal through midspinal column. **C:** Coronal through midspinal canal.

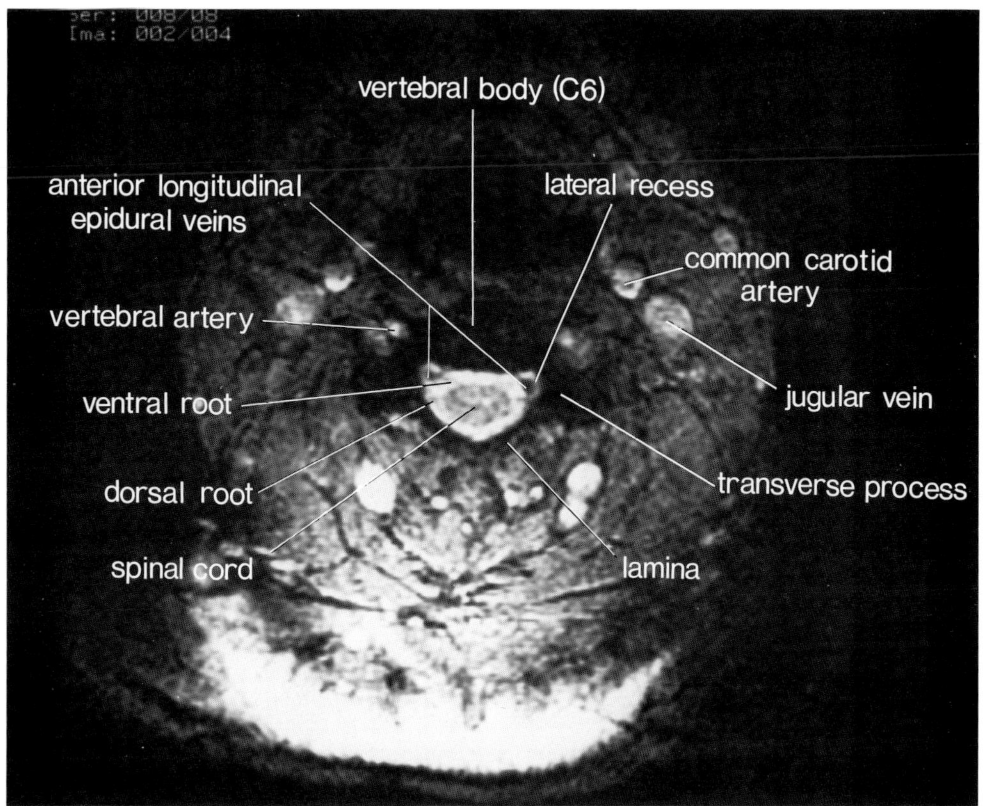

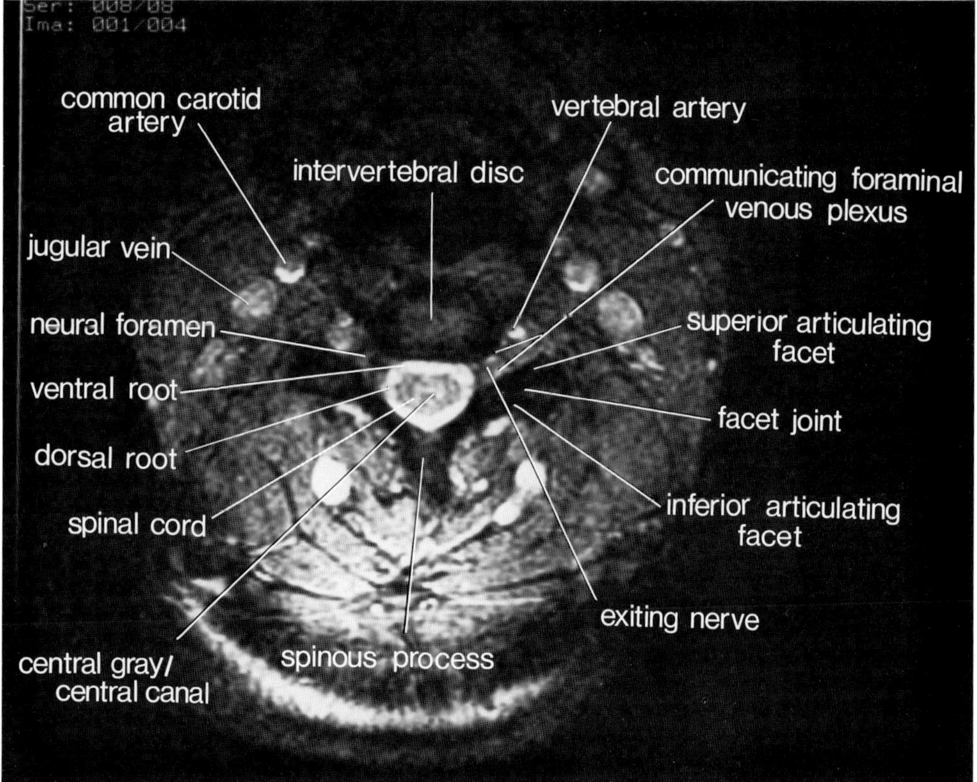

FIG. 5-6. Normal gradient-echo axial image (TR 200 msec, TE 20 msec, 12° flip angle) through (**A**) C6 vertebral body and (**B**) the sixth cervical interspace. This sequence delineates the spinal cord and nerve roots, CSF, intervertebral discs, and vertebral bodies well.

A,B

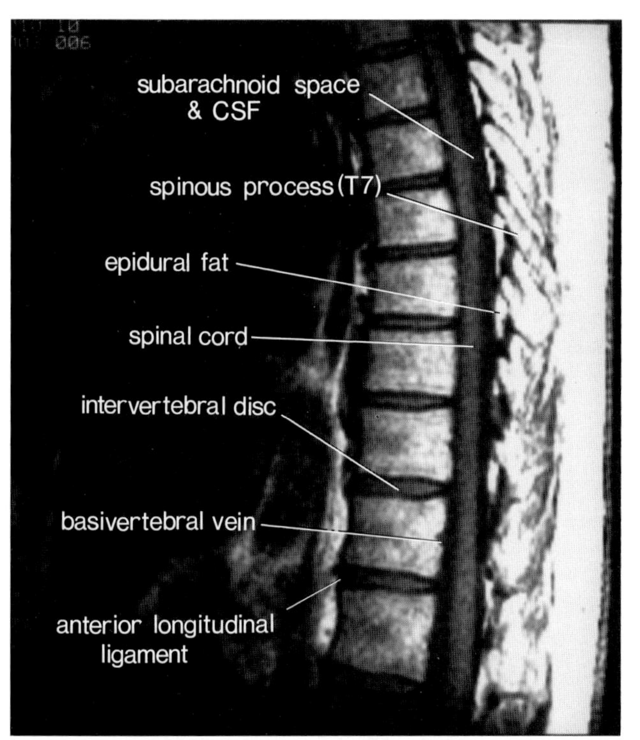

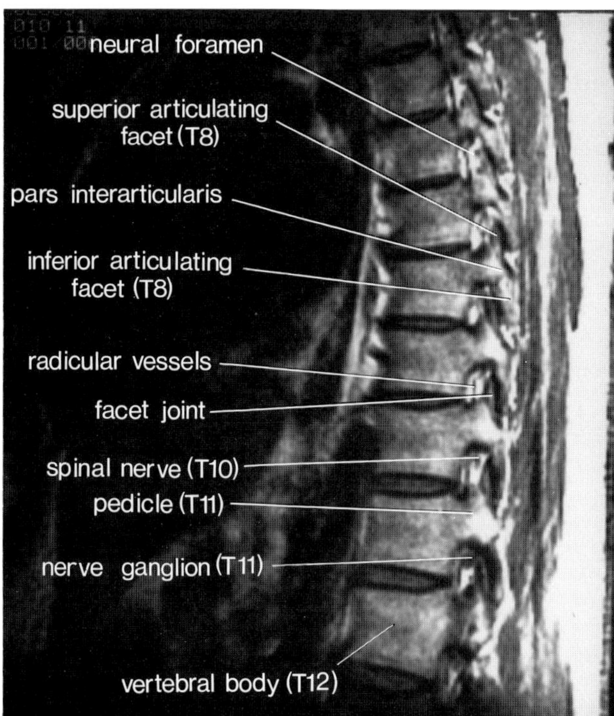

FIG. 5-7. **A:** Midline sagittal T1W image through the thoracic spinal canal using a 26 FOV (TR 500 msec, TE 20 msec). **B:** The anatomy of the intervertebral foramina is best depicted on lateral parasagittal sections (TR 500 msec, TE 20 msec).

A,B

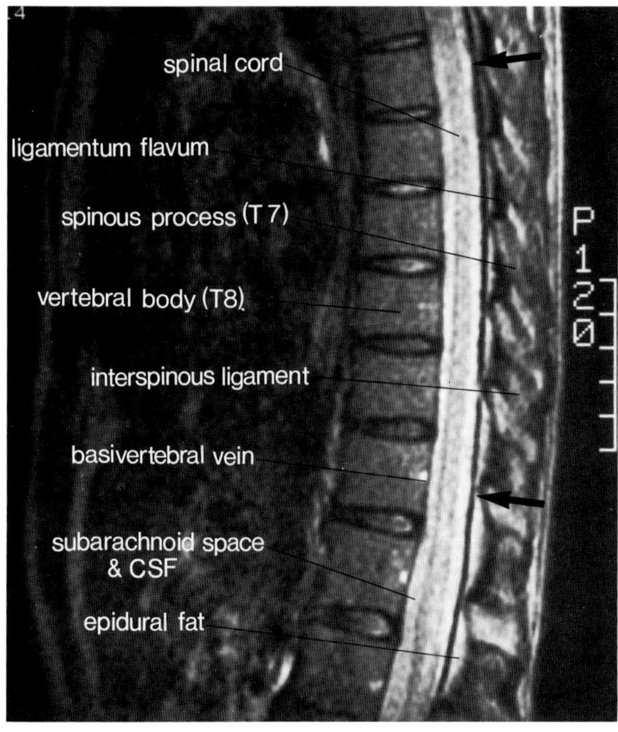

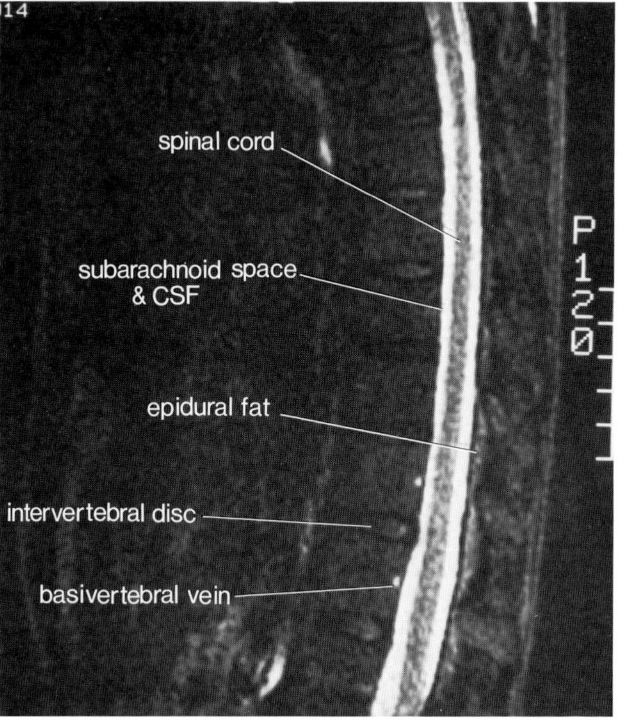

FIG. 5-8. Midline sagittal thoracic spinal canal with progressive T2 weighting. **A:** TR 1,500 msec, TE 70 msec. **B:** TR 1,500 msec, TE 140 msec. The CSF extradural interface is best seen in (**A**) (*arrows*), while the contrast between cord and CSF is best appreciated with more heavily T2 weighting. Both of these images were obtained using a combination of presaturation pulses, flow compensation gradients, and phase and frequency gradient reversal.

and below (20,78). The anterior margin of the foramen or canal is the posterior vertebral body and uncinate process. The articular masses and facet joints form the posterior margin. The ventral and dorsal roots are located within the inferior portion of the foramen, at and below the disc level (78). In the lumbar region, the superior and inferior borders of the neural foramen are again formed by the pedicles. The anterior margin is formed by the posterior vertebral body above and the posterior disc margin below. The facet joint and a small portion of the ligamentum flavum form the posterior border. The lumbar nerve roots are located within the superior portion of the foramen above the disc level.

The first two cervical vertebrae, the atlas and the axis, are different in morphology due to their specialized function of holding up the head and allowing for a variety of rotational and tilting motions (74). The atlas, or C1, is ring shaped and lacks a well-formed vertebral body. It has an anterior arch and a posterior arch that are connected by a lateral mass on each side. The superior articulating facets articulate with the occipital condyle at the base of the skull and the inferior articular facets articulate with the superior articulating facets on the axis. A long process extends from the superior surface of the body of the axis, which is called the odontoid process or the dens. It forms a synovial joint at its articulation with the posterior aspect of the anterior arch of C1, is held in place by a set of strong ligaments (which will be discussed later), and provides a pivot on which the atlas and skull can rotate (74).

The signal intensity of the vertebral bodies depends on the amount and type of marrow present. Normally, the proportion of red to yellow marrow is high so that the vertebral bodies show medium to high signal with T1W, intermediate to low signal with T2W, and low signal on gradient-echo sequences. The signal pattern may be homogeneous or inhomogeneous depending on the distribution of marrow fat and fibrous tissue. The end-plates demonstrate low signal on T1W, T2W, and partial flip angle sequences because of a combination of the composition (cortical bone covered with cartilage) and chemical shift artifact (79). The articular cartilage lining the facet joints usually demonstrates low signal intensity on T1W and T2W sequences and is difficult to distinguish from cortical bone (44). However, it demonstrates increased signal on gradient-echo sequences, distinct from the bone. Following radiation therapy, the vertebral bodies become brighter in intensity on T1W sequences when fat replaces the marrow elements (Fig. 5-14).

Intervertebral Discs

The intervertebral discs are interposed between adjacent vertebral bodies, hydrostatically cushioning the mechanical forces present. The disc consists of a central gelatinous nucleus pulposus that is believed to be the remnant of the primitive notochord and peripheral fibrocartilage (68,79). This fibrocartilage is arranged in a concentric lamellar pattern, which forms the annulus fibrosus, and is designed to withstand radial tension. Superiorly and inferiorly, collagenous (Sharpey's) fibers insert into the ring apophysis of the vertebral body end-plates. The superior and inferior portions of the disc are at least partially covered by a thin hyaline cartilage that is continuous with the cartilage over the adjacent vertebral body end-plates (74). Although these components are histologically separate in a normal disc, discrete border zones are not identified at pathology. Rather, the nucleus pulposus blends imperceptibly with the annulus fibrosus.

The MRI appearance of the intervertebral disc reflects its water content. Normal discs demonstrate low signal on T1W sequences and high signal on T2W and gradient-echo sequences. The decline in T2 signal radially from the nucleus pulposus out to the periphery of the disc parallels the normal decrease in water content seen at pathology. The water content, varying from very high (85–90%) in the nucleus to 70–80% in the innermost annulus, falls to its lowest concentration in the most peripheral portions of the disc (69). With MRI, the outermost annular fibers show low signal on T1W and T2W sequences, so distinction from the anterior and posterior longitudinal ligaments or the vertebral body end-plates is not possible. The transition zone from nucleus pulposus to annulus fibrosus is relatively sharp in the young but becomes less distinct with aging. A horizontal band of low signal on T2W sequences may be seen within the central portion of the disc on sagittal images, which can vary from a small notch to a complete partition (1,69,79,122). Its etiology is unclear. Some authors describe annular-like tissue in the region of the cleft at pathology, which is believed to represent degenerative fibrosis (1,122). Other researchers have failed to find a pathologic correlate (79).

With aging, there is progressive loss of water content in the nucleus pulposus and annulus fibrosus. Also, the biochemical structure of the nucleus pulposus changes, with replacement of the gelatinous matrix by disorganized fibrocartilage (68,69). Eventually, the degenerated nucleus blends imperceptibly with the annulus fibrosus on imaging and at pathology. The result is a progressive decrease in signal on T2W sequences as the disc becomes a dessicated degenerated structure that is mostly fibrocartilage.

Spinal Ligaments

The vertebral bodies and intervertebral discs are linked together by a variety of ligaments (74). The anterior longitudinal ligament extends from the base of the

Text continues on p. 101

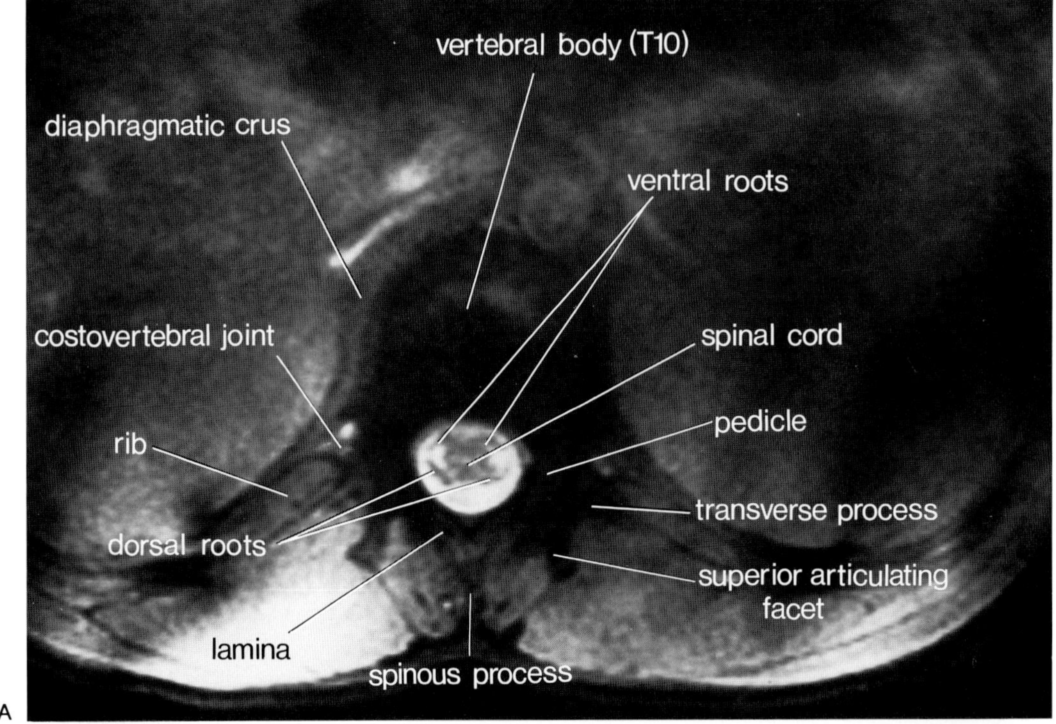

A

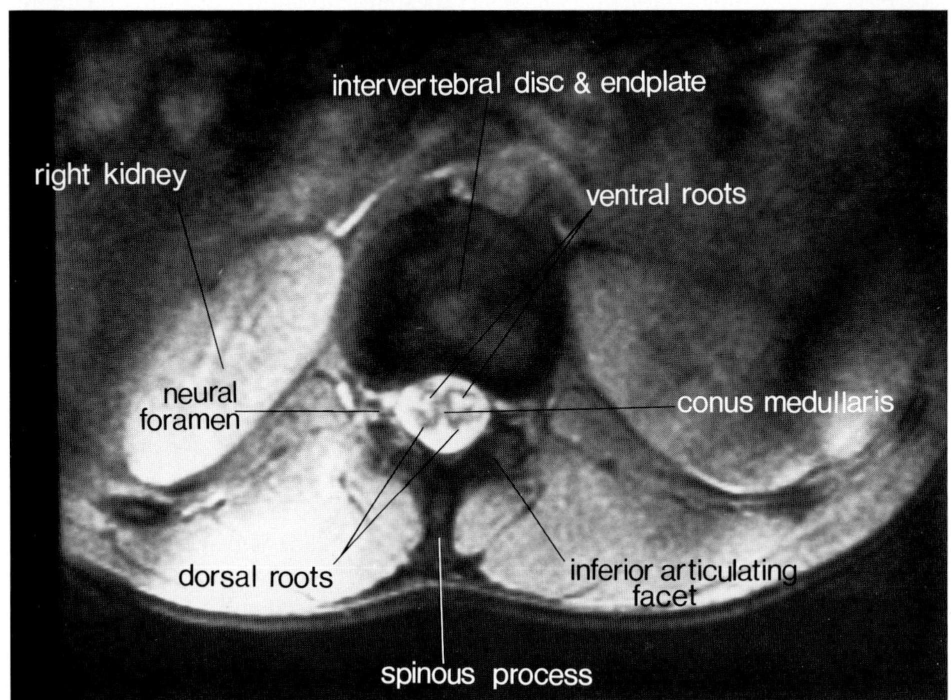

B

FIG. 5-9. Gradient-echo axial images through the distal spinal cord (**A**) and conus (**B**) and (**C**) using a 16 FOV. (TR 400 msec, TE 20 msec, 12° flip angle.)

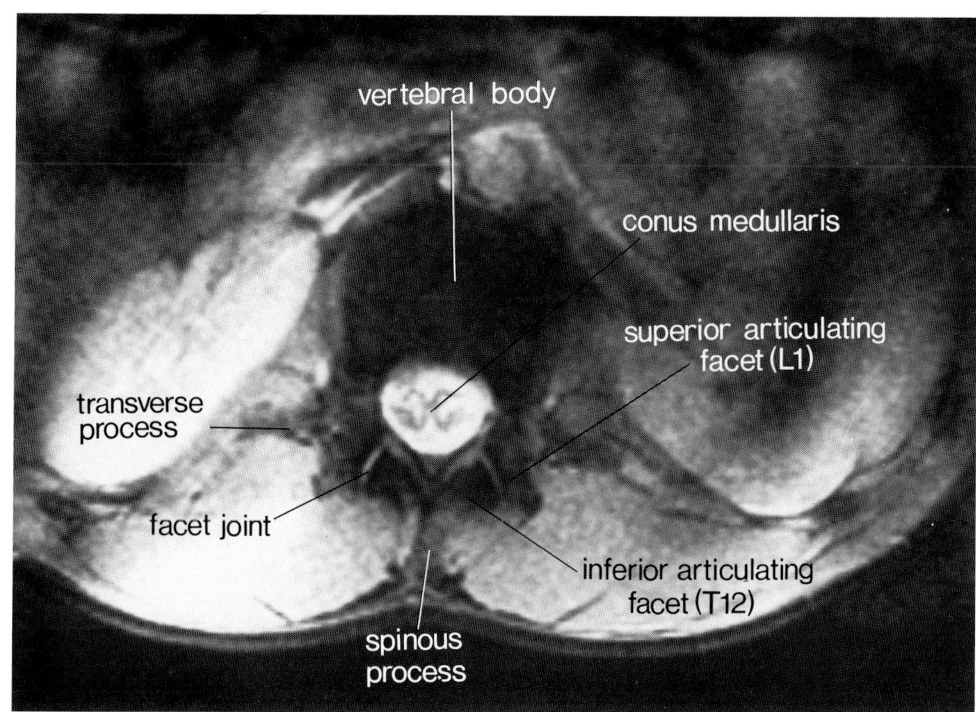

C **FIG. 9 (C).** *Continued.*

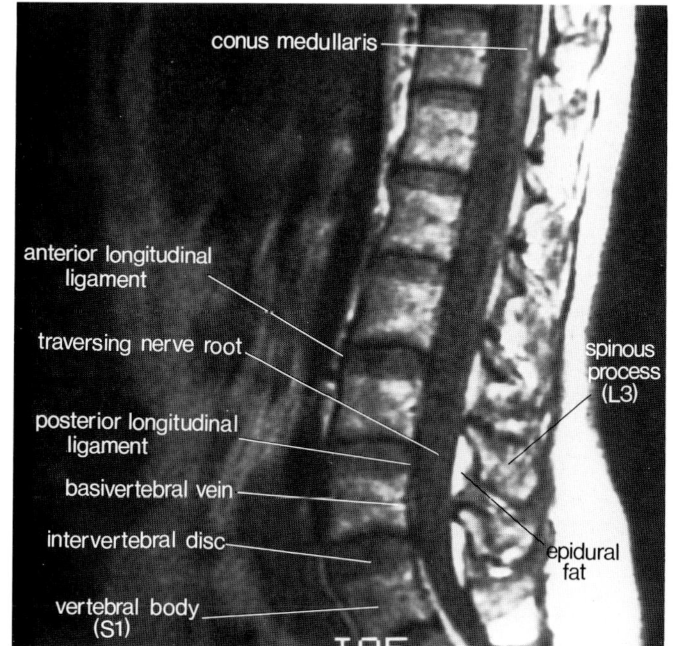

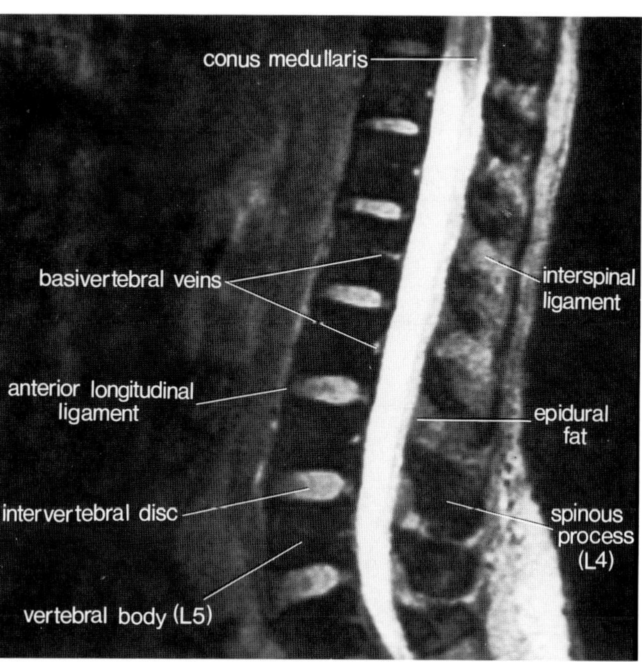

A,B

FIG. 5-10. Midline sagittal T1W (**A**) (TR 500 msec, TE 20 msec) and gradient-echo (**B**) (TR 300 msec, TE 20 msec, 12° flip angle) images in the lower thoracic and lumbar region using a 26 FOV. The distal spinal cord and conus can be evaluated, as well as the intervertebral discs, using this FOV. The CSF is very white in (**B**), which allows easy identification of intradural and extradural pathology.

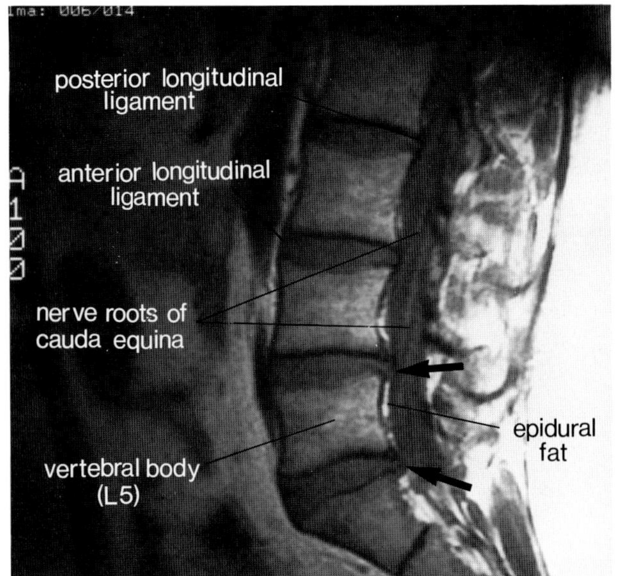

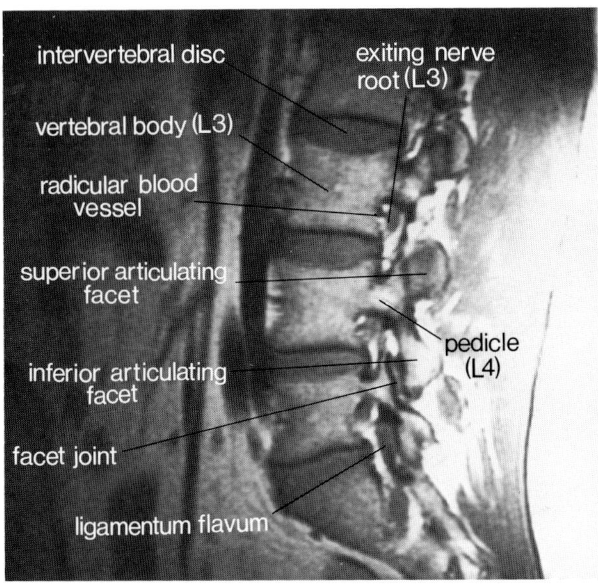

A,B

FIG. 5-11. More detailed evaluation of the lumbar region requires a smaller FOV to increase the resolution. The intervertebral discs, individual nerve roots, facet joints, and intervertebral foramina are best seen on these T1W sequences using a 16 FOV (TR 600 msec, TE 20 msec). **A:** Parasagittal image just to the left of midline. Note asymptomatic disc protrusions at L4 and L5 interspaces (*arrows*). **B:** Parasagittal image at the level of the neural foramen.

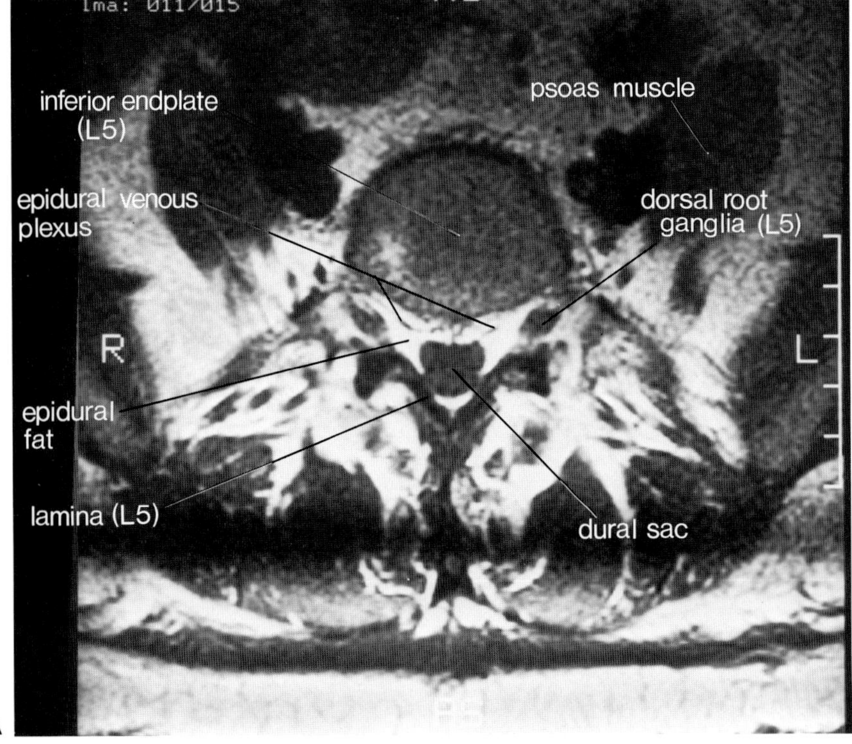

A

FIG. 5-12. T1W axial sequences through L5 interspace showing the normal relationship of the dural sac, nerve roots, and intraspinal/paraspinal fat at the various levels (TR 500 msec, TE 20 msec). **A:** L5 interspace at the level of the dorsal root ganglion. **B:** Inferior aspect of the neural foramen. **C:** S1 vertebral body level.

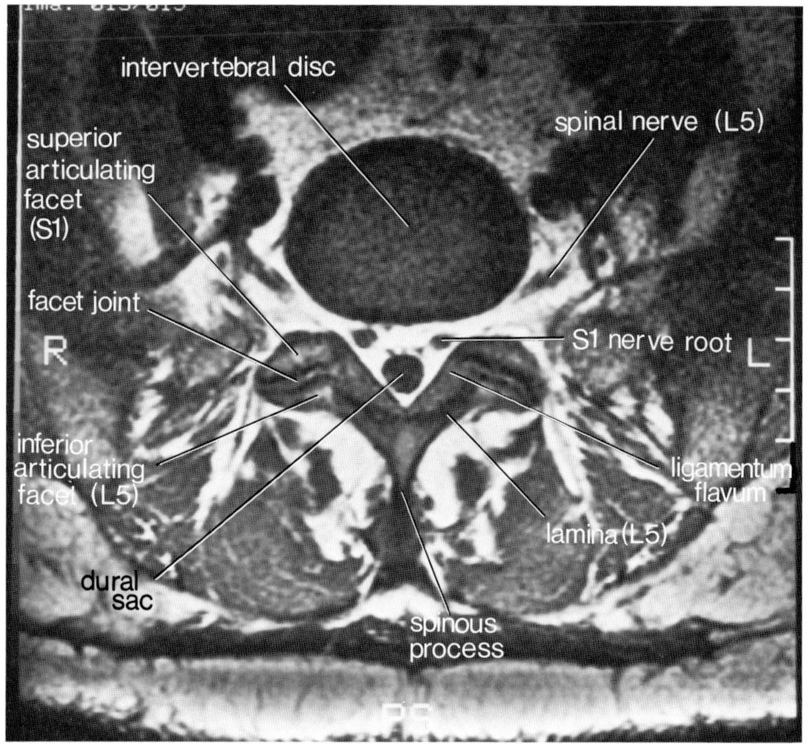

B

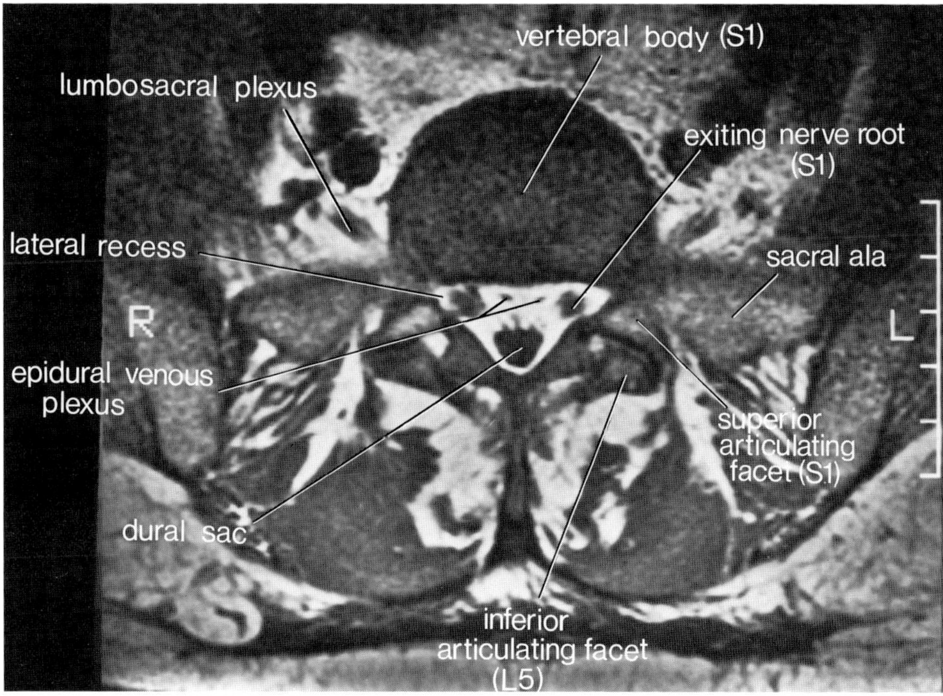

C

Fig. 5-12. *Continued.*

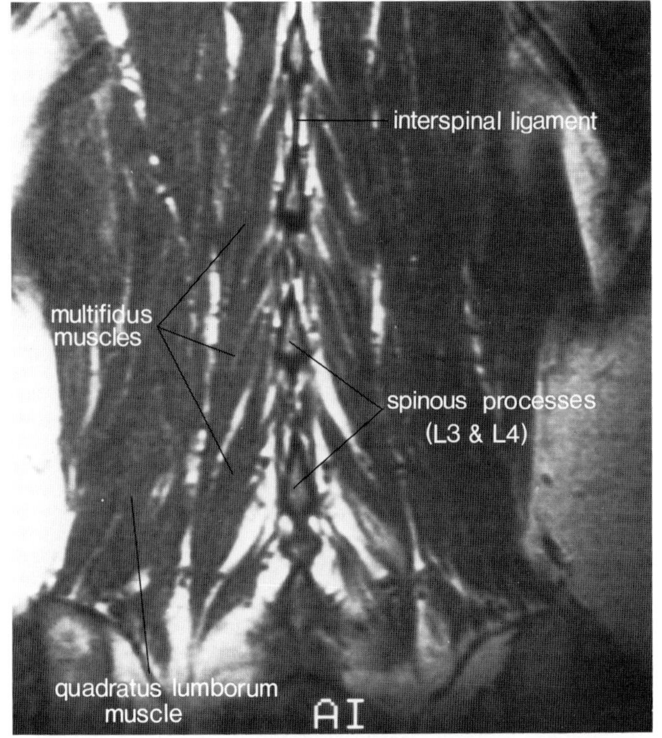

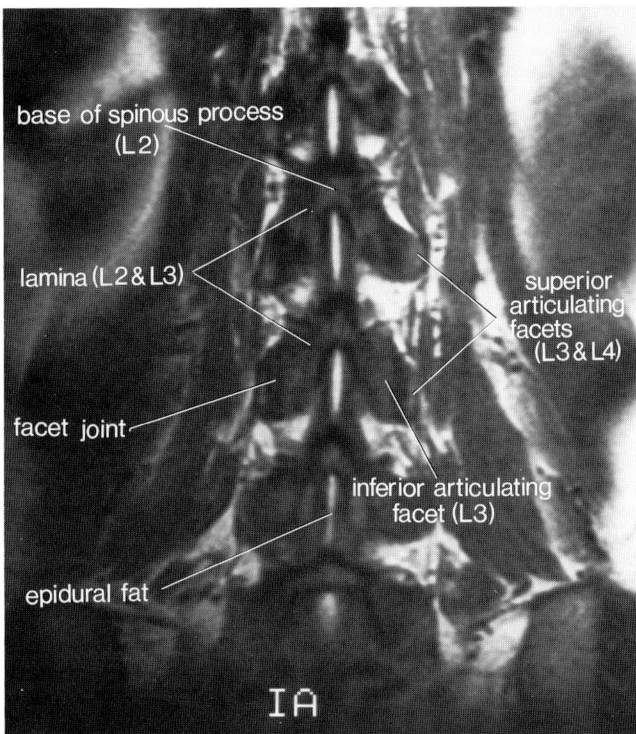

A,B

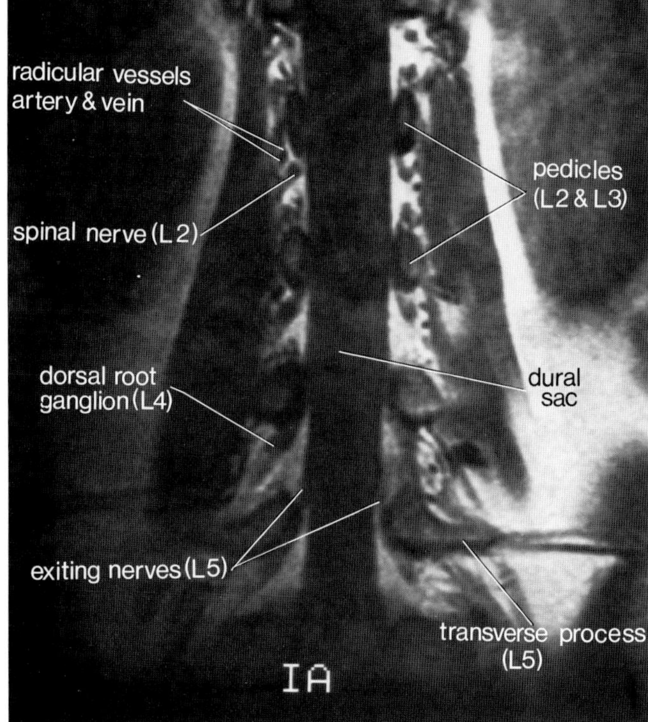

C

FIG. 5-13. Occasionally, coronal images of the lumbar spine provide additional information in the evaluation of intradural or extradural pathology. These images were obtained at the level of the spinous processes (**A**), posterior elements (**B**), and spinal canal (**C**).

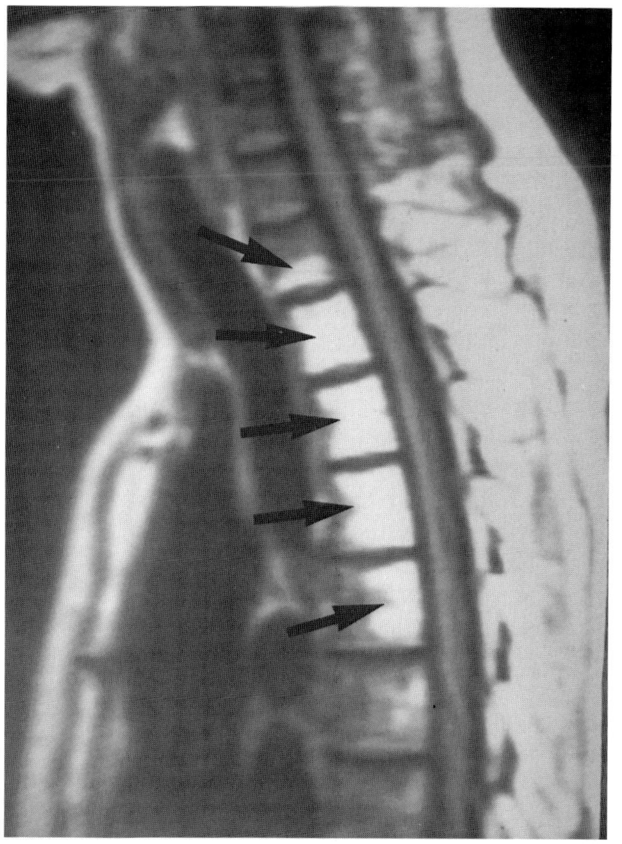

FIG. 5-14. Increased marrow fat signal is seen within these upper thoracic vertebral bodies (*arrows*) secondary to radiation therapy performed for breast carcinoma. Compare their signal intensity to that seen in the nonirradiated marrow above and below, and to that seen in Fig. 5-7A. (TR 500 msec, TE 20 msec.)

skull to the sacrum and is adherent to the anterior vertebral bodies and the anterior disc margins. A corresponding ligament, the posterior longitudinal ligament, extends from C2 to the sacrum. This ligament is firmly attached to the vertebral body end-plates and posterior disc margins but is separated from the midposterior vertebral body to allow room for the anterior internal epidural venous plexus and basivertebral veins. The superior extension of the posterior longitudinal ligament is the tectorial membrane that extends from C2 to the lower clivus. The laminae of each vertebral body are segmentally joined by the ligamentum flavum, which is named for its yellow color noted at surgery. The ligamentum flavum extends posterolaterally to merge with the facet joint. The interspinous ligament segmentally connects the spinous processes and the supraspinous ligament extends along the tips of the spinous processes.

Additional ligaments are present at the craniovertebral junction that stabilize the atlantoaxial and cranial cervical junction. The anterior atlanto-occipital membrane extends from the anterior margin of the foramen magnum to the anterior arch of the atlas. A corresponding posterior atlanto-occipital membrane extends from the posterior margin of the foramen magnum to the posterior arch of the atlas. An important ligament is the cruciform ligament, named for its crosslike shape. It has a horizontal portion that forms the transverse ligament and holds the dens to the ring of C1 and a vertical portion that, together with the tectorial membrane, attaches to the lower clivus. The apical ligament extends from the tip of the dens to the anterior margin of the foramen magnum and the alar ligaments extend laterally from the dens to each occipital condyle (74).

With MRI, most ligaments, with the exception of the ligamentum flavum, demonstrate low signal intensity, similar to bone, on all imaging sequences because of their high collagen content (43,44). The ligaments blend imperceptibly with cortical bone, the outer fibers of the annulus fibrosus, and the dura. The ligamentum flavum demonstrates intermediate signal on T1W and T2W sequences and high signal on gradient-echo sequences. The reason for this discrepancy is presumably related to its different biochemical composition. The ligamentum flavum contains only 20% collagen with 80% being elastin (44,47).

Spinal Cord and Nerves

The spinal cord begins as the caudal extension of the medulla oblongata at the level of the foramen magnum. Its distal extent is more variable and age dependent. The spinal cord and vertebral column are equal in length until the third fetal month. Thereafter, because of discordant growth between the cord and the spinal column, the tip of the conus "ascends" to lie opposite the L1 vertebral body in the adult, with a range from the eleventh thoracic interspace to the second lumbar interspace (101). The conus terminates in the filum terminale, which is less than 2 mm in diameter and extends to the first coccygeal segment (101).

The spinal cord varies in size depending on its level within the spinal canal. It is widest at the cervical enlargement (C5–C6), narrowest at the midthoracic region (T5–T9), and enlarges again in the lumbar region from T10 to the conus (101). The anteroposterior diameter of the cord remains relatively constant at 9–10 mm throughout the length of the spinal cord.

The spinal nerves are formed by the union of a dorsal sensory and a ventral motor root. There are eight pairs of cervical nerve roots but only seven cervical vertebral bodies. The first seven cervical nerves exit above the pedicles of their corresponding vertebral body level. For example, the C5 nerve root exits at the fourth cervical interspace level above the C5 pedicle. The C8 nerve root exits below the C7 pedicle at the seventh cervical interspace. Below T1, the remaining nerve roots exit inferior to their corresponding vertebral body levels, so that the

T1 nerve root exits at the first thoracic interspace, the T2 nerve root exits at the second thoracic interspace, and so on. In the cervical region, the nerve roots course relatively horizontal to exit their neural foramen. Because of the discrepancy between the length of the spinal cord and vertebral column, the course of the nerve roots becomes progressively more vertical throughout the thoracic region. Below the tip of the conus, the lumbar and sacral nerve roots have a rather long, parallel, vertical course that forms the cauda equina (74).

With MRI, the spinal cord has intermediate signal on T1 weighted sequences and low signal on T2 weighted and gradient-echo sequences. On high-resolution studies at high field strength, some internal architecture can be seen on T2W and gradient-echo sequences. This is particularly apparent on axial images where an "H"-shaped zone of slightly higher signal may be seen in the region of a central gray matter surrounded by the slightly lower signal of the white matter tracks (Fig. 5-6B). A corresponding longitudinal stripe of slightly higher signal is seen within the mid-spinal cord on the sagittal T2W and gradient-echo sequences (21) (Fig. 5-4B). This distinction between white and gray matter is thought to be secondary to a combination of the differences in water content between white and gray matter, the differences in relaxation times, and the presence or absence of myelin (21). This gray–white differentiation is not apparent on T1 weighted sequences. Individual nerve roots can sometimes be resolved as separate from the CSF if a small FOV is used (71).

Dural Coverings

The dural coverings of the spinal cord and nerve roots are in continuity with those in the cranial cavity. The dura and the arachnoid are closely adherent with only a potential space between the two. They form the outer boundary of the subarachnoid space. The inner boundary is formed by the pia mater, which is closely adherent to the spinal cord and nerve roots. Cerebral spinal fluid (CSF) circulates within the subarachnoid space and freely communicates with the cranial CSF spaces. It demonstrates low signal intensity (lower than spinal cord) on T1W sequences and cannot be distinguished from the dura or posterior longitudinal ligament. On gradient-echo and T2 weighted sequences, the CSF becomes high in signal, much greater than the spinal cord, demonstrating the myelogram effect.

Vascular

The blood supply to the spinal cord is via a larger anterior spinal artery, which supplies the anterior two-thirds to four-fifths of the spinal cord, and two small posterior spinal arteries, which supply the remainder of the cord (74). The anterior and posterior spinal arteries are asymmetrically and variably supplied at a few levels by multiple radiculomedullary arteries, which arise from the vertebrals, aortic intercostal arteries, and lumbar arteries. The anterior spinal artery is formed by the junction of paired medullary branches of the intracranial vertebral arteries. Additional arterial contribution is seen at two or three other cervical levels. The upper thoracic cord is poorly supplied with a watershed zone at approximately T4. The predominant arterial supply to the thoracolumbar region is the great anterior medullary artery, or the artery of Adamkiewicz. It arises on the left side 75% of the time and usually between T9 and L2 (85%) (101). It makes a characteristic hairpin bend as it forms the ascending and descending anterior spinal artery. The venous system roughly mirrors the arterial system with multiple medullary veins draining into pial veins that communicate with the prominant posterior spinal vein and smaller anterior spinal veins (74). Radicular veins coursing with the nerve roots drain the pial veins into the internal vertebral venous plexus, which is in the epidural space surrounded by fat (38). The internal vertebral venous plexus drains into the external vertebral venous plexus either via the basivertebral vein through the vertebral body or via paired anterior longitudinal epidural veins that drain through the neural foramen (74). The external vertebral venous plexus ultimately empties into the azygos system.

EXAMINATION TECHNIQUE

Surface coils must be used for the evaluation of the spine. They come in a variety of shapes and configurations, including special coils for the neck. In the cervical region, a special posterior neck coil works well. It is shaped to conform to the cervical lordotic curve and it is quite comfortable for the patient to lie on. If this is not available, a 7 inch by 11 inch rectangular "license plate" coil or a 5 inch round circular coil may be used. If more than one portion of the spine is being examined, a platform device, which allows the technician to move the coil without disturbing the patient, is useful (54) (Fig. 5-15). In general, at least three coil placements are necessary for evaluation of the spinal canal from the foramen magnum to the upper sacrum.

A T1W sagittal sequence is initially performed. A T2W or gradient-echo sagittal sequence is then added, depending on what is seen or what the clinical indication is. Gradient-echo sequences tend to work best in the evaluation of intradural and extradural disease in the cervical and lumbar region (34,35,51,117). They are quick and turn the CSF white, resulting in the myelogram effect. Unfortunately, the image quality in the thoracic region is often degraded by diaphragm motion (Fig. 5-16). T2W sagittal sequences take longer to per-

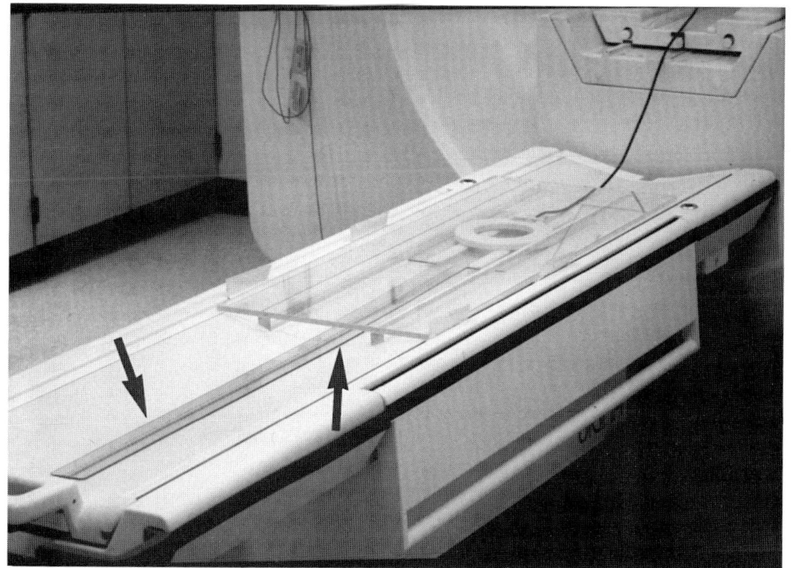

A

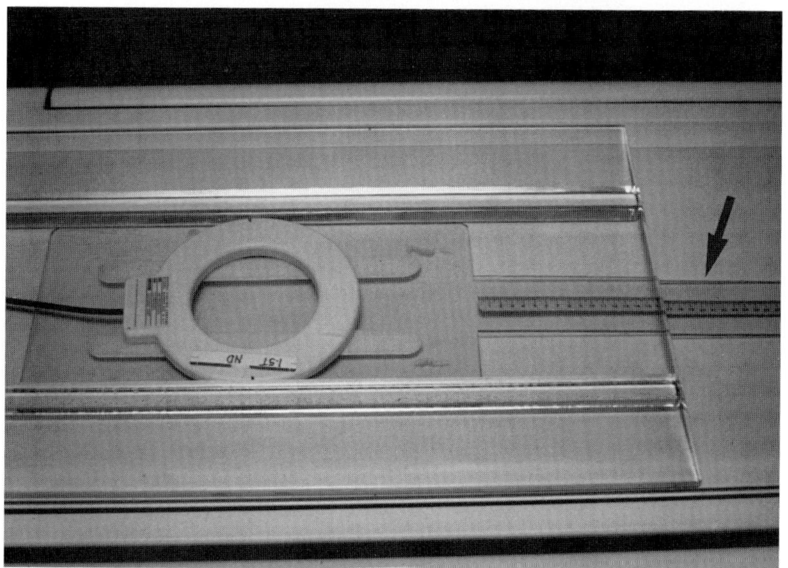

B

FIG. 5-15. A: This plexiglass platform was constructed by our Facilities and Engineering Department. Velcro strips attach a variety of surface coils (5 inch round coil pictured) to a movable paddle. A measuring device is attached to the paddle (*arrows*), which allows accurate movement of the coil by the technologist underneath the platform without disturbing the patient. **B:** Close-up view showing the detail of the platform and paddle.

form but demonstrate intradural pathology best in the thoracic region. In the evaluation of degenerative disc disease, axial sequences are performed next with the axial sections being parallel to the interspaces (Fig. 5-17). In the lumbar region, T1W sequences are used to take advantage of the sharp contrast between intraspinal fat and disc material, nerve roots, and bone. Gradient-echo axials are preferred in the cervical region because they tend to differentiate spinal cord, dural sac, disc material, and bone the best (34,35,117). Axial gradient-echo sequences work particularly well to confirm and further characterize intradural or intramedullary lesions seen on the sagittal sequences (51). They are also useful in excluding pathology when the findings on the sagittal sequences are equivocal. Intravenous contrast is then given and T1W sagittal and/or axial sequences are performed if intradural pathology is found or if the clinical indication suggests a meningeal process or a spinal vascular malformation.

Patients with scoliosis require special imaging considerations. Only small portions of the spinal canal and cord are imaged on each slice. Intradural pathology may be obscured with the pathology mimicking volume averaging. Repeating the T1W sequences in the coronal plane usually provides additional information. Also, the coronal and sagittal planes may be obliqued to allow imaging of a larger portion of the spine on any one slice. Contrast may be used more liberally to increase the conspicuousness of intradural lesions in a patient with a documented myelopathy.

There is no one correct way to image the spine. Multiple pulse sequences and imaging options are available. Motion compensation mechanisms must be used and not all options are available on each imager. The choice

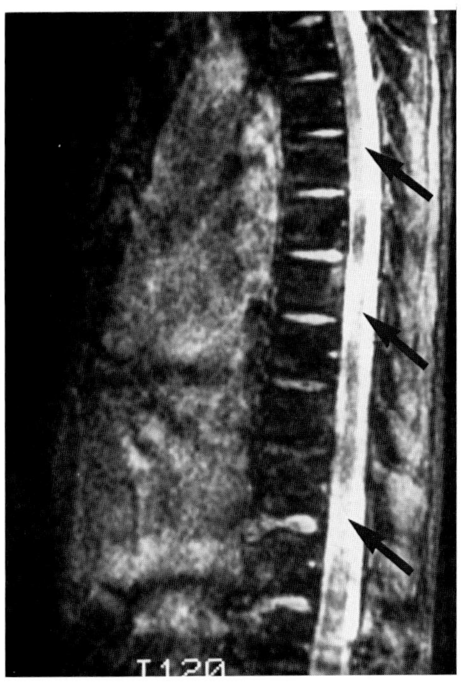

FIG. 5-16. Typical alternating bright bands of intensity across the spinal canal and cord (*arrows*) from diaphragm motion often encountered when using gradient-echo sequences in the thoracic region. (TR 250 msec, TE 20 msec, 12° flip angle.)

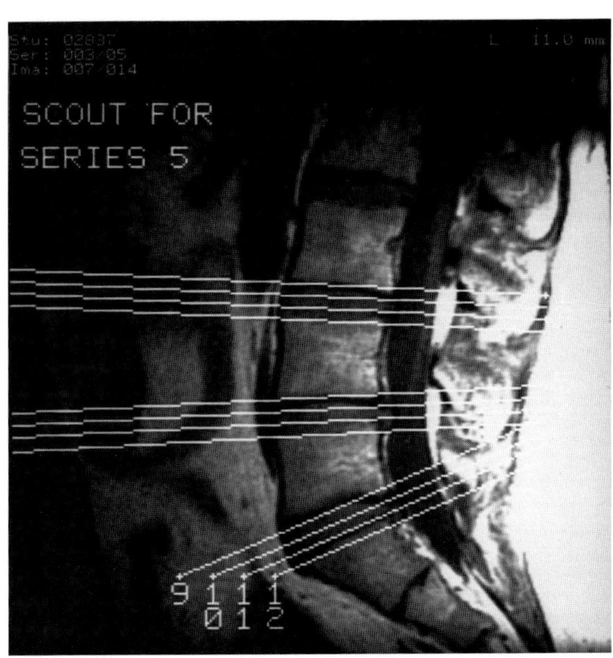

FIG. 5-17. This is a scout view from a lumbar spine exam performed for the evaluation of disc disease. The locations of the axial images are cross-referenced on this sagittal view. Note that the axial slices are obtained parallel to and at the level of the intervertebral discs.

TABLE 5-1.

Area	Coil	Plane	TR (msec)	TE (msec)	Flip angle	Views/ Nex	Thickness/ skip (mm)	FOV (cm)	Time (min)	Comments[a]
Cervical spine	Posterior neck or rectangular	SAG	500	20	—	192/2	4/0	20	4	NF, NP, ST
		SAG	200–300	20	12°	192/4	4/0	20	4	FC, NF, NP, (1)
		SAG	1,500	60/120	—	192/2	4/2	20	9	FC, NBW, NF, NP, ST, (2)
		Oblique axials	400–500	20	12°	192/4	4/0	20	6	FC, NF, NP, (3)
Thoracic spine	Rectangular	SAG	500	20	—	192/2	4/0	24–26	4	NF, NP, ST, (4)
		SAG	1,500	70/140	—	192/2	4/2	24–26	9	FC, NBW, NF, NP, ST, (4)
		Oblique axials	400–500	20	12°	192/4	4/0	20	6	FC, NF, NP, (5)
Lumbar spine	Rectangular	SAG	500	20	—	192/2	4/0	26	4	NF, NP, ST
		SAG	400	20	12°	192/4	4/0	26	4	FC, NF, NP
		Oblique axials	500	20	—	192/2	4/0	16	6–13	FC, NF, NP, (6)
		Oblique axials	400–500	20	12°	192/4	4/0	20	6	FC, NF, NP, (6), (7)

[a] Abbreviations: FC, flow compensation gradient; NBW, narrow bandwidth; NF, no frequency wrap function; NP, no phase wrap function; ST, presaturation pulse sequences applied superior, inferior, and anterior.

Notes: (1) radiculopathy indication; (2) myelopathy indication; (3) three or four slices through abnormal or suspected abnormal interspaces; (4) change phase direction to superior and inferior; (5) through abnormal or suspected abnormal areas; (6) four or five slices through lower three or four interspaces; (7) optional sequence.

of repetition times, echo times, and flip angles to achieve optimum contrast between spinal cord and CSF on T2W or gradient-echo sequences may vary, depending on the motion compensation mechanisms available (flow compensation and presaturation versus cardiac gating) and the type of magnet. A sample protocol is included in Table 5-1 that represents my own personal bias for obtaining optimum images of the spine.

MR CONTRAST AGENTS

The first agent released to the general medical community is gadolinium diethylenetriaminepentaacetic acid (Gd-DTPA). It is marketed under the trade name of Magnavist by the Berlex Corporation. Additional agents are expected to be released in the near future. Gd-DTPA is a paramagnetic metal ion chelate that has been approved by the FDA for spine imaging. In contrast to conventional iodinated material, where the agent itself is imaged, paramagnetic materials themselves do not produce signals. Rather, they alter the molecular environment of the tissue in which they reside, thus affecting the signal of the hydrogen nuclei present (98,118). The magnetic moment of the paramagnetic agent is considerably greater than the moment of the nearby hydrogen nuclei due to the presence of unpaired electrons. Paramagnetic agents are also designed in such a way to bind water molecules. The large magnetic moment of the paramagnetic agent enhances relaxation or shortens the relaxation time of the bound water protons, which are continually exchanging with free water. They enhance both the T1 and T2 relaxation. At the clinically effective dosage used, the T1 relaxation effect predominates, resulting in an area of increased signal on T1W sequences wherever the agent has accumulated (98,118).

The volume of distribution of Gd-DTPA in the CNS is similar to that of iodinated agents. Blood supply to the tissue and blood–brain barrier breakdown are required to allow accumulation of the agent. Gadolinium is excreted unchanged in the urine. Eighty percent is excreted within the first 6 hr with 90% being eliminated by 24 hr. The biologic half-life is about 90 min (9).

The most common side effect reported in preclinical trials was transient headache noted in 6.5% of patients (41). However, in approximately one-half of these patients it is unclear whether the headache was related to the drug or the patients' underlying condition. Injection site coldness (3.6%) and nausea (1.9%) were the other common complaints. Uncommon reactions, seen in less than 1% of patients, included localized pain, rash, transient hypotension or hypertension, fever, and seizures (41).

Gadolinium has been helpful or essential in the diagnosis and characterization of intraspinal neoplasms, meningeal abnormalities, inflammatory conditions, and postoperative failed back syndromes (97).

PATHOLOGIC CONDITIONS

Disc Diseases

Degenerative (Nonsurgical Lesions)

The single most common indication for MRI of the spine at our institution is degenerative disc disease. A normal sequela of aging, disc degeneration begins early in life. It begins as a loss of hydration, resulting in loss of disc height and diffuse disc bulging. Tears occur in the degenerating annulus fibrosus with three distinct types being identified at autopsy: concentric, radial, and transverse tears (123,124). Of these types, the concentric and transverse tears are thought to have no clinical significance. Whether the radial tears are clinically significant or not remains controversial. Radial tears result from rupture in all layers of the annulus between the nucleus pulposus and the disc surface without frank herniation of the nucleus pulposus. Slow leakage of nuclear material into the annulus fibrosus and spinal canal has been implicated as a cause of chronic low back pain, which has been termed "discogenic" pain (124). With MRI, areas of increased T2 signal within the radial tears of the annulus fibrosus of cadavers have been described (124), as well as areas of Gd-DTPA enhancement in living patients that corresponds to vascularized granulation tissue at surgery (89). However, studies addressing the clinical relevance of these findings are lacking.

With aging, the vertebral body end-plates undergo degeneration as well, which results in end-plate thinning, hyalinization, and fissuring. Granulation tissue may be noted within the end-plates and annulus in an attempt at healing. The end-plate changes associated with degenerative disc disease have been categorized into three main types (70). Type I changes have been observed in 4% of patients being evaluated for low back pain and are characterized by a decreased signal on T1W and increased signal on T2W sequences. Fissuring and disruption of the end-plates with vascularized fibrous tissue within the adjacent marrow have been observed at histology. These changes may mimic those of disc space infection on imaging (Fig. 5-18). Type I changes may be transient and have been observed to convert to type II. Type II changes are characterized by increased signal relative to normal bone marrow on T1W and a slight increased signal or isointensity on T2W sequences (Fig. 5-19). These changes have been observed in 16% of patients evaluated for low back pain and appear more stable. At histology, these end-plates show evidence of disruption with yellow marrow replacement. Type III end-plate changes are seen in end-stage degenerative disc disease and are characterized by decreased signal on both T1W and T2W sequences. These changes correspond to the dense sclerosis seen on plain films as the marrow fat becomes replaced by bone (Fig. 5-20). These

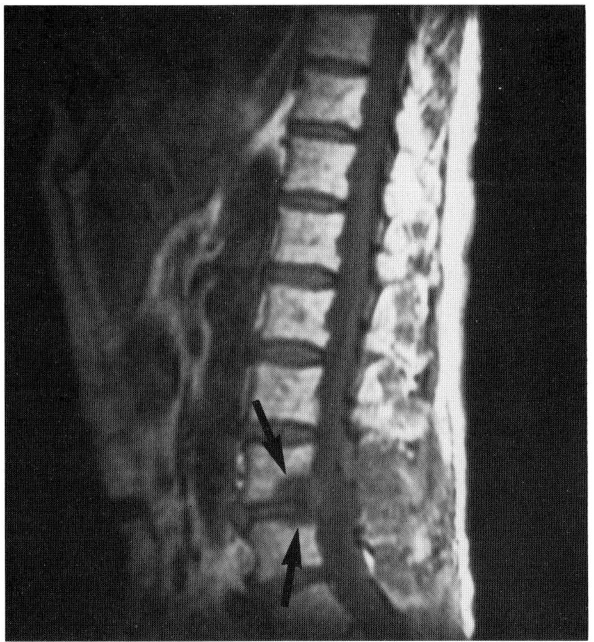
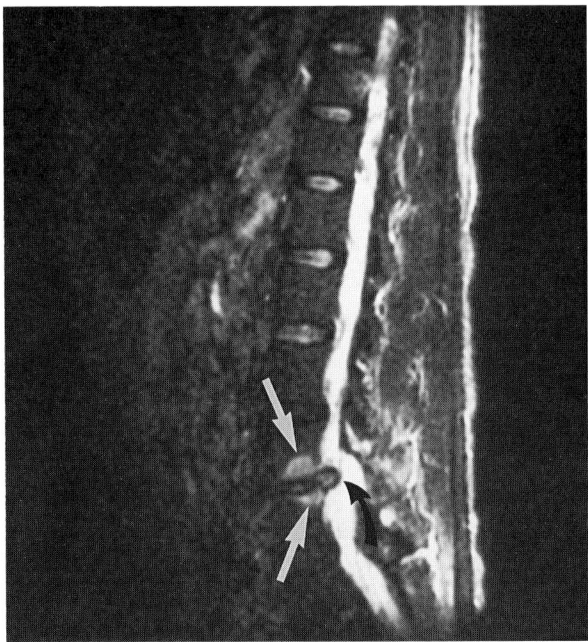

A,B

FIG. 5-18. Typical type I end-plate changes observed in a patient with a previous L4 laminectomy and a recurrent L4 disc protrusion (*curved arrow*). **A:** Note areas of signal loss within the inferior end-plate of L4 and the superior end-plate of L5 (*arrows*). (TR 400 msec, TE 20 msec.) **B:** Corresponding increased signal is seen with T2 weighting (*arrows*). (TR 1,700 msec, TE 120 msec.) These changes may be difficult to distinguish from infection. In this patient the disc itself is relatively preserved and there was no sign of a disc infection clinically or at reoperation.

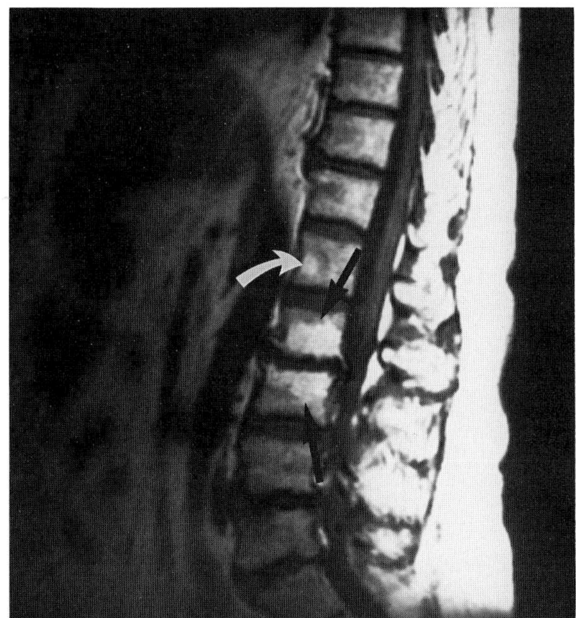
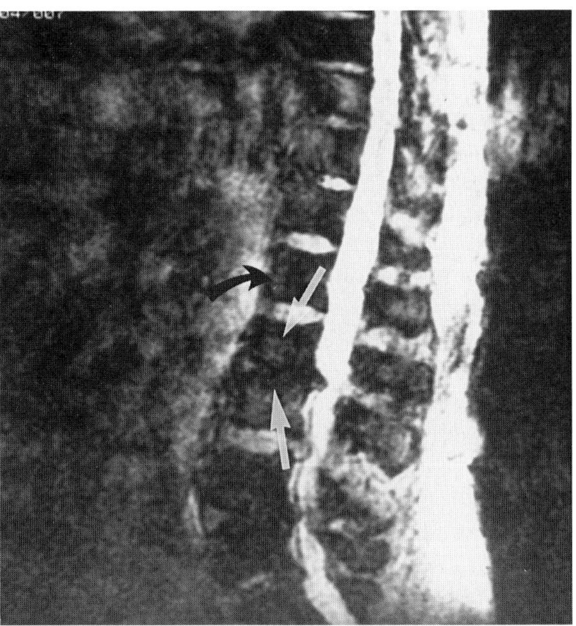

A,B

FIG. 5-19. Type II end-plate changes. **A:** Sagittal lumbar spine in a patient with advanced degenerative disc disease at multiple levels. At the fourth lumbar interspace, increased signal relative to bone marrow is identified within the adjacent end-plates (*arrows*). Note the presumed cavernous hemangioma (discussed later) within the anterior inferior aspect of L1 vertebral body (*white curved arrow*). (TR 500 msec, TE 20 msec.) **B:** These same end-plates (*arrows*) and the cavernous hemangioma (*curved arrow*) become isointense to normal bone marrow with T2 weighting. (TR 300 msec, TE 20 msec, 12° flip angle.)

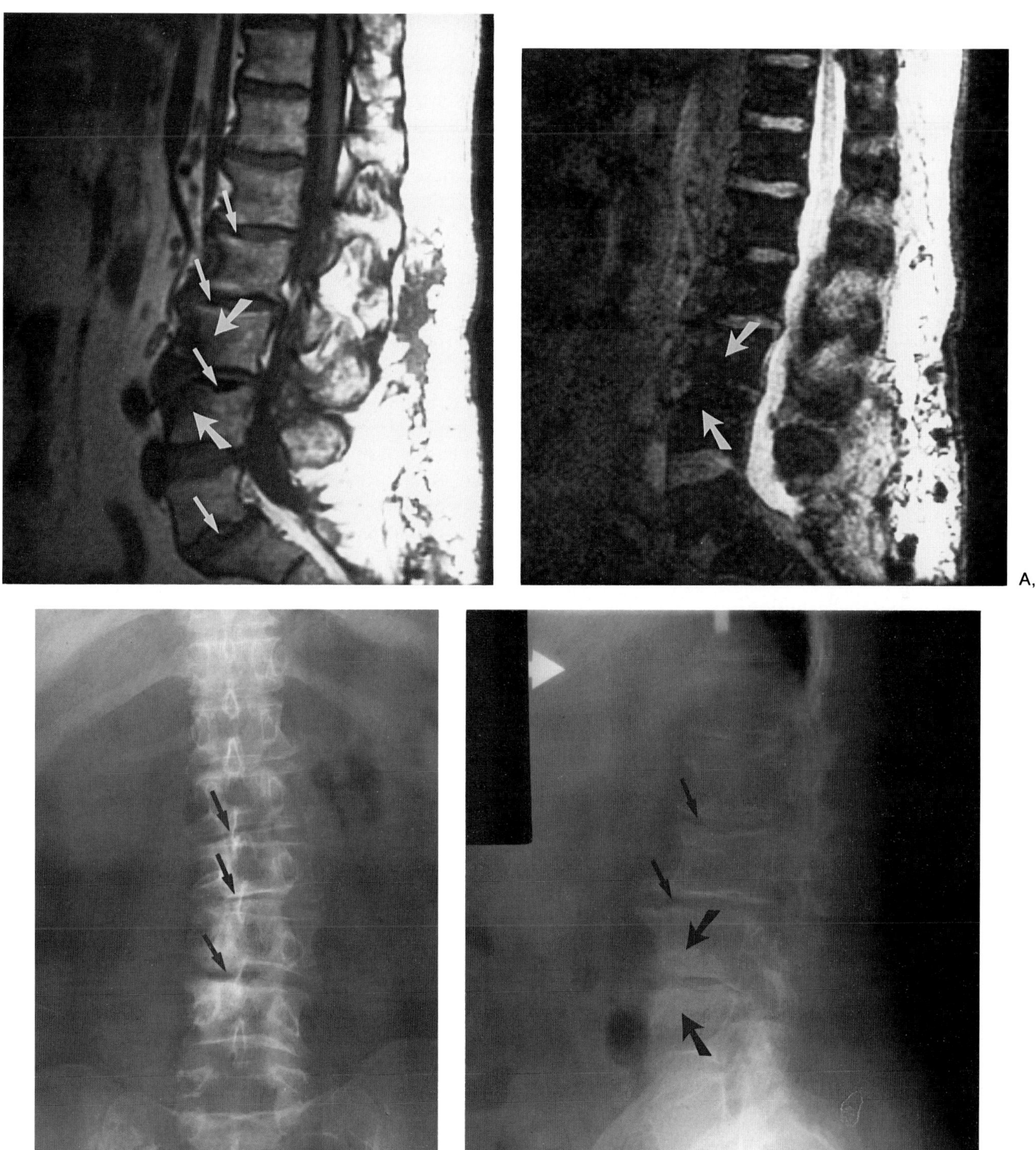

FIG. 5-20. Type III end-plate changes. **A:** Ill-defined zones of decreased signal intensity are seen within the end-plates adjacent to the third lumbar intervertebral disc (*thick arrows*). (TR 500 msec, TE 20 msec.) **B:** These end-plates become isointense to normal bone marrow with T2 weighting (*arrows*). (TR 250 msec, TE 20 msec, 12° flip angle.) **C, D:** The MR findings correspond to the dense bony sclerosis seen on AP (**C**) and lateral (**D**) (*thick arrows*) plain radiographs of the lumbar spine. Note linear areas of marked signal loss within the first, second, third, and fifth lumbar interspaces in (**A**) (*thin arrows*), which corresponds to intradiscal gas identified on the plain films (**C**) and (**D**) (*thin arrows*) and computed tomography (not illustrated).

three types of change observed may have no clinical correlation. However, it is important to recognize these changes as being degenerative so as to distinguish them from other etiologies such as neoplasm or infection.

Degenerative (Surgical Lesions)

The loss of disc space height associated with degeneration results in malalignment and altered mechanical stresses on the facet joints and ligaments. In an attempt at stabilization, facet joint hypertrophy, ligamentous laxity and hypertrophy, and lipping at adjacent endplates occur. This together with the diffuse bulging of the annulus fibrosus results in narrowing of the central spinal canal, lateral recesses, and/or neural foramina. This process, called spondylosis, may affect multiple levels and may progress to result in significant nerve root or cauda equina compression. On MRI, dorsal and ventral extradural defects are evident at the level of the interspaces (Fig. 5-21). These changes are most prominent posteriorly. Axial T1W and T2W images are essential for determining the degree of stenosis present because sagittal images can be misleading. Sagittal T1W sequences tend to underestimate the degree of stenosis, while sagittal T2W or gradient-echo images tend to overestimate it. Because of a magnetic susceptibility effect, axial gradient-echo sequences may also overestimate the degree of stenosis (Fig. 5-22). Similar changes of spondylosis can be observed in the cervical region, with the result being a compressive cervical myelopathy of varying degrees. As in the lumbar spine, these changes usually involve multiple levels and predominantly involve the mid and low cervical interspaces (Fig. 5-23). With chronic compression, areas of increased T2 signal have been observed within the cord parenchyma from myelomalacia (83,112). This finding has some prognostic significance because patients with myelomalacia (increased T2 signal) respond less favorably to surgical or medical management than those without it (112). Cystic necrosis and atrophy are seen in the late stages of myelomalacia. These patients have a poor prognosis regardless of management.

Studies have shown that MRI identifies more abnormalities, particularly in the cervical region, than CT myelography. Most of these changes are minimal and have no clinical correlation. Teresi et al. have observed asymptomatic "significant" spinal cord impingement in 16–26% of patients referred for MR examinations of the larynx (114). These studies underscore the importance of proper triage and clinical correlation of the imaging findings. Because of the ease in obtaining a MR image and its noninvasive nature, the MR examination may be performed in lieu of a good neurologic examination in patients with nonspecific symptoms. Caution is advised in interpreting these studies to avoid subjecting patients to unnecessary operations.

Nevertheless, severe central canal stenosis can usually be diagnosed by MRI. A substantial number of patients, however, have mild to moderate stenosis, where correlation of the radiologic degrees of stenosis with the severity of clinical signs or symptoms is difficult or impossible. A myelogram may provide additional information in these instances. At fluoroscopy, the degree of obstruction to the flow of contrast material can be evaluated, as well as the presence or absence of dilated vessels and redundant nerve roots, which are additional criteria that may be used for operation, particularly in patients with less specific clinical syndromes.

Herniated Nucleus Pulposus

Focal disc herniations result from rupture of the annulus fibrosus with extrusion of the nucleus pulposus out of the disc space. The herniations are most commonly posteriorly into the spinal canal, where they may be midline in location or extend to the right or left. Midline disc herniations are often asymptomatic unless they are large and result in considerable compromise of the central canal. More often, the posterior disc herniations extend to the right or left of midline where they cause symptoms of radiculopathy as they compress the traversing nerve root of the vertebral body segment below. Ten to fifteen percent of all disc herniations are lateral in location with extension of disc material within or beyond the neural foramen (101). These herniations are more subtle and may be confused with diffuse bulging of the annulus fibrosus unless the herniated fragment is large. Lateral disk herniations, because they compress the exiting nerve roots, cause radiculopathies of the nerve roots of the same vertebral body segments. Other locations of herniations include central herniations with extension of disc material into adjacent vertebral bodies (Schmorl's nodules) (Fig. 5-24) and anterior locations with extension of disc material anterior to the vertebral bodies (50,76). Whether or not these herniations are clinically significant is controversial. Jinkins et al. (50) hypothesized a vertebrogenic symptom complex of local and referred pain and autonomic reflex dysfunction within lumbosacral zones of the head from anterior and central disc herniations compressing afferent sensory fibers. Currently, these findings have no surgical significance.

In our practice, we use the term disc protrusion to imply a surgically significant herniation of the nucleus pulposus that is still confined by the outermost annular layers. On sagittal and axial images, the disc material is seen only at the level of the interspace. Once the nucleus has ruptured completely through the annulus (disc extrusion), it is free to extend above, or more commonly below, the level of the interspace. It may still be contained by the posterior longitudinal ligament or extend through the ligament to become a free disc fragment.

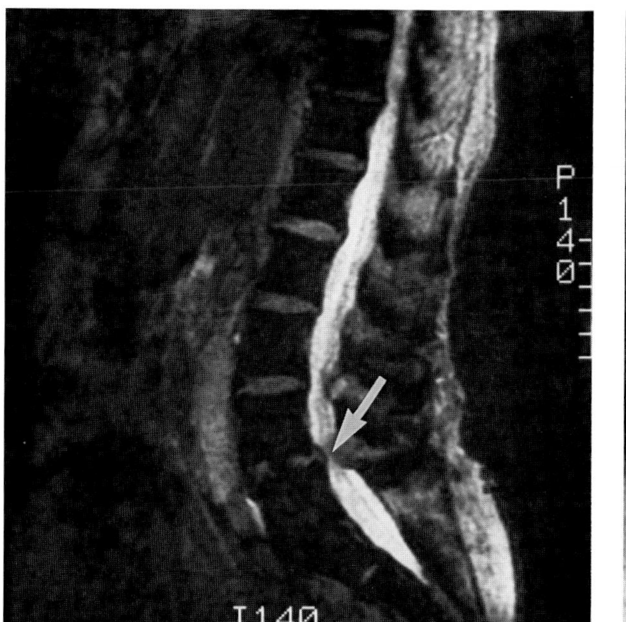

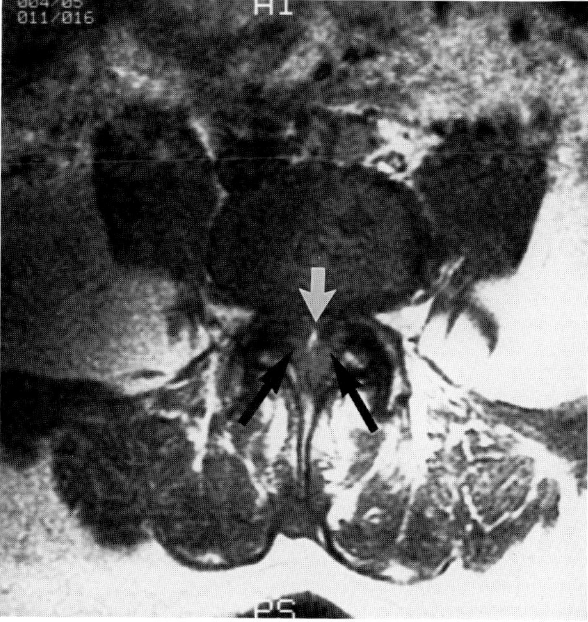

A,B

FIG. 5-21. A: Sagittal lumbar spine shows hypertrophy of the ligamentum flavum and mild bulging annulus at the fourth lumbar interspace, resulting in narrowing of the subarachnoid space (*arrow*). These changes are superimposed on slight degenerative subluxation of L4 on L5. (TR 400 msec, TE 20 msec, 12° flip angle.) **B:** The central canal stenosis is confirmed on this axial section (*white arrow*), which shows facet joint hypertrophy and thickening of the ligamentum flavum (*arrows*). (TR 600 msec, TE 20 msec.)

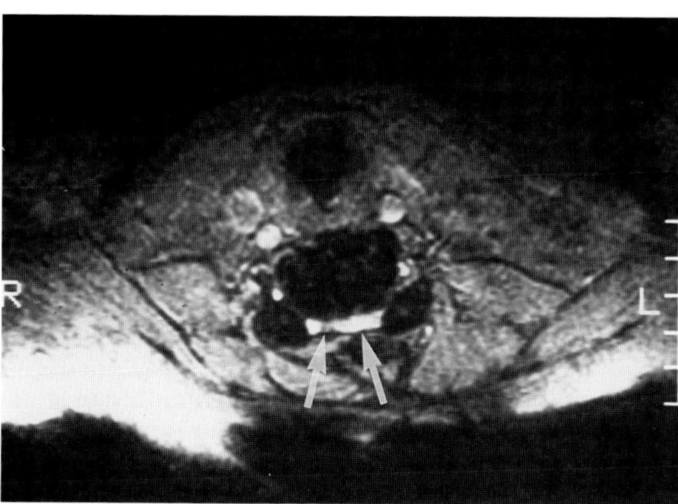

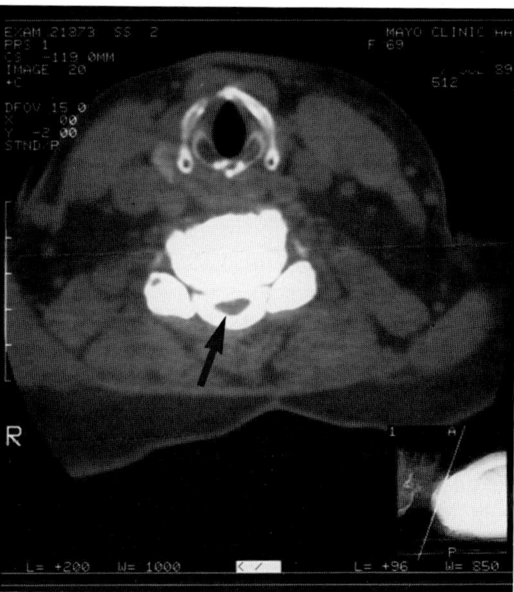

A,B

FIG. 5-22. A: Apparent recurrent central canal stenosis (*arrows*) is seen at the fifth cervical interspace in this patient who has had a previous cervical decompressive laminectomy. The spinal cord cannot be distinguished from the CSF because of increased T2 signal from myelomalacia. (TR 500 msec, TE 20 msec, 12° flip angle.) **B:** Postmyelographic CT section at the same level shows only atrophy of the spinal cord (*arrow*) and no recurrent stenosis. This is the most severe overestimation of stenosis that we have encountered.

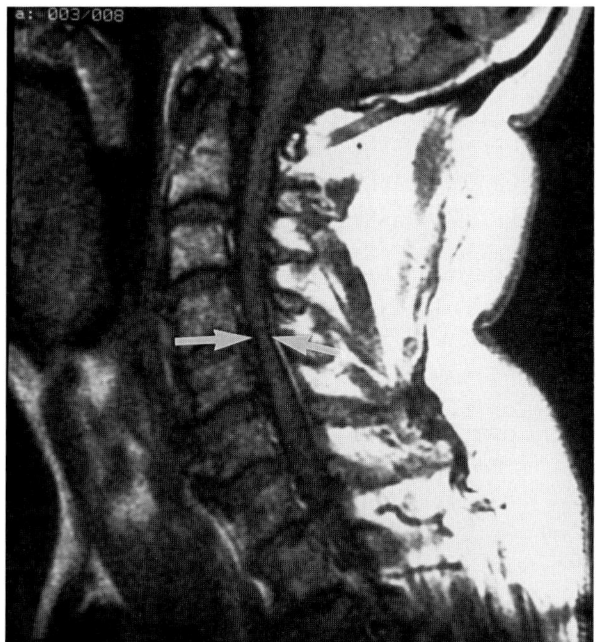

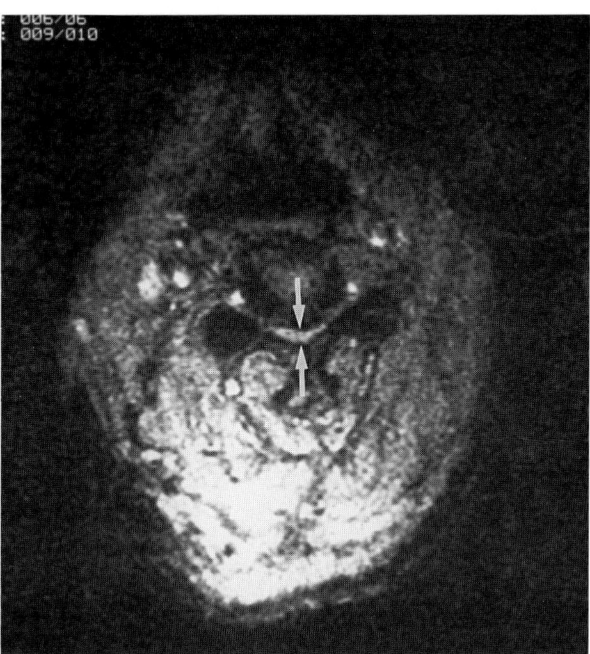

A,B

FIG. 5-23. A: Sagittal cervical spine demonstrates changes of spondylosis with the midcervical spine superimposed on a congenitally small canal. The changes are most marked at the fourth cervical interspace level where they result in AP compression of the underlying spinal cord (*arrows*). (TR 500 msec, TE 20 msec.) **B:** Axial gradient-echo sequence confirms the presence of severe central canal stenosis here with marked flattening of the underlying cord (*arrows*). Note how the degree of stenosis is greater than predicted in (**A**). (TR 500 msec, TE 20 msec, 12° flip angle.)

Disc fragments no longer maintain their attachment to the parent disc and may extend several millimeters above or below the interspace.

Not all disc herniations are surgical lesions (119). Due to the ubiquitous nature of degenerative disc disease and disc herniations (central, anterior, midline), many asymptomatic lesions are found on imaging studies. To be surgically significant, the herniated disc must be large enough and in the correct location (posterior right or left, lateral) to compress the appropriate nerve root or roots that correspond to a defined clinical syndrome.

With MRI, lumbar disc herniations may be suspected on sagittal images but must be confirmed on axial sequences. Similar criteria as used in CT myelography are applied. Posterior disc herniations result in a focal bulge in the disc contour, resulting in compression of epidural fat and mass effect with displacement of the traversing nerve root if the disc extends to the right or left. Relatively acute free fragments may signal greater than the parent disc on T2W sequences, presumably secondary to inflammation (60) (Fig. 5-25). Post Gd T1W axial images may better delineate the herniated disc fragment from the dural sac as the peripheral portion of the disc may enhance, presumably secondary to ingrowth of new vessels in an attempt at repair (90) (Fig. 5-26). Lateral disc herniations are more difficult to image. A soft tissue mass within the neural foramen is seen that obliterates the foraminal fat (Fig. 5-27). Under ideal circumstances, MRI has been shown to be equal to myelography in the diagnosis of disc herniations in the lumbar region (66). However, in our experience, many times the examinations are suboptimal for a number of reasons (motion, patient factors, and asymmetric positioning), particularly in older patients who tend to have a paucity of intraspinal fat. In these circumstances, a confident diagnosis of a clinically significant disc herniation cannot be made, so a myelogram is always performed.

In the cervical region, many studies show MRI to be more or less equal to CT myelography in diagnosing disc herniations (13,46,67), particularly if the herniated fragment is large or has a midline component (Fig. 5-28). However, due to the small size of the structures being imaged, small slice thicknesses and small fields of view are necessary to evaluate the neural foramen. This pushes the technique beyond the limits of its resolution, so that small disc herniations may be overlooked or overdiagnosed. While CT myelography suffers from similar limitation, the spatial resolution is still better and the combination of a cervical myelogram with follow-up CT affords the best chance at the diagnosis of clinically significant small cervical herniations.

Disc herniations may also occur in the thoracic region as well (Fig. 5-29). Many of these lesions may have no clinical/surgical significance, unless they are large and result in spinal cord compression (99). Similar imaging criteria, as used in the cervical or lumbar region, are

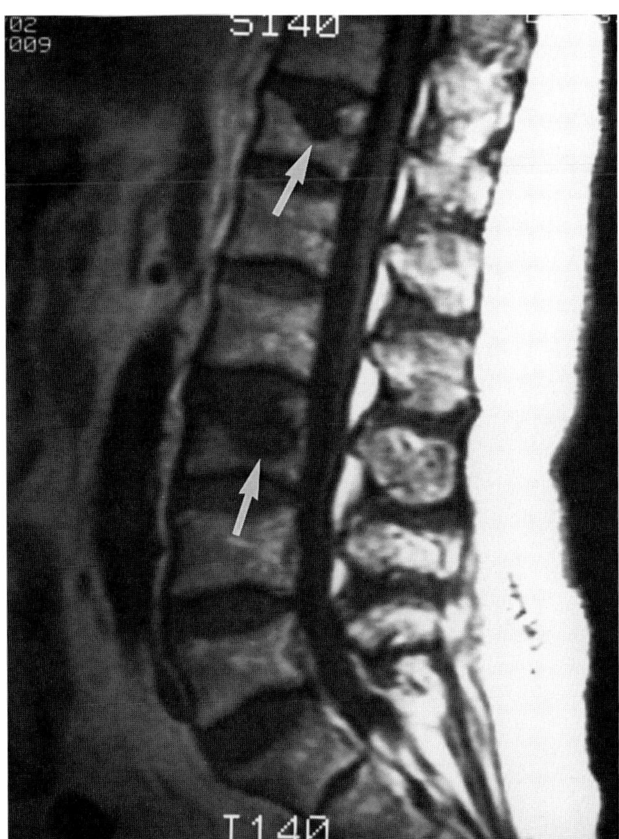

FIG. 5-24. Central herniation of disc material through the superior end-plates of T12 (*arrows*) and L3 (*curved arrows*). This is the typical appearance of Schmorl's nodules. (TR 500 msec, TE 20 msec.)

applied here (91). Axial views are necessary to determine the degree of cord compression, if present.

Postoperative Evaluation

Causes of persistent pain or the failed back syndrome include mechanical low back pain from altered stresses and spinal instability, as well as arachnoiditis, dural scarring, and recurrent disc herniation. Often these conditions cannot be differentiated clinically and imaging evaluation is requested. Imaging evaluation of the postlaminectomy patient with recurrent pain is difficult but clinically important because the patients with recurrent disc herniation may benefit from reoperation, whereas in the other conditions listed, symptoms may actually worsen because further laminectomies may make the spine more unstable and increase the amount of arachnoiditis and dural scarring. MRI may be useful in the differentiation of recurrent disc from dural scarring (14,39,48,49,85–87,106).

In arachnoiditis, the nerve roots of the cauda equina either clump together or migrate to the periphery of the dural sac where they become incorporated into the dural wall, resulting in a thick rind of dura, nerve roots, and scar tissue. Individual nerve roots may be visualized by MRI, and the imaging appearance of arachnoiditis has been described in the literature (88). The findings are best seen on T1W axial images and are similar to those seen on the CT myelogram with clumping of individual nerve roots, peripheral migration to the edges of the dural sac, and thickening of the dura. However, no large well-controlled, pathologically confirmed studies comparing the sensitivity and specificity of MRI versus myelo CT in the diagnosis of arachnoiditis exist.

Postcontrast MRI is showing promise in the differentiation of recurrent discs from dural scarring (49,86). This differentiation has always been difficult since not even myelo CT or post-intravenous contrast CT (10,37,113) can reliably distinguish between the two. In both of these conditions, anterior soft tissue mass may be present at the level of the interspace, resulting in obliteration of the epidural fat and nonvisualization of the nerve root or roots on the noncontrast MRI. This soft tissue may or may not appear to be continuous with the laminectomy site. Sometimes the signal of the tissue may be different from the dural sac, disc margin, and nerve roots on T1W or T2W sequences, so a diagnosis of scar tissue can be made with confidence. However, more often the signal of the soft tissue mass cannot be differentiated from normal neural structures. Intravenous gadolinium administration has been most valuable in these conditions. In theory, scar tissue enhances because it is vascular, whereas disc material is avascular and should not enhance (at least not initially) (49,85,86). T1W axial sequences performed immediately following contrast infusion demonstrate enhancement of the scar tissue, allowing it to be differentiated from the dural sac, nerve roots, and disc material (Fig. 5-30). If the epidural soft tissue enhances and the traversing or exiting nerve root can be well visualized and not displaced on postcontrast images, a confident diagnosis of dural scarring can be made (Fig. 5-31). If a nonenhancing anterior soft tissue mass persists that displaces or compresses the nerve root, a recurrent disc herniation is suspect (Fig. 5-32). Some combination of enhancing scar and nonenhancing disc material may be present (Fig. 5-33). However, confusion still exists if there is soft tissue enhancement and mass effect with displacement of the nerve roots. We have observed surgically proven disc fragments that enhanced immediately following contrast administration on MRI, as well as nerve roots being tethered and displaced by dural scar (Fig. 5-34).

Neoplasms

Spinal neoplasms are best characterized by their location relative to the dural sac and spinal cord. Three main compartments can be identified: extradural, intradural

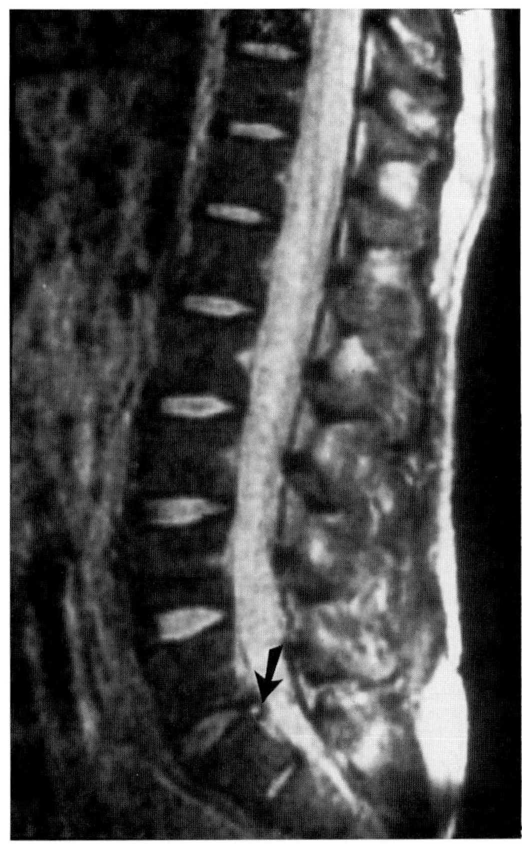

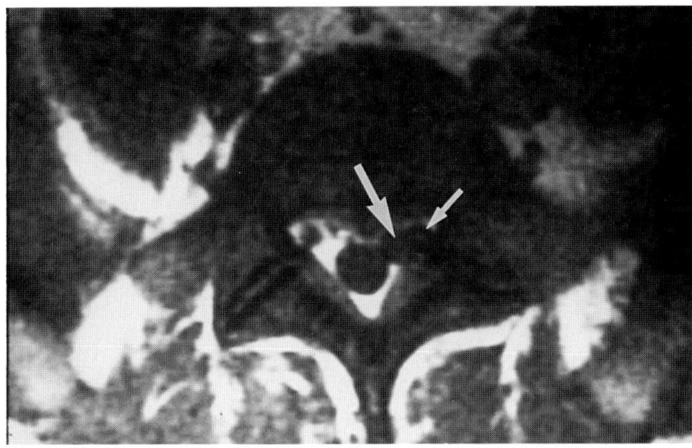

A,B

FIG. 5-25. A: A small disc extrusion at the lumbosacral level is identified on this midline view. The disc material that extends below the level of the interspace demonstrates increased T2 signal relative to the parent disc (*arrow*). (TR 1,500 msec, TE 60 msec.) **B:** The presence of a disc fragment at the lumbosacral level on the left is confirmed on this axial view (*large arrow*), which has lodged between the dural sac and the left S1 nerve root (*small arrow*). (TR 500 msec, TE 25 msec.)

extramedullary, and intramedullary (101). The extradural compartment contains the bony spinal canal and ligaments, epidural space and venous plexus, and the intervertebral discs. The pia, arachnoid, CSF, blood vessels, and nerve roots comprise the intradural extramedullary compartment. The intramedullary compartment includes the spinal cord parenchyma and the filum terminale. The differential diagnosis of spinal neoplasms depends on which compartment the neoplasm arises within since characteristic lesions are seen at each location.

Extradural Lesions

Extradural neoplasms may be primary bone tumors (chordoma, sarcoma), focal or diffuse marrow infiltrative disorders (multiple myeloma, lymphoma), or, more commonly, metastatic lesions. Unlike CT or plain films, MRI studies do not directly image the bone but rather the bone marrow. Bony neoplasms are identified best on T1W sequences by a loss of the normal marrow fat signal (Fig. 5-35). Increased signal on T2W or gradient-echo sequences may be seen (4,22,62,104). It appears that MRI is more sensitive than a radionuclide bone scan in the detection of spinal metastasis (4,62). The benign cavernous hemangioma is the only lesion that shows increased signal relative to normal marrow on T1W sequences and variable signal (increased, decreased, isointense) relative to normal marrow on T2W or gradient-echo sequences (Fig. 5-36). The differential diagnosis of bone neoplasms and marrow infiltrative disorders are discussed in more detail in Chapters 12 and 14, respectively.

One major advantage of MRI over CT, plain films, and myelography is its ability to noninvasively image epidural extension of neoplasm directly (16,81). This is best seen on T2 weighted/gradient-echo sequences, where associated spinal cord or nerve root compromise can be identified and the levels of involvement determined for surgical or radiation therapy planning (Fig. 5-37). Unfortunately, many of these patients with significant epidural disease are in severe pain, making the MRI study suboptimal or nondiagnostic. In a prospective study comparing MRI to myelopathy in cancer patients with suspected epidural disease, Quint et al. (81)

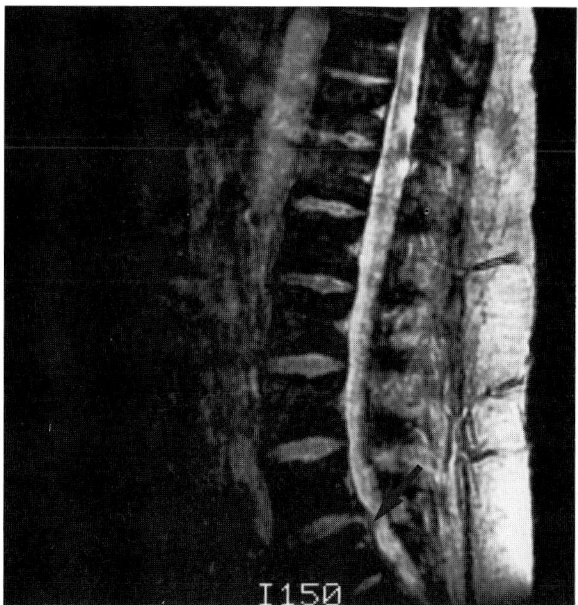

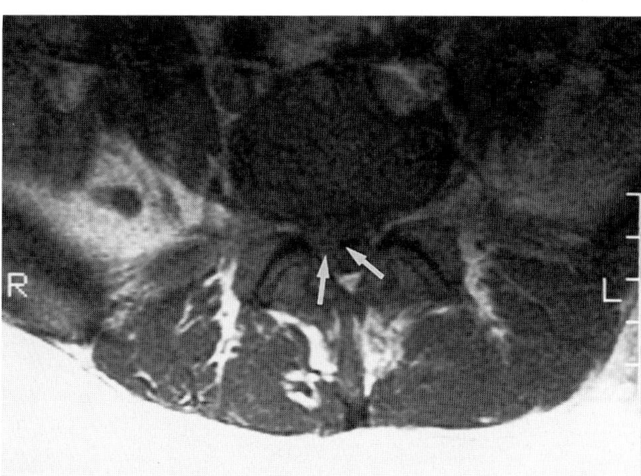

A,B

C

FIG. 5-26. A: Sagittal lumbar spine demonstrates a disc extrusion at the fifth lumbar interspace with inferior migration of disc material over S1 (*arrow*). (TR 300 msec, TE 20 msec, 12° flip angle.) **B:** This axial view confirms its presence on the right (*arrows*). (TR 500 msec, TE 20 msec.) **C:** The margins of this disc fragment enhance following gadolinium administration, which increases its conspicuousness (*arrows*). Also note that the disc fragment slightly enhances since its signal intensity is greater than that of the parent disc. (TR 500 msec, TE 20 msec.)

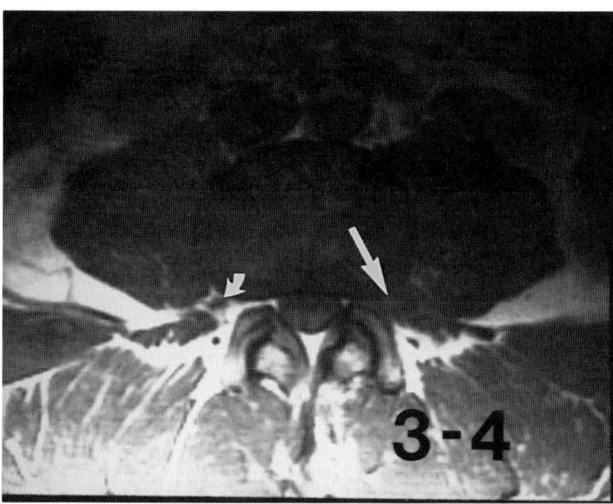

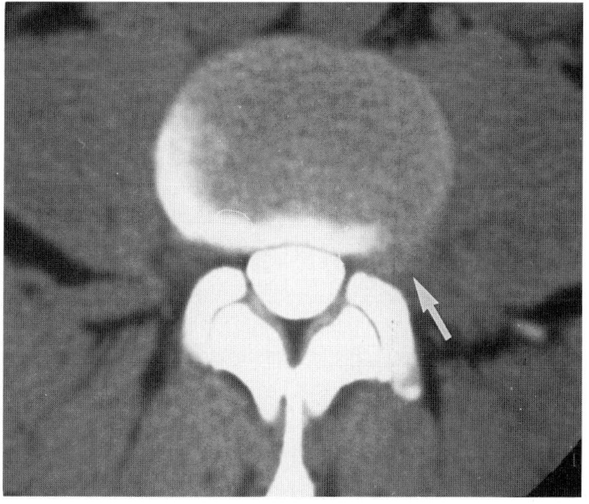

A,B

FIG. 5-27. A: Axial image at the third lumbar interspace demonstrates obliteration of the paraspinal fat within and lateral to the intervertebral foramen on the left (*arrow*). The left L3 nerve root cannot be visualized as a separate structure as is seen on the right (*short curved arrow*). (TR 650 msec, TE 20 msec.) **B:** Postmyelogram CT at the same level showing the same findings (*arrow*) in this patient with a surgically proven lateral disc fragment.

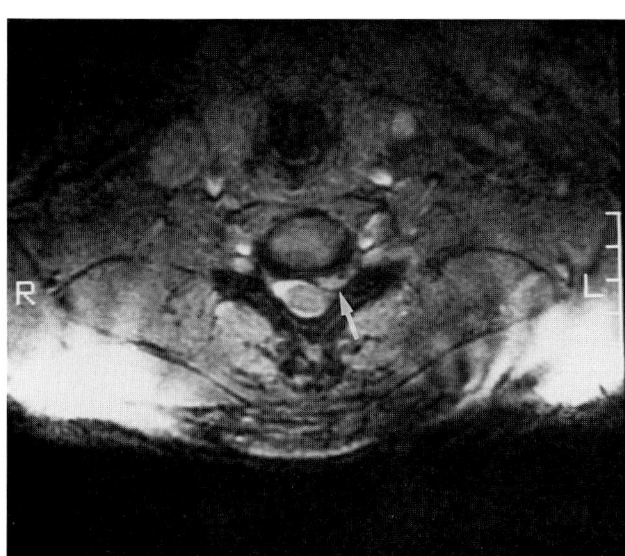

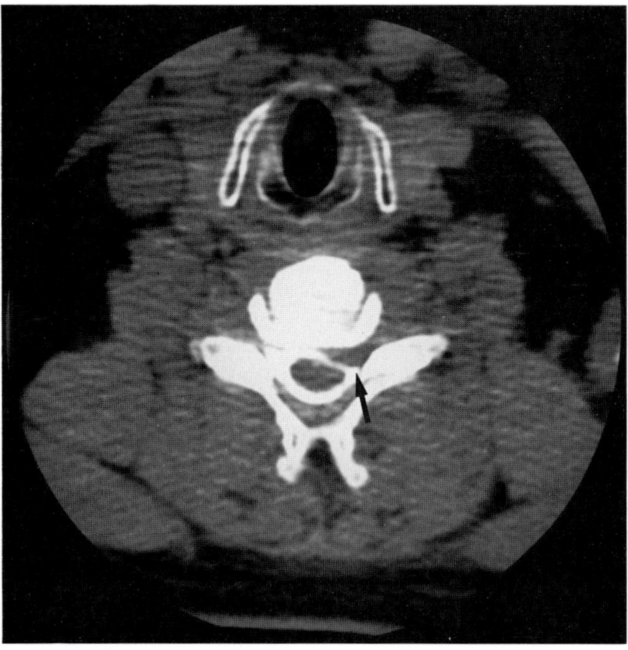

A,B

FIG. 5-28. A: This axial image was obtained at the sixth cervical interspace level. It shows a disc extrusion on the left that effaces the subarachnoid space and partially fills the neural foramen (*arrow*). (TR 600 msec, TE 20 msec, 20° flip angle.) **B:** Postmyelogram CT at the same level confirms these findings.

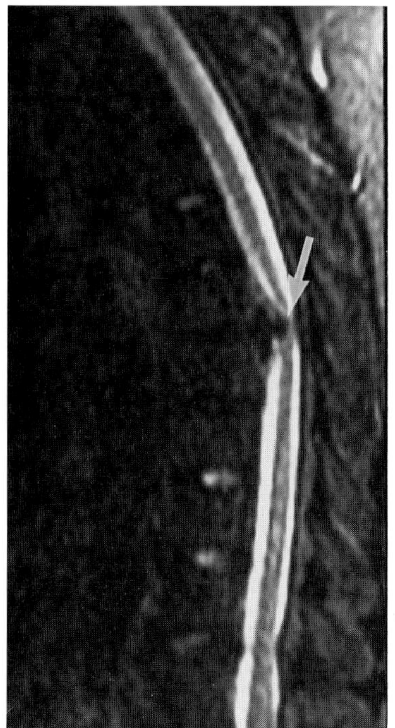

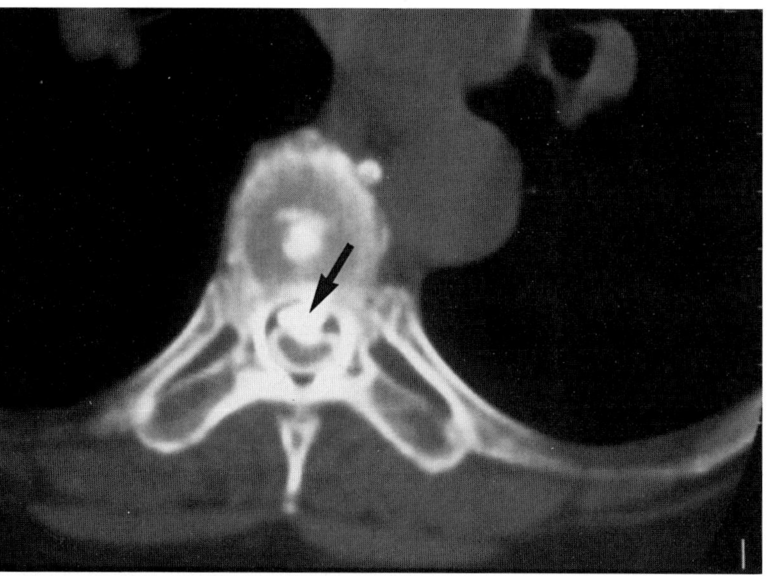

A,B

FIG. 5-29. A: Sagittal thoracic spine shows a large midline disc herniation at the sixth thoracic interspace that narrows the spinal canal and compresses the spinal cord (*arrow*). This disc demonstrates signal loss, indicating a calcified composition. (TR 1,500 msec, TE 140 msec.) **B:** Postmyelogram CT section at this level confirms the presence of a heavily calcified disc fragment within the spinal canal (*arrow*). Note that the degree of central canal narrowing and spinal cord compression is overestimated on the MR illustrated in (**A**).

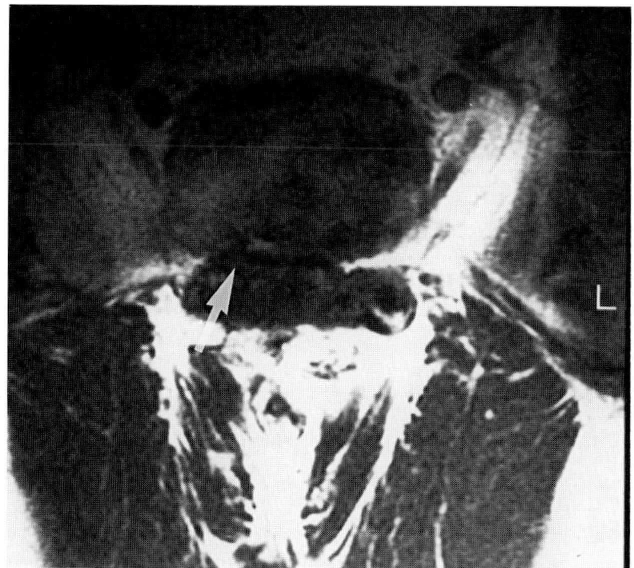

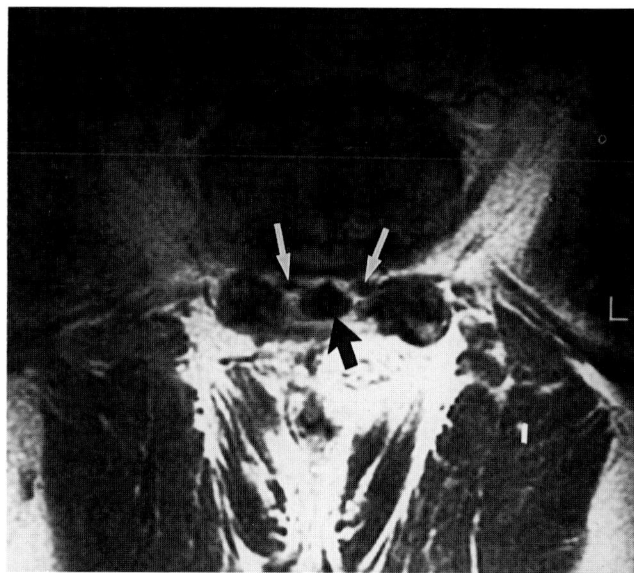

A,B

FIG. 5-30. A: Axial section through the fourth lumbar interspace in a patient with a prior decompressive laminectomy and recurrent low back pain. Intraspinal contents are obscured at this level and the question of a recurrent disc protrusion on the right is raised (*arrow*). (TR 300 msec, TE 20 msec.) **B:** Postcontrast image at the same level demonstrates enhancement of epidural scar tissue so that the dural sac (*thick black arrow*) and L5 nerve roots (*thin white arrows*) are seen as separate structures. There is no evidence of recurrent herniation on this view. (TR 300 msec, TE 20 msec.)

found 40% of the MRI exams performed to be nondiagnostic despite sedatives. A myelogram may ultimately be needed for definitive evaluation.

MRI contrast agents such as Gd-DTPA may provide additional information in the evaluation of extradural neoplasm. However, contrast-enhanced only studies should not be performed as screening sequences because contrast enhancement can be confusing and may actually obscure pathology (11,111). We have observed bony metastases that enhanced isointense normal bone marrow, making them undetectable on postcontrast T1W sequences (Fig. 5-38). These sequences should only be used as an adjuvant after noncontrast T1 and T2 weighted/gradient-echo weighted sequences have been performed. In cases where extension of epidural neoplasm is not clear, postcontrast images have been useful because the epidural component enhances, allowing differentiation from dural sac and surrounding bony ligamented structures (Fig. 5-39).

Intradural Extramedullary Lesions

Meningiomas and neurogenic tumors (neurilemoma and neurofibroma) are the most common intradural extramedullary neoplasms encountered. Less common lesions include lipomas, which may or may not be clinically significant, and intradural metastases.

Meningiomas

Meningiomas most commonly occur in the thoracic region in middle-aged females, lie posterior to the spinal cord, and compress the posterior columns. A few may be located anteriorly. Typically, on MRI they present as a well-circumscribed thoracic intradural mass that can be separated from the spinal cord parenchyma. They are usually isointense to cord parenchyma on T1W and T2W or gradient-echo sequences. Coarse or linear areas of decreased signal relative to the cord parenchyma may also be observed within these lesions on T2W sequences, which corresponds to calcification seen at pathology (Fig. 5-40). Because these lesions lack a blood–brain barrier, homogeneous enhancement following gadolinium administration is observed on postcontrast T1W studies (27,77,108). There may be a broad base of attachment to the dura (Fig. 5-41).

Neurogenic Tumor

In contrast to meningiomas, neurogenic tumors can occur anywhere in the spinal canal. There is no sex predilection and they tend to occur in a slightly younger population. The presenting symptoms depend on their location (cervical, thoracic, lumbar) and may be similar

Text continues on p. 121

A,B

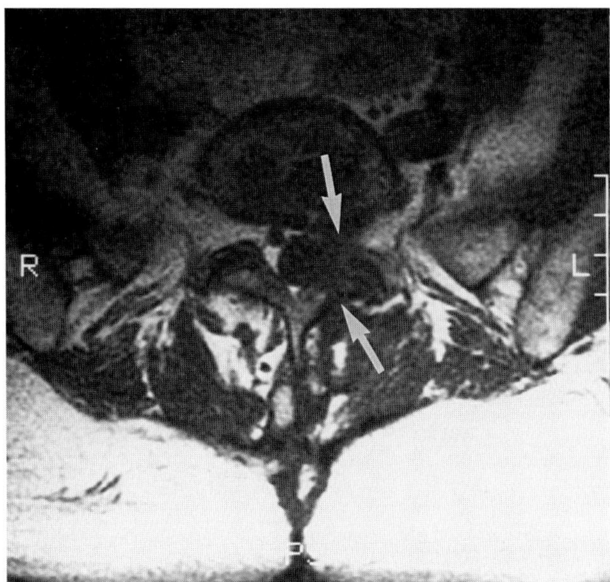

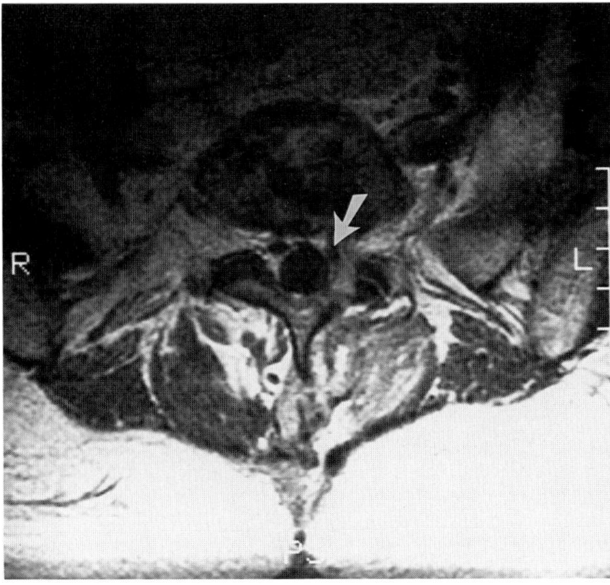

FIG. 5-31. **A:** Axial section through the lumbosacral level in a patient with a prior left L5 laminectomy is indeterminate for recurrent disc herniation. Soft tissue is seen on the left, which extends from the laminectomy site to the posterior disc margin (*arrows*). The left S1 nerve root is not identified. (TR 500 msec, TE 20 msec.) **B:** This postcontrast study at the same level as in (**A**) demonstrates enhancing epidural scar that extends to the posterior disc margin and surrounds the left S1 nerve root (*arrow*), which is not displaced. The changes seen in (**A**) can all be accounted for on the basis of dural scarring. (TR 400 msec, TE 20 msec.)

A,B

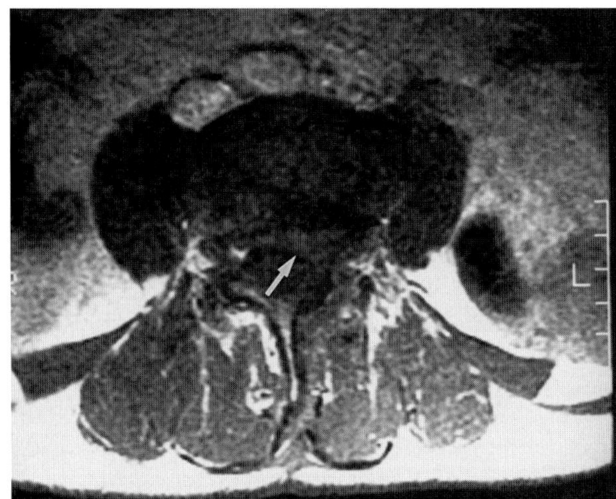

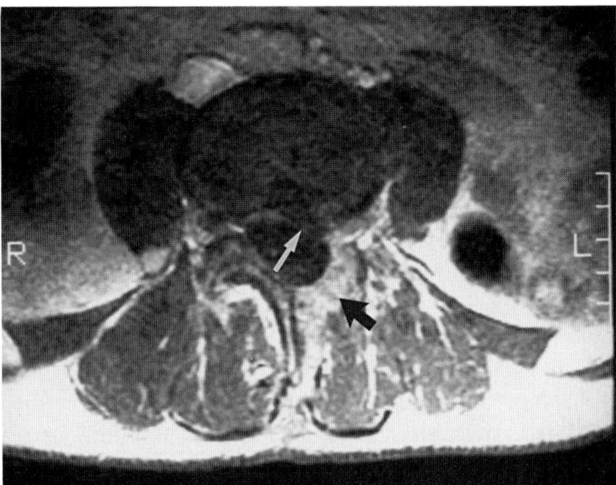

FIG. 5-32. **A:** This is a precontrast image through the fourth lumbar interspace of the patient illustrated in Fig. 5-18. A recurrent disc protrusion is suspected on the left (*arrow*). However, this anterior epidural soft tissue mass blends imperceptibly with the tissue at the laminectomy site. **B:** Following contrast administration, the epidural scar on the left (*thick black arrow*) enhances, clearly delineating the dural sac, while the disc protrusion does not (*thin white arrow*). A diagnosis of recurrent disc protrusion can be made with greater confidence. (TR 500 msec, TE 30 msec.)

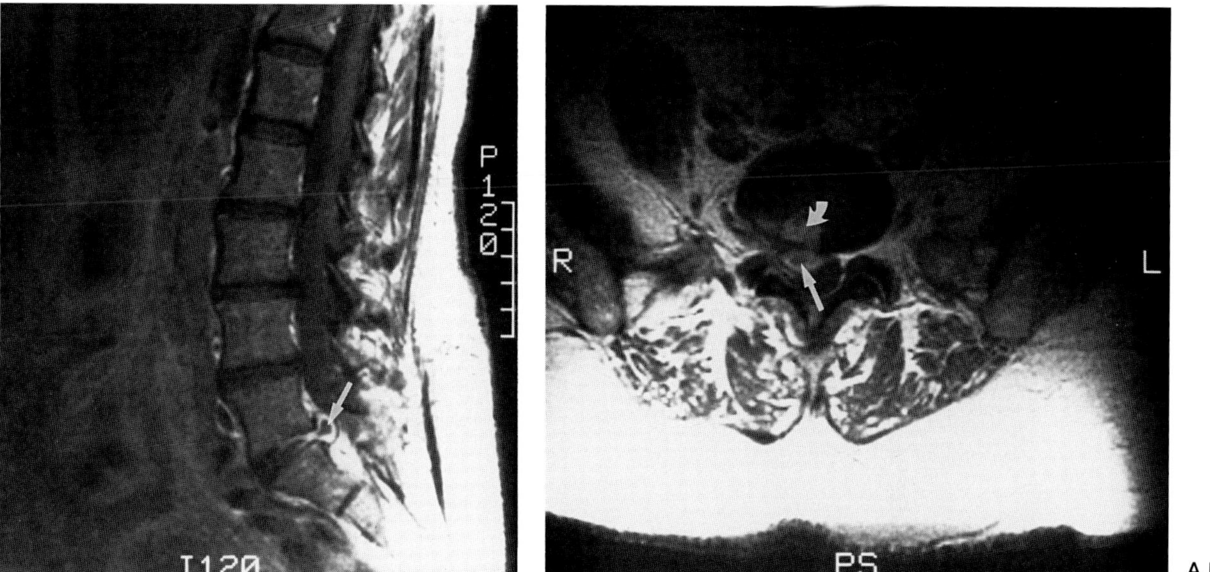

FIG. 5-33. **A:** This postcontrast sagittal lumbar spine demonstrates the coexistence of epidural scarring and recurrent disc protrusions. Enhancing scar tissue is seen around a nonenhancing recurrent disc fragment (*arrow*). (TR 800 msec, TE 30 msec.) **B:** Similar findings can be seen on this enhanced axial image at the fifth interspace (*arrow*). Note extension of enhancement into the posterior aspect of the intervertebral disc on the right, which is presumably secondary to ingrowth of new vessels in a repairative attempt (*short curved arrows*). (TR 600 msec, TE 20 msec.)

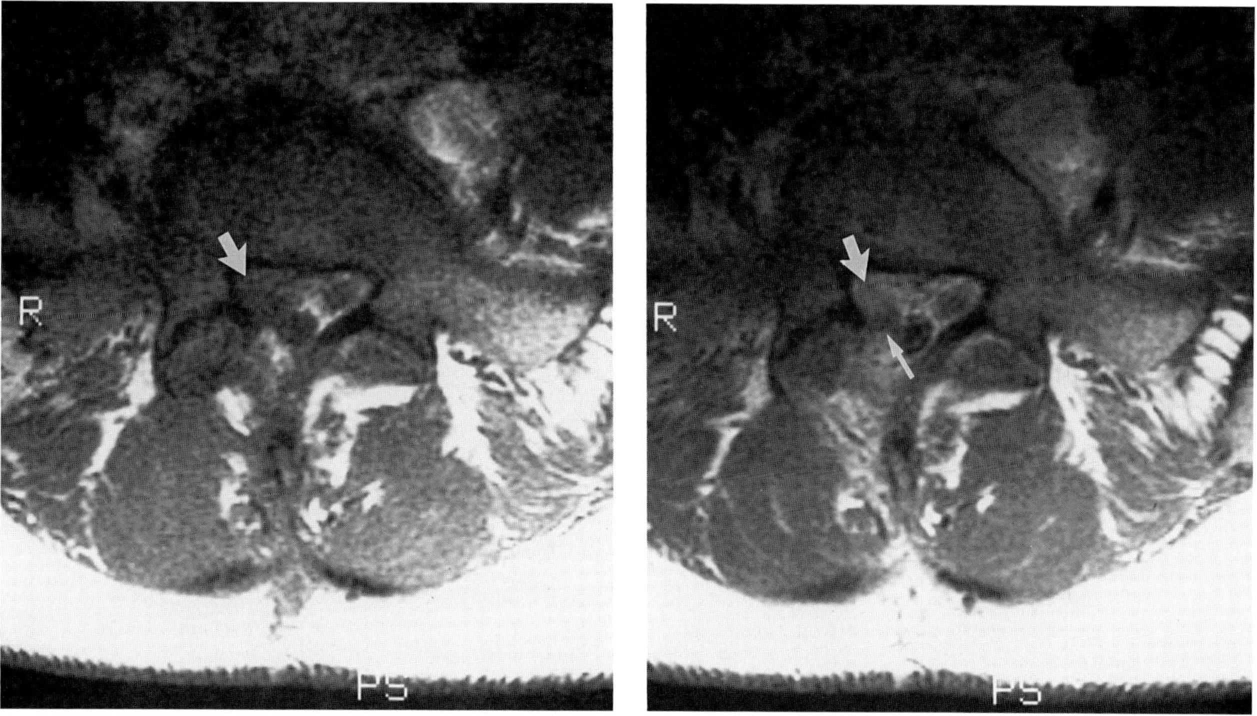

FIG. 5-34. **A:** A large anterior epidural soft tissue mass is seen at the lumbosacral level on the right in this patient with a prior right L5 laminectomy (*arrow*). (TR 600 msec, TE 20 msec.) **B:** This image was obtained at the same level as (**A**) immediately following contrast administration. The epidural soft tissue mass enhances similar in degree to the scar tissue identified at the laminectomy site, implying epidural scar (*arrow*). The right S1 nerve root is displaced posteriorly (*thin arrow*). This patient was reoperated at this level because of a high clinical suspicion of a recurrent disc fragment, which was confirmed at surgery. This case and Fig. 5-26 illustrate the point that not everything that enhances is scar. (TR 600 msec, TE 20 msec.)

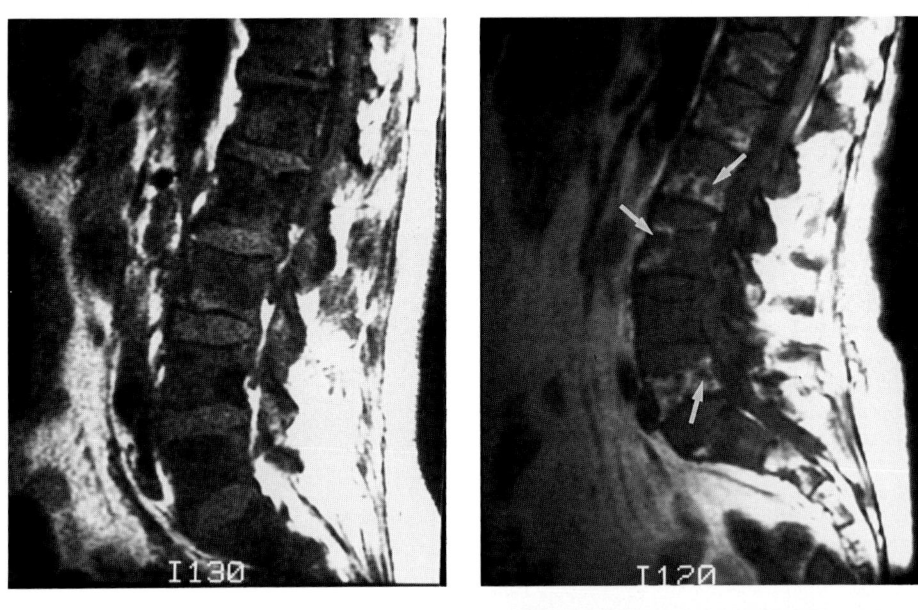

A,B

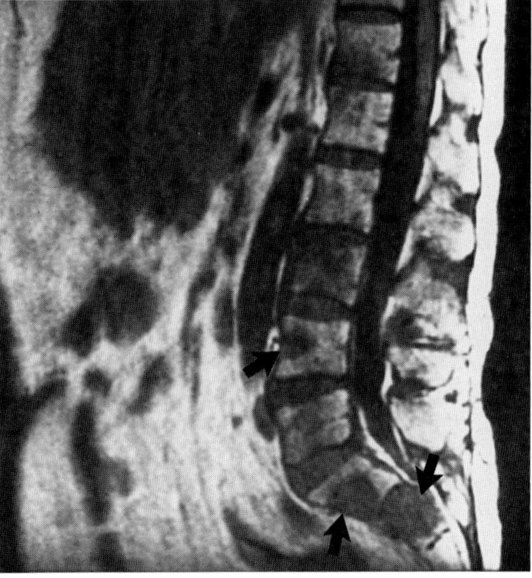

C

FIG. 5-35. Loss of the normal marrow fat signal is seen on these sagittal images of the lumbar spine in three patients with (**A**) metastatic prostate carcinoma, (**B**) multiple myeloma, and (**C**) metastatic hepatocellular carcinoma. The changes are diffuse in (**A**), focal (*arrows*) and diffuse in (**B**), and focal (*arrows*) in (**C**). Compare these images to Fig. 5-10, which illustrates the normal marrow fat signal. (TR 500 msec, TE 20 msec.)

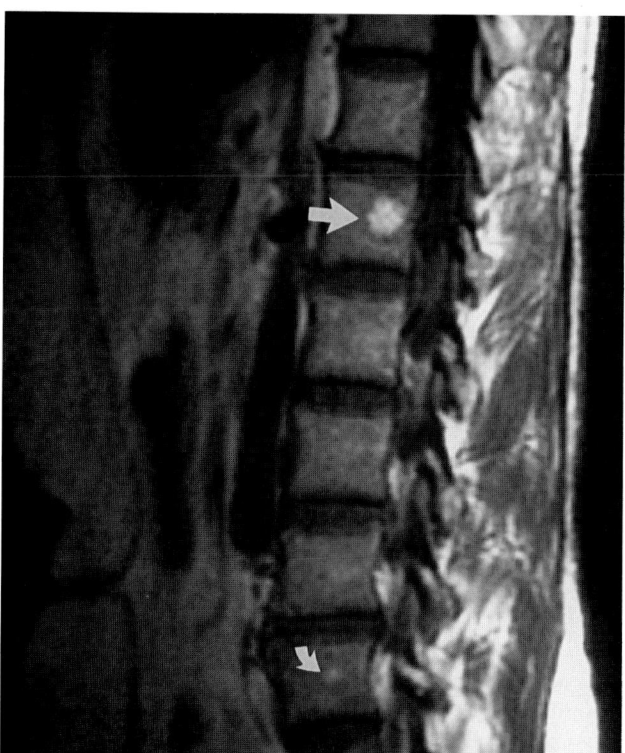

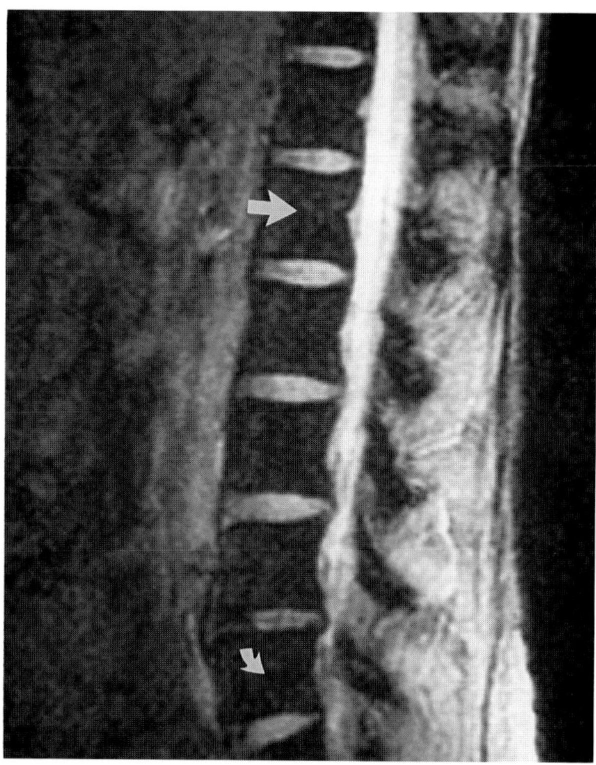

A,B

FIG. 5-36. A: A well-circumscribed lesion of increased signal intensity is seen within the posterior aspect of the L1 vertebral body (*arrow*). A similar appearing but much smaller lesion is seen within L5 (*small curved arrows*). (TR 500 msec, TE 20 msec.) **B:** These lesions, presumably benign cavernous hemangiomas, become isointense to normal bone marrow on this gradient-echo sequence. (TR 350 msec, TE 20 msec, 12° flip angle.)

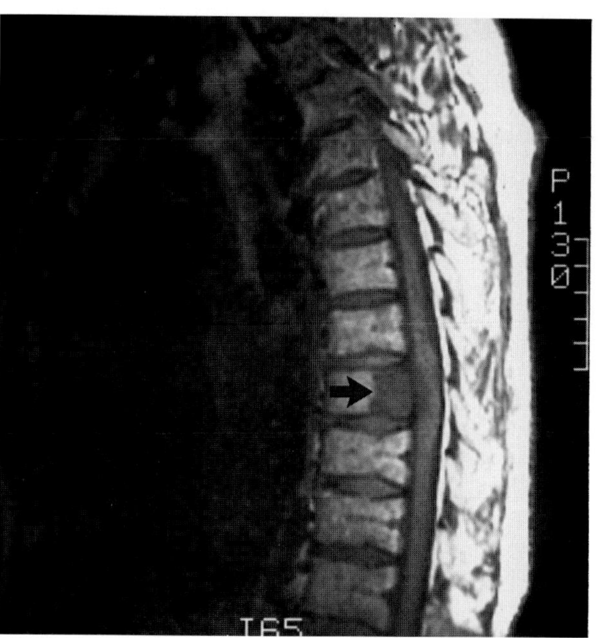

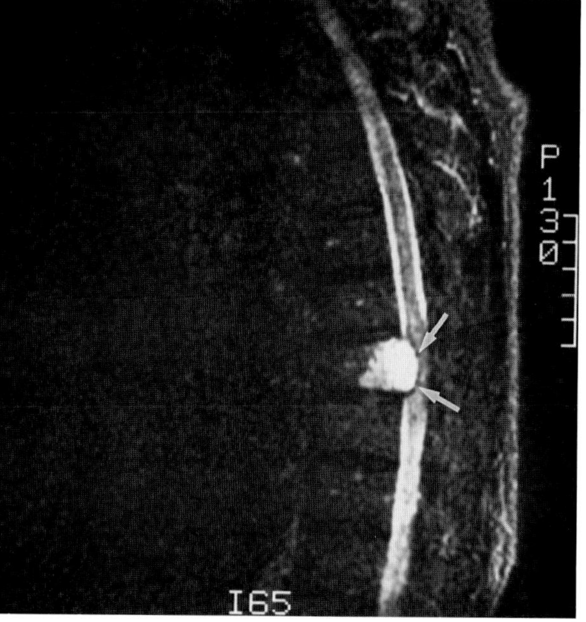

A,B

FIG. 5-37. A: A T9 bony metastasis from known cranial chordoma is seen as a loss of the normal marrow fat in this patient with a thoracic myelopathy (*arrow*). (TR 500 msec, TE 20 msec.) **B:** An associated epidural soft tissue component is seen to better advantage with T2 weighting (*arrows*), resulting in spinal canal narrowing and compression of the thoracic spinal cord. (TR 1,500 msec, TE 140 msec.)

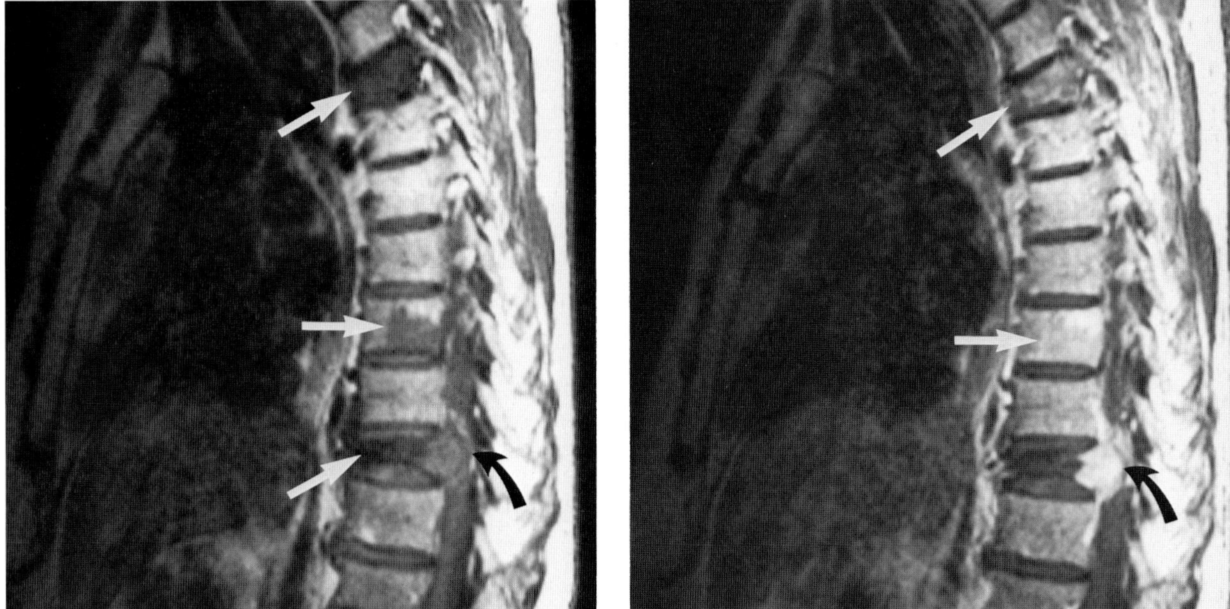

FIG. 5-38. **A:** Sagittal thoracic spine illustrates loss of normal marrow fat signal within T4, T8, and T10 vertebral bodies from transitional cell carcinoma metastasis (*arrows*) and intraspinal extension at T10 (*curved arrow*) (TR 500 msec, TE 25 msec) **B:** After contrast administration, the bony metastatic lesions at T4 and T8 enhance similar to normal bone marrow (*arrows*) and thus are not evident. Note that the epidural extension of tumor at T10 (*curved arrow*) enhances and compresses the spinal cord (TR 500 msec, TE 25 msec).

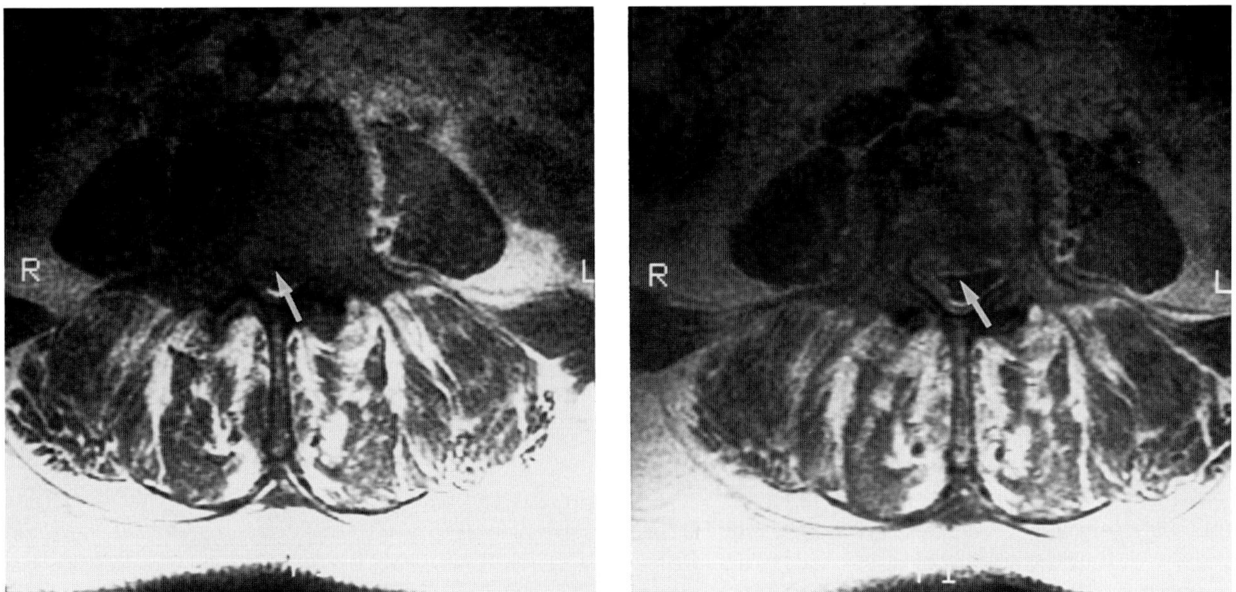

FIG. 5-39. **A:** This is an axial image at the L4 vertebral body level from the patient illustrated in Fig. 5-35B. The question of epidural spread of disease is raised anteriorly and on the right (*arrow*). (TR 500 msec, TE 20 msec.) **B:** Following contrast administration, intraspinal extension of neoplasm is more apparent as the epidural component enhances, allowing it to be distinguished from the dural sac (*arrows*). (TR 550 msec, TE 20 msec.)

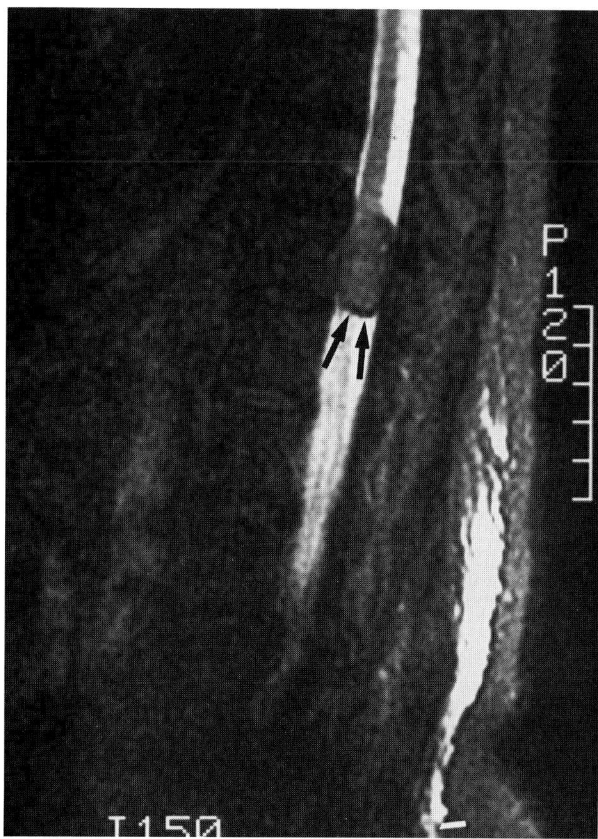

FIG. 5-40. This well-circumscribed intradural extramedullary mass at T10 proved to be a meningioma at surgery. Note the linear area of signal loss at the periphery of the mass (*arrows*), which corresponded to calcifications noted at pathology. (TR 1,500 msec, TE 140 msec.)

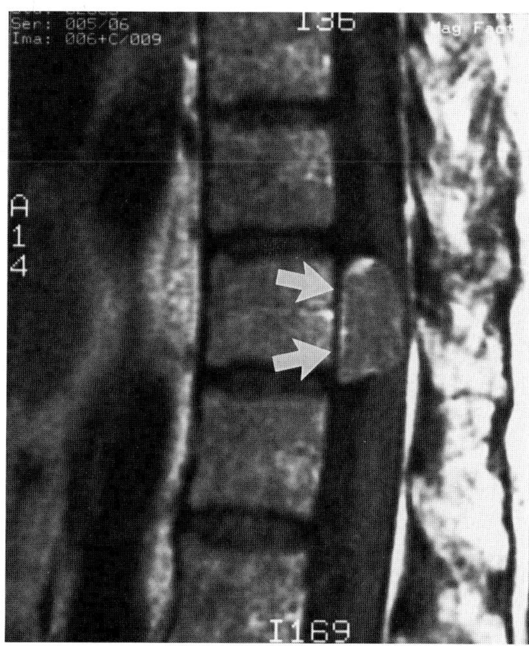

FIG. 5-41. Postcontrast sagittal thoracic spine shows a homogeneously enhancing intradural extramedullary mass at T11 level. The mass is located anteriorly within the spinal canal and has a broad base of attachment to the anterior dura (*arrows*). This too was a meningioma at operation. (TR 500 msec, TE 20 msec.)

to that seen in meningiomas or disc disease. They are also more likely to be multiple. Neurofibromas are neoplasms of the nerves themselves and occur only in association with neurofibromatosis. Nerve sheath tumors—neurilemomas—are the most common neurogenic tumors encountered in the nonneurofibromatosis patient.

The typical MRI appearance of a neurogenic tumor is that of a well-circumscribed, slightly lobulated intradural extramedullary mass that is located lateral or posterolateral to the spinal cord. Sixteen percent have an extradural component that extends through the neural foramen into the paraspinal soft tissues (dumbbell tumor) (101). The extradural component may be quite prominent and may widen the neural foramen. As in meningiomas, neurogenic tumors tend to be isointense to spinal cord parenchyma on T1W and T2W or gradient-echo sequences. However, their MRI appearance is more variable (15,116) because neurogenic tumors have a propensity to undergo cystic degeneration and central necrosis, which makes them hypointense on T1W sequences and hyperintense on T2W or gradient-echo sequences, more similar to CSF. If large areas of cystic degeneration or necrosis are present, they may be difficult to identify on noncontrast sequences, especially if a large field of view is used. As with meningiomas, neurogenic tumors lack a blood–brain barrier. Their appearance on postcontrast T1W sequences varies because they may enhance homogeneously, inhomogeneously, or peripherally, depending on the degree of cystic degeneration (Fig. 5-42).

Lipoma

Intraspinal lipomas demonstrate the typical MRI appearance of fat, being hyperintense to cord parenchyma on T1W sequences and hypointense on T2W or gradient-echo sequences, similar to bone marrow and paraspinal fat (Fig. 5-43). The normal bright T1 signal can be confused with enhancement if only postcontrast studies are obtained and lead to an erroneous diagnosis of meningioma or neurogenic tumor. These uncommon intraspinal lesions can occur anywhere in the spinal canal and do not have an age or sex predilection. Tending to be well circumscribed, these slightly lobulated tumors usually do not deform the spinal cord. Some may cause symptoms if large; others are found incidentally in patients being evaluated for nonspinal indications. Contrast-enhanced sequences offer no additional information.

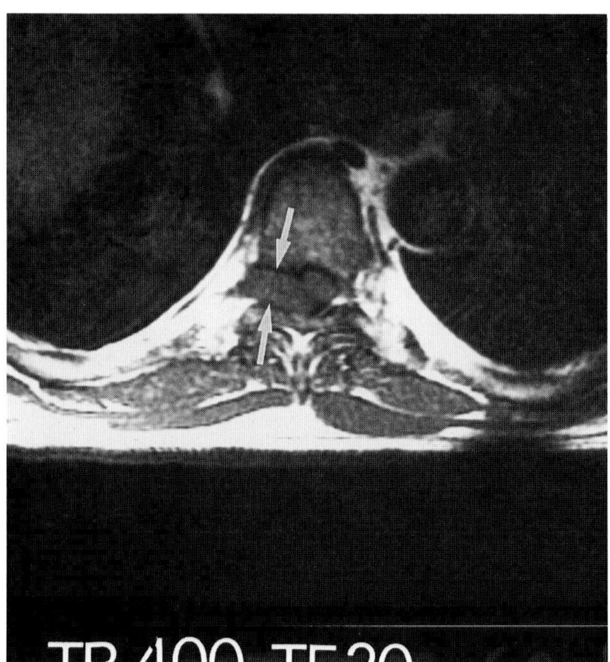

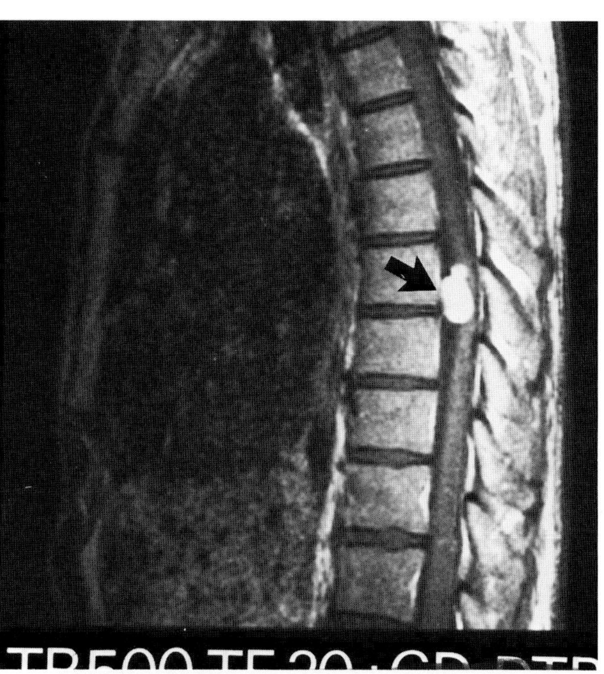

A,B

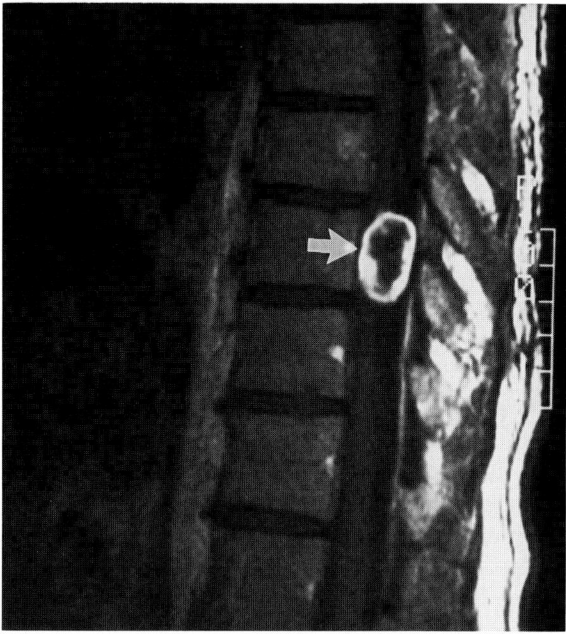

C

FIG. 5-42. A: This axial image, obtained at the eighth thoracic interspace, demonstrates an oval-shaped right-sided intraspinal mass that extends through an expanded T8 neural foramen (*arrows*). This neurilemoma was both intradural and extradural in location at operation. (TR 400 msec, TE 20 msec.) **B:** Postcontrast midline sagittal thoracic spine in another patient with a slightly lobulated homogeneously enhancing intradural extramedullary mass centered at the eighth thoracic interspace (*arrow*). This too was a neurilemoma at surgery. (TR 500 msec, TE 20 msec.) **C:** Another postcontrast sagittal thoracic spine demonstrates a large peripherally enhancing cystic or necrotic intradural extramedullary mass at T9 (*arrow*). A partially necrotic neurilemoma was found at surgery. (TR 500 msec, TE 20 msec.) These three cases illustrate the variety of appearances of neurilemomas encountered.

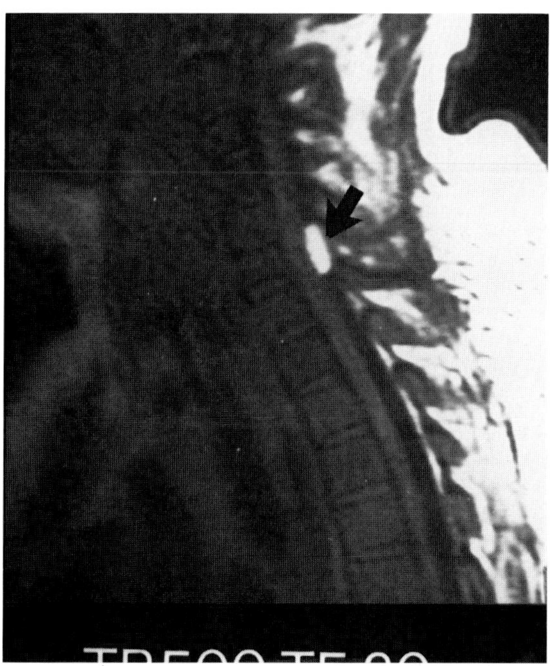

FIG. 5-43. A well-circumscribed, oval-shaped intraspinal mass is seen at C6 posteriorly on this sagittal view (*arrow*). It is characterized by increased signal, similar to the paraspinal and subcutaneous fat. (TR 500 msec, TE 20 msec.) This lipoma was an incidental finding in this neurologically normal patient.

Intradural Metastasis

Intradural metastases may be dropped metastases from midline primary CNS tumors (pineal tumors, ependymomas, medulloblastomas, glioblastoma), local invasion from primary spinal cord neoplasms (ependymomas), or hematogenously disseminated neoplasms to the CSF from aggressive nonneurologic primary neoplasms (breast, lung, melanoma). Unless large, these deposits of tumor are not visualized on noncontrast MRI sequences (7,55) (Fig. 5-44). The MRI findings are similar to that seen on myelography (53). Nodular enhancement along the spinal cord surface or enhancing nodules attached to the nerve roots of the cauda equina are seen on enhanced T1W sequences (Fig. 5-45). Some researchers report increased detectability of leptomeningeal tumor spread on contrast-enhanced MRI compared to myelography (108). However, we have observed one case in which the myelogram was positive and the postcontrast MRI was, at best, equivocal (Fig. 5-46). CSF cytology remains the mainstay for diagnosing intradural metastases.

Intramedullary Lesions

Ependymoma

Of the primary cord neoplasms, ependymomas are the most common tumors (60–70%) (101). They occur predominantly at the conus/filum terminale but can be seen anywhere in the spinal cord. There is no sex predilection and they most often occur from the third through the sixth decades of life. They are slow growing, benign, well-circumscribed lesions that may be focal or involve long segments of the cord and may be associated with bony remodeling of the spinal canal. The tumor may contain areas of prior hemorrhage, cystic degeneration, or calcium. Often, there is an associated spinal cord cyst that widens the cord above and/or below the neoplasm.

MRI features include fusiform intramedullary expansion of the spinal cord parenchyma in conjunction with decreased signal relative to the cord on T1W sequences and increased signal on T2W or gradient-echo sequences. If the ependymoma arises from the filum terminale, an intradural mass separate from the conus can be seen that cannot be differentiated from neurogenic tumor (Fig. 5-47). The signal changes are often complex, depending on the presence or absence of hemorrhage, calcium, or necrosis. The presence of an associated spinal cord cyst often complicates the picture (42). The cysts usually contain a high protein fluid, appear solid, and are difficult to distinguish from the neoplasm. Associated edema may have a similar appearance, adding to the confusion. Postcontrast T1W sequences are essential in the evaluation of any intramedullary neoplasm (11,27,77,107,110,116). The margins of the tumor enhance, allowing it to be separated from the edema or spinal cord cyst (Fig. 5-48). This allows for exact localization of the tumor within the spinal cord, limiting the size of the laminectomy required. The ependymoma may be disproportionately small relative to the length of the cord cyst and difficult to identify on noncontrast studies (Fig. 5-49).

Astrocytoma

Astrocytomas comprise 30–40% of primary cord neoplasms, present at a slightly earlier age than ependymomas (30–40 years), and lack a sex predilection (101). They can be low- or high-grade lesions. Higher grades of malignancy tend to afflict patients who present at the younger ages. The MRI appearance resembles ependymomas because they have a variety of appearances and may undergo necrosis and may be associated with spinal cord cysts or edema (77,110,116). In the young, these tumors tend to be infiltrative lesions, involve long segments of the spinal cord, and may have a more homogeneous appearance on MRI (Fig. 5-50). As in ependymomas, postcontrast T1W sequences are needed to define the extent of the neoplasm.

Hemangioblastoma

Hemangioblastomas are uncommon, benign, primary spinal cord neoplasms often associated with von Hip-

A,B

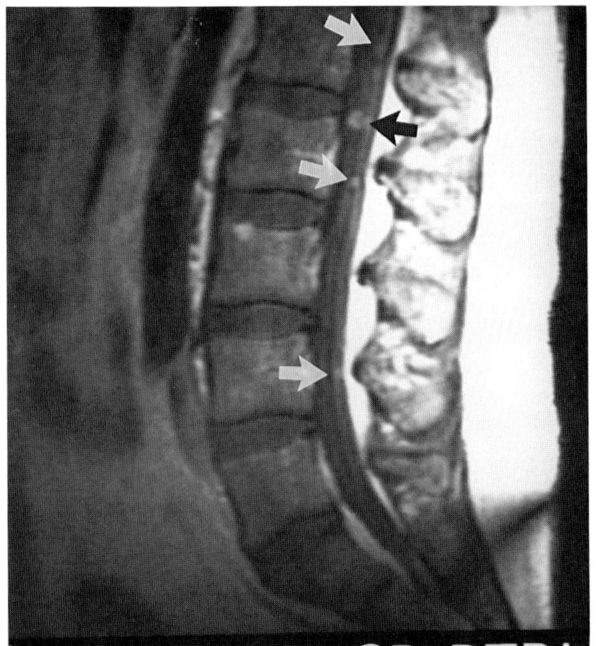

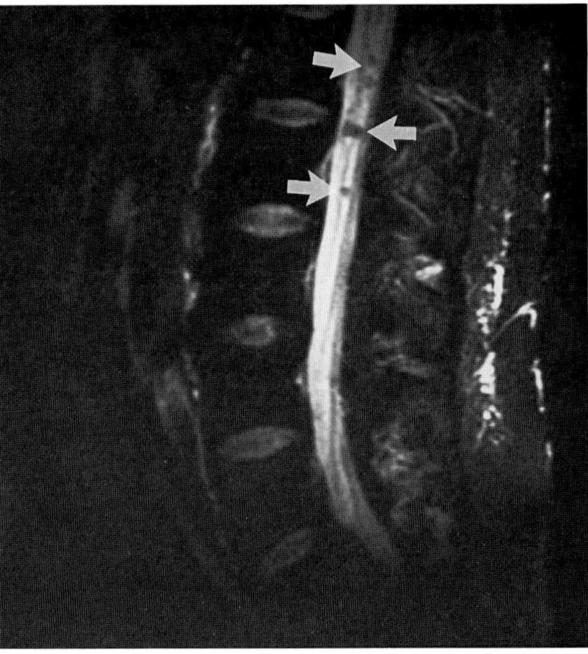

FIG. 5-44. A: Multiple high-intensity intradural nodules involving the nerve roots of the cauda equina are seen on this enhanced sagittal lumbar spine (*arrows*). CSF cytology was positive for metastatic melanoma. Presumably, these nodules are hyperintense because of the paramagnetic effect of melanin rather than enhancement. A precontrast study was not performed. (TR 500 msec, TE 20 msec.) **B:** These nodules can also be identified with T2 weighting (*arrows*). (TR 1,700 msec, TE 120 msec.)

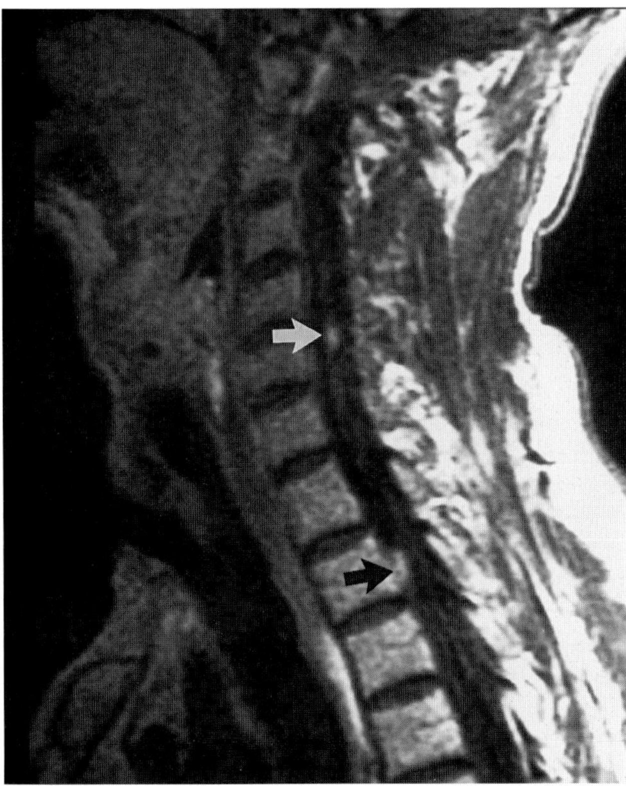

FIG. 5-45. Two enhancing intradural metastatic deposits are seen in this patient with a high-grade fourth ventricular glial mesenchymal tumor and positive CSF cytology (*arrows*). (TR 500 msec, TE 20 msec.)

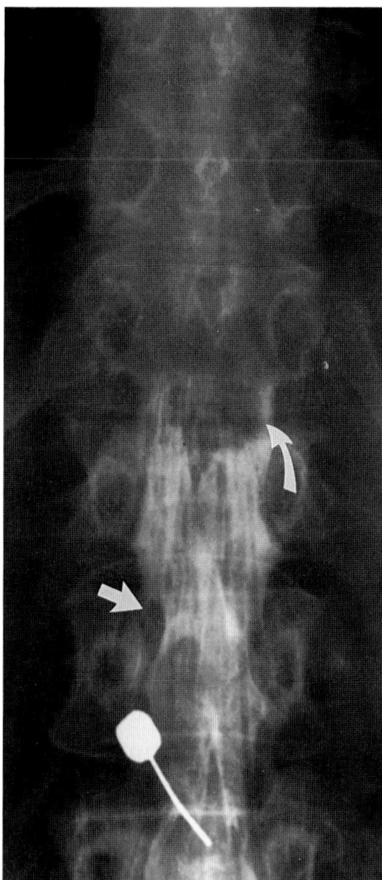

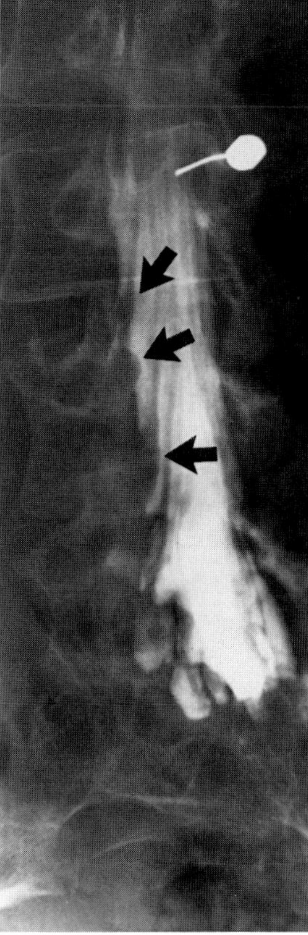

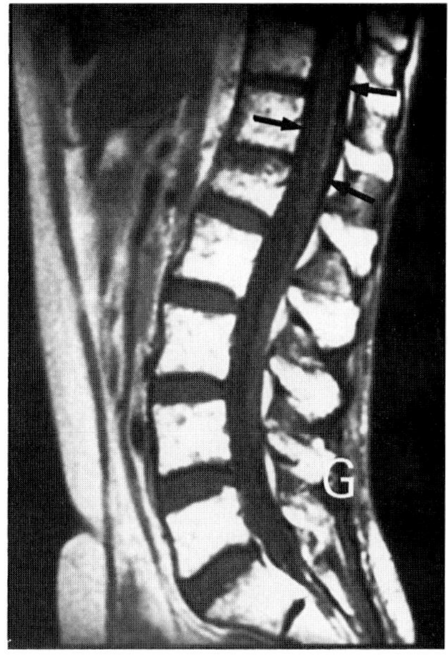

A,B,C

FIG. 5-46. AP (**A**) and oblique (**B**) myelograms obtained for detection of intradural metastasis in a patient with a recurrent fourth ventricular neoplasm and a polyradiculopathy. These views demonstrate beading of multiple nerve roots of the cauda equina (*arrows*) and a metastatic deposit at the conus (*curved arrow*) from diffuse meningeal metastases. **C:** Sagittal enhanced MR image obtained hours after the myelogram. The meningeal metastatic lesions are not evident. Only equivocal pial enhancement of the cord surface is identified (*arrows*). Note increased signal within the marrow of the lower thoracic and lumbar vertebral bodies from prior radiation. (TR 525 msec, TE 20 msec.) From *Mayo Clinic Proceedings* 1989;64:986–1004, with permission.)

pel–Lindau disease. They may be solitary or multiple, most often affect the cervical cord, and present as long areas of intramedullary expansion secondary to a spinal cord cyst or edema. The cystic component may be septated. The neoplasm itself presents as a small mural nodule, which may be eccentric within the cyst wall and may not be visible on noncontrast studies. Postcontrast T1W sequences demonstrate intense enhancement of the nodule (27,77,110) (Figs. 5-51 and 5-52). Associated findings include a dilated posterior pial venous plexus draining the tumor nodule seen as serpentine flow voids along the dorsal aspect of the cord. The combination of abnormal vasculature and a cystic intramedullary mass with an enhancing nodule is fairly diagnostic of a hemangioblastoma. In the absence of a cystic intramedullary mass, the differential diagnosis would include an intramedullary arteriovenous malformation (AVM) (Fig. 5-53).

Metastasis

Intramedullary metastases are uncommon, occurring in only 1–3% of tumor patients (29). As in intradural metastases, these lesions may be from primary CNS neoplasms spread via CSF pathways or hematogenously spread from non-CNS primary tumors. They may be associated with intradural metastases, particularly if the primary tumor is a CNS neoplasm. The metastatic deposits may be singular or multiple, causing fusiform or irregular cord enlargement or no enlargement at all. The involved cord often shows decreased signal on T1W and increased signal on T2W sequences predominantly secondary to edema. Oftentimes, the metastatic deposit itself is small, asymmetrically involving only a portion of the cord parenchyma, which may only be distinguished from the surrounding edema on postcontrast studies (Fig. 5-54).

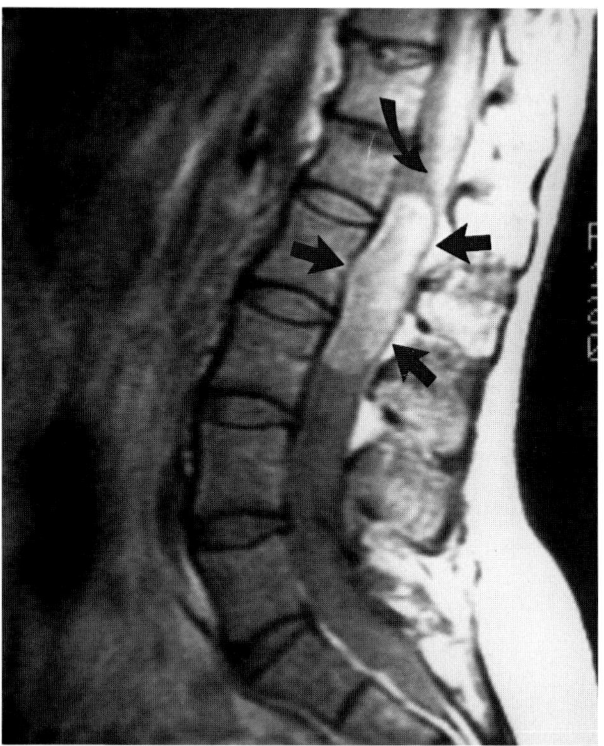

FIG. 5-47. A well-circumscribed, oval-shaped intradural mass is seen on this midsagittal lumbar exam (*arrows*). This mass is separate from the tip of the conus (*curved arrow*). This was an ependymoma arising from the filum terminale at surgery. The differential diagnosis would include an intradural neurilemoma. (TR 1,500 msec, TE 30 msec.)

Inflammatory Conditions

Both the spinal column and the spinal cord may be involved by inflammatory processes. Inflammatory diseases of the spinal column include disc space infection, osteomyelitis of the vertebral bodies, paraspinal abscess, and epidural inflammation or abscess. These patients present with a wide variety of symptoms including sepsis, localized pain and tenderness, and paraplegia. MRI is particularly suited for evaluation of suspected spinal infection since myelography risks iatrogenic meningitis.

Pyogenic Discitis

Disc space infection may be localized to one disc space or uncommonly may involve multiple spaces. Hematogenous pyogenic organisms from remote septic foci spread to the spinal column initially at the vertebral body end-plates. From there, these organisms gain access to the intervertebral discs. The discs are relatively avascular and are unable to mount an inflammatory reaction, which allows the organisms uninhibited growth. This together with the proteolytic enzymes released results in rapid destruction of the intervertebral disc. The adjacent end-plate is then quickly invaded. Depending on the time course and the virulence of the organism, the entire vertebral body can be involved with

A,B

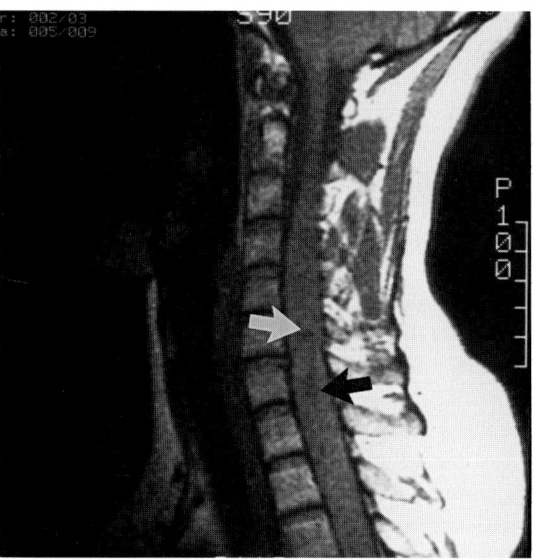

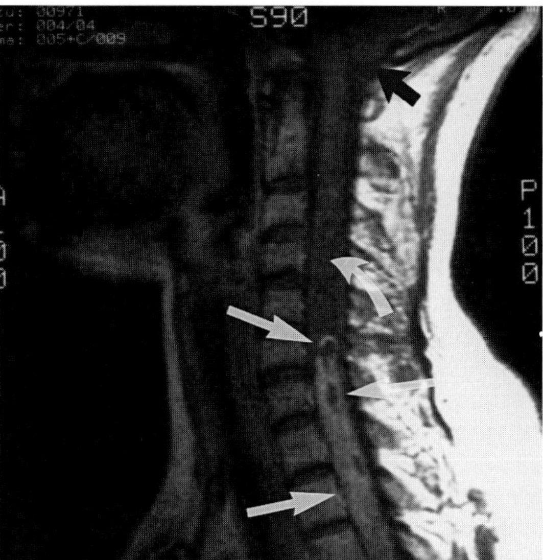

FIG. 5-48. A: Sagittal cervical spine demonstrates fusiform intramedullary widening of a long segment of the spinal cord beginning at C3 and extending below T3. Areas of decreased signal are seen within this lesion (*arrows*). (TR 500 msec, TE 20 msec.) **B:** Postcontrast image at the same level demonstrates an enhancing intramedullary mass, an ependymoma, which begins at C6 (*arrows*). The enlarged cord above the ependymoma was the result of an associated syrinx (*curved arrow*). The lower portion of the tumor is not included on this image. The low attenuation areas noted in (**A**) are seen to better advantage after contrast and represented necrosis at surgery. The cerebellar tonsils are low in position but still maintain a normal rounded configuration (*short black arrow*). (TR 500 msec, TE 20 msec.)

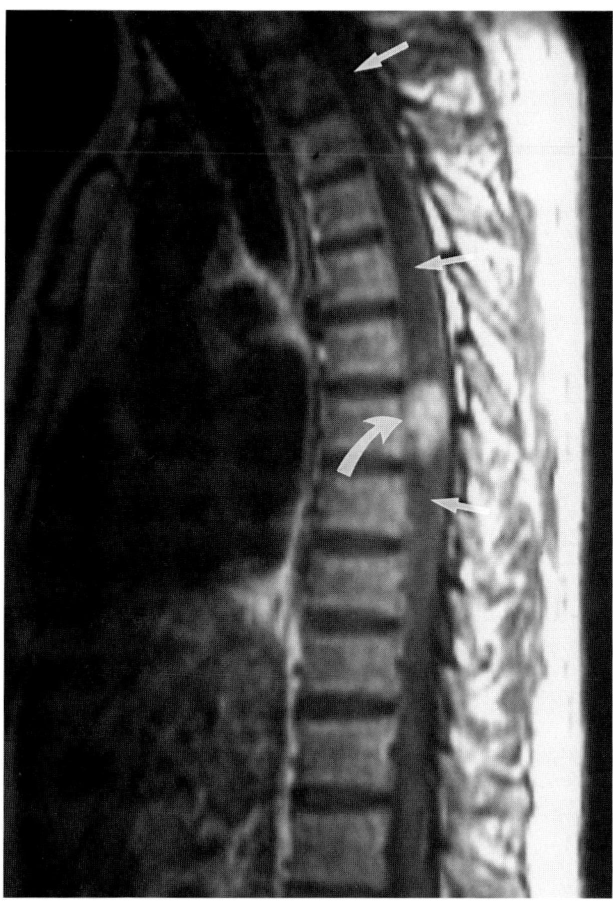

FIG. 5-49. Postcontrast sagittal view of the thoracic spine shows intramedullary expansion of the spinal cord secondary to a long syrinx cavity (*arrows*) that extends from approximately T9 superiorly into the cervical region. A homogeneously enhancing solid intramedullary mass is identified opposite T7 vertebral body (*curved arrow*). A spinal angiogram performed to exclude the possibility of a hemangioblastoma was negative. A limited laminectomy was performed over the enhancing mass, which was determined to be an ependymoma at operation. (TR 600 msec, TE 20 msec.) From *Mayo Clinic Proceedings* 1989;64:986–1004, with permission.)

osteomyelitis. There may an associated paraspinal or epidural abscess. Once the infection has spread to the epidural space, it is free to extend above and below the involved interspace for several segments. The epidural component may consist of inflammatory reaction or abscess. If large, it may cause spinal cord compromise, resulting in a compressive myelopathy or cord infarction from thrombophlebitis of epidural spinal veins.

The MRI findings in pyogenic disc space infection have been well described (24,65). On T1W sequences, decreased signal intensity within the involved intervertebral disc, loss of disc space height, and loss of normal marrow signal within the adjacent vertebral body end-plates are seen. The vertebral body changes may be minimal or extensive, depending on the degree of associated osteomyelitis. With T2 weighting, increased signal is seen within the intervertebral disc and adjacent end-plates (Fig. 5-55). These same areas enhance following the administration of Gd-DTPA. These findings are thought to be fairly specific for pyogenic infection since metastasis rarely involves the intervertebral discs.

Paraspinal/Epidural Abscess

Paraspinal abscesses are best seen on axial T1W or T2W sequences as soft tissue masses or fluid collections that may be loculated or enhance following contrast administration (Fig. 5-56). Hematogenously disseminated pyogenic organisms may primarily infect the epidural space. MRI is ideal to evaluate for the presence and extent of epidural disease, which is best identified on T2W sequences as an extradural mass whose signal intensity is greater than CSF (3,28) (Fig. 5-57). However, the epidural abscess may be difficult to distinguish from CSF in the presence of spinal meningitis. Donovan Post et al. (28) described three patients with surgically proven epidural abscesses where MRI was unable either to diagnose the abscess (one patient) or to determine the true extent of the lesions (two patients). While MRI should be the initial screening procedure in patients with spinal infection, occasionally myelography with CT may be needed as a supplemental study in patients with a nondiagnostic MR exam.

Tuberculous Spondylitis

Tuberculous spondylitis is uncommon and differs from pyogenic discitis and osteomyelitis clinically and on MRI (25,102,103). It has an insidious onset with symptoms ranging from months to years as opposed to days to months in patients with pyogenic infections. The MRI findings, which resemble those for neoplasm, include widespread destruction of the vertebral bodies and relative preservation of the disc spaces. The anterior inferior aspect of the vertebral body is classically affected first, resulting in a gibbous deformity. The entire vertebral body may be involved, including the posterior elements. The infection tends to spread subligamentously, often affecting multiple vertebral bodies (25,102,103). Extension into the paraspinal soft tissues with abscess formation is common. Differentiation from neoplasm may be impossible on the basis of MR images alone.

Spinal Cord Infection/Inflammation

Inflammatory diseases of the spinal cord parenchyma are exceedingly rare. Cord infections and inflammation from pyogenic organisms, fungi, TB, cysticercosis, and sarcoidosis have been reported (17,33,52,73). The MRI appearance of these lesions is limited to individual case

A,B

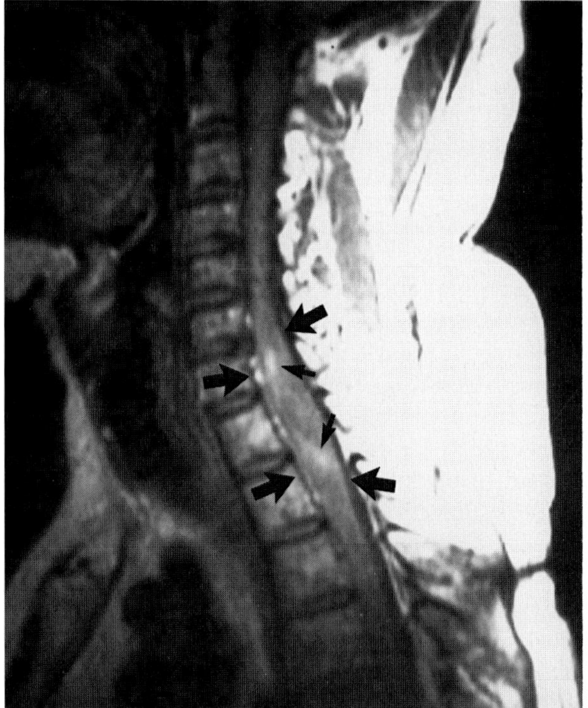

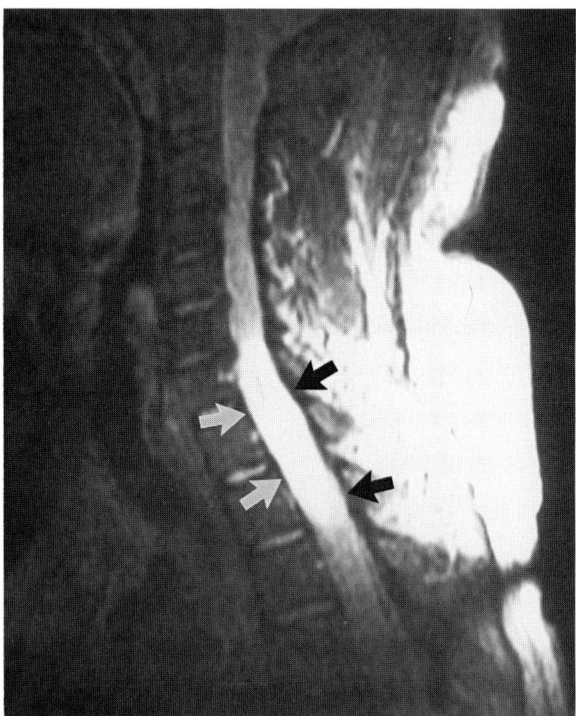

FIG. 5-50. **A:** Segmental intramedullary expansion of the spinal cord is seen that extends from C6 to T3 (*large arrows*). Areas of increased signal are seen within the lesion that may represent subacute hemorrhage (*small arrows*). Unfortunately, gadolinium was not available at our institution at the time of this study. (TR 500 msec, TE 20 msec.) **B:** A corresponding zone of increased signal is seen on this T2W sequence. This proved to be an infiltrative astrocytoma at operation. (TR 1,500 msec, TE 80 msec.)

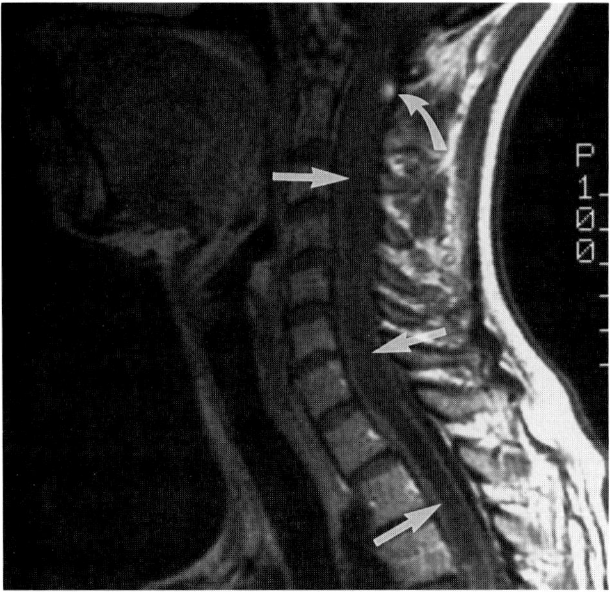

FIG. 5-51. Postcontrast sagittal cervical spine demonstrates intramedullary expansion of the spinal cord by a long syrinx cavity that extends from C1 to at least T4 (*arrows*). The lower extent of the syrinx is not included on this image. A homogeneously enhancing tiny nodule is identified within the posterior aspect of the spinal cord at the first cervical interspace (*curved arrow*). This proved to be a hemangioblastoma at operation in this patient with von Hippel–Lindau disease. (TR 500 msec, TE 20 msec.)

reports. In general, these lesions show nonspecific intramedullary mass effect with decreased signal on T1W and increased signal on T2W sequences within the cord parenchyma. Postcontrast studies help localize areas of active inflammation, granuloma, or abscess formation, differentiating them from the surrounding edema. We have observed patchy intramedullary enhancement and linear leptomeningeal enhancement in both tuberculosis (Fig. 5-58) and sarcoid myelitis (Fig. 5-59). Although it is difficult, or impossible, to distinguish cord infections from neoplasm, their extensive nature, patchy enhancement following contrast administration, and propensity for leptomeningeal involvement may suggest an inflammatory or infectious etiology.

Transverse Myelitis

Transverse myelitis is an inflammatory condition of the spinal cord of indeterminate etiology. It may present in a variety of different clinical settings and be related to an allergic, viral, or paraneoplastic type process. The most common clinical presentation is that of an acute onset of ascending paresthesias, which may be associated with pain or weakness. The midthoracic cord is commonly involved. The MR scan may be normal initially. Long segmental intramedullary expansion may be

Text continues on p. 133

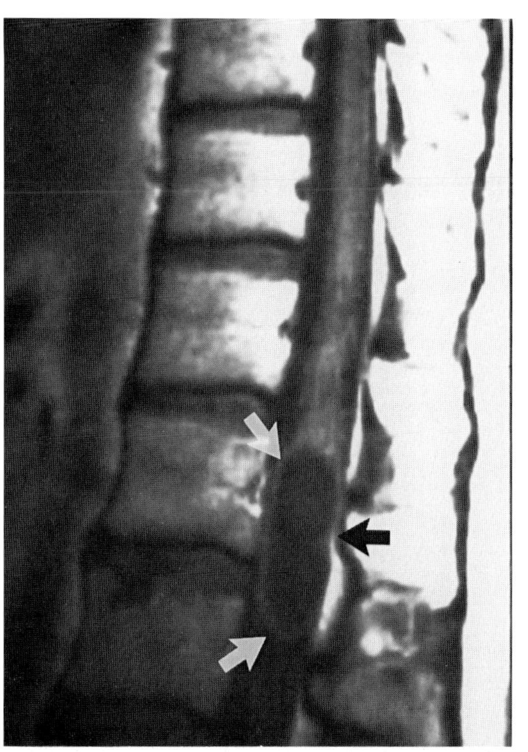

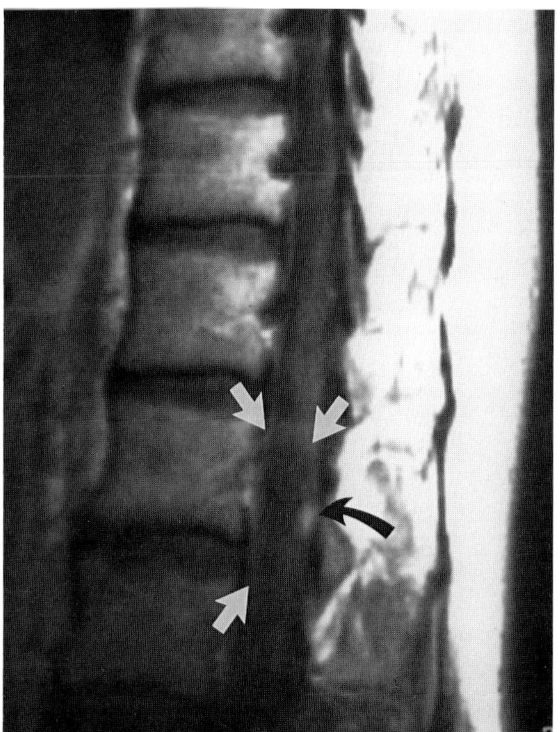

A,B

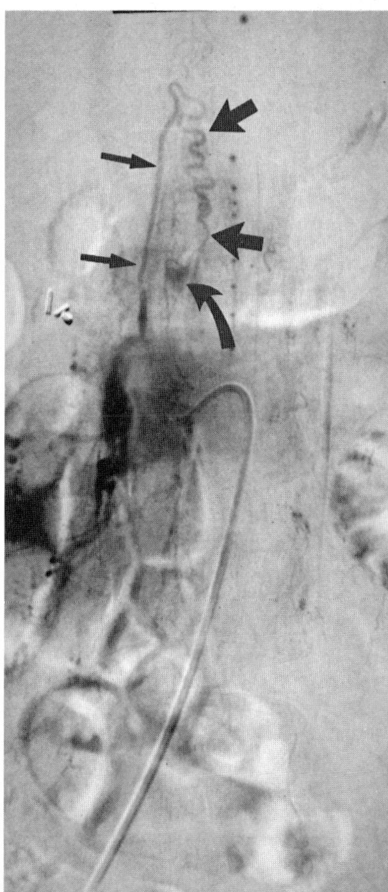

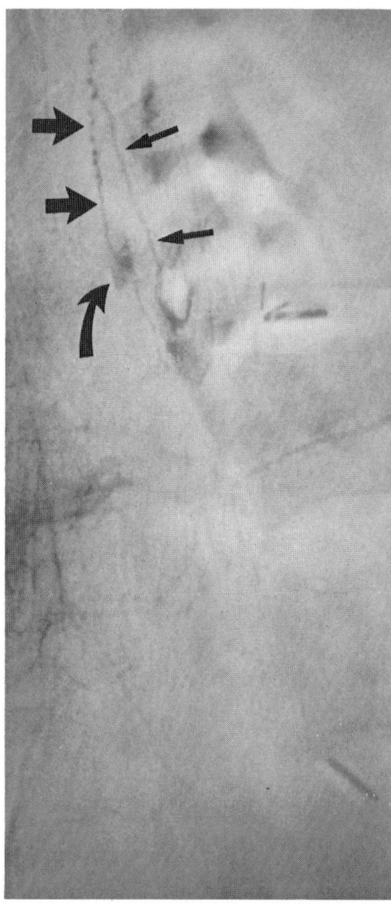

C,D

FIG. 5-52. Contrast-enhanced sagittal images of the lower spinal cord and conus demonstrate intramedullary expansion of the distal spinal cord by a cystic mass in (**A**) (*arrows*). A tiny enhancing mural nodule is seen in (**B**) (*curved arrow*) within the superior and posterior aspect of the cyst. (TR 600 msec, TE 22 msec.) Subtraction views of the midarterial phase from an AP (**C**) and lateral (**D**) spinal angiogram with selective injection into the right L2 intercostal artery demonstrate a tiny vascular tumor nodule (*curved arrows*) that stains intensely. The blood supply is via a hypertrophied left posterior spinal artery (*thick arrows*), which is fed from a medullary branch (*thin arrows*) from the right L2 intercostal artery.

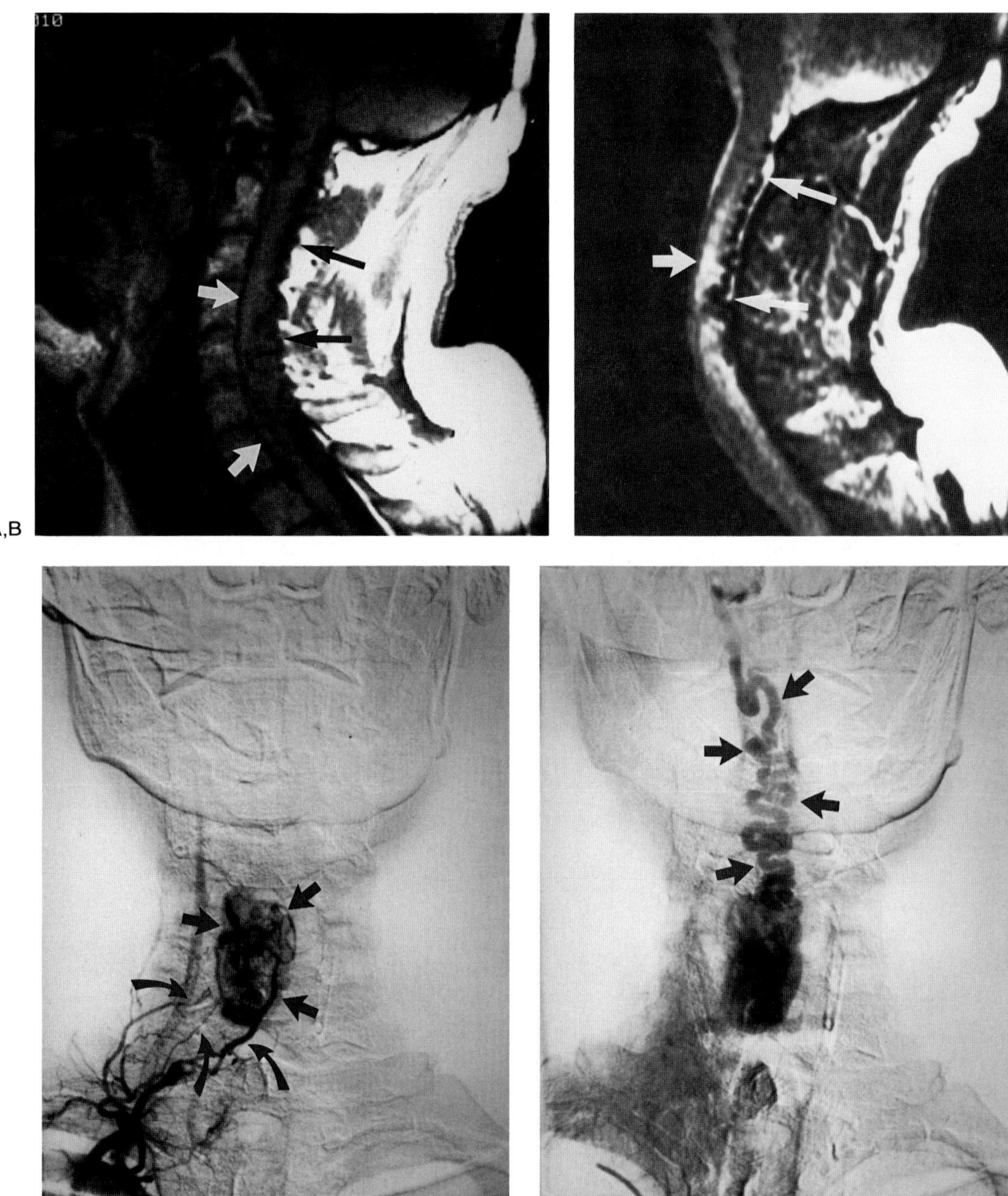

FIG. 5-53. **A:** Sagittal cervical spine demonstrates ill-defined intramedullary expansion of the cord from C4 to C7 (*thick arrows*). Serpentine flow voids (*thin arrows*) are seen posteriorly. Unfortunately, gadolinium was not available at our institution at the time of this study. (TR 400 msec, TE 20 msec.) **B:** This sequence shows nonspecific increased signal within the spinal cord parenchyma (*thick arrow*). The abnormal enlarged vasculature posterior to the spinal cord is seen to better advantage (*thin arrows*). An intraspinal vascular malformation was considered, as well as a vascular cord tumor. (TR 1,500 msec, TE 120 msec.) **C:** AP view from a right subclavian angiogram, early arterial phase, demonstrates intense tumor staining and vascular lakes (*arrows*) within a cord neoplasm. The blood supply is via ascending cervical branches (*curved arrows*) of the thyrocervical trunk. A right vertebral angiogram (not illustrated) demonstrated additional blood supply from the right vertebral artery. **D:** Venous phase of the right subclavian angiogram demonstrates persistence of intense tumor stain and venous drainage into enlarged veins (*arrows*) of the posterior pial plexus above the level of the tumor, which corresponds to the abnormal vasculature noted on the MR image. The angiographic findings are classic for a hemangioblastoma, which was proven at surgery.

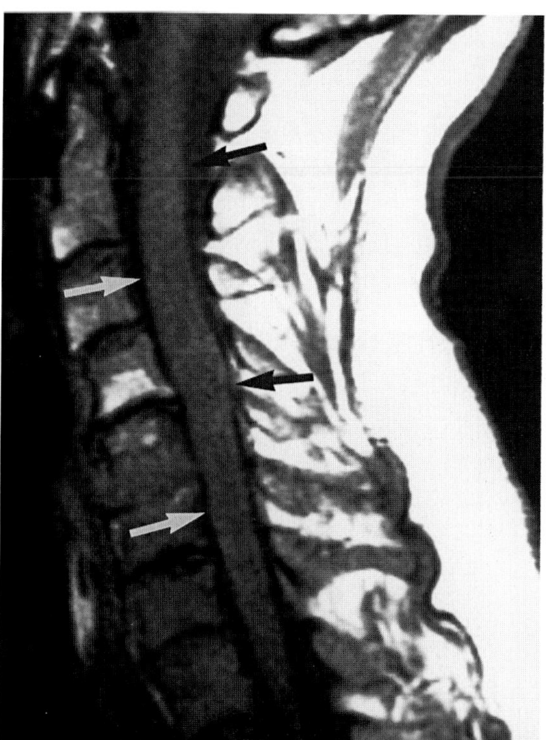
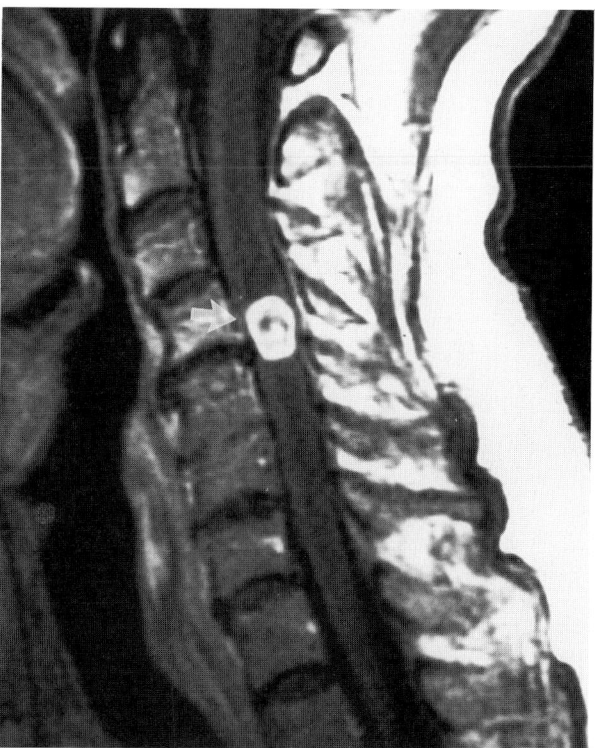

A,B

FIG. 5-54. A: Nonenhanced sagittal cervical spine shows nonspecific intramedullary expansion of a long segment of the cervical spinal cord (*arrows*). (TR 500 msec, TE 20 msec.) **B:** Following contrast administration, an intensely enhancing partially necrotic intramedullary mass is seen opposite the fourth cervical interspace (*arrows*). This lesion cannot be identified on the precontrast images. At surgery, an adenocarcinoma metastasis was found. The intramedullary expansion of the cord above and below the level of the lesion was attributed to cord edema. (TR 500 msec, TE 20 msec.)

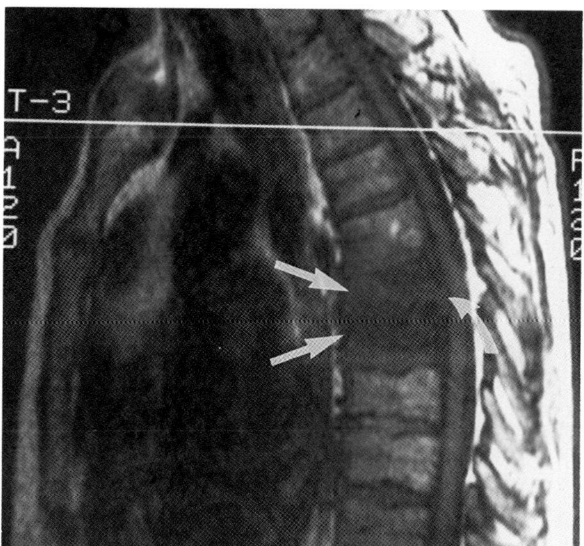

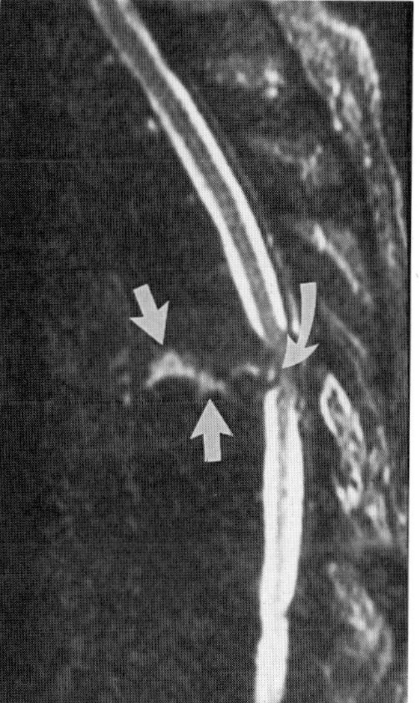

A,B

FIG. 5-55. A: There is loss of the normal marrow fat signal of the T6 and T7 vertebral bodies (*arrows*). The sixth thoracic disc cannot be identified as a separate structure. This combination is fairly specific for a pyogenic disc space infection. Note the epidural extension of inflammation (*curved arrow*). (TR 500 msec, TE 20 msec.) **B:** With T2 weighting, increased signal is seen within the T6 disc and adjacent vertebral body end-plates (*arrows*). The epidural component is seen to better advantage where it narrows the spinal canal and causes some compression of the spinal cord (*curved arrow*). (TR 1,500 msec, TE 140 msec.)

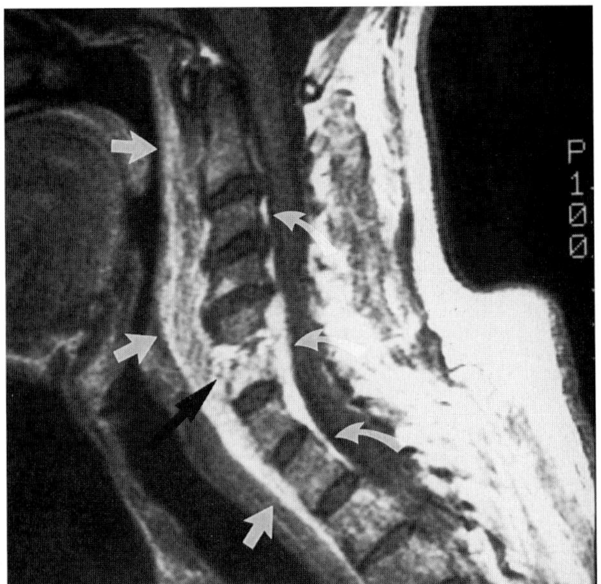

FIG. 5-56. This is a postcontrast sagittal view in a patient with a pyogenic disc space infection at the fifth cervical interspace. There is intense enhancement of the intervertebral disc (*arrows*) and entire T6 vertebral body. Note the enhancing prevertebral (*short arrows*) and epidural (*curved arrows*) abscesses. (TR 500 msec, TE 20 msec.)

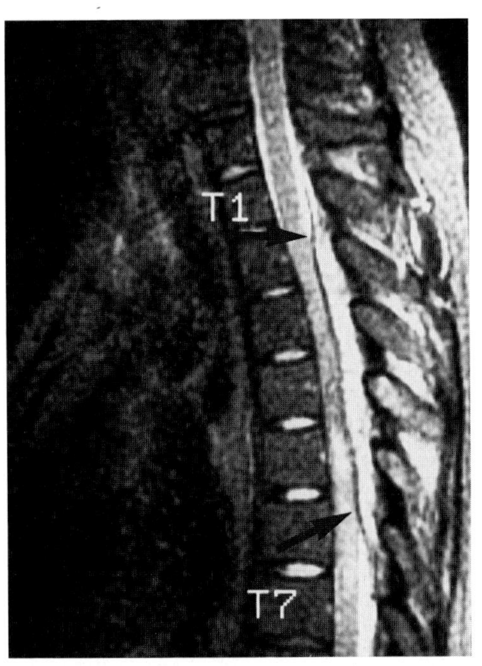

FIG. 5-57. Sagittal thoracic spine in an intravenous drug abuser who presents with fever, chills, and a thoracic myelopathy. An extensive epidural mass is identified posterior to the spinal cord (*arrows*), which was an epidural abscess at surgery. (TR 1,800 msec, TE 100 msec.) From *Mayo Clinic Proceedings* 1989;64:986–1004, with permission.)

A,B

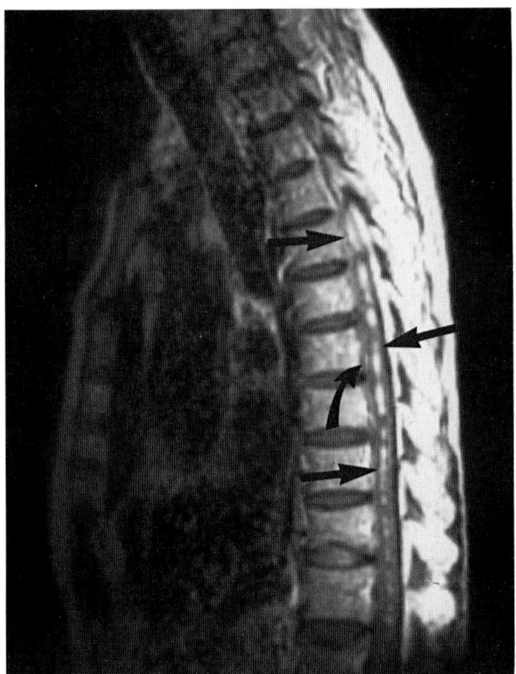

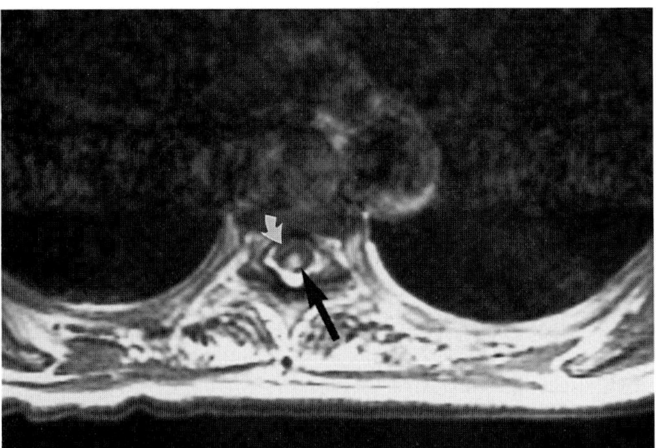

FIG. 5-58. A: Contrast-enhanced sagittal thoracic spine in a patient with a progressive thoracic myelopathy. Note intramedullary expansion of the spinal cord and unusual nodular and linear enhancement of the cord parenchyma (*arrows*), which extends from T11 to at least T6. Also note subtle leptomeningeal enhancement along the ventral cord surface (*curved arrow*). (TR 500 msec, TE 20 msec.) **B:** Postcontrast axial image in the lower thoracic region confirms nodular enhancement within the dorsal aspect of the cord parenchyma (*arrow*). Subtle leptomeningeal enhancement is also seen at the cord surface (*curved arrow*). An open biopsy performed for diagnosis demonstrated acid fast bacilli consistent with tuberculosis. The patient improved following antituberculosis treatment. (TR 550 msec, TE 20 msec.)

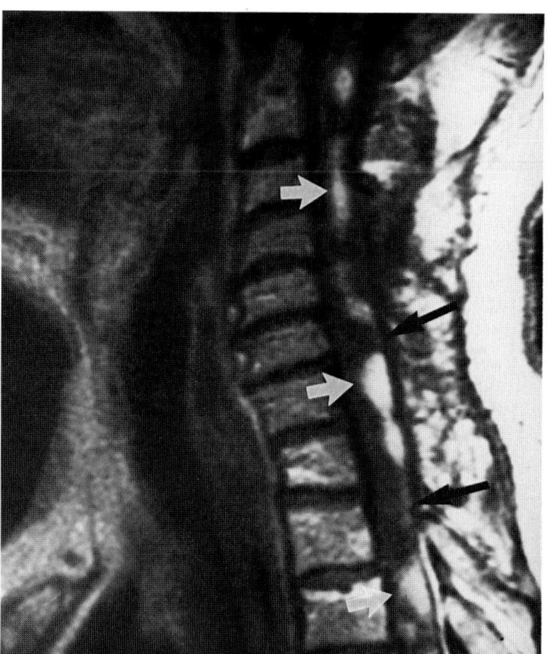

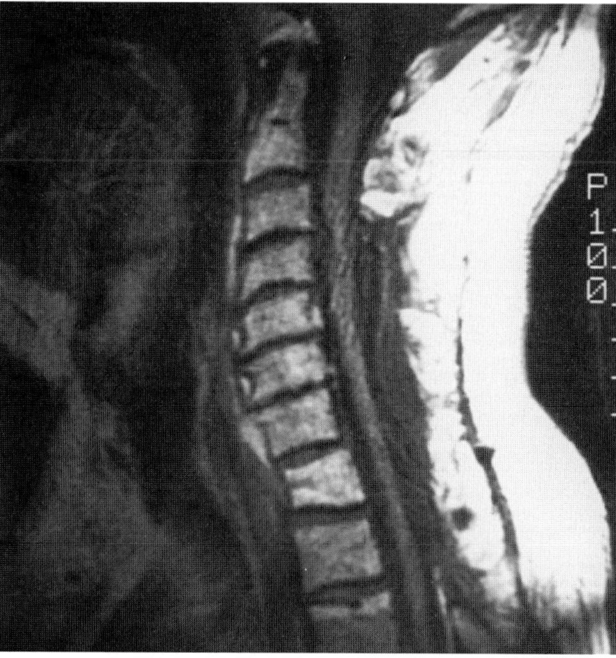

A,B

FIG. 5-59. A: This enhanced sagittal cervical spine demonstrates intramedullary cord expansion and patchy enhancement of the cord parenchyma, which is broad based to the cord's surface (*short arrows*). The enhancing lesions do not extend the full cord thickness. Subtle linear leptomeningeal enhancement is also appreciated (*long arrows*). An open biopsy of an enhancing lesion demonstrated noncaseating granulomas consistent with sarcoid myelitis. Note the extensive decompressive laminectomy performed elsewhere for presumed compressive myelopathy. (TR 500 msec, TE 20 msec.) **B:** This postcontrast sagittal image was obtained following steroid therapy after the patient had clinically improved. The intramedullary expansion and abnormal enhancement seen in (**A**) has since resolved. (TR 500 msec, TE 20 msec.) From ref. 73, with permission.)

seen with decreased signal on T1W and increased signal on T2W sequences, which is indistinguishable from neoplasm (Fig. 5-60). The MRI abnormalities are often more extensive than predicted clinically (33). This disparity, as well as the relative acute onset of symptoms, helps distinguish this condition from neoplasm clinically. The MRI characteristics following contrast administration have not been described.

Demyelinating Disease

MRI is the modality of choice in evaluating patients for the presence of spinal cord demyelinating plaques. In fact, MRI is the only modality that allows direct visualization of these lesions. Although the clinical diagnosis of multiple sclerosis (MS) is well established in many patients at the time of imaging, a cord plaque may be the presenting symptom in a patient with a cervical myelopathy of indeterminate etiology.

Optimum MRI technique is particularly important in demyelinating conditions because many of these lesions are small, which necessitates good quality, artifact-free, high-resolution T2W images. The typical MRI appearance is that of a focal area of increased signal on T2W sequences within the mid or upper cervical spinal cord. The lesion usually asymmetrically involves the dorsal or lateral aspects of the cord (57,59,110). Rarely, the full cord diameter is involved (Fig. 5-61). No signal changes are seen on T1W sequences unless the lesion is fairly large or acute. Plaques may be multiple or may involve a long segment of the cord. There may be focal intramedullary expansion present as well, particularly if the plaque is acute. Sometimes, these cord lesions cannot be distinguished from neoplasms, particularly in patients with equivocal clinical or laboratory evidence of MS. In these cases, MR examination of the head may be useful because many patients will have additional intracranial periventricular lesions that may be clinically silent (Fig. 5-62). Occasionally, a biopsy may be necessary to exclude the possibility of neoplasm.

The enhancement characteristics of MS plaques following contrast administration has not been studied. In two small series of MS patients with cord plaques by Sze et al. (110) (three patients) and Larsson et al. (57) (five patients), enhancement was noted within the plaque on postcontrast T1W sequences in three patients with active disease referable to the cord lesions. The remaining five patients showed no enhancement. Four of these five patients were clinically stable or had improved at the

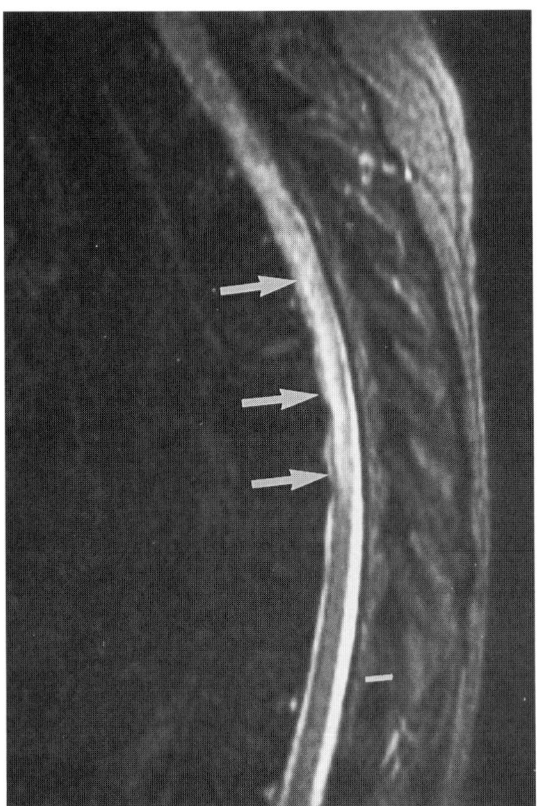

FIG. 5-60. Subtle intramedullary expansion and abnormal T2 signal involve a long segment of the upper and midthoracic spinal cord in this patient with a clinical diagnosis of transverse myelitis (*arrows*). An open biopsy performed to exclude neoplasm demonstrated only inflammation. (TR 1,500 msec, TE 140 msec.)

time of the MRI. The last patient, without enhancement, had clinically active disease referable to the cord plaque. These findings would imply that the enhancement characteristics of cord plaques may parallel those seen in the head, where enhancement indicates active lesions. The lack of enhancement does not necessarily imply inactivity, however. Interestingly, Larsson et al. (57) noted that the enhancement was maximal on delayed images obtained 45–60 min postcontrast infusion. This characteristic is different from intraspinal neoplasms, where enhancement is usually, but not always, maximal immediately following injection (109).

Congenital Spinal Abnormalities

Congenital spinal abnormalities encompass a wide variety of conditions including spinal dysraphism, sacral anomalies and caudal regression, vertebral body abnormalities and congenital scoliosis, and the Arnold–Chiari malformation. There is considerable overlap among these conditions, which may occur by themselves or in association with the others. MRI is the imaging modality of choice for the noninvasive evaluation of patients with known or suspected congenital abnormalities.

Spinal Dysraphism

Spinal dysraphism is a general term that denotes incomplete midline fusion of mesenchymal, bone, and neural elements. Spina bifida refers to failure of fusion of the vertebral column, which may be occult or obvious with a prominent skin defect and exposure of neural elements. The latter condition is referred to as spina bifida aperta and encompasses a variety of conditions including meningocele, myelocele, meningomyelocele, and myelocystocele. In meningocele, only the meninges and subarachnoid spaces protrude through the skin defect. A myelocele is a condition where the distal spinal cord terminates in a neural placode with neural tissues being exposed at the skin surface. The protruding myelocele may be surrounded by the meninges and subarachnoid space, forming a meningomyelocele. In myelocystocele, there is cystic dilatation of the distal spinal cord central canal, which protrudes through the defect. This condition may be difficult to distinguish from meningomyelocele. However, in myelocystocele, the cystic cavity is lined by ependymal cells rather than arachnoid.

Spinal bifida occulta or occult spinal dysraphism denotes a group of skin-covered abnormalities that may be minimal, with isolated failure of fusion of the posterior elements of a vertebral body, or severe. More severe forms of occult spinal dysraphism include tethered cord, thickened filum terminale, dorsal dermal sinus, diastematomyelia, and spinal lipomas. An abnormal skin patch, nevus, or dimple may signify the presence of more severe intraspinal abnormalities.

MRI is particularly useful for the noninvasive evaluation of patients with known or suspected spinal dysraphism (2,7,23,82) (Fig. 5-63). In addition to the risk of ionizing radiation and contrast reaction, the presence of a congenital abnormality increases the morbidity of the myelogram because a spinal tap from the lumbar route risks puncture of a low-lying spinal cord and a cervical puncture risks quadriparesis or death from intraspinal hematoma or inadvertent cord puncture. In spinal dysraphism, the level of the neural placode or conus medullaris can easily be identified as well as the presence and nature of any associated intraspinal masses (Fig. 5-64). MRI is particularly well suited for the screening of patients with suspected occult spinal dysraphism because the location of the conus medullaris can usually be determined on sagittal or coronal T1W images (Fig. 5-65). In questionable cases, axial T1 sequences can be performed for precise localization. The conus medullaris usually reaches the adult level sometime during the first few months of life, with the level of termination

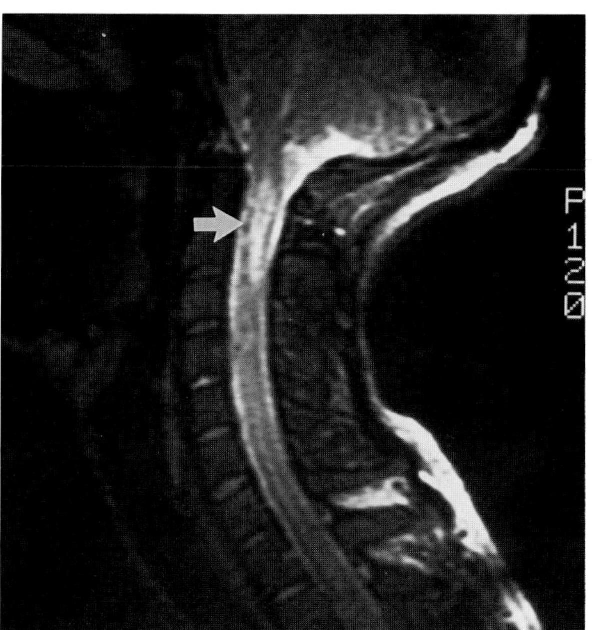

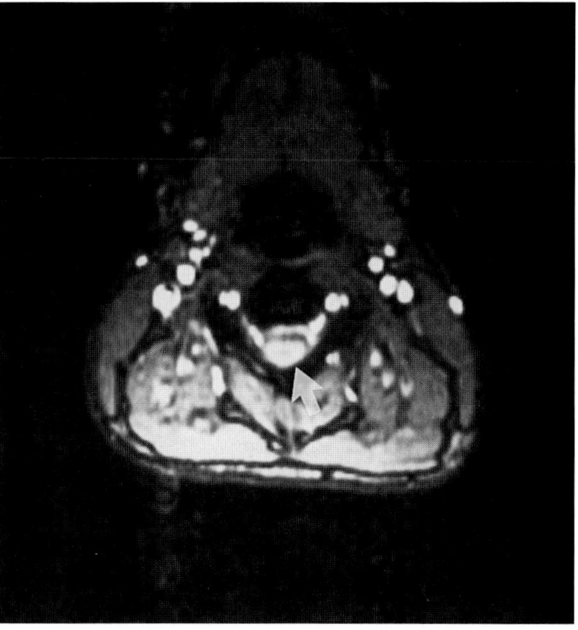

A,B

FIG. 5-61. **A:** Sagittal cervical spine in a patient with a high cervical myelopathy and no prior history of illness. It demonstrates subtle intramedullary expansion of the upper cervical cord and abnormal T2 signal changes that extend from C1 to C3 (*arrow*). (TR 2,000 msec, TE 80 msec.) **B:** This axial image confirms abnormal signal changes within the cord parenchyma that do not involve the entire cord thickness (*arrow*). The diagnosis of MS was suspected but could not be confirmed clinically. A spinal cord biopsy performed to exclude neoplasm disclosed a typical demyelinating plaque consistent with MS. (TR 21 msec, TE 12 msec, 10° flip angle.)

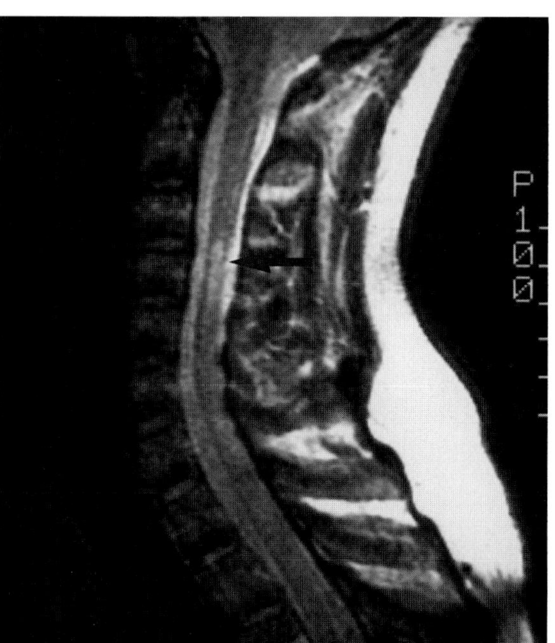

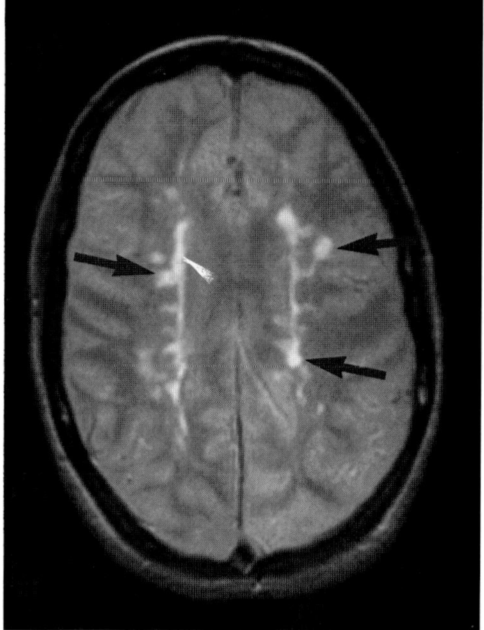

A,B

FIG. 5-62. **A:** This patient has a clinical diagnosis of MS and a new cervical myelopathy. This midline sagittal image shows abnormal T2 signal within the cord parenchyma opposite C4 vertebral body without intramedullary expansion (*arrow*). The MR findings are consistent with a demyelinating spinal cord plaque. (TR 1,800 msec, TE 100 msec.) **B:** This axial image of the head at the midventricular level demonstrates the presence of multiple intracranial demyelinating plaques predominately involving the periventricular white matter of both cerebral hemispheres (*arrows*). (TR 2,000 msec, TE 40 msec.)

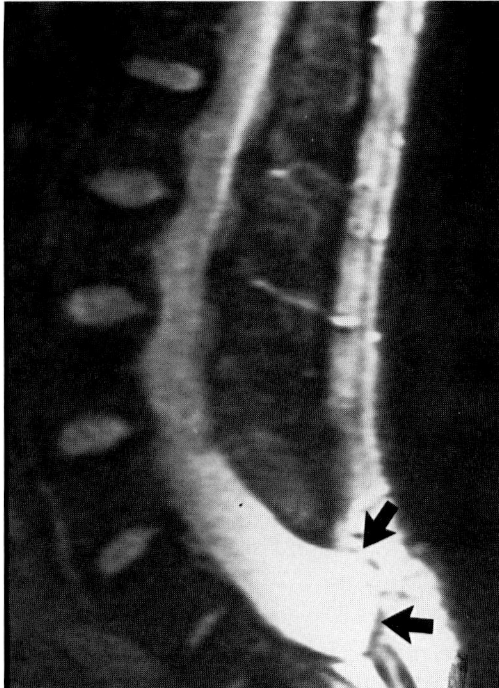

FIG. 5-63. Sagittal lumbar spine in a patient with a meningocele repaired at birth. Note extension of the meninges and subarachnoid space through a bony defect in the upper sacrum (*arrows*). (TR 2,000 msec, TE 70 msec.)

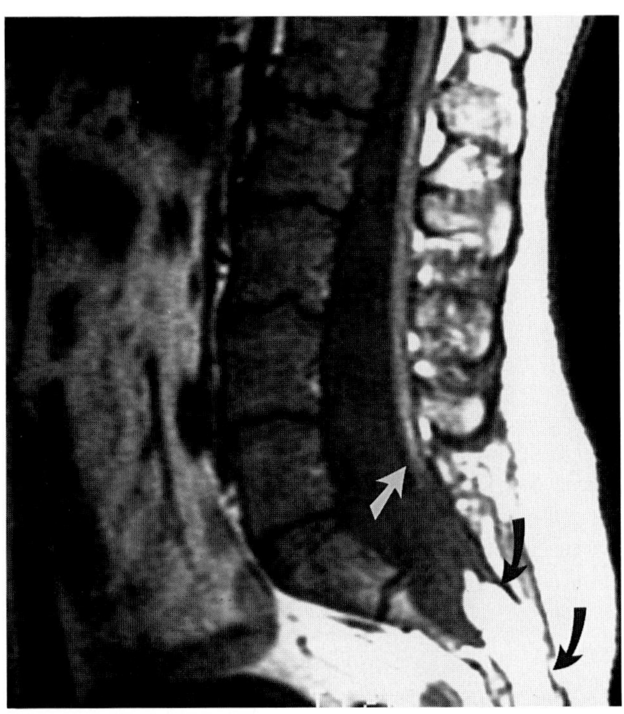

FIG. 5-64. This patient had a myelomeningocele repaired at birth. The cord ends opposite L5 vertebral body (*arrow*). Note the absence of the posterior elements of the sacrum, as well as the presence of a high signal intensity mass (lipoma) within the sacral spinal canal (*curved arrows*). (TR 600 msec, TE 20 msec.)

A,B

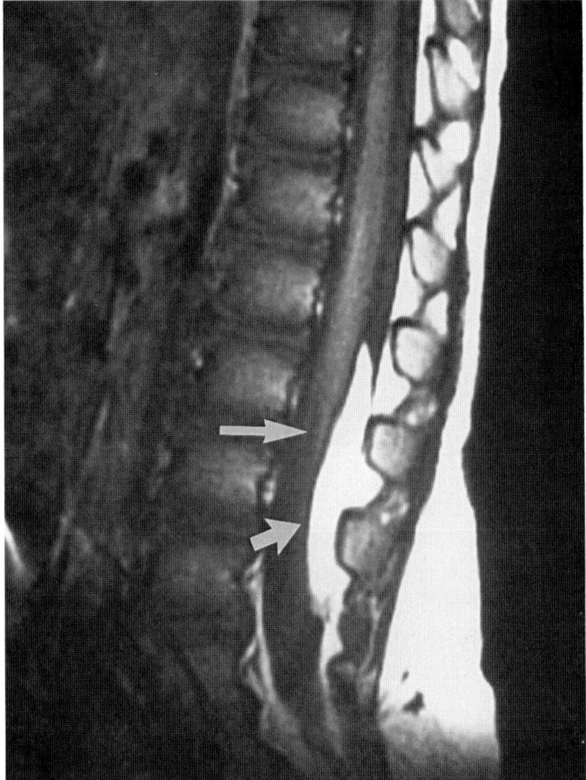

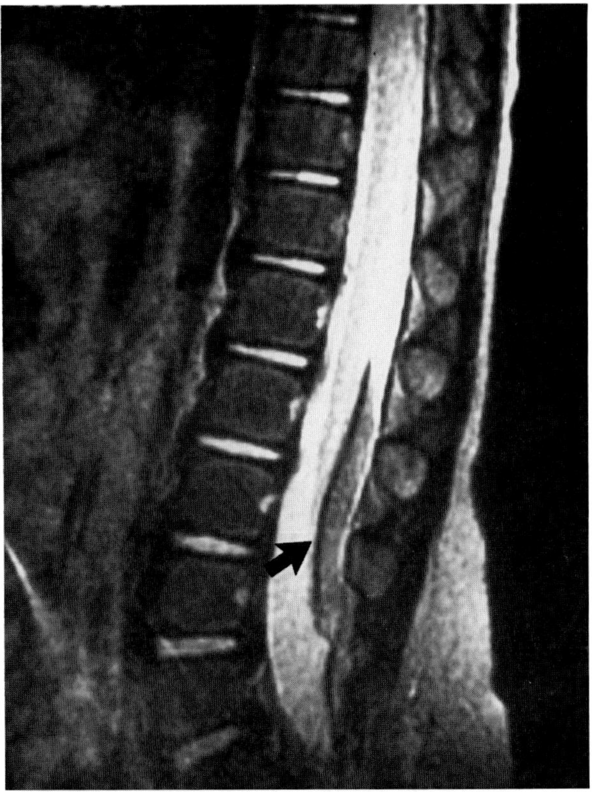

FIG. 5-65. A: This patient was being evaluated for occult spinal dysraphism. The tip of the conus is low in position, ending at the L2 interspace (*arrow*). It is being tethered here by a high signal intensity mass—lipoma—within the posterior spinal canal (*short arrow*). (TR 500 msec, TE 20 msec.) **B:** The intraspinal mass turns dark on this sequence, similar to subcutaneous fat, confirming its fatty composition. (TR 1,800 msec, TE 100 msec.)

above the second lumbar interspace being normal. A conus termination at or below the third lumbar interspace is abnormal at any age. A termination at L3 is abnormal in adults but indeterminate in the pediatric population (120). When the thickness of the filum terminale exceeds 2 mm, it is abnormal. The presence or absence of a tethering mass, as well as its composition (fatty or fibrous), can easily be determined.

Congenital Scoliosis

Segmentation abnormalities of the vertebral bodies such as hemivertebrae, butterfly vertebrae, and block vertebrae result in congenital scoliosis. Intraspinal abnormalities seen in patients with congenital scoliosis include Chiari I and II malformations, syrinx, spinal cord tumor, tethered cord, myelomeningocele, and diastematomyelia (75) (Fig. 5-66). The bony abnormalities of congenital scoliosis are best evaluated by plain films, while the presence or absence of associated intraspinal disorders is best evaluated by MRI. Unfortunately, these patients are difficult to image by MR because only small portions of spinal cord and canal are included on any one section. Multiple oblique sagittal and coronal planes are needed for complete evaluation (Fig. 5-67). Contrast agents may have a role in the evaluation of congenital scoliosis by increasing the conspicuousness of an associated intraspinal mass as small lesions may be missed without contrast.

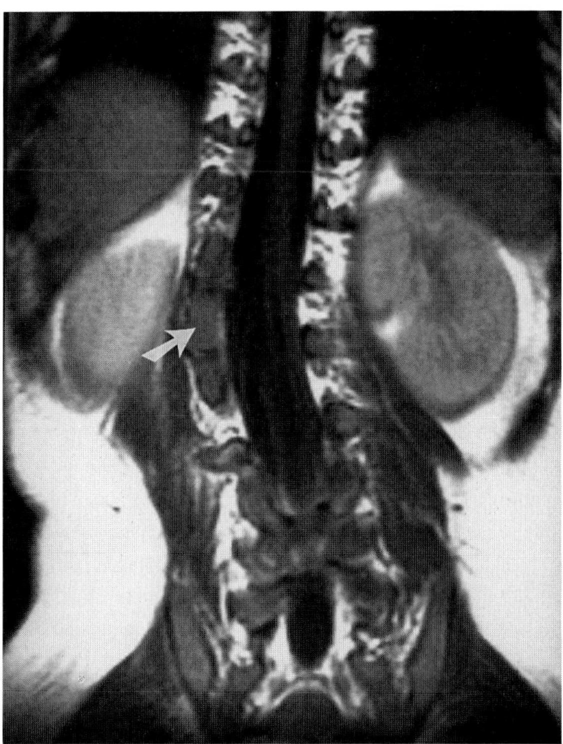

FIG. 5-67. The coronal plane can be useful in the evaluation of patients with scoliosis. A long segment of the spinal canal can be imaged on one section. Note the hemivertebra at L1 (*arrow*). (TR 500 msec, TE 20 msec.)

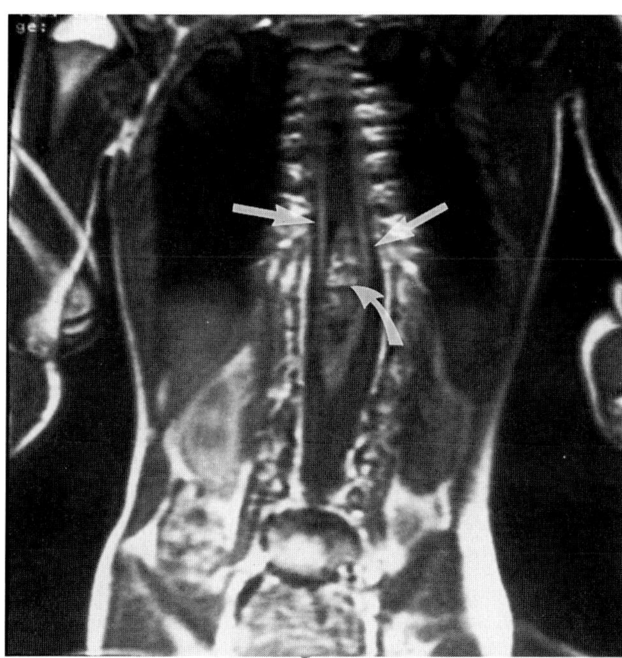

FIG. 5-66. Coronal image through the spinal canal in an infant with congenital scoliosis. A diagnosis of diastematomyelia with diplomyelia can easily be made because two spinal cords are seen (*arrows*) being separated by a bony spur that contains marrow (*curved arrow*). The hemicords unite inferior to the bony spur. (TI 900 msec, TR 2,000 msec, TE 40 msec.) (From *Mayo Clinic Proceedings* 1989;64:986–1004, with permission.)

Caudal Regression Syndrome

Sacral anomalies in the caudal regression syndrome cover a wide spectrum, ranging from minimal with absence of the coccyx to severe with absence of the distal spinal column, anal atresia, and malformation of the external genitalia. Associated conditions include tethered cord, meningocele, myelocele, and meningomyelocele (5).

When suspected, imaging the lower lumbar and sacral regions should be performed to verify the diagnosis of caudal regression. The level of vertebral regression, the presence of central spinal stenosis, and vertebral dysraphic anomalies can be determined. A characteristic wedge-shaped (longer dorsally) cord terminus has been described (5).

Chiari Malformation

Arnold–Chiari malformations are complex hindbrain developmental abnormalities that are divided into three types, depending on the degree of deformity present. Type I, the adult type, is characterized by inferior displacement of the cerebellar tonsils and medulla through the foramen magnum into the upper spinal canal. The cerebellar tonsils have an abnormal configuration, being pointed or beak-shaped, indicating compression. There may be some associated brain stem kinking or angulation present at the junction between the spinal cord and medulla or a spinal cord syrinx, which may be septated. The fourth ventricle is near its normal position (Fig. 5-68). Normally, the cerebellar tonsils may project at or slightly below the posterior margin of the foramen magnum. However, in these instances, the normal rounded configuration of the tonsils is preserved, which helps differentiate this condition from a mild type I malformation (see Fig. 5-48).

More severe hindbrain abnormalities are present in the type II malformation, which presents in childhood. Caudal displacement of the medulla, cerebellar tonsils, and vermis is seen through the foramen magnum, with inferior displacement of the fourth ventricle. Brain stem kinking is a constant feature. Spinal dysraphism, such as meningocele or meningomyelocele, and hydrocephalus nearly always coexist. Other associated spinal abnormalities include syrinx and diastematomyelia. The type III malformation is the most severe, with caudal displacement of nearly the entire cerebellar hemisphere into an upper cervical or occipital encephalocele.

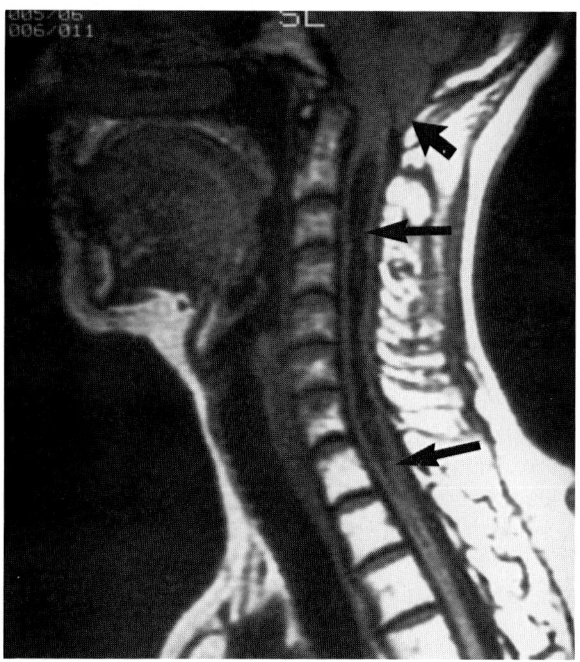

FIG. 5-68. Sagittal cervical spine in a patient with a type I Arnold–Chiari malformation. Note the low position of the cerebellar tonsils (*short arrow*) and the associated intramedullary cord syrinx that extends from C2 to T2 (*long arrows*). (TR 500 msec, TE 20 msec.)

Abnormalities of the craniovertebral junction, such as the Chiari malformations, are best imaged with MRI using sagittal or coronal T1W sequences that allow accurate determination of the location of the cerebellar tonsils. The presence or absence of associated conditions, such as syringohydromyelia and spinal dysraphism, can also be determined (32,100,105,121).

Trauma

MRI has been used successfully in the evaluation of both acute and chronic trauma (40,56,64,80). While plain films and CT satisfactorily evaluate the spinal column and ligaments in the acute setting, MRI is the best way to noninvasively evaluate for spinal cord injuries. However, significant logistical hurdles exist, which limits the usefulness of MRI in the acute spinal cord injury patient. These include limited off-hours availability of scanning time, limited availability of MRI-compatible life-support systems, limited access to the patient by support staff while in the scanner, and lack of MRI-compatible immobilization or traction devices. Many vendors have currently developed or are developing MRI-compatible systems that will increase the utility of MRI in the acute setting.

In clinically stable patients, MRI is useful as an alternative to the myelogram. Traumatic cord avulsions or cord compression from bone fragments or traumatic disc protrusions can be visualized directly (64). In addition, MRI can provide valuable information about the cord parenchyma that is not available on the myelogram. Intraparenchymal hematoma can be distinguished reliably from spinal cord edema on the basis of signal characteristics on T2W sequences (18,45,56). Hours after the traumatic event, acute hematomas demonstrate decreased signal on T2W sequences, presumably secondary to deoxyhemoglobin and intracellular methemoglobin. Cord edema and contusion demonstrate increased signal. No corresponding signal changes can be seen on T1W sequences, which only demonstrate cord enlargement. The distinction between acute hematomas and cord contusion has important prognostic significance (56). Patients with cord hemorrhage usually have severe or complete lesions and are unlikely to recover neurologic function. Patients with edema or cord contusion usually have incomplete or less severe neurologic deficits and may recover significant neurologic function. Mixed patterns of cord hemorrhage and edema have also been described. The prognosis of these patients depends on the initial neurologic deficit and the size of the hematoma seen (56).

MRI has been particularly useful in the evaluation of the chronically injured spine (40,80). Patients with a spinal cord injury and a new or progressive neurologic deficit months to years after the initial injury are best assessed by this technique. Etiologies of post-traumatic progressive myelopathy include spinal cord cysts, which may extend cephalad or caudad from the level of the injury, and myelomalacia. MRI more accurately distinguishes myelomalacia from spinal cord cysts than myelography with delayed CT (40,80). Lesions that parallel the intensity of CSF on T1W, intermediate weighted, and T2W sagittal sequences most likely represent a cord cyst (Figs. 5-69 and 5-70). This distinction has important neurosurgical implications as patients with an ascending myelopathy and a spinal cord cyst above the level of the initial injury are likely to benefit from a cyst-to-subarachnoid space shunt procedure, particularly if the cyst is large. Similarly, patients with incomplete neurologic deficits, a descending myelopathy, and a spinal cord cyst extending below the level of the injury may also benefit. Patients with myelomalacia tend to have a poor response to therapy of any kind (40,80).

The utility of MRI in the evaluation of traumatic nerve root avulsions or dural tears has not yet been determined. Presently, myelography with a follow-up CT remains the best diagnostic procedure (72).

Vascular

Spinal vascular malformations are divided into three types, depending on the location of the nidus. The nidus may be located within the cord parenchyma (medullary arteriovenous malformation), within the pia/arachnoid (perimedullary arteriovenous fistula), or within the dura (dural arteriovenous fistula) (84). The clinical features

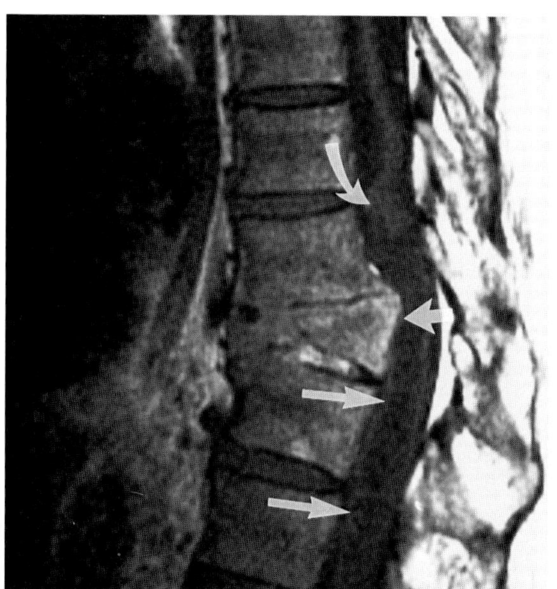

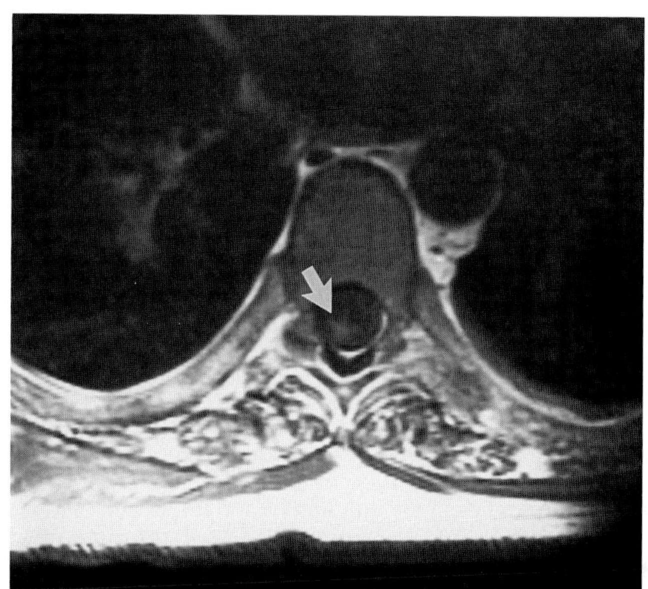

A,B

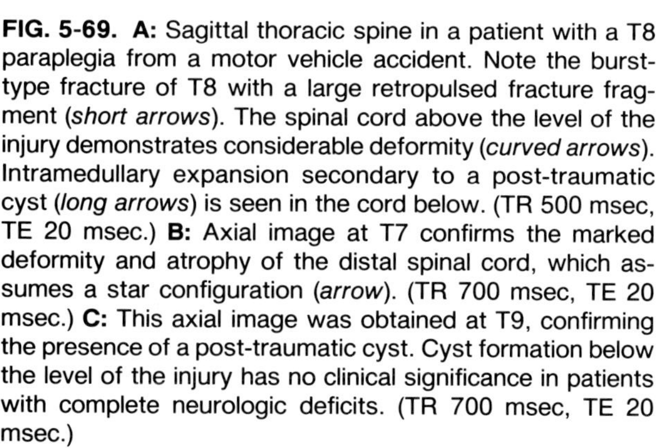

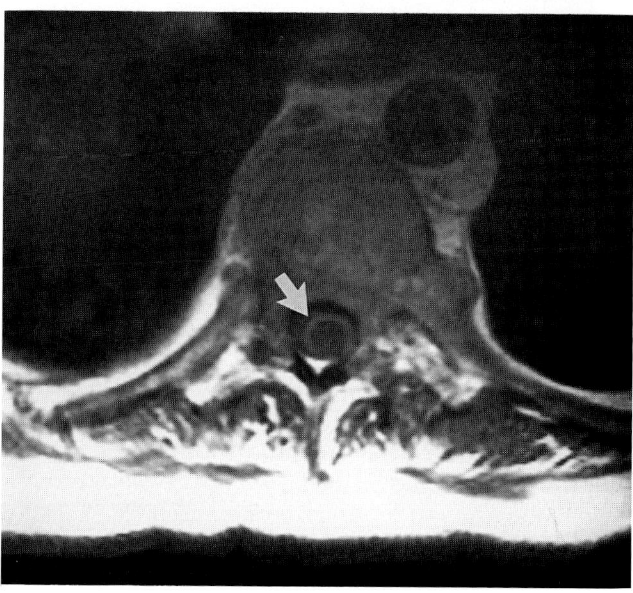

C

FIG. 5-69. A: Sagittal thoracic spine in a patient with a T8 paraplegia from a motor vehicle accident. Note the burst-type fracture of T8 with a large retropulsed fracture fragment (*short arrows*). The spinal cord above the level of the injury demonstrates considerable deformity (*curved arrows*). Intramedullary expansion secondary to a post-traumatic cyst (*long arrows*) is seen in the cord below. (TR 500 msec, TE 20 msec.) **B:** Axial image at T7 confirms the marked deformity and atrophy of the distal spinal cord, which assumes a star configuration (*arrow*). (TR 700 msec, TE 20 msec.) **C:** This axial image was obtained at T9, confirming the presence of a post-traumatic cyst. Cyst formation below the level of the injury has no clinical significance in patients with complete neurologic deficits. (TR 700 msec, TE 20 msec.)

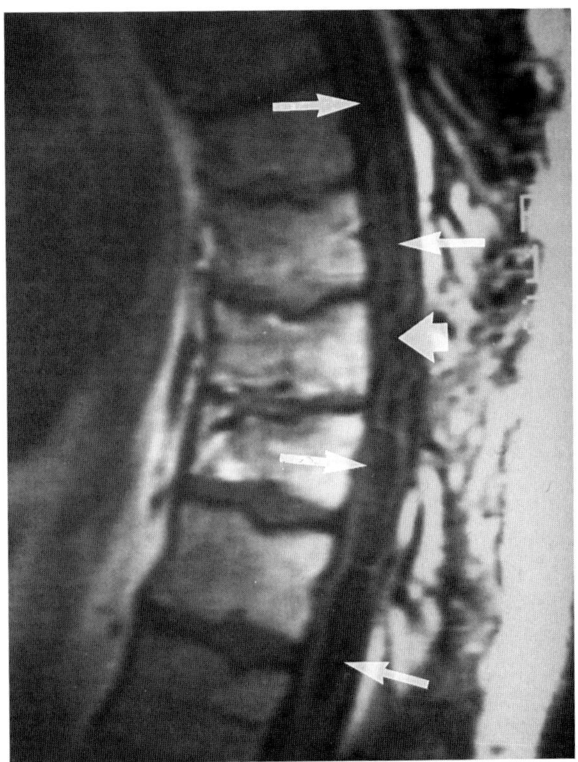

FIG. 5-70. This patient presents with an ascending myelopathy months following a diving accident. Compression of multiple midthoracic vertebral bodies is seen, as well as near complete cord transsection (*thick arrow*). There is intramedullary expansion of the spinal cord above and below the level of the transsection by a post-traumatic cyst (*thin arrows*). (TR 500 msec, TE 20 msec.) (From *Mayo Clinic Proceedings* 1989;64:986–1004, with permission.)

and age of presentation are different between the medullary arteriovenous malformations (AVMs) and the dural arteriovenous (AV) fistula. The perimedullary AV fistula has features similar to both of the other two groups. MRI has been particularly useful as the first examination in the screening for intramedullary AVMs but may fail to diagnose dural and perimedullary AV fistulae since the MRI may be normal or the finding so subtle that clinically important lesions may be missed.

Dural Arteriovenous Fistula

Dural AV fistulae are the most common spinal vascular malformations encountered. These patients present between the ages of 40 and 70 years of age. Pain is the most common initial symptom, which may be radicular in nature. A progressive thoracic myelopathy follows with subjective and objective sensory disturbances preceding progressive motor weakness. Bowel and bladder dysfunction can also occur in the late stages (115). The symptoms are chronic, confusing, and may lead to ill-advised lumbar laminectomies unless the patient is carefully evaluated.

These lesions are thought to be acquired. The nidus of the fistula is located in the neural foramen within the dura surrounding the nerve root. The blood supply to the nidus is via a meningeal branch of the dorsal ramus of an aortic intercostal artery. The AV fistula subsequently drains retrograde into a radicular vein communicating with the posterior pial plexus, which dilates due to the elevated pressure and increased flow. Clinical symptoms are thought to result from venous hypertension-induced spinal cord ischemia (31,61).

The MRI findings of dural AV fistula have been well described and include direct signs such as visualization of the dilated posterior pial venous plexus, indirect signs of cord ischemia, or a normal MRI. The posterior pial plexus may be seen as serpentine flow voids posterior to the thoracic spinal cord and conus on sagittal T1W and T2W sequences (30,61). This finding may be seen on T2W sequences (Fig. 5-71). However, CSF pulsation artifacts can both obscure or simulate this (93). Minute scalloping of the posterior cord margin has been described on T1W sequences because the dilated vessels lie immediately adjacent to the cord surface (63). Sequences obtained in the coronal plane may show the vessels to better advantage. Intravenous contrast administration has also been used in the diagnosis of dural AV fistula and subtle enhancement of the pial plexus along the posterior cord surface has been described (27) (Fig. 5-72A).

A long area of increased signal within the spinal cord and conus on T2W sequences has been described as an indirect sign of dural AV fistula (31,61). This may be present as the only MRI abnormality and is thought to represent ischemic change. However, this finding alone cannot be differentiated from neoplasm or infection (Fig. 5-72B).

A supine myelogram continues to be more sensitive than MRI in detecting dural AV fistula. Serpentine defects are seen within the contrast column along the dorsal aspect of the cord. Spinal angiography is necessary for definitive diagnosis and to determine the location of the nidus for surgical excision or endovascular embolization (Fig. 5-72C–E).

Medullary Arteriovenous Malformation

Medullary AVMs are less common than dural AV fistulae and are thought to be congenital lesions. Most patients present with symptoms of acute intraparenchymal spinal cord hemorrhage or spinal subarachnoid hemorrhage prior to 30 years of age (115). The nidus is located within the cord parenchyma and may be large or small in size, superficial or deep in location, or involve only one side of the cord. These lesions are always fed by the spinal arteries: the anterior spinal artery (including the artery of Adamkiewicz) if the nidus is anterior to the cord or one or both posterior spinal arteries if the nidus

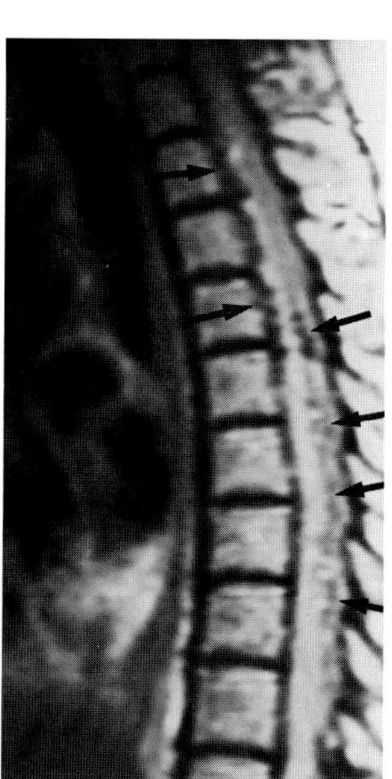

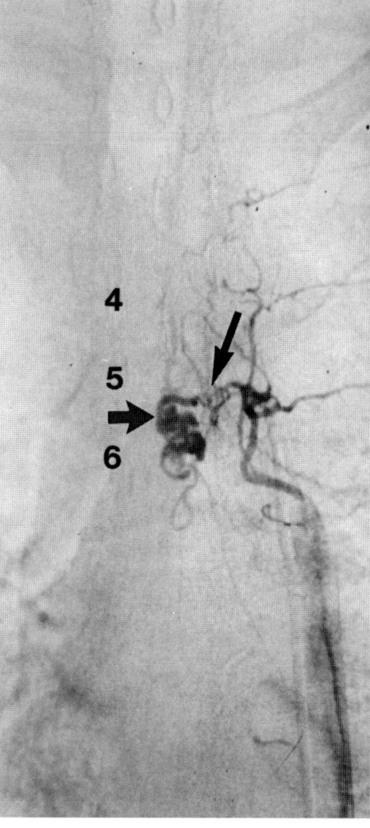

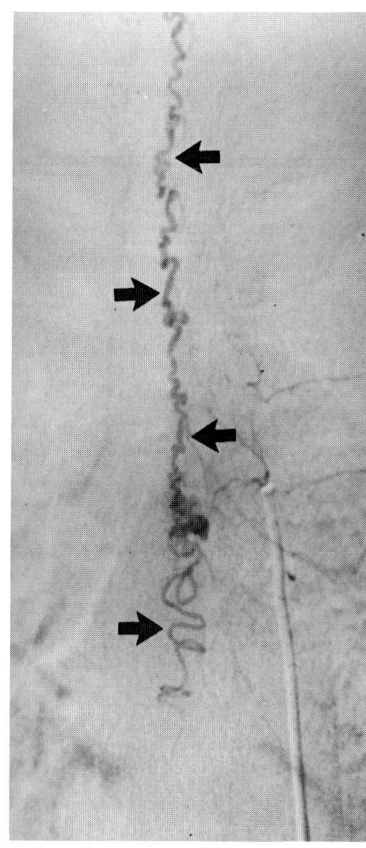

A,B,C

FIG. 5-71. **A:** Serpentine enlarged vessels are seen posterior and anterior (*arrows*) to the spinal cord in this patient with a progressive thoracic myelopathy. (TR 1,500 msec, TE 70 msec.) **B:** A spinal angiogram performed confirms the presence of a dural AV fistula with the nidus located inferior to the left T5 pedicle (*long arrow*). This fistula subsequently drains into the pial venous plexus of the spinal cord (*short arrow*). **C:** This is a slightly later image from the spinal angiogram confirming the presence of an enlarged pial vein (*arrows*), which corresponds to the abnormal vasculature identified in (**A**). (From *Mayo Clinic Proceedings* 1989;64:986–1004, with permission.)

extends posteriorly (84). If the nidus of the AVM is small, there may only be one medullary arterial feeder, which arises from the dorsal rami of the aortic intercostal artery. If the nidus is large and extensive, several aortic intercostal arteries may contribute blood supply.

MRI is the screening modality of choice for clinically suspected intramedullary AVMs. Localized intramedullary enlargement of the spinal cord at the site of the nidus has been described. Serpentine flow voids can be identified within the cord parenchyma, as well as within the posterior pial venous plexus (26,30,31,63). The degree of pial plexal enlargement can be more prominent than that seen with the dural AV fistula if the nidus is large (Fig. 5-73). Intraparenchymal cord hematoma may be present, particularly if the patient presents with acute symptoms of paraplegia or quadraplegia. The signal changes seen depend on the age of the hematoma, with acute hematomas demonstrating no signal change on T1W and decreased signal on T2W sequences, subacute hematomas changing to increased signal on T1W and T2W sequences, and chronic hematomas showing a well-defined ring of decreased signal on T2W or gradient-echo sequences from hemosiderin deposition. Associated spinal cord edema may be present in the acute phase as an area of decreased signal on T1W and increased signal on T2W sequences. Acute hemorrhage into the nidus may partially or completely obliterate it, particularly if it is small. In these instances, an enlarged posterior venous plexus may not be a prominent feature and the differential diagnosis would include hemorrhage into a neoplasm (Fig. 5-74). Ultimately, the diagnosis of intramedullary AVM is made on spinal angiography or at surgery if the nidus has been obliterated by the hemorrhage.

Perimedullary Arteriovenous Fistula

Perimedullary AV fistulae are the rarest type of spinal vascular malformations encountered. The fistula is usually located within the posterior pia mater, although the nidus may be located anteriorly. There may be intramedullary extension of the fistula. The imaging, age at presentation, and clinical symptoms vary and overlap

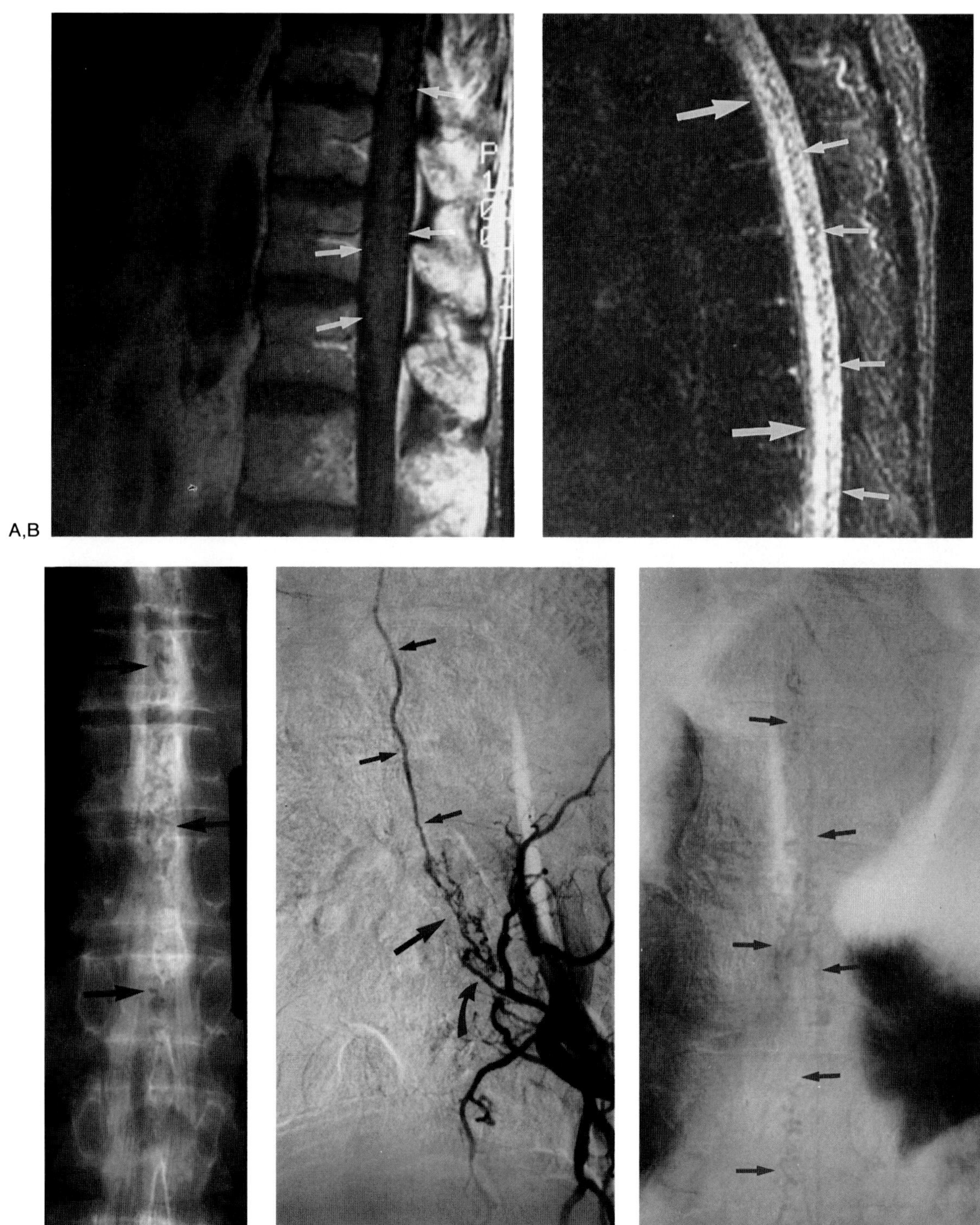

FIG. 5-72. A: Postcontrast sagittal image through the distal spinal cord and conus demonstrates subtle abnormal vasculature posterior and anterior to the spinal cord and tiny punctate vascular enhancement (*arrows*). (TR 500 msec, TE 20 msec.) **B:** Abnormal T2 signal can be identified within a long segment of the thoracic spinal cord (*long arrows*), as well as abnormal serpentine vasculature posterior to the spinal cord (*short arrows*). (TR 1,500 msec, TE 140 msec.) **C:** Lower thoracic supine myelogram confirms the presence of abnormal dilated veins (*arrows*). **D:** AP view from selective left iliac angiogram performed during the course of spinal angiography confirms the presence of a dural AV fistula. The fistula is located within the dural sleeve of the left S1 nerve root immediately inferior to the left S1 pedicle (*long arrow*). The blood supply to the fistula is via the left superior lateral sacral artery (*curved arrow*) with subsequent drainage into an enlarged medullary vein (*short arrows*). **E:** This is a slightly later phase of the iliac angiogram in (**D**) centered over the thoracic spine. Abnormal drainage into a dilated pial venous plexus is confirmed (*arrows*).

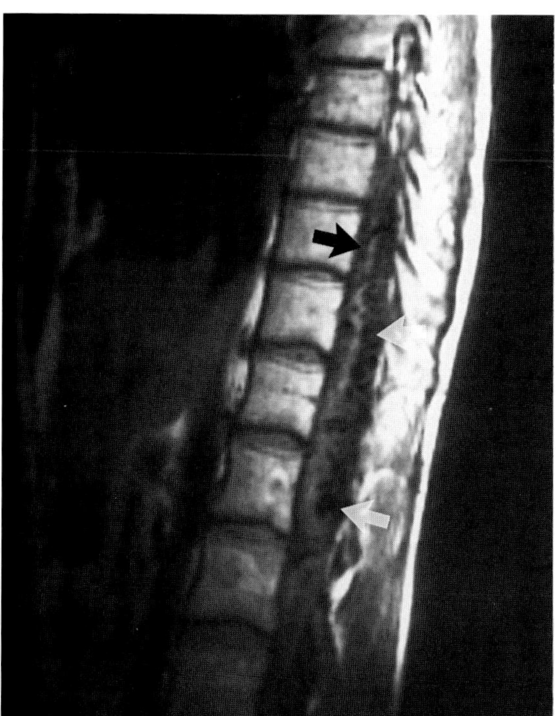

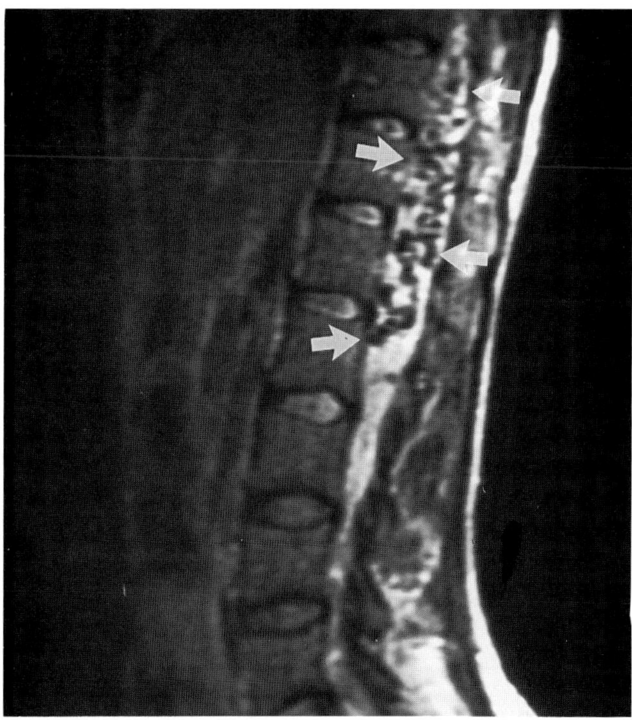

A,B

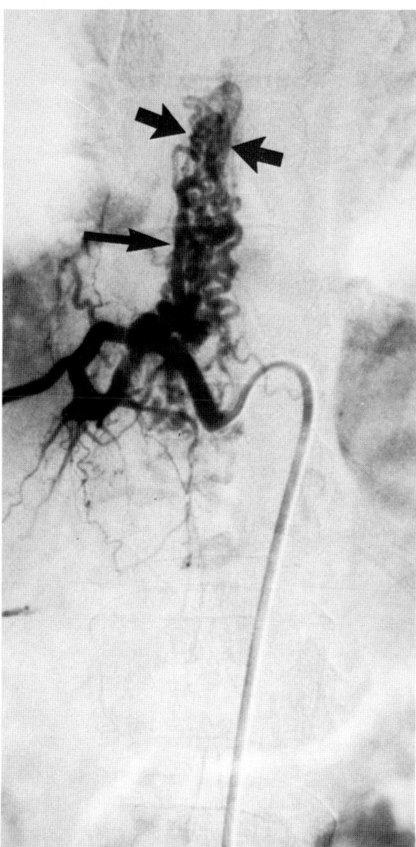

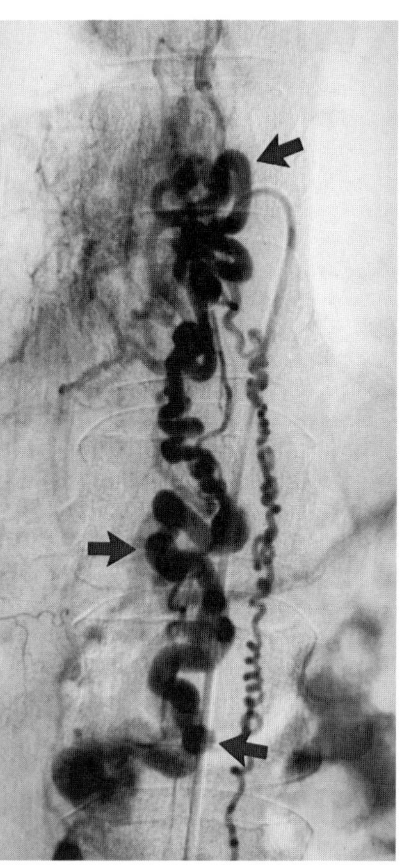

C,D

FIG. 5-73. A: Large abnormal vessels are seen in the region of the conus medullaris on this sagittal image (*arrows*). Some of these vessels appear to be within the cord parenchyma. (TR 500 msec, TE 20 msec.) **B:** The enlarged vessels are seen best on this T2W sequence (*arrows*). (TR 1,500 msec, TE 80 msec.) **C:** AP view from a spinal angiogram with injection of the right T11 intercostal artery confirms the presence of an intramedullary AVM (*short arrows*) that is fed by an enlarged left posterior spinal artery (*long arrow*). **D:** This slightly later phase of the spinal angiogram in (**C**) demonstrates the enlarged spinal veins (*arrows*) that correspond to the vessels on the MR image in (**A**).

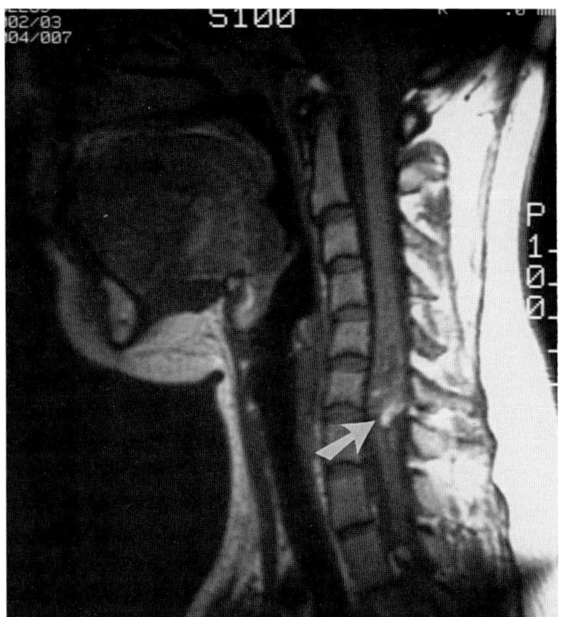

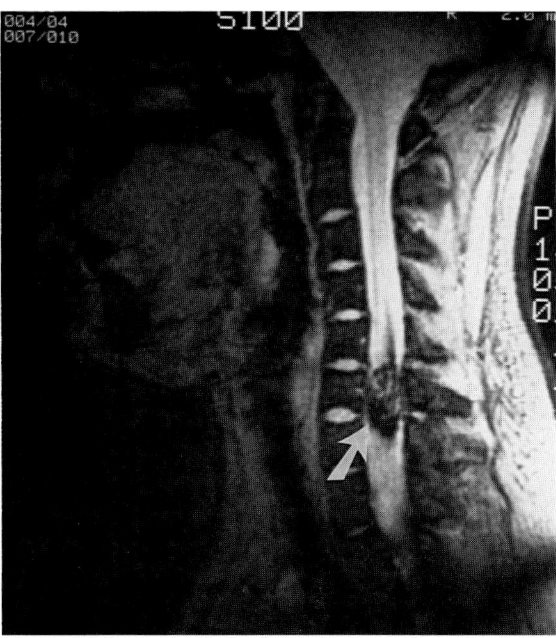

A,B

FIG. 5-74. Sixteen-year-old female who presents with an acute onset of paraplegia. This sagittal cervical spine MR image obtained a month after the initial event demonstrates intramedullary expansion of the spinal cord from C5 through C7. Areas of increased signal within the cord parenchyma are seen, consistent with extracellular methemoglobin (*arrow*). (TR 400 msec, TE 20 msec.) **B:** A large zone of signal loss—hemosiderin deposition—is best seen on this gradient-echo sagittal view (*arrow*), consistent with a subacute/chronic intraparenchymal cord hematoma. A cervical laminectomy performed for the exclusion of hemorrhagic neoplasm confirmed the presence of an intraparenchymal hematoma and a small medullary AVM. No enlarged draining veins are identified on the MR study because the hemorrhage resulted in near complete obliteration of the AVM nidus. (TR 500 msec, TE 15 msec, 20° flip angle.)

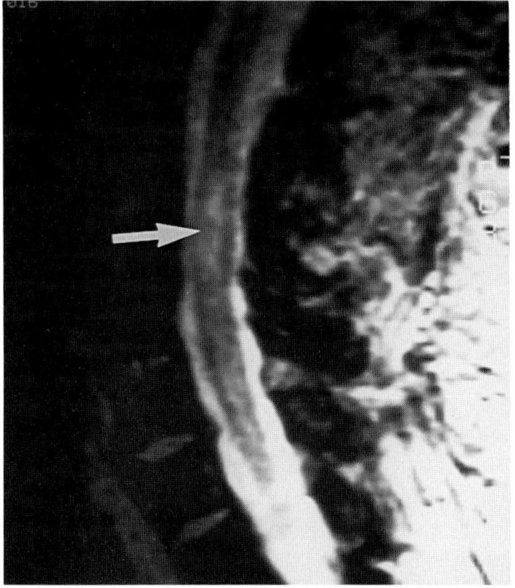

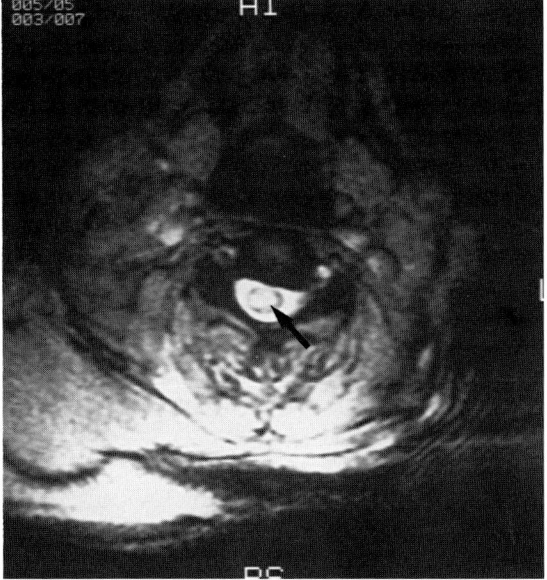

A,B

FIG. 5-75. A: This patient has a long history of steroid-dependent systemic lupus, acute quadriplegia, and a clinical diagnosis of spinal cord infarct. This sagittal cervical spine demonstrates subtle intramedullary expansion of the spinal cord at C3 with abnormal T2 signal (*arrow*). (TR 700 msec, TE 14 msec, 15° flip angle.) **B:** Axial view through the lesion confirms increased signal within the central portion of the cord (*arrow*). (TR 300 msec, TE 20 msec, 15° flip angle.)

considerably with the medullary AVMs and the dural AV fistulae (84). These patients may present at a young age with acute symptoms from hemorrhage or later in life with symptoms of progressive thoracic myelopathy from chronic venous spinal cord ischemia. They are always supplied by spinal arteries like the medullary AVMs. The blood supply may come from one or multiple aortic intercostal arteries.

Infarct

The MRI appearance of spinal cord infarcts has not been described satisfactorily. In fact, little appears in the imaging literature and only isolated case reports are found (27,33). Spinal cord infarcts are difficult to document by any imaging modality or to confirm histologically even though the diagnosis is clinically suspected. They occur in the clinical setting of abdominal aortic aneurysm repair procedures from inadvertent occlusion of an intercostal artery supplying a spinal artery, in severe atherosclerotic disease from stenosis of an intercostal artery supplying a spinal artery, in patients with a vasculitis, or from thrombosis of an intraspinal vascular malformation (27). The MRI may be normal or there may be medullary expansion of the segment of infarcted cord. Normal signal on T1W sagittal sequences and increased signal on T2W sequences, secondary to spinal cord edema has been described (Fig. 5-75). Acute infarcts may show enhancement following contrast administration, mimicking a neoplasm (27). The spinal cord may become atrophic in the chronic stage of infarction, with abnormal signal changes persisting from gliosis .

ACKNOWLEDGMENT

I wish to thank Dr. O. Wayne Houser for his contributions to this chapter, as well as Debbie L. Roach for her assistance in the preparation and typing of the manuscript.

REFERENCES

1. Aguila LA, Piraino DW, Modic MT, Dudley AW, Duchesneau PM, Weinstein MA. The intranuclear cleft of the intervertebral disk: magnetic resonance imaging. *Radiology* 1985;155:155–158.
2. Altman NR, Altman DH. MR imaging of spinal dysraphism. *AJNR* 1987;8:533–538.
3. Angtuaco EJC, McConnell JR, Chadduck WM, Flanigan S. MR imaging of spinal epidural sepsis. *AJNR* 1987;8:879–883.
4. Avrahami E, Tadmor R, Dally O, Hadar H. Early MR demonstration of spinal metastases in patients with normal radiographs and CT and radionuclide bone scans. *J Comput Assist Tomogr* 1989;13:598–602.
5. Barkovich AJ, Raghavan N, Chuang S, Peck WW. The wedge-shaped cord terminus: a radiographic sign of caudal regression. *AJNR* 1989;10:1223–1231.
6. Barloon TJ, Yuh WTC, Yang CJC, Schultz DH. Spinal subarachnoid tumor seeding from intracranial metastasis: MR findings. *J Comput Assist Tomogr* 1987;11:242–244.
7. Barnes PD, Lester PD, Yamanashi WS, Prince JR. MRI in infants and children with spinal dysraphism. *AJR* 1986;147:339–346.
8. Bellon EM, Haacke EM, Coleman PE, Sacco DC, Steiger DA, Gangarosa RE. MR artifacts: a review. *AJR* 1986;147:1271–1281.
9. Brasch RC. Safety profile of gadopentetate dimeglumine. *MRI Decisions* 1989;3(6):13–17.
10. Braun IF, Hoffman JC Jr, Davis PC, Landman JA, Tindall GT. Contrast enhancement in CT differentiation between recurrent disk herniation and postoperative scar: prospective study. *AJR* 1985;145:785–790.
11. Breger RK, Williams AL, Daniels DL, et al. Contrast enhancement in spinal MR imaging. *AJNR* 1989;10:633–637.
12. Bronskill MJ, McVeigh ER, Kucharczyk W, Henkelman RM. Syrinx-like artifacts on MR images of the spinal cord. *Radiology* 1988;166:485–488.
13. Brown BM, Schwartz RH, Frank E, Blank NK. Preoperative evaluation of cervical radiculopathy and myelopathy by surface-coil MR imaging. *AJNR* 1988;9:859–866.
14. Bundschuh CV, Modic MT, Ross JS, Masaryk TJ, Bohlman H. Epidural fibrosis and recurrent disk herniation in the lumbar spine: MR imaging assessment. *AJNR* 1988;9:169–178.
15. Burk DL Jr, Brunberg JA, Kanal E, Latchaw RE, Wolf GL. Spinal and paraspinal neurofibromatosis: surface coil MR imaging at 1.5 T. *Radiology* 1987;162:797–801.
16. Carmody RF, Yang PJ, Seeley GW, Seeger JF, Unger EC, Johnson JE. Spinal cord compression due to metastatic disease: diagnosis with MR imaging versus myelography. *Radiology* 1989;173:225–229.
17. Castillo M, Quencer RM, Donovan Post MJ. MR of intramedullary spinal cysticercosis. *AJNR* 1988;9:393–395.
18. Chakeres DW, Flickinger F, Bresnahan JC, Beattie MS, Weiss KL, Miller C, Stokes BT. MR imaging of acute spinal cord trauma. *AJNR* 1987;8:5–10.
19. Czervionke LF, Czervionke JM, Daniels DL, Haughton VM. Characteristic features of MR truncation artifacts. *AJNR* 1988;9:815–824.
20. Czervionke LF, Daniels DL, Ho PSP, et al. Cervical neural foramina: correlative anatomic and MR imaging study. *Radiology* 1988;169:753–759.
21. Czervionke LF, Daniels DL, Ho PSP, et al. The MR appearance of gray and white matter in the cervical spinal cord. *AJNR* 1988;9:557–562.
22. Daffner RH, Lupetin AR, Dash N, Deeb ZL, Sefczek RJ, Schapiro RL. MRI in the detection of malignant infiltration of bone marrow. *AJR* 1986;146:353–358.
23. Davis PC, Hoffman JC Jr, Ball TI, Wyly JB, Braun IF, Fry SM, Drvaric DM. Spinal abnormalities in pediatric patients: MR imaging findings compared with clinical, myelographic, and surgical findings. *Radiology* 1988;166:679–685.
24. Deeb ZL, Schimel S, Daffner RH, Lupetin AR, Hryshko FG, Blakley JB. Intervertebral disk-space infection after chymopapain injection. *AJR* 1985;144:671–674.
25. de Roos A, van Persijn van Meerten EL, Bloem JL, Bluemm RG. MRI of tuberculous spondylitis. *AJR* 1986;146:79–82.
26. Di Chiro G, Doppman JL, Dwyer AJ, et al. Tumors and arteriovenous malformations of the spinal cord: assessment using MR. *Radiology* 1985;156:689–697.
27. Dillon WP, Norman D, Newton TH, Bolla K, Mark A. Intradural spinal cord lesions: Gd-DTPA-enhanced MR imaging. *Radiology* 1989;170:229–237.
28. Donovan Post MJ, Quencer RM, Montalvo BM, Katz BH, Eismont FJ, Green BA. Spinal infection: evaluation with MR imaging and intraoperative US. *Radiology* 1988;169:765–771.
29. Donovan Post MJ, Quencer RM, Green BA, Montalvo BM, Tobias JA, Sowers JJ, Levin IH. Intramedullary spinal cord metastases, mainly of nonneurogenic origin. *AJNR* 1987;8:339–346.
30. Doppman JL, Di Chiro G, Dwyer AJ, Frank JL, Oldfield EH. Magnetic resonance imaging of spinal arteriovenous malformations. *J Neurosurg* 1987;66:830–834.

31. Dormont D, Gelbert F, Assouline E, et al. MR imaging of spinal cord arteriovenous malformations at 0.5 T: study of 34 cases. *AJNR* 1988;9:833–838.
32. El Gammal T, Mark EK, Brooks BS. MR imaging of Chiari II malformation. *AJNR* 1987;8:1037–1044.
33. Enzmann DR, DeLaPaz RL, Rubin JB. *Magnetic resonance of the spine.* St. Louis, MO: CV Mosby, 1990.
34. Enzmann DR, Rubin JB. Cervical spine: MR imaging with a partial flip angle, gradient-refocused pulse sequence. Part I. General considerations and disk disease. *Radiology* 1988;166:467–472.
35. Enzmann DR, Rubin JB. Cervical spine: MR imaging with a partial flip angle, gradient-refocused pulse sequence. Part II. Spinal cord disease. *Radiology* 1988;166:473–478.
36. Enzmann DR, Rubin JB, Wright A. Use of cerebrospinal fluid gating to improve T2-weighted images. Part I. The spinal cord. *Radiology* 1987;162:763–767.
37. Firooznia H, Kricheff II, Rafii M, Golimbu C. Lumbar spine after surgery: examination with intravenous contrast-enhanced CT. *Radiology* 1987;163:221–226.
38. Flannigan BD, Lufkin RB, McGlade C, et al. MR imaging of the cervical spine: neurovascular anatomy. *AJNR* 1987;8:27–32.
39. Frocrain L, Duvauferrier R, Husson J-L, Noel J, Ramee A, Pawlotsky Y. Recurrent postoperative sciatica: evaluation with MR imaging and enhanced CT. *Radiology* 1989;170:531–533.
40. Gebarski SS, Maynard FW, Gabrielsen TO, Knake JE, Latack JT, Hoff JT. Posttraumatic progressive myelopathy: clinical and radiologic correlation employing MR imaging, delayed CT metrizamide myelography, and intraoperative sonography. *Radiology* 1985;157:379–385.
41. Goldstein HA, Kashanian FK, Blumetti RF, Holyoak WL, Hugo FP, Blumenfield DM. Safety assessment of gadopentetate dimeglumine in U.S. clinical trials. *Radiology* 1990;174:17–23.
42. Goy AMC, Pinto RS, Raghavendra BN, Epstein FJ, Kricheff II. Intramedullary spinal cord tumors: MR imaging, with emphasis on associated cysts. *Radiology* 1986;161:381–386.
43. Grenier N, Greselle J-F, Vital J-M, et al. Normal and disrupted lumbar longitudinal ligaments: correlative MR and anatomic study. *Radiology* 1989;171:197–205.
44. Grenier N, Kressel HY, Schiebler ML, Grossman RI, Dalinka MK. Normal and degenerative posterior spinal structures: MR imaging. *Radiology* 1987;165:517–525.
45. Hackney DB, Asato R, Joseph PM, et al. Hemorrhage and edema in acute spinal cord compression: demonstration by MR imaging. *Radiology* 1986;161:387–390.
46. Hedberg MC, Drayer BP, Flom RA, Hodak JA, Bird CR. Gradient echo (GRASS) MR imaging in cervical radiculopathy. *AJNR* 1988;9:145–151.
47. Ho PSP, Yu S, Sether LA, Wagner M, Ho K-C, Haughton VM. Ligamentum flavum: appearance on sagittal and coronal MR images. *Radiology* 1988;168:469–472.
48. Hochhauser L, Kieffer SA, Cacayorin ED, Petro GR, Teller WF. Recurrent postdiskectomy low back pain: MR–surgical correlation. *AJNR* 1988;9:769–774.
49. Hueftle MG, Modic MT, Ross JS, et al. Lumbar spine: postoperative MR imaging with Gd-DTPA. *Radiology* 1988;167:817–824.
50. Jinkins JR, Whittemore AR, Bradley WG. The anatomic basis of vertebrogenic pain and the autonomic syndrome associated with lumbar disk extrusion. *AJNR* 1989;10:219–231.
51. Katz BH, Quencer RM, Hinks RS. Comparison of gradient-recalled-echo and T2-weighted spin-echo pulse sequences in intramedullary spinal lesions. *AJNR* 1989;10:815–822.
52. Kelly RB, Mahoney PD, Cawley KM. MR demonstration of spinal cord sarcoidosis: report of a case. *AJNR* 1988;9:197–199.
53. Kim KS, Ho SU, Weinberg PE, Lee C. Spinal leptomeningeal infiltration by systemic cancer: myelographic features. *AJR* 1982;139:361–365.
54. Krol G, Sze G, Amster J. Table-top support plate for imaging the entire spine with surface-coil MR. *AJNR* 1988;9:396–397.
55. Krol G, Sze G, Malkin M, Walker R. MR of cranial and spinal meningeal carcinomatosis: comparison with CT and myelography. *AJNR* 1988;9:709–714.
56. Kulkarni MV, McArdle CB, Kopanicky D, Miner M, Cotler HB, Lee KF, Harris JH. Acute spinal cord injury: MR imaging at 1.5 T. *Radiology* 1987;164:837–843.
57. Larsson E-M, Holtas S, Nilsson O. Gd-DTPA-enhanced MR of suspected spinal multiple sclerosis. *AJNR* 1989;10:1071–1076.
58. Levy LM, Di Chiro G, Brooks RA, Dwyer AJ, Wener L, Frank J. Spinal cord artifacts from truncation errors during MR imaging. *Radiology* 1988;166:479–483.
59. Maravilla KR, Weinreb JC, Suss R, Nunnally RL. Magnetic resonance demonstration of multiple sclerosis plaques in the cervical cord. *AJR* 1985;144:381–385.
60. Masaryk TJ, Ross JS, Modic MT, Boumphrey F, Bohlman H, Wilber G. High-resolution MR imaging of sequestered lumbar intervertebral disks. *AJNR* 1988;9:351–358.
61. Masaryk TJ, Ross JS, Modic MT, Ruff RL, Selman WR, Ratcheson RA. Radiculomeningeal vascular malformations of the spine: MR imaging. *Radiology* 1987;164:845–849.
62. Mehta RC, Wilson MA, Perlman SB. False-negative bone scan in extensive metastatic disease: CT and MR findings (case report). *J Comput Assist Tomogr* 1989;13:717–719.
63. Minami S, Sagoh T, Nishimura K, et al. Spinal arteriovenous malformation: MR imaging. *Radiology* 1988;169:109–115.
64. Mirvis SE, Geisler FH, Jelinek JJ, Joslyn JN, Gellad F. Acute cervical spine trauma: evaluation with 1.5-T MR imaging. *Radiology* 1988;166:807–816.
65. Modic MT, Feiglin DH, Piraino DW, Boumphrey F, Weinstein MA, Duchesneau PM, Rehm S. Vertebral osteomyelitis: assessment using MR. *Radiology* 1985;157:157–166.
66. Modic MT, Masaryk TJ, Boumphrey F, Goormastic M, Bell G. Lumbar herniated disk disease and canal stenosis: prospective evaluation of surface coil MR, CT, and myelography. *AJR* 1986;147:757–765.
67. Modic MT, Masaryk TJ, Mulopulos GP, Bundschuh C, Han JS, Bohlman H. Cervical radiculopathy: prospective evaluation with surface coil MR imaging, CT with metrizamide, and metrizamide myelography. *Radiology* 1986;161:753–759.
68. Modic MT, Masaryk TJ, Ross JS, Carter JR. Imaging of degenerative disk disease. *Radiology* 1988;168:177–186.
69. Modic MT, Pavlicek W, Weinstein MA, Boumphrey F, Ngo F, Hardy R, Duchesneau PM. Magnetic resonance imaging of intervertebral disk disease. *Radiology* 1984;152:103–111.
70. Modic MT, Steinberg PM, Ross JS, Masaryk TJ, Carter JR. Degenerative disk disease: assessment of changes in vertebral body marrow with MR imaging. *Radiology* 1988;166:193–199.
71. Monajati A, Wayne WS, Rauschning W, Ekholm SE. MR of the cauda equina. *AJNR* 1987;8:893–900.
72. Morris RE, Hasso AN, Thompson JR, Hinshaw DB Jr, Vu LH. Traumatic dural tears: CT diagnosis using metrizamide. *Radiology* 1984;152:443–446.
73. Nesbit GM, Miller GM, Baker HL Jr, Ebersold MJ, Scheithauer BW. Spinal cord sarcoidosis: a new finding at MR imaging with Gd-DTPA enhancement. *Radiology* 1989;173:839–843.
74. Netter FH. In: Brass A, ed. *Nervous system. Part I. Anatomy and physiology.* Volume 1: The CIBA Collection of Medical Illustrations. West Caldwell, NJ: CIBA Pharmaceutical Company, 1986.
75. Nokes SR, Murtagh FR, Jones JD III, Downing M, Arrington JA, Turetsky D, Silbiger ML. Childhood scoliosis: MR imaging. *Radiology* 1987;164:791–797.
76. Osborn AG, Hood RS, Sherry RG, Smoker WRK, Harnsberger HR. CT/MR spectrum of far lateral and anterior lumbosacral disk herniations. *AJNR* 1988;9:775–778.
77. Parizel PM, Baleriaux D, Rodesch G, et al. Gd-DTPA-enhanced MR imaging of spinal tumors. *AJNR* 1989;10:249–258.
78. Pech P, Daniels DL, Williams AL, Haughton VM. The cervical neural foramina: correlation of microtomy and CT anatomy. *Radiology* 1985;155:143–146.
79. Pech P, Haughton VM. Lumbar intervertebral disk: correlative MR and anatomic study. *Radiology* 1985;156:699–701.
80. Quencer RM, Sheldon JJ, Donovan Post MJ, Diaz RD, Montalvo BM, Green BA, Eismont FJ. MRI of the chronically injured cervical spinal cord. *AJR* 1986;147:125–132.
81. Quint DJ, Patel SC, Sanders WP, Hearshen DO, Boulos RS. Importance of absence of CSF pulsation artifacts in the MR detection of significant myelographic block at 1.5 T. *AJNR* 1989;10:1089–1095.

82. Raghavan N, Barkovich AJ, Edwards M, Norman D. MR imaging in the tethered spinal cord syndrome. *AJNR* 1989;10:27–36.
83. Ramanauskas WL, Wilner HI, Metes JJ, Lazo A, Kelly JK. MR imaging of compressive myelomalacia. *J Comput Assist Tomogr* 1989;13:399–404.
84. Riche MC, Reizine D, Melki JP, Merland JJ. Classification of spinal cord vascular malformations. *Radiat Med* 1985;3(1):17–24.
85. Ross JS, Blaser S, Masaryk TJ, et al. Gd-DTPA enhancement of posterior epidural scar: an experimental model. *AJNR* 1989;10:1083–1088.
86. Ross JS, Delamarter R, Hueftle MG, et al. Gadolinium-DTPA-enhanced MR imaging of the postoperative lumbar spine: time course and mechanism of enhancement. *AJNR* 1989;10:37–46.
87. Ross JS, Masaryk TJ, Modic MT, Bohlman H, Delamater R, Wilber G. Lumbar spine: postoperative assessment with surface-coil MR imaging. *Radiology* 1987;164:851–860.
88. Ross JS, Masaryk TJ, Modic MT, Delamater R, Bohlman H, Wilbur G, Kaufman B. MR imaging of lumbar arachnoiditis. *AJNR* 1987;8:885–892.
89. Ross JS, Modic MT, Masaryk TJ. Tears of the anulus fibrosus: assessment with Gd-DTPA-enhanced MR imaging. *AJNR* 1989;10:1251–1254.
90. Ross JS, Modic MT, Masaryk TJ, Carter J, Marcus RE, Bohlman H. Assessment of extradural degenerative disease with Gd-DTPA-enhanced MR imaging: correlation with surgical and pathologic findings. *AJNR* 1989;10:1243–1249.
91. Ross JS, Perez-Reyes N, Masaryk TJ, Bohlman H, Modic MT. Thoracic disk herniation: MR imaging. *Radiology* 1987;165:511–515.
92. Rubin JB, Enzmann DR. Harmonic modulation of proton MR precessional phase by pulsatile motion: origin of spinal CSF flow phenomena. *AJR* 1987;148:983–994.
93. Rubin JB, Enzmann DR. Imaging of spinal CSF pulsation by 2DFT MR: significance during clinical imaging. *AJR* 1987;148:973–982.
94. Rubin JB, Enzmann DR. Optimizing conventional MR imaging of the spine. *Radiology* 1987;163:777–783.
95. Rubin JB, Enzmann DR, Wright A. CSF-gated MR imaging of the spine: theory and clinical implementation. *Radiology* 1987;163:784–792.
96. Rubin JB, Wright A, Enzmann DR. Lumbar spine: motion compensation for cerebrospinal fluid on MR imaging. *Radiology* 1988;166:225–231.
97. Runge VM, Carollo BR, Wolf CR, Nelson KL, Gelblum DY. Gd DTPA: a review of clinical indications in central nervous system magnetic resonance imaging. *RadioGraphics* 1989;9:929–958.
98. Runge VM, Clanton JA, Lukehart CM, Partain CL, James AE Jr. Paramagnetic agents for contrast-enhanced NMR imaging: a review. *AJR* 1983;141:1209–1215.
99. Ryan RW, Lally JF, Kozic Z. Asymptomatic calcified herniated thoracic disks: CT recognition. *AJNR* 1988;9:363–366.
100. Samuelsson L, Bergstrom K, Thuomas K-A, Hemmingsson A, Wallensten R. MR imaging of syringohydromyelia and Chiari malformations in myelomeningocele patients with scoliosis. *AJNR* 1987;8:539–546.
101. Shapiro R. *Myelography,* 4th ed. Chicago: Year Book Medical Publishers, 1984.
102. Sharif HS, Aideyan OA, Clark DC, et al. Brucellar and tuberculous spondylitis: comparative imaging features. *Radiology* 1989;171:419–425.
103. Smith AS, Weinstein MA, Mizushima A, Coughlin B, Hayden SP, Lakin MM, Lanzieri CF. MR imaging characteristics of tuberculous spondylitis vs vertebral osteomyelitis. *AJNR* 1989;10:619–625.
104. Smoker WRK, Godersky JC, Knutzon RK, Keyes WD, Norman D, Bergman W. The role of MR imaging in evaluating metastatic spinal disease. *AJNR* 1987;8:901–908.
105. Smoker WRK, Keyes WD, Dunn VD, Menezes AH. MRI versus conventional radiologic examinations in the evaluation of the craniovertebral and cervicomedullary junction. *RadioGraphics* 1986;6:953–994.
106. Sotiropoulos S, Chafetz NI, Lang P, Winkler M, Morris JM, Weinstein PR, Genant HK. Differentiation between postoperative scar and recurrent disk herniation: prospective comparison of MR, CT, and contrast-enhanced CT. *AJNR* 1989;10:639–643.
107. Stimac GK, Porter BA, Olson DO, Gerlach R, Genton M. Gadolinium-DTPA-enhanced MR imaging of spinal neoplasms: preliminary investigation and comparison with unenhanced spin-echo and STIR sequences. *AJNR* 1988;9:839–846.
108. Sze G, Abramson A, Krol G, Liu D, Amster J, Zimmerman RD, Deck MDF. Gadolinium-DTPA in the evaluation of intradural extramedullary spinal disease. *AJNR* 1988;9:153–163.
109. Sze G, Bravo S, Krol G. Spinal lesions: quantitative and qualitative temporal evolution of gadopentetate dimeglumine enhancement in MR imaging. *Radiology* 1989;170:849–856.
110. Sze G, Krol G, Zimmerman RD, Deck MDF. Intramedullary disease of the spine: diagnosis using gadolinium-DTPA-enhanced MR imaging. *AJNR* 1988;9:847–858.
111. Sze G, Krol G, Zimmerman RD, Deck MDF. Malignant extradural spinal tumors: MR imaging with Gd-DTPA. *Radiology* 1988;167:217–223.
112. Takahashi M, Yamashita Y, Sakamoto Y, Kojima R. Chronic cervical cord compression: clinical significance of increased signal intensity on MR images. *Radiology* 1989;173:219–224.
113. Teplick JG, Haskin ME. Intravenous contrast-enhanced CT of the postoperative lumbar spine: improved identification of recurrent disk herniation, scar, arachnoiditis, and diskitis. *AJR* 1984;143:845–855.
114. Teresi LM, Lufkin RB, Reicher MA, et al. Asymptomatic degenerative disk disease and spondylosis of the cervical spine: MR imaging. *Radiology* 1987;164:83–88.
115. Tobin WD, Layton DD Jr. The diagnosis and natural history of spinal cord arteriovenous malformations. *Mayo Clin Proc* 1976;51:637–646.
116. Valk J. Gd-DTPA in MR of spinal lesions. *AJNR* 1988;9:345–350.
117. VanDyke C, Ross JS, Tkach J, Masaryk TJ, Modic MT. Gradient-echo MR imaging of the cervical spine: evaluation of extradural disease. *AJNR* 1989;10:627–632.
118. Weinmann H-J, Brasch RC, Press W-R, Wesbey GE. Characteristics of gadolinium-DTPA complex: a potential NMR contrast agent. *AJR* 1984;142:619–624.
119. Weinreb JC, Wolbarsht LB, Cohen JM, Brown CEL, Maravilla KR. Prevalence of lumbosacral intervertebral disk abnormalities on MR images in pregnant and asymptomatic nonpregnant women. *Radiology* 1989;170:125–128.
120. Wilson DA, Prince JR. MR imaging determination of the location of the normal conus medullaris throughout childhood. *AJNR* 1989;10:259–262.
121. Wolpert SM, Anderson M, Scott RM, Kwan ESK, Runge VM. Chiari II malformation: MR imaging evaluation. *AJNR* 1987;8:783–792.
122. Yu S, Haughton VM, Lynch LK, Ho K-C, Sether LA. Fibrous structure in the intervertebral disk: correlation of MR appearance with anatomic sections. *AJNR* 1989;10:1105–1110.
123. Yu S, Haughton VM, Sether LA, Wagner M. Anulus fibrosus in bulging intervertebral disks. *Radiology* 1988;169:761–763.
124. Yu S, Sether LA, Ho PSP, Wagner M, Haughton VM. Tears of the anulus fibrosus: correlation between MR and pathologic findings in cadavers. *AJNR* 1988;9:367–370.

MRI of the Musculoskeletal System, 2nd Edition, edited by T. H. Berquist. Raven Press, Ltd., New York © 1990.

CHAPTER 6

Pelvis, Hips, and Thighs

Thomas H. Berquist

Technique, 149
Pelvis and Sacroiliac Joints, 149
Hips, 162
Thighs, 162
Anatomy, 162
Osseous Anatomy, 162
Muscular Anatomy, 163
Neurovascular Anatomy, 170
Pitfalls, 172
Applications, 174
Osteonecrosis, 174
Transient Osteoporosis or Edema, 181
Trauma, 181
Neoplasms, 186
Arthropathies, 189
Infection, 190
Pediatric Disorders, 190
References, 192

Magnetic resonance imaging (MRI) of the pelvis and hips has achieved wide acceptance as an imaging technique. This is largely due to the sensitivity and specificity of MRI for early detection of avascular necrosis (AVN) (7,9,10). However, as with other musculoskeletal regions, the applications for MRI of the pelvis, hips, and thighs continue to expand and have replaced many of the previously accepted studies, including CT, for evaluation of both bone and soft tissue pathology.

Many patients are referred for MRI of the pelvis and hips because of nonspecific pain, largely to exclude AVN. However, there are numerous causes of symptoms about the hip. Therefore, it is important to thoroughly evaluate this region and screen for problems other than AVN. The anatomy and techniques for evaluating various types of pathology are discussed in this chapter.

TECHNIQUE

The image planes and pulse sequences chosen for evaluation of the pelvis, hips, and thighs depend on the clinical indication. Specific techniques are discussed later; however, there are certain standard techniques that can be used for screening examinations.

T. H. Berquist: Mayo Medical School and Mayo Clinic, Rochester, Minnesota 55905.

Pelvis and Sacroiliac Joints

Examinations for suspected pathology of the pelvis and/or sacroiliac joints can be accomplished using the body coil. A coronal scout image is obtained with the patient in the supine position. Every effort should be made to be certain the patient is properly positioned with the hips at the same level. If a soft tissue abnormality is suspected posteriorly, the patient may be placed in the prone position. This reduces compression of the soft tissues and anatomic distortion. After the initial scout image, axial images are obtained using 1 cm thick slides with either a 5 or 2.5 mm skip and a double-echo T2 weighted sequence (TE 20-30/60-80, TR 2,000). The field of view (FOV) selected varies with patient size but generally 40–42 cm is adequate. A matrix of 256 × 256 with 1 acquisition (Nex) is obtained. Respiratory compensation techniques should be used to reduce motion artifact in the upper pelvis (Fig. 6-1). Thinner slices can be used if a more defined area of the anatomy is to be studied. After the initial images have been evaluated, a second pulse sequence is obtained in either the axial or coronal plane (Figs. 6-2 and 6-3). This is generally performed using a T1 weighted (SE 500/20) sequence. The same slice thickness is used if the images are performed in the same image plane. This allows more accurate comparison of T1 and T2 weighted sections. When the coronal or sagittal plane is used, the slice thickness

Text continues on p. 162

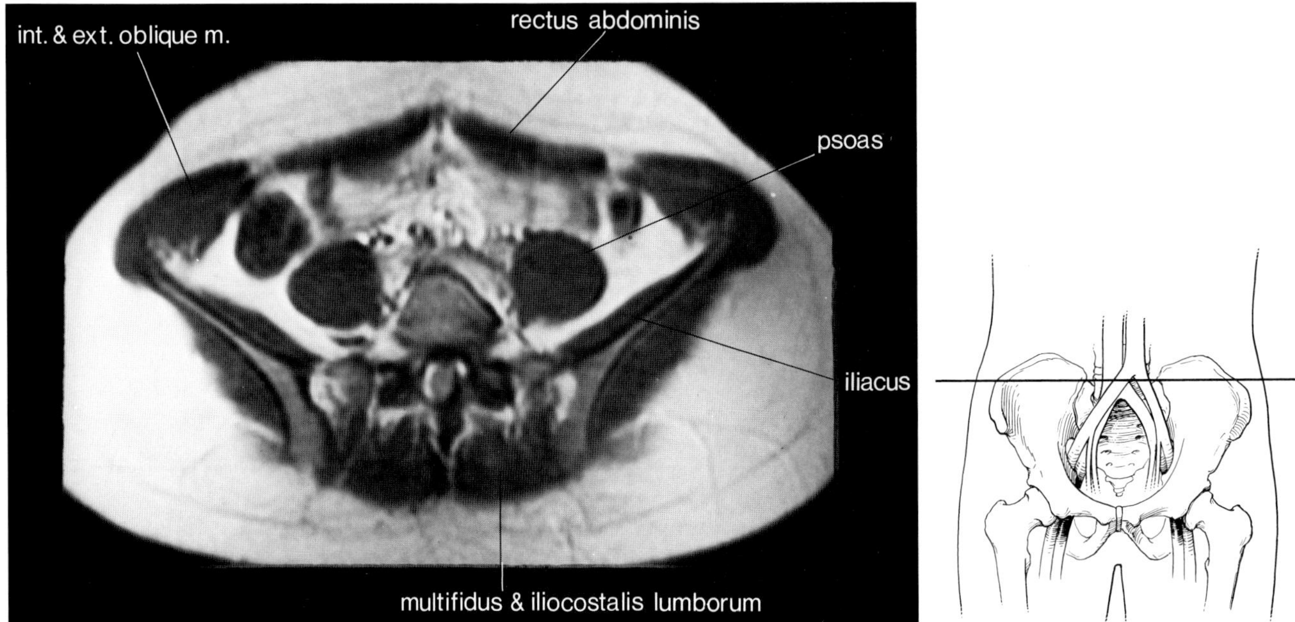

FIG. 6-1. Axial MR images (SE 2,000/30) of the pelvis, hips, and upper thighs. **A:** Axial image through the upper pelvis.

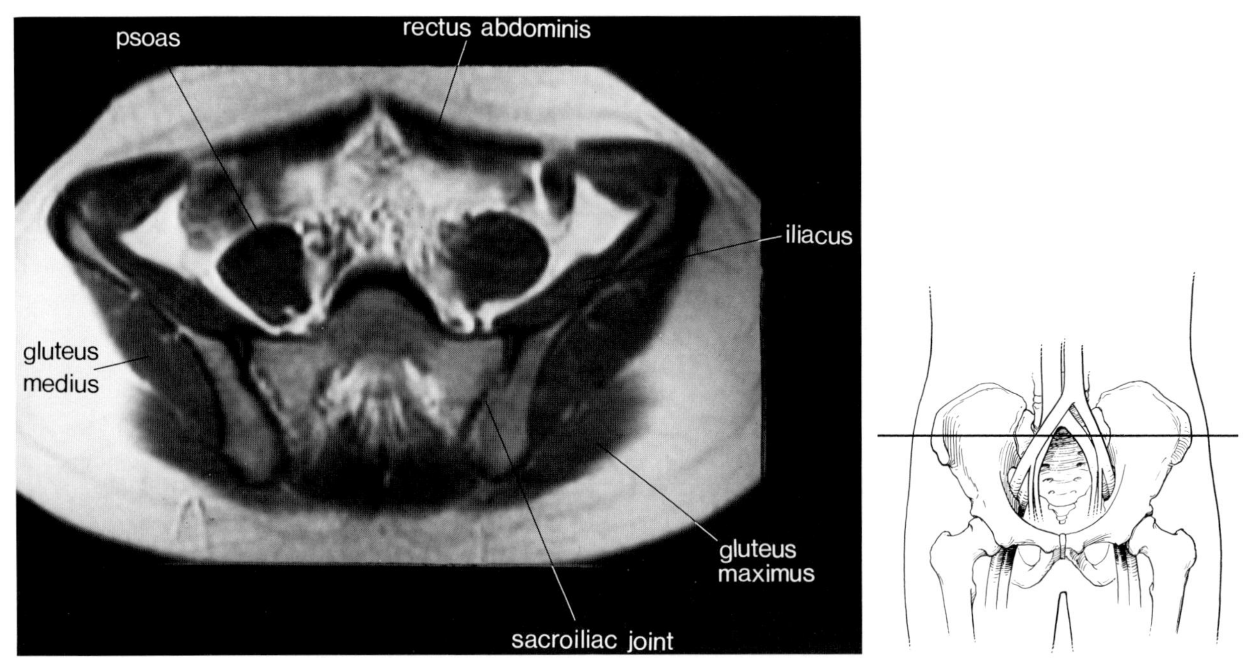

FIG. 6-1. B: Axial image through the upper sacrum.

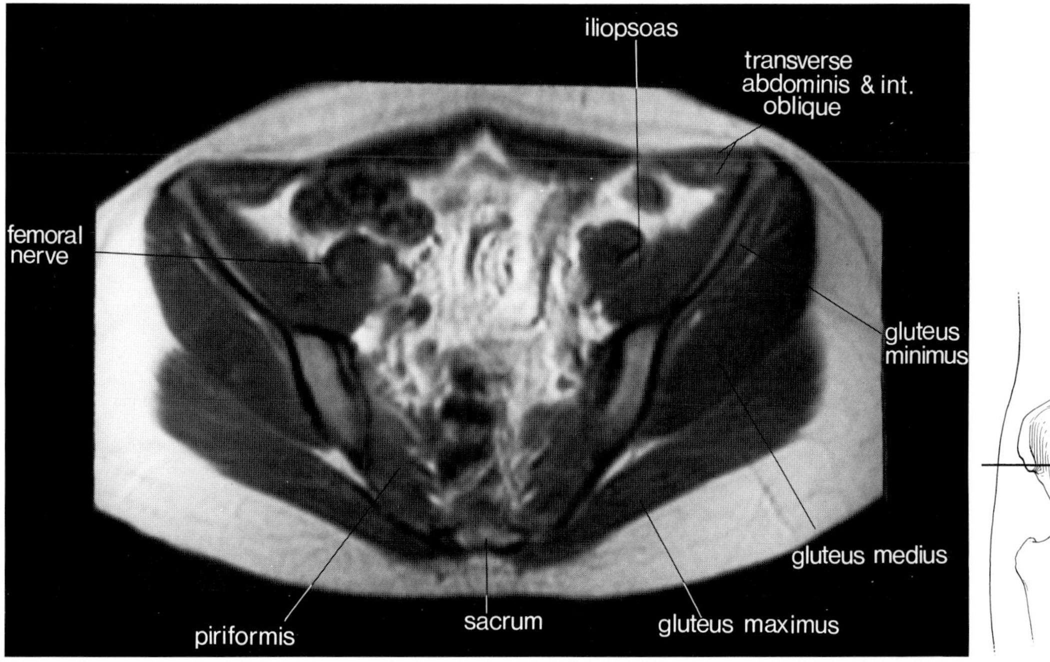

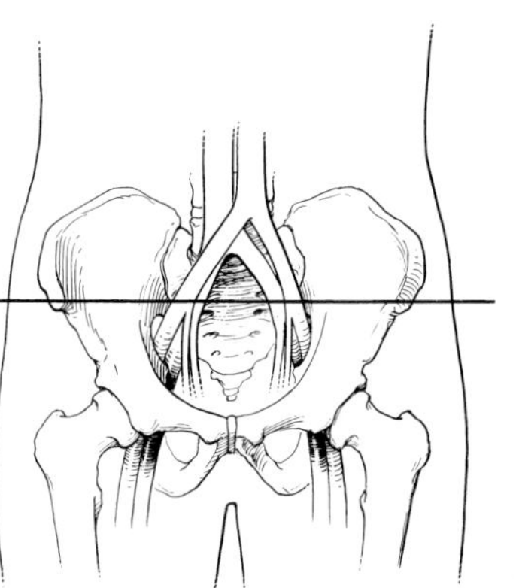

FIG. 6-1. C: Axial image through the lower SI joint.

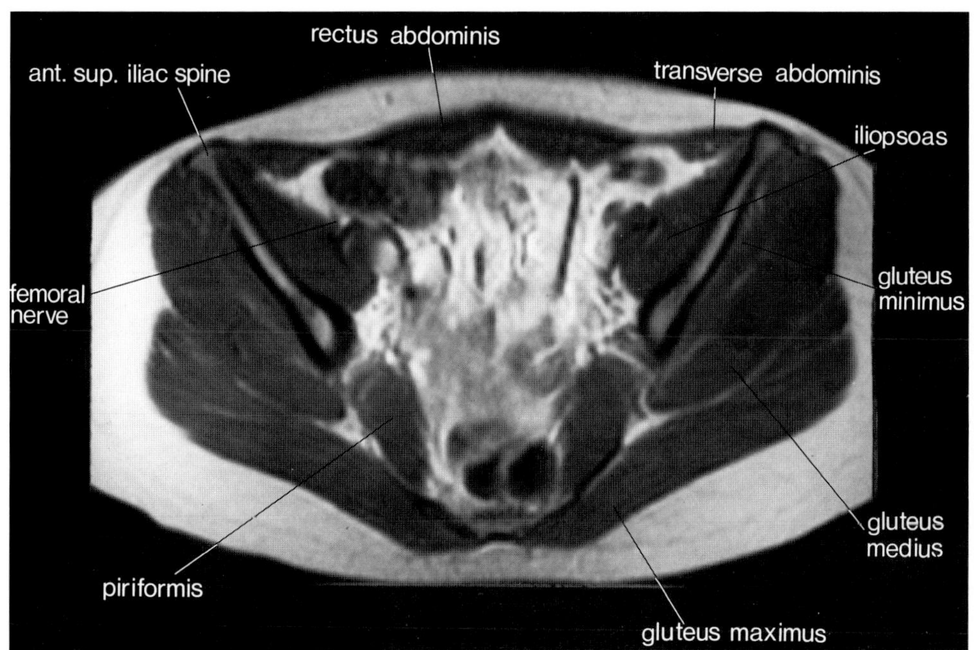

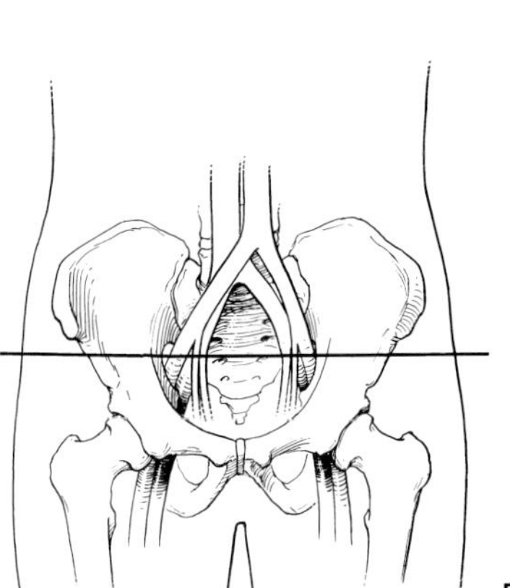

FIG. 6-1. D: Axial image through the sciatic notch.

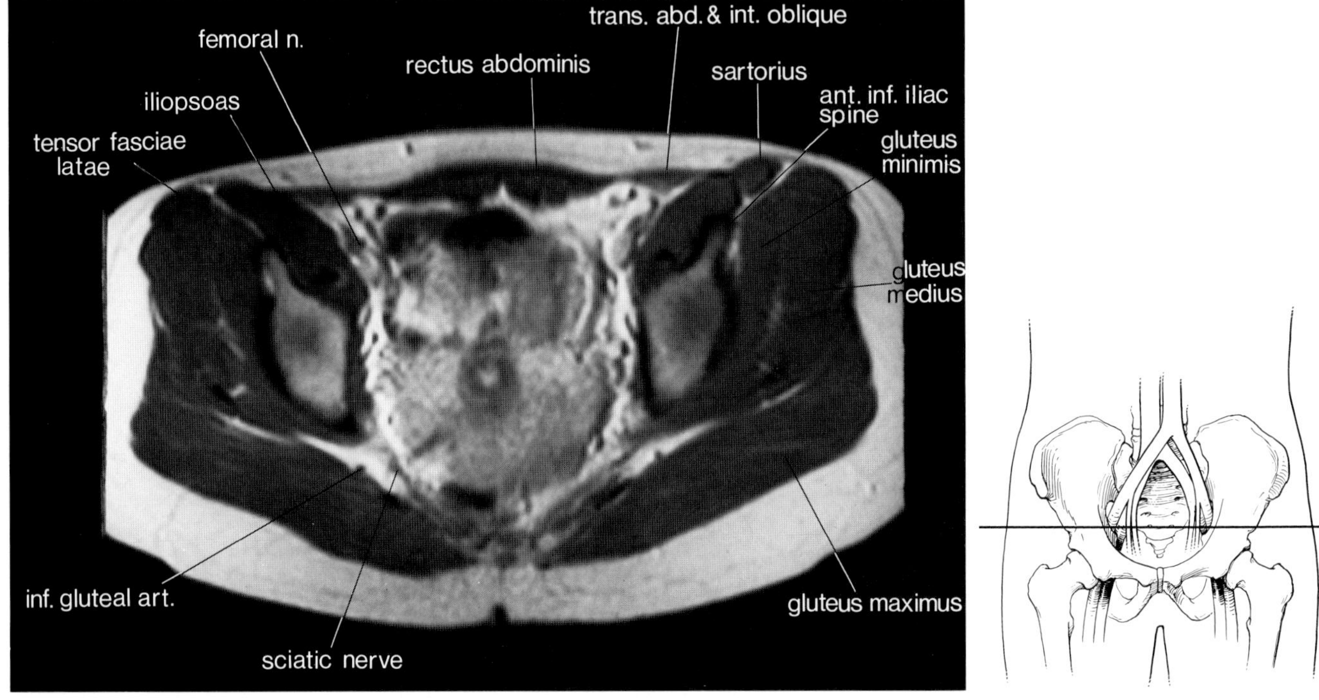

FIG. 6-1. E: Axial image through the anterior inferior iliac spine.

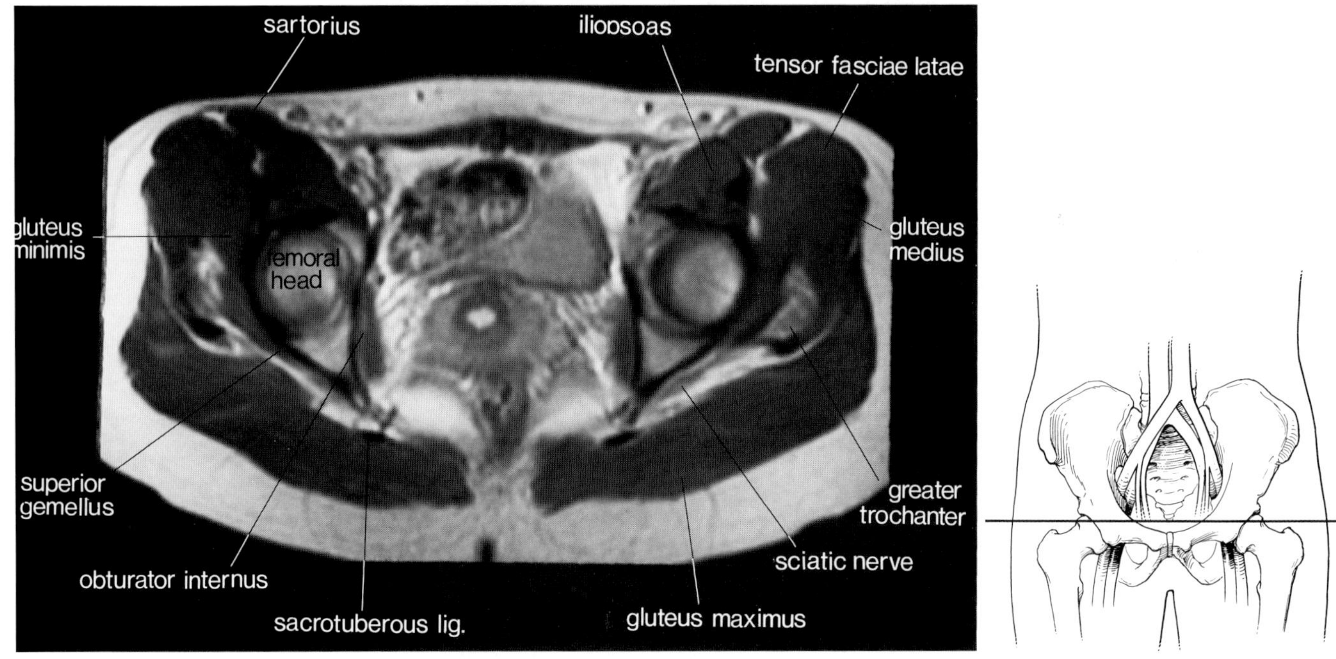

FIG. 6-1. F: Axial image through the upper femoral head.

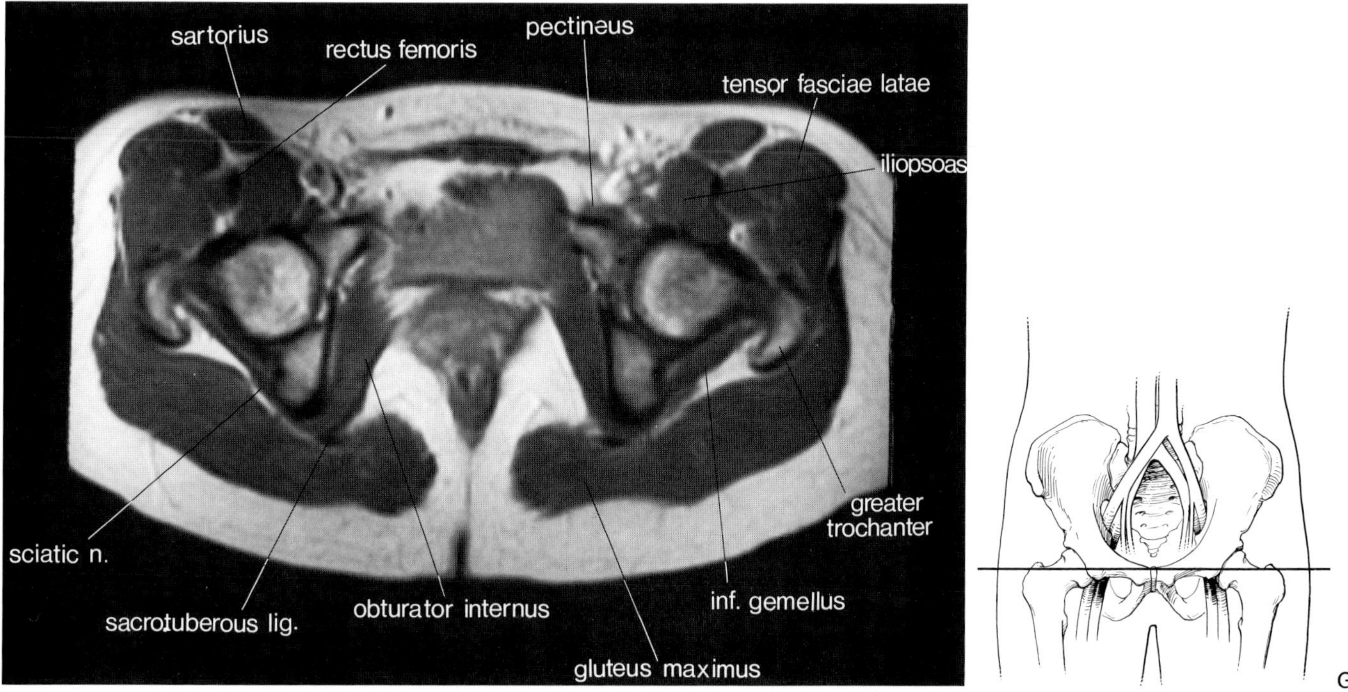

FIG. 6-1. G: Axial image through the femoral head and greater trochanter.

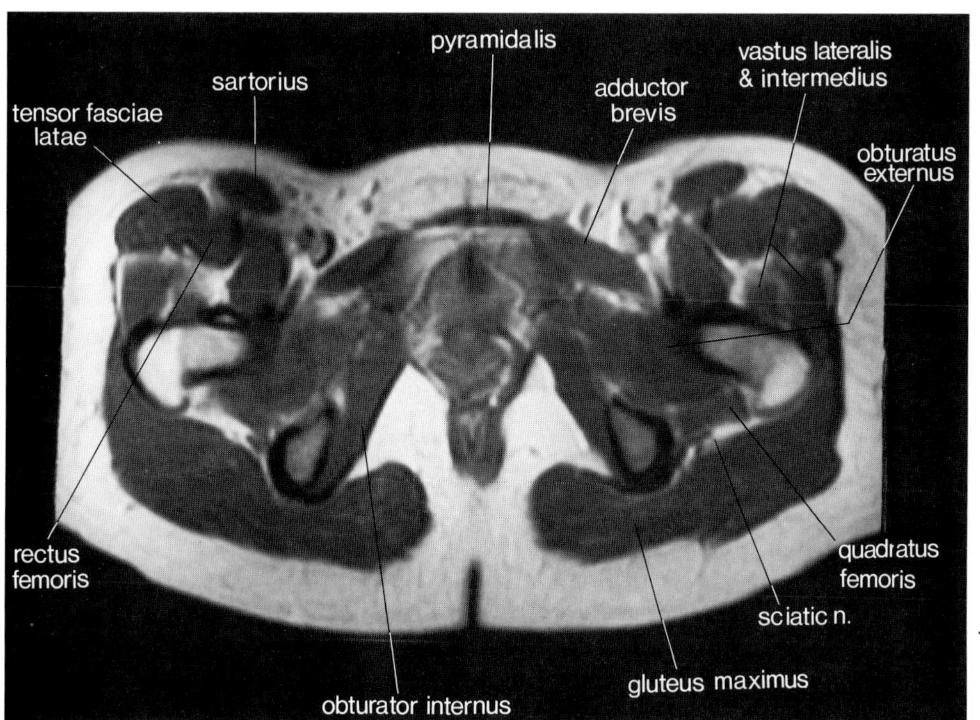

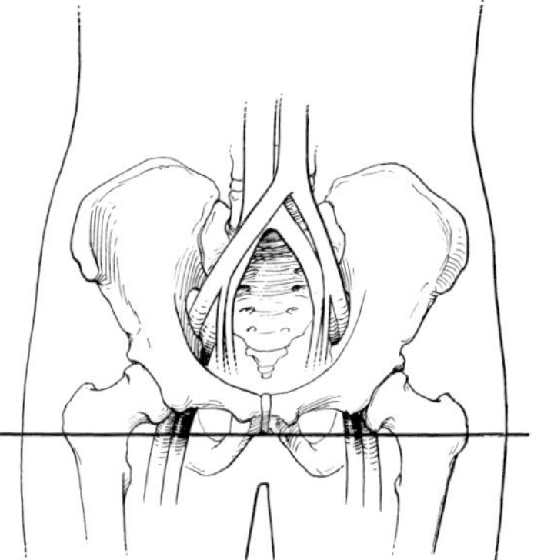

FIG. 6-1. H: Axial image through the femoral neck.

I

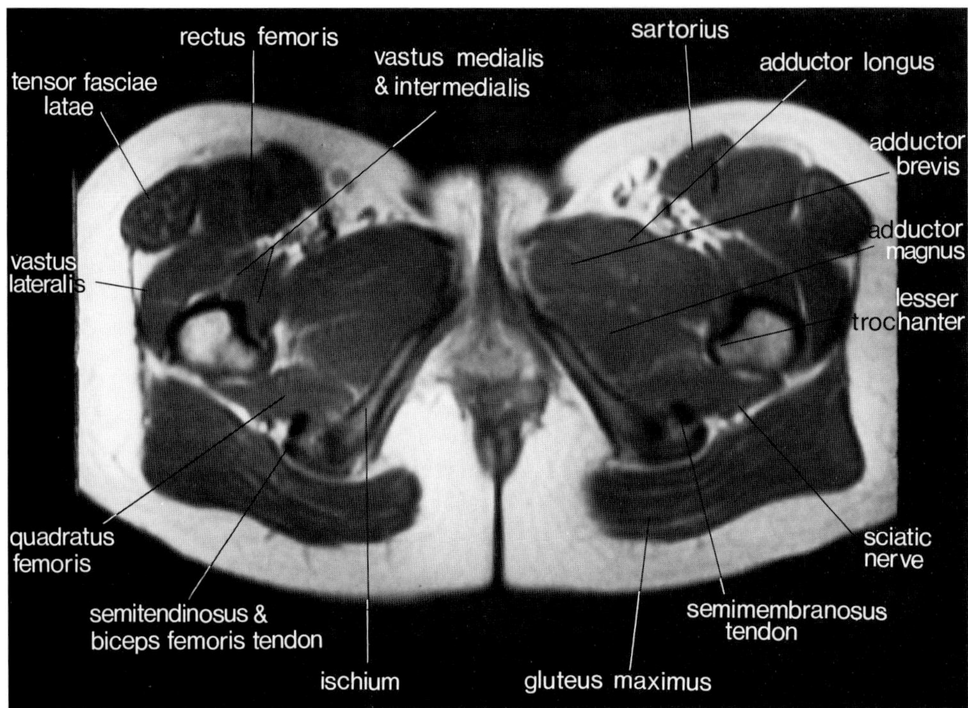

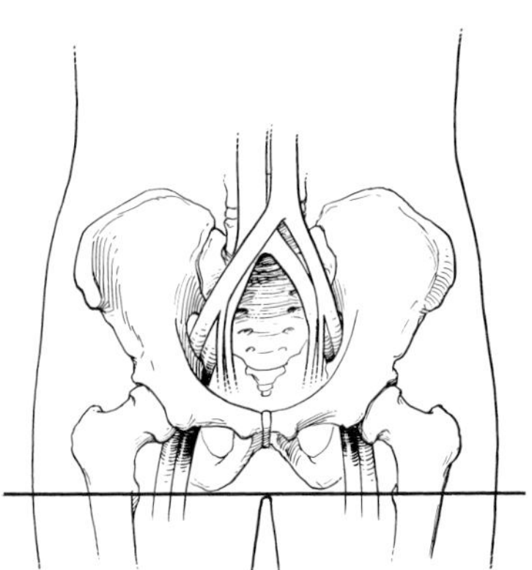

FIG. 6-1. I: Axial image through the lesser trochanter.

J

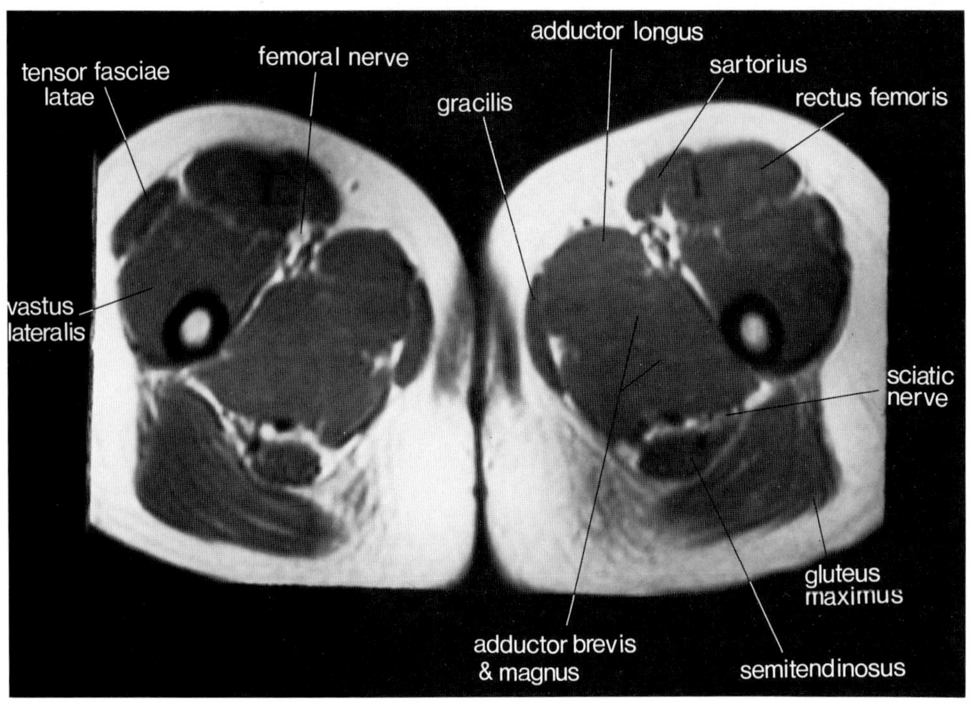

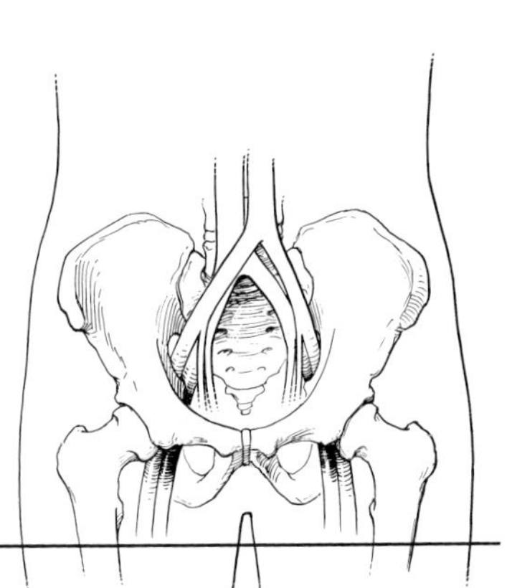

FIG. 6-1. J: Axial image through the upper femur.

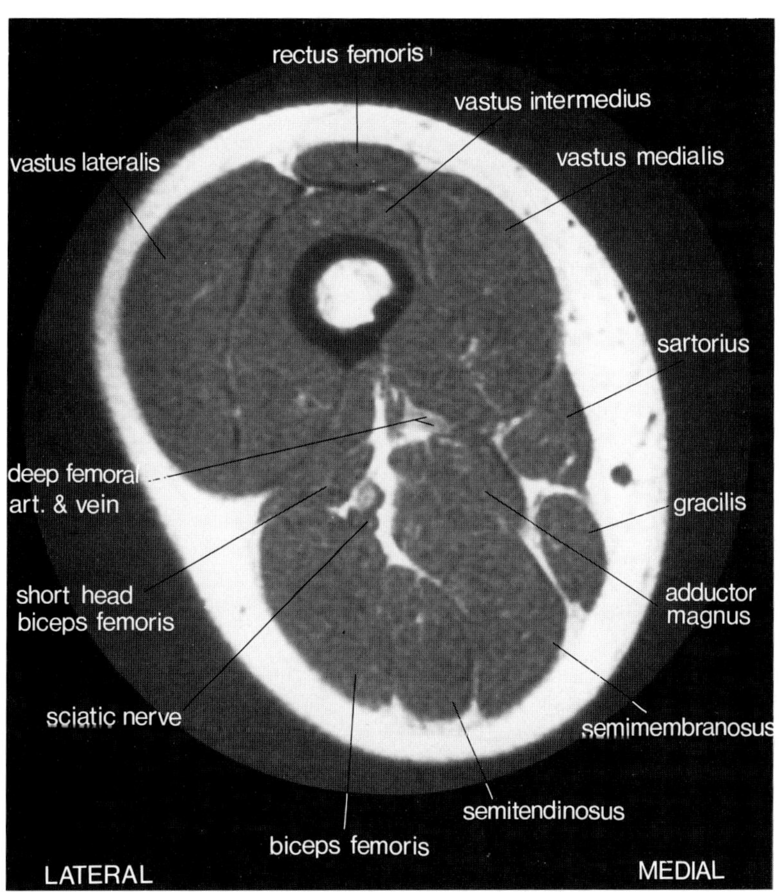

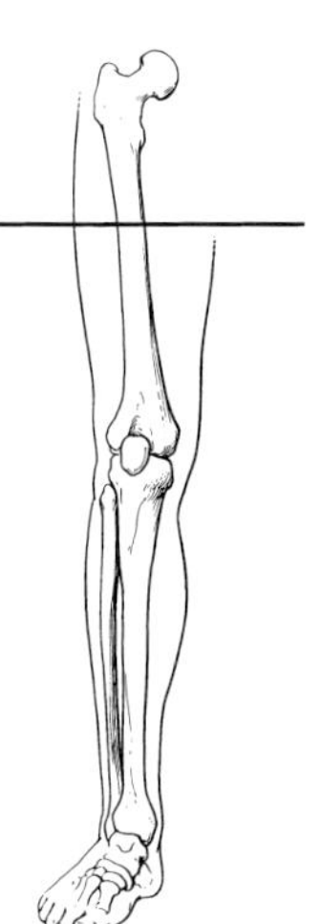

FIG. 6-1. K: Axial image through the upper thigh.

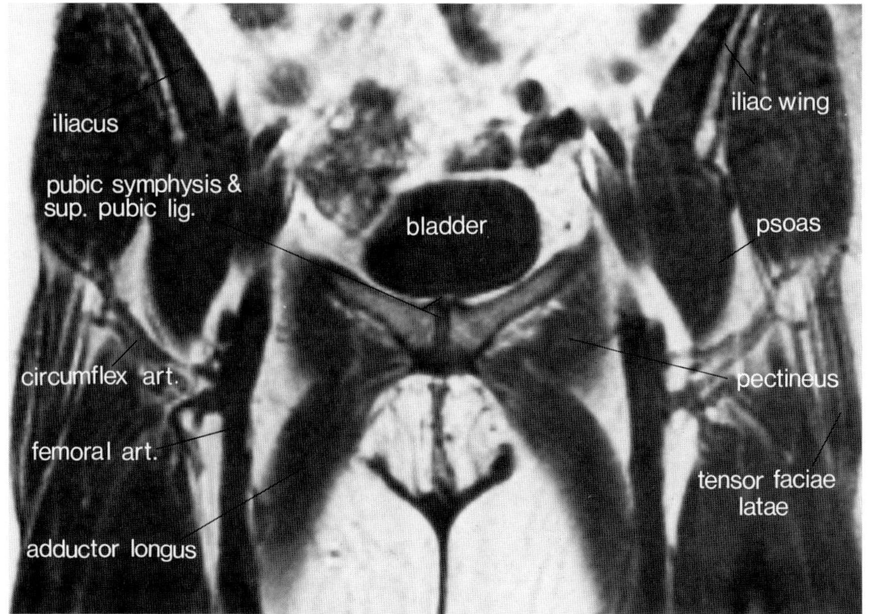

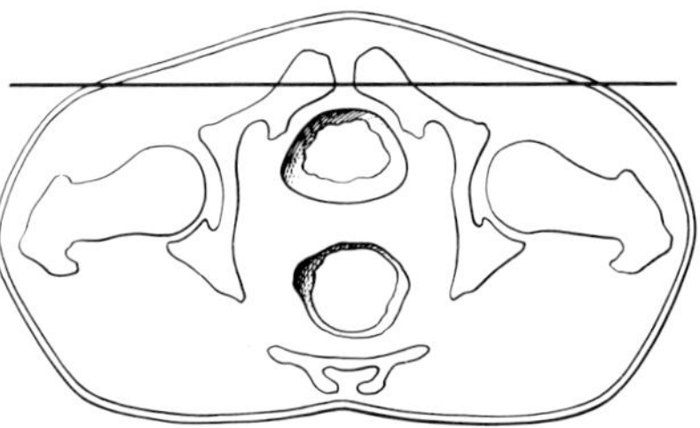

A

FIG. 6-2. Coronal MR images (SE 500/20) of the pelvis, hips, and thighs. **A:** Coronal image through the pubic symphysis.

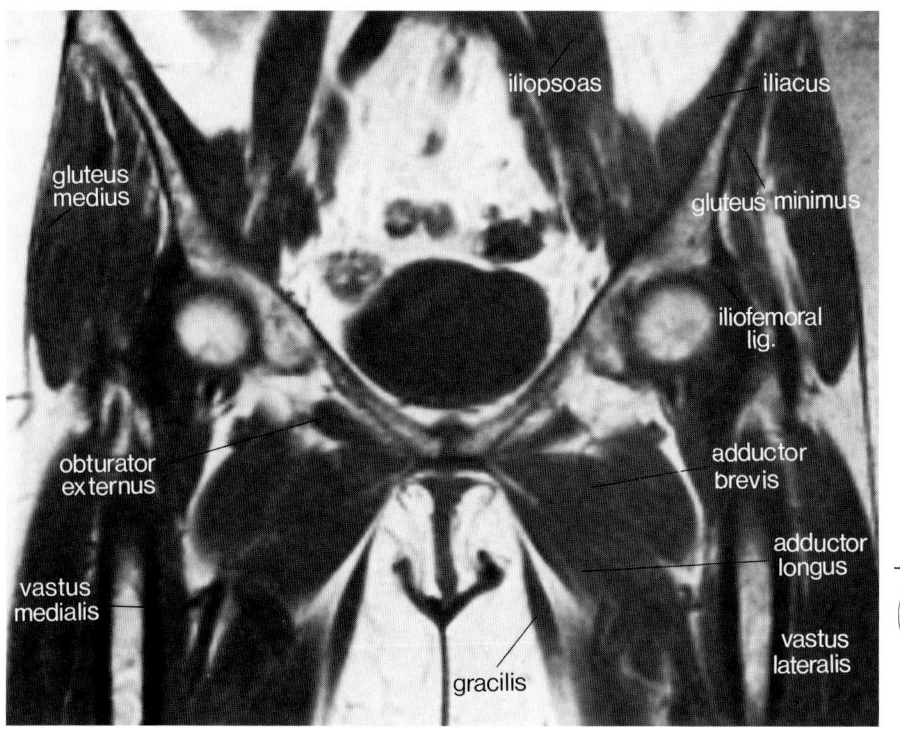

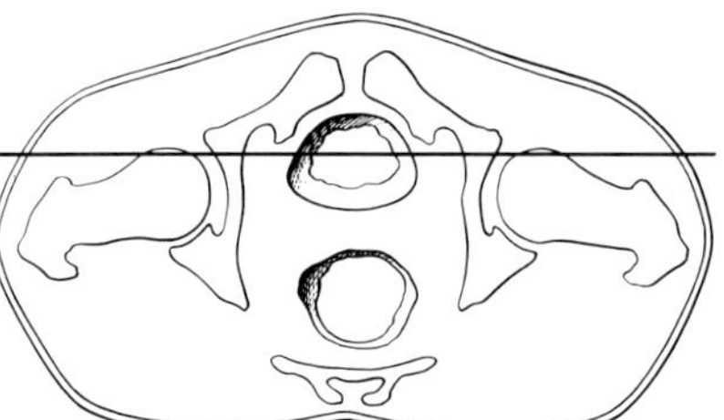

B

FIG. 6-2. **B:** Coronal image through the anterior aspect of the hips.

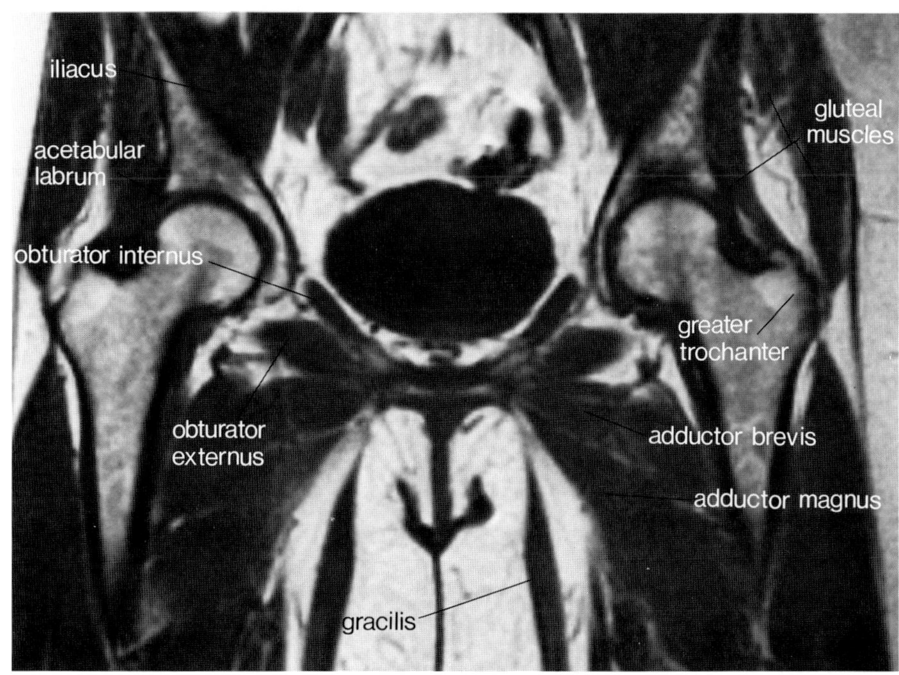

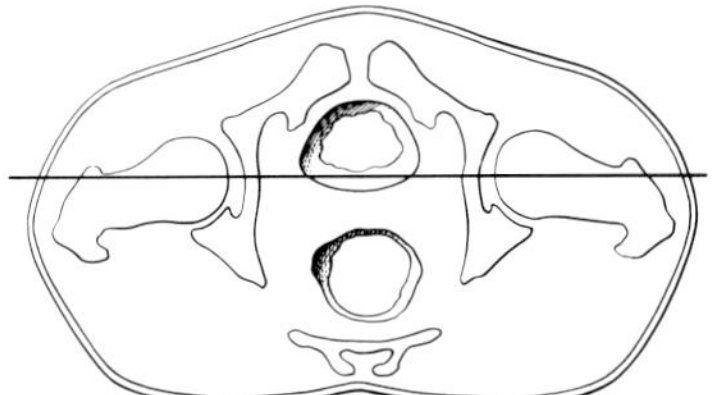

FIG. 6-2. C: Coronal image through the midhip.

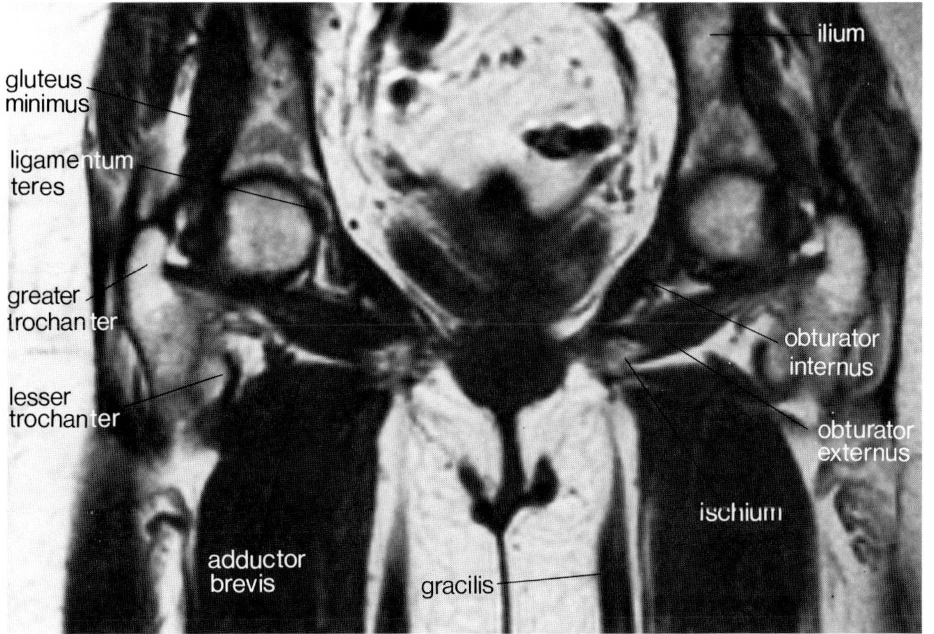

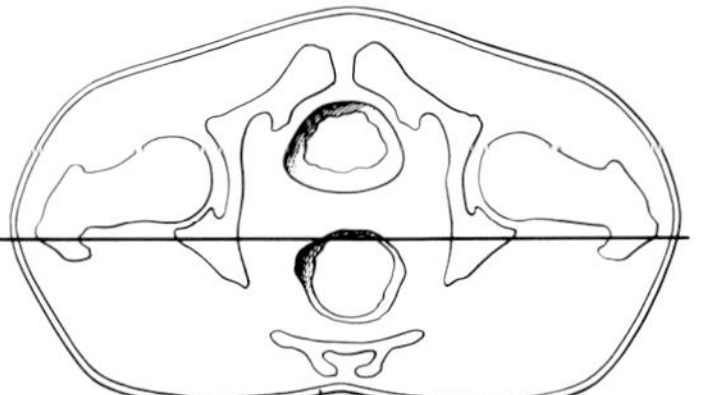

FIG. 6-2. D: Coronal image through the greater trochanteric level of the hips.

E

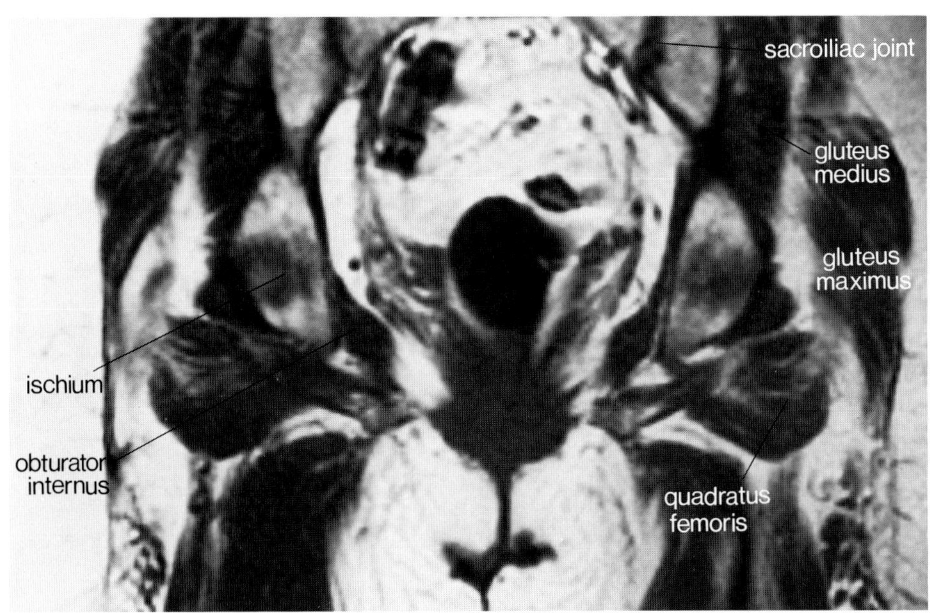

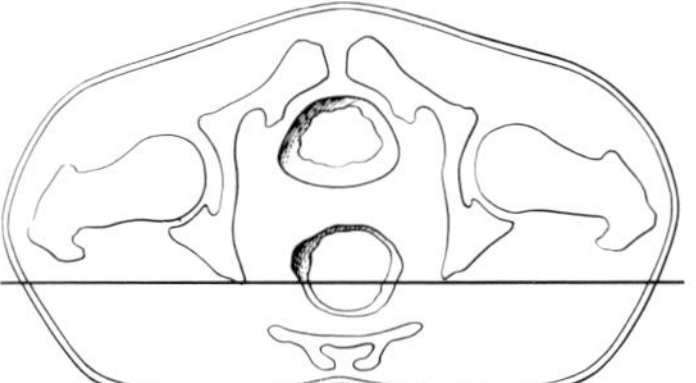

FIG. 6-2. E: Coronal image through the ischium.

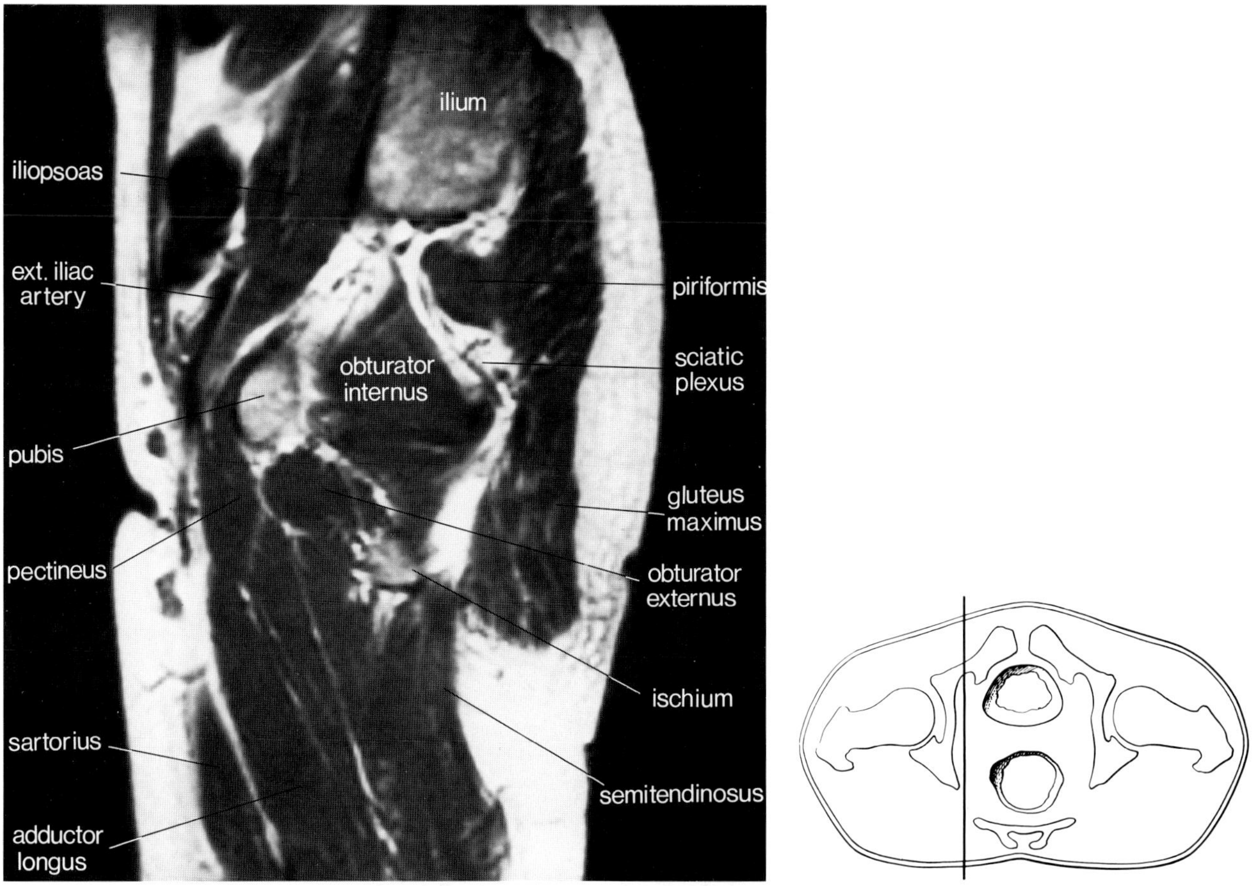

FIG. 6-3. Sagittal MR images (SE 500/20) of the pelvis, hips, and thighs progressing from the midline laterally. **A:** Sagittal image through the medial ilium near the sciatic notch.

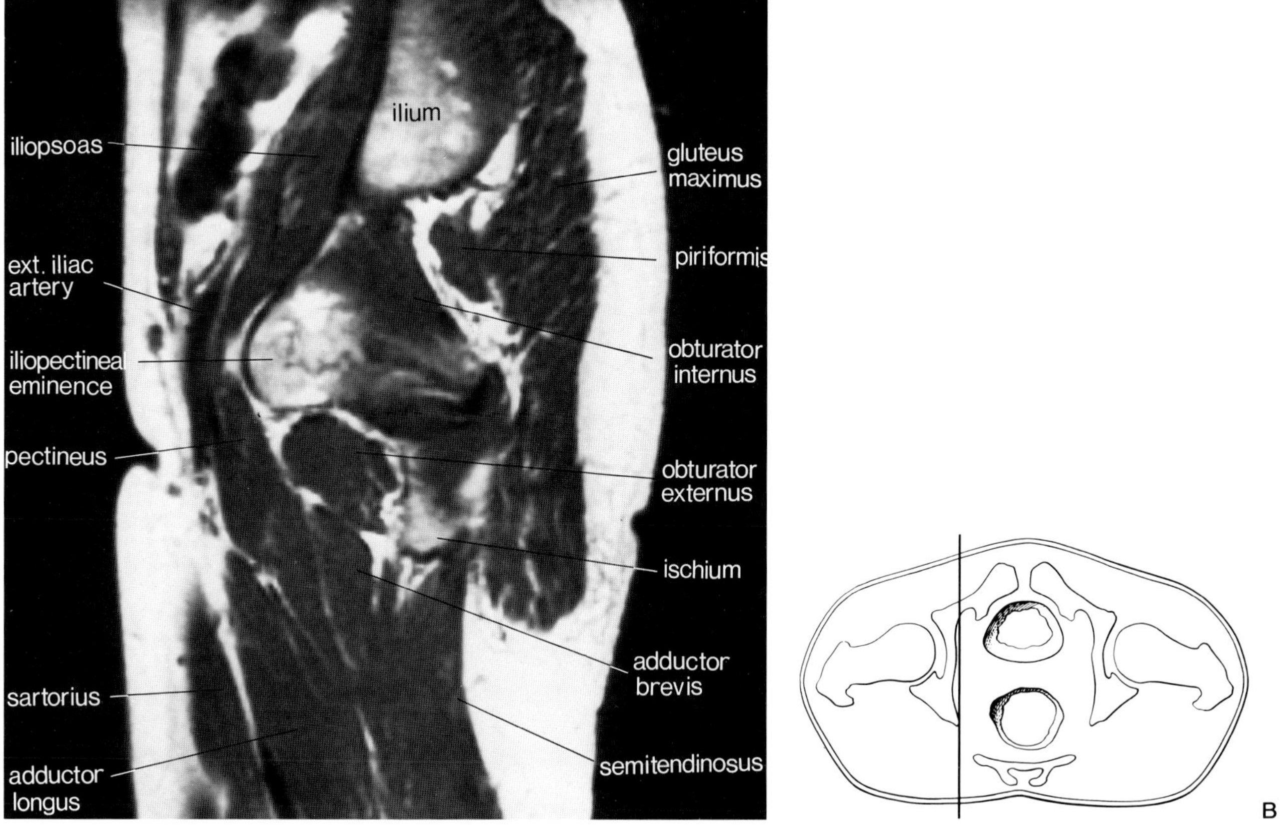

FIG. 6-3. B: Sagittal image through the level of the iliopectineal eminence.

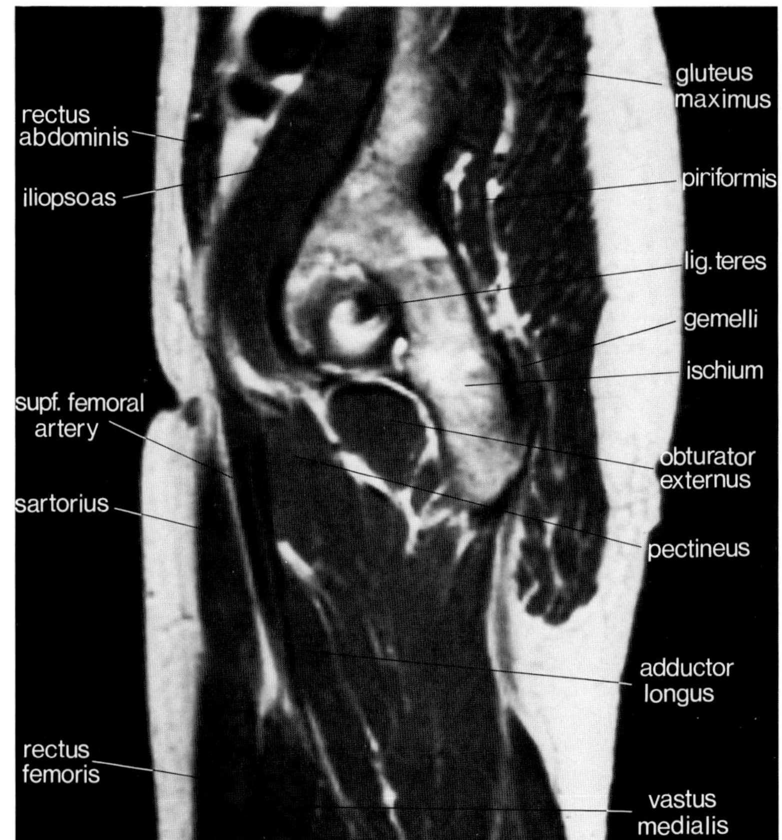

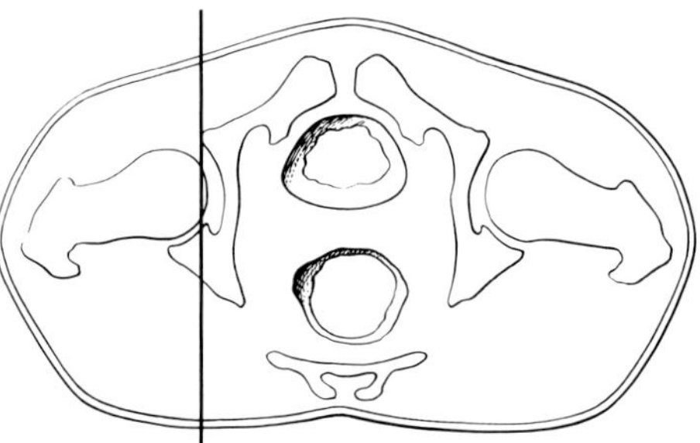

FIG. 6-3. C: Sagittal image through the medial acetabulum.

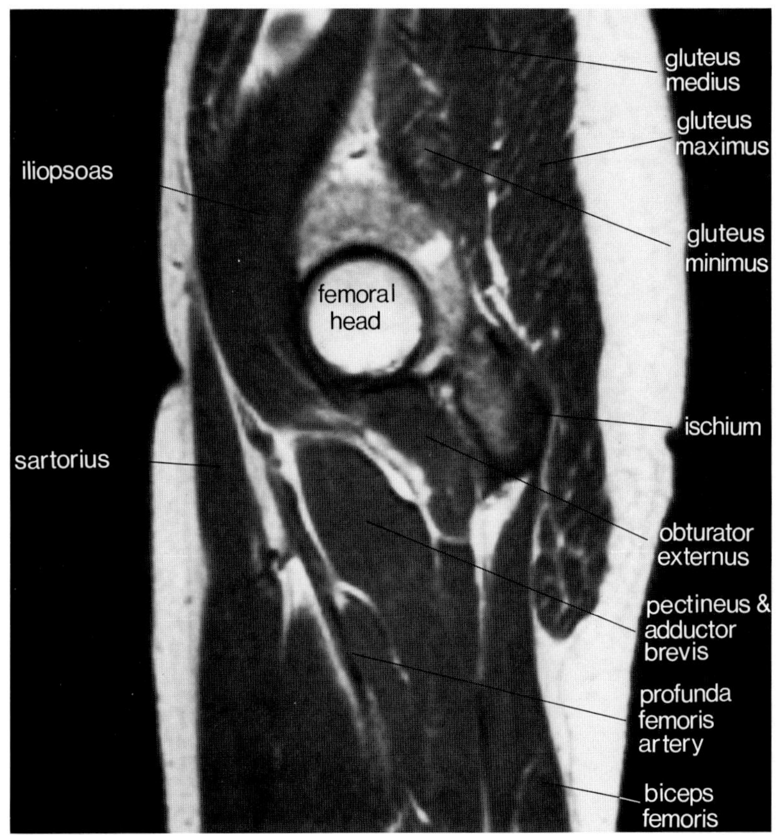

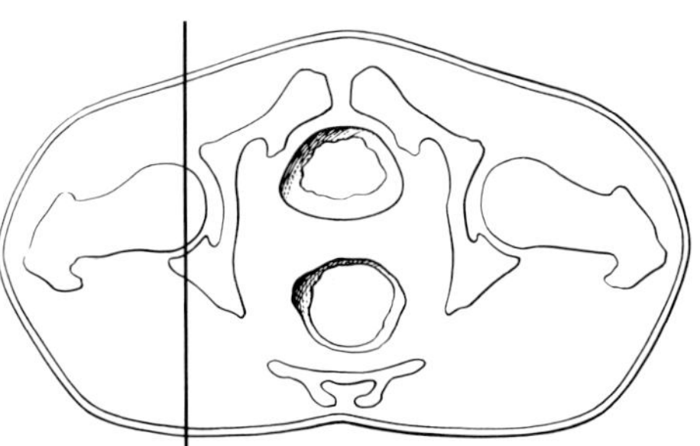

FIG. 6-3. D: Sagittal image through the medial femoral head.

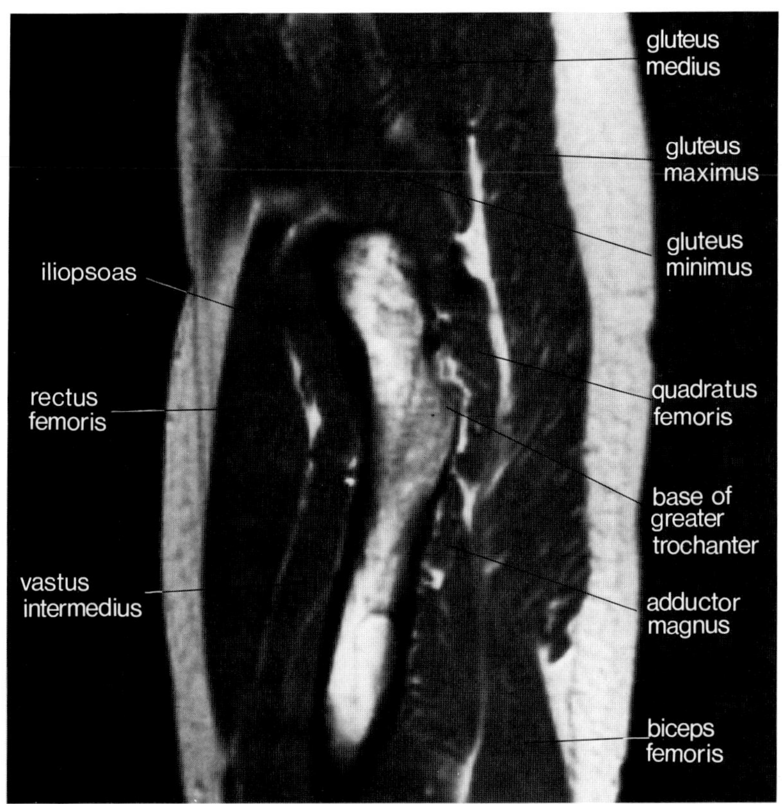

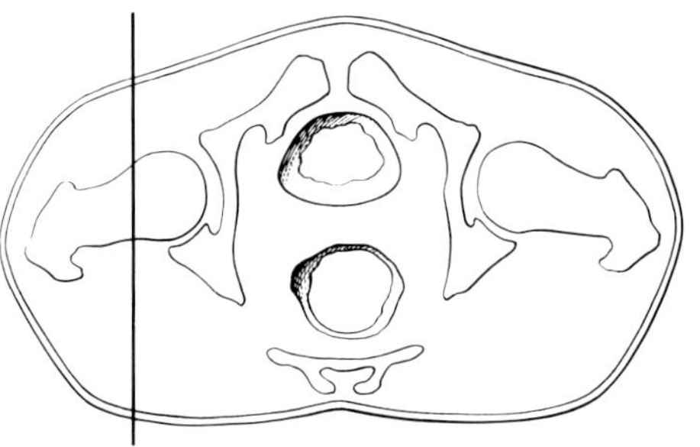

FIG. 6-3. E: Sagittal image through the femur.

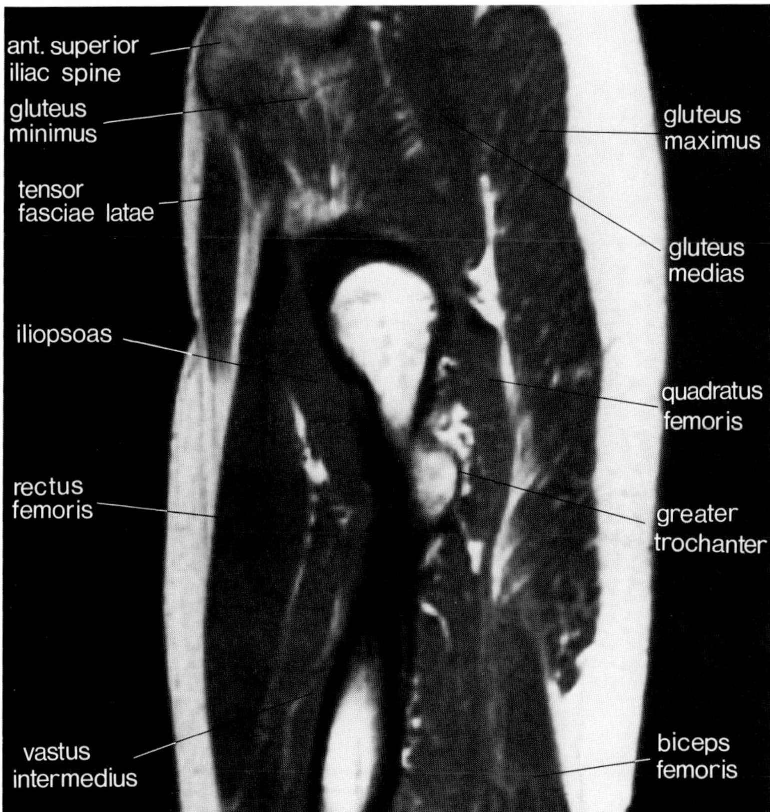

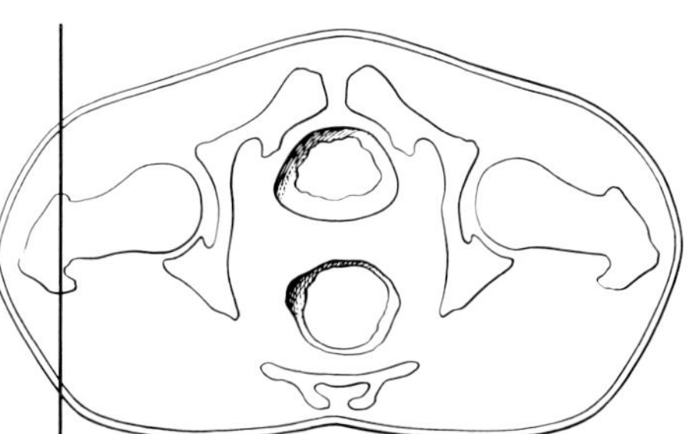

FIG. 6-3. F: Sagittal image through the level of the greater trochanter and anterior superior iliac spine.

TABLE 6-1. *MR examinations of the pelvis, hips, and thighs*

	Pulse sequence	Slice thickness	Matrix	Field of view (FOV) (cm)	Acquisitions (Nex)	Image time
Pelvis–SI Joints						
Coronal scout	SE 400/20	Three 1 cm slices	128 × 256	42	1	51 sec
Axial	SE 2,000/60, 20	1 cm/skip 2.5 mm or 5 mm/skip 2.5 mm	256 × 256	30–42[a]	1	8 min 56 sec
Coronal, sagittal, or axial	SE 500/20	1 cm/skip 2.5 mm or 5 mm/skip 2.5 mm	256 × 256	30–42[a]	1	2 min 8 sec
					Total =	11 min 54 sec
Hips						
Axial scout	SE 400/20	Three 1 cm slices	128 × 256	42	1	51 sec
Coronal	SE 500/20	5 mm/no skip	256 × 256	30–42[a]	1	2 min 8 sec
Axial	SE 2,000/60, 20	1 cm/skip 2.5 mm or 5 mm/skip 2.5 mm	256 × 256	30–42[a]	1	8 min 56 sec
					Total =	11 min 54 sec
Thighs						
Coronal scout	SE 400/20	Three 1 cm slices	128 × 256	42	1	51 sec
Axial	SE 2,000/60, 20	1 cm/skip 2.5 mm or 5 mm/skip 2.5 mm	256 × 256	30–42[a]	1	8 min 56 sec
Axial, coronal, or sagittal	SE 500/20	1 cm/skip 2.5 mm or 5 mm/skip 2.5 mm	256 × 256	30–42[a]	1	2 min 8 sec
					Total =	11 min 54 sec

[a] Varies with patient size and area of interest.

varies depending on the tissue volume of the area to be studied. Typically, 5 mm/skip 2.5 mm or 1 cm contiguous sections are obtained. The other parameters are the same as those used for the T2 weighted sequence described above. These two sequences and image planes generally provide an adequate screening examination (Table 6-1). In certain circumstances, which are discussed later, further pulse sequences and image planes may be indicated.

Hips

Evaluation of patients with symptoms more defined to the hip region are performed with a slightly different technique. An axial scout image is obtained through the level of both hips. Using this sequence as a guide, a T1 weighted coronal sequence (SE 500/20) is performed using 5 mm thick sections with no interslice gap. This technique will usually define AVN and other obvious marrow abnormalities in the hips. When there is no evidence of AVN or if other abnormalities are suspected, a second T2 weighted (SE 2,000/20-30, 60-80) axial sequence is performed similar to the one described above (pelvis and sacroiliac joints) (Table 6-1). In certain situations, such as AVN or subtle osteochondral abnormalities of the femoral heads, it may be of benefit to use a surface coil or dual coupled coils to improve image quality. Sagittal images may also be useful to provide more information regarding surface area involvement of the femoral head. In this setting a small FOV (16–20 cm) should be used (66).

Thighs

Generally, both T1 and T2 weighted sequences are required to fully evaluate the soft tissues of the thighs and the upper femurs. Again, a coronal scout through the hip and thigh region is generally obtained from which T2 weighted axial images are selected. Depending on the findings noted with the T2 weighted images, a second series of T1 weighted images is performed in either the axial plane or coronal or sagittal plane. The second sequence is important in characterizing the nature of the lesion. Two different planes are essential if the extent of a lesion is important to define, such as for a neoplasm, abscess, or hematoma.

New angiographic software or conventional GRASS images are useful when vascular abnormalities are suspected in the pelvis or thighs. Variations in techniques are discussed more fully later with specific clinical applications.

ANATOMY

It is essential that the anatomy of the bone and soft tissue structures be clearly understood in all image planes typically used with MRI (Figs. 6-1 to 6-3) (35).

Osseous Anatomy

The pelvis is formed by the two innominate bones that articulate posteriorly with the sacrum at the sacroiliac joints and anteriorly at the pubic symphysis. Each innominate bone is composed of an ilium, ischium, and pubis. The acetabulum is formed by the junction of all three of these osseous structures. The posterior acetabulum is stronger and, along with the dome, comprises the weight-bearing portion of the acetabulum (1,37). The margin of the acetabulum is surrounded by a fibrocartilaginous labrum. Identification of the shape of this labrum, its relationship to the femoral head, and whether the structure is intact are important in infants, children, and adults (39). Special image planes may be required to demonstrate the entire labrum. These techniques are discussed later in this chapter.

Further discussion of the articulations in the pelvis is important, because these areas are easily assessed with MRI. Anteriorly, the pubic symphysis is formed by the junction of the two pubic bones. The osseous structures are attached by ligaments (superior pubic ligament and arcuate pubic ligament), which encase a fibrocartilaginous disc that lies between the two pubic bones (Fig. 6-2A) (1,16,37). The sacroiliac joint is a synovial joint with posterior and anterior ligamentous support. The posterior ligaments are stronger than the anterior ligaments, which allows some anterior motion. In addition, there are several accessory ligaments that assist in the support of the sacroiliac joint. These include the sacrotuberous ligament, which extends from the inferolateral margin of the sacrum to the ischial tuberosity, the sacrospinous ligament, which extends from the lower margin of the sacrum to the ischial spine, and the iliolumbar ligament, which extends from the anterior inferior transverse process of L5 and passes inferiorly to blend with the anterior sacroiliac ligament along the base of the sacrum. These ligamentous structures appear dark or have no signal intensity on MR images. The synovial cavity of the sacroiliac joint contains only a small amount of fluid, which is most easily identified on axial T2 weighted MR images (Fig. 6-1) (1,16,37,50).

The hip is a ball and socket joint. The fibrous capsule of the hip joint is lined with synovial membrane, and hyaline cartilage covers the articular surfaces of the acetabulum and femoral head (Fig. 6-4). There are several important intra-articular structures that should be identified on MR images. Ligamentum teres is a firm ligament extending from the fovea of the femoral head to the acetabulum. The ligament enters a small notch in the medial acetabular wall where it is surrounded by fat (Figs. 6-2E, F and 6-4). A fibrocartilaginous acetabular labrum surrounds the acetabular rim. This structure is clearly defined on MR images. Axial, coronal (Figs. 6-1 and 6-2), or radial images may be necessary to completely define this structure. Inferiorly, the labrum is incomplete but connected by the transverse ligament (Fig. 6-4). This ligament has an elliptical configuration and should not be confused with an acetabular labral tear. The ligaments that surround the capsule of the hip

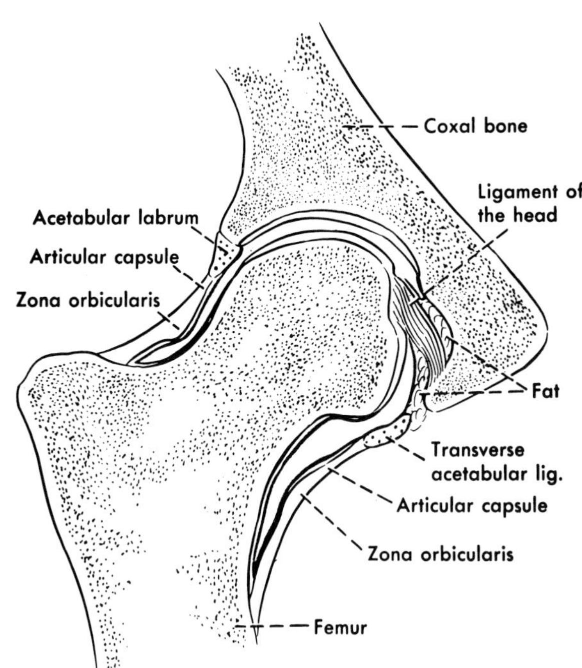

FIG. 6-4. Coronal illustration of the hip, demonstrating the major articular components and capsule. (From ref. 37, with permission.)

blend with the capsule and are not easily defined using MRI. Major ligaments (Fig. 6-5) include the pubofemoral ligament, which arises from the body of the pubis close to the acetabulum, passes anterior to the lower part of the femoral head, blends with the lower limb of the iliofemoral ligament as it attaches to the lower margin of the femoral neck. The iliofemoral ligament is thicker and probably the strongest of the supporting ligaments of the hip. It is more triangular, with its apex attached to the lower part of the anterior inferior iliac spine and body of the ilium. The base of this triangular ligament attaches to the intertrochanteric line (Fig. 6-5). The ischiofemoral ligament, the thinnest of the three major ligaments, arises from the ischium behind and below the acetabulum. Its upper fibers are horizontal; its lower fibers extend upward and laterally and attach to the upper posterior neck at the junction of the greater trochanter. The vascular supply of the hip and femoral head is important, especially in the etiology of avascular necrosis. This is discussed more thoroughly later in the section on avascular necrosis (1,4,37).

Muscular Anatomy

The anatomy of the muscles acting on the pelvis, hips, and thighs in axial, coronal, sagittal, and even oblique planes must be thoroughly understood to interpret MR images and evaluate symptoms related to these areas. The muscles acting on the hip joint per se are numerous.

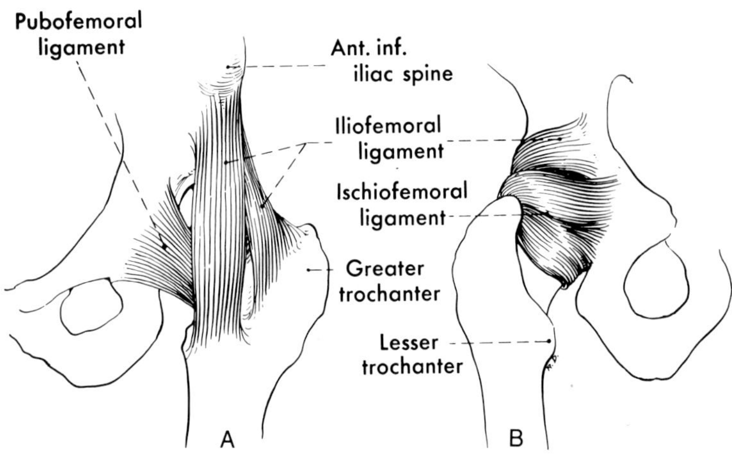

FIG. 6-5. Illustration of the supporting ligaments of the hip from anterior (**A**) and posterior (**B**). (From ref. 37, with permission.)

Therefore, it is simplest to discuss them based on their function (1,16,37,39,50).

The chief extensors of the hip include the gluteus maximus and posterior portion of the adductor magnus (Fig. 6-6). Extension is also accomplished to some degree by assistance from the semimembranosus, semitendinosus, biceps femoris, gluteus medius, and gluteus minimus (1,37) (Table 6-2).

The primary flexor of the hip is the iliopsoas muscle (Fig. 6-7). However, the pectineus, tensor fasciae latae, adductor brevis, and sartorius also function in this regard. Accessory flexors include the adductor longus, adductor magnus, gracilis, and gluteus minimus (37).

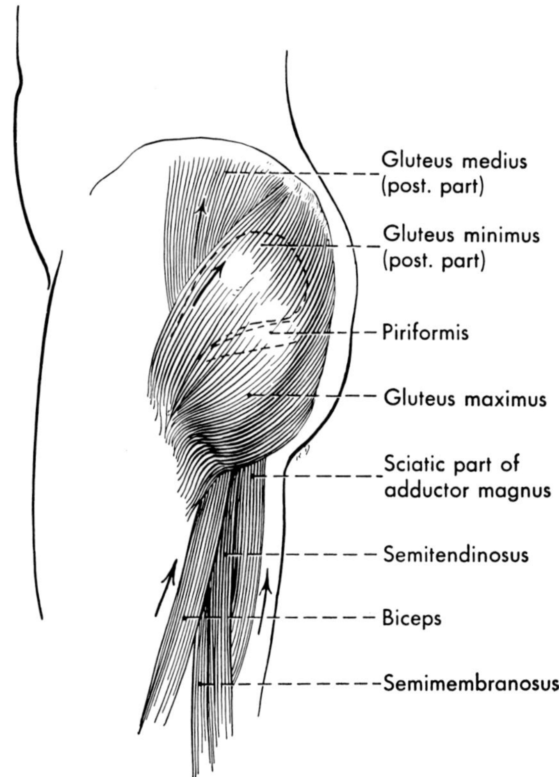

FIG. 6-6. Illustration of the extensors of the thigh. (From ref. 37, with permission.)

Adduction of the femur and thigh is primarily accomplished by the adductor group and gracilis (Figs. 6-1 and 6-3). The adductor group includes the adductor brevis, adductor longus, and adductor magnus. Accessory adductors include the gluteus maximus, pectineus, and obturator externus. The hamstring muscles also assist slightly in this regard (Fig. 6-8). Medial or internal rotation of the hip is primarily accomplished by the gluteus medius and minimus and the tensor fasciae latae. Semitendinosus, semimembranosus, and to some degree the gracilis also participate in internal rotation. External rotation of the hip is accomplished by the gluteus maximus and the short rotators of the gluteal region or the piriformis, obturator internus, and the gemelli muscles (Fig. 6-9) (1,37).

Table 6-2 summarizes the muscles of the pelvis and hips along with their origins, insertions, and functions. Identification of these muscles in all planes is essential in properly evaluating the pelvis, hips, and thighs with MRI. It is also important to know the relationships of these muscles to the various neurovascular structures.

The gluteus maximus (Table 6-2) is a large oblique muscle that largely contributes to the shape of the buttock (Figs. 6-1, 6-3, and 6-9B). This muscle arises from the posterior ilium and dorsal surface of the sacrum and coccyx. The gluteus maximus has both superficial and deep insertions. Portions of the insertion blend with the tendinous fibers of the fasciae latae and form a portion of the iliotibial tract. The deeper part of the muscle inserts into the gluteal tuberosity of the femur. This lies below the level of the trochanters along the posterior margin of the femur. A subcutaneous bursa frequently lies over the superficial portion of the tendon at the level of the greater trochanter. There is a larger bursa that typically lies between the tendon and the greater trochanter (1,37,50). When inflamed, these bursae are seen as well-defined high-intensity lesions near the insertions (T2 weighted sequences).

TABLE 6-2. *Muscles of the pelvis, hips, and thighs* (1,37)

Muscle	Origin	Insertion	Function	Innervation
Gluteus maximus	Posterior ilium, dorsolateral sacrum and coccyx	Gluteal tuberosity of femur, iliotibial tract	Hip extensor, external rotator	Inferior gluteal nerve (L5–S2)
Gluteus medius	Posterior ilium below crest	Posterolateral greater trochanter	Hip abductor	Superior gluteal nerve (L4–S1)
Gluteus minimus	Posterior mid-ilium	Anterior greater trochanter	Hip abductor	Superior gluteal nerve (L4–S1)
Tensor fasciae latae	Anterior iliac crest	Iliotibial tract	Flexor, internal rotator, abductor	Superior gluteal nerve (L4–S1)
Piriformis	Anterolateral sacrum S2–S4	Superior border greater trochanter	External rotator, abductor	S1, S2
Obturator internus	Pubic and ischial margins	Medial greater trochanter	External rotator	L5–S2
Superior gemellus	Posterior ischial spine	Obturator internus tendon	External rotator	L5–S2
Inferior gemellus	Ischial tuberosity	Obturator internus tendon	External rotator	L5–S2
Quadratus femoris	Lateral ischial tuberosity	Posterior femur below intertrochanteric line	External rotator, adductor	L4–S1
Iliopsoas				
Psoas major	Lateral margin T12–L5	Lesser trochanter	Thigh flexor, accessory adductor	L2–L4
Psoas minor	Lateral margin T12–L1	Iliopectineal eminence	Tilt pelvis upward	T12–L2
Iliacus	Inner iliac surface below crest	Lesser trochanter	Thigh flexor	L2–L4
Sartorius	Anterior superior iliac spine	Proximal anteromedial tibia	Thigh flexor, accessory external rotator	Femoral nerve (L2–L3)
Quadriceps femoris				
Rectus femoris	Anterior inferior iliac spine	Upper patella	Extensor of knee, accessory thigh flexor	Femoral nerve (L3–L4)
Vastus lateralis	Upper lateral and posterolateral femur	Upper lateral patella	Extensor of knee	L3–L4
Vastus medialis	Medial posterior femur	Medial tendon of rectus femoris	Extensor of knee	L3–L4
Vastus intermedius	Anterior midfemur	Upper posterior patella	Extensor of knee	L3–L4
Pectineus	Superior pubic ramus	Pectineal line femur	Thigh flexor	Femoral nerve (L2, L3)
Adductor longus	Anterior pubic bone	Medial linea aspera	Thigh adductor	Obturator nerve (L2–L3)
Adductor brevis	Pubic bone and inferior ramus	Upper linea aspera	Thigh adductor	Obturator nerve (L2–L3)
Adductor magnus	Ischium and inferior pubic ramus	Linea aspera, adductor tubercle	Thigh adductor	Obturator and tibial nerves (L3–L5)
Gracilis	Inferior pubic ramus near symphysis	Upper anterior tibia	Thigh adductor, medial rotator thigh	Obturator nerve (L3–L4)
Obturator externus	Outer margins of obturator foramen	Intertrochanteric fossa	Lateral rotator	Obturator nerve (L3–L4)
Semitendinosus	Posteromedial ischial tuberosity	Upper anterior tibia	Thigh extensor, knee flexor	Tibial side of sciatic (L5–S1)
Biceps femoris	Long head: posteromedial ischial tuberosity; short head: lateral lip linea aspera	Fibular head	Extend thigh, flex knee	Long head: tibial side of sciatic nerve (L5–S1); short head: peroneal side of sciatic nerve (L5–S2)
Semimembranosus	Posterolateral ischial tuberosity	Posteromedial upper tibia	Thigh extensor, accessory medial rotator and thigh adductor	Tibial side of sciatic nerve (L5–S2)

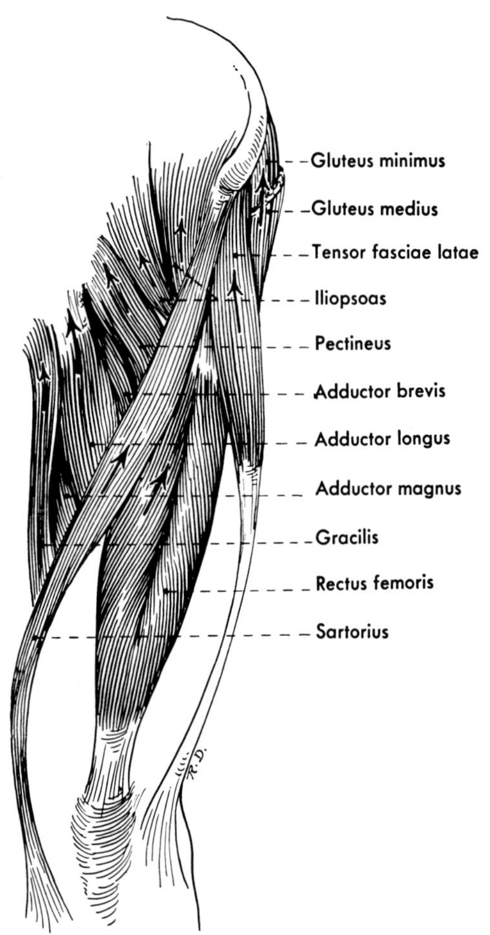

FIG. 6-7. Illustration of the flexors of the thigh. (From ref. 37, with permission.)

The gluteus medius (Fig. 6-9B) arises from a large area on the posterior wing of the ilium, below the iliac crest. It extends inferiorly and laterally to insert on the greater trochanter along its posterolateral surface. An additional bursa typically lies between the anterior fibers and the adjacent trochanter. Major fibers of the superior gluteal nerve and vessels lie between the gluteus medius and minimus (Figs. 6-1 and 6-16). The gluteus minimus is also a fan-shaped muscle arising from a more inferior aspect of the posterior ilium and extending along a similar course to insert in the upper anterior surface of the greater trochanter. There is also a bursa between this muscle and the trochanter. These two muscles combine to form the major abductors of the hip. The muscles are innervated by the superior gluteal nerve (1,37).

The tensor fasciae lata (Fig. 6-10) arises from the anterior-most aspect of the iliac crest and passes posteriorly and inferiorly inserting in the anterior part of the iliotibial tract. It is innervated by the superior gluteal nerve and serves primarily as a flexor, internal rotator, and abductor of the thigh (1,37).

The piriformis (Figs. 6-9B and 6-10) is the most superior of the small muscles in the gluteal region and plays a significant role in vascular disorders in the gluteal region. This muscle largely fills the greater sciatic notch through which the sacral plexus and associated neurovascular structures pass. The superior gluteal nerve and vessels typically lie along the upper border of this muscle, while the pudendal nerve and vessels and inferior gluteal nerve and vessels along with the sciatic nerve typically lie along its lower margin (Fig. 6-16). In up to

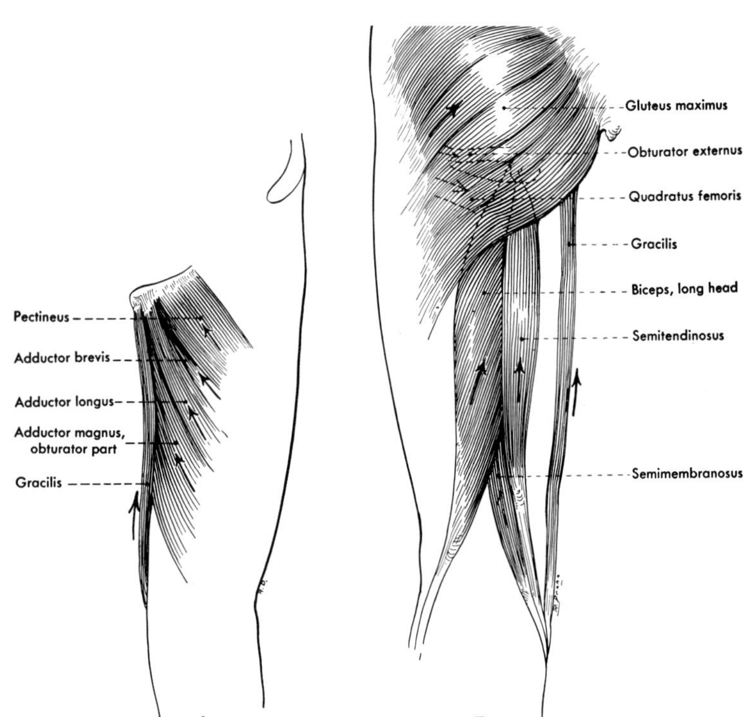

FIG. 6-8. Illustration of the adductors of the thigh seen anteriorly (**A**) and posteriorly (**B**). (From ref. 37, with permission.)

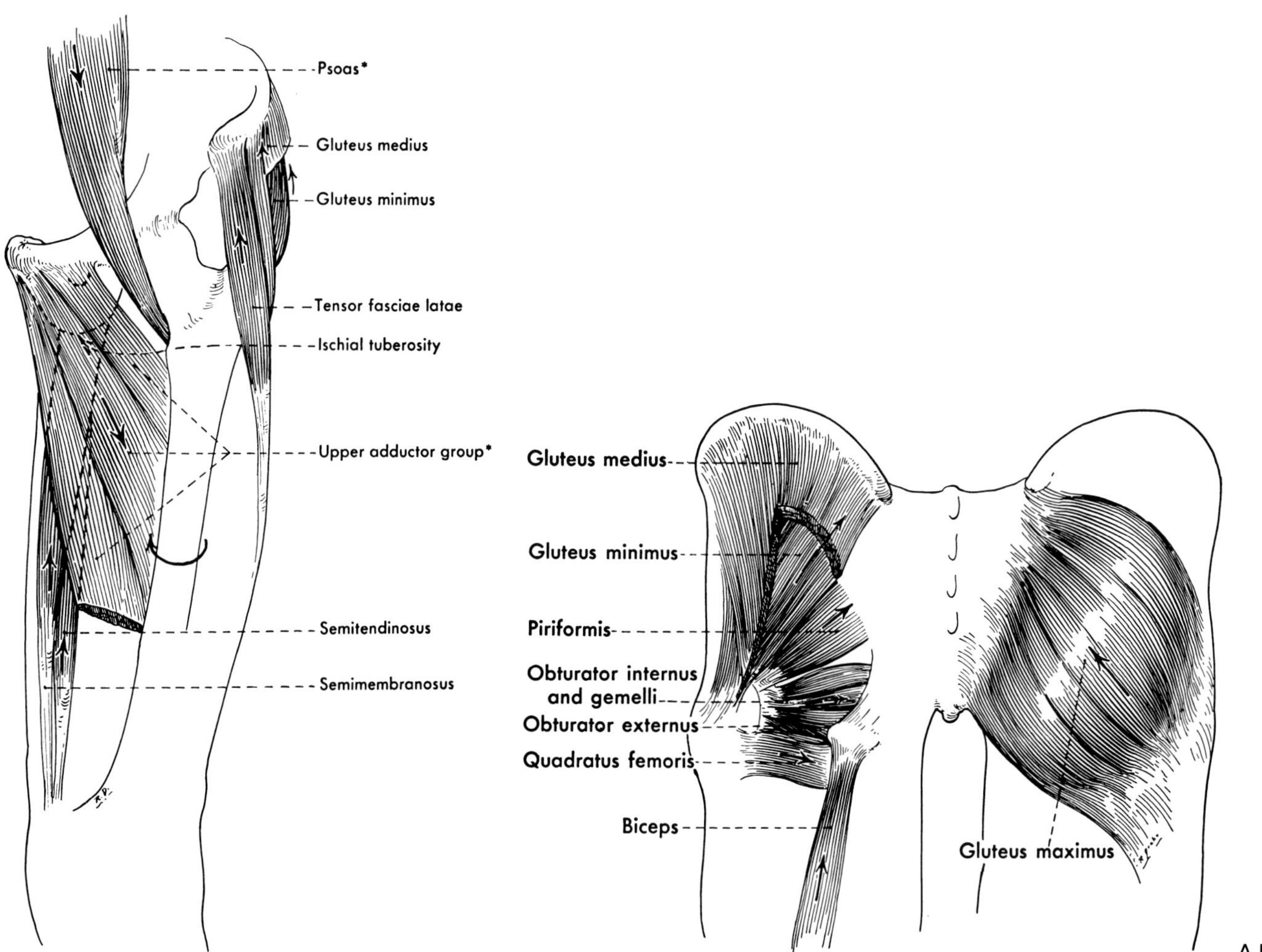

FIG. 6-9. Illustration of the rotators of the thigh. **A:** Anterior illustration of the rotators of the thigh. Internal rotation includes all muscles except the iliopsoas and gluteus medius, which are external rotators. **B:** Posterior illustration of the external rotators. The gluteus minimus is often excluded from this group. (From ref. 37, with permission.)

10% of patients the piriformis is actually perforated by the sciatic nerve or its branches. The muscle arises from the lateral aspect of the sacrum at the level of the second through fourth sacral segments and extends laterally and posterior to the hip joint to insert on the posterior aspect of the greater trochanter (1,16,37).

The obturator internus takes its origin from the internal pelvic wall of the bones forming the obturator foramen (Figs. 6-1 and 6-3). The muscle passes laterally through the lesser sciatic foramen, posterior to the lesser sciatic notch of the ischium, running posterior to the hip joint to insert on the medial surface of the greater trochanter just above the trochanteric fossa. Again, a bursa typically separates the tendon from the bone in this region (1,16,37). This bursa is typically not identified on MR images unless inflamed and distended with fluid.

The superior and inferior gemelli muscles (Fig. 6-9B) lie above and below the obturator internus, respectively. Superior gemellus originates from the posterior ischial spine and the inferior gemellus from the upper part of the ischial tuberosity. Both muscle bundles converge to insert with the obturator internus tendon and assist this muscle in external rotation of the hip (1,37).

The final muscle in the external rotator group is the quadratus femoris. This muscle takes its origin from the lateral aspect of the ischial tuberosity and inserts on the posterior aspect of the femur just below the intertrochanteric line (Figs. 6-2 and 6-9B).

The anterior muscles of the thigh (Fig. 6-11), with which we include the iliopsoas, are the sartorius and the four segments of the quadriceps muscle. The pectineus muscle is also included in this muscle group (37).

The iliopsoas as it appears in the thigh is a combination of two muscles, the iliacus and the psoas major (Fig. 6-11). The psoas major arises in the retroperitoneum at the lateral margin of the T12 through L5 lumbar vertebrae. This muscle passes inferiorly and slightly laterally, where it joins the iliacus to insert on the lesser tro-

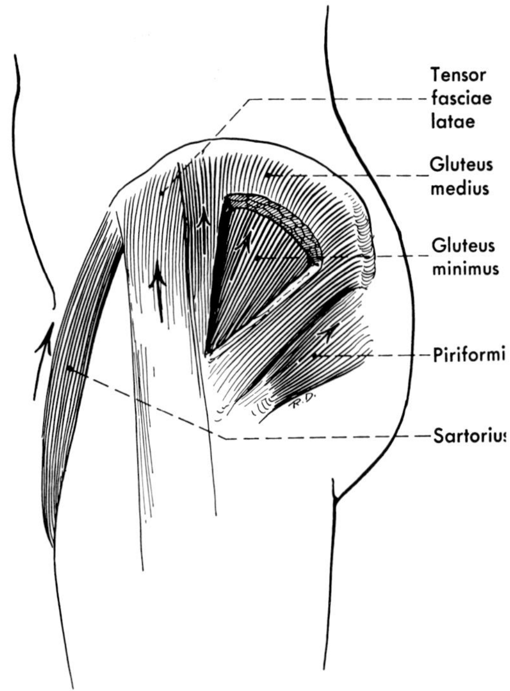

FIG. 6-10. Illustration of the abductors of the thigh. (From ref. 37, with permission.)

chanter (1,37). The psoas minor is an inconsistent muscle that typically arises from the adjacent borders of the last thoracic and first lumbar vertebrae and extends along the anterolateral margin of the psoas major to insert on the iliopectineal eminence of the innominate bone. The iliacus takes its origin from the internal surface of the ilium below the iliac crest and passes slightly obliquely anterior to the hip joint, inserting with the psoas muscle in the lesser trochanter (Fig. 6-11). An important bursa (which can cause clinical symptoms and local hip pain) is the iliopectineal bursa, which lies beneath the iliopsoas muscle just as it crosses the anterior surface of the hip joint. This bursa may approach 3–7 cm in length and 2–4 cm in width. The bursa communicates with the hip joint in up to 15% of patients (1,10,37).

The sartorius is a long straplike muscle that originates from the anterior superior iliac spine, passing obliquely and medially to run along the inner thigh. Below the level of the knee joint it inserts on the anteromedial aspect of the upper tibia (Fig. 6-11). At its insertion it lies largely above the gracilis and semitendinosus. The combination of these three tendons forms the pes anserinus tendon. A bursa typically lies deep to the insertion of the sartorius. This bursa tends to separate it from the insertions of the gracilis and semitendinosus (1,37).

The quadriceps femoris is composed of four muscles. These include the rectus femoris, vastus lateralis, vastus intermedius, and vastus medialis, all of which blend at their patellar insertions (Figs. 6-1, 6-2, and 6-11). The most anterior muscle of the group is the rectus femoris, which arises from the anterior inferior iliac spine. This muscle has the distinction of being the only member of the quadriceps group that crosses the hip joint as it passes along its anterior superficial course to insert with the other muscles in the quadriceps tendon, which inserts in the upper border of the patella. A second, more inconsistent, origin is also noted from the upper margin of the acetabulum. This is important in that a bursa typically lies deep to this reflected tendon of the rectus femoris. The quadriceps tendon, with the patella, continues to form the patellar ligament, which inserts on the tibial tuberosity (1,37).

The vastus lateralis is a large member of the quadriceps group which is covered anteriorly by the rectus femoris and tensor fasciae latae (Fig. 6-1). The muscle itself lies anterior and lateral to the vastus intermedius. Its origin is from the femur just below the greater trochanter and posterolaterally along the margin of the linea aspera and intermuscular septum. The vastus intermedius inserts along the upper lateral margin of the patella, forming a portion of the quadriceps tendon. The vastus medialis makes its origin from just below the lesser trochanter anteriorly and the medial and posterior aspect of the femur. It extends inferiorly and inserts into the medial aspect of the rectus femoris tendon. The vastus intermedius covers a major portion of the front, medial, and lateral aspects of the femur (Fig. 6-11) (1,16,37). It is completely covered superficially by the vastus lateralis and medialis on its sides and the rectus femoris anteriorly. Distally, its fibers fuse with the vastus medialis and lateralis to insert in the posterior upper surface of the patella (1,37,50).

The pectineus arises from the superior anterior aspect of the superior pubic ramus and extends obliquely in an inferolateral direction to insert along the pectineal line of the femur, which extends inferiorly from the lesser trochanter to the linea aspera (Fig. 6-11) (1,16,37).

Anatomists often include the adductor brevis, adductor longus, adductor magnus, gracilis, and obturator externus in the anterior medial muscle group because all these muscles are innervated by the obturator nerve (37) (Table 6-2). In the axial plane, the adductor longus is the most anterior of the adductor muscles in the upper thigh (Fig. 6-1). The adductor longus takes its origin from the pubic bone superiorly near the pubic symphysis and extends in a triangular fashion inferiorly and laterally to insert along the medial aspect of the linea aspera at the level of the midfemur. This muscle forms the floor of the femoral triangle along with the pectineus and iliopsoas muscle. The adductor brevis arises from a broad tendon from the body and inferior ramus of the pubis and expands in a triangular fashion to insert in the upper half of the linea aspera. It is typically seen between the adductor longus and magnus on the axial views with the

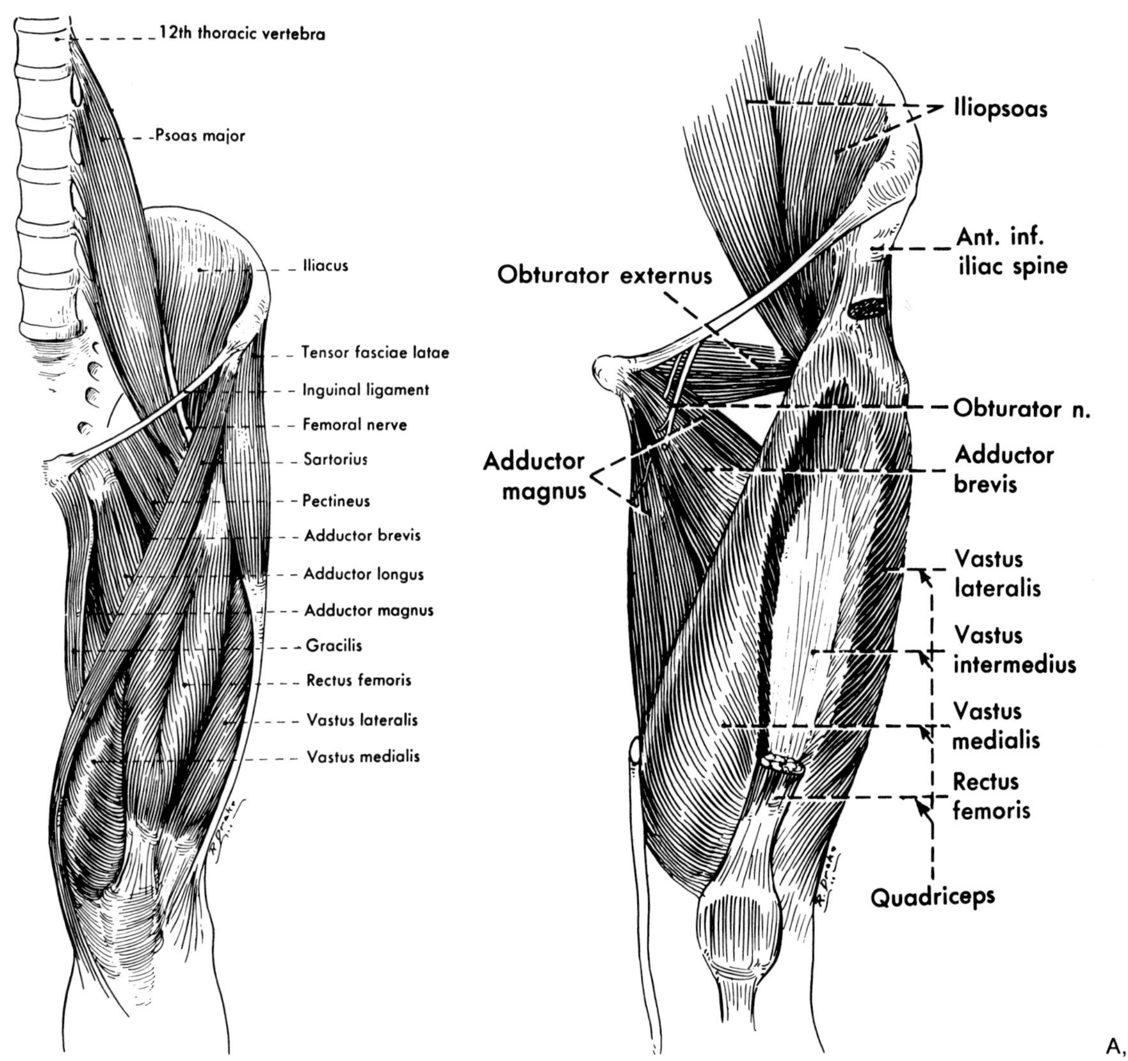

FIG. 6-11. Illustration of the anterior muscles of the thigh. Superficial group (**A**) and deep muscles (**B**). (From ref. 37, with permission.)

gracilis running along its medial aspect (Fig. 6-1) (1,16,37,50).

The adductor magnus, like the other adductor muscles, is triangular but much larger (Fig. 6-11). It arises from the lower part of the inferior pubic ramus and the entire length of the ramus of the ischium. As it courses inferiorly and laterally, the upper portion inserts on the linea aspera with lower fibers inserting in the adductor tubercle just above the medial femoral condyle (1,16,37).

The gracilis is a long thin muscle that arises from the inferior aspect of the pubic bone close to the symphysis (Figs. 6-1, 6-2, and 6-11). It passes medially along the thigh, superficial to the adductor muscles (Fig. 6-12). Near the knee it lies first between the sartorius and semimembranosus and then between the sartorius and semitendinosus. Below the knee the tendon curves anteriorly and inserts in the upper medial anterior tibia with a bursa termed the anserine bursa intervening between gracilis, sartorius, and semitendinosus tendons and the tibia (1,37).

The obturator externus (Figs. 6-1, 6-2, and 6-11) is the most deeply placed muscle in the adductor group. This muscle arises from the external margins of the obturator foramen, namely, the superior pubic ramus, inferior pubic ramus, and upper margin of the ischium, and extends laterally and posterior to the hip to insert at the base of the femoral neck adjacent to the greater trochanter (trochanteric fossa) (Fig. 6-2). As the muscle passes posterior to the hip capsule, it may be separated from the capsule proper by a bursa. The obturator internus functions primarily as a lateral rotator (1,37).

The posterior muscles of the thigh, commonly referred to as the hamstring muscles, include the semitendinosus, the biceps femoris, the semimembranosus, and a portion of the adductor magnus that arises from the ischial tuberosity (Fig. 6-13). All the hamstring muscles take their origin from the ischial tuberosity except for

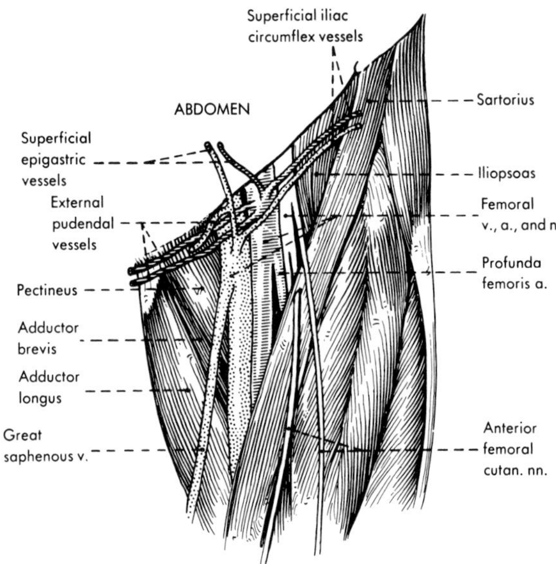

FIG. 6-12. Illustration of the neurovascular structures and muscular boundaries of the femoral triangle. (From ref. 37, with permission.)

the short head of the biceps femoris. The semitendinosus arises from the posteromedial aspect of the ischial tuberosity. Its origin is fused with the long head of the biceps. Just above the medial condyle the tendinous portion of the muscle continues posterior to the knee and forward along the medial aspect to insert in the upper anterior tibia, just posterior to the insertions of the gracilis and sartorius. As noted previously, this is, along with the above tendons, a part of the pes anserinus complex (1,37).

The biceps femoris has two heads, a short and long head (Fig. 6-13). The long head of the biceps arises from the posteromedial aspect of the inferior aspect of the ischial tuberosity in common with the semitendinosus tendon. The short head of the biceps originates from the lower lateral aspect of the linea aspera. This muscle lies lateral to the belly of the long head as it extends inferiorly, and at the level of the knee joint a common tendon forms that crosses the knee and inserts into the head of the fibula (1,37).

The semimembranosus arises from a long flat tendon at the posterolateral aspect of the ischial tuberosity, which is lateral to the common origin of the biceps femoris and semitendinosus (Fig. 6-13). The muscle becomes tendinous posterior to the medial femoral condyle with its straight part attaching to the medial meniscus as it crosses the knee. At the level of the joint it gives off an oblique expansion that also attaches to the medial collateral ligament. Its insertion is the posterior medial aspect of the upper tibia just below the knee (1,16,37,50).

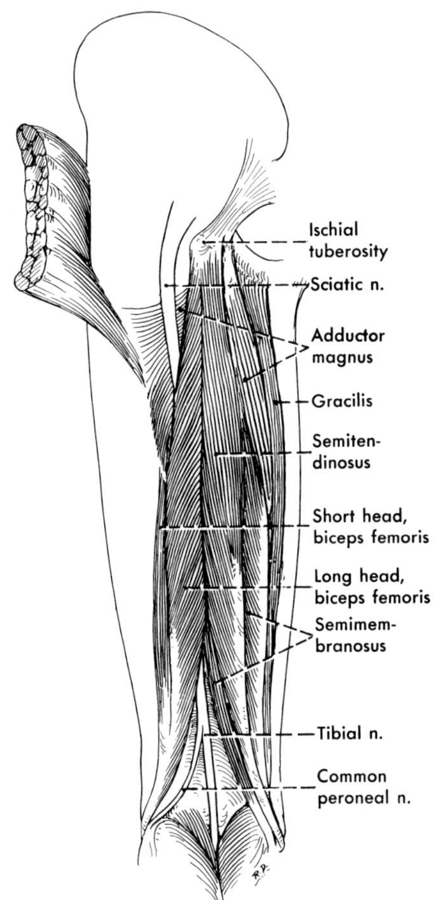

FIG. 6-13. Illustration of the hamstring muscle group. (From ref. 37, with permission.)

Neurovascular Anatomy

The neurovascular anatomy of the pelvis, hips, and thigh is complex, and the relationships of these structures to the above muscles are important in evaluating pathology along the course of the neurovascular bundles. Demonstration of these structures can be accomplished using axial planes (Fig. 6-1) but may be difficult with coronal and sagittal planes because of the difficulty in following the changes in the course of the neurovascular structures (Figs. 6-2 and 6-3).

The abdominal aorta usually bifurcates at the L4 level, forming the iliac arteries. The iliac arteries divide at the level of the sacroiliac joints to form the internal and external iliac vessels (Fig. 6-14). The internal iliac artery gives off the superior and inferior gluteal arteries, which supply the posterior or buttock muscles (Fig. 6-16). These vessels and their branches are difficult to define on conventional orthogonal MR images. The common femoral artery is a continuation of the external iliac below the inguinal ligament. The circumflex arteries and branches of the obturator artery (via ligamentum

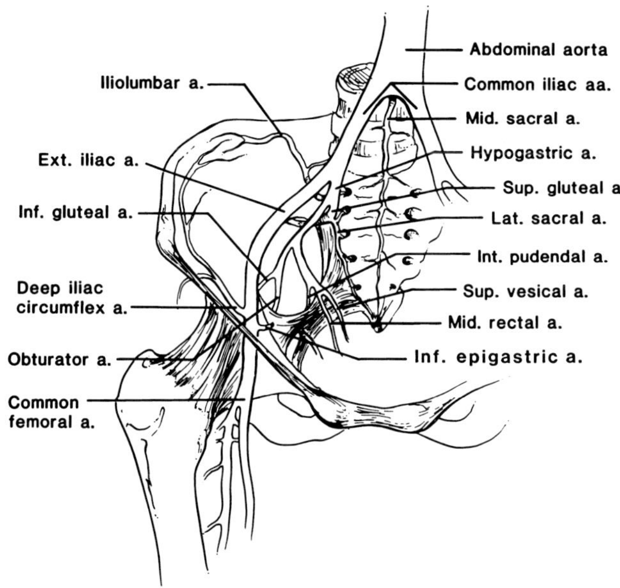

FIG. 6-14. Illustration of the major vessels to the pelvis and thighs. (From ref. 10, with permission.)

teres) supply the hip. The superficial femoral and deep femoral (profunda) arteries form slightly distal to this level (Figs. 6-12 and 6-14) (4,10,37). They branch at about the same level as the superficial femoral and saphenous veins (Fig. 6-12). The course of the major arteries and companion veins is easily followed on contiguous axial MR images (Fig. 6-1). In the upper thigh (Fig. 6-12) the superficial femoral artery lies anterior to the adductor longus and deep to the sartorius. The profunda femoris artery and vein lie more laterally between the adductor longus and magnus near the linea aspera of the femur (Fig. 6-1). Perforating branches are usually identifiable between the adductor magnus and hamstring muscles just posterior and slightly lateral to the linea aspera of the femur (1,16,37).

The major neural structures are derived from the lumbosacral plexus (L1–S2) (Fig. 6-15) (10). Portions of the T12 and S3 ventral rami also contribute to this plexus. The sacral branches exit the ventral foramina along with the L4–L5 segments for the sciatic nerve (L4–S3). The sciatic nerve exits the pelvis posteriorly and lies just posterior to the hip. This is best seen on axial MR images (Fig. 6-1) (1,10,37,50).

The sciatic nerve enters the buttock below the piriformis (Fig. 6-16) in about 85% of patients. In some cases the sciatic nerve may pass through the piriformis or its peroneal and tibial segments may be separated by this muscle (37). The nerve lies posterior to the obturator externus, gemelli, and quadriceps femoris and it passes distally (Figs. 6-1 and 6-16). The posterior femoral cutaneous branch also exits below the piriformis but is less easily identified on MR images. The superior gluteal nerve lies between the gluteus minimus and medius

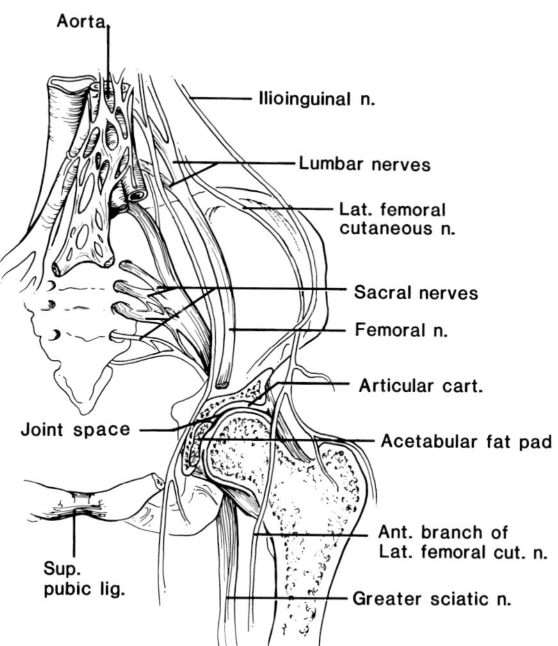

FIG. 6-15. Illustration of the major neural structures of the pelvis and hips. (From ref. 10, with permission.)

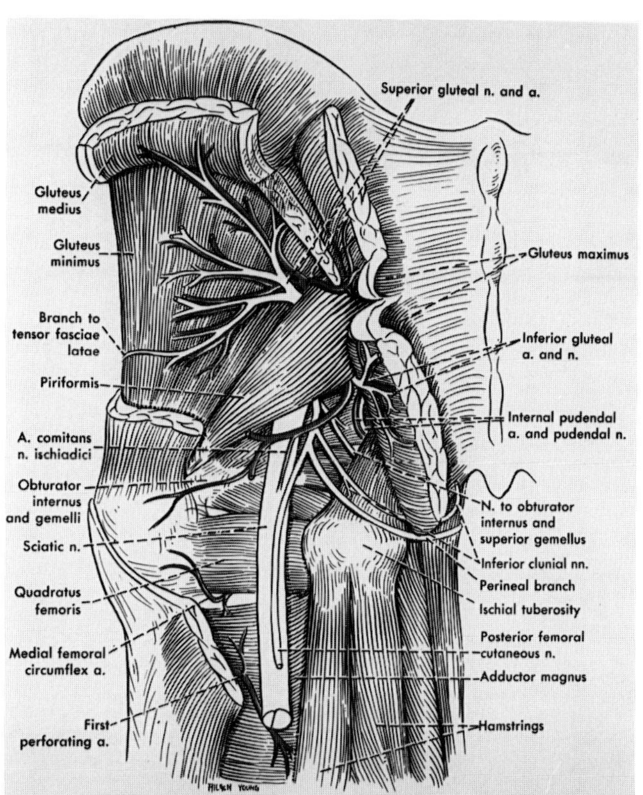

FIG. 6-16. Neurovascular anatomy of the gluteal region. (From ref. 37, with permission.)

above the level of the piriformis (Fig. 6-16). In the posterior thigh the sciatic nerve lies posterior to the adductor magnus and deep to the biceps femoris (Fig. 6-1). The nerve branches innervate the hamstring group. Just above the knee the sciatic nerve generally divides into common peroneal and tibial branches (1,37).

The anterior muscles of the pelvis and thigh are innervated by either the obturator or femoral nerve (Table 6-1). Both are derived from the L2–L4 segments. The femoral nerve lies just lateral to the artery and vein in the femoral triangle (Fig. 6-12). In the upper portion of the femoral triangle it divides into muscular and cutaneous branches (Figs. 6-17 and 6-18) (1,37). The largest branches may be identified on MR images. These branches (saphenous nerve and nerve to the vastus medialis) lie anterior to the adductor group and deep to the sartorius (Fig. 6-1) (1,16,37). The obturator nerve enters the thigh through the obturator canal, deep to the pectineus (Fig. 6-11B). Its anterior branch lies between the adductor longus and brevis and the posterior branch posterior to the adductor brevis (1,16,37).

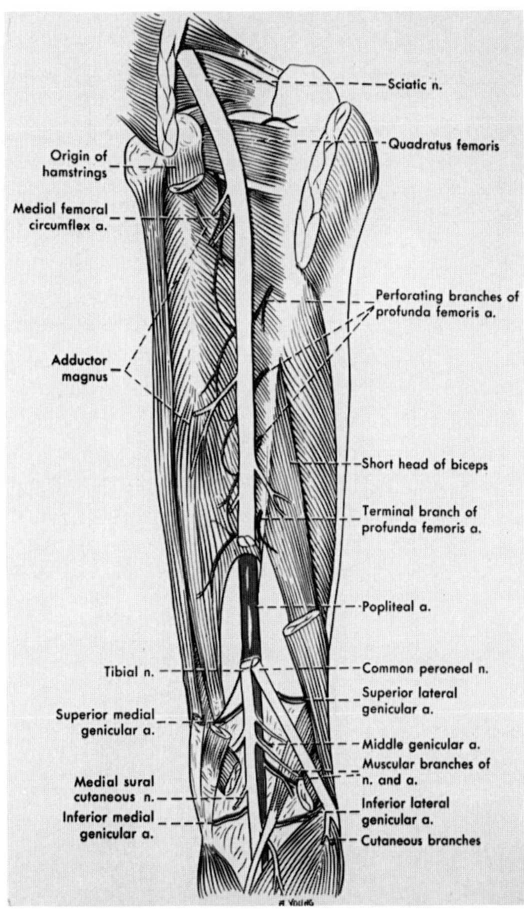

FIG. 6-17. Illustration of sciatic nerve and its muscular branches in the posterior thigh. (From ref. 37, with permission.)

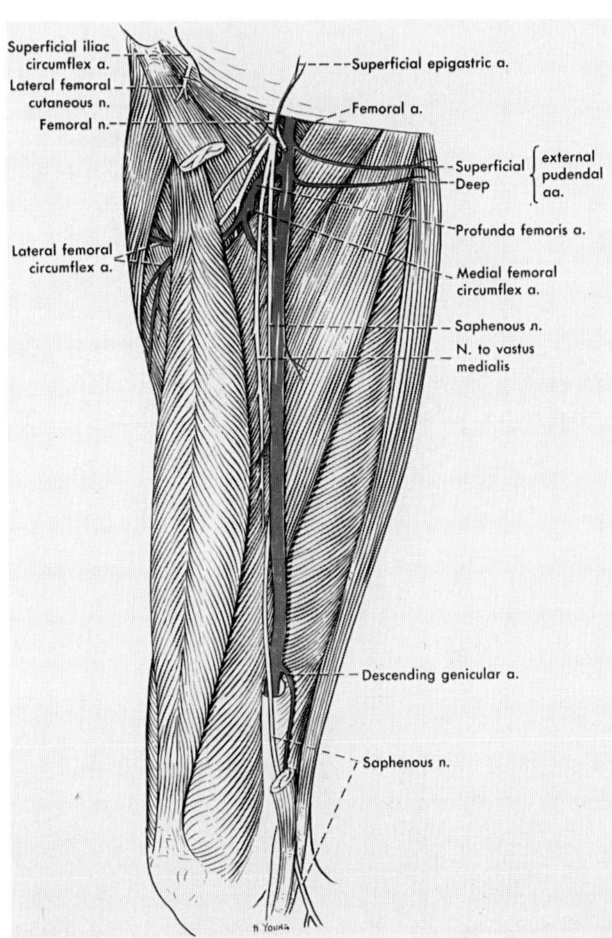

FIG. 6-18. Illustration of the anteromedial neurovascular supply to the thigh. (From ref. 37, with permission.)

PITFALLS

Pitfalls in MRI of the pelvis, hips, and thighs do not differ significantly from other areas in regard to hardware and software artifacts. However, certain bone and soft tissue variants do require further discussion.

Soft tissue variants are important when evaluating patients with suspected neoplasm or sciatic nerve pathology (10,37,83). Knowledge of the normal variants in the sciatic–piriformis muscle anatomy are important in patients with suspected piriformis syndrome. As noted above, the sciatic nerve typically passes deep to the piriformis muscle, but it may pass through the muscle or the tibial and peroneal tracts may be separated by the muscle (1,37). Inflamed bursae should not be confused with neoplasms. Most of these bursae were described in the anatomy section of this chapter. However, infrequently bursae may develop between the piriformis and the femur, between the gluteal muscles, and over the ischial tuberosities (37). When present, these bursae appear as well-marginated, high-intensity lesions of variable size

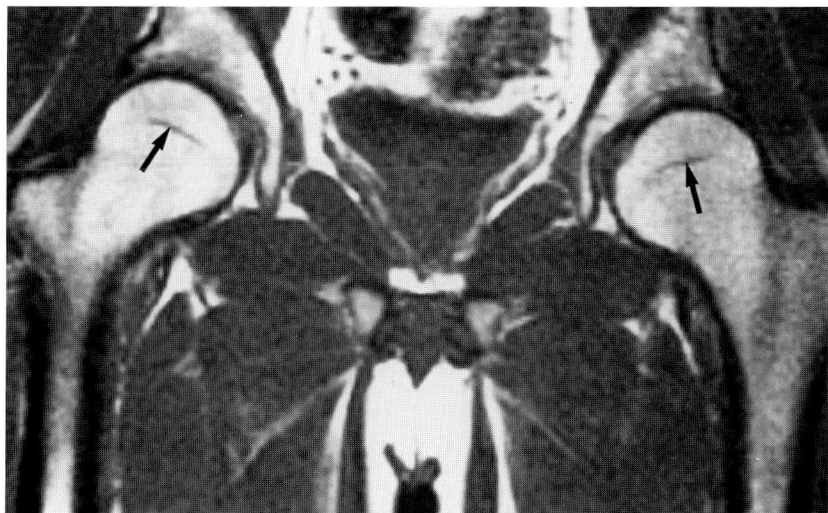
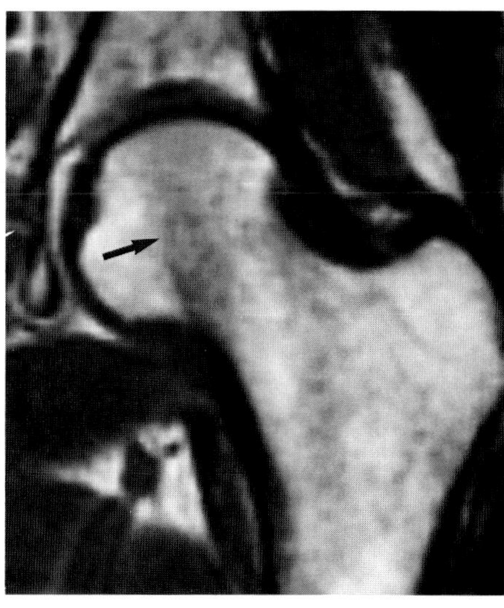

A,B

FIG. 6-19. Adult hips. **A:** SE 500/30 image of the pelvis and hips, demonstrating predominantly fatty marrow in the femoral heads and necks. The physeal scars (*arrows*) should not be confused with AVN. **B:** Coronal SE 500/20 image of the left hip. The low-intensity region (*arrow*) created by the trabecular pattern in the femoral neck is normal.

on T2 weighted sequences and are low intensity on T1 weighted sequences.

Variations in marrow patterns in the pelvis, hips, and femurs and focal areas of abnormality in the femoral head can be very confusing (9,10,57,80,81). A more thorough discussion of marrow imaging is presented in Chapter 14. However, certain common problems and variants deserve mention here.

The transition from hematopoietic to fatty marrow occurs normally with age. This may be partially related to decreased medullary blood flow (58,80). In younger patients the capital epiphysis and greater trochanter are typically composed of fatty marrow, resulting in high signal intensity on T1 weighted sequences. With age the hematopoietic marrow in the intertrochanteric region becomes replaced with fatty marrow so that after age 50 most of the marrow in this region is fatty (Fig. 6-19) (53). The compressive and tensile trabeculae in the femoral head and neck are seen as linear areas of low signal intensity on both T1 and T2 weighted sequences (Fig. 6-19B) (10,80). Lack of familiarity with the changes normally seen in the marrow of the acetabulum and femur can lead to false positive diagnosis such as avascular necrosis (AVN) or metastasis.

Well-defined areas of abnormal signal intensity may be noted in the femoral neck. These herniation pits are due to mechanical effects of the anterior capsule. The result is a focal cortical defect that allows soft tissue erosion into the femoral neck. These defects are noted in about 5% of the adult population (57,61). Radiographically, these defects are nearly always in the anterior outer quadrant of the femoral neck (Fig. 6-20). They are generally 1 cm in diameter with sclerotic well-defined margins. Multilobulated herniation pits have also been described (57,61,80). On MR images the appearance is also typical. The location and typical low intensity on

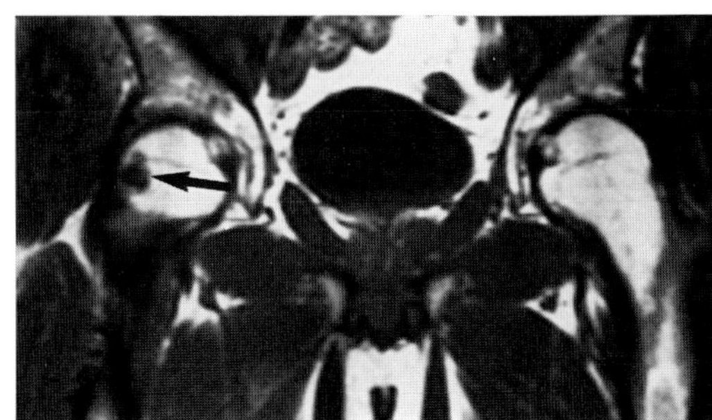
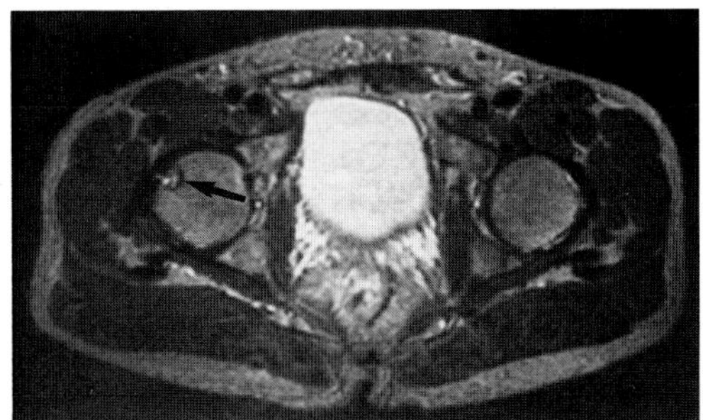

A,B

FIG. 6-20. Coronal SE 500/20 (**A**) and axial SE 2,000/60 (**B**) images of the pelvis, demonstrating a typical herniation pit (*arrows*).

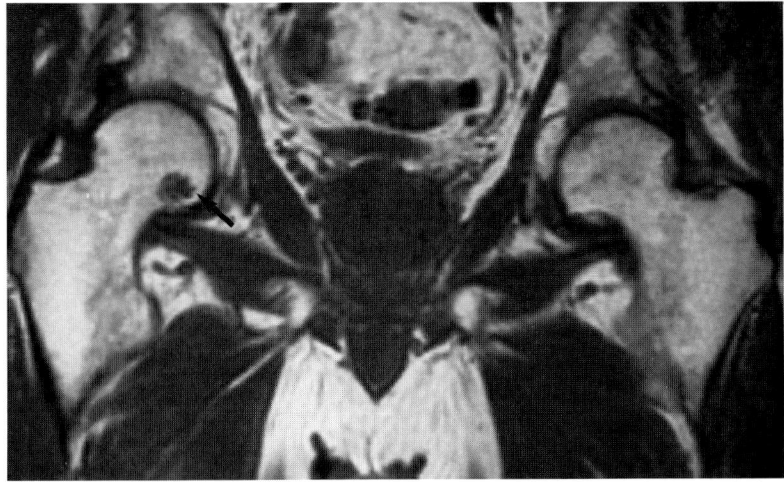
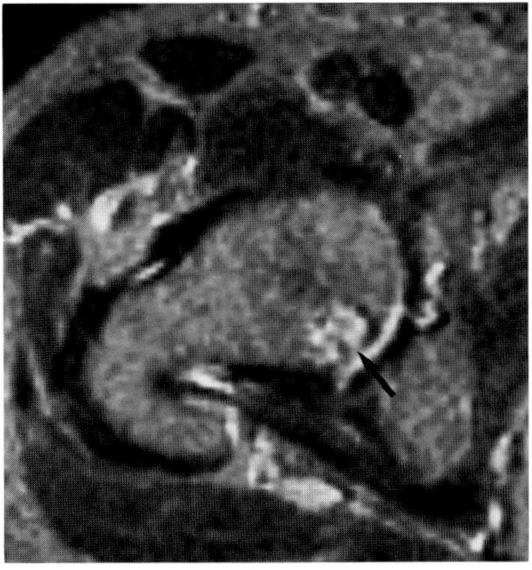

A,B

FIG. 6-21. Coronal SE 500/20 (**A**) and axial SE 2,000/60 (**B**) images of a synovial herniation posteromedially (*arrows*).

T1 weighted images and high intensity with a low-intensity margin on T2 weighted images should not be confused with AVN, metastasis, or interosseous ganglia (57). Comparison with radiographs will confirm the diagnosis when MR features seem atypical (Fig. 6-21).

APPLICATIONS

Most patients referred for musculoskeletal MRI examinations of the pelvis, hips, and thighs present with pain or suspected soft tissue or skeletal neoplasms. There are numerous causes of hip pain; however, because of its sensitivity and specificity, MRI has progressed most rapidly in evaluating patients with suspected AVN of the femoral heads (7,9,32).

Osteonecrosis

Osteonecrosis is a general term applied to conditions resulting in necrosis of bone and marrow elements. The term avascular necrosis is most commonly applied when the epiphysis or subchondral bone is involved. Osteonecrosis of the metaphyseal or diaphyseal bone is commonly referred to as a bone infarct (56,73).

Bone necrosis occurs when flow is disrupted by thrombosis, external compression, vessel wall disease, or traumatic disruption of vessels. The numerous causes of osteonecrosis are summarized in Table 6-3. Though osteonecrosis can occur in any area of the skeleton, it is a frequent and significant problem in the femoral head. Therefore, the major discussion here is on pathophysiology and MR features. A more brief discussion will be included in the other anatomic chapters.

Susceptibility to AVN in the hip is due in part to the vascular anatomy. The foveal artery supplies only the area of the femoral head immediately adjacent to the fovea (Fig. 6-22). Distally, the medial and lateral femoral circumflex arteries supply the remainder of the femoral head and neck (Figs. 6-22 and 6-23). Their location makes them particularly susceptible to damage with femoral neck fractures (10,37).

Early diagnosis and selection of the most appropriate therapy have been particularly challenging in patients with AVN of the hips (3,5,9,34,60). Early diagnosis allows more conservative therapy such as nonweight bearing with crutches and core decompression. Use of core decompression is controversial, even in early AVN, but many surgeons feel the technique is effective if diagnosis is established early (9,10,38). Reports have demonstrated gradual decrease in flow to the femoral head when systemic corticosteroids are used. Flow gradually returns to normal following core decompression (82). Later stages of AVN do not respond to core decompression. These patients usually require hip arthroplasty (10). Camp and Colwell (15) reported progression of AVN in 60% of patients treated with core decompression. Hopson and Siverhus (38) reported healing in 40% of patients with stage I and II AVN treated by core

TABLE 6-3. *Etiology of osteonecrosis* (73)

Trauma
Corticosteroids
Sickle cell disease
Alcoholism
Gaucher's disease
Nitrogen narcosis
Radiation
Collagen disease
Pancreatitis
Idiopathic

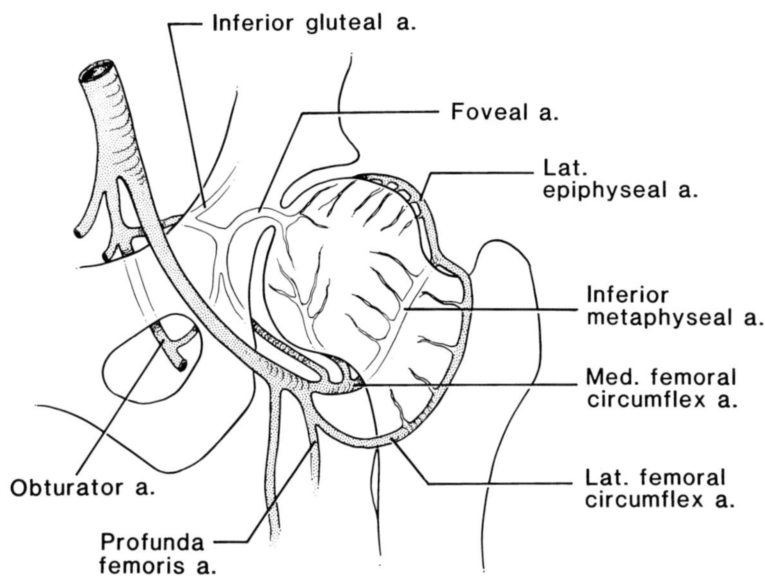

FIG. 6-22. Illustration of the vascular anatomy of the hip. (From ref. 10, with permission.)

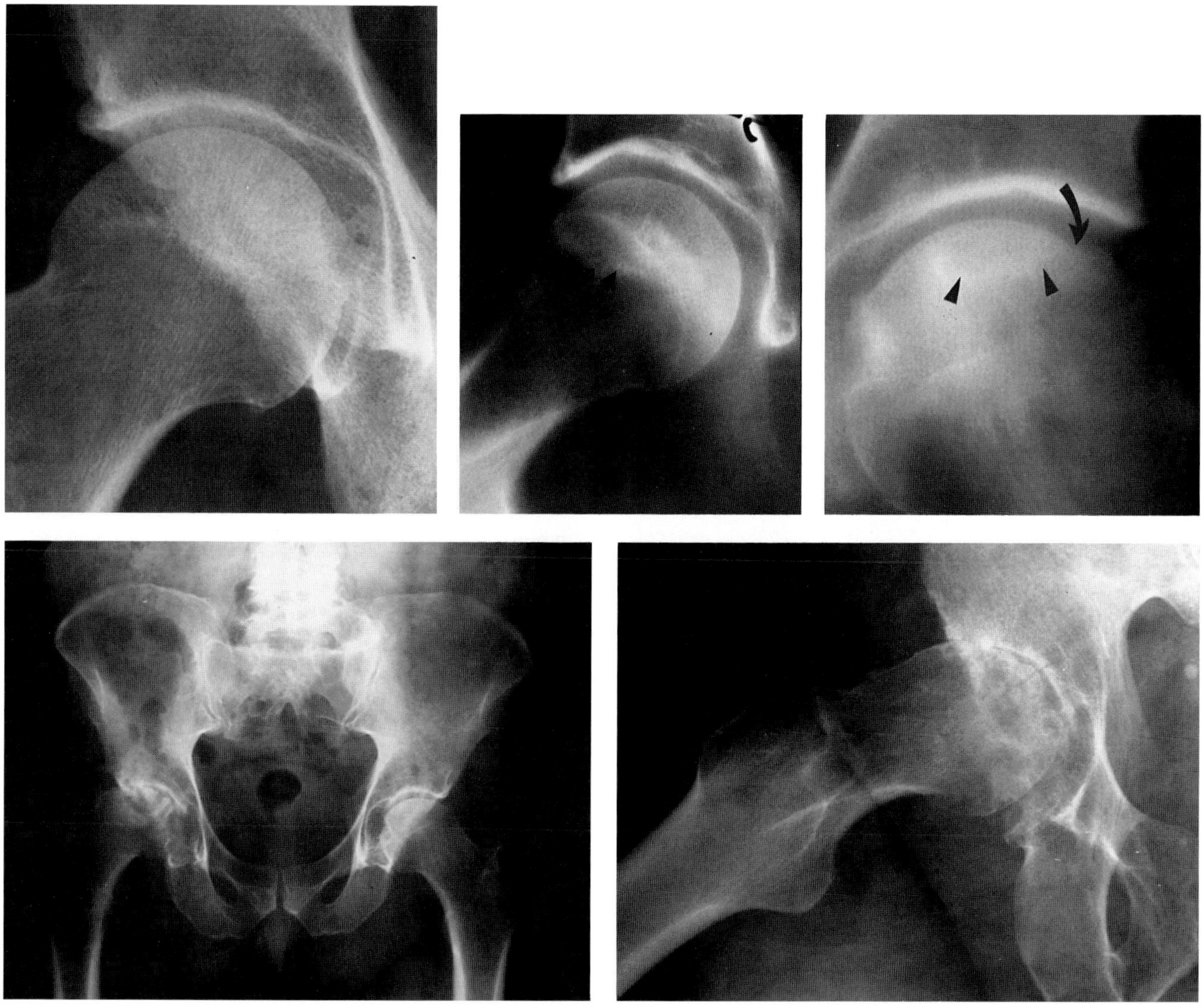

A,B,C

D,E

FIG. 6-23. Radiographic features of AVN. **A:** Normal AP view of the hip; stage 0–I AVN. **B:** Oblique tomogram demonstrates a normal joint space and the articular surface of the femoral head is normal. There is a lucent area with marginal sclerosis (*arrow*) due to AVN; stage II AVN. **C:** AP tomogram demonstrating a lucent area (*arrowheads*) with articular collapse (*curved arrow*); stage III AVN. **D:** AP view of the pelvis and oblique view of the hip (**E**) show advanced articular collapse with osteoarthritis; stage IV AVN.

decompression. Sixty percent of patients required further surgery within 9.2 months of core decompression.

Early detection of AVN with imaging techniques has been challenging despite the use of computed tomography and isotope studies (9,33). Radiographs are often normal in early stages of AVN. Changes may be subtle even during stage II disease. Detection at this time (Table 6-4) may require tomography or CT in addition to AP and oblique radiographs. Isotope studies have been very useful at this stage. However, early changes can be difficult to evaluate with radionuclide scans as well. Comparison with the opposite hip may not be useful since the disease is bilateral in up to 81% of patients (9,33,71).

Ficat (25) and Ficat and Arlet (26) described the stages of AVN of the femoral head based on radiographic and clinical features. This staging is also useful in evaluating MR images (Table 6-4). Stages 0 and I have no radiographic findings, and clinical symptoms are subtle. Stage II changes are often overlooked on routine radiographs but consist of focal areas of subchondral lucency or sclerosis. Stages III and IV are usually easily detected on radiographs due to the crescent sign and progressive subchondral collapse and degenerative joint disease (Table 6-4).

Before discussing the corresponding MR features, we should discuss some specific aspects of technique which were not fully discussed in the introductory technique section of this chapter. When positive, coronal T1 weighted (SE 500/20) images are adequate for diagnosis of AVN (3,9,23,31,51,52,55,76). This sequence can be performed quickly (2–4 min) using a 32–40 cm FOV, 1 Nex, and a 256 × 256 matrix. We also perform sagittal images of both hips to further define the articular surface of the joint and better map the area of femoral head involvement (Fig. 6-24). In subtle cases, the involved hip should be studied using surface coils to improve image quality. These images are especially useful for defining the joint space, subtle articular changes, and subchondral fractures (66). It is also important to evaluate the healing process or progression of disease (51). Therefore, a T2 weighted sequence in either the coronal or axial plane is essential. The utility of this sequence becomes even more important in difficult cases or in patients with no evidence of AVN. There are numerous causes of hip pain. Other lesions that may mimic AVN or present with similar clinical symptoms are discussed later.

The earliest MR findings of AVN may be difficult to interpret or separate from edema seen in conditions such as transient osteoporosis of the hip (77). The MR signal intensity in the femoral head and neck depends on the presence of fat cells, hematopoietic cells, and trabecular bone (9,11,23,30). Fat cells become necrotic about 48 hr after the initial ischemic episode. Hematopoietic elements become necrotic over the next several days (76). Early animal studies show MR images remain normal until about the seventh day. Beginning on the seventh day an inhomogeneous loss of signal intensity can be demonstrated on T1 weighted images. These changes correspond histologically to lymphocytic infiltration (14). This inhomogeneity progresses over the first 16 days until day 20, when a more homogeneous loss of signal intensity in the femoral head becomes evident (Fig. 6-25). This correlates with increased lymphocyte infiltration and early fibrosis. As expected, radiographs remain normal during this time period (14) (Table 6-4). Early uniform loss of signal intensity in the femoral head and neck, which is similar to transient

TABLE 6-4. *Staging of avascular necrosis of the hip* (9,14,15,25,26,76)

Stage	Clinical	Radiograph	Isotope	MRI	Pathology
0	No symptoms	Normal	±	?	Hematopoietic cell necrosis after several days; fat cell necrosis after 48 hr
I	May have symptoms	Normal or may have patchy osteoporosis (see Fig. 6-23A)	Uniform uptake	Signal intensity T1 (see Fig. 6-25), inhomogeneous signal intensity	Sinus congestion, fibroblasts, hypoplastic marrow, empty lacunae
II	Pain, stiffness	Osteoporosis, mixed osteoporosis and sclerosis, cystic changes (may require tomography) (see Fig. 6-23B)	Nonuniform uptake	Wedge-shaped crescent sign (x-ray stage III) (see Figs. 6-26 and 6-27)	Necrotic central tissue, margin fibrous with revasculation and new bone on dead trabeculae
III	Stiffness, groin and knee pain	Crescent sign sequestra, cortical collapse, joint preserved (see Fig. 6-23C)	Photon deficient (cold spot)	Crescent sign sequestra, cortical collapse, joint preserved	Necrosis surrounded by granulation tissue
IV	Pain and limp may be severe	Stage III plus degenerative changes with narrowed joint space (see Fig. 6-23D,E)		Stage III plus degenerative changes with narrowed joint space (see Fig. 6-30)	Changes of stage III exaggerated

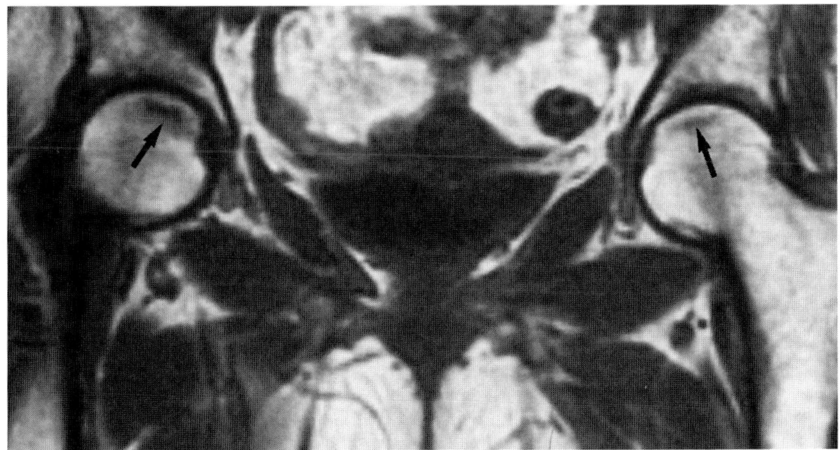

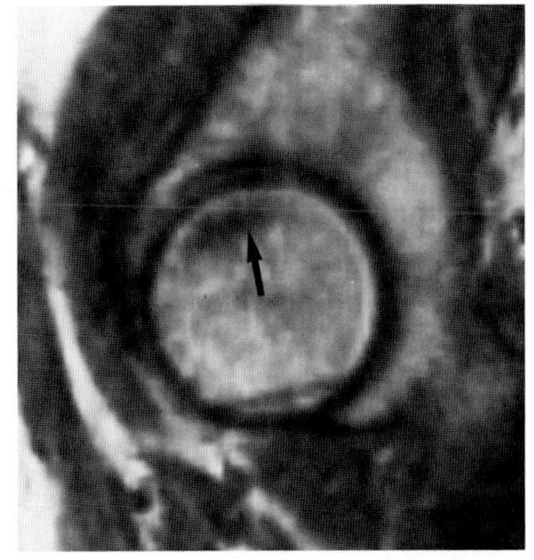

A,B

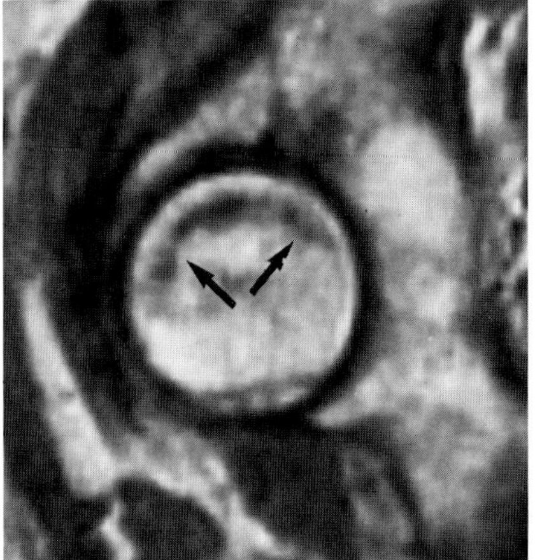

C

FIG. 6-24. SE 500/20 images of the hips in a patient with early AVN. Radiographs were normal. **A:** Coronal image demonstrating small linear subchondral defects (*arrows*). **B:** Sagittal image of the right hip more clearly defines the extent of involvement (*arrow*). **C:** Sagittal image of the left hip demonstrates that changes (*arrows*) are more advanced than appreciated on the coronal image.

osteoporosis of the hip, has also been reported (51). Conservative management is employed in either condition. However, follow-up studies are important in clarifying which disorder is present and to exclude other inflammatory diseases, specifically infection.

Also during the early phase a low-intensity line of demarcation may be evident at the margin of the necrotic zone. This is easily appreciated on T1 weighted coronal images (Fig. 6-26). The signal intensity of the necrotic zone may be indistinguishable from normal

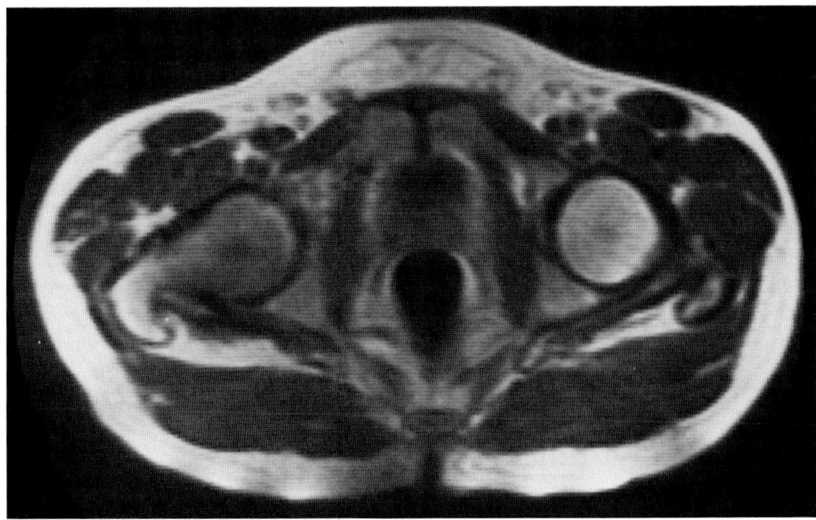

FIG. 6-25. Axial SE 500/20 image demonstrating signal intensity loss in the right femoral head due to early AVN.

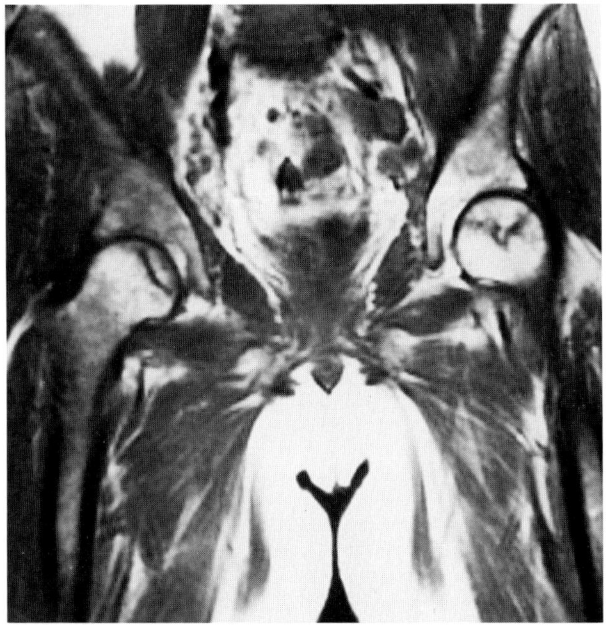

FIG. 6-26. Coronal SE 500/20 image of the hips in early AVN. There is a low-intensity margin around the necrotic area. The necrotic area maintains its normal signal intensity.

marrow (9,23). During early phases this low-intensity zone is most likely due to hyperemia. During this phase of AVN the radiographs are typically normal though slight sclerosis or lucency may be evident with early stage II AVN (Fig. 6-27) (7,9,23,52) (Table 6-4). Cold spots may be evident on radionuclide scans at this point (Fig. 6-28) (52).

Gradually (>2 weeks), the cells around the necrotic zone modulate into fibroblasts, which have low signal

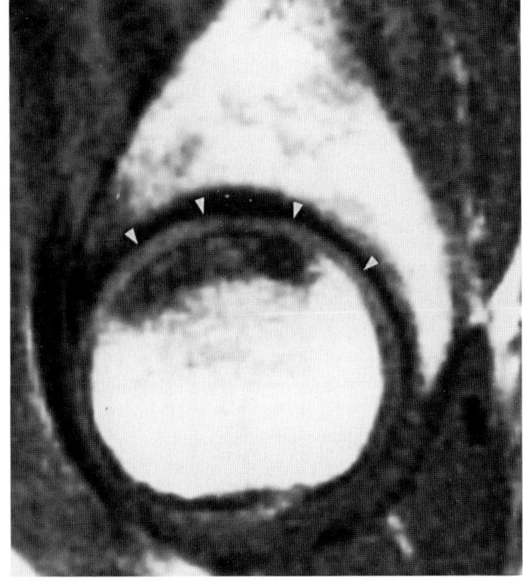

FIG. 6-27. Sagittal SE 500/20 image demonstrating a focal area of AVN. The articular cartilage (*arrowheads*) is intact.

intensity on T1 weighted sequences. Hyperemia will cause mixed low and high signal intensity margins on T2 weighted images (9,52). Little progression is evident on radiographs or isotope scans at this point (23).

Reinforcement of trabeculae and persistent hyperemia lead to widening of the low-intensity margin on both T1 and T2 weighted sequences (Fig. 6-29). The hyperemia remains high intensity on T2 weighted lesions. At this stage a clear stage II radiographic picture (Fig. 6-23B) is usually evident: namely, a lucent area surrounded by bony sclerosis (9,23,68).

With progression, the subchondral bone collapses, resulting in stage III AVN or the crescent sign on radiographs (Fig. 6-23C). This can be seen as a subchondral low-intensity line on T1 weighted sequences or a high-intensity area on T2 weighted sequences. The latter may be more easily appreciated due to the high contrast between the dark cortical bone and high signal seen with T2 weighted sequences (40). Early subchondral collapse may only be seen with coronal and sagittal surface coil images.

Once stage IV AVN (Table 6-4) has been reached, the appearance of the MR images and radiographs are more similar. Effusions are more obvious on MR images at this stage (17,54). However, subtle joint space changes are definitely more easily assessed with radiographs (Fig. 6-23D, E) or tomography than with conventional body coil MR images of the hip (Fig. 6-30).

The MR patterns of AVN, though imperfect, are useful in understanding the histologic phases of AVN (23,43). Mitchell et al. (52) correlated the MR signal intensity with radiographic features. Signal intensity was evaluated on both T1 and T2 weighted spin-echo sequences (Table 6-5). When signal intensity was similar to fat or marrow, the symptoms and radiographic features were generally early (stage I or II). Signal intensity that corresponded to fluid or fibrous tissue (Table 6-5) was nearly always associated with more advanced (stage III or IV) disease. Beltran et al. (5) also described MRI patterns and divided stages into early, intermediate, and late (Fig. 6-31). We prefer comparing MRI and histologic changes with the more commonly used Ficat classification (Table 6-4). A thorough understanding of these histologic changes and the morphologic patterns of AVN makes this technique both sensitive and specific. When compared with radiography, CT, and isotope scans, MRI is clearly the technique of choice for diagnosis and follow-up evaluation (9,11,23,52,55). Glickstein et al. (32) reported specificity of 98% and sensitivity of 97% in differentiating AVN from normal hips. MRI was 91% sensitive in differentiating AVN from other types of hip pathology. The sensitivity of MRI was 96% compared to 86% for radionuclide scans (74). Also, false negative isotope studies have been reported in up to 18% of patients with biopsy-proven AVN (11).

MRI is also useful in evaluating early stages of AVN

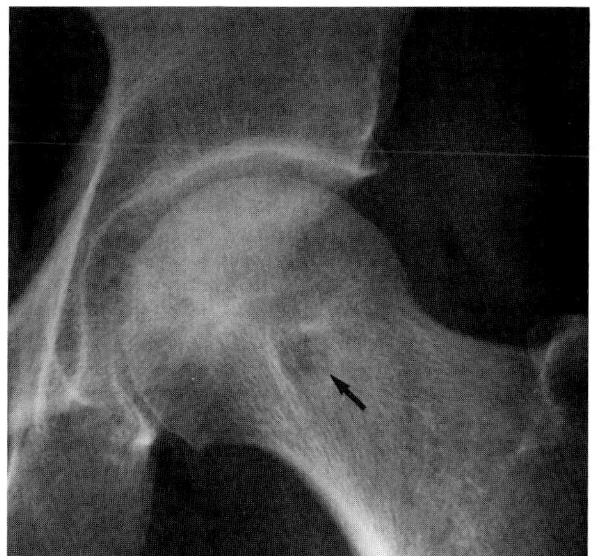

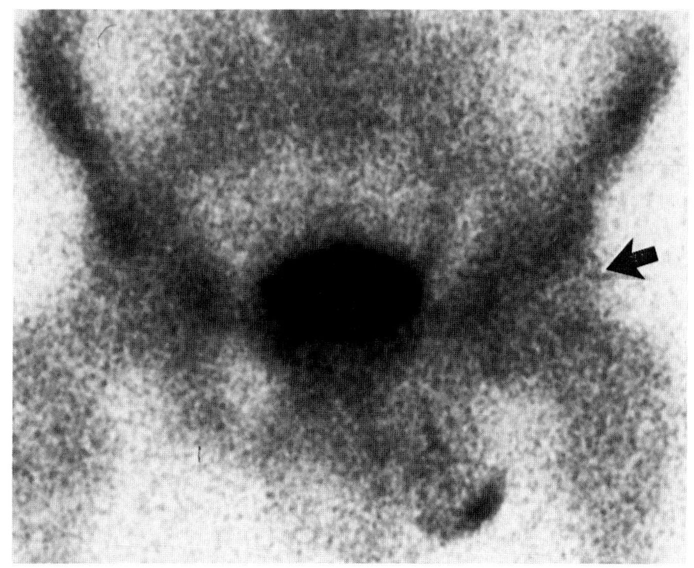

A,B

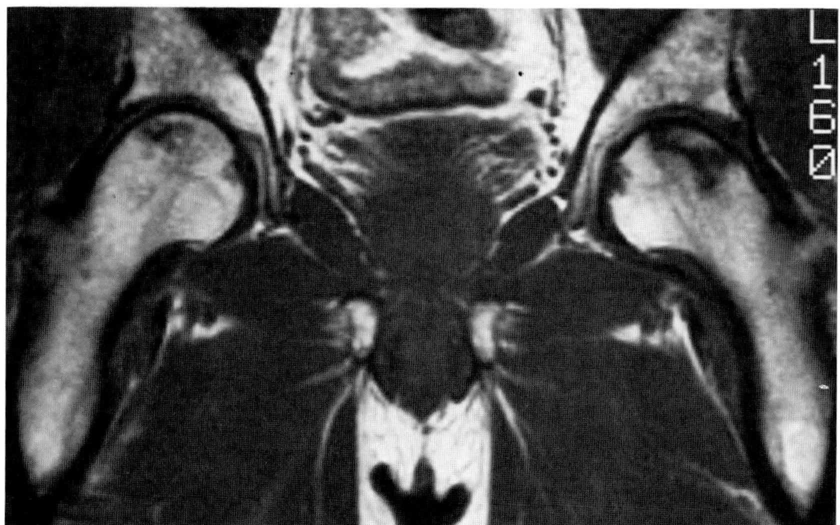

C

FIG. 6-28. Patient with left hip pain. **A:** Routine radiograph shows a herniation pit (*arrow*) but no definite AVN. **B:** Radionuclide scan shows a photopenic area (*arrow*) on the left. **C:** Coronal SE 500/20 image shows bilateral AVN greater on the left.

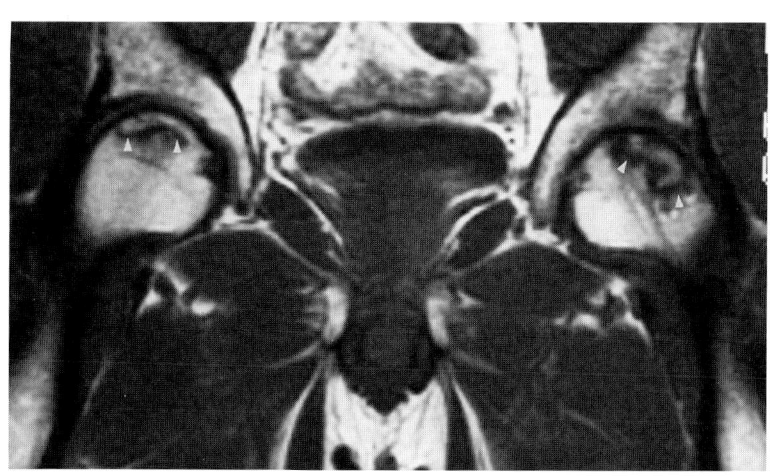

FIG. 6-29. Coronal SE 500/20 image with early AVN on the right and a thin marginal low-intensity zone (*arrowheads*). The changes on the left have progressed to trabecular reinforcement, leading to a widening of the reactive zone (*arrowheads*).

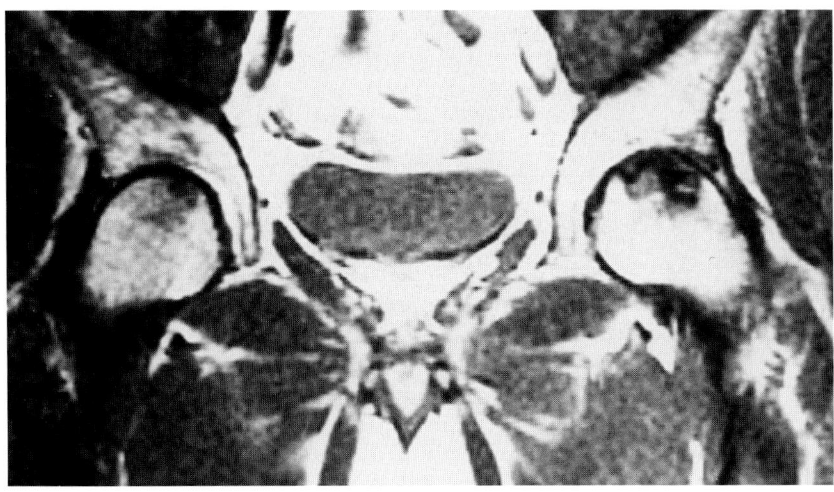

FIG. 6-30. Coronal SE 500/20 image of the pelvis and hips with early AVN on the right. There is joint space narrowing on the left, indicating stage IV disease (see Table 6-4).

for selection of patients suitable for conservative management with nonweight bearing (crutches) or core decompression (9,52,60). Until recently, the radiographic stage was used to determine treatment of AVN (52). Patients with stage I and II disease were considered as potential candidates for core decompression. Stage III and IV changes usually require arthroplasty (9,52,60). As noted above, the MR features can roughly be correlated with histologic change and are evident earlier than radiographic features. Previous studies using radiography have demonstrated progression of AVN after core decompression in the majority of patients (15). However, our early experience suggests the progression is frequently arrested by core decompression in patients with normal radiographs but early MRI abnormalities (Fig. 6-32). Further investigation in this regard may clarify the controversy concerning core decompression in treatment of early AVN.

Bone infarcts in the pelvis and upper femurs also have a very typical MRI appearance (9,23,56). Radiographic, CT, and radionuclide features of bone infarcts may be nonspecific, appear more aggressive than bone infarction (i.e., malignancy or infection), or be totally unremarkable (23,56). MR images show an area of low intensity in the diaphysis or metaphysis. This may have a well-defined serpiginous margin and multiple areas of abnormality are frequent. On T2 weighted sequences (SE 2,000/60-80) the margins are more clearly defined and form a "double line" of low and high signal intensity. This appearance may be due to chemical shift artifact—in which case, the high intensity will be on opposite sides of the dark line—or due to hyperemia and new bone formation or calcification—in which case, the high-intensity zone remains along the same margin of the lesion throughout (17). Bone sclerosis and calcification appear as areas of low intensity on both T1 and T2 weighted sequences and are usually seen in chronic infarcts (56). (See Chapter 7 for examples of bone infarction.)

TABLE 6-5. *MR signal intensity in AVN of the femoral head* (52)

Signal intensity		Signal intensity analogous to	Radiologic stage
Short TR/TE	Long TE/TR		
High	Intermediate	Fat	I–II
High	High	Blood	I–II
Low	High	Fluid	III–IV
Low	Low	Fibrous tissue, bone	III–IV

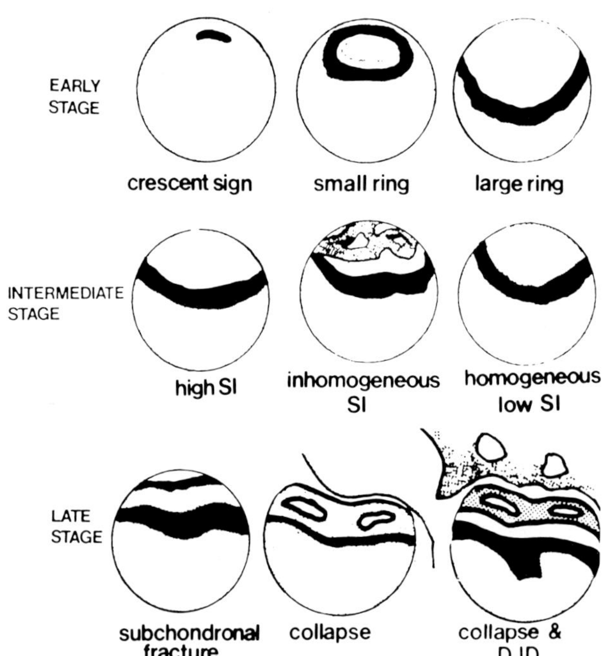

FIG. 6-31. Illustration of patterns and signal intensity changes in AVN of the femoral head. (From ref. 5, with permission.)

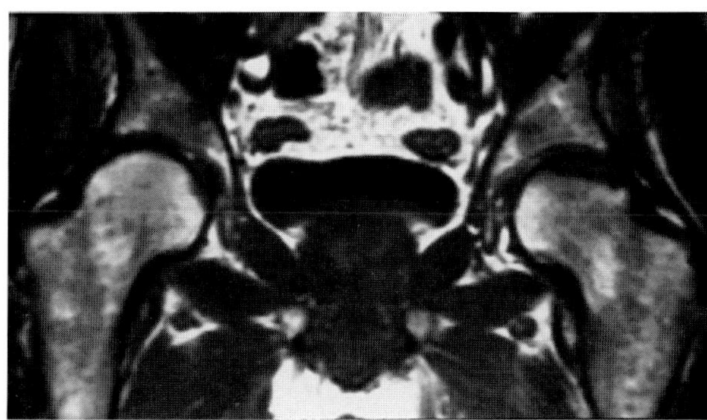

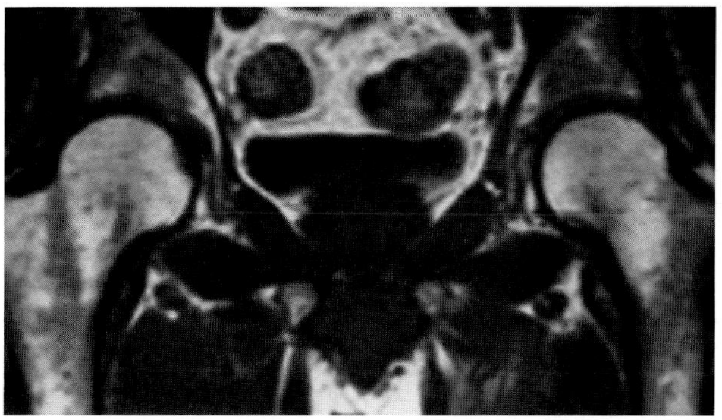

A,B

FIG. 6-32. Patient with AVN treated with nonweight bearing and crutches. **A:** Initial coronal SE 500/20 image shows early AVN in the left femoral head. **B:** Coronal SE 500/20 image is normal 5 months after conservative therapy.

Transient Osteoporosis or Edema

Transient osteoporosis or edema is a painful condition that typically occurs in young to middle-aged men. When the condition occurs in women, the process almost always involves the left hip. Pain is usually localized to the hip, but it may be referred to the knee (12).

Image features have been described with routine radiographs, radionuclide scans, and MRI (12,85). Radiographs are generally normal. However, osteopenia is noted in some cases. Radionuclide scans show increased uptake in the femoral head and upper femur. The patterns described with MRI include reduced signal intensity in the femoral head and neck on T1 weighted sequences and normal to high signal intensity on T2 weighted sequences (Fig. 6-33). Joint effusions have also been described. Signal intensity in the acetabulum is normal (12,85). Similar features could be appreciated with migratory osteoporosis, reflex sympathetic dystrophy, and osteoporosis. However, avascular necrosis, bone infarction, metastases or primary tumor, stress fractures, and osteomyelitis must also be considered in the differential diagnosis. Osteomyelitis is generally more focal and soft tissue inflammation is common. Both the femoral head and acetabulum are abnormal in the presence of joint space infection (9,10). Stress fractures are also usually more focal and changes are usually confined to the femoral neck (see Fig. 6-35). Infiltrative malignancies such as lymphoma or leukemia can have a similar appearance, but primary and metastatic lesions are usually inhomogeneous and well defined. The pattern of AVN is geographic and confined to the femoral head. However, associated edema in the upper femur can be identified in some patients (Fig. 6-34).

Trauma

MRI has become an effective tool for detection of osseous, articular, and soft tissue trauma in the pelvis, hips, and thighs (9,20,27,69). Generally, MRI is not requested for skeletal injuries because routine radiography, CT, and isotope studies are more commonly employed (9). However, subtle fractures, such as stress

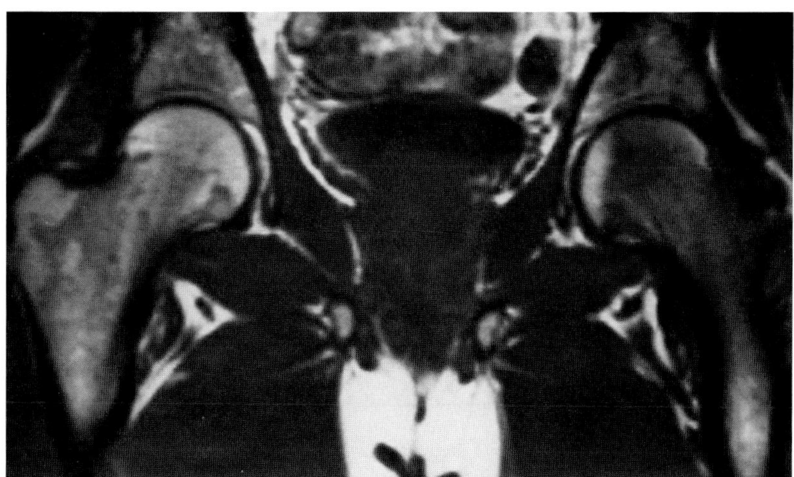

FIG. 6-33. Transient osteoporosis of the hip. SE 500/20 coronal image shows reduced signal intensity in the upper femur. The process extends into the neck. Acetabular signal intensity is normal.

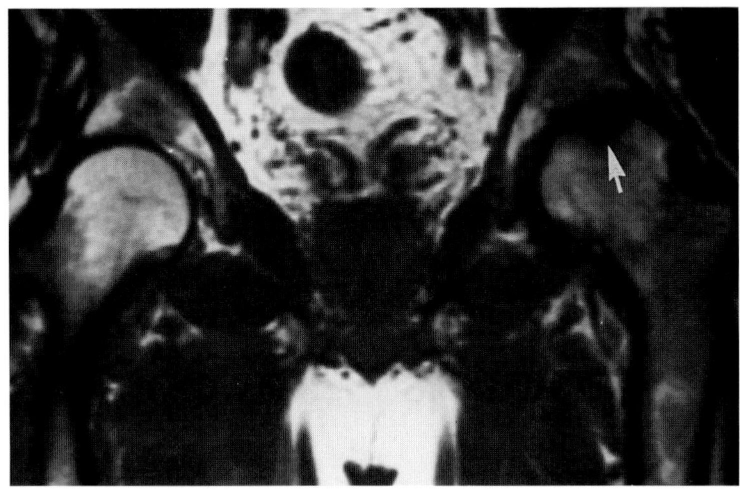

FIG. 6-34. Coronal SE 500/20 image of the pelvis and hips. There is a focal lesion (*arrow*) in the femoral head due to AVN. The signal intensity in the upper femur is reduced due to edema.

fractures (Fig. 6-35), and unsuspected fractures can be defined using MRI (20,21). Deutsch et al. (20) reported detection of hip fractures by MRI in 9/9 patients with normal radiographs. Subtle insufficiency fractures in the pelvis and complex pelvic fractures are more effectively imaged with CT (9,10). Fracture healing (bony union, non-union, fibrous union) and complications of fractures (Fig. 6-36) can also be assessed with MRI.

MRI is ideally suited to evaluate soft tissue and many articular disorders in the hip and thigh region (9,27,36,83,87). Injuries to the thigh muscles and their pelvic attachments (Fig. 6-37) are common in trained and untrained athletes (2,48,49,58,59). Up to 30% of soccer injuries involve the thigh, usually hematomas or muscle strains (28,42,63). The hamstring muscles are injured most frequently (Fig. 6-38), but tears in the quadriceps (Fig. 6-39) and adductor muscles (Fig. 6-40) also occur. Fortunately, most tears are first or second degree strains, which heal in approximately 20 weeks (2,9). First degree strains are minor tears with injury to

A

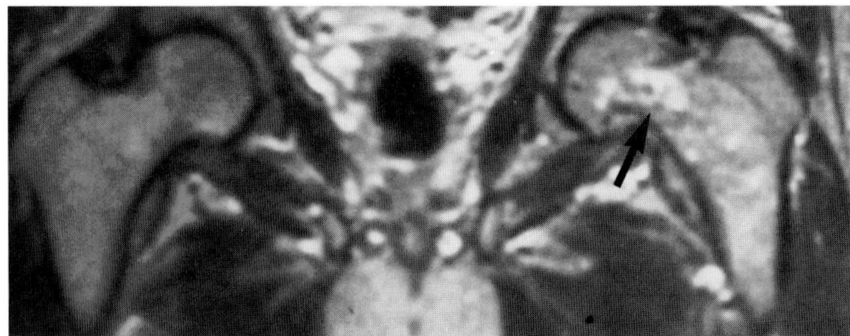

B

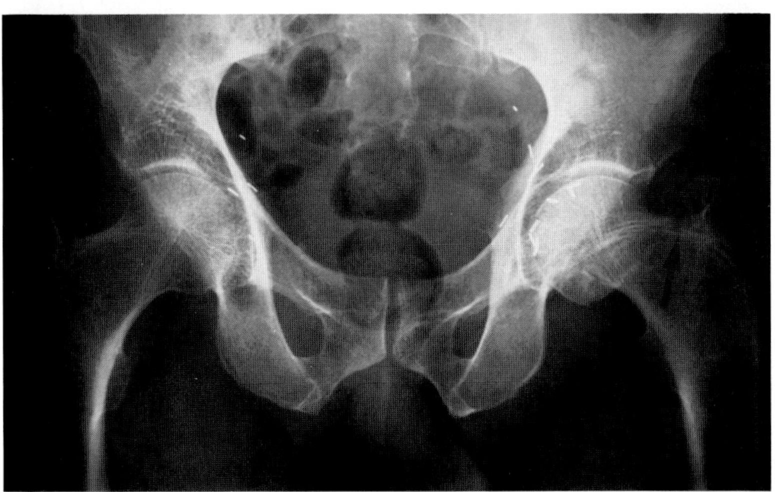

FIG. 6-35. A: Coronal SE 2,000/60 image of the pelvis demonstrates a focal area of increased signal intensity in the left femoral neck (*arrow*). **B:** A radiograph obtained several weeks later demonstrates Paget's disease with an incomplete fracture (*arrow*) of the femoral neck.

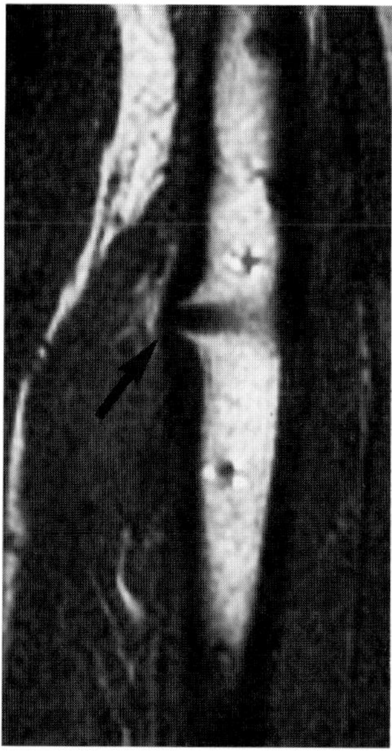
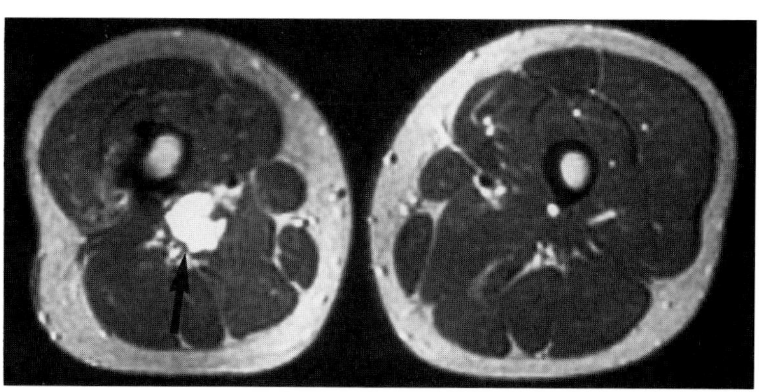

A,B

FIG. 6-36. Old femoral fracture with removal of the plate and screws due to pain. Sagittal SE 500/20 image (**A**) shows cortical distortion due to the previous screw, which had penetrated the cortex (*arrow*). Axial SE 2,000/60 images of the thighs (**B**) demonstrate a high signal intensity mass (*arrows*) adjacent to the cortical defect. Post-traumatic neuroma.

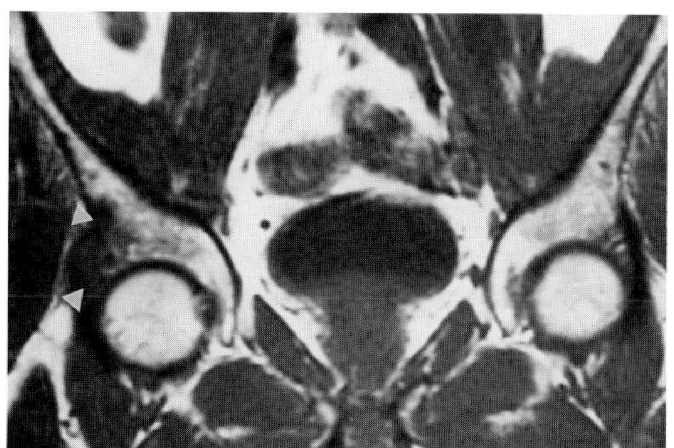
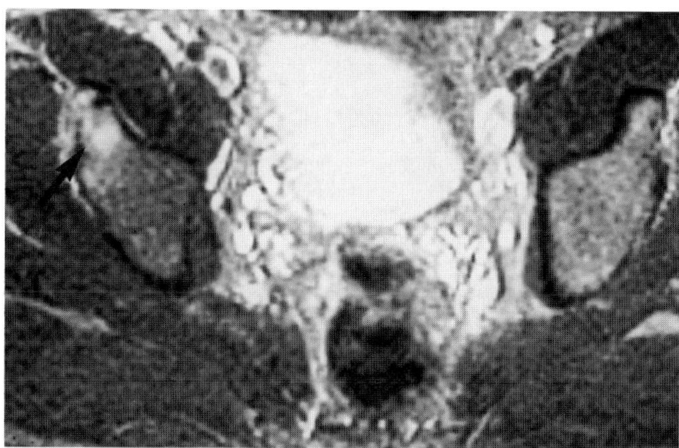

A,B

FIG. 6-37. Avulsion stress injury of the anterior inferior iliac spine at the rectus femoris origin. **A:** Coronal SE 500/20 image of the hips shows an area of soft tissue swelling and reduced signal intensity in the marrow (*arrowheads*). **B:** Axial T2 weighted SE 2,000/60 image shows increased signal intensity in the anterior inferior iliac spine (*arrow*).

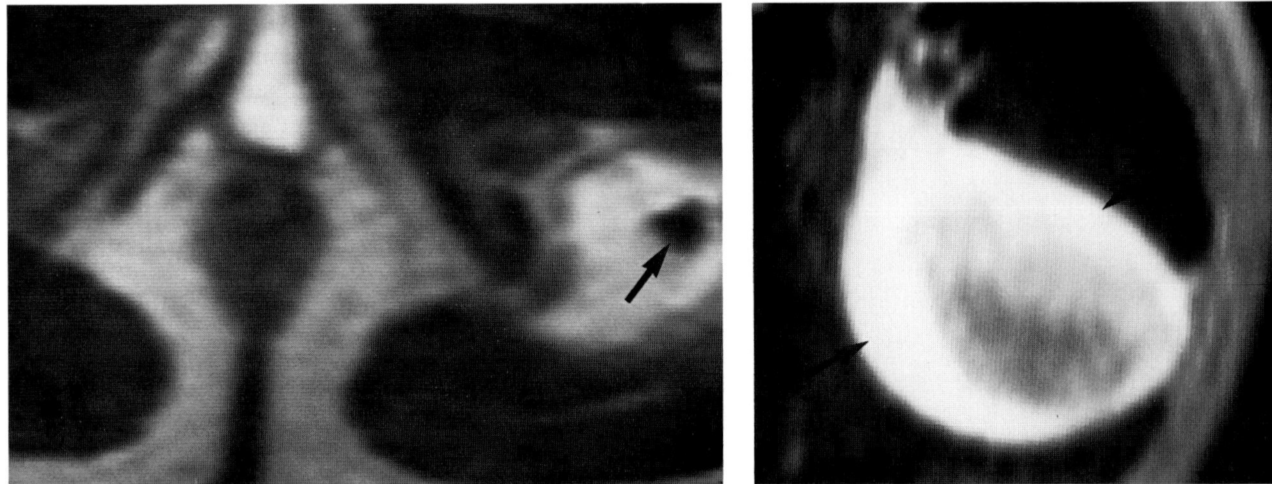

A,B

FIG. 6-38. Axial SE 2,000/60 images at the ischial origin (**A**) and more inferiorly (**B**), showing a grade 3 hamstring tear with a large high signal intensity hematoma (*arrows* in **B**). Note the displaced tendon (*arrow* in **A**).

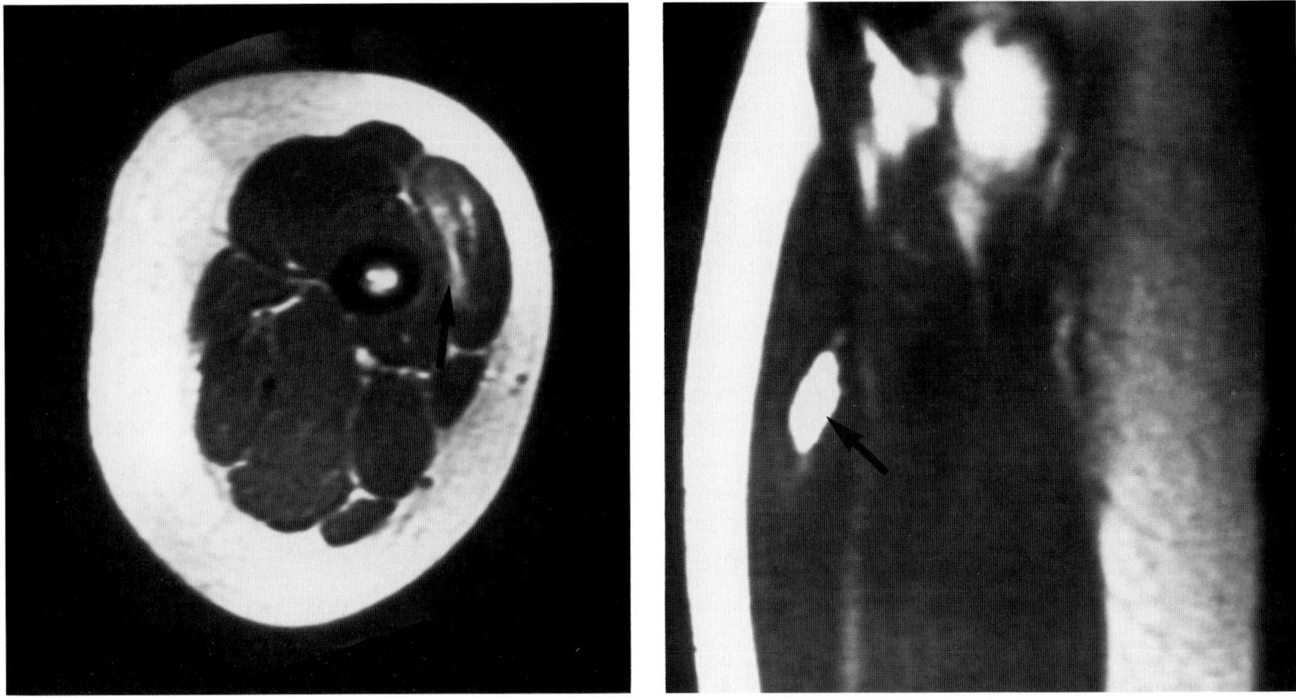

A,B

FIG. 6-39. Axial (**A**) and sagittal (**B**) SE 2,000/30 images of the thigh, demonstrating high signal intensity (*arrow*) in the vastus medialis due to a grade 1–2 muscle tear.

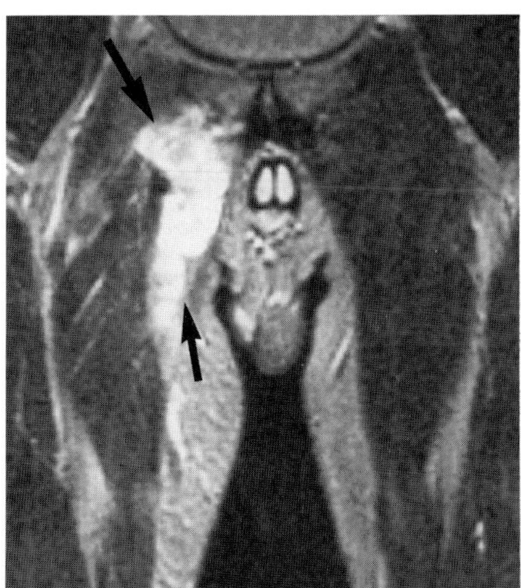

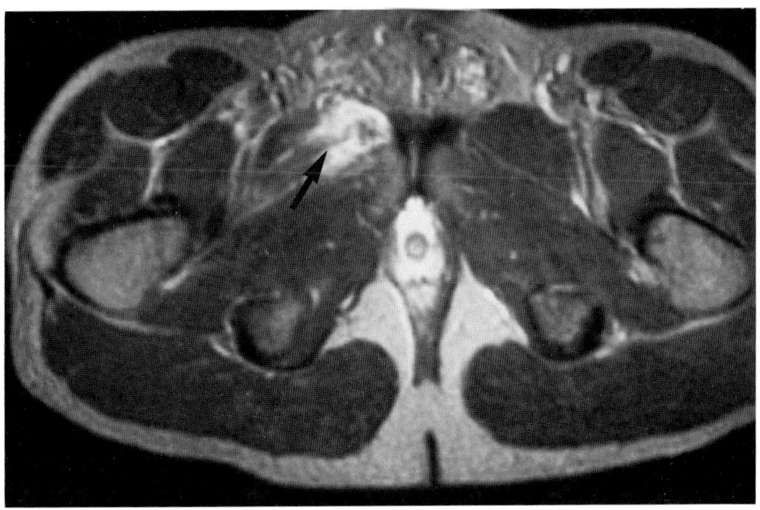

A,B

FIG. 6-40. Coronal (**A**) and axial (**B**) SE 2,000/60 images demonstrating an adductor origin tear with hematoma formation (*arrows*).

only a few fibers. Second degree strains result in disruption of about 50% of the muscle fibers. Third degree strains are complete tears (58,59). Both second and third degree tears can lead to large organized hematomas, which tend to heal more slowly with a more guarded prognosis.

Direct or indirect nerve injuries may result in femoral and/or sciatic nerve palsies. MRI is also ideal for following patients with muscle and tendon injury. Effective therapy will result in healing and return of muscle and tendon signal to normal. Clinical symptoms usually resolve before images return to normal. Re-injury is seen as a new area of increased signal intensity. Scar tissue formation is seen as an area of low signal intensity on both T1 and T2 weighted sequences.

Compartment syndromes are more common in the lower leg (see Chapter 8); however, they have been reported in the posterior thigh (62). Persistent pain and circulatory compromise occur due to increased intracompartment pressure. If not properly diagnosed and treated, the changes may progress to myonecrosis and fibrous replacement (59,62). Exercise induced rhabdomyolysis may also occur due to overuse (Fig. 6-41). This process results from loss of integrity of cell membranes, which allows cell fluids to escape into extracellular space. Early diagnosis and evaluation of the extent of the process are important. Sequelae include renal failure, hyperkalemia, and hypocalcemia. Enzyme studies (CK, LDH, GOT) are elevated (67,79,87). Early diagnosis can be accomplished using radionuclide scans (47). Recently, MRI has been used to evaluate the extent of the process (22,27,36,87).

Evaluation of the extent of muscle, tendon, and associated nerve injuries is most easily accomplished with T2 weighted sequences using two planes. We generally use either axial–sagittal or axial–coronal combinations. Lesions due to edema or hemorrhage in muscle can be completely overlooked on T1 weighted sequences (Fig. 6-41).

Other post-traumatic conditions such as iliopsoas inflammation (Fig. 6-42), bursitis, and acetabular labral tears can also be clearly identified with MRI (9,83). The

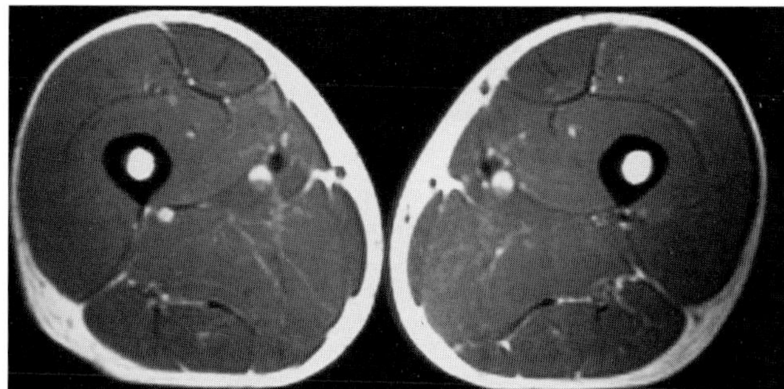

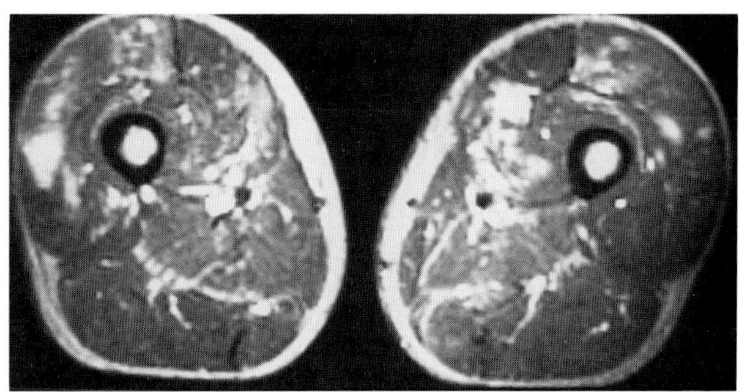

A,B

FIG. 6-41. Rhabdomyolysis due to overuse in a bicycle racer. **A:** Axial SE 500/20 image is normal. **B:** Axial SE 2,000/60 image at the same level shows diffuse edema and hemorrhage in both thighs, especially in the adductors and quadriceps muscle groups.

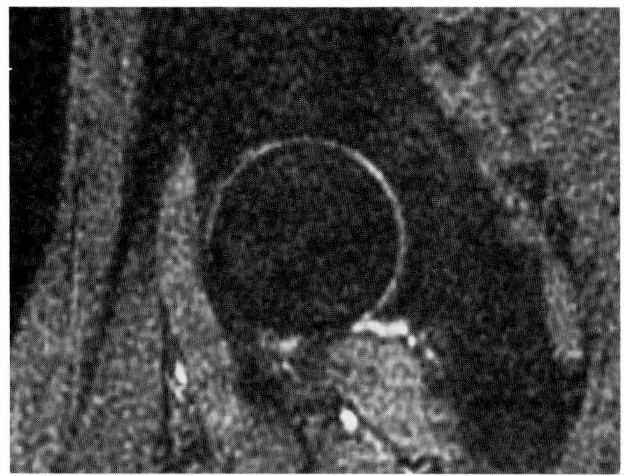
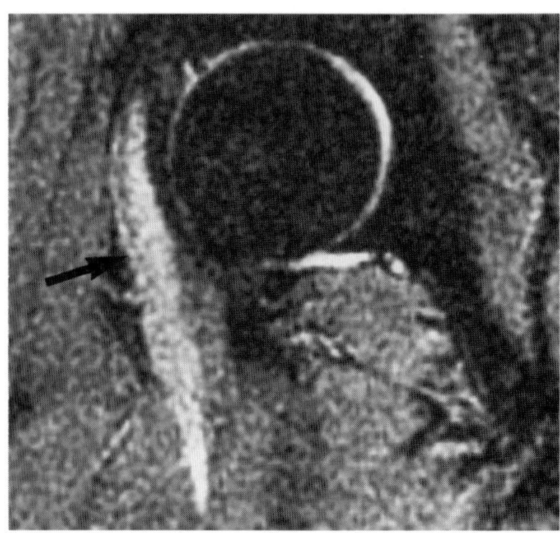

A,B

FIG. 6-42. Radial GRIL (GRASS–interleaved) images of the hips. The right iliopsoas (**A**) is normal. Note the increased signal (*arrow* in **B**) on the left due to inflammation after trauma.

latter are difficult to define with arthrography alone or in combination with CT or tomography. Radial GRIL images are best suited for evaluating acetabular labral tears since the labrum can be viewed tangentially (Fig. 6-43). Normally, the labrum should be a triangular low-intensity structure. Changes in configuration or tears, seen as areas of high signal intensity on T2 weighted images, can cause pain and clicking with hip motion (7). Surgical therapy is generally indicated to repair these defects.

Neoplasms

MRI examinations of the pelvic region are frequently requested to evaluate patients with suspected musculoskeletal neoplasms. Metastatic disease is common in this location (8,19,88). Chapter 12 discusses musculoskeletal neoplasms more fully; however, certain neoplasms and imaging considerations in the pelvis deserve mention.

Table 6-6 summarizes the skeletal and soft tissue neoplasms in the pelvic region (19,24). The appearance of

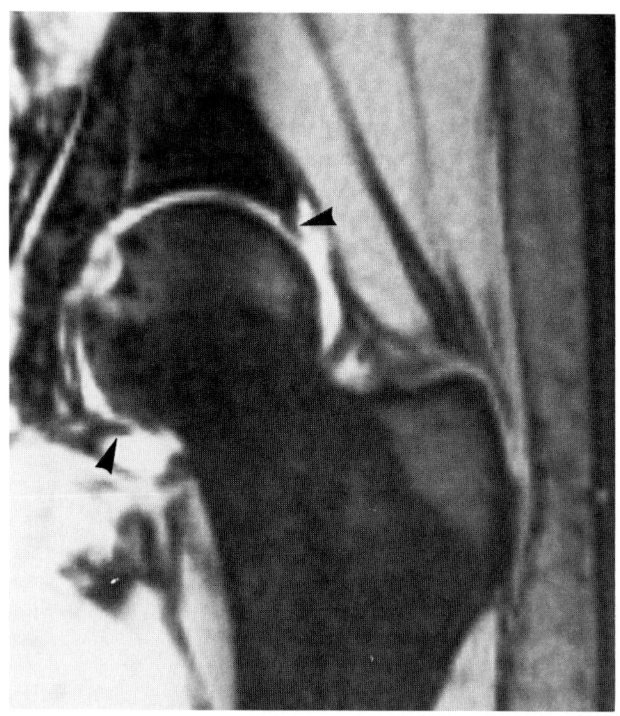
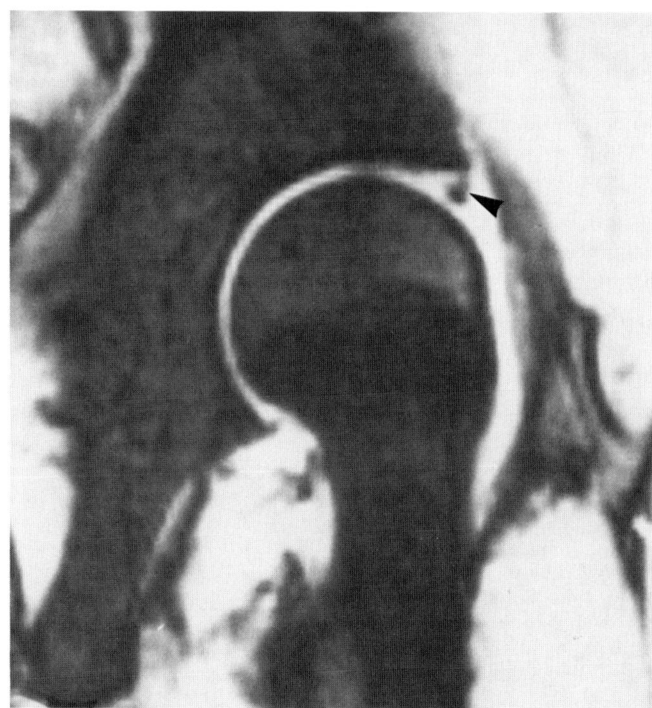

A,B

FIG. 6-43. Acetabular labral tear. Radial GRIL (GRASS–interleaved) images show normal (**A**) superior and inferior labrum (*arrows*) with high signal intensity joint fluid. The labrum on the opposite side (**B**) is partially separated superiorly (*arrow*).

TABLE 6-6. *Bone and soft tissue neoplasms about the pelvis, hips, and upper thighs* (19,24)

Bone tumors	
Metastasis	
Malignant primary tumors	(number/8,542 cases)
Chondrosarcoma	241
Osteosarcoma	187
Lymphoma	146
Chordoma	133
Ewings	131
Myeloma	114
Fibrosarcoma	54
Postradiation sarcoma	25
Benign	
Osteochondroma	115
Osteoid osteoma	80
Giant cell tumor	67
Chondroma	23
Chondroblastoma	19
Soft tissue tumors	
Liposarcoma	130
Desmoids	67
Alveolar sarcoma	42
Synovial sarcoma	22
Epithelioid sarcoma	22

soft tissue lesions does not differ significantly according to location. Benign lesions tend to be homogeneous and well marginated and do not cause neurovascular encasement (see Chapter 12). Exceptions are hemangiomas (Fig. 6-44) and desmoids, which have more inhomogeneous signal intensity with irregular margins (8,9). Lesions that become necrotic can also cause confusion (Fig. 6-45). Synovial sarcomas can appear more benign and cystic. This is an important factor to consider due to their significant incidence about the pelvis (8,24). As a rule, malignant soft tissue masses are inhomogeneous, have irregular margins, and more often encase neurovascular structures.

An enlarged iliopsoas bursa (Fig. 6-46) can be confused with neoplasm clinically. These lesions are palpable and can be symptomatic. CT and arthrography can be used for diagnosis. Communication with the hip joint is common. T2 weighted MR images clearly demonstrate the nature of the lesion as communication with the joint can be demonstrated, especially in the axial plane. Lesions also have homogeneous high signal intensity with well-defined margins, which is typical of a periarticular cyst.

Soft tissue neoplasms are more easily characterized than skeletal tumors. The marrow pattern in the pelvis and upper femurs is often inhomogeneous due to the trabecular patterns and variations in fatty and hematopoietic marrow (18,40,70) (see Chapter 14). When one evaluates skeletal neoplasms it is imperative to have routine radiographs for comparison. Radiographs are useful in characterizing the lesions. Also, blastic lesions (Fig. 6-47) and subtle lesions such as osteoid osteomas (Figs. 6-47 and 6-48) may be confused with other conditions

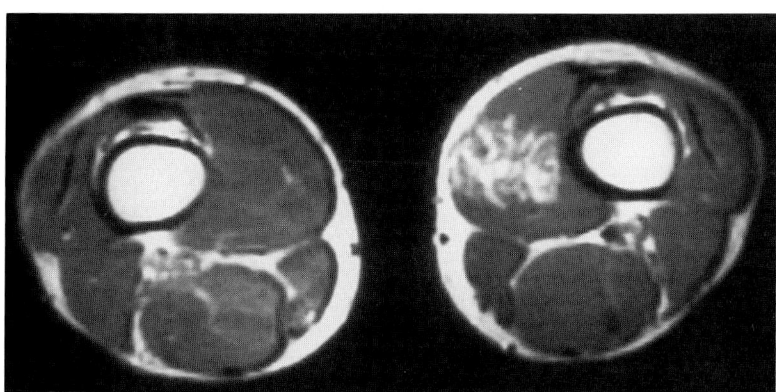

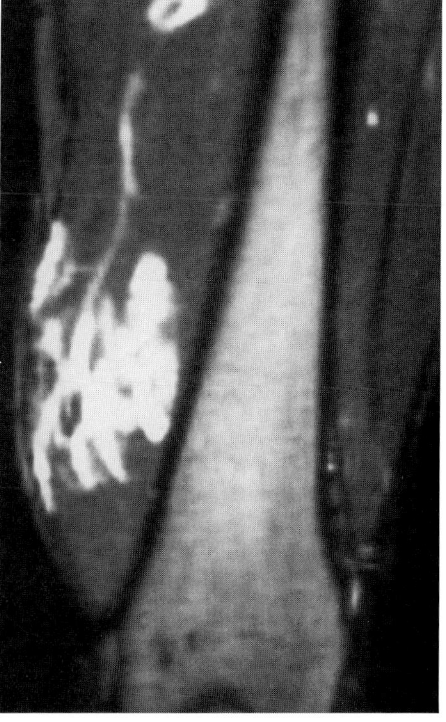

A,B

FIG. 6-44. Hemangioma in the medial left thigh. Axial SE 2,000/30 (**A**) and coronal GRASS (**B**) images demonstrate a large high signal intensity soft tissue lesion with numerous vessels typical of hemangioma. GRASS sequences are particularly useful in defining the vascularity of these lesions.

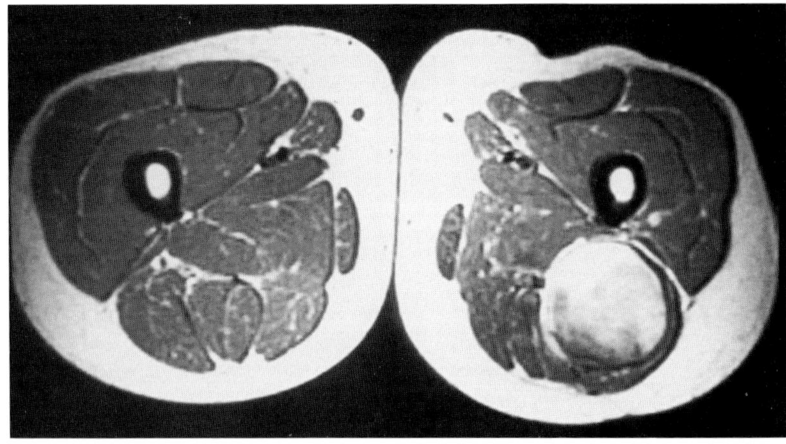
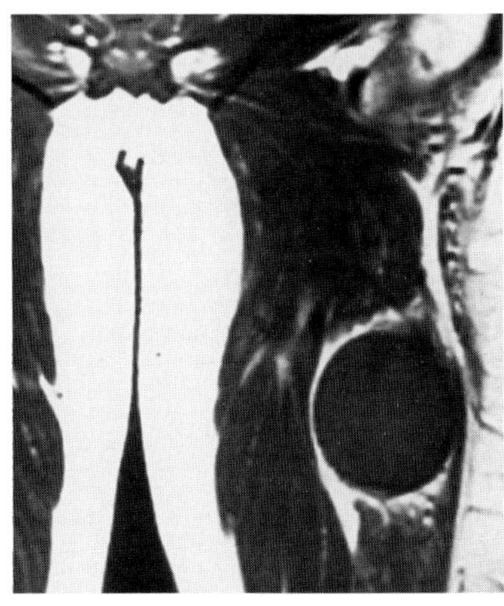

A,B

FIG. 6-45. Necrotic neurofibroma. Axial SE 2,000/30 (**A**) and coronal SE 500/20 (**B**) images demonstrate a well-marginated mass in the region of the sciatic nerve. The lesion has inhomogeneous signal intensity on the more T2 weighted sequence (**A**), which is common with malignant lesions.

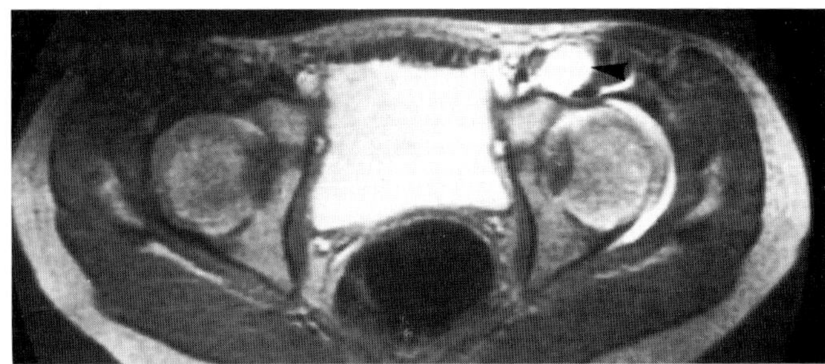
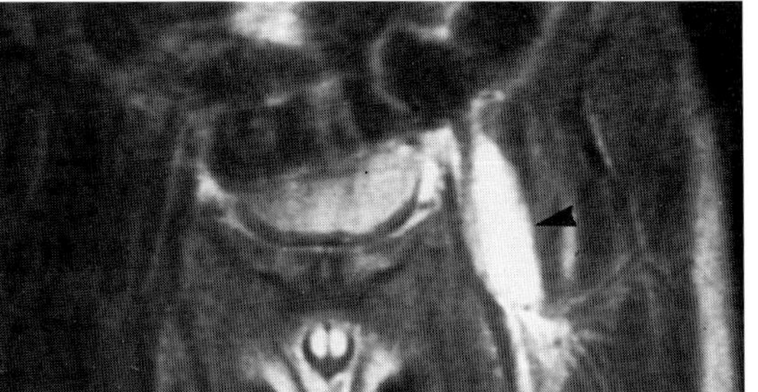

A,B

FIG. 6-46. Axial (**A**) and coronal (**B**) SE 2,000/60 images of the pelvis demonstrate a well-defined high signal intensity mass anterior to the left hip (*arrowheads*). Appearance and location are typical of an enlarged iliopsoas bursa.

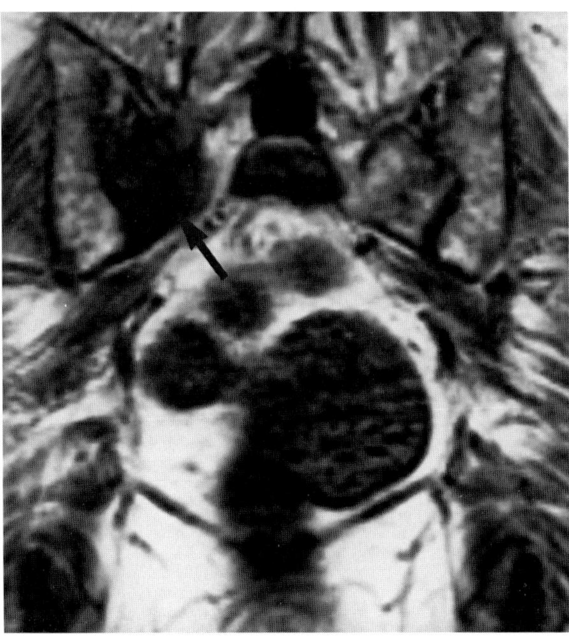
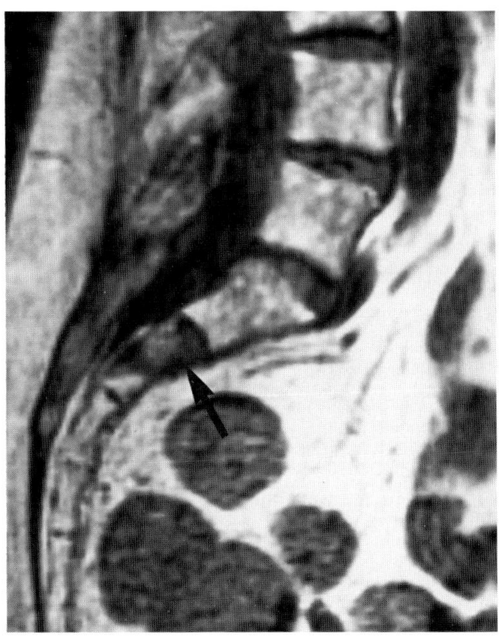

A,B

FIG. 6-47. Coronal (**A**) and sagittal (**B**) SE 500/20 images of the sacrum, demonstrating a blastic metastasis in the upper sacrum (*arrow* in **A**) and mixed blastic and lytic lesion (inhomogeneous lesion—*arrow* in **B**) in the second sacral segment.

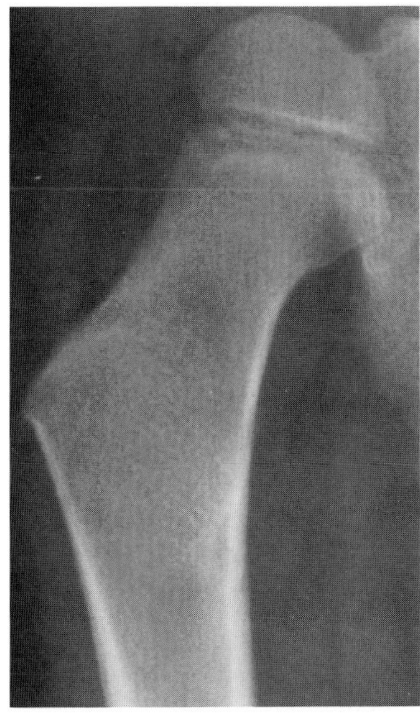

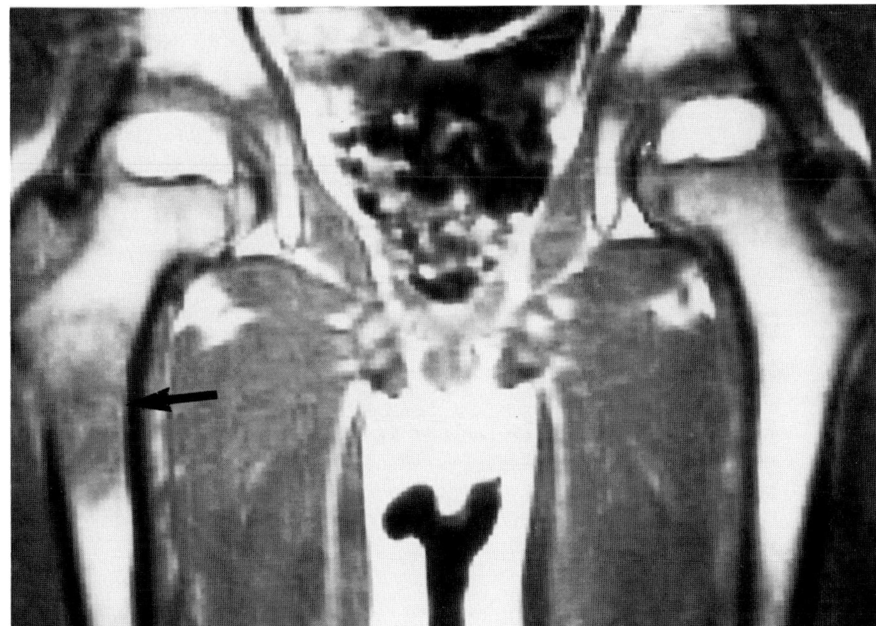

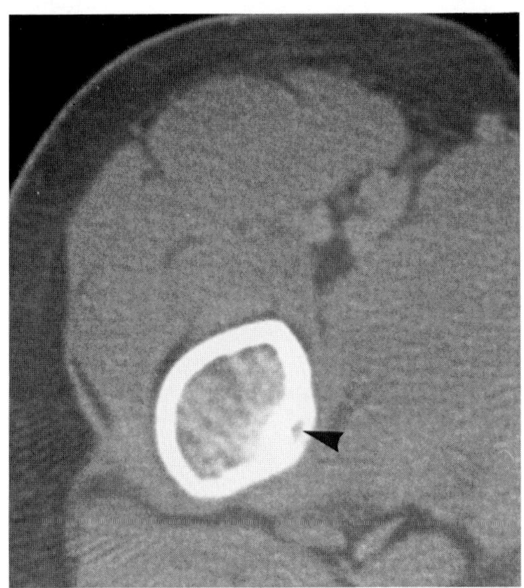
C

FIG. 6-48. A: AP radiograph of the upper femur is normal. No lytic or blastic lesions are identified. **B:** Coronal SE 500/20 image shows a large area of low signal intensity (*arrow*) in the upper right femur. This is nonspecific and could be infection, tumor, or reaction due to a stress fracture. **C:** CT scan demonstrates cortical thickening with a lucent nidus (*arrowhead*) typical of osteoid osteoma.

such as benign bone islands and Paget's disease (Fig. 6-49). MRI is generally reserved for staging suspected malignancy and evaluating the extent of lymphoma or other infiltrative processes (Fig. 6-50) (9,72,88). Generally, T1 and T2 weighted sequences are used to define the extent and nature of lesions in marrow and cortical bone. However, especially in the pelvis, STIR images may be very useful to evaluate subtle changes in bone marrow, cortical bone, and soft tissues.

Arthropathies

A more complete discussion of the role of MRI in evaluating arthropathies can be found in Chapter 15. However, there have been several reports in the MR literature on the grading and evaluation of hip arthropathies, specifically osteoarthritis. Osteoarthritis is most often evaluated with routine radiography. Occasionally, CT, conventional tomography, or arthrography are required to evaluate subtle changes and exclude other causes of hip pain (9,10,69). The role of MRI is not clear at this time. However, the ability to evaluate articular cartilage may prove useful in patients with early osteoarthritis (13,44,45). In addition, this condition is frequently encountered when evaluating the hips. Therefore, it is important to be familiar with the MR features of this process.

Li et al. (45) correlated MRI, radiographic, and functional factors in ten patients with osteoarthritis. The correlations are useful in understanding the role of MRI

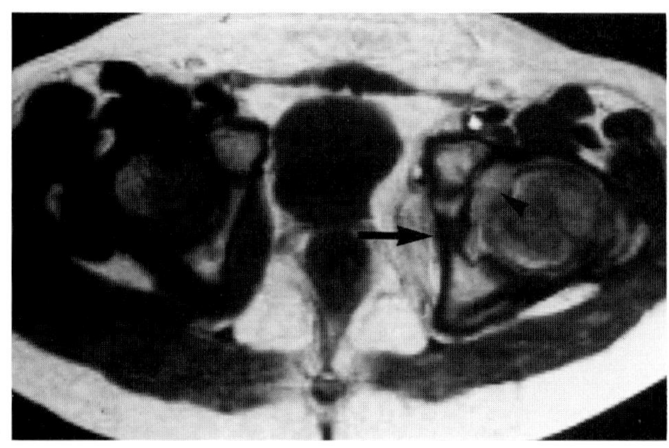
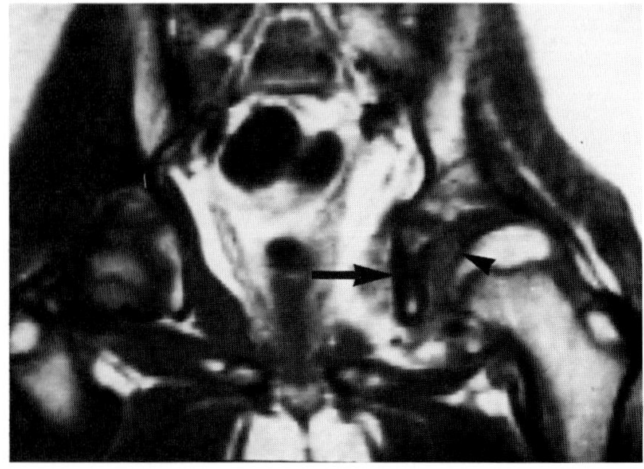

A,B

FIG. 6-49. Axial (**A**) and coronal (**B**) SE 500/20 images of the hips show synovial hypertrophy (*arrowheads*) and bone sclerosis (*arrows*) typical of osteoid osteoma. This lesion can easily be overlooked if the proper image planes and sequences are not used. A T2 weighted sequence would confirm the sclerotic nature of the bone changes. Most physicians are more familiar with the CT appearance of osteoid osteomas (see Fig. 6-48C).

in evaluating patients with osteoarthritis. Table 6-7 compares the grading systems for radiographs and MRI. MR features compare favorably with patients' symptoms in the early stages of disease but do not provide much utility in more advanced stages. The role of MRI in evaluating osteoarthritis requires further investigation before it can be suggested that it replace more conventional imaging techniques.

Synovial and cartilage changes in other inflammatory arthropathies can also be detected earlier with MRI than conventional imaging studies (6,9,65,86). Changes are frequently not specific and the role of MRI has not been clearly established (see Chapter 15).

Infection

MRI is a sensitive technique for early detection of osteomyelitis and for differentiating osseous from soft tissue infection (9,29,46,78,84). The latter is often difficult with radionuclide imaging. MRI is particularly useful in detecting early infection in children (9,29). Marrow signal intensity in the hip region is frequently inhomogeneous. Therefore, both T1 and T2 weighted sequences are usually required to properly characterize the pathology (Fig. 6-51). Short TI inversion recovery sequences (STIR) are particularly useful in this region. Signal intensity of fatty marrow is suppressed and the area of abnormality is clearly seen as an area of high signal intensity. This is useful in cortical bone and soft tissue as well (see Chapter 13).

Pediatric Disorders

MRI of pediatric disorders will be more completely discussed in Chapter 15. However, since pediatric hip disorders present a common orthopedic problem, we

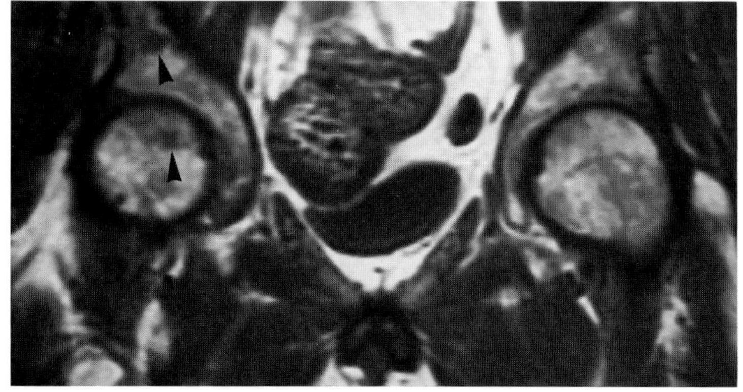
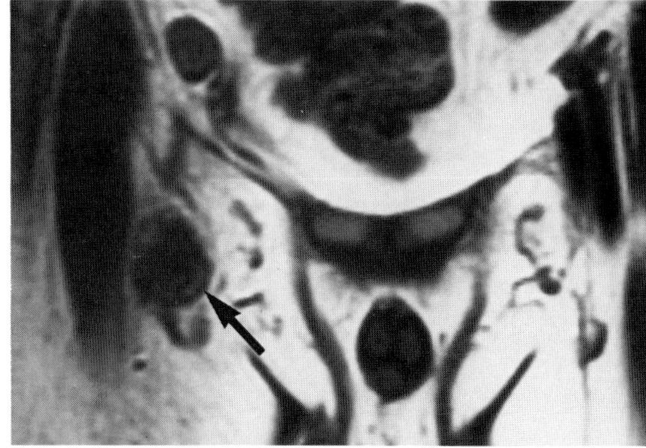

A,B

FIG. 6-50. Coronal SE 500/20 images of the hips (**A**) and inguinal region (**B**) in a patient with lymphoma. There are focal areas of decreased signal intensity in the marrow (*arrowheads*) and enlarged inguinal nodes (*arrow*).

TABLE 6-7. *Osteoarthritis radiographic and MRI stages*

Grade	Radiographic staging	MRI staging (coronal images)
0	Normal	Normal
1	Joint space narrowing (?) and subtle osteophytes	Inhomogeneous high signal intensity in cartilage (T2WI)[a]
2	Definite joint space narrowing, osteophytes, and sclerosis, especially in acetabular region	Inhomogeneity with areas of high signal intensity in articular cartilage (T2WI); indistinct trabeculae or signal intensity loss in femoral head and neck (T1WI)[b]
3	Marked joint space narrowing, osteophytes, cyst formation, and deformity of femoral head	Criteria of stages 1 and 2 plus indistinct zone between femoral head and acetabulum; increasing subchondral signal loss (both T1WI and T2WI) due to bone sclerosis
4	Gross loss of joint space with above features plus large osteophytes and increased deformity of the femoral head and acetabulum	Above criteria plus deformity of femoral head

[a] T2WI, T2 weighted image.
[b] T1WI, T1 weighted image.

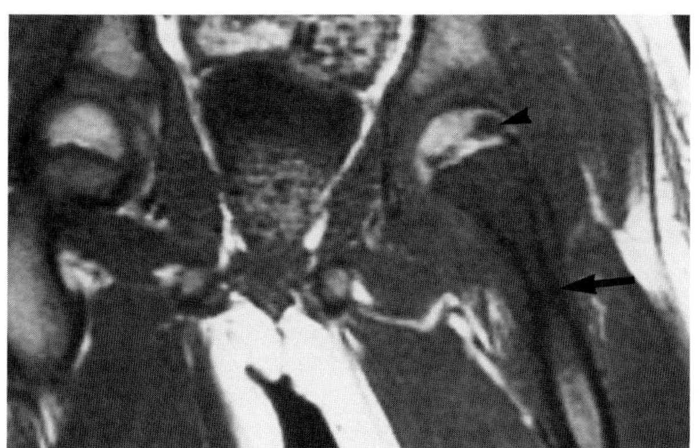
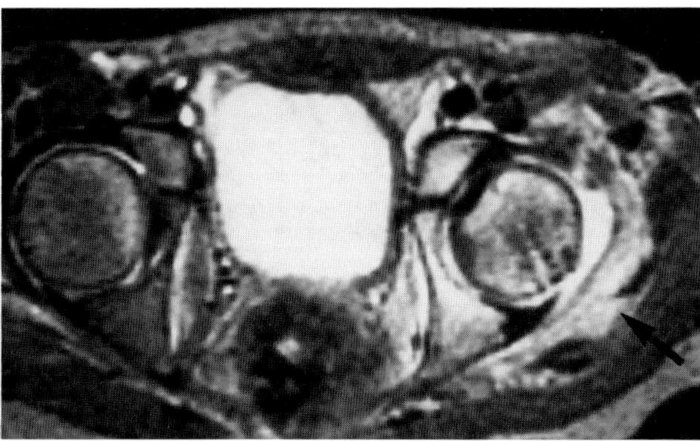

A,B

FIG. 6-51. Joint space infection and osteomyelitis. **A:** Coronal SE 500/20 image shows the left hip is abducted due to discomfort. There is reduced signal intensity in the epiphysis (*arrowhead*) and upper femur (*arrow*). The joint space is also widened. **B:** Axial SE 2,000/60 image shows an effusion and inflammation (*arrow*) of the periarticular soft tissues.

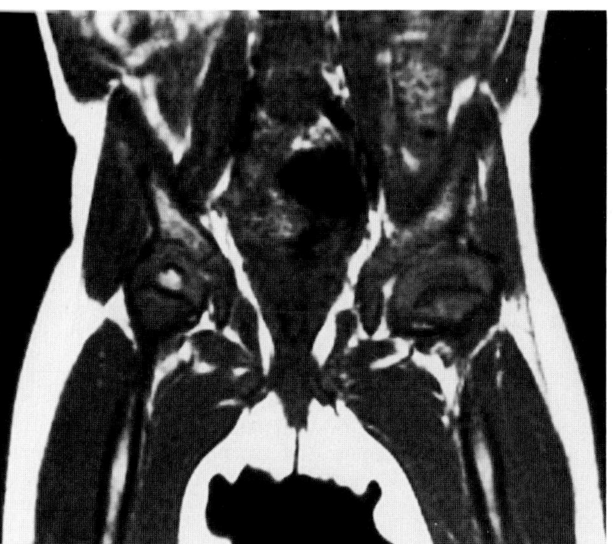
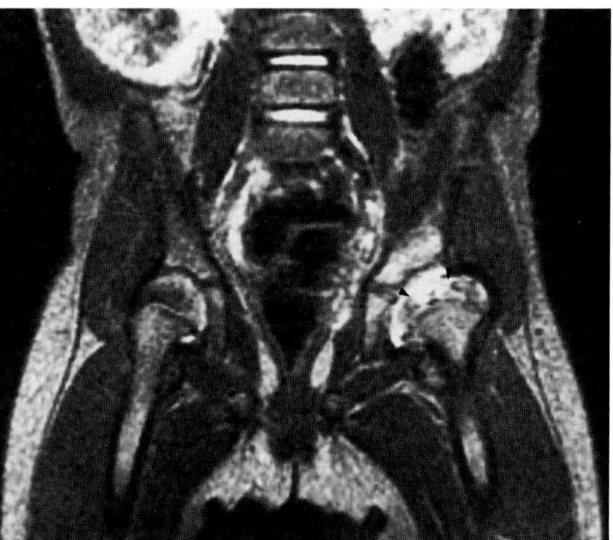

A,B

FIG. 6-52. Coronal SE 500/20 (**A**) and SE 2,000/60 (**B**) images in a patient with Legg–Calvé–Perthes disease. There is marked deformity of the femoral head with an effusion and areas of necrosis and deformity (*arrowheads*) in the epiphysis.

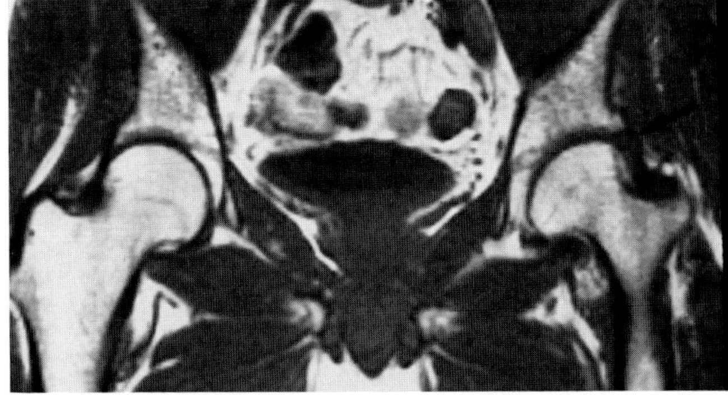

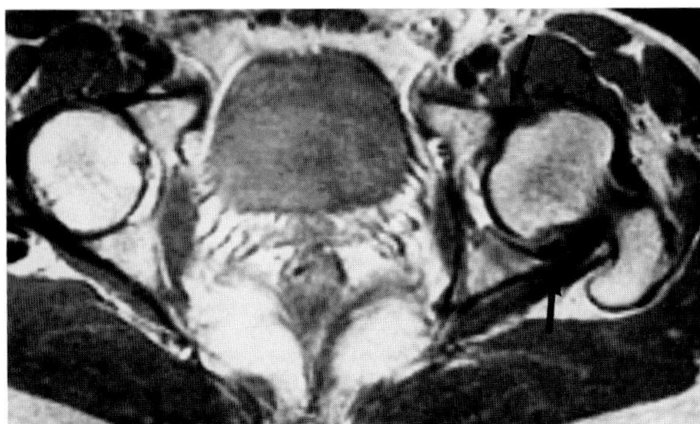

A,B

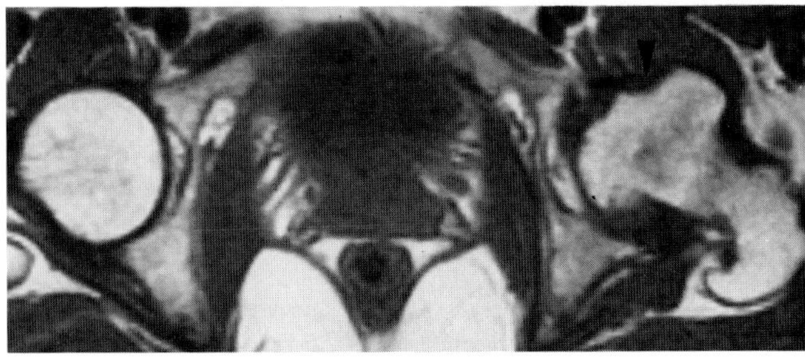

C

FIG. 6-53. Congenital hip disease. **A:** Coronal SE 500/20 image shows deformity of the left femoral head and increase in the acetabular angle. The labrum (*arrow*) is deformed but covers the femoral head. **B, C:** Axial images demonstrate the anterior and posterior labrum (*arrows*) and show an unsuspected deformity in the articular surface of the femoral head anteriorly (*arrowhead*).

discuss the utility of MRI in evaluating congenital hip disease and Legg–Calvé–Perthes disease in this section.

Routine radiographs, CT, and arthrography have been used to evaluate pediatric hip diseases. More recently, ultrasound has played an important role in evaluating congenital hip disease (41). MRI can define the osseous, soft tissue, and cartilage (articular and labral) anatomy of the hip. Definition of the capsular and labral anatomy is particularly important for planning conservative or operative therapy. Also, the ability to select and vary the image planes is very useful for evaluating hip disorders in children (39,75).

Multiple image planes are usually required to fully evaluate the changes in congenital hip disease and Legg–Calvé–Perthes disease (64). Most often coronal and axial planes are selected. Both T1 and T2 weighted sequences are usually required. In some cases radial GRIL images may be needed to define the acetabular labrum to best advantage.

In patients with these conditions (Figs. 6-52 and 6-53) the MR features are valuable in defining anatomy, the extent of osteonecrosis, and in differentiating these conditions from transient synovitis, infection, and other causes of hip pain.

REFERENCES

1. Anderson JE. *Grant's atlas of anatomy,* 8th ed. Baltimore: Williams & Wilkins, 1983.
2. Baker BE. Current concepts in diagnosis and treatment of musculotendinous injuries. *Med Sci Sports Exerc* 1984;16:323–327.
3. Bassett LW, Gold RH, Reicher M, Bennett LR, Tooke SM. Magnetic resonance imaging in the early diagnosis of ischemic necrosis of the femoral head. *Clin Orthop* 1987;214:237–248.
4. Baum PA, Matsumoto AH, Teitelbaum GP, Zuurbier RA, Barth KA. Anatomic relationship between the common femoral artery and vein: CT evaluation and clinical significance. *Radiology* 1989;173:775–777.
5. Beltran J, Burk JM, Herman LJ, Clark RN, Zuelzer WA, Freddy MR, Simon S. Avascular necrosis of the femoral head: early MRI detection and radiological correlation. *Magn Reson Imaging* 1987;5:431–442.
6. Beltran J, Caudill JL, Herman LA. Rheumatoid arthritis: MR imaging manifestations. *Radiology* 1987;165:153–157.
7. Beltran J, Herman LJ, Burk JM, et al. Femoral head avascular necrosis: MR imaging and clinical–pathologic and radionuclide correlation. *Radiology* 1988;166:215–220.
8. Berquist TH. MRI of musculoskeletal neoplasms. *Clin Orthop* 1989;244:101–118.
9. Berquist TH, Ehman RL, Richardson ML. *Magnetic resonance of the musculoskeletal system.* New York: Raven Press, 1987.
10. Berquist TH, Coventry MB. The pelvis and hips. In: Berquist TH, ed. *Imaging of orthopedic trauma and surgery.* Philadelphia: Saunders, 1986:181–279.
11. Bieber E, Hungerford D, Leunox DW. Factors in the diagnosis of avascular necrosis of the femoral head. *Adv Orthop Surg* 1985;147:221–226.
12. Bloem JL. Transient osteoporosis of the hip: MR imaging. *Radiology* 1988;167:753–755.
13. Bongartz G, Bock E, Horback T, Requard H. Degenerative cartilage lesions in the hip—magnetic resonance evaluation. *Magn Reson Imaging* 1989;7:179–186.
14. Brody AS, Strong M, Babikian S, Seidel FG, Kuhn JP. Early avascular necrosis: MRI and histological examination in an animal model. Presented at the Society for Pediatric Radiology, New Orleans, 1989.
15. Camp JF, Colwell CW. Core decompression of the femoral head for osteonecrosis. *J Bone Joint Surg* 1986;68A:1313–1319.
16. Carter BL, Morehead J, Walpert SM, Hammerschlag SB, Griffiths HJ, Kahn PC. *Cross-sectional anatomy: computed tomography and ultrasound correlation.* New York: Appleton-Century-Crofts, 1977.
17. Cohen JM, Hodges SC, Weinreb JC, Muschler G. MR imaging of iliopsoas bursitis and concurrent avascular necrosis of the femoral head. *J Comput Assist Tomogr* 1985;9:969–971.
18. Daffner RH, Lupetin AR, Dash N, Deeb ZL, Sefczek RJ, Schapiro RL. MRI in the detection of malignant infiltration of bone marrow. *AJR* 1986;146:353–358.

19. Dahlin DC, Unni KK. *Bone tumors: general aspects and data on 8,542 cases,* 4th ed. Springfield, IL: CC Thomas, 1986.
20. Deutsch AL, Mink JH, Waxman AD. Occult fractures of the proximal femur: MR imaging. *Radiology* 1989;170:113–116.
21. Deutsch AL, Mink JH. Musculoskeletal trauma. *Top Magn Reson Imaging* 1989;1(4):53–66.
22. Dooms GC, Fisher MR, Hricak H, Higgins CB. MR imaging of intramuscular hemorrhage. *J Comput Assist Tomogr* 1985;9:908–913.
23. Ehman RL, Berquist TH, McLeod RA. MR imaging of the musculoskeletal system: a 5-year appraisal. *Radiology* 1988;166:313–320.
24. Enzinger FM, Weiss SW. *Soft tissue tumors.* St. Louis, MO: Mosby, 1983.
25. Ficat RF. Treatment of avascular necrosis of the femoral head. *Hip* 1983;2:279–295.
26. Ficat RF, Arlet J. Bone necrosis of known etiology. In: Hungerford P, ed. *Ischemia and necrosis of bone.* Baltimore: Williams & Wilkins, 1980.
27. Fleckenstein JL, Canby RC, Parkey RW, Peschock RM. Acute effects of exercise on MR imaging of skeletal muscles in normal volunteers. *AJR* 1988;151:231–237.
28. Fleckenstein JL, Weatherall PT, Parkey RW, Payne JA, Peshock RM. Sports-related muscle injuries: evaluation with MR imaging. *Radiology* 1989;172:793–798.
29. Fletcher BD, Scoles PV, Nelson AD. Osteomyelitis in children: detection by magnetic resonance. *Radiology* 1984;150:57–60.
30. Genez BM, Wilson MR, Houk RW, Weiland FL, Unger HR, Shields NN, Rugh KS. Early osteonecrosis of the femoral head: detection in high-risk patients with MR imaging. *Radiology* 1988;168:521–524.
31. Gillespy T, Genant H, Helms CA. Magnetic resonance imaging of osteonecrosis. *Radiol Clin North Am* 1986;24:193–208.
32. Glickstein MF, Burk DL Jr, Schiebler ML, Cohen EK, Dalinka MK, Steinberg ME, Kressel HY. Avascular necrosis versus other diseases of the hip: sensitivity of MR imaging. *Radiology* 1988;169:213–215.
33. Greiff J, Lang S, Hoilund-Carlsen PF, Karle AK, Uhrenholt A. Early detection of ^{99}Tc-SN-pyrophosphate scintigraphy of femoral head necrosis following femoral neck fractures. *Acta Orthop Scand* 1980;51:119–125.
34. Hauzeur JP, Pasteels JL, Schoutens A, Hinsenkamp M, Appelboom T, Chochrad I, Perlmutter N. The diagnostic value of magnetic resonance imaging in non-traumatic osteonecrosis of the femoral head. *J Bone Joint Surg* 1989;71A:641–648.
35. Heiken JP, Lee JKT. MR imaging of the pelvis. *Radiology* 1988;166:11–16.
36. Herfkens BJ, Sievers R, Kaufman L. Nuclear magnetic resonance imaging of infarcted muscle: a rat model. *Radiology* 1983;147: 761–764.
37. Hollinshead WH. *Anatomy for surgeons,* Vol 3, 3rd ed. New York: Harper & Row, 1982:563–583.
38. Hopson CN, Siverhus SW. Ischemic necrosis of the femoral head: treatment by core decompression. *J Bone Joint Surg* 1988;70: 1048–1051.
39. Johnson ND, Wood BP, Noh KS, Jackman KV, Westesson P, Katzberg RW. MR imaging anatomy of the infant hip. *AJR* 1989;153:127–133.
40. Kaplan PA, Asleson RJ, Klassen LW, Duggan MJ. Bone marrow patterns in aplastic anemia: observations with 1.5-T MR imaging. *Radiology* 1987;164:441–444.
41. Keller MS, Weltin GG, Rattner Z, Taylor KJW, Rosenfield NS. Normal instability of the hip in the neonate: US standards. *Radiology* 1988;169:733–736.
42. Kent JA, Bolinger L, Strear CM, Elliott M, Leigh JS, Chance B. Proton image T1 measurements in human calf muscle during exercise. Presented at the Society of Magnetic Resonance in Medicine, Amsterdam, The Netherlands, 1989.
43. Lang P, Jergesen HE, Moseley ME, Block JE, Chafetz NI, Genant HK. Avascular necrosis of the femoral head: high-field-strength MR imaging with histologic correlation. *Radiology* 1988;169: 517–524.
44. Lehner KB, Rechl HP. Normal morphology and degeneration of hyaline articular cartilage in MR imaging: an *in vitro* study in bovine patellae and human arthritic femoral heads. Presented at the Society of Magnetic Resonance in Medicine, Amsterdam, The Netherlands, 1989.
45. Li KC, Higgs J, Aisen AM, Buckwalter KA, Martel W, McCune WJ. MRI in osteoarthritis of the hip: gradiation of severity. *Magn Reson Imaging* 1988;6:229–236.
46. Mason MD, Zlatkin MB, Esterhai JL, Dalinka MK, Velchik MG, Kressel HY. Chronic complicated osteomyelitis of the lower extremity: evaluation with MR imaging. *Radiology* 1989;173:355–359.
47. Matin P, Lange G, Caretta R, Simon G. Scintigraphic evaluation of muscle damage following extreme exercise. Concise communication. *J Nucl Med* 1983;24:308–311.
48. McKeag DB. The concept of overuse: the primary care aspects of overuse syndromes in sports. *Primary Care* 1984;11:43–59.
49. McMaster PE. Tendon and muscle ruptures. *J Bone Joint Surg* 1933;15A:705–722.
50. Middleton WD, Lawson TL. *Anatomy and MRI of the joints: a multiplanar atlas.* New York: Raven Press, 1989.
51. Mitchell DG. Using MR imaging to probe the pathophysiology of osteonecrosis. *Radiology* 1989;171:25–26.
52. Mitchell DG, Rao VM, Dalinka MK, et al. Femoral head avascular necrosis: correlation of MR imaging, radiographic staging, radionuclide imaging, and clinical findings. *Radiology* 1987;162:709–715.
53. Mitchell DG, Rao VM, Dalinka M, et al. Hematopoietic and fatty bone marrow distribution in the normal and ischemic hip: new observations with 1.5-T MR imaging. *Radiology* 1986;161:199–202.
54. Mitchell DG, Rao V, Dalinka M, et al. MRI of joint fluid in the normal and ischemic hip. *AJR* 1986;146:1215–1218.
55. Mitchell MD, Kunkel HL, Steinberg ME, Kressel HY, Alavi A, Axel L. Avascular necrosis of the hip: comparison of MR, CT, and scintigraphy. *AJR* 1986;147:67–71.
56. Munk PL, Helms CA, Holt RG. Immature bone infarcts: findings of plain radiographs and MR scans. *AJR* 1989;152:547–549.
57. Nokes SR, Vogler JB, Spritzer CE, Martinez S, Herfken RJ. Herniation pits of the femoral neck: appearance at MR imaging. *Radiology* 1989;172:231–234.
58. Oakes BW. Hamstring muscle injuries. *Aust Fam Physician* 1984;13:587–591.
59. O'Donoghue DH. *Treatment of injuries to athletes,* 4th ed. Philadelphia: Saunders, 1984.
60. Petty W. Osteonecrosis. *J Bone Joint Surg* 1986;68A:1311–1312.
61. Pitt MJ, Graham AR, Shipman JH, Birkby W. Herniation pits of the femoral neck. *AJR* 1982;138:1115–1121.
62. Raether PM, Lather LD. Recurrent compartment syndrome in the posterior thigh. A report of a case. *Am J Sports Med* 1982;10:40–43.
63. Renström D. Swedish research on traumatology. *Clin Orthop* 1984;191:144–158.
64. Rush BH, Bramson RT, Ogden JA. Legg–Calvé–Perthes disease: detection of cartilaginous and synovial changes with MR imaging. *Radiology* 1988;167:473–476.
65. Sanchez RB, Quinn SF. MRI of inflammatory synovial processes. *Magn Reson Imaging* 1989;7:529–540.
66. Shuman WP, Castagno AA, Baron RL, Richardson ML. MR imaging of avascular necrosis of the femoral head: value of small-field-of-view sagittal surface-coil images. *AJR* 1988;150:1073–1078.
67. Siegel AJ, Silverman LM, Holman BL. Elevated creatinine kinase MG isoenzyme levels in marathon runners. *JAMA* 1981;246: 2049–2051.
68. Simmons DJ, Daum WJ, Totty W, Murphy WA. Correlation of MRI images with histology in avascular necrosis in the hip. A preliminary study. *J Arthroplasty* 1989;4:7–14.
69. Smith DK, Totty WG. Magnetic resonance imaging of articular disorders of the hip. *Top Magn Reson Imaging* 1989;1(3):29–41.
70. Smith SR, Williams CE, Davies JM, Edwards RHT. Bone marrow disorders: characterization with quantitative MR imaging. *Radiology* 1989;172:805–810.
71. Springfield DS, Enneling WJ. Surgery for asceptic necrosis of the femoral head. *Clin Orthop* 1978;130:175–178.
72. Sundarum M, McDonald DJ. The solitary tumor or tumor-like lesion of bone. *Top Magn Reson Imaging* 1989;1(4):17–29.

73. Sweet DE, Madewell JE. Pathogenesis of osteonecrosis. In: Resnick D, Niwayama G, eds. *Diagnosis of bone and joint disorders.* Philadelphia: Saunders, 1988.
74. Thickman D, Axel L, Kressel HY, et al. Magnetic resonance imaging of avascular necrosis of the femoral head. *Skeletal Radiol* 1986;15:133–140.
75. Toby EB, Koman LA, Bechtold RE. Magnetic resonance imaging of pediatric hip disease. *J Pediatr Orthop* 1985;5:665–671.
76. Totty WG, Murphy WA, Ganz WI, Kamar B, Davin WJ, Siegel BA. Magnetic resonance imaging of the normal and ischemic femoral head. *AJR* 1984;143:1273–1280.
77. Turner DA, Templeton AC, Selzer PM, Rosenberg AG, Petasnick JP. Femoral capital osteonecrosis: MR finding of diffuse marrow abnormalities without focal lesions. *Radiology* 1989;171:135–140.
78. Unger E, Maldofsky P, Gatenby R, Hartz W, Broter G. Diagnosis of osteomyelitis MR imaging. *AJR* 1988;150:605–610.
79. Vesely TM. Exercise-induced rhabdomyolysis. Case of the week for Department of Diagnostic Radiology, Mayo Clinic, 1988.
80. Vogler JB, Murphy WA. Bone marrow imaging. *Radiology* 1988;168:679–693.
81. Vogler JB, Helms CA, Callen PW. *Normal variants and pitfalls in imaging.* Philadelphia: Saunders, 1986.
82. Wang GJ, Dughman SS, Reger SI, Stamp WG. The effect of core decompression on femoral head blood flow in steroid-induced avascular necrosis of the femoral head. *J Bone Joint Surg* 1985;67A:121–124.
83. Weinreb JC, Cohen JM, Maravilla KR. Iliopsoas muscles: MR study of normal anatomy and disease. *Radiology* 1985;156:435–440.
84. Wilson AJ. Nonarticular soft tissues. *Top Magn Reson Imaging* 1989;1(4):1–16.
85. Wilson AJ, Murphy WA, Hardy DC, Totty WG. Transient osteoporosis: transient bone marrow edema? *Radiology* 1988;167:757–760.
86. Yulish BS, Lieberman JM, Newman AJ, Bryan PJ, Mulopulos GP, Modic MT. Juvenile rheumatoid arthritis: assessment with MR imaging. *Radiology* 1987;165:149–152.
87. Zagoria RJ, Karstaedt N, Koubek TD. MR imaging of rhabdomyosis. *J Comput Assist Tomogr* 1986;10:268–270.
88. Zimmer WD, Berquist TH, McLeod RA. Bone tumors: magnetic resonance versus computed tomography. *Radiology* 1985;155: 709–718.

MRI of the Musculoskeletal System, 2nd Edition, edited by T. H. Berquist.
Raven Press, Ltd., New York © 1990.

CHAPTER 7

The Knee

Thomas H. Berquist and Richard L. Ehman

Techniques, 195
Anatomy, 198
Bone and Articular Anatomy, 198
Muscles About the Knee, 212
Neurovascular Supply of the Knee, 214
Pitfalls, 214
Applications, 219
Meniscal Tears, 219
Meniscal Cysts, 224
Discoid Menisci, 226
Ligament Injuries, 227
Plicae, 233
Patellar Disorders, 236
Loose Bodies, 238
Fractures, 238
Osteochondritis Dissecans, 240
Osteonecrosis and Osteochondrosis, 242
Musculoskeletal Neoplasms and Soft Tissue Masses, 244
Arthritis and Synovial Diseases, 247
References, 248

Although the value of MRI for evaluating musculoskeletal conditions such as tumors and osteonecrosis processes was apparent almost immediately after the introduction of this modality in the early 1980s, early studies of knee imaging with MRI were inconclusive (10,11,57). Knee imaging is a technically demanding application of MRI, and the capabilities of the early low-field systems were simply insufficient to adequately and reliably depict knee anatomy.

With the introduction of special closely coupled extremity RF coils, high-field systems, and other technical advances, this situation has changed dramatically (8,16,28). These new-found capabilities have made knee imaging one of the fastest growing applications of MRI. MRI has now largely replaced arthrography in the evaluation of knee pathology (57,66,68).

TECHNIQUES

The techniques used for evaluating the knee should be tailored to the clinical indication and the imaging system that is employed. Although many techniques and image planes may be used, the discussion here is oriented toward the routine screening examination that is commonly used to evaluate most articular and periarticular disorders of the knee. More specific techniques are discussed later in the applications section as they apply to a given clinical setting.

Typically, the patient is placed in the supine position, with the knee placed in a closely coupled extremity coil (Fig. 7-1). The knee is externally rotated 15°–20° in order to facilitate visualization of the anterior cruciate ligament on sagittal images (10,54,55,66).

In choosing pulse sequences, the physician now has many options, ranging from spin-echo sequences to various gradient-echo sequences (Table 7-1). The contrast requirements in knee imaging are mixed. Meniscal tears are best imaged with MR sequences that are neither purely T1 or T2 weighted. Other structures such as ligaments are best evaluated with T2 weighted images.

A technical requirement that should not be underestimated is the need to use an adequate image geometry. The menisci and the cruciate ligaments are complex structures, and it is unreasonable to expect to be able to reliably evaluate them using a single slice orientation.

The pulse sequences that are now widely available for knee imaging are spin-echo techniques and gradient-echo techniques, both slice selective and three-dimensional FT versions.

T. H. Berquist and R. L. Ehman: Mayo Medical School and Mayo Clinic, Rochester, Minnesota 55905.

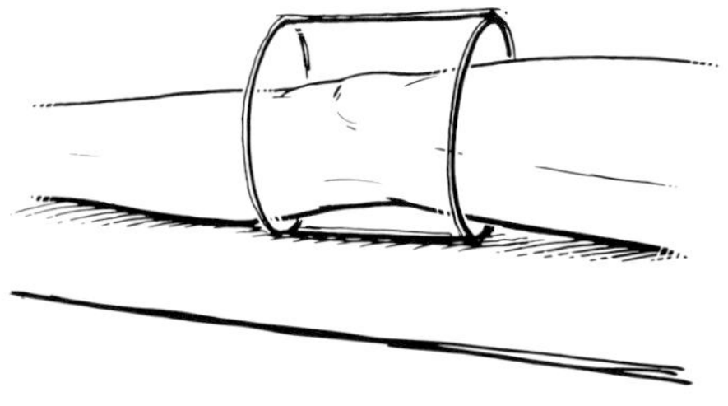

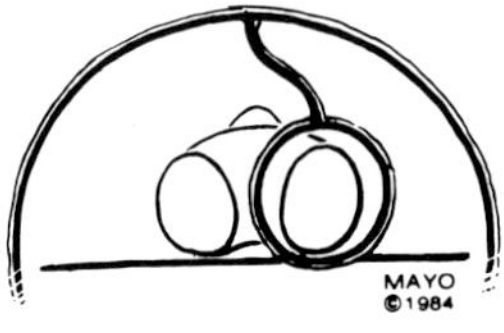

FIG. 7-1. Illustration of the knee positioned in a volume coil.

In the spin-echo category, we can consider short TR/TE sequences and long TR multiecho sequences. At this time, there seems to be little to recommend the sole use of short TR/TE spin-echo sequences for knee imaging. Although they are technically undemanding, rapidly acquired, and sensitive for medullary bone lesions, they only provide low contrast for meniscal lesions, they are not well suited for demonstrating acute ligamentous injuries or the interface between joint fluid and articular cartilage, and they require special windowing during photography.

Long TR, multiecho spin-echo sequences are very effective for knee imaging. A short, first echo provides intermediate contrast, which is excellent for identifying meniscal lesions, and a second, long echo provides T2 weighted contrast, which is critical for evaluation of the cruciate ligaments and other structures (19–22,66).

An excellent approach for knee imaging would be to perform sagittal and coronal spin-echo acquisitions (Fig. 7-2) (8,16,66). The exact technical approach will depend on the imaging hardware used. We have found the following parameters to be efficient and reliable using with a 1.5 T imager: TE 20/60 msec, TR 2,000 msec, 1 Nex, 192 views, 3 mm slices with 1.5 mm gaps, 16 cm field of view. These acquisitions require only 7.3 min each (Table 7-1).

Long TR multiecho sequences have the advantages of high slice throughput (in terms of images per unit time) and favorable contrast characteristics. They have the disadvantage of requiring longer acquisition times, and the long TE T2 weighted images are technically demanding in terms of imager performance (26).

Gradient-echo techniques have seen increasing use for musculoskeletal imaging in the last several years. They provide interesting capabilities in terms of contrast and speed. These techniques can broadly be divided into

TABLE 7-1. *Screening examination of the knee*

	Pulse sequence	Slice thickness	Field of view (cm)	Matrix	Acquisitions (Nex)	Image time
Image plane routine						
Axial scout	SE 200/20	1 cm/skip 0	16	128 × 256	1	26 sec
Coronal T1WI[a]	SE 500/20	5 mm/skip 0	16	256 × 256	1	2 min 8 sec
Coronal T2WI[b]	SE 2,000/60,20	3–5 mm/skip 1.5 mm	16	256 × 256	1	8 min 32 sec
Sagittal T1WI	SE 500/20	5 mm/skip 0	16	256 × 256	1	2 min 8 sec
Sagittal T2WI	SE 2,000/60,20	3–5 mm/skip 1.5 mm	16	256 × 256	1	8 min 32 sec
						Sagittal–coronal T1WIs 4 min 16 sec
						T1WI coronal, T2WI sagittal 10 min 40 sec
						T2WI coronal and sagittal 17 min 4 sec
Authors' technique						
Axial scout	SE 200/20	1 cm/skip 0	16	128 × 256	1	26 sec
Radial GRIL, medial and lateral meniscus (see Fig. 7-3)	SE 700/31,12 flip angle 25°	5 mm/skip 0 (10 slices with 18° separation; see Fig. 7-7)	16	192 × 256	2	5 min
Radial GRIL, sagittal	SE 2,000/60,20	3 mm/skip 1.5 mm	16	192 × 256	1	7 min 18 sec
					Total	12 min 44 sec

[a] T1WI, T1 weighted image.
[b] T2WI, T2 weighted image.

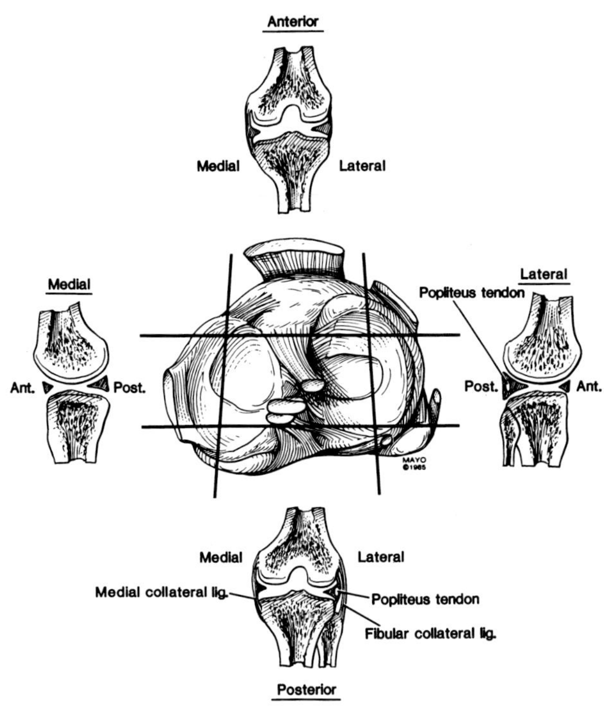

FIG. 7-2. Illustration of the axial anatomy of the knee and selected coronal and sagittal sections.

"steady-state" sequences, such as GRASS and FISP, and "spoiled" sequences, such as FLASH and Spoiled GRASS (see Chapter 2) (26,47,81,98).

Multislice gradient-echo acquisitions can be performed in two ways: (a) sequentially acquire each slice individually or (b) acquire the slices in an interleaved fashion similar to multislice spin-echo imaging. In the first alternative, the TR must be very short so that the total imaging time to acquire the entire set of slices will not be excessively long.

It turns out that for knee imaging with gradient echoes, the short TR, sequential single slice approach is less favorable than a long TR, multislice approach. In the specific application of knee imaging, the longer TR of the interleaved approach has the effect of improving the contrast and signal-to-noise characteristics of the images, compared with short TR gradient echoes (Table 7-1).

These long TR, medium TE gradient echoes provide excellent contrast for delineating meniscal tears. An advantage of this technique is that special windowing of the images is not required at photography. Long TR gradient-echo sequences can provide very pronounced T2 weighted contrast for depicting ligamentous lesions. Long TR gradient-echo images seem to have special capabilities for depicting chondral and osteochondral lesions as shown in these images, but these have not been fully explored as yet.

An interesting and valuable variation of the long TR, multislice gradient-echo technique is radial imaging. The structure of the meniscus is such that a radially oriented set of slices placed at the center of each semicircular meniscus is a geometrically advantageous imaging approach. The slices in a conventional spin-echo acquisition cannot be crossed for a good reason: there would be severe signal loss in the region of intersection. The special properties of gradient-echo sequences allow them not to have this limitation. In other words, a long TR multislice gradient-echo acquisition with this kind of geometry can have very little signal loss in the region where the slices intersect (Fig. 7-3).

It is possible to set up an acquisition of 18 or 20 images, which are radially oriented about both menisci, and perform the acquisition in 8 min or less. The technical details will vary, but typically the starting point is a transverse scout image at the joint line. The center of each tibial plateau is identified and a set of radial images are graphically prescribed. Initially, we utilized separate radial acquisitions for medial and lateral menisci. These each consisted of double-echo interleaved GRASS sequences (GRIL) (TE 12/31 msec, TR 600–700 msec, 2 Nex, flip angle 25°, 192 views, 5 mm slice thickness, 16 cm field of view, 10 sections at 18° rotational increments radiating from the central point). These acquisitions require about 5 min each.

More recently, we have used a single acquisition to obtain both sets of radial images. The acquisition is graphically prescribed from a transverse scout. A single echo interleaved GRASS sequence with a TE of 15 msec provides excellent results (TR 600 msec, 2 Nex, flip angle 15°, 192 views, 5 mm slice thickness, 16 cm field of view, two radially oriented sets of 9 sections at 20° rotational increments). This complete radial acquisition sequence for both menisci takes less than 4 min.

The radial geometry is not suitable for delineation of the cruciate ligaments. Because spin-echo images seem to provide slightly better depiction of ligamentous injuries, we follow the radial examination of the menisci with a sagittal spin-echo acquisition as described earlier. This yields a high-quality examination of the knee with a total imaging time of 12–14 min (Table 7-1).

The advantages of the radial acquisition technique are the excellent contrast characteristics, advantageous image geometry, and the short acquisition times. The only disadvantage is that the contrast characteristics and image orientation may be initially unfamiliar to radiologists who are accustomed to spin-echo methods.

An interesting MR technique for knee imaging is the three-dimensional FT acquisition (93). The great attraction of this technique is that a high-resolution volume data set can be processed retrospectively to generate any arbitrarily oriented plane of section. For instance, a radial image can be produced using suitable software (37,38,70,77,87,104).

Three-dimensional acquisitions are only practical with fast-scan sequences. A typical high-resolution ac-

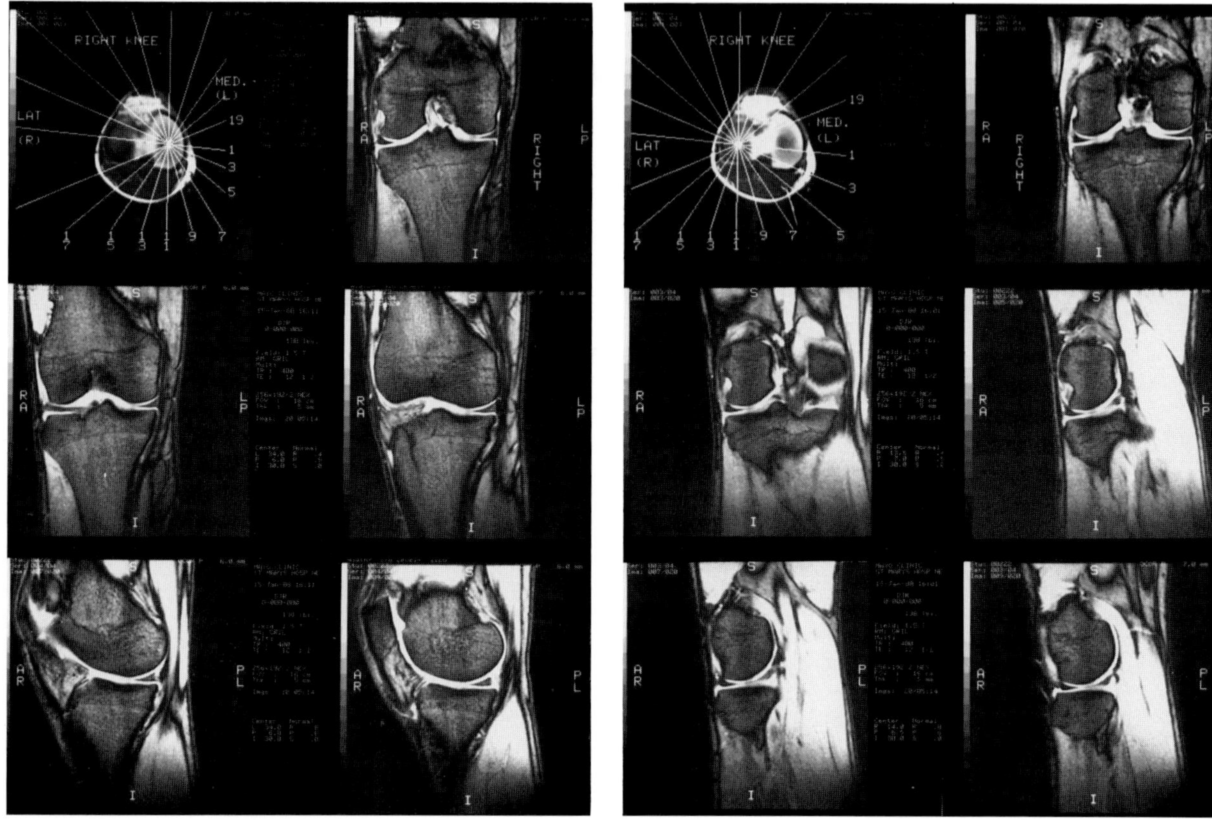

FIG. 7-3. Radial grill images of the knee set up for evaluation of the medial (**A**) and lateral (**B**) menisci.

quisition of the knee would use a GRASS sequence with a matrix of 128 × 192 × 256 and would take about 12 min to acquire. These would typically be reconstructed into a set of 128 sagittal images, each less than 1 mm in thickness.

To achieve the full potential of this technique, it is necessary to have a computerized display system, specially designed to manipulate three-dimensional data sets, preferably in real time. There are a number of open questions regarding the utility of three-dimensional acquisitions in knee MRI. The most important of these is the question of image quality.

The advantages of three-dimensional imaging are the ability to acquire thin sections without gaps and the potential for three-dimensional rendering and reformatting. The disadvantage of three-dimensional FT imaging is that the costs include a significantly larger requirement for resources such as computing power, memory, display, and storage. Other, less well established, concerns are that the examinations may take longer to interpret, given that more sections must be viewed, and that there may be a penalty in signal-to-noise and contrast, which accompanies the requirement for isotropic resolution in three-dimensional imaging. This is imposed by the short repetition time that must be used. Depending on the specific technical approach, this could result in somewhat lower image quality in comparison to two-dimensional acquisitions (37,48,81,87,94,104).

Gadolinium-DTPA has also been used to evaluate the knee. However, the need for intra-articular contrast medium for examinations of the knee has not been established (115).

In summary, there are many good approaches for imaging the knee. The technical advances of the last few years have provided numerous opportunities for manipulating the contrast, resolution, and signal to noise of knee studies. Some of these opportunities have yet to be fully explored (101,102).

ANATOMY

The multiple image planes that are used to evaluate the knee increase the need to completely understand the articular and periarticular anatomy of the knee in all image planes (Figs. 7-4 to 7-7) (62,90). In addition, a thorough knowledge of this anatomy is essential in order to select special image planes to properly demonstrate certain anatomic structures (61).

Bone and Articular Anatomy

The knee is formed by the femoral and tibial condylar articulations (2,17). The tibiofibular articulation (Fig.

Text continues on p. 209

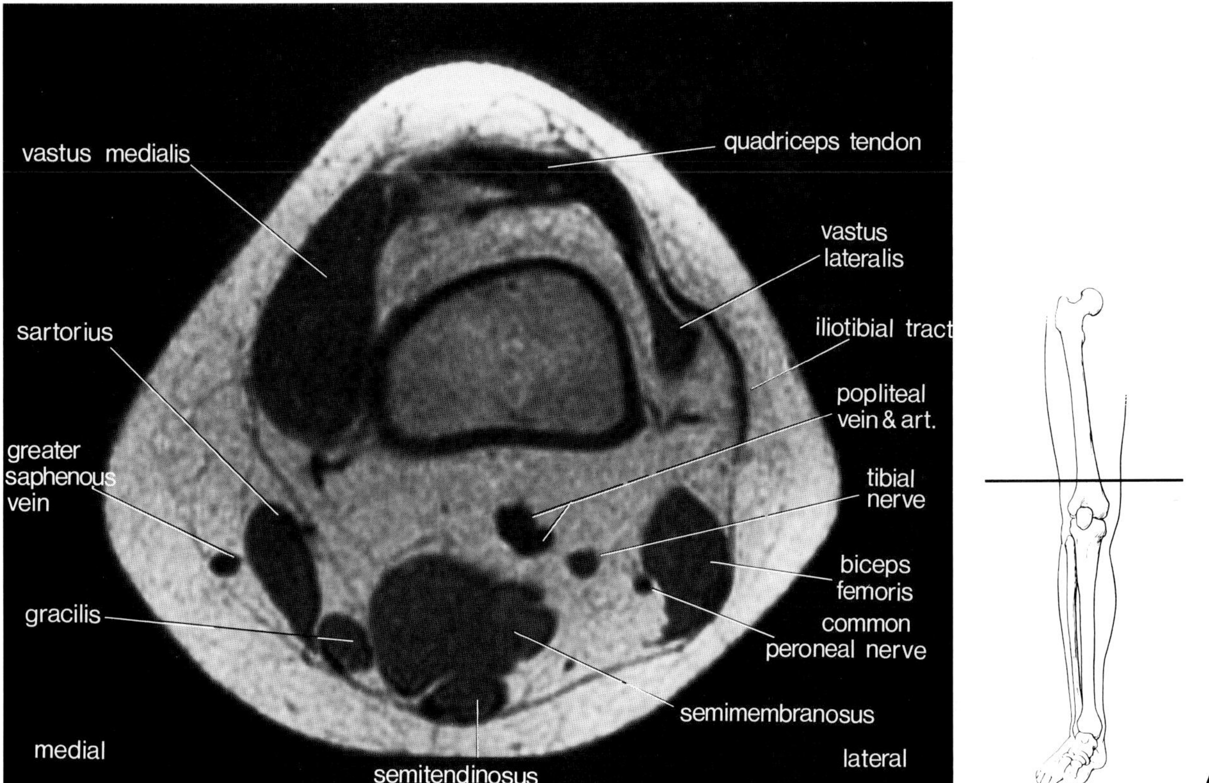

FIG. 7-4. Axial SE 500/20 MR images through the knee. **A:** Axial image through the distal femoral shaft above the patella.

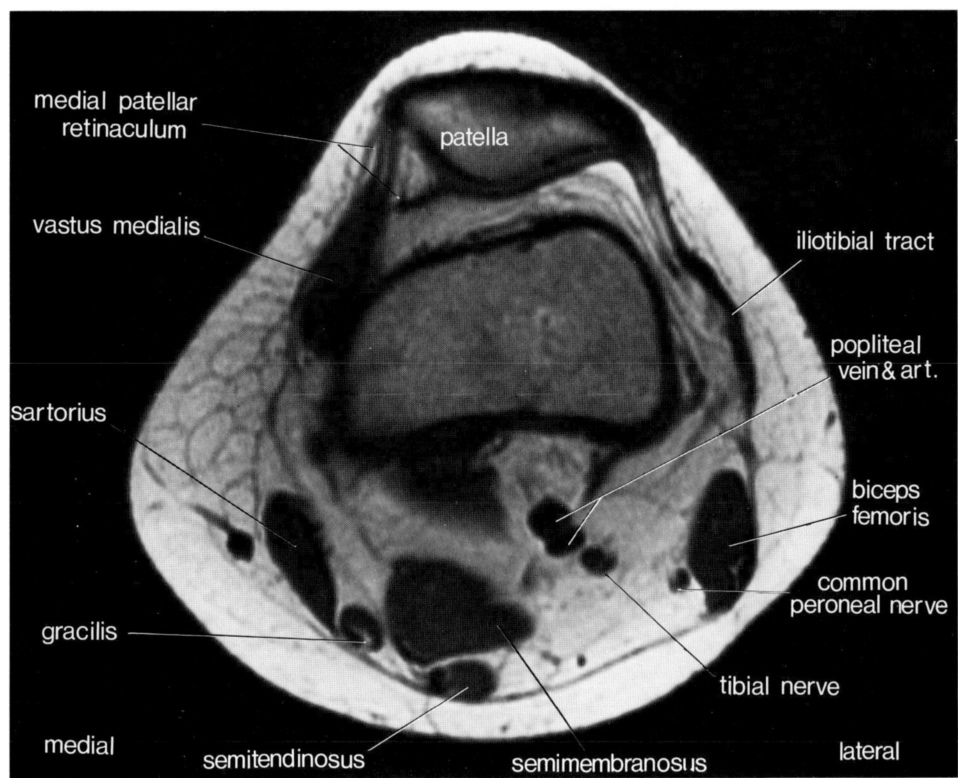

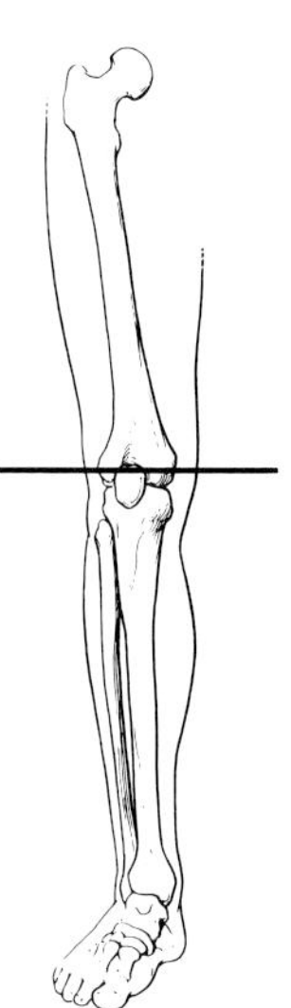

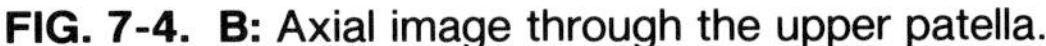

FIG. 7-4. B: Axial image through the upper patella.

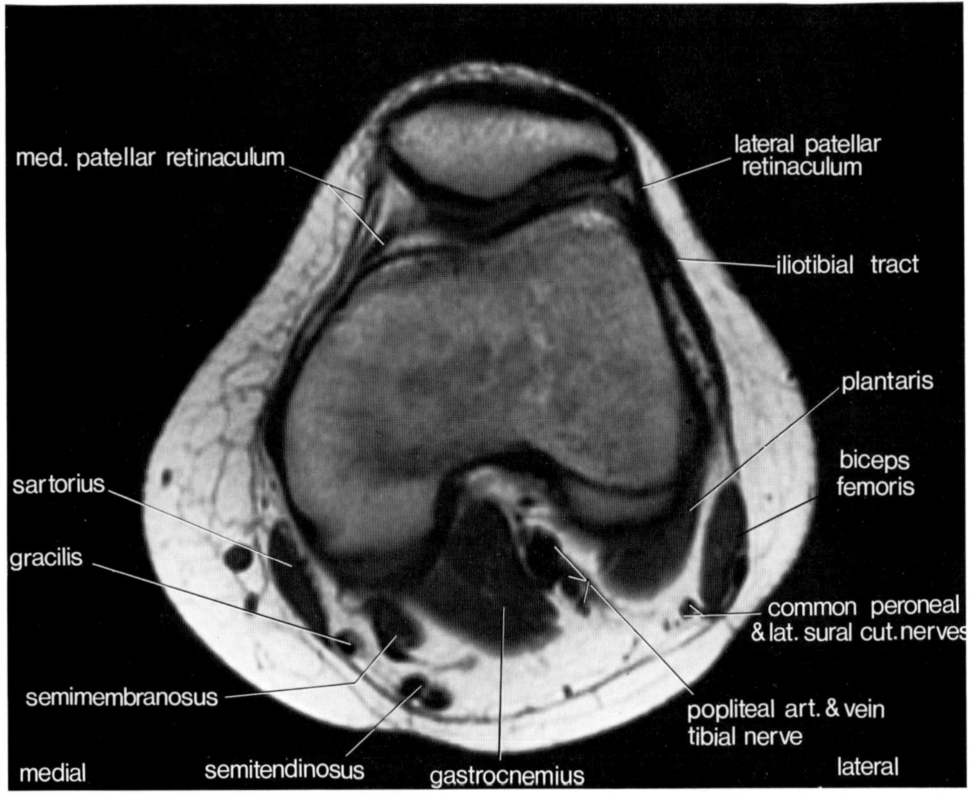

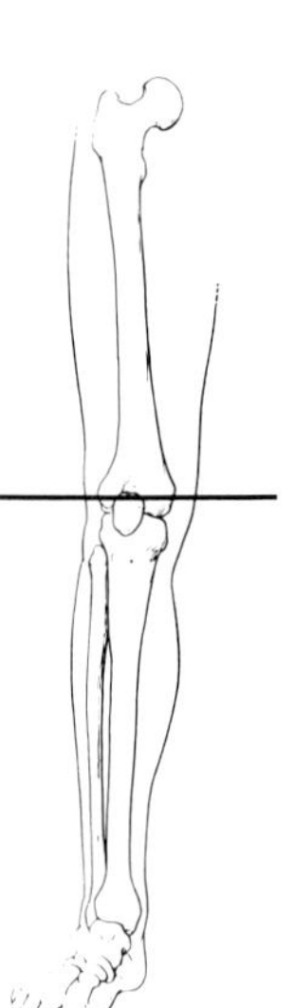

FIG. 7-4. C: Axial image through the upper femoral condyles and patella.

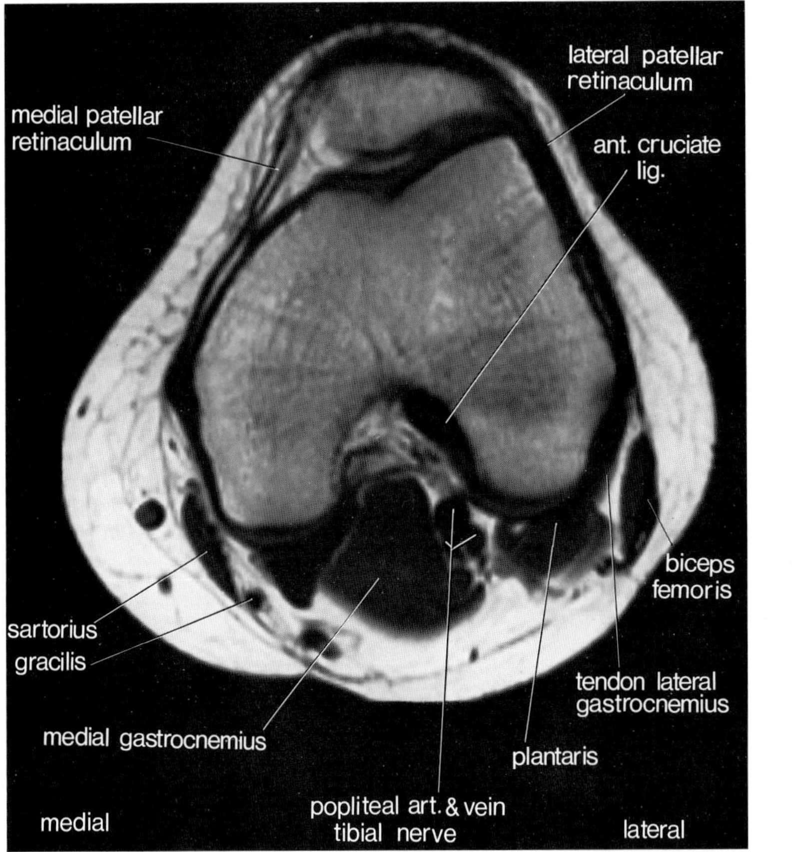

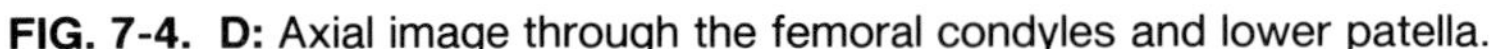

FIG. 7-4. D: Axial image through the femoral condyles and lower patella.

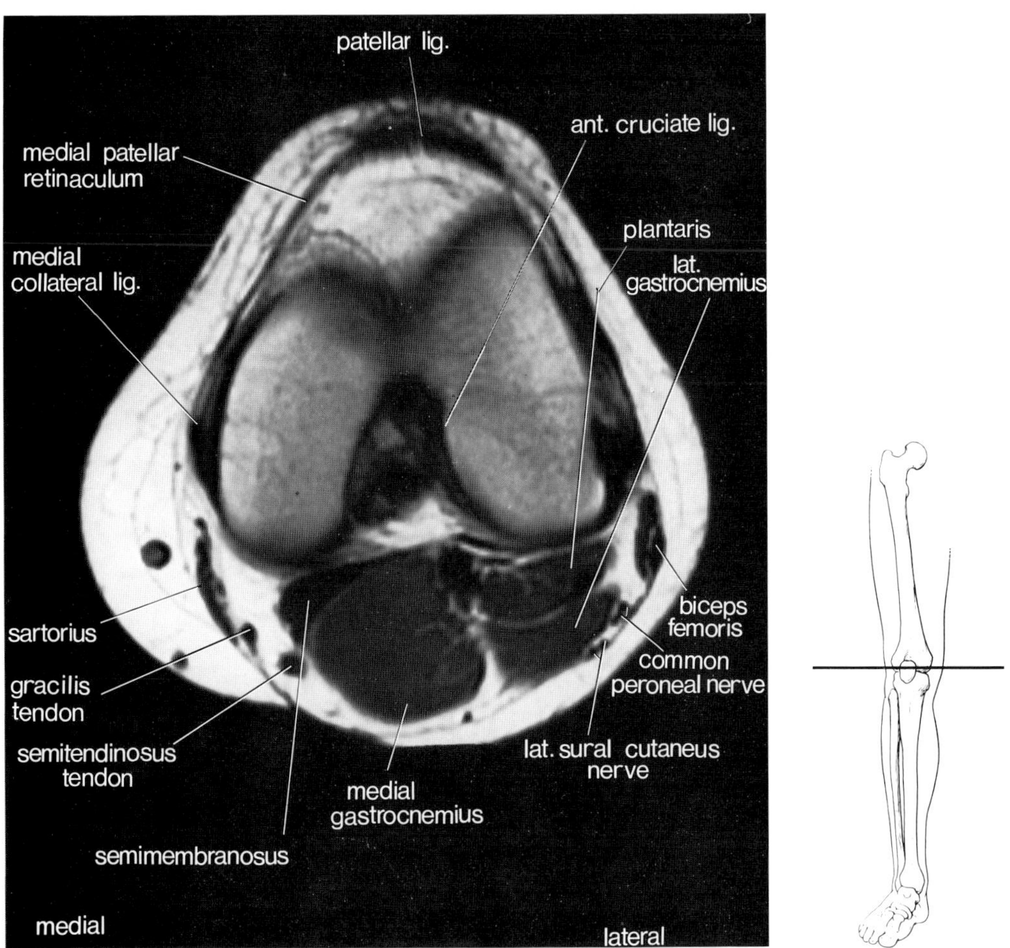

FIG. 7-4. E: Axial image through the lower femoral condyles.

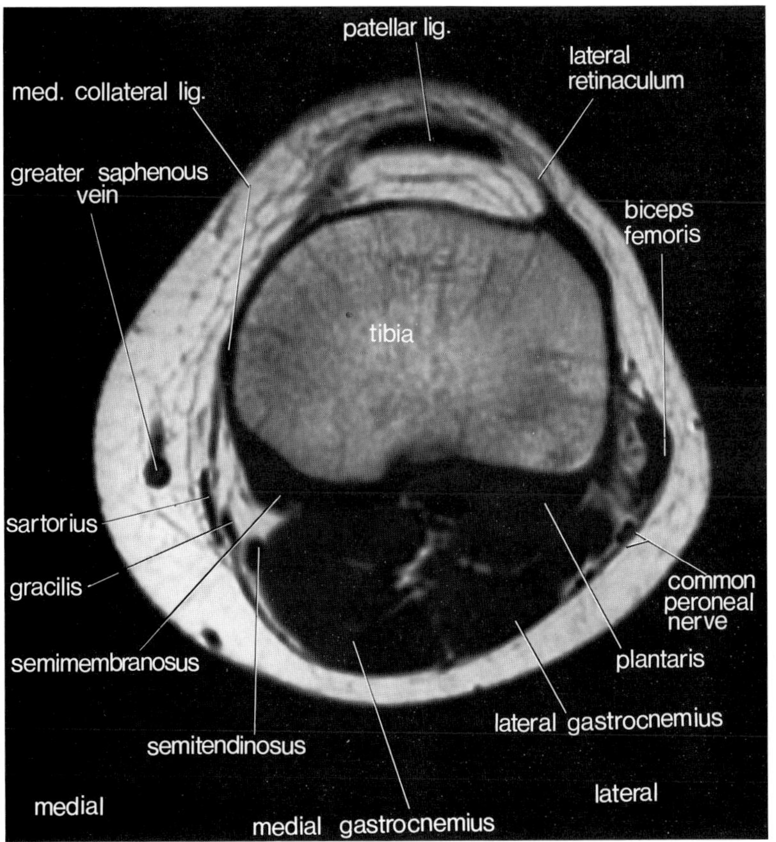

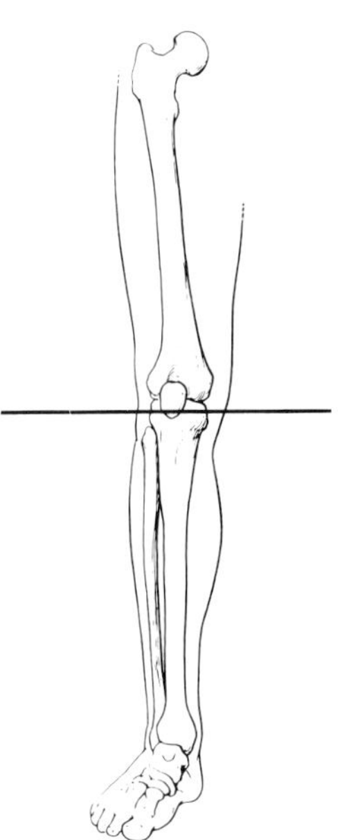

FIG. 7-4. F: Axial image through the upper tibia.

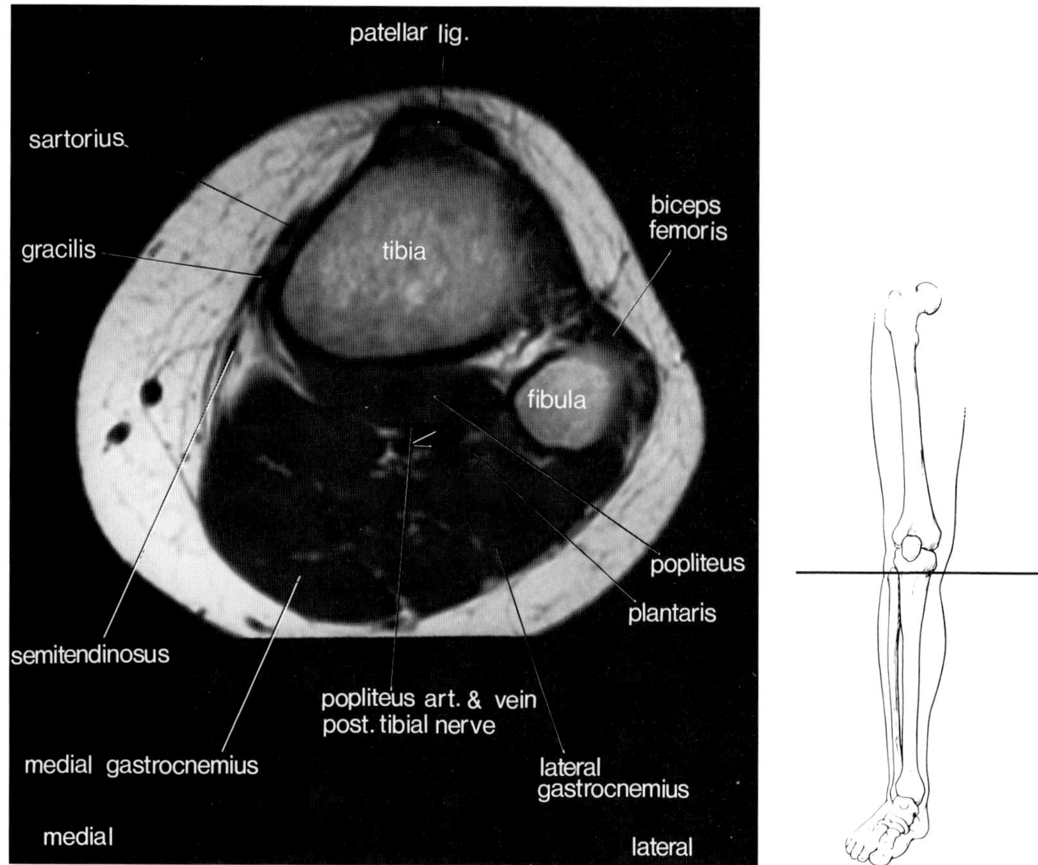

FIG. 7-4. G: Axial image through the tibia and fibular head.

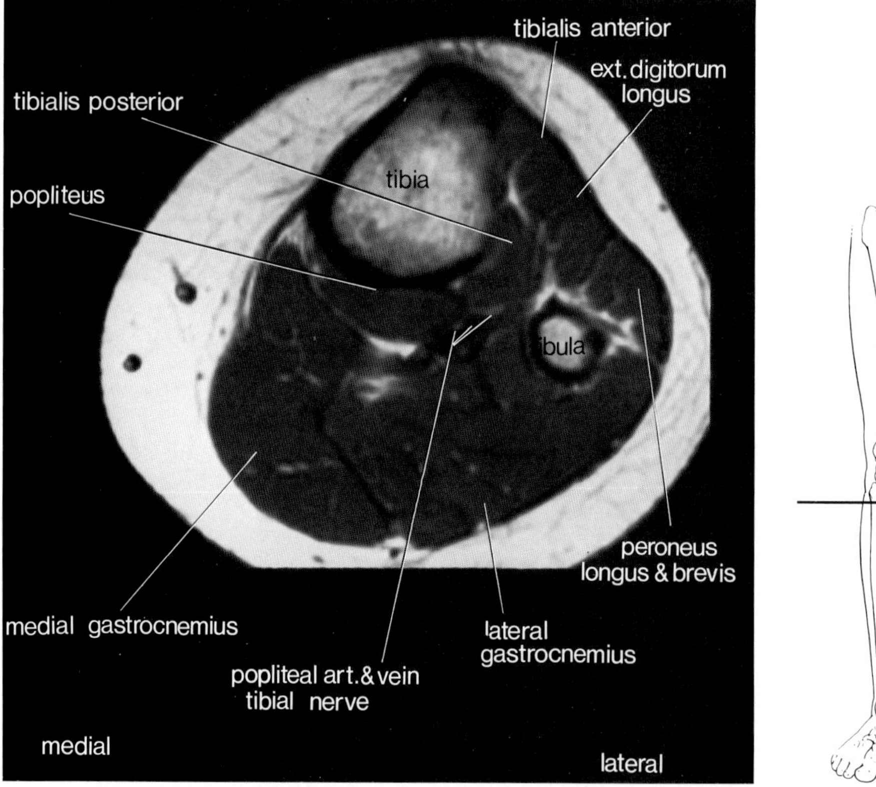

FIG. 7-4. H: Axial image through the upper tibia and fibula.

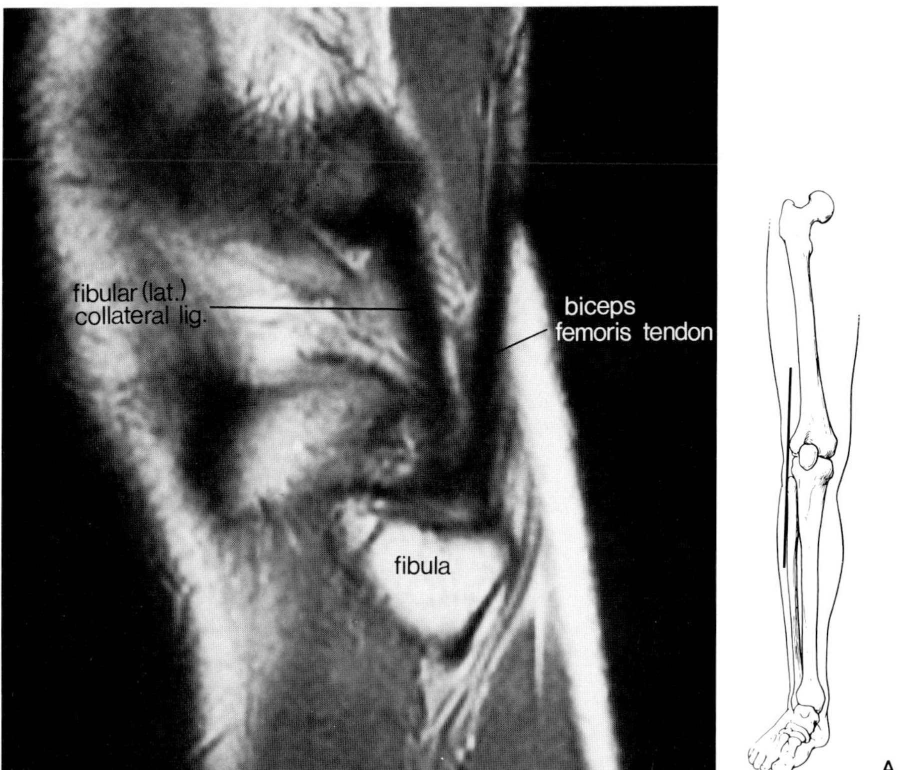

FIG. 7-5. Sagittal SE 500/20 images of the knee from lateral to medial. **A:** Sagittal image through the lateral margin of the fibular head.

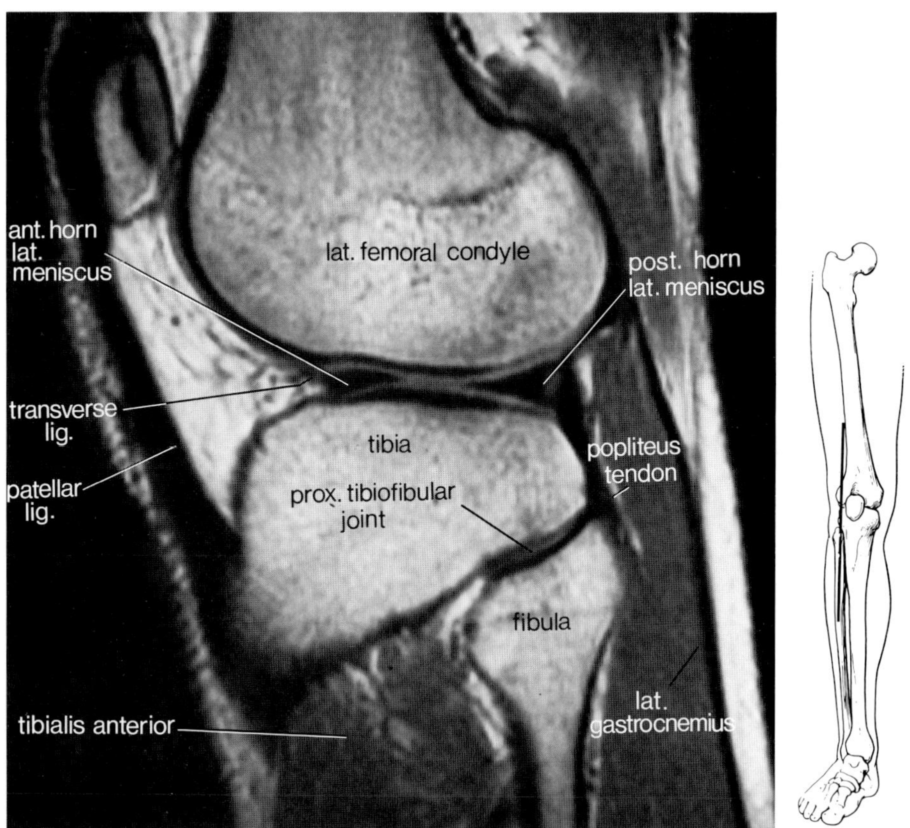

FIG. 7-5. B: Sagittal image through the tibiofibular articulation.

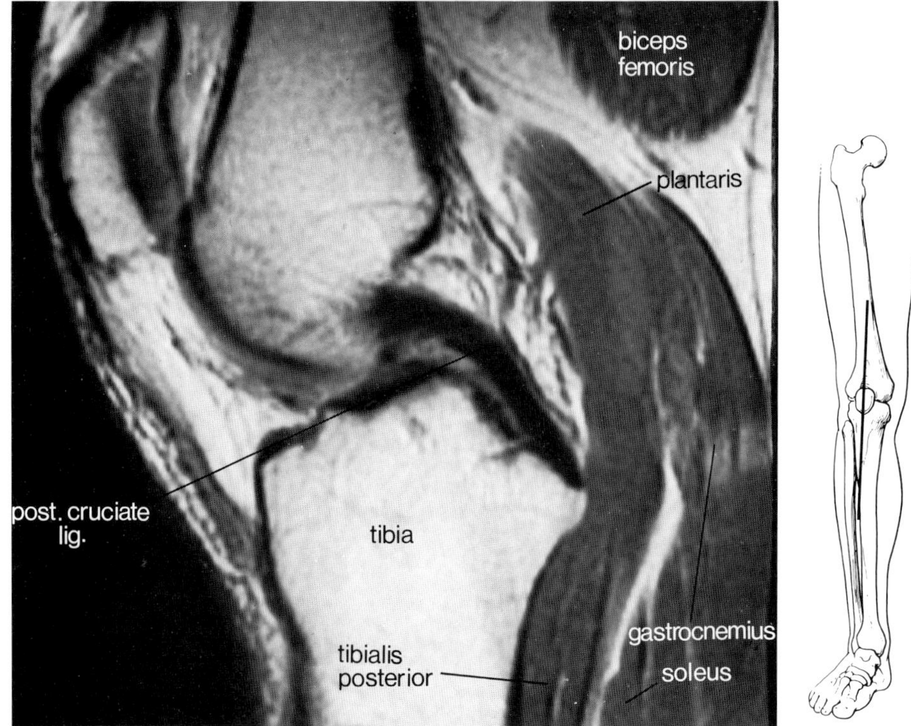

FIG. 7-5. C: Sagittal image through the posterior cruciate ligament.

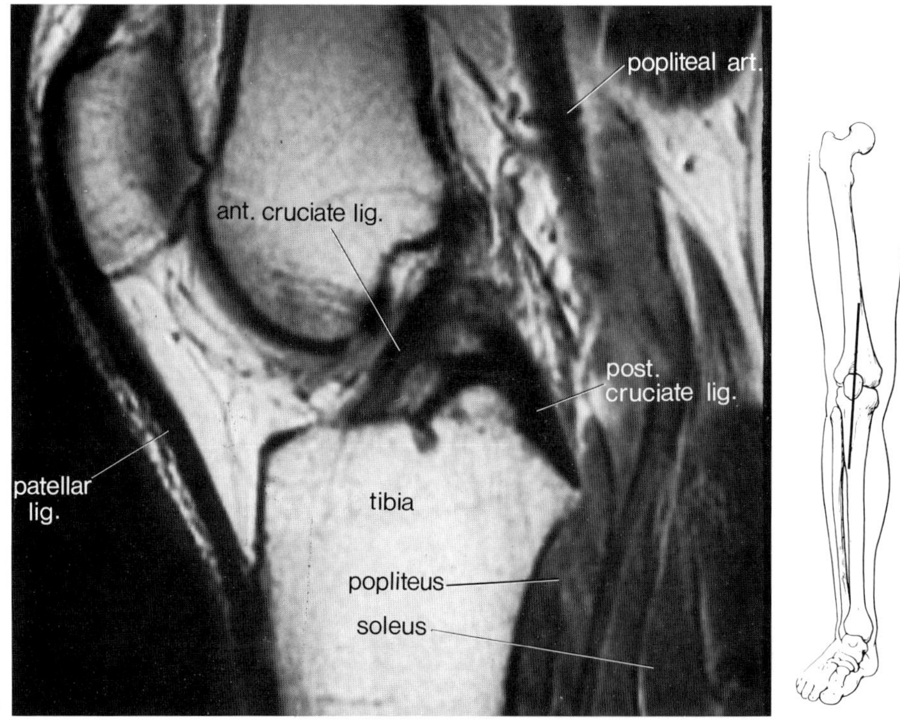

FIG. 7-5. D: Sagittal image through the anterior cruciate ligament.

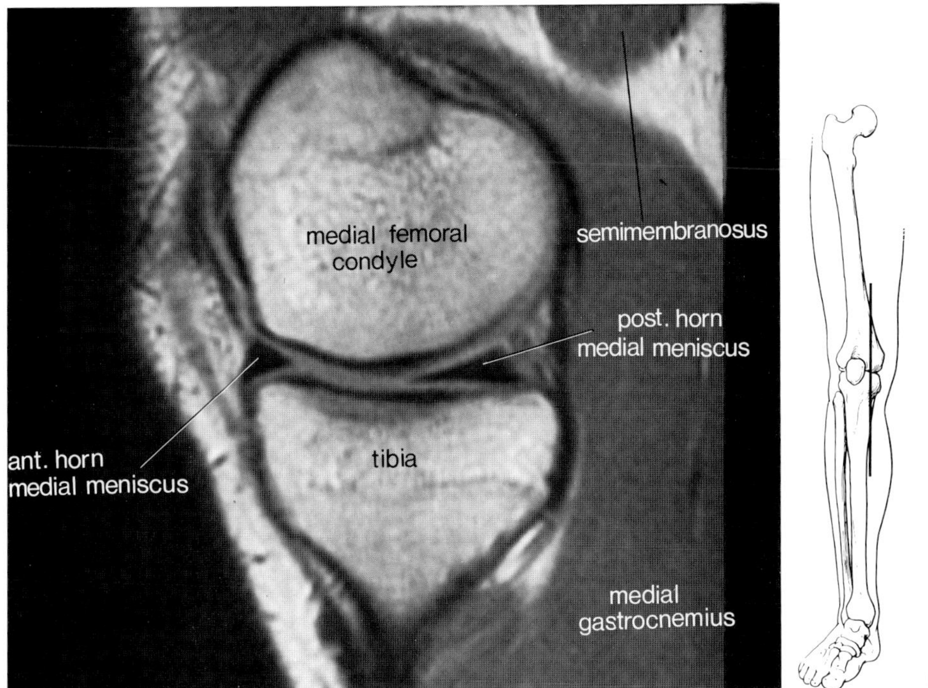

FIG. 7-5. E: Sagittal image through the medial compartment.

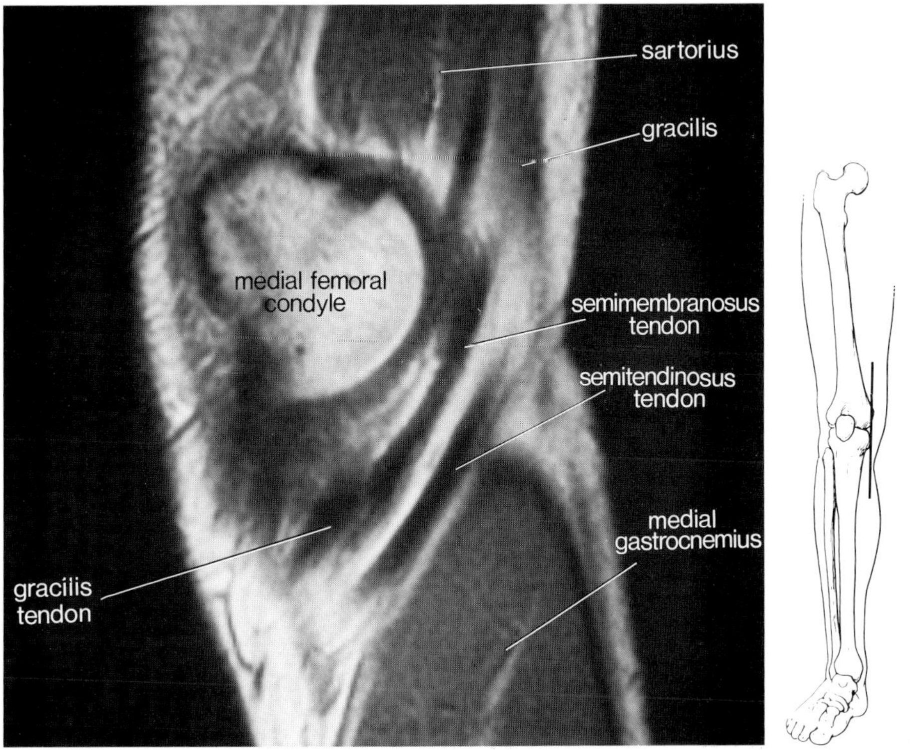

FIG. 7-5. F: Sagittal image through the medial soft tissues and margin of the femoral condyle.

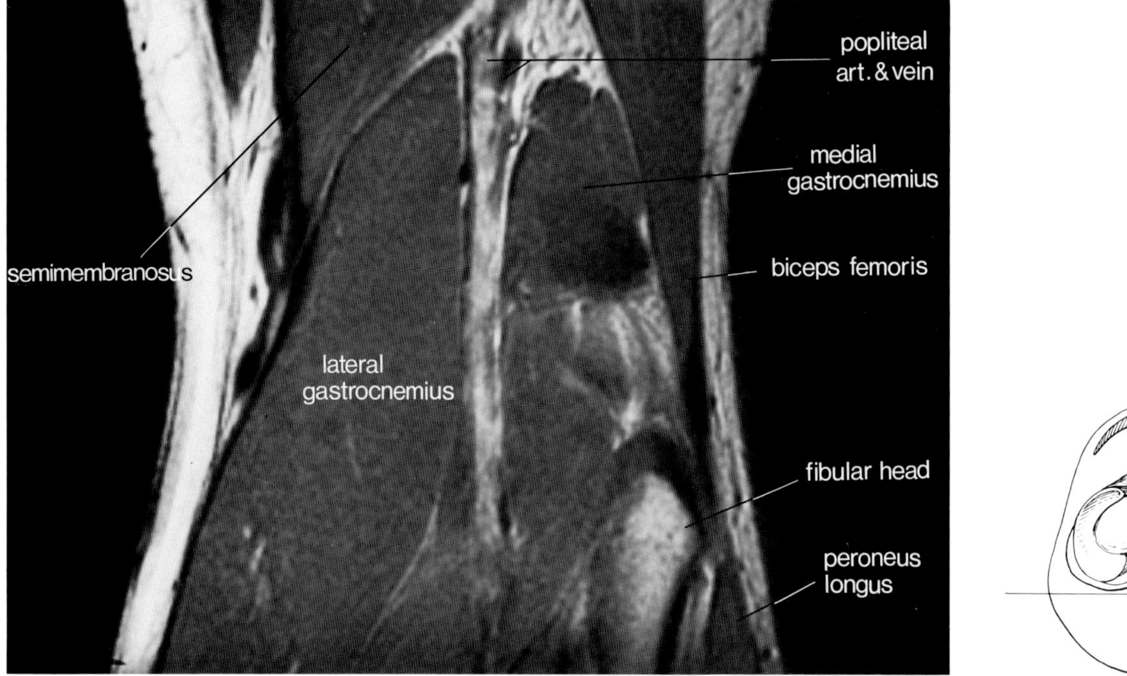

FIG. 7-6. Coronal SE 500/20 images of the knee from posterior to anterior. **A:** Coronal image through the posterior soft tissues.

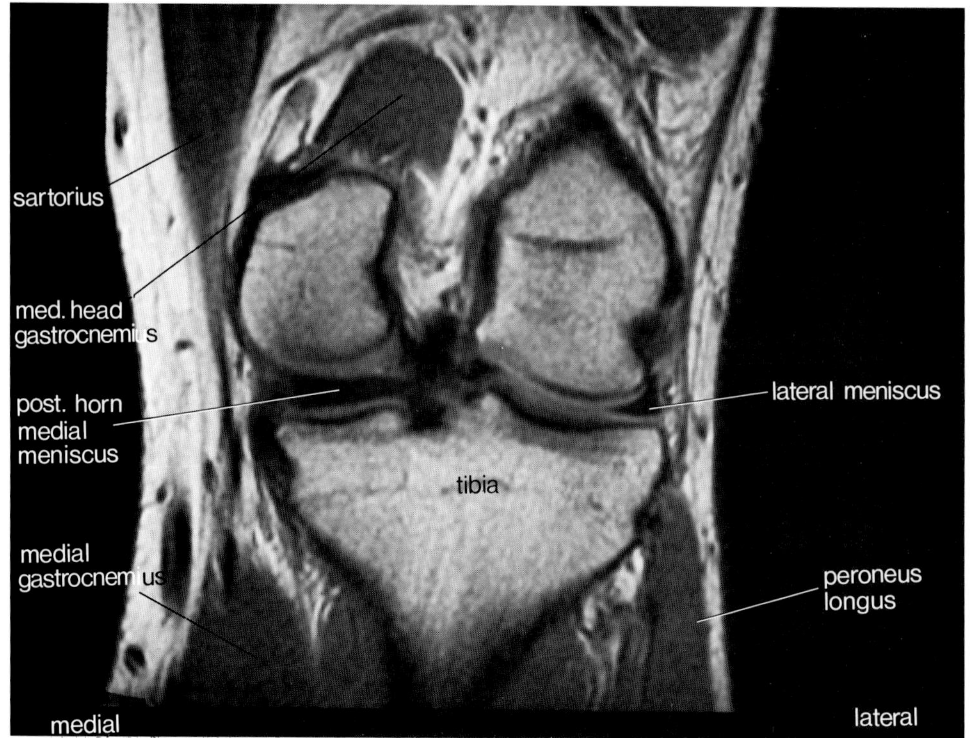

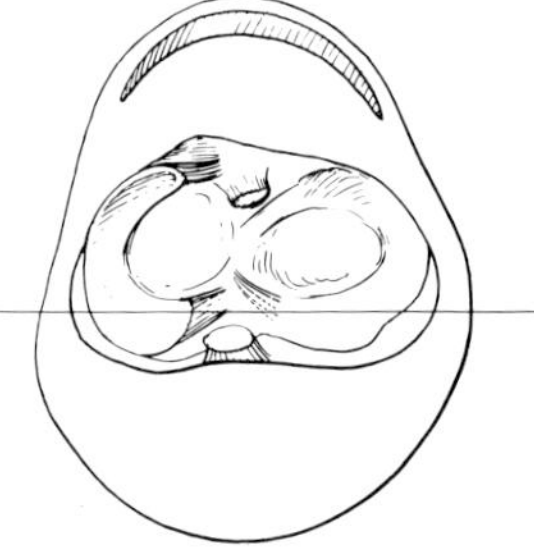

FIG. 7-6. B: Coronal image through the posterior tibia and femoral condyles.

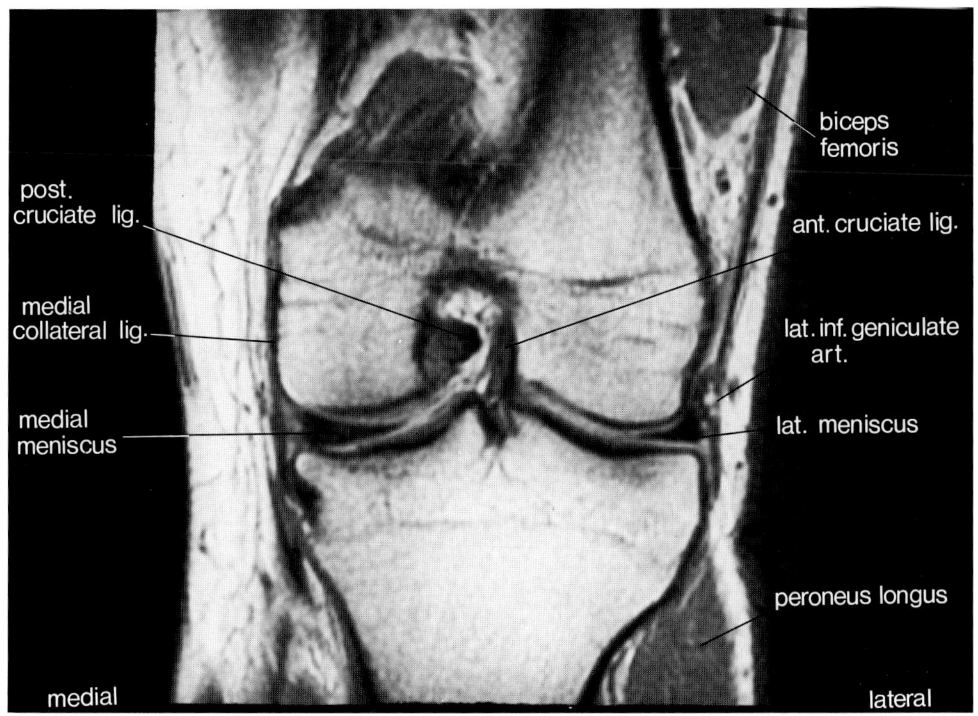

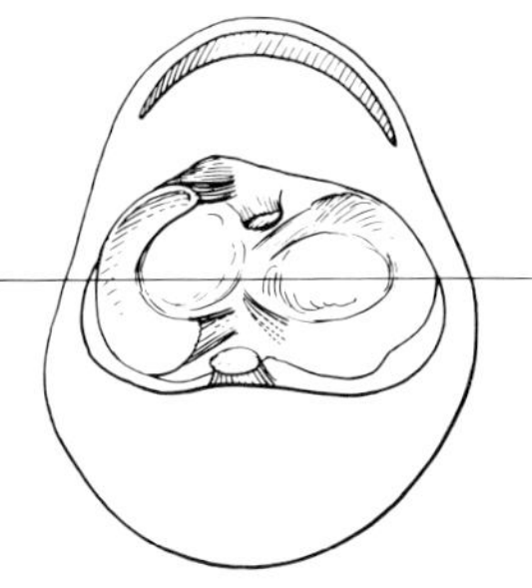

FIG. 7-6. C: Coronal image through the midjoint.

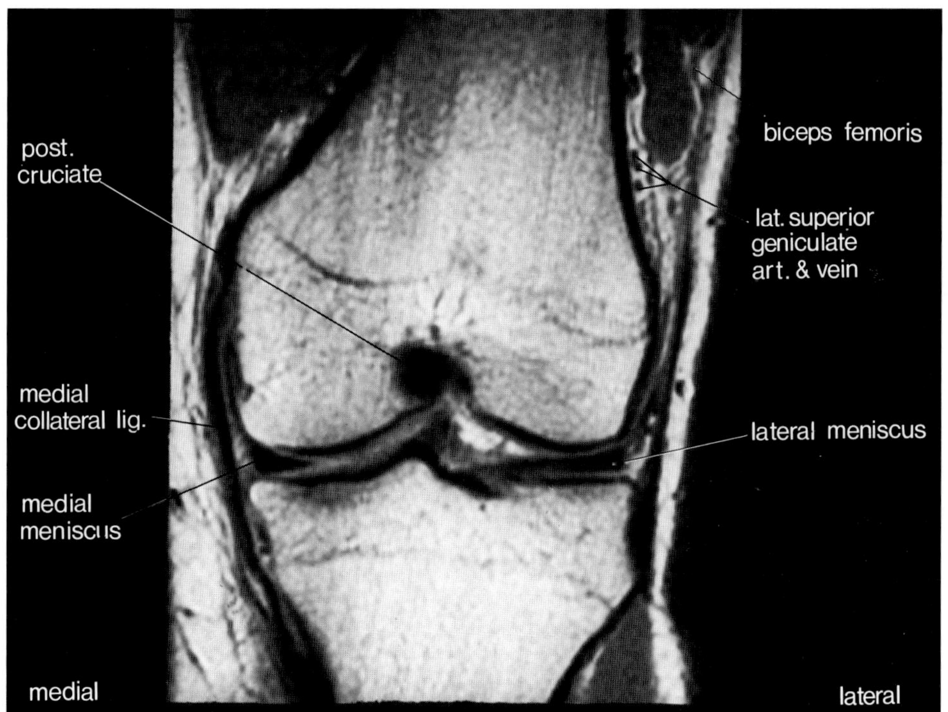

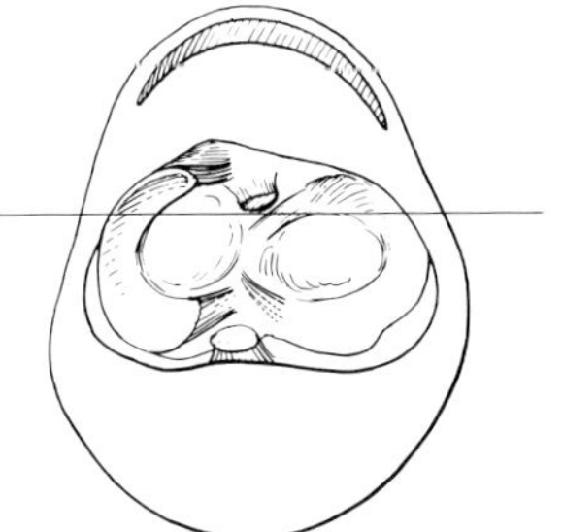

FIG. 7-6. D: Coronal image through the anterior joint.

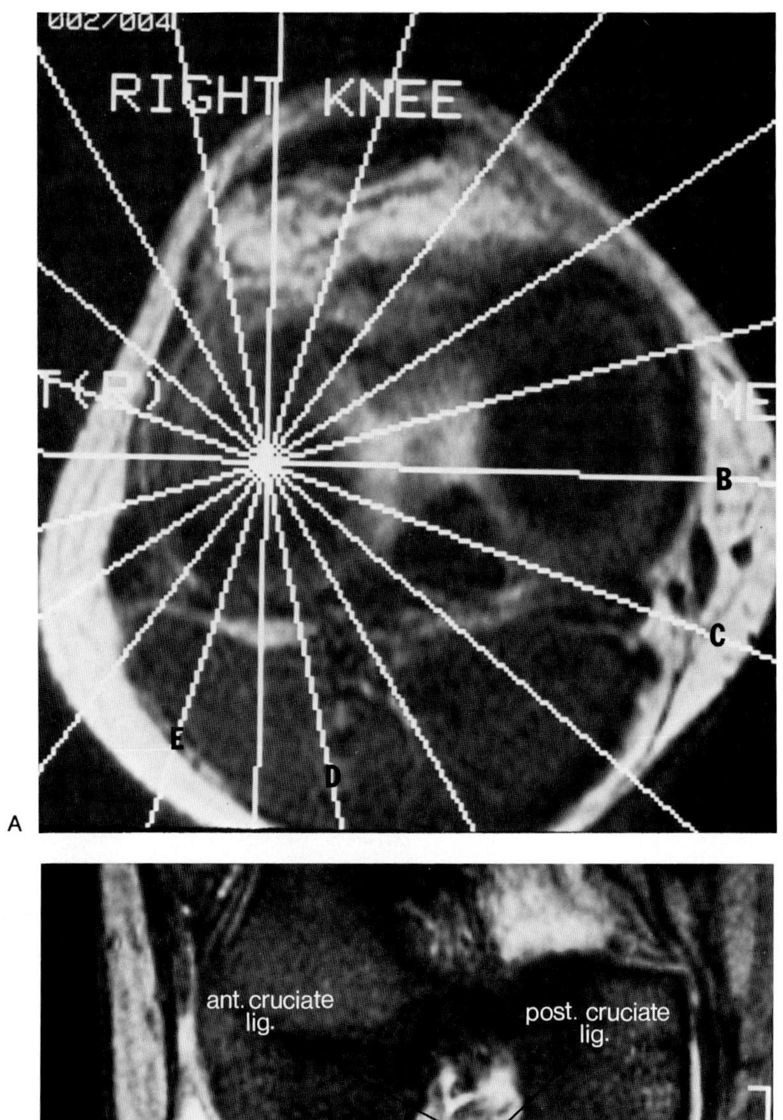

A

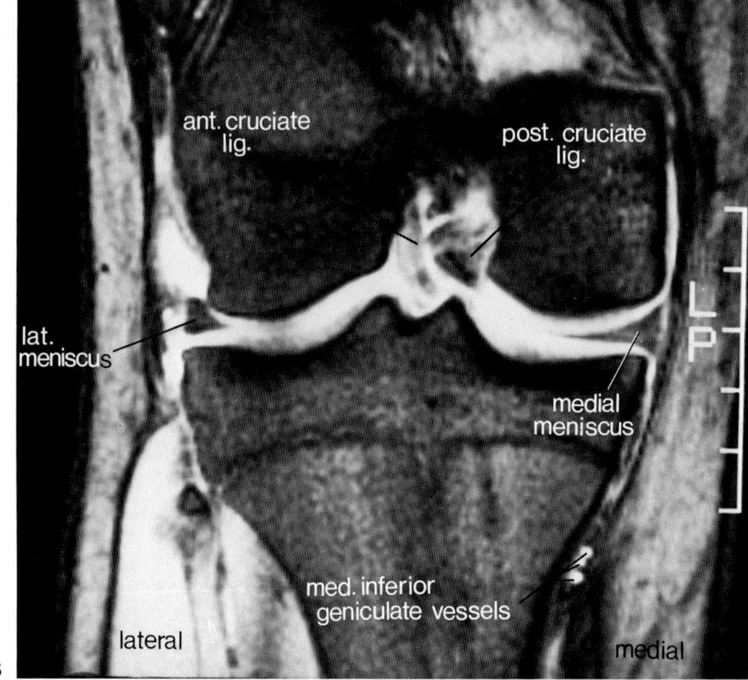

B

FIG. 7-7. Radial GRIL (MPGR) (TR 700, TE 12, flip angle 25°, FOV 16 cm, matrix 192 × 256, Nex 2) images of the knee centered on the lateral meniscus. **A:** Axial scout image showing image planes for MPGR images and levels for Figs. 7-7B–E. **B:** MPGR image through the midlateral meniscus and just posterior to the midbody of the medial meniscus. **C:** MPGR image through the anterior body of the lateral meniscus and posterior to the medial meniscus. **D:** MPGR image through the lateral meniscus, anterior and posterior horns. **E:** MPGR image through the lateral meniscus, anterior and posterior horns.

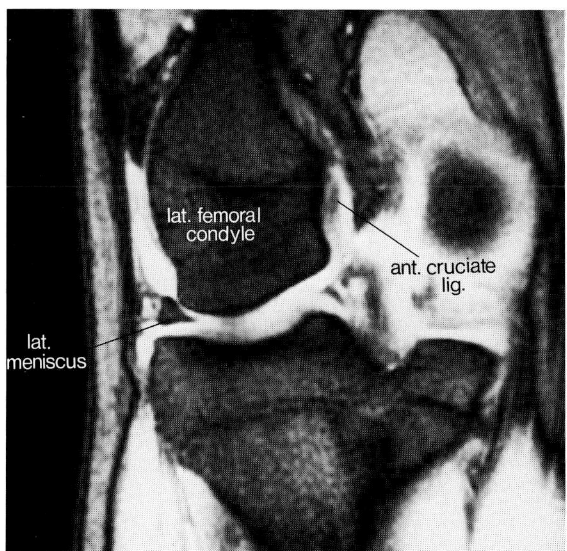

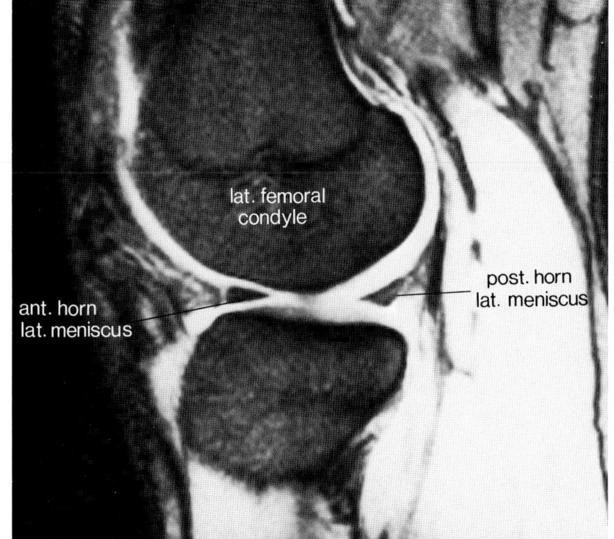

C,D

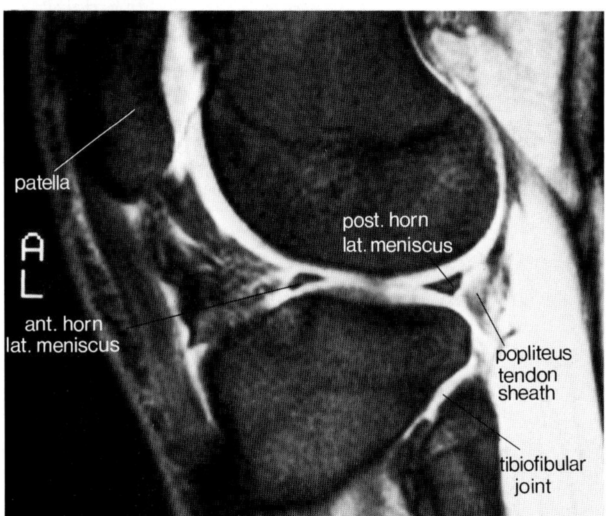

E

FIG. 7-7. *Continued.*

7-5B), though often considered a part of the knee, is in fact not a portion of the true knee joint (75). The knee is primarily a hinge joint that is protected anteriorly and posteriorly by muscles with special ligamentous attachments to the capsule. The articular surfaces of both the femoral condyles and tibial condyles are covered with hyaline cartilage. The femoral condyles are oval anteriorly and rounded posteriorly to provide increased stability in extension and increased motion and rotation in flexion (Fig. 7-4) (75). The medial femoral condyle is larger and important in load transmission across the knee. Medial and lateral tibial condyles form the expanded articular portion of the tibia. These condyles are separated by the intracondylar area, which serves for cruciate attachment and restricts translation. Between the tibial condyles are raised areas, known as the intercondylar eminence, that have medial and lateral tubercles (Fig. 7-6). The weight-bearing surfaces of the tibial and femoral condyles are separated by the fibrocartilaginous menisci, which are triangular when viewed tangentially and thicker laterally than medially (Fig. 7-6) (2,17,43,75).

The patella is the largest sesamoid bone in the body and develops in the tendon of the quadriceps (extensor mechanism) (Figs. 7-4 and 7-5). The patellar retinacula, which are formed by expansions in the quadriceps tendon and fascia lata, extend from the sides of the patella to the femoral and tibial condyles (Fig. 7-4). The patella is divided into several Wiberg types. The medial and lateral facets are of equal size in type I. Type II, the most common configuration, has a smaller medial than lateral facet (Fig. 7-4). Type III has a very small medial facet that is convex and a large concave lateral facet. Both facets are covered with hyaline cartilage and are most easily seen on axial MR images (Fig. 7-4) (43,75,113).

The capsule of the knee is lined by synovial membrane, which is subdivided into several communicating compartments (17,43). Anteriorly, the synovial membrane is attached to the articular margins of the patella. From the medial and lateral sides, the synovium extends circumferentially, in contact with the retinacula (Fig. 7-4). From the inferior aspect of the patella, the synovial membrane extends downward and backward and is separated from the patellar ligament by the intrapatellar fat pad (Fig. 7-8A,B). At the lower margin of the patella there is a central fold, the intrapatellar synovial fold, which is also sometimes referred to as the ligamentum mucosum (Fig. 7-8C). This is joined by two lesser alar folds or plicae that extend down from the sides of the patella. As the synovial fold extends into the femoral notch, it attaches to the intracondylar fossa of the femur anteriorly (Fig. 7-9A). The membrane fans out at its sides medially and laterally so that it covers the front and sides of the femoral attachment of the posterior cruciate ligament (Fig. 7-8D). Inferiorly, the synovial membrane continues down to the intracondylar area of the tibia, covering the attachment of the anterior cruciate ligament (Figs. 7-8D and 7-9A). Due to the fact that the fold attaches to both the femur and the tibia, it in fact divides the knee into medial and lateral synovial cavities separated by the extrasynovial space that houses the cruciate ligaments (2,17,43).

The synovial membrane extends superiorly from the upper margin of the patella for a variable distance and is closely applied to the quadriceps muscle (Fig. 7-9A). It then reflects onto the anterior aspect of the femur. This forms the suprapatellar bursa, which lies between the quadriceps and the front of the femur. Along the medial, lateral, and posterior aspects of the capsule, the synovial membrane attaches to the femur at the edges of the articular surfaces posteriorly (Fig. 7-8). Medially and laterally it passes from the articular margins inferiorly to attach to the articular margins of the tibial condyles (Fig. 7-9B). The intrasynovial space, which extends from the intracondylar fossa superiorly to the intracondylar area of the tibia inferiorly, houses the cruciate ligaments. The cruciate ligaments are therefore covered superiorly, medially, laterally, and anteriorly by synovial membrane but not posteriorly (Fig. 7-8D). Posterolaterally, the synovial membrane is separated from the fibrous capsule by the popliteus tendon (Figs. 7-5, 7-6, and 7-9B). It is not unusual to identify a bursa along the popliteus tendon which communicates with the joint space posterolaterally. The other common bursae about the knee are listed in Table 7-2 (2,17,43).

The fibrous capsule and periarticular ligaments of the knee are important in support and must be understood if one is to completely evaluate MR images of the knee (65,69,94,99). Anteriorly the knee capsule is essentially replaced by the quadriceps and its tendon, the patella, and the patellar ligament and retinacula (Fig. 7-10). Medially and laterally the capsule is attached to the femur just outside the synovial membrane and extends from the articular margin of the femoral condyles to the articular margin of the tibial condyles (Fig. 7-8). Laterally the main ligamentous support is provided by the lateral or fibular collateral ligament, which is clearly separated from the capsule (Fig. 7-10). The medial capsule is supported by the medial or tibial collateral ligament. Unique medial features include the fact that the medial collateral ligament blends with the capsule and the medial meniscus is attached to the capsule (Fig. 7-10A). The posterior capsule is supported by the oblique popliteal ligament and arcuate ligament. The oblique popliteal ligament is formed by an expansion from the semimembranosus tendon that turns superiorly and laterally to run across the joint of the lateral condyle of the femur. This ligament helps resist extreme hyperextension of the knee. The arcuate popliteal ligament extends laterally and inferiorly, where it is attached to the head of the fibula (43,75).

The coronary ligament is the portion of the capsule to which the meniscus is attached to the tibia (Fig. 7-10A). This ligament has some laxity, which allows slight motion of the menisci on the tibia (43,75).

The cruciate ligaments are intra-articular but lie outside the synovial compartment of the knee and are covered by synovial membrane anteriorly, medially, and laterally, but not posteriorly. The anterior cruciate ligament arises from the anterior nonarticular surface of the intracondylar area of the tibia adjacent to the medial condyle. It extends obliquely, superiorly, and posteriorly to attach the medial side of the lateral femoral condyle. The anterior cruciate ligament has significant variability in its appearance and is typically more slender and longer than the posterior cruciate. This and its oblique course account for some of the difficulty encountered in evaluating this structure with MRI (Fig. 7-10) (10,17,43,75).

The posterior cruciate ligament arises from the posterior intercondylar area and passes obliquely upward and forward in a nearly sagittal plane to attach to the anterior intercondylar fossa of the lateral surface of the medial femoral condyle (Figs. 7-6 and 7-10). The posterior cruciate, because of its larger transverse diameter and more straight sagittal course, is consistently identified on sagittal MR images (Fig. 7-6) (10,66).

The fibrocartilaginous menisci have a differing shape, with the medial meniscus being larger and thicker in transverse diameter posteriorly than anteriorly (Figs. 7-5 to 7-7 and 7-10A). The lateral meniscus is more C shaped and uniform in width (Fig. 7-10A). There are several ligamentous attachments that may cause confusion on MR images. For example, the posterior horn of the lateral meniscus is closely applied to the posterior cruciate ligament and may give off a band of fibers, termed the meniscofemoral ligament, that follows the posterior cruciate ligament to its attachment on the femur. Between the anterior horns of the medial and

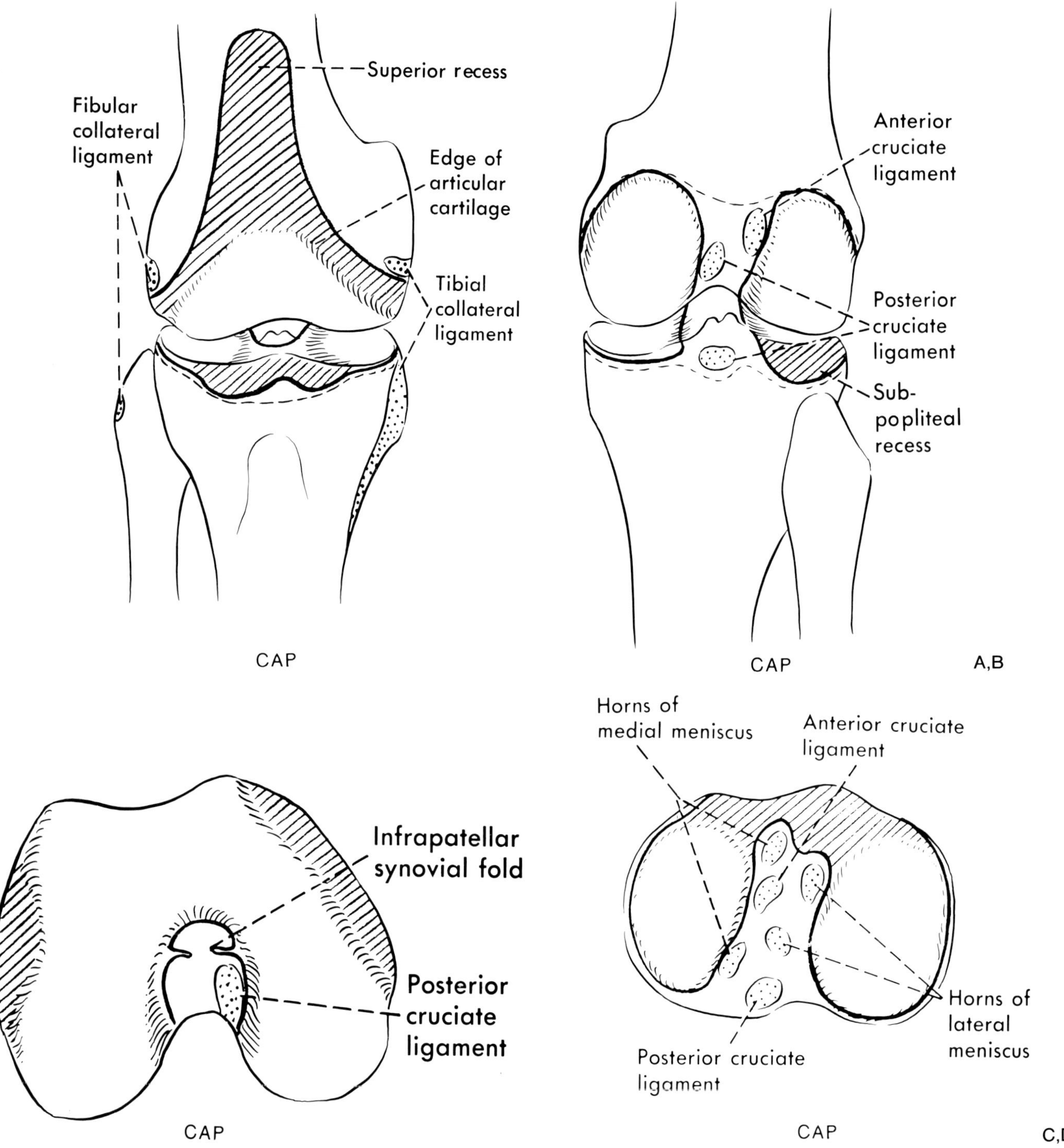

FIG. 7-8. Illustration of the synovial lining and capsular attachments of the knee. From (**A**) anterior, (**B**) posterior, (**C**) femoral articular, and (**D**) tibial articular surfaces. (From ref. 43, with permission.)

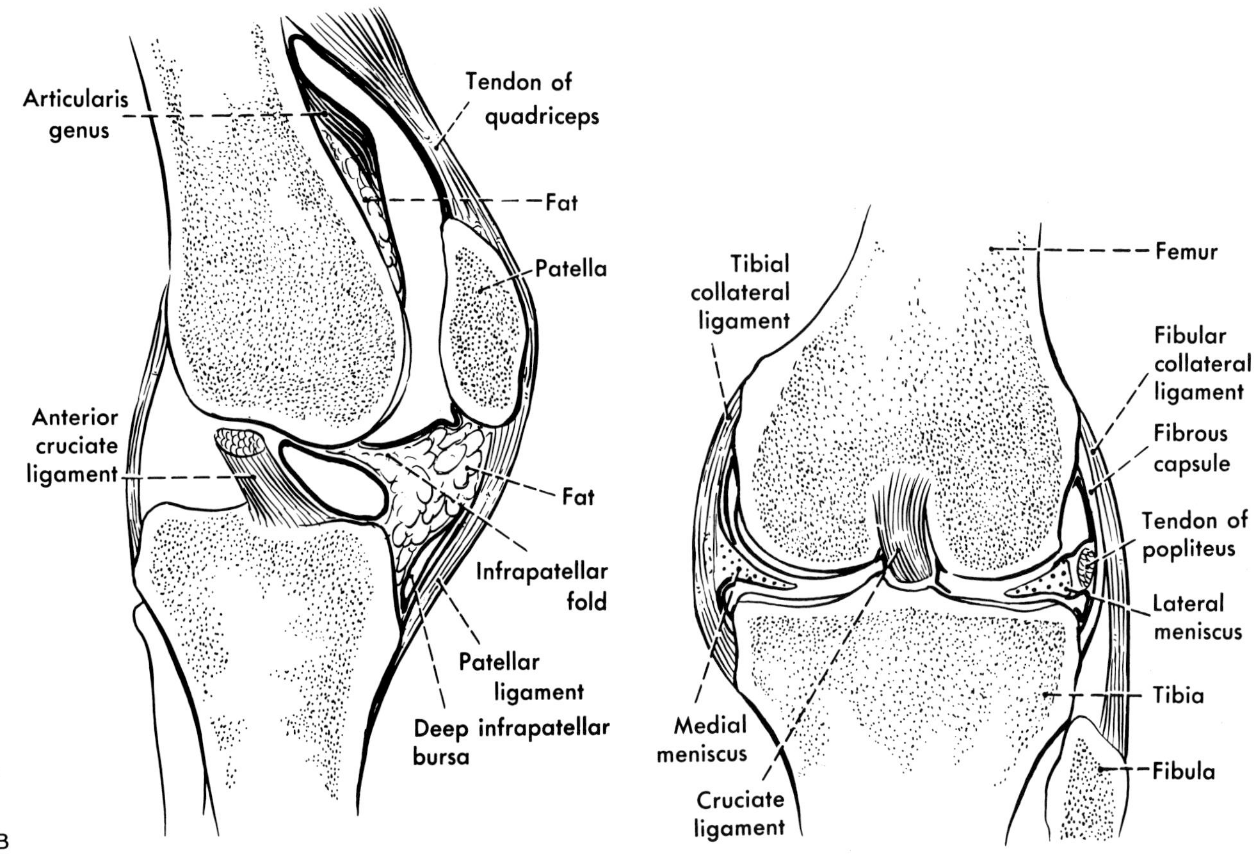

FIG. 7-9. Illustrations of the sagittal (**A**) and coronal (**B**) capsule, synovial lining, and major supporting ligaments of the knee. (From ref. 43, with permission.)

TABLE 7-2. *Bursae about the knee* (17,43)

Anterior	
Prepatellar	Between patella and skin
Retropatellar	Between patellar ligament and upper tibia
Pretibial	Between tibial tuberosity and skin
Suprapatellar[a]	Between quadriceps and femur (communicates with joint)
Lateral	
Gastrocnemius	Between lateral gastrocnemius and capsule
Fibular	Between fibular collateral ligament and biceps tendon
Fibulopopliteal	Between fibular collateral ligament and popliteus tendon
Popliteal[a]	Between popliteus tendon and lateral femoral condyle (communicates with joint)
Medial	
Gastrocnemius[a]	Between medial head of gastrocnemius and capsule (often communicates with joint)
Pes anserine	Between tibial collateral ligament and gracilis, sartorius, and semitendinosus tendons

[a] Communicating bursae.

lateral meniscus there is a transverse band of fibers termed the transverse ligament of the knee. This can easily be confused with an anterior meniscal tear, especially on the medial side (Fig. 7-11) (43,66,75).

Muscles About the Knee

The muscles of the thigh, calf, and foot and ankle have been discussed in Chapters 6 and 8. Therefore, a thorough review of their origins and insertions would be redundant. However, it is important to review the muscles about the knee, their neurovascular and biomechanical functions. Chief movements at the knee are those of flexion and extension. Mild rotation, however, can occur. If one starts from the flexed position (Fig. 7-12), the posterior condyles of the femur are in contact with the posterior horns of both menisci. The medial and lateral collateral ligaments are also relaxed in this position. In full flexion, both anterior and posterior cruciate ligaments are taut. In this flexed position more rotary motion is allowed. As one goes from the flexed to the extended position, the femoral condyles shift, such

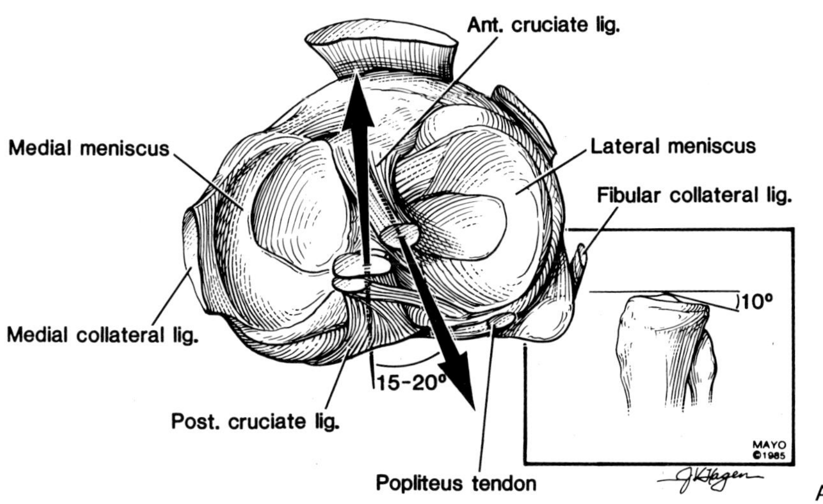

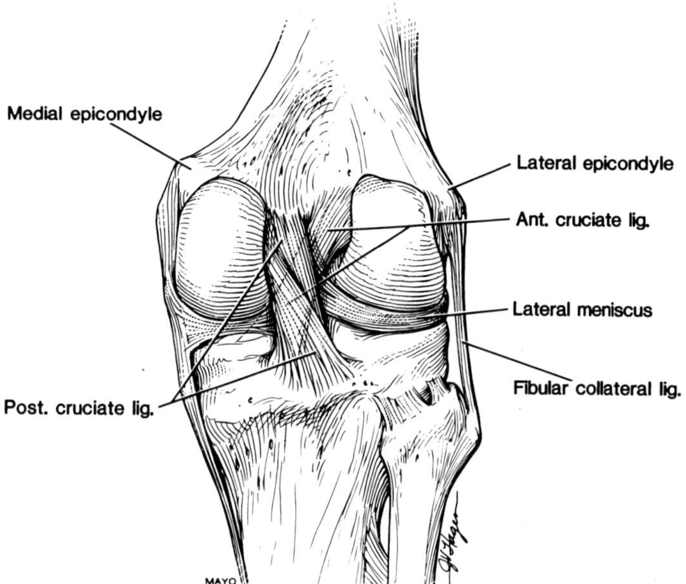

FIG. 7-10. Axial (**A**), coronal (**B**), and sagittal (**C**) illustrations of the ligaments and menisci of the knee.

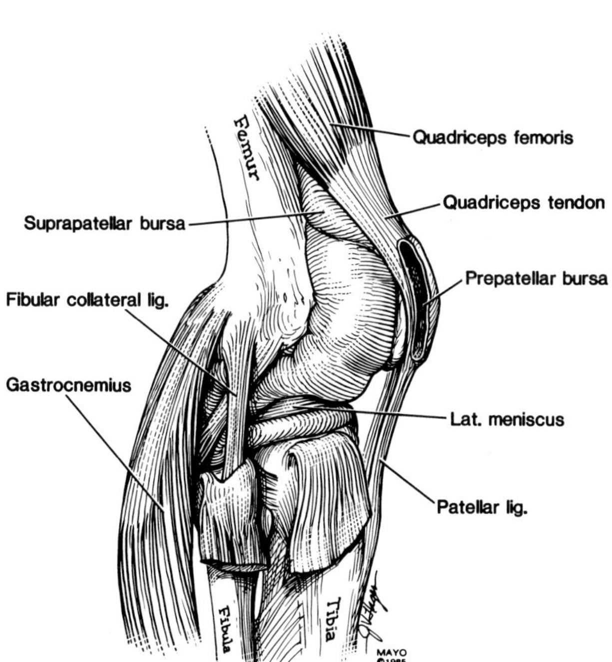

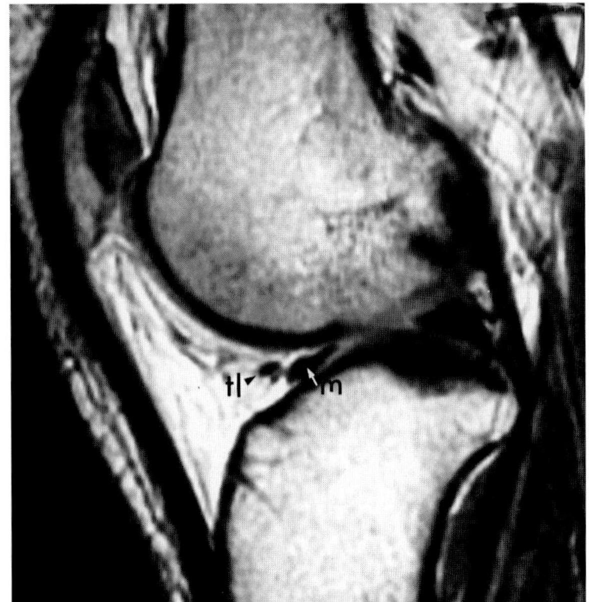

FIG. 7-11. Sagittal SE 500/20 image of the knee, demonstrating a normal anterior horn of the medial meniscus (m) and the transverse ligament (tl). This should not be confused with a meniscal tear.

that the more anterior parts of the menisci and tibial condyles are now in contact (Fig. 7-12) (43,75).

The primary flexors of the knee are the hamstring muscle group (semimembranous, semitendinous, and biceps femoris) along with the gracilis and sartorius (Fig. 7-13). The popliteus muscle has some significance in the early phases of flexion due to its rotary action on the femor or tibia (Table 7-3). In the nonweight-bearing state, the gastrocnemius muscle is also used in flexion of the knee. The quadriceps group is the chief extensor of the knee (Fig. 7-14 and Table 7-3) (17,43,103).

Neurovascular Supply of the Knee

The arterial supply about the knee is primarily via branch vessels of the distal superficial femoral and popliteal arteries (Fig. 7-15). Superiorly there are medial and lateral genicular arteries as well as muscular branches at the level of the knee joint. Inferiorly, medial and lateral inferior genicular arteries supply the knee. There are numerous anastomoses that interconnect this vascular supply.

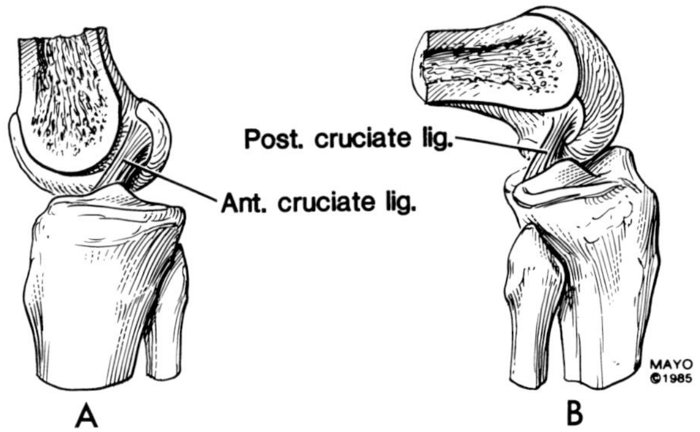

FIG. 7-12. Sagittal illustrations of the knee and cruciate ligaments in the extended (**A**) and flexed (**B**) positions.

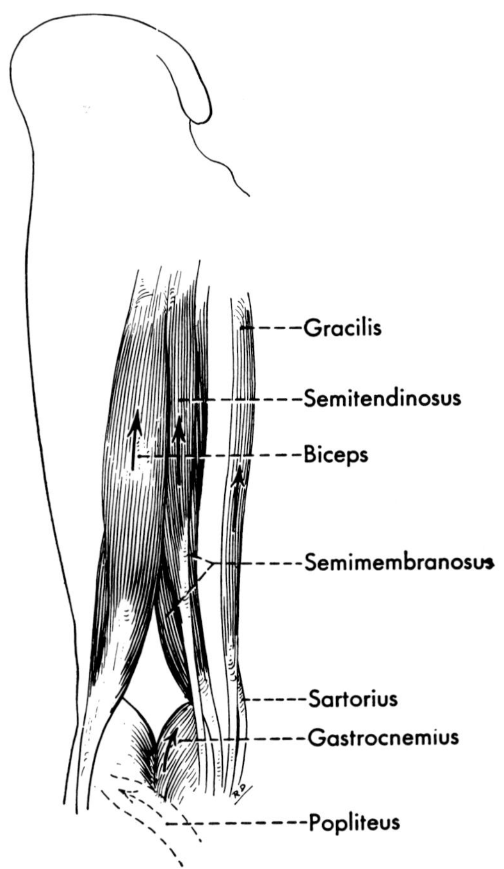

FIG. 7-13. Illustration of the flexors of the knee. (From ref. 43, with permission.)

Innervation of the knee (see Table 7-3) is primarily by branches of the femoral, obturator, and sciatic nerves. Posterolaterally, recurrent branches of the peroneal nerve also supply the knee (17,43).

PITFALLS

The majority of the pitfalls in evaluating the knee are related to normal anatomy or variants and artifacts created by flow, motion, and software problems (66, 110,111). Partial volume effects must also be considered when evaluating the knee.

Problems with flow artifacts occur less frequently during examination of the knee than in the more peripheral extremities, where vascular structures per unit area are more numerous (see Chapters 3 and 11). The largest problem with flow artifact occurs in the sagittal plane, where the midline anatomy can be distorted by flow

TABLE 7-3. *Knee flexors and extensors* (43)

Muscle	Origin	Insertion	Innervation
Flexors			
Semitendinosus	Posteromedial ischial tuberosity	Medial tibia posterior to gracilis and sartorius	Tibial nerve (L5–S1)
Biceps femoris	Two heads: long head with semitendinosus, short head with midlinea aspera	Fibular head	Peroneal (L5–S1)
Semimembranosus	Posterolateral ischial tuberosity, medial meniscus	Proximal medial tibia	Tibial (L5–S1)
Gracilis	Inferior pubic ramus near symphysis	Medial upper tibia between sartorius and semitendinosus	Obturator (L3–L4)
Sartorius	Anterior superior iliac spine	Upper medial tibia above gracilis and semitendinosus	Femoral (L3–L4)
Extensors—quadriceps			
Rectus femoris	Anterior inferior iliac spine	Quadriceps tendon to patella	Femoral (L3–L4)
Vastus lateralis	Below greater trochanter	Quadriceps tendon to patella	Femoral (L3–L4)
Vastus medialis	Below lesser trochanter	Quadriceps tendon to patella	Femoral (L3–L4)
Vastus intermedius	Midfemur	Quadriceps tendon to patella	Femoral (L3–L4)

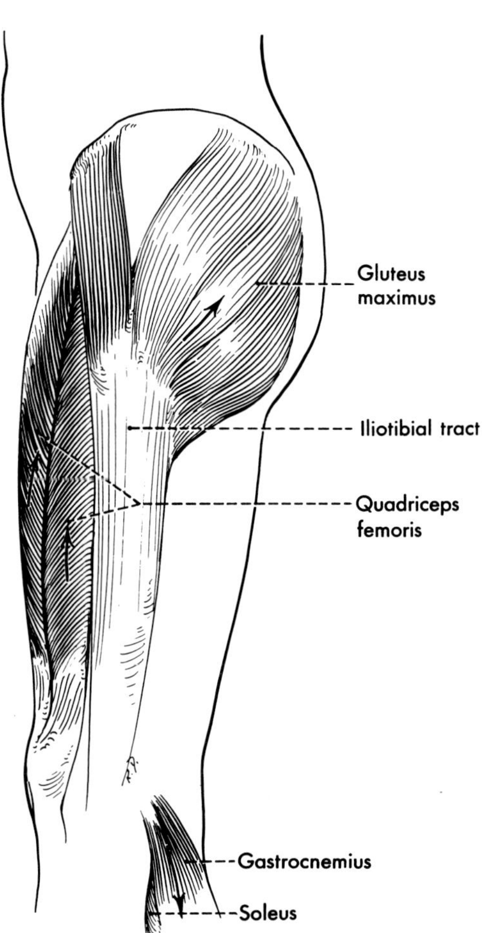

FIG. 7-14. Illustration of extensors of the knee. (From ref. 43, with permission.)

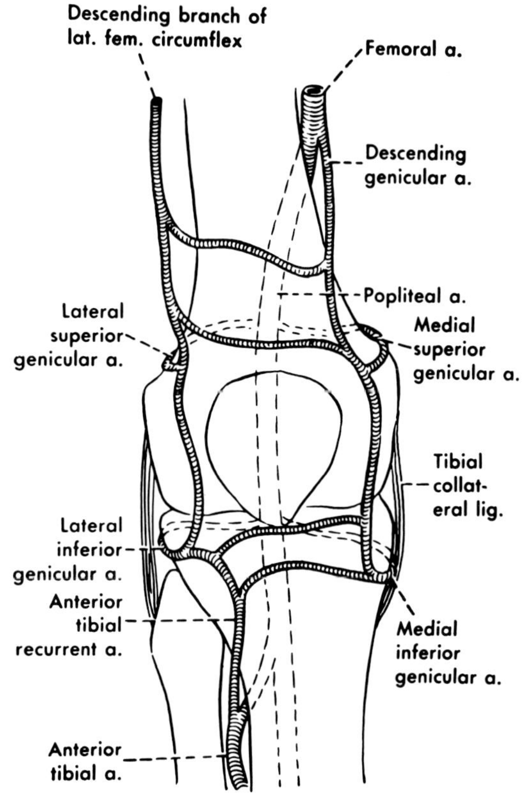

FIG. 7-15. Illustration of the vascular anatomy of the knee. (From ref. 43, with permission.)

artifact from the popliteal artery (Fig. 7-16). This can be corrected by swapping the phase to the superior inferior direction instead of the transverse direction. The artifact can also be reduced to some degree by placing the patient prone. In the latter situation, the pulsatile effect of the popliteal artery does not create as much motion artifact as when the patient is supine.

Flow artifact can create false positive interpretations if the phase direction is not considered. For example, when patellofemoral disease is being evaluated in the axial plane, the phase should be in the "X" or transverse direction (Fig. 7-17). This prevents the artifact from entering the area of interest.

There are two artifacts noted consistently on images performed using the radial MPGR (multiplanar GRASS) techniques. One is a small, low-intensity, circular artifact that is seen at the crossover point (see Fig. 7-6A) (11) and can be confused with a loose body (Fig. 7-18). The location remains the same on each radial image, which is useful in differentiating this artifact from a loose body. The second is a marrow artifact that is seen as a "blotchy" appearance in the femur and tibia (Fig. 7-19). This always occurs in a linear fashion from superior to inferior. This should not be confused with an infiltrative marrow process.

A significant number of interpretation errors are related to lack of familiarity with normal anatomy and

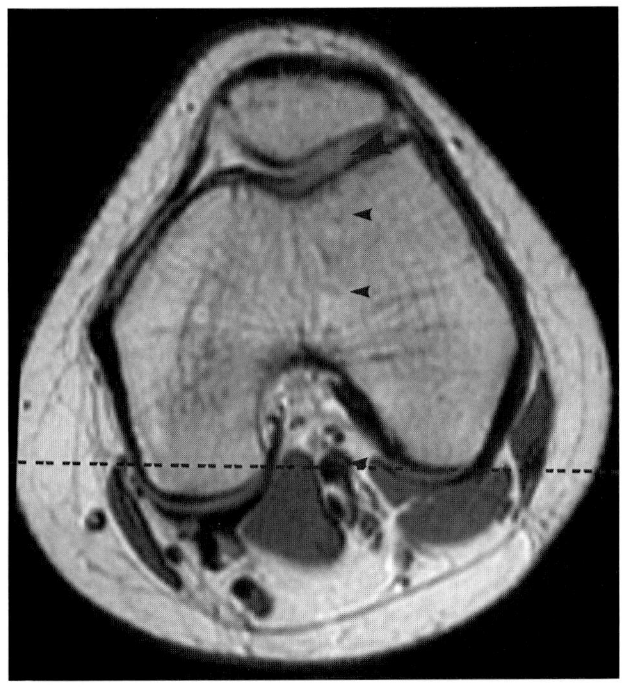

FIG. 7-17. Axial SE 2,000/20 image in a patient referred for patellofemoral pain. The local defect in the lateral femoral condyle (*large arrowhead*) is due to flow artifact (*small arrowheads*). This should not be confused with an articular defect. This problem can be avoided by swapping phase direction to the transverse (*dotted line*) plane.

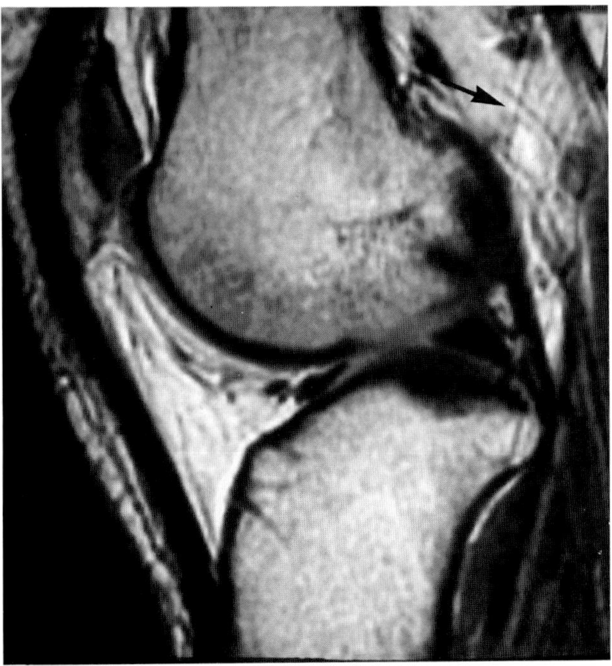

FIG. 7-16. Sagittal SE 2,000/20 image of the knee, demonstrating pulsatile motion artifact (*arrows*) from the popliteal artery.

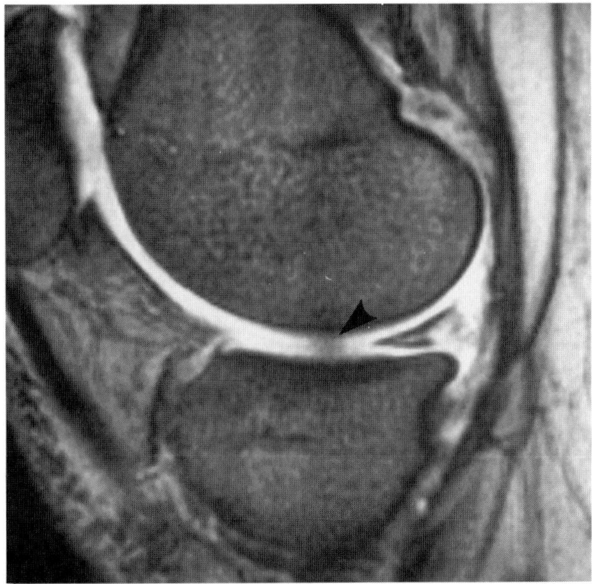

FIG. 7-18. Radial gradient-echo (MPGR) image of the knee (TE 700, TR 12, FA 20°). The "cross artifact" (*arrowhead*) should not be confused with a loose body. This is always at the central point where the radial images cross and it maintains this position on all the radial images for the side selected. (See Fig. 7-7A.)

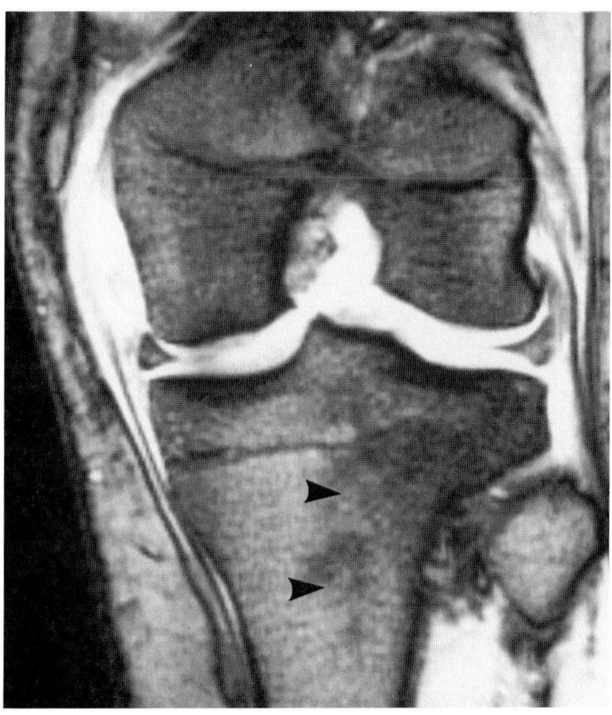

FIG. 7-19. Oblique gradient-echo (MPGR) image of the knee in a patient with a medial collateral ligament tear. Note the marrow artifact (*arrowheads*). This should not be confused with an infiltrative marrow disease.

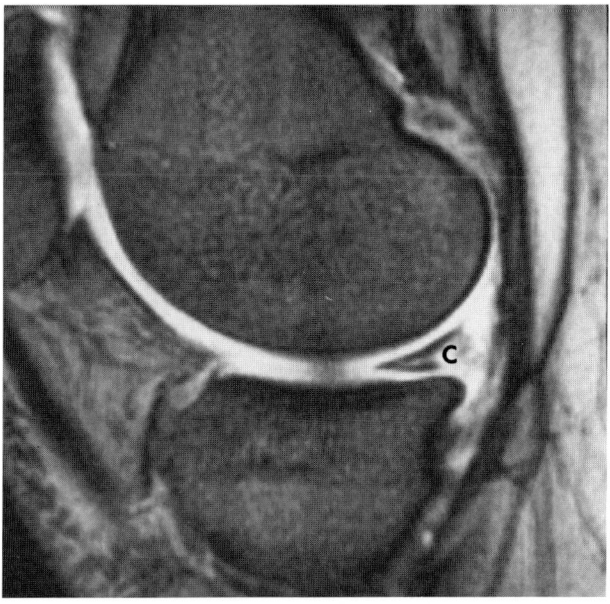

FIG. 7-20. Sagittal gradient-echo (MPGR) image of the posterior medial meniscus, demonstrating the concave meniscosynovial junction (C), which can be confused with a tear. There is also a linear area of increased signal intensity (grade 2) in the meniscus that does not communicate with the articular surface.

anatomic variants (110,111). The majority of these pitfalls are related to normal variants in the appearance of the menisci and/or variation in lesser known ligaments associated with the menisci. There is vascular tissue and variable amounts of fat and synovial tissue near the attachment of the menisci, especially the posterior medial meniscus (41,66,75). This is a more difficult problem on nontangential sagittal and coronal images as tissue is projected between the meniscus and the margin of the capsule. This should not be confused with a peripheral tear in the meniscus (Fig. 7-20). Typically, this tissue has the appearance of fat or signal intensity similar to fat on T1 and T2 weighted images. Meniscal tears are seen as an area of high signal intensity, similar to fluid. As with arthrography, evaluation of the posterior lateral meniscus can be difficult due to the popliteus tendon and its sheath, which pass between the capsule and meniscus posteriorly. This should not be mistaken for a meniscal tear (Fig. 7-21) (66,110,111). Additional anatomic structures that can cause confusion are the inferior lateral geniculate vessels that course along the margin of the lateral meniscus anteriorly. The signal intensity of these vessels can give the appearance of a peripheral detachment (Figs. 7-14 and 7-22) (41). The transverse meniscal ligament is seen anteriorly and can be confused with a horizontal tear in the anterior horn of the meniscus (Fig. 7-11).

Variations in the cruciate ligaments and collateral ligaments may also cause confusion. The main problem with the anterior cruciate is its oblique course (Fig. 7-10A). This can result in incomplete visualization of the ligament. Further oblique views should be obtained when the ligament is not completely identified. Normal

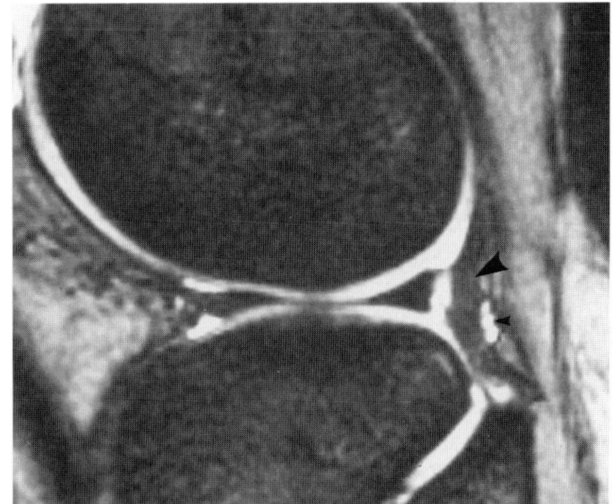

FIG. 7-21. Sagittal MPGR image of the knee. The popliteus tendon (*large arrowhead*) and tendon sheath pass between the lateral meniscus and capsule. This should not be confused with a tear. The small areas of high signal intensity (*small arrowhead*) are due to the inferior genicular vessels.

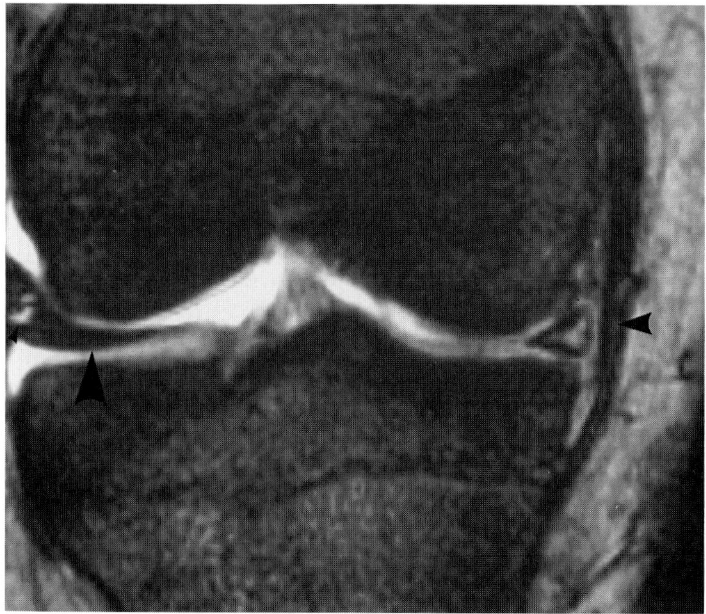

FIG. 7-22. Coronal MPGR image of the knee, demonstrating a discoid lateral meniscus (*large arrowhead*). Note the inferior geniculate vessels (*small arrowhead*), which should not be confused with a tear. Medially (*arrowhead*) there is fat between the fibers of the medial collateral ligament, which is normal.

variations in the posterior ligaments can be confused with partial tears in the posterior cruciate ligament. The meniscal femoral ligament extends from near the posterior capsular attachment of the lateral meniscus to the medial femoral condyle and may have two branches. The most common segment is the ligament of Wrisberg, which is seen just posterior to the posterior cruciate ligament (Fig. 7-23). This is evident in 23–32.5% of sagittal MR images and should not be confused with a partial tear (41,66,110,111). The anterior bundle of this ligament or the ligament of Humphrey is seen in 34% of patients (Fig. 7-24) (110,111). This lies just anterior to the posterior cruciate ligament.

There is frequently a linear collection of fat (Fig. 7-22) between the fibers of the medial collateral ligament and between the lateral collateral ligament and capsule (110,111). These areas can be confused with tears. However, the fat signal is suppressed on T2 weighted sequences. Fluid and blood from a tear should have high signal intensity. Using double-echo sequences is useful

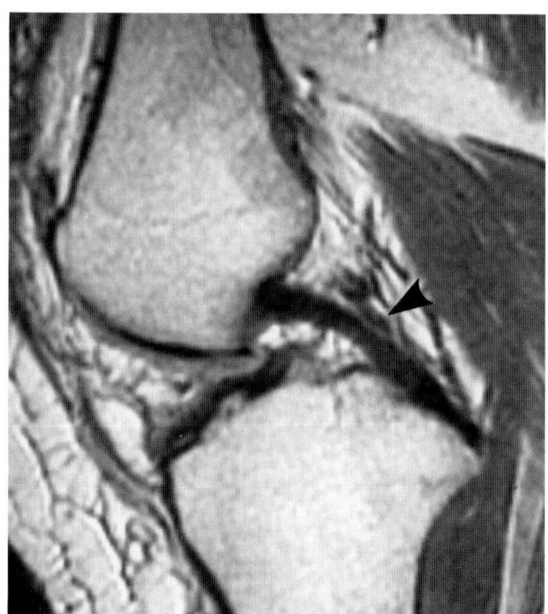

FIG. 7-23. Sagittal SE 2,000/30 image demonstrating a normal posterior cruciate ligament. The ligament of Wisberg (*arrowhead*) should not be confused with a posterior cruciate defect.

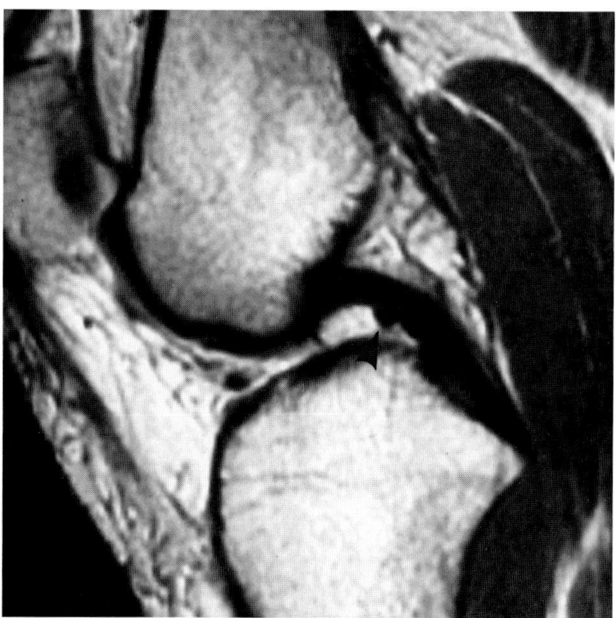

FIG. 7-24. Sagittal, SE 2,000/20 image of the posterior cruciate ligament. Note the ligament of Humphrey (*arrowhead*) anteriorly.

because fat signal is suppressed on the second echo and the signal intensity of fluid increases.

Discoid menisci can cause significant problems if one does not consider this variant. Discoid menisci are more common laterally and occur in 1–2% of arthrographic and 2–5% of surgical series. The meniscus has a wafer-like appearance on the coronal and radial MPGR images (Fig. 7-22) and projects farther into the joint space on sagittal images. These menisci are more prone to tears and are important to recognize (92).

Familiarity with the anatomic variations and normal ligamentous attachments in the knee is critical in evaluating MR images so that false positive interpretations do not occur.

APPLICATIONS

MRI provides excellent soft tissue contrast and is capable of evaluating the soft tissue and bony structures of the knee in multiple image planes, which provides it with significant advantages over conventional arthrography, CT, and other imaging techniques. The major application for MRI of the knee has been evaluation of patients with trauma or suspected internal derangement of the knee (30,58).

Most patients are referred for MRI of the knee to exclude tears in the menisci or ligamentous structures. Prior to the acceptance of MRI, arthrography was the imaging technique of choice for evaluation of the menisci. Accuracy of arthrography, specifically using the double-contrast technique, approaches 95% for medial meniscal tears and approximately 90% for the lateral meniscus (35,61,75,78). However, this technique does have shortcomings in evaluating the collateral ligaments and cruciate ligaments, and the accuracy is reduced when large effusions or hemarthrosis are present (75). Arthroscopy is considered the gold standard for evaluating the accuracy of imaging techniques. However, keep in mind that the accuracy of arthroscopy varies from 69 to 98% depending on the experience of the examiner (65).

Meniscal Tears

The most common causes of knee pain and disability are tears in the medial and/or lateral menisci. Pain due to meniscal tears can be mediated via the neurovascular bundle, which is in the outer third of the meniscus, or can occur when innervated synovium invaginates into a tear. Patients may also present with "locking," which is usually related to a bucket handle tear, or "giving way," which is more often related to pain (75).

Prior to discussing the MR features of meniscal tears it is essential to review certain anatomic and pathophysiology aspects of meniscal injury. The lateral meniscus is C shaped and thicker than the medial meniscus. The transverse diameter is similar in the body, posterior, and anterior horns (Fig. 7-25). The lateral meniscus is also less firmly attached to the capsule and is, in fact, separated posteriorly by the popliteus tendon and tendon sheath (Figs. 7-21, 7-25, and 7-26). The horns of the meniscus attach to the tibia in the intercondylar region (Figs. 7-8D and 7-27). The medial meniscus is more firmly attached to the capsule. The anterior horn attaches to the intercondylar eminence anterior to the anterior cruciate ligament (Figs. 7-8D and 7-27). The transverse diameter of the anterior horn is smaller (Fig. 7-25) than the posterior horn. The posterior horn attaches to the intercondylar eminence anterior to the posterior cruciate ligament (43,66,75).

Tears in the menisci may result from acute trauma or repetitive trauma and progressive degeneration (66,75,102,105). Acute tears are usually due to athletic injuries with crushing of the meniscus between the tibia and femoral condyles. Chronic repetitive trauma is more common in the nonathlete and with aging. In this setting, chondrocyte necrosis and increase in mucoid ground substance lead to meniscal tears (25,66).

Examination techniques (see Techniques section) vary depending on the software and preferences of the examiner. Throughput and ease of lesion detection are

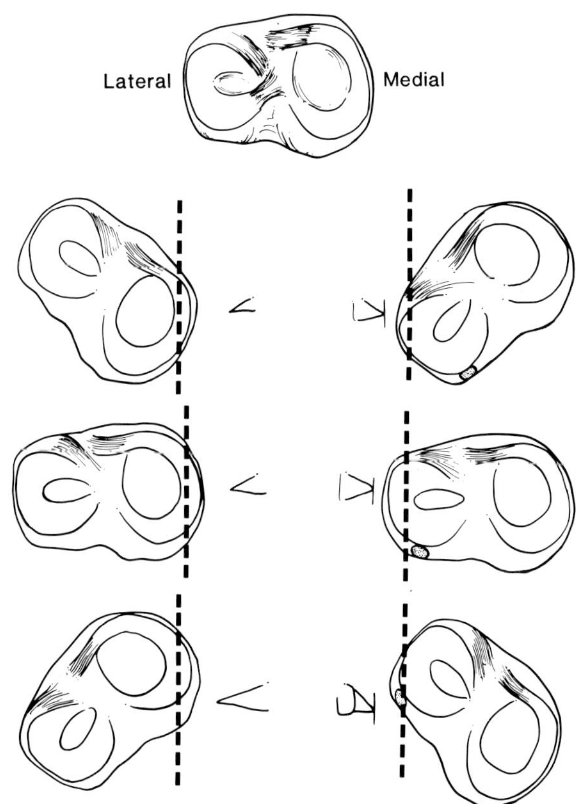

FIG. 7-25. Illustration of tangential sections of the medial and lateral menisci. (From ref. 75, with permission.)

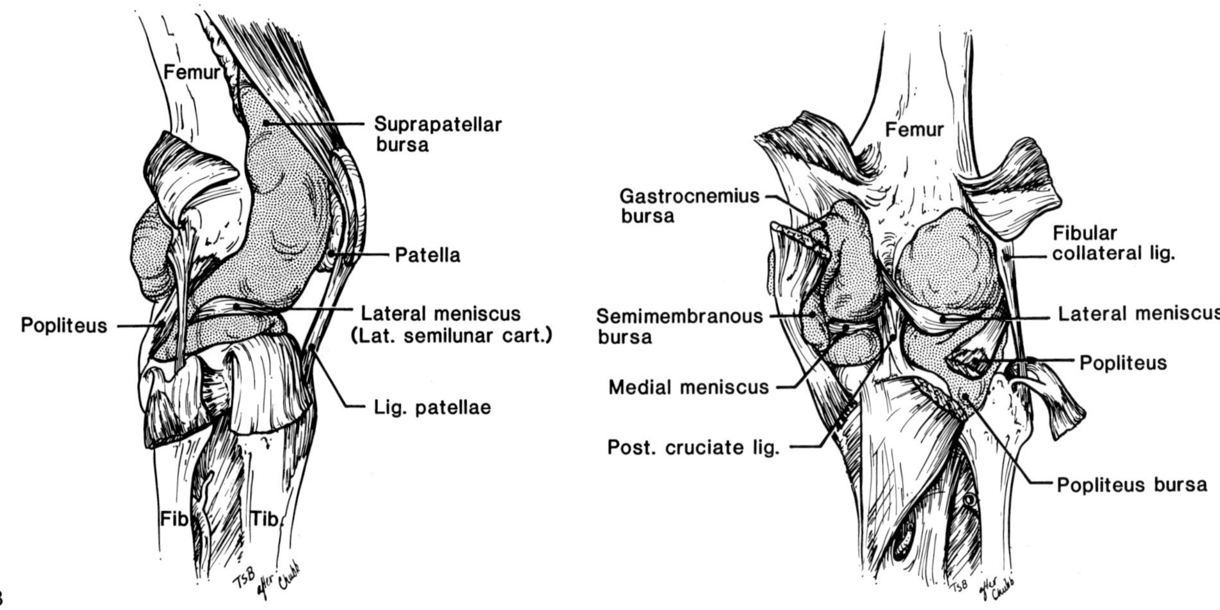

FIG. 7-26. Lateral (**A**) and posterior (**B**) illustration of the knee, demonstrating the joint space and associated ligament and muscular anatomy. (From ref. 75, with permission.)

both important (Table 7-1). We prefer T2 weighted spin-echo or gradient-echo sequences. The contrast of lesions (high signal intensity) compared to the normal low signal intensity (black) of the menisci allows defects to be appreciated more easily. Some authors prefer T1 weighted sequences or three-dimensional gradient-echo sequences (7,14,39,66,77,79,91,94,104). The use of intra-articular contrast medium has also been investigated. Hajek et al. (33,34) reviewed the effects of air, blood, saline, Renografin 60, and Gd-DTPA as contrast material for MRI (Fig. 7-28). T1 weighted sequences can be used, which affords excellent anatomy in less time than long TE, TR T2 weighted sequences. However, the examination becomes invasive and more expensive. The time required for injection would likely negate or increase examination time gained by using T1 weighted sequences. Also, newer gradient-echo sequences achieve the same degree of contrast compared to T2 weighted sequences and they can be performed in about the same amount of time as a T1 weighted spin-echo sequence. Therefore, to date, contrast media are not frequently used to examine the knee.

The appearance of normal menisci and meniscal tears has been well documented in the MRI literature (Fig. 7-29). Increased signal intensity has been noted on T1, T2, and gradient-echo sequences (20–23,25). These changes can be seen with mucoid degeneration as well as meniscal tears. Grading systems for meniscal tears have been described by Stoller et al. (99), Crues et al. (20–22), and Mink et al. (66) based on pathologic findings in cadaver specimens (Fig. 7-29). A grade 1 meniscal lesion is globular in nature and does not communicate with the articular surface (Fig. 7-29C). Histologically this stage correlates with early mucoid degeneration. It is felt that these changes are not symptomatic but represent a response to mechanical stress and loading, which result in increased production of mucoid polysaccharide ground substance (66,99).

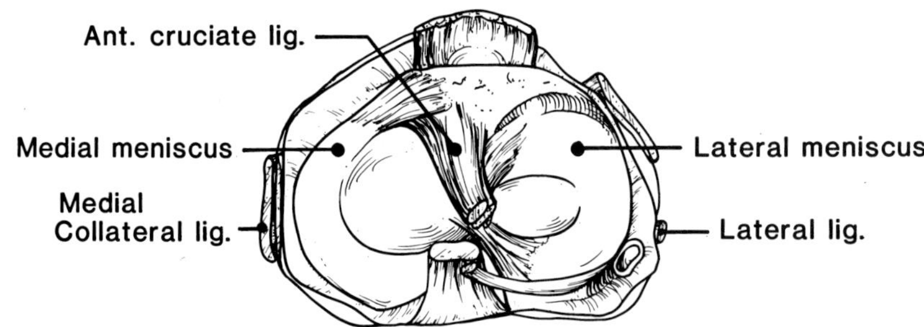

FIG. 7-27. Illustration of the menisci and their attachments and associated ligament and tendon anatomy. (From ref. 75, with permission.)

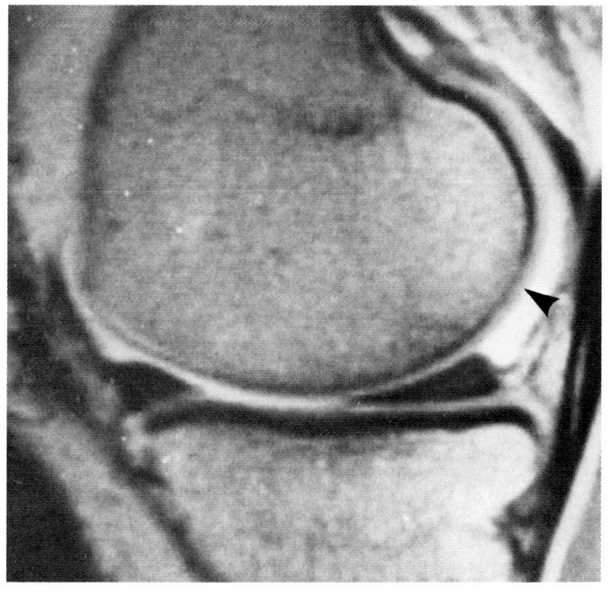

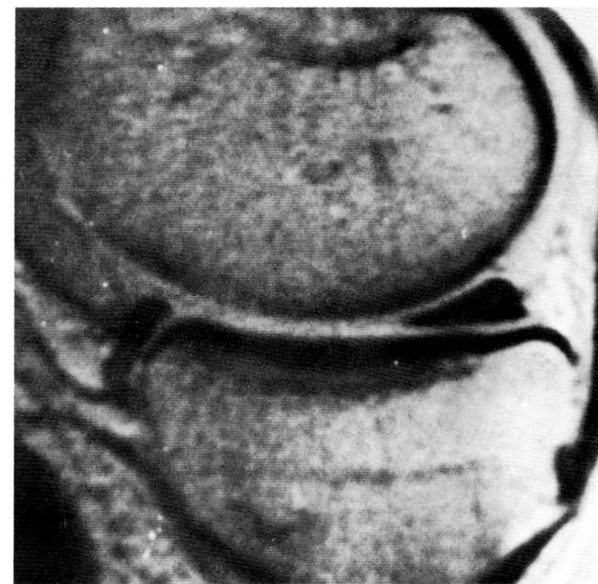

A,B

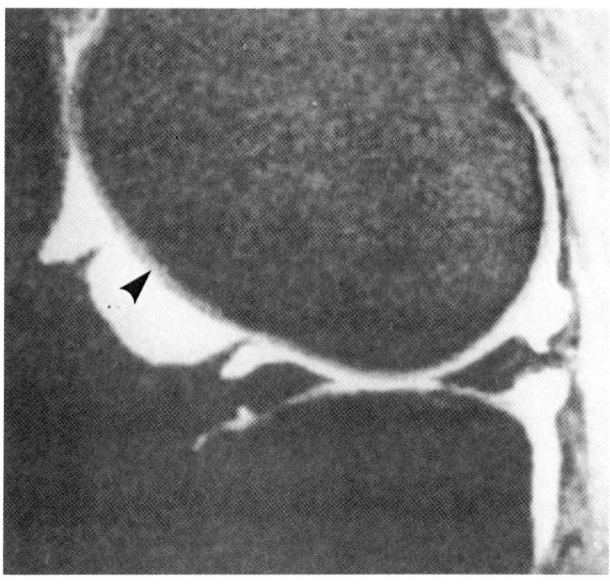

C

FIG. 7-28. Sagittal images of the knee using different pulse sequences and contrast media. **A:** SE 600/25 image after 5 ml Gd-DTPA injection. The articular cartilage (*arrowhead*) is easily differentiated from the contrast medium. **B:** SE 600/25 image after injection of saline. The cartilage is not as well demonstrated compared to Gd-DTPA. **C:** SE 2,000/70 image after Renografin 60 injection. Cartilage and fluid (*arrowhead*) anteriorly are easily identified. (From ref. 34, with permission.)

Grade 2 signal intensity is linear in nature and remains within the substance of the meniscus (Fig. 7-29D). Once again there is no evidence of communication with the articular surface of the meniscus. Histologically these changes are characterized by more extensive bands of mucoid degeneration. Most feel that stage 2 changes represent progression of stage 1. It is felt that stage 2 lesions are precursors to complete tears (25,66,99).

With grade 3 tears there is increased signal intensity within the meniscus that extends to the articular surface (Fig. 7-29E). Mink et al. (66) have further divided grade 3 into two subcategories. Grade 3A signal intensity is a linear intermeniscal signal that abuts the articular margin (Fig. 7-29F). Grade 3B is a more irregular area of signal intensity that abuts the articular margin (Fig. 7-29H). The grade 3B lesions are most often associated with more extensive degenerative change in the adjacent areas of the meniscus associated with the tear.

Grade 4 menisci are distorted (Figs. 7-29 and 7-30) in addition to changes described with grade 3 (25).

The MR appearance of different types of meniscal tear is similar to those that have been described with arthrography (Fig. 7-31). Vertical tears are usually traumatic compared with horizontal tears, which are more often degenerative. Degenerative fraying of the surface of the meniscus may also be evident on MR images and is demonstrated as areas of irregular increased signal intensity on the meniscal surface compared to the normal dark or low intensity of the body of the meniscus (Fig. 7-32). Radial tears may be somewhat difficult to diagnose but are typically seen as areas of increased signal in the inner margin of the menisci (Fig. 7-33). Bucket handle tears are vertical tears with displacement

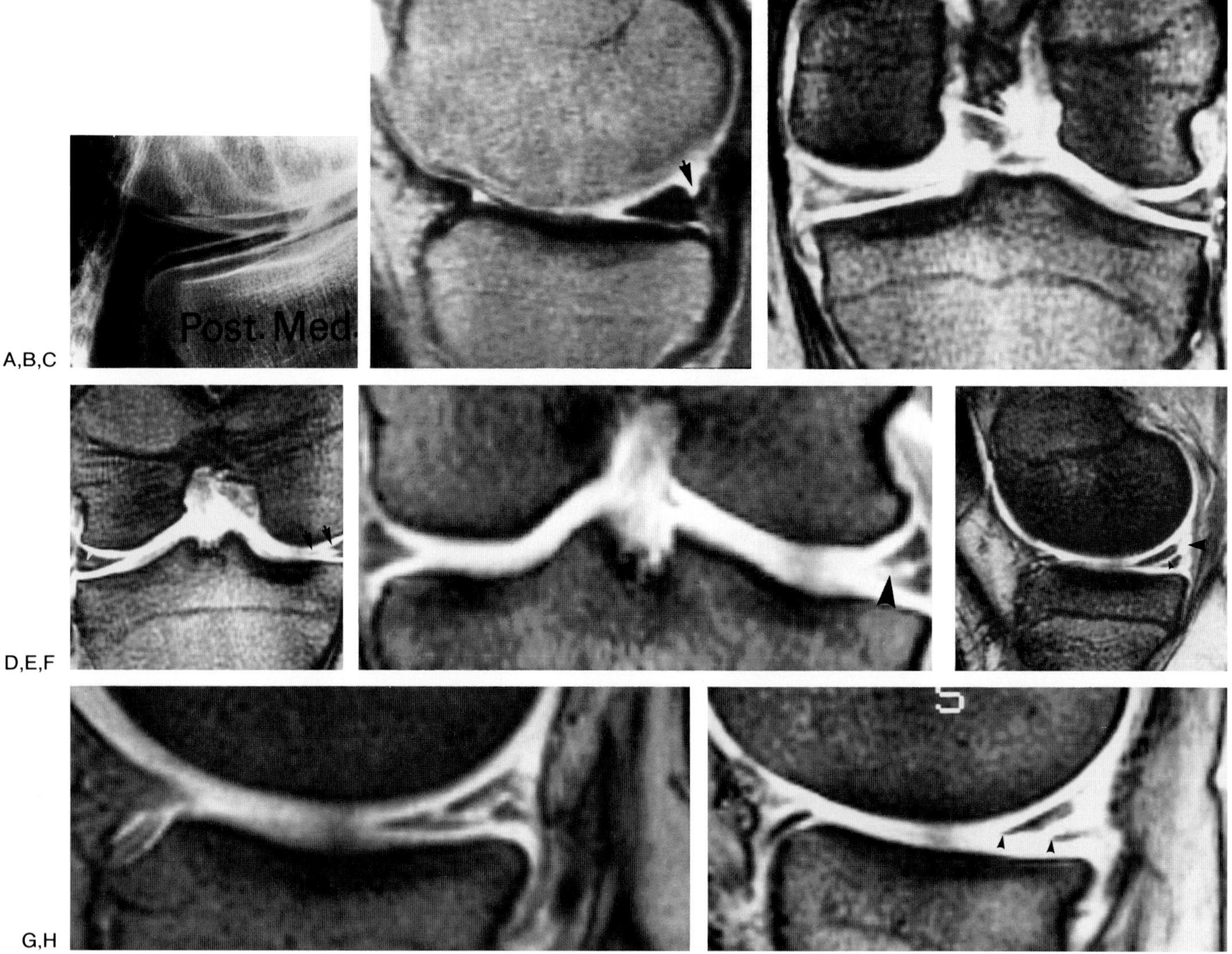

FIG. 7-29. Normal and abnormal menisci. **A:** Normal medial meniscus on a double-contrast arthrogram. **B:** Normal sagittal SE 2,000/60 image of the medial meniscus. There is no signal in the meniscus. Note the normal superior recess (*arrow*). **C:** Grade 1—globular increased signal intensity in both menisci on a coronal radial (MPGR) image. **D:** Grades 2 and 4—coronal GRIL image demonstrating a linear area of increased signal laterally (*white arrowhead*) and a bucket handle tear with meniscal deformity (*black arrows*) medially. **E:** Grade 3—gradient-echo (MPGR) image demonstrating a linear area of increased signal intensity (*arrowhead*) communicating with the articular surface (horizontal tear). **F:** Sagittal MPGR image demonstrating a grade 3A tear (*small arrowhead*) with an associated meniscal cyst (*large arrowhead*). **G:** Sagittal MPGR image demonstrating a more complex linear tear in the posterior horn of the medial meniscus. **H:** Grade 3B meniscal tear with a broad area of articular involvement (*arrowheads*).

of the inner fragment for variable distances (Figs. 7-31B–D and 7-35).

When bucket handle tears are identified, one must search carefully to be certain that the entire displaced fragment is identified (Fig. 7-35). Loose bodies or fragments of menisci in the intercondylar regions are not uncommon (25,66,75). These lesions may be very subtle such that reduction in the size of the meniscus may be the only finding (Figs. 7-31 and 7-35). Parrot beak tears (Fig. 7-34) are horizontal tears with vertical or radial components at the meniscal margin. These lesions are most common at the junction of the body and posterior horn of the lateral meniscus (25,66). Peripheral tears or separations in the meniscus can also be identified. These are usually easily diagnosed with arthrography but can be subtle on MR images due to vascular tissue and synoviomeniscal junction along the margins of the meniscus (Figs. 7-20, 7-22, and 7-35). It is important to clearly define the location (medial, lateral, inner margin, peripheral) and type of tear when possible. Grade 1 and 2 lesions will not be identified arthroscopically (21,22,49,80). Certain lesions are stable and can heal

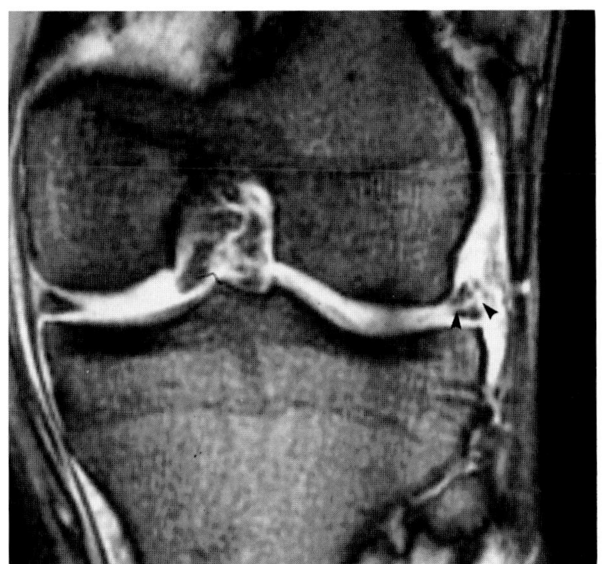

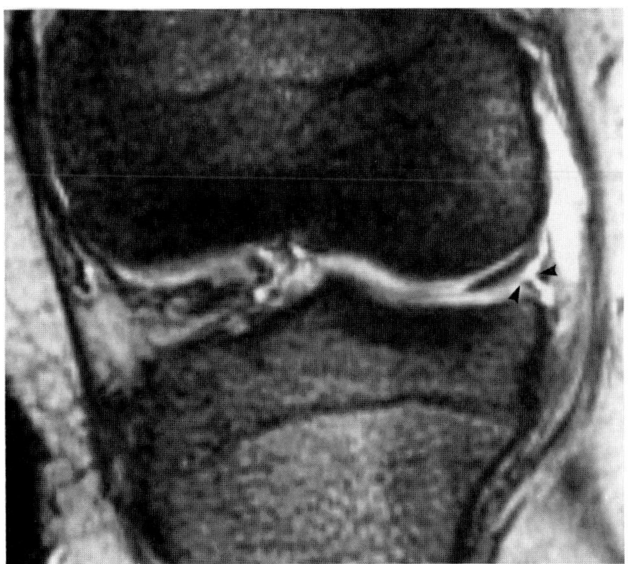

A,B

FIG. 7-30. Grade 4 meniscal tears. **A:** Complex degenerative tear in the lateral meniscus (*arrowheads*) on a coronal gradient-echo (MPGR) sequence. **B:** Oblique MPGR image demonstrating a complex (*arrowheads*) meniscal tear.

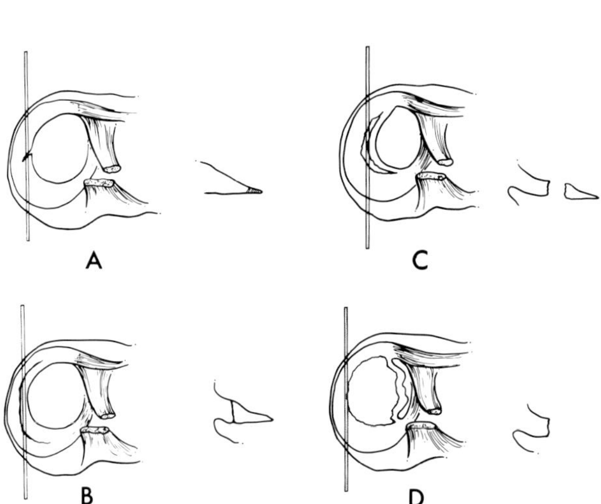

FIG. 7-31. Illustration of a radial tear (**A**) and bucket handle tears (**B–D**) with variable degrees of displacement. (From ref. 75, with permission.)

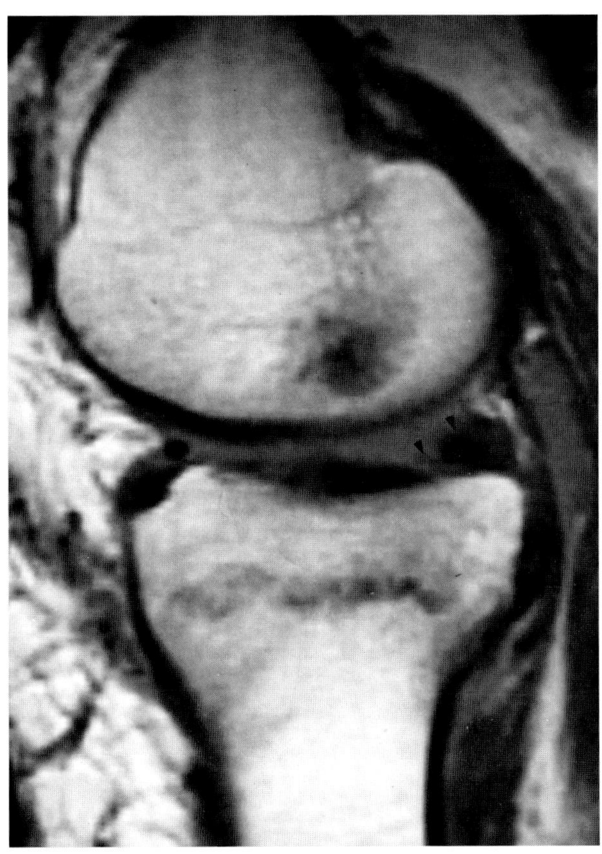

FIG. 7-32. SE 2,000/20 image demonstrating degeneration of the inner margin and dorsal articular surface of the posteromedial meniscus (*arrowheads*).

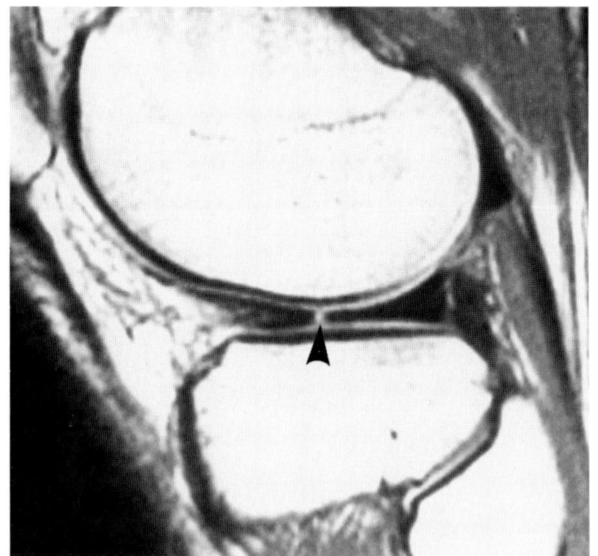

FIG. 7-33. Sagittal SE 2,000/20 image of the lateral meniscus, demonstrating a small radial tear in the margin of the body of the meniscus (*arrowhead*).

with conservative therapy so arthroscopy may be avoided. The vascular tissue along the periphery of the menisci may allow healing to occur (Fig. 7-36) (112).

Several reports in the MR literature have described the accuracy for MRI in identification of meniscal tears (29,95,104) (see Table 7-4). Sensitivity for MRI in detecting meniscal tears seen at arthroscopy ranges from 75 to 100%. Reicher et al. (80), using meniscal grading systems, reported a specificity of 92% and sensitivity of 89% for detection of meniscal lesions with MRI compared to arthroscopy. These same groups found the negative predicted value of MRI approached 100%. Review of our data demonstrated a sensitivity of 99%, specificity of 90%, accuracy of 90%, positive predictive value of 96%, and negative predicted value of 98% for the medial meniscus. MRI of the lateral meniscus showed a 97% sensitivity, 97% specificity, and 91% accuracy.

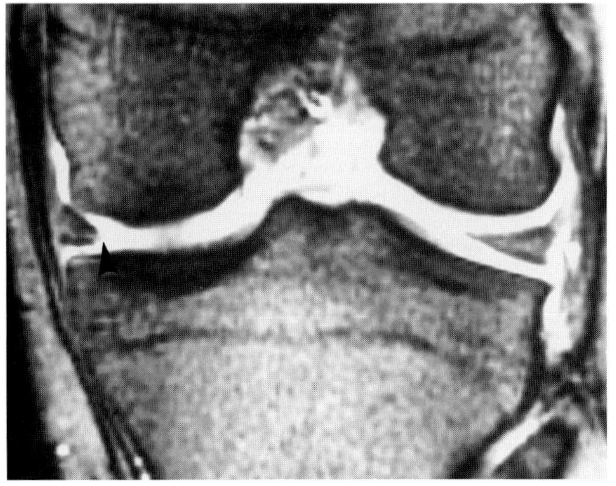

FIG. 7-34. Coronal MPGR image showing grade 1 signal intensity in the lateral meniscus. There is a horizontal tear in the medial meniscus and the meniscus is shortened with the inner margin (*arrowhead*) absent. Parrot beak or bucket handle?

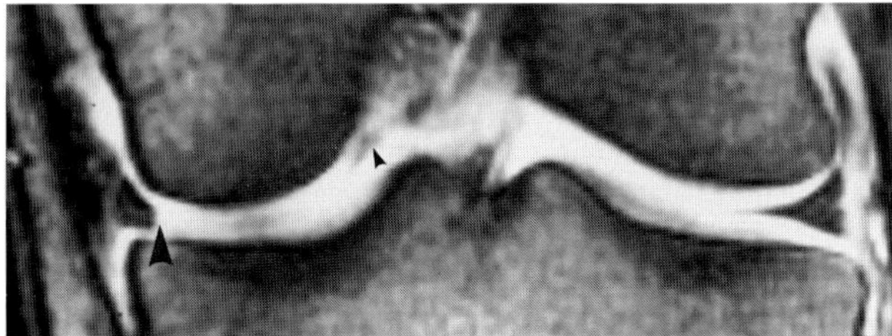

FIG. 7-35. Bucket handle tear with shortening of the medial meniscus (*large arrowhead*) and marked displacement of the inner fragment (*small arrowhead*).

One could consider arthrography as an equally effective tool in evaluating only meniscal lesions (accuracy 91% medial meniscus, 81% lateral meniscus), although it is clearly not as valuable in evaluating the other structures in the knee (66,75). However, even in this setting there are two situations where MRI is clearly superior and a more effective technique. This would include children with knee pain and patients with acute trauma and hemarthrosis.

MRI is also of value in studying patients who have had either partial or complete meniscectomy or arthroscopic repairs of the meniscus. Patients who have been treated in this manner are generally referred to exclude residual fragments, remnants of a tear that was not completely resected, or new tears. Interpretation of MR images following surgery for meniscal tears should not be approached differently than for MR images performed on nonoperated knees. Signal intensity changes noted within the menisci are similar and unless communication with the articular surface is identified, a tear should not be suggested.

Meniscal Cysts

MRI is also of value in detecting other pathology such as meniscal cysts. Meniscal cysts have been reported in up to 1% of patients undergoing meniscectomy. Most cysts are located in the lateral meniscus, but they may occur along the margin of either meniscus (Fig. 7-29F) (15,18). The patients typically present with localized tenderness and occasionally swelling along the joint line. Similar presentations can be noted in patients with periarticular ganglion cysts. Ganglion cysts may or may not have a clearly defined connection with the joint. They may also occur along the periarticular tendon sheaths and tibiofibular joint (15). Popliteal cysts are typically located posteromedially near the medial head of the gastrocnemius (15,43). Distinction between these conditions is important as operative management of menis-

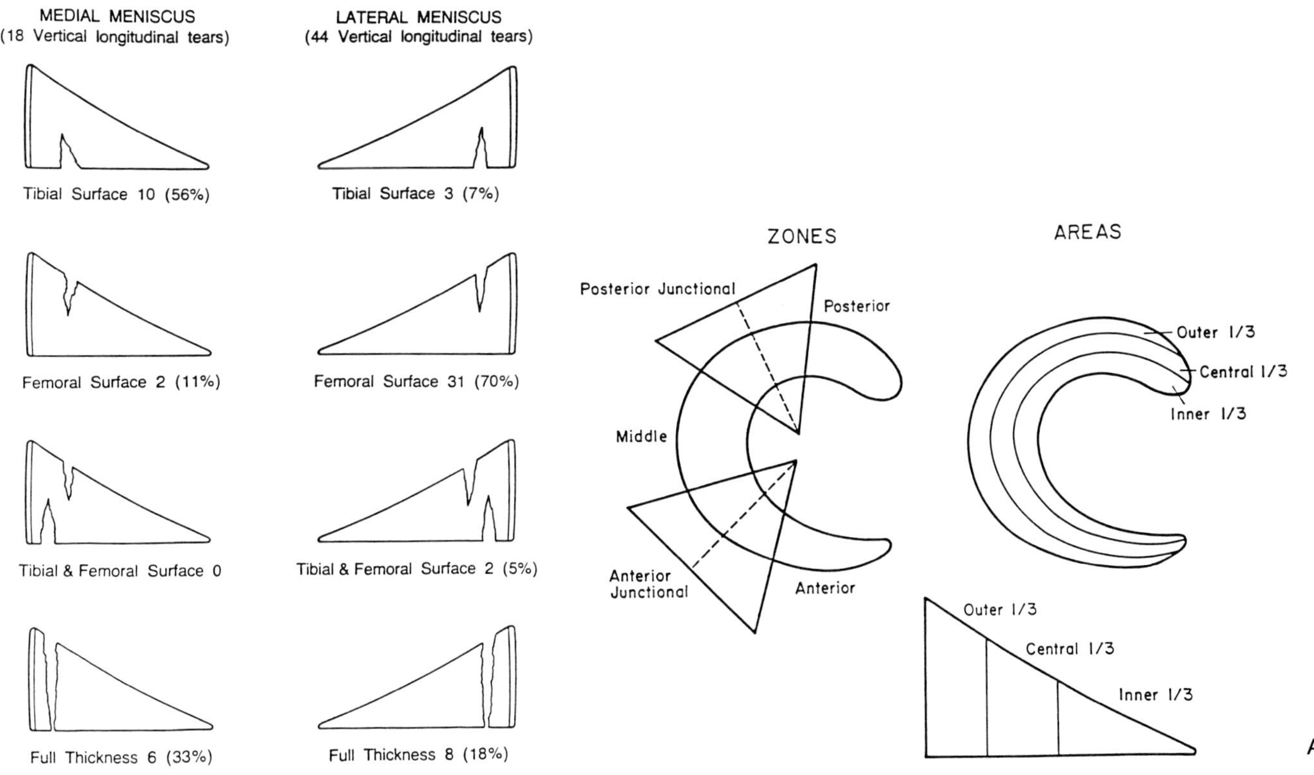

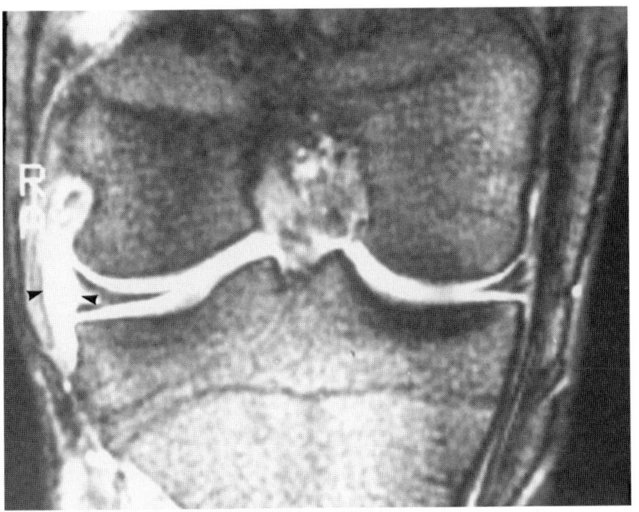

FIG. 7-36. **A:** Illustration of stable peripheral meniscal tears. **B:** Illustration of zones and areas of the meniscus that are important to use when describing meniscal tears. (From ref. 112, with permission.) **C:** Coronal MPGR image demonstrating a peripheral detachment. Note the high signal zone (*arrowheads*) separating the meniscus from the capsule.

TABLE 7-4. *MRI of meniscal tears*

	Mayo series		Reicher et al. (78,79)		Glashow et al. (29)	Crues et al. (19,20)		Polly et al. (74)		Munk et al. (68)	
	MM[a]	LM[b]	MM	LM	Both menisci	MM	LM	MM	LM	MM	LM
Number of cases	129	129	69	69	50	144	144	54	54	242	242
Accuracy	90%	91%	77%	78%	—	89%	94%	98%	90%	94%	92%
Sensitivity	99%	97%	84%	58%	83%	87%	88%	95.8%	66.7%	97%	92%
Specificity	90%	97%	80%	100%	84%	91%	98%	100%	95.1%	89%	91%
Positive predictive value	96%	76%	84%	92%	75%	93%	96%	—	—	—	—
Negative predictive value	98%	99%	69%	86%	90%	84%	92%	—	—	—	—

[a] MM, medial meniscus.
[b] LM, lateral meniscus.

cal cysts is more commonly required. Popliteal ganglion cysts, however, if persistently symptomatic may also require resection. Medial cysts, though less common, frequently tend to be asymptomatic even though they may be larger than cysts in the lateral meniscus (15,18,66).

The etiology of meniscal cysts is controversial. Various theories have been proposed including chronic infection, hemorrhage, and mucoid degeneration. Since the fluid is similar to synovial fluid, it is hypothesized that a tear in the meniscus may lead to fluid accumulation within the meniscal tear itself leading to cyst formation (Fig. 7-29F). It is likely that the etiology is multifactorial; however, most authors exclude hemorrhage and infection as causes (15,66).

MRI features of meniscal cysts and ganglia are easily appreciated on T2 weighted and gradient-echo sequences (Fig. 7-37). Both are well-marginated, high-intensity lesions. Meniscal cysts tend to be within or at the margin of the meniscus while ganglion cysts may extend from the capsule or be located in the periarticular soft tissues (Fig. 7-38) (15,18).

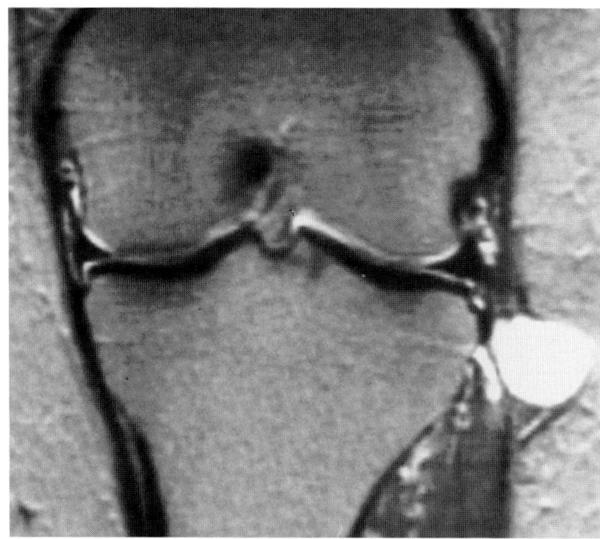

FIG. 7-38. Ganglion cyst. Coronal SE 2,000/60 image demonstrating a well-defined, high signal intensity lesion below the lateral joint line. The meniscus is normal.

Discoid Menisci

Discoid menisci are uncommon and are reported in 1.5–15.5% of lateral menisci (35,66). Discoid medial menisci are rare. Both the etiology and classification of discoid menisci are controversial. Hall (35) has described an arthrographic classification that we prefer to use.

Discoid menisci are typically broad and disk shaped. This configuration and the extension into the joint make this meniscus more susceptible to tearing. Type 1 discoid menisci are thick, slablike menisci with parallel superior and inferior surfaces. Type 2 are more slablike with a thin central portion. Type 3 discoid menisci are only slightly larger than normal menisci (Fig. 7-22). Type 4 are asymmetric with the anterior horn extending farther into the joint than the posterior horn. Type 5 is between normal and slab type and type 6 is any of the above with an associated tear (Fig. 7-39) (35,75).

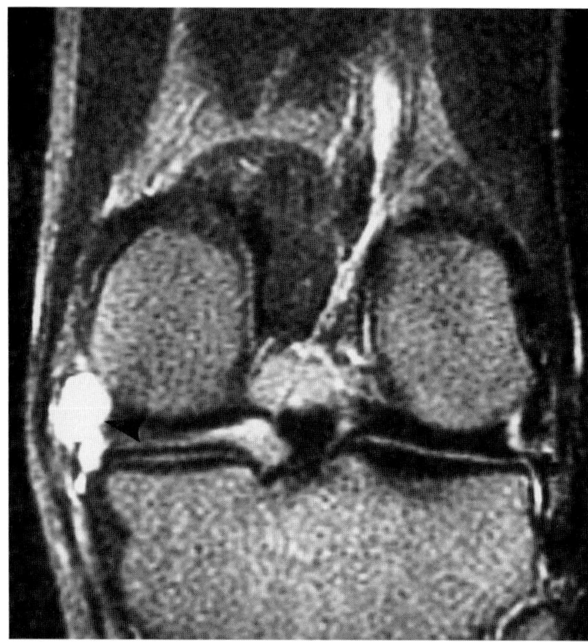

FIG. 7-37. Coronal gradient-echo (MPGR) image demonstrating a medial meniscal cyst (*arrowhead*).

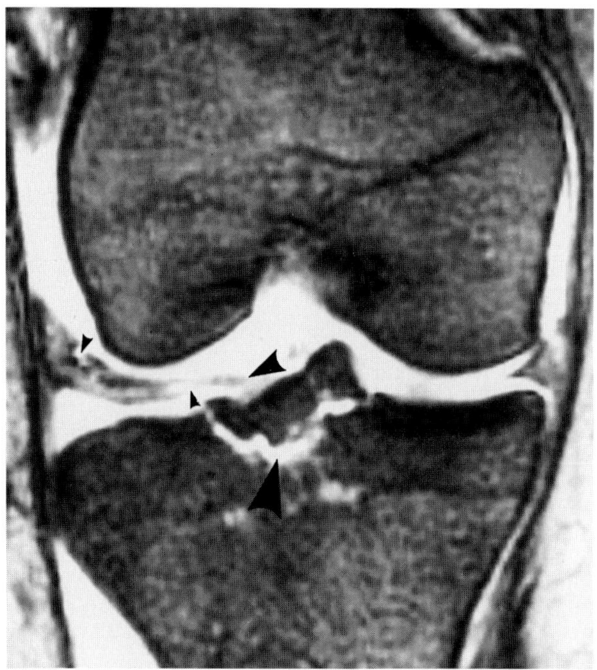

FIG. 7-39. Gradient-echo (MPGR) image demonstrating a large discoid lateral meniscus extending into the midjoint space (*arrowhead*). There are multiple tears (*small arrowheads*) and a tibial spine fracture (*large arrowhead*).

Clinically patients with a discoid meniscus present with symptoms of snapping and occasionally pain as these menisci are more prone to tear. Though there is no large series of MR findings in discoid menisci, Hartzman et al. (40) and Mink et al. (66) did report a series describing the MR findings. The transverse diameter of the normal meniscus is approximately 10–11 mm and, therefore, the increased transverse diameter of a discoid meniscus can result in typical findings on both coronal and sagittal MR images. For example, on sagittal 5 mm slices, only two slices should demonstrate the meniscus. Visualization of the meniscus in more than three slices is indicative of a discoid meniscus. Coronal and radial images of the meniscus are perhaps more useful in that the true extension into the joint can be better demonstrated (Figs. 7-22 and 7-39) (66,75).

Ligament Injuries

Complete evaluation of the capsule, medial, and lateral collateral ligaments and cruciate ligaments in the knee has been difficult with conventional arthrography and arthrotomography. Multiplanar MRI provides significant improvement in our ability to assess these structures. The anatomy of the ligaments of the knee was discussed in the initial section of this chapter; however, some review is necessary in discussing the technical aspects for evaluating these structures. The anterior cruciate ligament, because of its oblique course (Fig. 7-10A), can be more difficult to identify and in early studies, prior to oblique off-axis imaging, the ability to completely demonstrate the anterior cruciate ligament in a given slice was significantly hindered. Our initial review demonstrated that incomplete evaluation of the anterior cruciate ligament occurred in up to 30% of cases. Improved positioning (15°–20° external rotation) and software developments have greatly improved our ability to demonstrate the ligaments of the knee (Fig. 7-40) (10,54,65,67,78,86).

The anterior cruciate, through its oblique course, is intra-articular but extrasynovial (43,108). This ligament is one of the main stabilizers of the knee, preventing excessive anterior displacement of the femur on the tibia (75). Typically the anatomic appearance on MR images varies with the anterior cruciate having multiple fibers that are seen as linear areas of low signal intensity compared to the thicker and more uniform low signal intensity of the posterior cruciate ligament (Fig. 7-41). Though oblique sagittal or externally rotated (20°–30°) true sagittal images are optimal, the anterior cruciate ligament (ACL) should also be studied in other image planes (Figs. 7-42 and 7-43). Tears in the ACL occur with internal rotation of the femur on the tibia with the knee extended. Up to 70% of patients have other intraarticular injuries, most often the posteromedial meniscus (66,75). The posterior cruciate ligament is thicker and has a midline sagittal course and is therefore not difficult to visualize on MR sagittal images (10,66,75). This ligament serves as a stabilizer of the knee in flexion, extension, and internal rotation (75). Tears of the PCL occur with posterior force to the flexed knee or forced hyperextension (69).

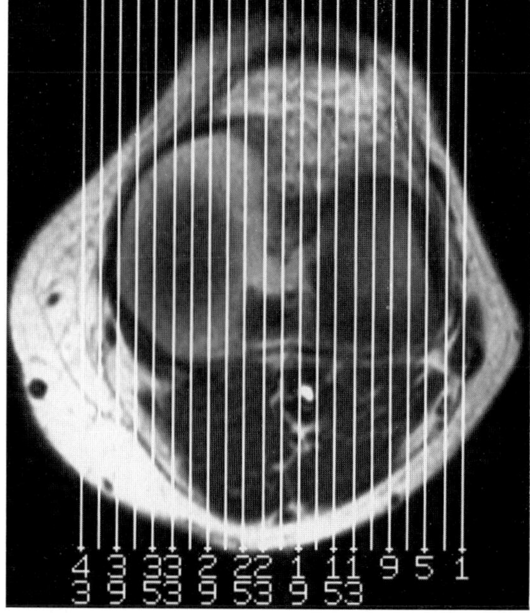

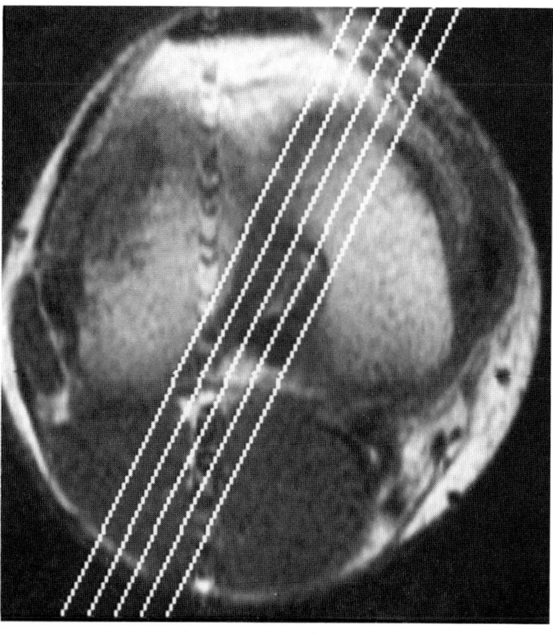

A,B

FIG. 7-40. Scout image with typical sagittal selections (**A**) and oblique sagittal plane selection (**B**) to demonstrate the cruciate ligament.

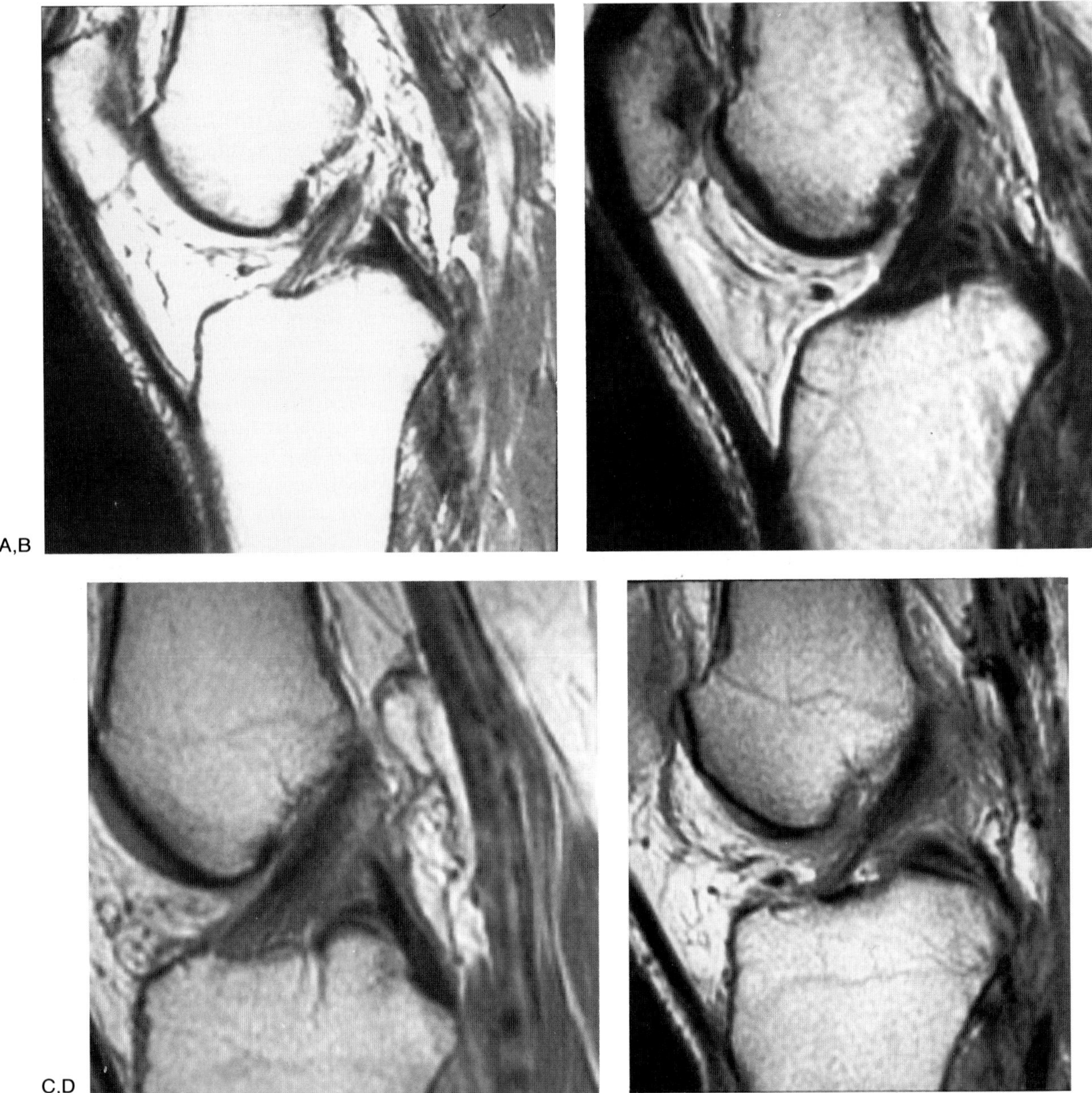

FIG. 7-41. Variations in appearance of the normal anterior cruciate ligament. **A:** SE 500/20 sagittal image demonstrating the normal course of the cruciate ligament even though the femoral attachment is not completely seen. Note the thin low-intensity fibers with interspersed bands of intermediate signal intensity. **B:** Sagittal SE 500/20 image demonstrating a thicker low-intensity normal anterior cruciate ligament. The entire structure is visualized. (**C, D**) SE 2,000/30 sagittal images demonstrating normal anterior cruciate ligaments with variable degrees of signal intensity and low-intensity fibrous bands.

Technique for routine examination of the knee was described above and is generally adequate for evaluation of the cruciate ligaments and medial and lateral collateral ligaments. In certain cases, the anterior cruciate ligament may be incompletely seen, in which case repeat oblique images can easily be obtained. One should strive to demonstrate both cruciate ligaments completely on a single slice to more easily assess abnormalities (Fig. 7-40).

MRI findings with disruption of either the anterior or posterior cruciate ligament are similar (Table 7-5). The appearance or signal intensity will, of course, vary with the age of the lesion. We prefer T2 weighted images for assessment of the cruciate ligaments because the high signal intensity seen with acute lesions provides excellent contrast compared to the normally low signal intensity (black) ligaments (Fig. 7-44). Mink et al. (66) found T2 weighted sequences to be more sensitive and

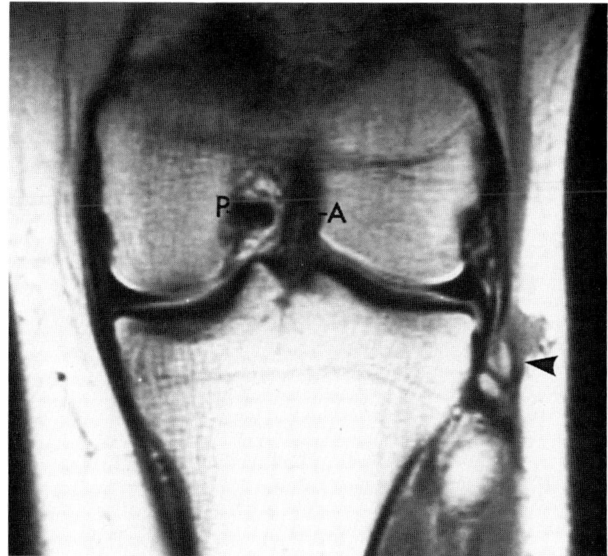

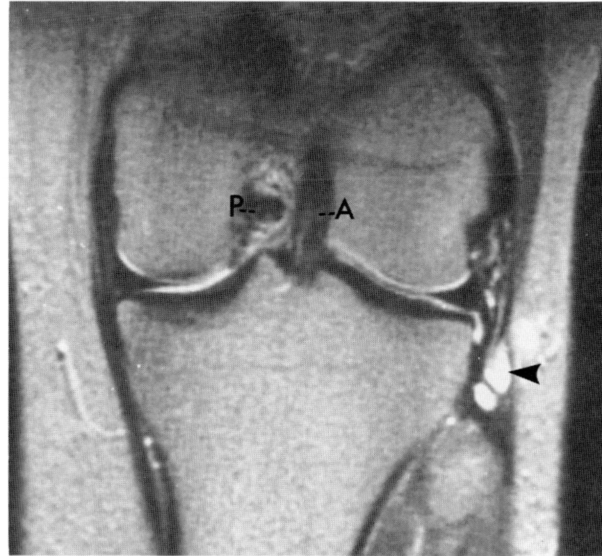

FIG. 7-42. Coronal SE 500/20 (**A**) and SE 2,000/60 (**B**) images demonstrate normal posterior (P) and anterior (A) cruciate ligaments. Note the capsular defect and post-traumatic cyst laterally (*arrowhead*).

accurate than T1 weighted sequences. Sensitivity was 85%, specificity 95%, and accuracy 94% using T1 weighted sequences compared to 100%, 91%, and 97%, respectively, for T2 weighted sequences. We prefer the double-echo (SE 2,000/60,20) technique because increasing signal intensity on the second echo (SE 2,000/60) confirms the acute nature of the injury (Fig. 7-45). Acute tears are seen as areas of high signal intensity in the tendons, usually at either the tibial or femoral attachments. Disruption at the femoral attachment is more common (Fig. 7-46) (25). With complete tears, the signal intensity extends throughout the width of the tendon and there is usually separation of the tendon ends at the site of the tear with laxity or loss of the normal straight appearance of the anterior cruciate ligament (Figs. 7-44 to 7-46). Chronic tears are seen as areas of intermediate signal intensity, typically with tendon thickening and associated ligament laxity (Fig. 7-47). The MRI findings in posterior cruciate tears are similar to anterior cruciate tears except that the course of the ligament is not as useful because the posterior cruciate ligament typically has a more curved appearance with convexity of its upper surface (Fig. 7-48). Changes in the

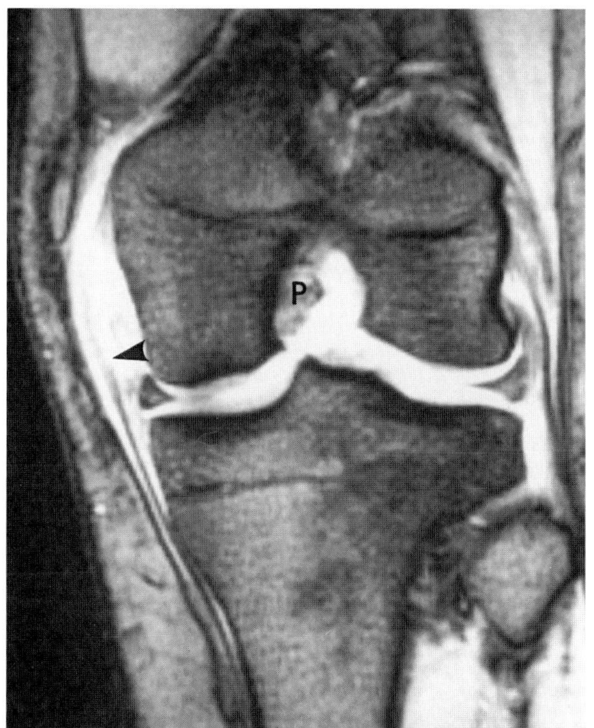

FIG. 7-43. Gradient-echo (MPGR) image in a patient with a medial collateral ligament tear (*arrowhead*). The posterior cruciate is seen in the medial aspect of the notch (P). There is no anterior cruciate ligament. Compare to Fig. 7-42.

TABLE 7-5. *Criteria for anterior cruciate ligament tears* (54,65,66)

Acute—complete
1. Discontinuity with increased signal intensity between segments or at femoral attachment on T2 weighted sequences.
2. Flat or horizontal distal (tibial segment) with high signal intensity near the femoral attachment.
3. Wavy ligament or curved course.
4. Acute angulation of an intact posterior cruciate ligament.

Acute—incomplete
1. Areas of increased signal intensity and thickening on T2 weighted sequences.

Chronic
1. Thickening with slight increase in signal intensity that does not increase on second echo of T2 weighted (SE 2,000/60,20) sequence.
2. Irregularity and atrophy.

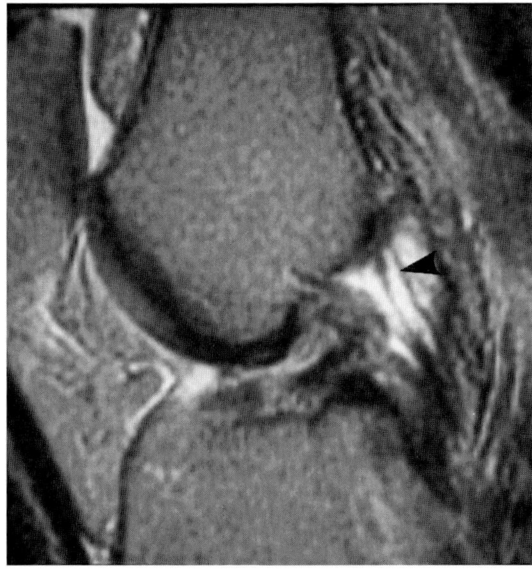

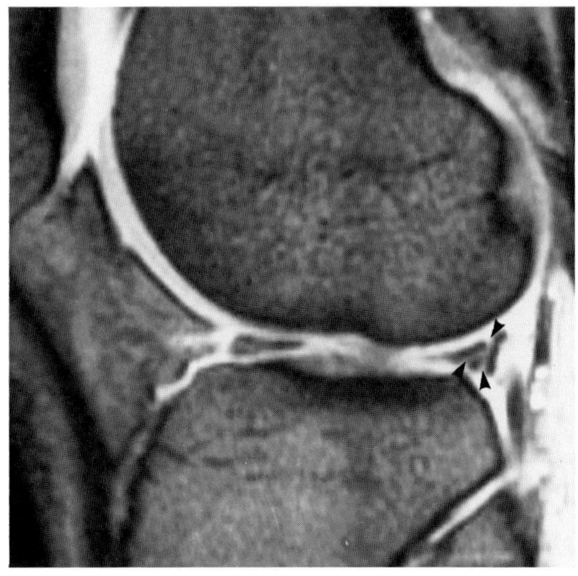

A,B

FIG. 7-44. Acute anterior cruciate ligament tear with a complex tear of the posterior horn of the lateral meniscus (*small arrowheads*). **A:** Sagittal SE 2,000/60 image shows increased signal intensity at the femoral attachment (*arrowhead*). **B:** No anterior cruciate ligament is identified on this section.

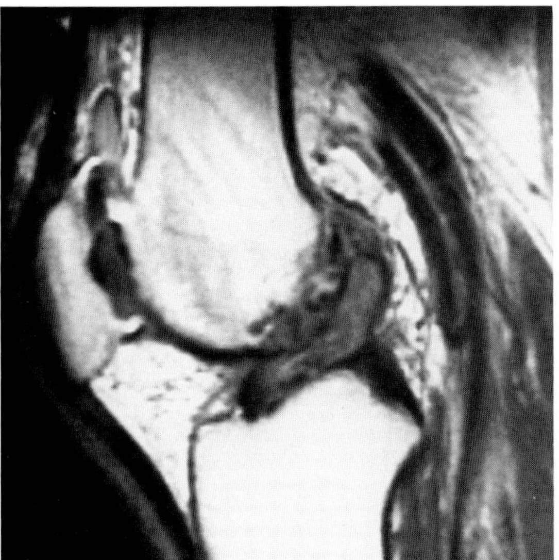

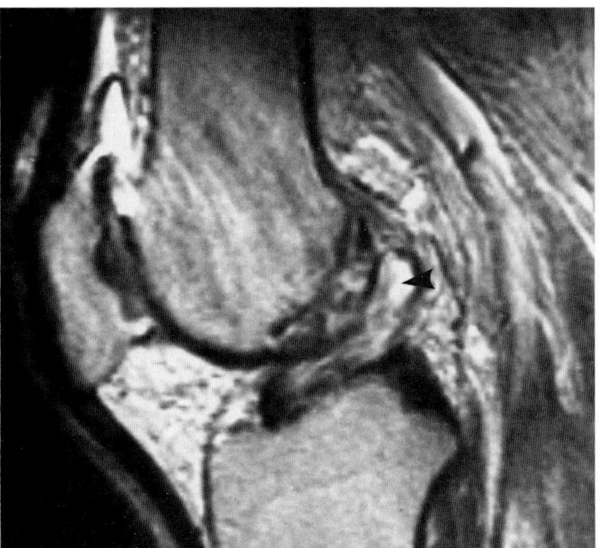

A,B

FIG. 7-45. SE 2,000/20 (**A**) and SE 2,000/60 (**B**) images show thickening, an S-shaped course, and increased signal intensity (*arrowhead*) at the femoral attachment due to an ACL tear. The motion artifact is more evident on the second echo (**B**).

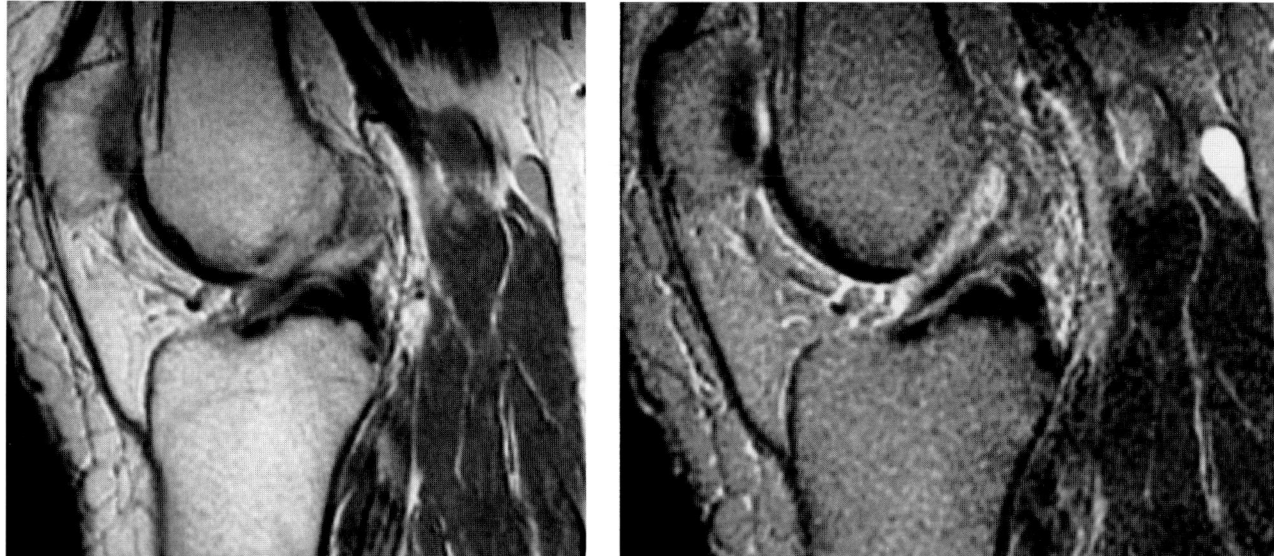

A,B

FIG. 7-46. ACL tear. SE 2,000/20 (**A**) and SE 2,000/60 (**B**) sagittal images demonstrate a thin irregular anterior cruciate with increased signal intensity at the femoral attachment.

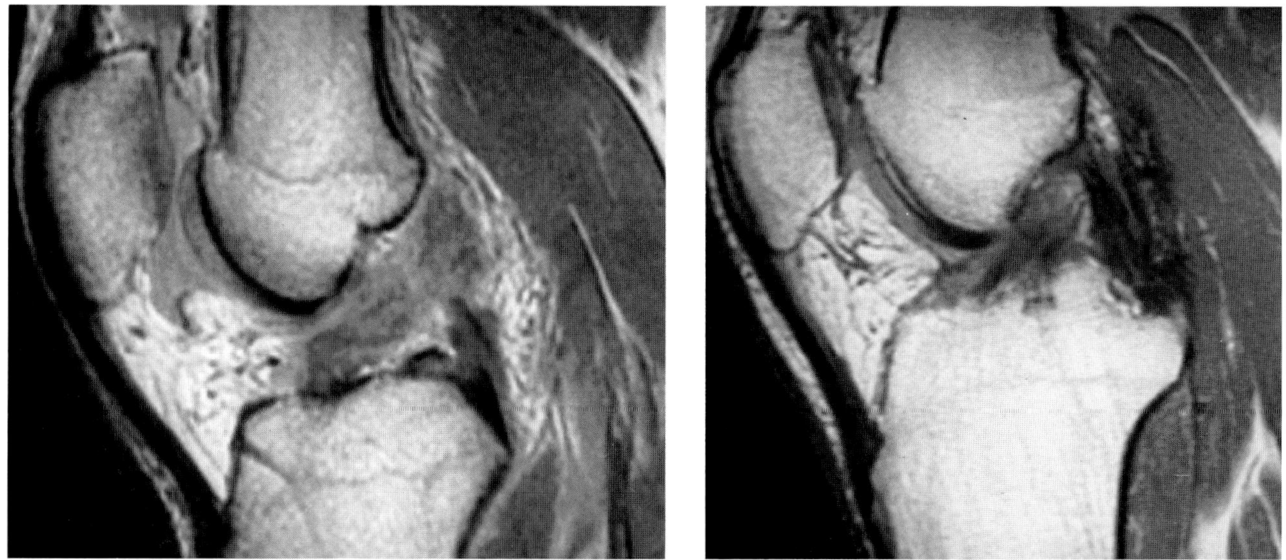

A,B

FIG. 7-47. Chronic ACL injuries. Sagittal images (SE 2,000/20) show thickening and irregularity of the ACL (**A**) and involvement of both ligaments (**B**).

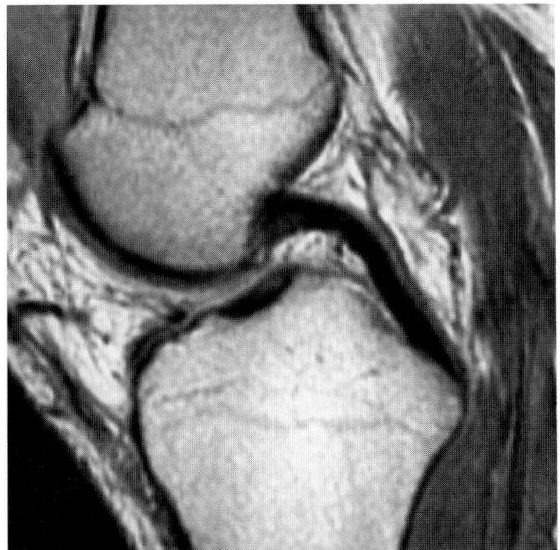

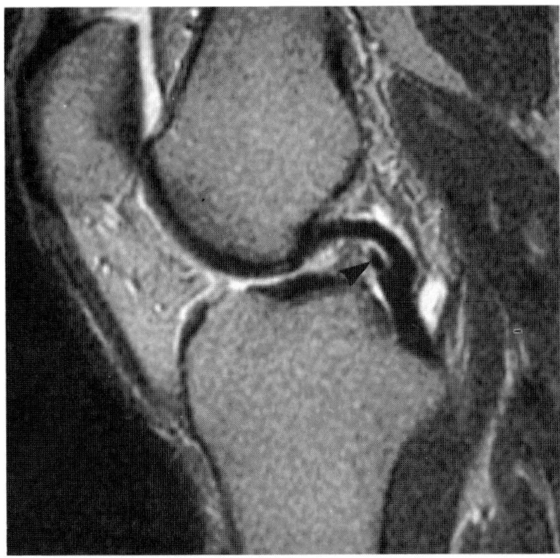

A,B

FIG. 7-48. Normal posterior cruciate ligaments. **A:** Sagittal SE 2,000/20 showing the normal slightly curved course and thickness of the PCL. **B:** Sagittal SE 2,000/60 image showing a normal PCL with the ligament of Humphrey anteriorly (*arrowhead*).

configuration of the posterior cruciate ligament are useful as a secondary sign of anterior cruciate ligament disruption (Fig. 7-49). An acute angle in the upper portion of the posterior cruciate ligament forming a question mark configuration suggests a positive drawer sign due to anterior cruciate ligament tear (Fig. 7-50).

Early and recent arthrographic studies of these ligaments indicate an accuracy of 91% for evaluation of the posterior cruciate ligament but only 50% for the anterior cruciate ligament using conventional arthrography or CT arthrography. Accuracy of the anterior cruciate ligament may be increased by using stressed crosstable lateral techniques (75). MRI is more accurate than arthrographic techniques. Using the criteria in Table 7-5, Mink et al. (64–66) found MRI correlated with arthroscopy in 95% of cases. Our data demonstrated an accuracy of 95%, specificity of 98%, positive predictive value of 88%, and a negative predictive value of 96%.

Evaluation of cruciate repairs can be more difficult with MRI (66,83). The technique used may involve metal staples or bone plugs fixed with screws, causing significant metal artifact. If metal is not present, the tendon or ligament grafts used have a similar appearance to the normal ligament (86). The tunnel, integrity,

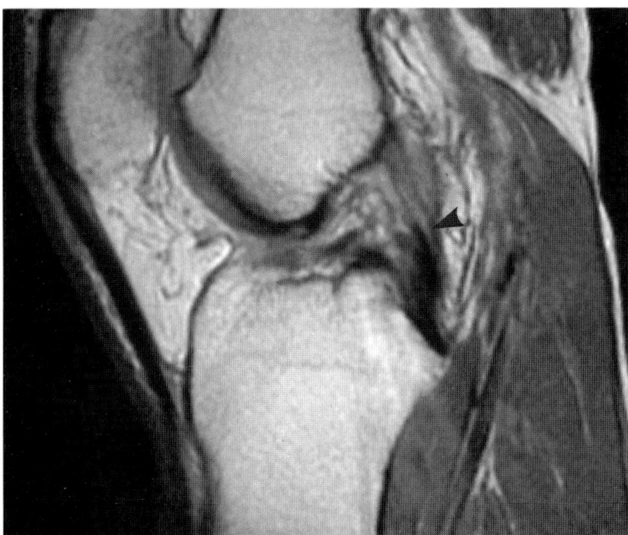

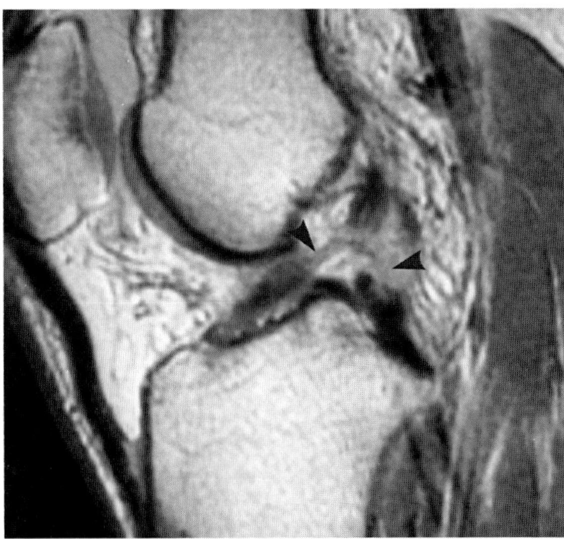

A,B

FIG. 7-49. Sagittal SE 2,000/20 images demonstrating tears in the PCL (*arrowhead*) (**A**) and both the ACL (*arrowhead*) and PCL (*arrowhead*) (**B**).

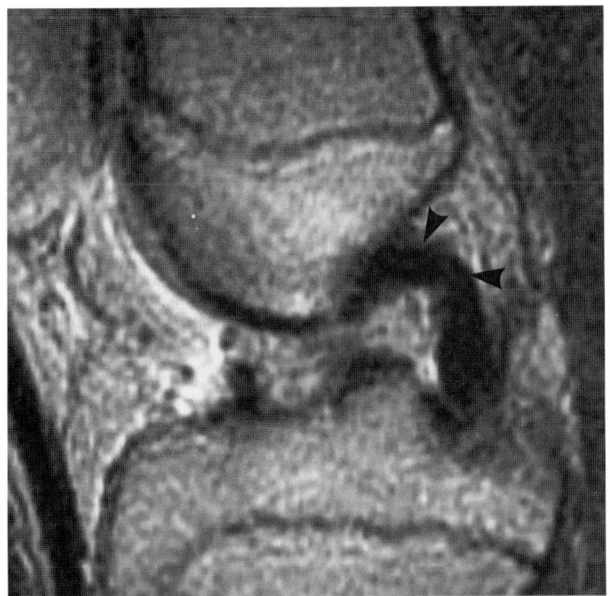

FIG. 7-50. Sagittal SE 2,000/60 image in a patient with an ACL tear and buckling of the PCL (*arrowhead*) and a positive drawer sign.

and the course of the ligament can be assessed with MRI (Fig. 7-51).

Evaluation of the medial and lateral collateral ligaments is generally easily accomplished using the routine MR examination. However, in some cases additional axial and coronal slices may be necessary to more clearly define subtle lesions. The medial collateral ligament is typically divided into superficial and deep bands (Figs. 7-6 and 7-9B). The superficial portion of the ligament typically arises from the medial femoral condyle and passes distally to insert approximately 5 cm below the joint line. Superficial fibers are separated from the deep fibers by a bursa, which may be inflamed and enlarged and should not be confused with a tear in the medial collateral ligament (Fig. 7-22). The deep ligament is firmly attached to the capsule (Fig. 7-10) and midportion of the medial meniscus and attaches to the femur and tibia more nearly adjacent to the joint. The medial collateral ligament is a stabilizer that resists external rotation and anterior forces and is more often injured than its lateral counterpart. Tears of the anterior cruciate ligament are frequently noted in association with MCL tears (30%) (Figs. 7-10 and 7-52) (75).

The lateral or fibular collateral ligament (Fig. 7-10) originates from the lateral epicondyle above the popliteus tendon and courses posteriorly and inferiorly to join the biceps femoris tendon and together they insert on the fibular head. These structures, along with the iliotibial band, fabellofibular ligament, and arcuate ligament, provide the lateral support for the knee (66,75). The fibular collateral ligament is not immediately associated with the capsule and is much less frequently injured than the medial collateral ligament. When the ligament is disrupted it is not uncommon to identify associated tears in the posterior cruciate ligament.

Acute incomplete tears result in areas of increased signal intensity in the soft tissues and within the normally dark appearing ligaments. When an incomplete tear is present, the joint space is normal and the course of the ligament unchanged. Care should be taken not to misinterpret the medial collateral ligament bursa or fat between its superficial and deep fibers as an incomplete injury. Complete tears in either ligament are identified by increased signal intensity at the site of the tear with lack of continuity of the ligament and typically retraction of the torn ends (Fig. 7-52). Secondary findings, such as joint space widening, are not unusual (10,25,75).

Assessment of the quadriceps tendon and patellar ligament is easily accomplished on sagittal MR images (Fig. 7-53) (10). Thus, routine knee screening examination is adequate. Inflammation and acute disruption have been detected with MRI (12,23,31). When a tear in either of these structures is identified, it is important to obtain axial images so that classification of the tear can be more accurately completed. Again, T2 weighted or gradient-echo sequences are preferred to identify and classify these injuries. These injuries are usually more evident clinically and can often be palpated. Therefore, MRI may not be necessary except to define the exact extent of the lesion.

MRI of the knee has progressed rapidly as a clinical imaging technique because of its ability to accurately screen for meniscal, ligament, bony, and periarticular soft tissue injuries. It has become the technique of choice for evaluation of knee injuries and has largely replaced arthrography in diagnosis of knee trauma. This is especially true in children and in patients with acute hemarthrosis. In a traumatic setting, there is little need to perform arthrography. The only indication for arthrography of the knee would be to confirm needle position prior to aspiration or injection following trauma. Arthrography and specifically aspiration of the knee may be indicated in other clinical settings (25,66,75).

Plicae

The significance of synovial plicae was not fully recognized prior to the advent of arthroscopy (4,75). Plicae are embryonic synovial remnants that may be present in an asymptomatic knee. During fetal development there are thin membranes that divide the knee into medial, lateral, and suprapatellar compartments. During development these membranes involute, resulting in a single cavity in the knee. When the membrane or a portion of it persists into adult life it is termed a plica. These remnants are reported in up to 20% of the population

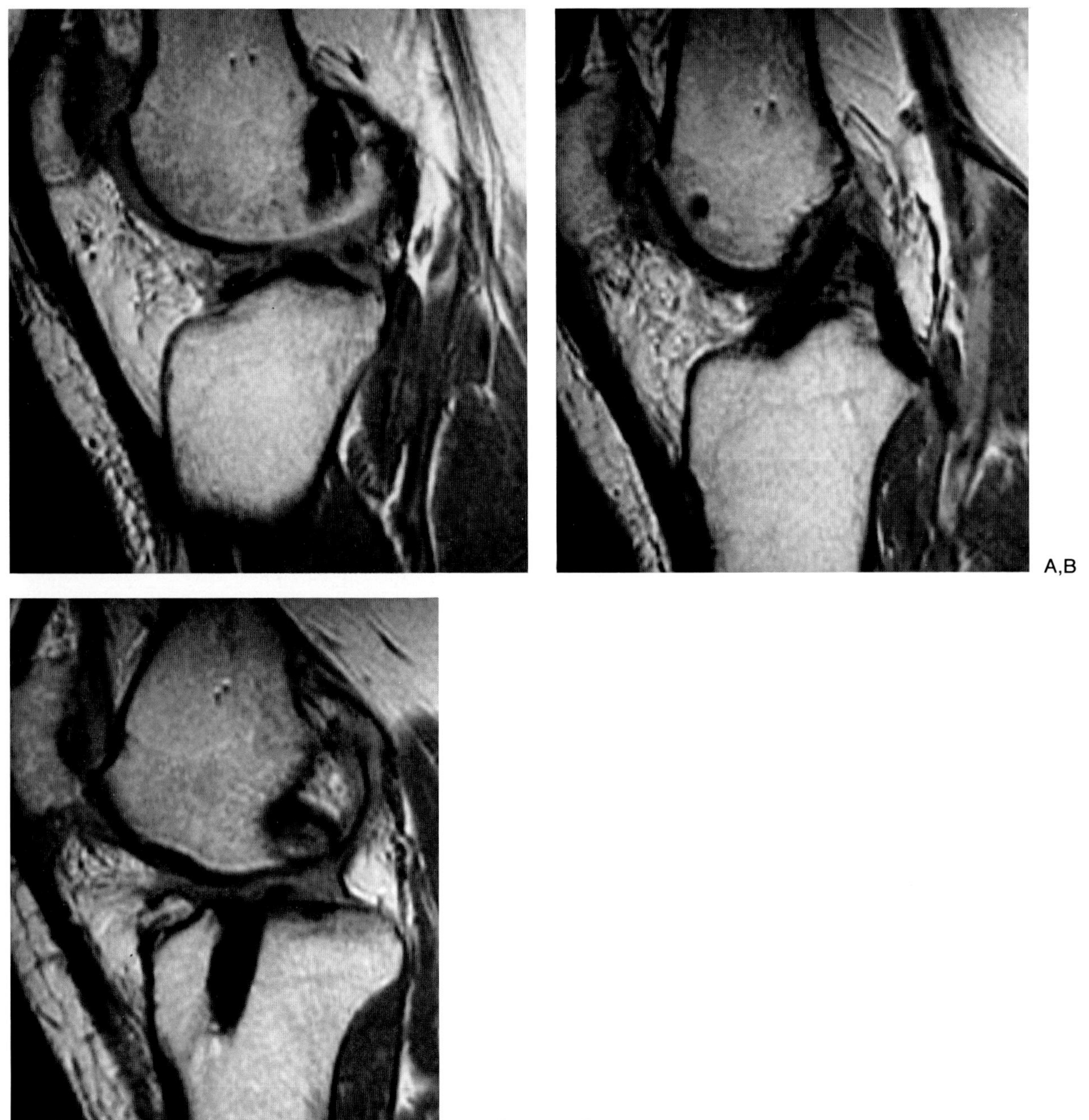

A,B

C

FIG. 7-51. Sequential sagittal images (**A–C**) after ACL repair, demonstrating the intact ligament graft and osseous tunnels.

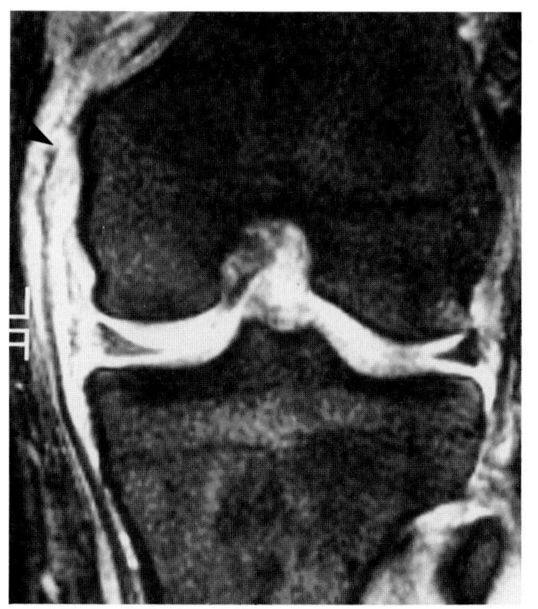

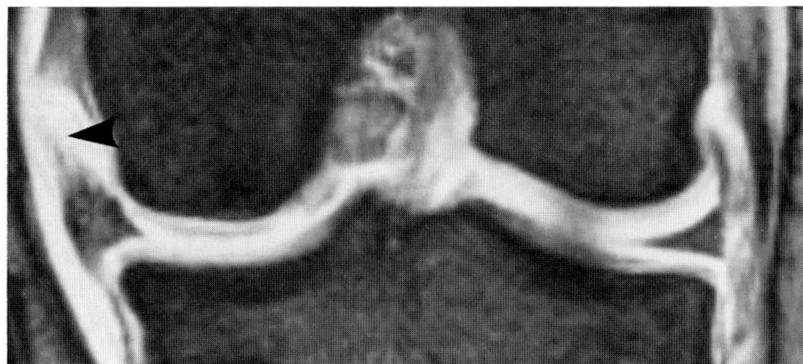

A,B

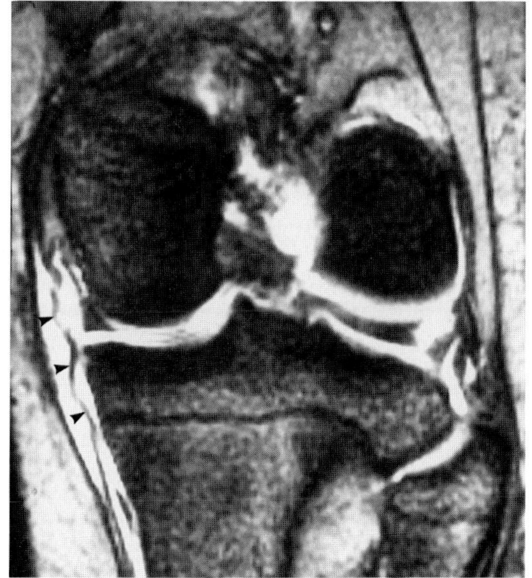

C

FIG. 7-52. Medial collateral ligament (MCL) tears demonstrated on gradient-echo MPGR images. **A:** Coronal image with increased signal along the MCL and a complete tear (*arrowhead*) near the femoral origin. **B:** Complete tear of the capsule and MCL (*arrowhead*) just above the meniscus. **C:** Wavy MCL (*arrowheads*) due to a complete tear proximally.

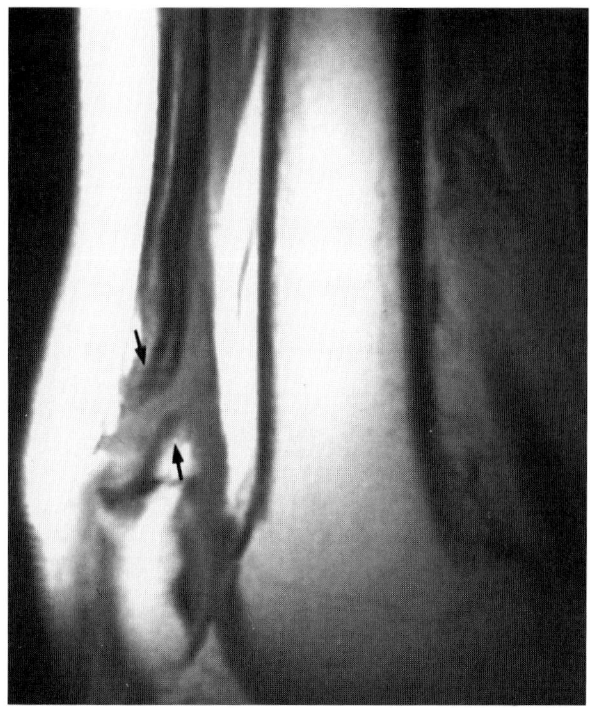

FIG. 7-53. Sagittal SE 2,000/20 image of the knee, demonstrating a complete tear (*arrows*) in the quadriceps tendon.

(36,71). These plicae (Fig. 7-54) are classified as suprapatellar, mediopatellar, and infrapatellar based on the location of the original fetal membrane (71).

The suprapatellar plica is the remnant that separated the suprapatellar bursa from the medial and lateral compartments (Fig. 7-54). Several forms have been observed: a transverse septum with a small central communication and medial or lateral remnants (Fig. 7-54). The medial suprapatellar plica is the most common. On sagittal MR or CT images this can be seen as a fold of soft tissue extending through the suprapatellar bursa above the patella.

The mediopatellar plica begins above the patella medially and progresses distally to insert on the synovium above the infrapatellar fat pad (Fig. 7-54) (4,36).

The infrapatellar plica is detected most frequently. This plica follows a course along the upper margin of the anterior cruciate ligament. It is rarely symptomatic (4,36).

With chronic inflammation these membranes can become thickened and cause clicking or snapping as they pass over the femoral condyles. When left untreated, synovitis and cartilage damage can occur (36,71). The exact etiology is unclear but trauma and other associated conditions, such as osteoarthritis and loose bodies, may be evident (36,78). Most patients (90%) present with tenderness above the joint near the superior pole of the patella. A snap can be demonstrated in 71% of patients. Symptoms are generally due to thickening of the mediopatellar plica; however, the suprapatellar plica has been implicated in patellar tracking abnormalities (36). Arthroscopic or open synovectomy may be necessary to relieve symptoms (36).

When patients present with symptoms suggesting plicae syndrome (snapping, peripatellar pain), the MR examination must be modified. The T2 weighted sagittal images are adequate for identification of the suprapatellar and infrapatellar plicae. However, axial T1 weighted or T2 weighted images are indicated to identify the mediopatellar plicae. In the presence of an effusion, a T2 weighted sequence or gradient-echo sequence is preferred. The low signal intensity plica is more easily seen with the high signal intensity synovial fluid.

Patellar Disorders

Patellofemoral pain syndromes are commonly related to chondromalacia or instability due to abnormalities in the extensor mechanism (75). Imaging of patellofemoral disorders has been attempted with patellar views in 0°–60° of flexion, arthrography, CT, arthrotomography and, more recently, MRI (75,89,119).

Chondromalacia patella is a disorder of young adults. The patellar articular changes may result from subluxation, fracture, or repetitive microtrauma with disruption of the vertical collagen fibers (119).

Currently, arthroscopy is the technique of choice for evaluating the patellar surface (75,119). However, MRI has recently proved to be useful in classification of chondromalacia (51,66). Correlation with arthroscopic findings (focal cartilage swelling, irregularity, thinning, and areas of base bone) has been achieved, especially in the more advanced stages (81,119). Table 7-6 summarizes the arthroscopic and corresponding MRI stages of chondromalacia (75,119).

MRI techniques in the axial (Fig. 7-55) and sagittal (Fig. 7-56) planes have been reported (25,66,119). T1, T2, and gradient-echo sequences have all been employed to evaluate chondromalacia. Gadolinium-DTPA has also been advocated for more accurate delineation of articular cartilage (25,36,81,119). T2 weighted sequences provide a high signal intensity interface between the femoral and patellar articular surfaces. This allows subtle changes to be more easily detected. Gradient-echo sequences provide similar information and excellent tissue contrast between the high signal intensity of the articular cartilage and low intensity of subchondral bone (81). Axial images are most useful. A volume coil and small field of view (16 cm) are also important.

Patellofemoral instability is potentially complex and can be difficult to image accurately with consistent reproducibility. Normally the apex of the patella should be centered between the medial and lateral femoral condyles. This position should be maintained when chang-

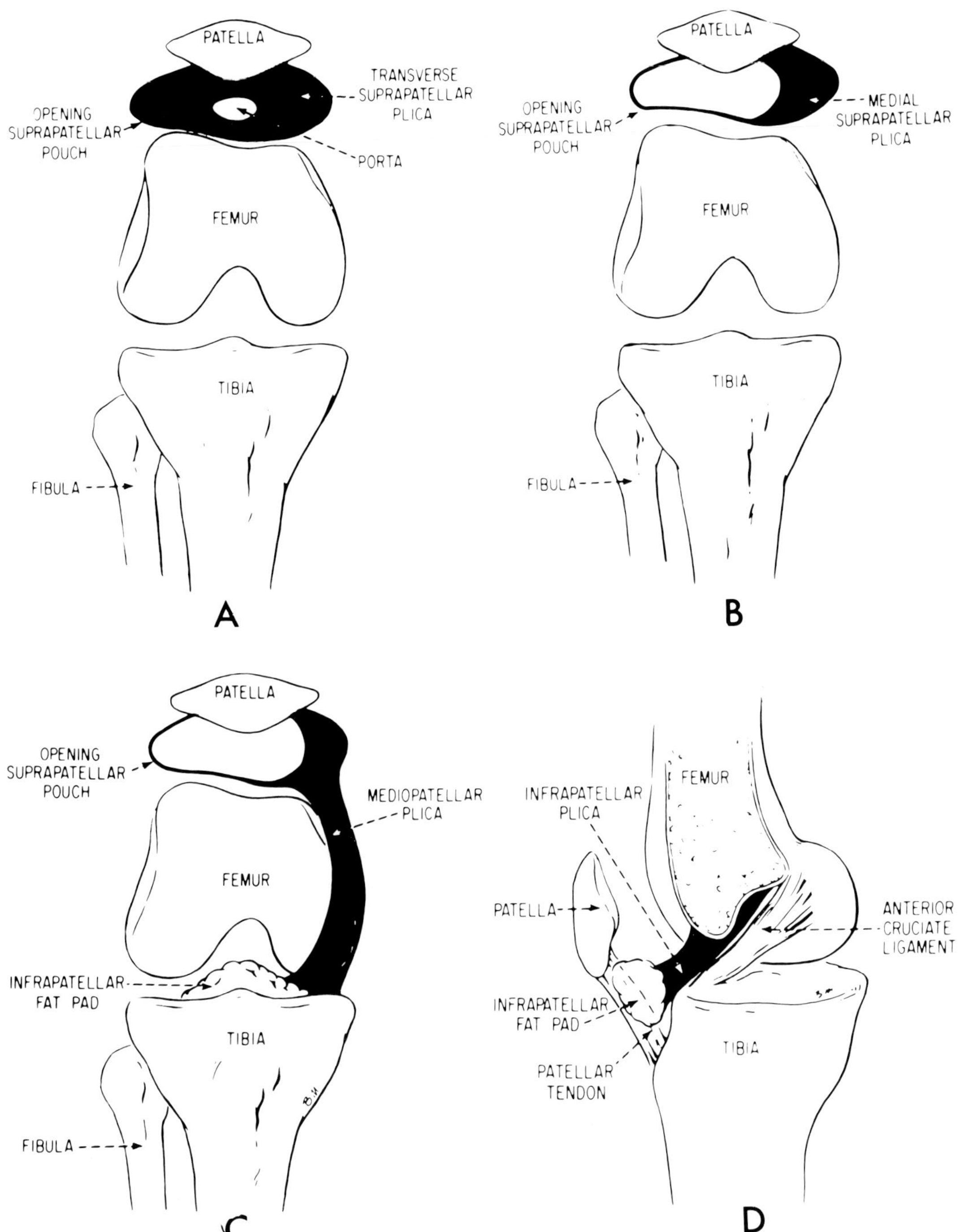

FIG. 7-54. Illustration of plicae of the knee. **A:** Transverse suprapatellar plica with porta, anterior view. **B:** Medial suprapatellar plica, anterior view. **C:** Mediopatellar plica. **D:** Infrapatellar plica, lateral view. (From ref. 36, with permission.)

TABLE 7-6. *Arthroscopic and MR classification of chondromalacia patellae* (88,119)

Arthroscopic classification		MRI classification and image features	
Grade 1	Softening of articular cartilage	Stage 1	Focal areas of swelling with decreased signal intensity on T1 and T2 weighted sequences
Grade 2	Blisterlike swelling		
Grade 3	Surface irregularity and areas of thinning	Stage 2	Irregularity and focal thinning
Grade 4	Ulceration and bone exposure	Stage 3	Focal bone exposure

ing from the extended to flexed (up to 30°) position (75,89). Translation and rotation or progressive asymmetry of the relationships of the medial and lateral facets with relation to the femoral condyles need to be assessed in the extended and flexed positions (Fig. 7-57). Conditions that may be detected are listed below (75,89).

Lateral subluxation—lateral translation of the patella so the patellar facet extends beyond the articular margin of the femoral condyle.

Excessive lateral pressure syndrome—lateral facet joint narrowed or patella tilted with no subluxation.

Medial subluxation—medial translation of the patella so the patellar facet extends beyond the articular margin of the femoral condyle.

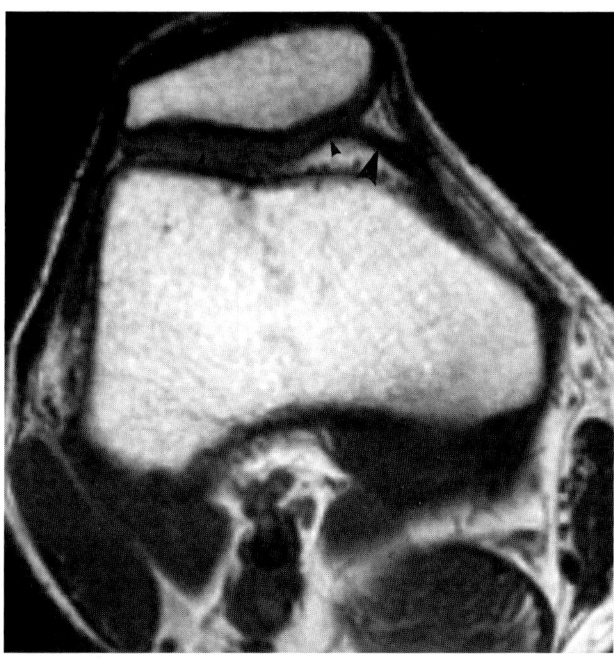

FIG. 7-55. Axial SE 500/20 image shows normal patellar cartilage (*small arrowhead*). The thickened posterior patellar retinacula (*large arrowhead*) should not be confused with a plica.

Lateral-medial subluxation—the patella starts in lateral subluxation but shifts to medial subluxation during flexion.

Dislocation—complete loss of articular interface with the femoral condyles (89).

Imaging of instability requires motion or flexion of the knee. Both knees should be examined simultaneously for comparison purposes. Therefore, the body coil is used with the patient supine. The knees should be imaged in extension and up to 30° of flexion at 5°–10° increments. This can be most effectively performed using gradient-echo sequences to reduce image time (89). Cine loop motion studies are also useful in following patellar movement.

Loose Bodies

Detection of osseous or cartilaginous fragments in the joint can be difficult. Loose bodies can develop following fracture, meniscal tears, and in patients with osteochondromatosis, synovial chondromatosis, and osteochondritis dissecans (66,75,84). Patients generally present with pain, recurrent effusions, locking, or restricted motion (75).

Identification of loose bodies has been accomplished using arthrography with or without conventional or computed tomography and arthroscopy (75). Routine radiographs can detect calcified or osseous bodies, but it is difficult to determine if the lesion is a loose body or calcification or ossification in the cruciate ligament or attached to the capsule. Technically, a loose body should move in the joint and on arthrograms should be surrounded by contrast material (75).

MRI can also identify loose bodies (Figs. 7-58 to 7-60). Calcification or ossification has low signal intensity even though osseous loose bodies may actually contain marrow. Cartilage or chronic synovial proliferation may have a similar low signal intensity on both T1 and T2 weighted sequences. T2 weighted and gradient-echo sequences are generally used to identify loose bodies because these lesions are more easily detected in the presence of high signal intensity synovial fluid. However, there are numerous structures that can cause confusion. These include the transverse ligament anteriorly, the ligament of Wisberg and Humphrey posteriorly, and areas of synovial hypertrophy (10,110,111). Comparison with radiographs is very useful in evaluating loose bodies. Ossification near the tibia spines is common and should not be confused with a loose body.

Fractures

Routine radiography, tomography, and isotope scans are typically used to identify fractures and stress frac-

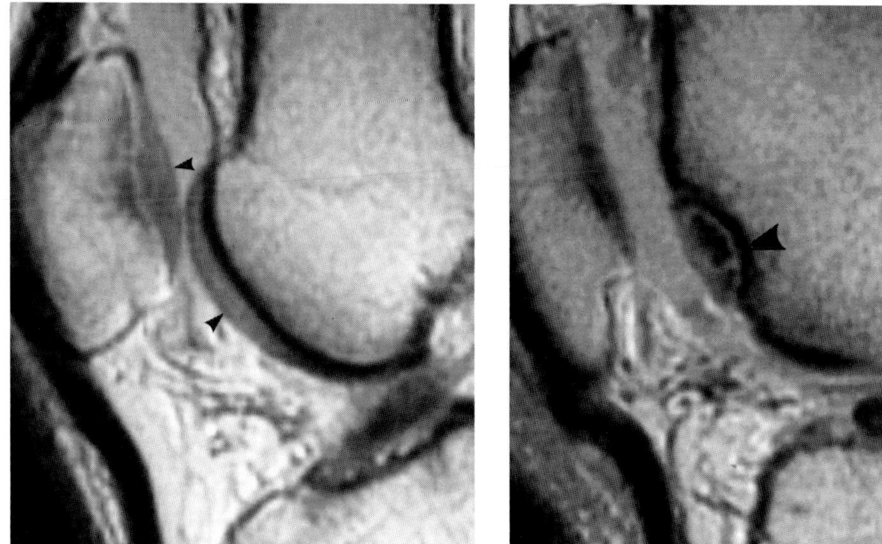

FIG. 7-56. Sagittal SE 2,000/20 images showing normal articular cartilage (*arrowheads*) (**A**) and loss of articular cartilage (**B**) with an osteochondral fragment in the femoral condyle (*arrowhead*).

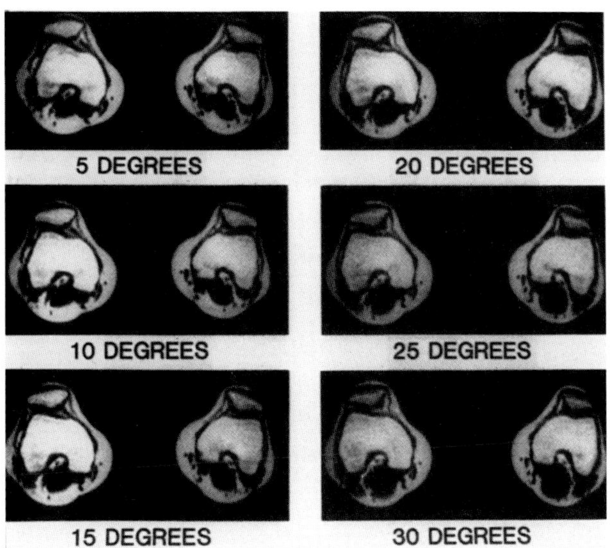

FIG. 7-57. Axial 5 mm thick images of the knee obtained with varying degrees of flexion. There is slight lateral translation of the left patella but it reduces in 15% of flexion. The translation is more obvious in the right patella. (From ref. 89, with permission.)

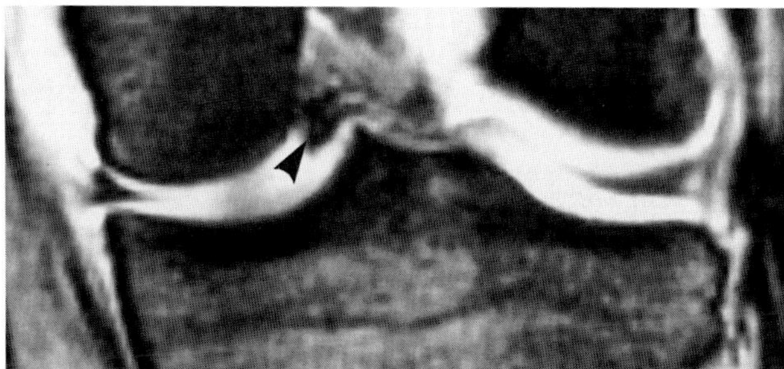

FIG. 7-58. Coronal gradient-echo image demonstrating a loose fragment (*arrowhead*) adjacent to the intercondylar eminence.

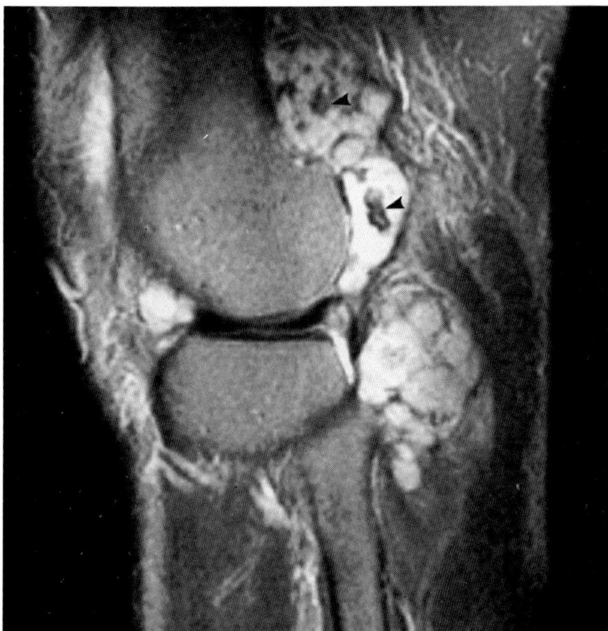

FIG. 7-59. Sagittal SE 2,000/60 image in a patient with synovial chondromatosis. The chondromatous bodies are seen as areas of low signal intensity (*arrowheads*).

tures about the knee. Subtle fractures may be evident with MRI. Also, MRI can be useful for evaluating intraarticular fractures, the joint space, and articular cartilage integrity. During the early stages of development MRI was considered primarily a soft tissue imaging technique. As use of MRI expanded, especially for evaluating patients with suspected internal derangement or other

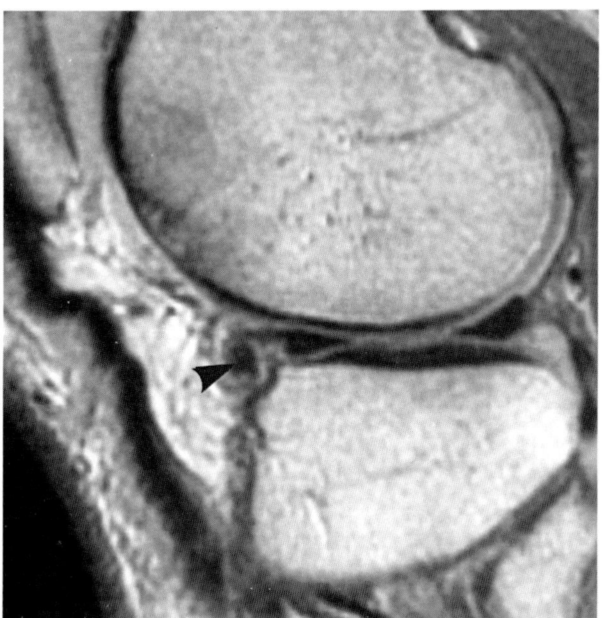

FIG. 7-60. Sagittal SE 2,000/20 image demonstrates a well-defined loose body anterior to the meniscus (*arrowhead*).

soft tissue injuries of the knee, it became apparent that subtle bone lesions could be identified that had not been identified on routine radiographs. Several types of injury have been identified (57,64,107).

Stress fractures are not uncommon in the upper tibia. MRI features of stress fractures are usually easily appreciated, even in the presence of normal radiography (97). T1 weighted images demonstrate linear or irregular areas of low signal intensity. The frature may be high intensity on T2 weighted sequences. This is usually due to reactive changes along the fracture line. Compressed trabeculae are low intensity on T1 and T2 weighted sequences (Fig. 7-61) (9,116,117).

Similar findings are noted with subtle osteochondral fractures, plateau fractures, and incomplete fractures (Fig. 7-62). Growth plate fractures are also easily identified (53,57).

A more unique fracture, the "bone bruise," has a different appearance on MR images. Radiographs are normal. This injury is more geographic, with low signal intensity on T1 weighted sequences and high signal intensity on T2 weighted and gradient-echo sequences. These injuries occur in either the tibia or femoral condyles and are geographic or stellate in nature (57,64,66). Twisting, varus, and valgus stress injuries with tears in the cruciate ligament or collateral ligaments are commonly associated with bone bruises (64).

Osteochondritis Dissecans

Osteochondritis dissecans is a disease of teenagers. The average age of onset is 15 years (63). Males outnumber females by a 3:1 ratio. The lesion most commonly involves the lateral aspect of the medial femoral condyle, but the lateral condyle, patella, and other areas in the knee can also be involved (60,75). The right knee is involved slightly more commonly than the left and bilateral involvement is reported in up to 25% of cases (1,60). The etiology is unclear but the disease is probably related to repetitive trauma and/or ischemia (1,75).

Symptoms, such as pain or instability, and the radiographic appearance dictate whether conservative (rest), arthroscopic, or open surgery treatment is required. Therefore, it is important to assess the size, location, position, and cartilaginous articular surface of the lesion (60,75). Mesgarzadeh et al. (60) found that lesions greater than 0.8 cm^2 and with sclerotic margins greater than 3 mm tended to be unstable. Lesions can usually be identified on routine radiographs. However, evaluation of the position and articular cartilage requires further study.

Arthrography with or without tomography has been used in the past. However, MRI provides an ideal technique for evaluating these lesions. Both coronal and sagittal images are needed to fully evaluate the size and

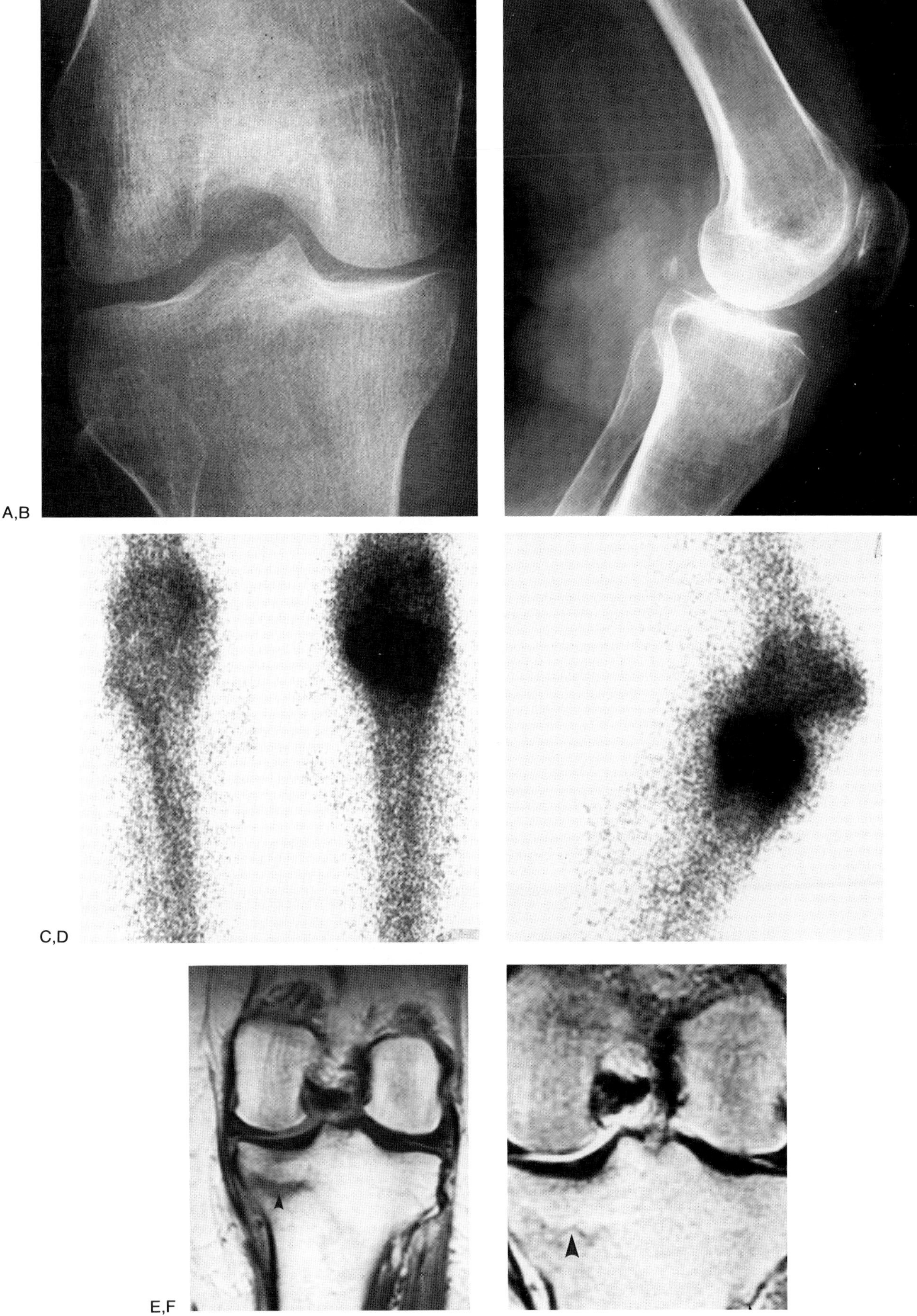

FIG. 7-61. Fifty-three-year-old female with knee pain. AP (**A**) and lateral (**B**) radiographs are normal. Radionuclide scans show increased uptake in the tibia on frontal (**C**) and lateral (**D**) views. Osteonecrosis or metastasis? Coronal SE 500/20 (**E**) and SE 2,000/60 (**F**) images demonstrate a stress fracture (*arrowheads*). There is also buckling of the lateral cortex (*arrow*).

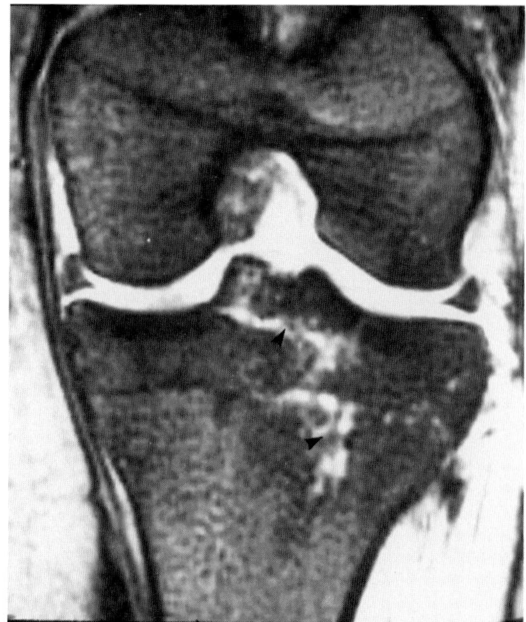

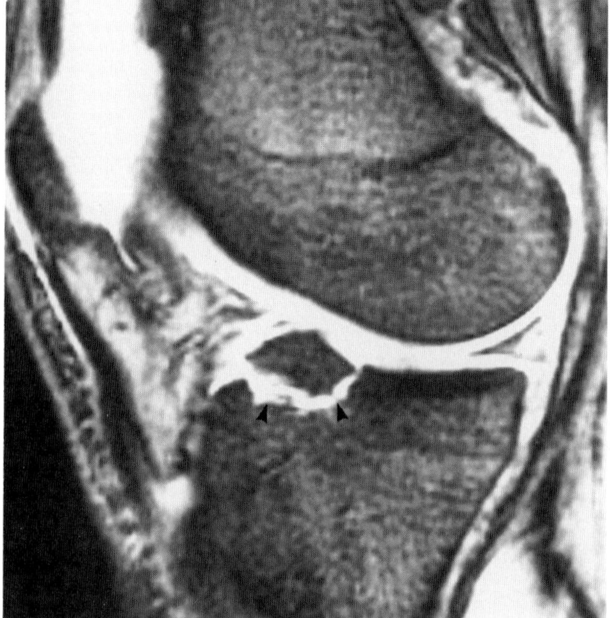

A,B

FIG. 7-62. Coronal (**A**) and sagittal (**B**) gradient-echo (MPGR) images in a patient with a plateau fracture (*arrowheads*).

position of the lesion. Gradient-echo or T2 weighted sequences are most useful. Loose fragments may be displaced or simply have a linear fluid collection (high intensity on T2 weighted sequences between the native bone and osteochondral fragment). MRI is also effective in assessing the cartilage and whether it is intact or completely covers the lesion (Fig. 7-63).

Osteonecrosis and Osteochondrosis

Osteonecrosis, including the histologic changes and pathophysiology, is discussed in Chapter 6. However, although the etiology and MRI appearance of AVN in the knee are similar, there are certain differences that should be emphasized.

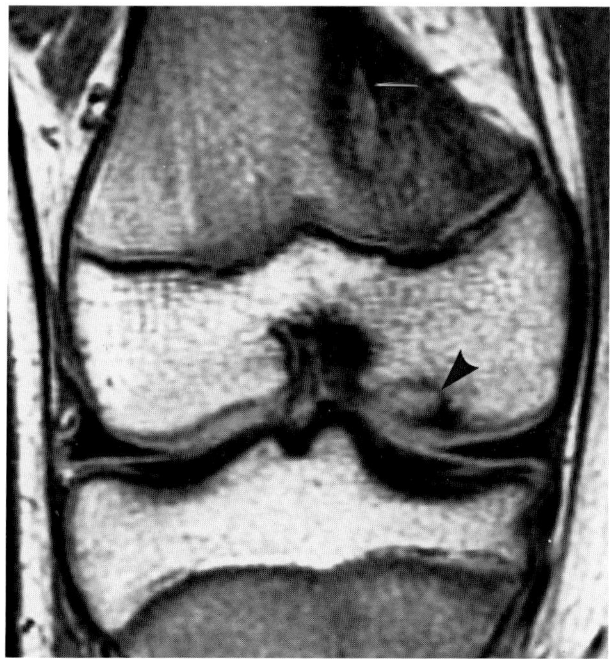

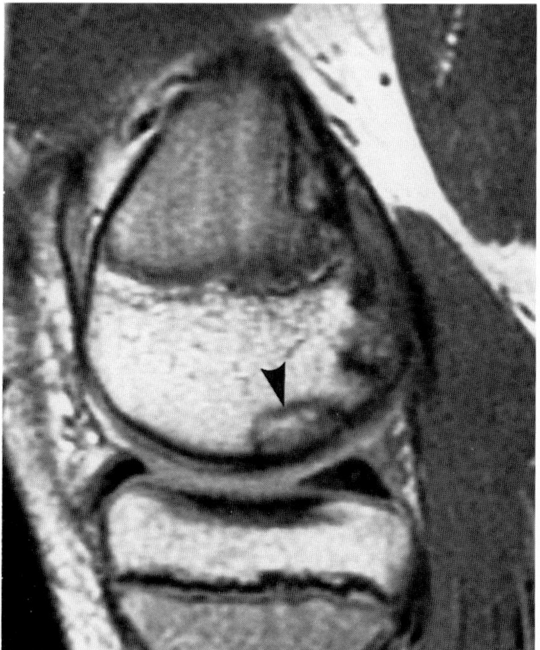

A,B

FIG. 7-63. Osteochondritis dissecans. Coronal (**A**) and sagittal (**B**) SE 2,000/20 images define the defect (*arrowhead*) and show intact articular cartilage over the lesion.

The incidence of avascular necrosis in the femoral condyles follows the hip and shoulder (66). MRI features are also similar and the stages described in Chapter 6 (Table 6-4) can be applied to the knee as well as the hip (Fig. 7-64). There are several variations peculiar to the knee. These include spontaneous osteonecrosis, which typically involves the medial femoral condyle but can also involve the lateral femoral condyle and medial tibial plateau, and osteochondrosis (40,73,74,86).

Acute or spontaneous osteonecrosis is a condition associated with females 50 years of age or older. The primary disorder is of unknown etiology but most likely is ischemic in nature. Patients on steroids (secondary) may develop changes in similar sites (73). The medial femoral condyle is most frequently involved. However, the lateral femoral condyle and tibial plateau can also be affected. The clinical history is similar regardless of location. Patients present with acute pain and tenderness over the affected area. The pain, often worse at night, progresses for 6–8 weeks before subsiding.

Radiographs are normal in early stages of the disease (Table 7-7). Isotope scans will demonstrate increased uptake. However, this is nonspecific and often not useful in patients of this age group (56,66,109). MRI features are more useful and appear earlier than radiographic changes (Fig. 7-65 and Table 7-7) (56). As with AVN of the hip, the MRI and radiographic features are more easily correlated in the later stages of the disease. An additional advantage of MRI is the ability to differentiate spontaneous osteonecrosis from other conditions that may have similar clinical presentations, such as meniscal tears, pes anserine bursitis (Fig. 7-66), and simple osteoarthritis (Fig. 7-67) (66).

Two common osteochondroses involving the knee are Blount's disease and Osgood–Schlatter disease. Blount's disease presents in infantile and adolescent forms. The infantile variety is seen as a varus deformity of the knee with progressive bowing. The adolescent form presents from 8 to 15 years of age and, unlike the infantile type, is often unilateral with pain in the involved knee (66,82,87).

Clinical features and radiographic changes have been sufficient for diagnosis of this disorder. However, early experience with MRI would indicate that demonstration of early changes, especially in the unossified epiphysis, can be more fully evaluated. The coronal plane, using a double-echo (TR 2,000/60,20) T2 weighted sequence, is best suited for this purpose.

Osgood–Schlatter disease is a common problem in adolescent males. The condition is frequently bilateral and occurs in active or athletic patients. Patients present with pain and swelling over the tibial tuberosity. The clinical presentation and demonstration of fragmentation of the tuberosity on radiographs usually are sufficient to confirm the diagnosis (82). Sagittal T2 weighted MR images are useful in evaluating the patellar tendon and associated soft tissue changes (Fig. 7-68). However, MRI is probably not indicated unless the normal resolution of the process with rest is not achieved or other complications are suspected.

A,B

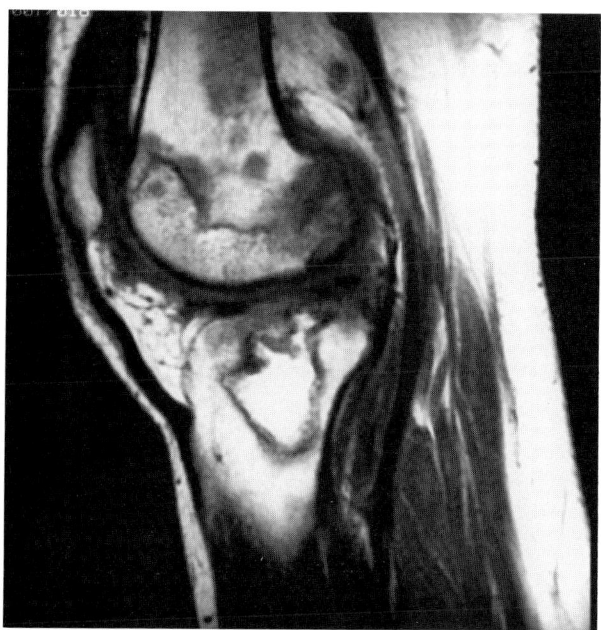

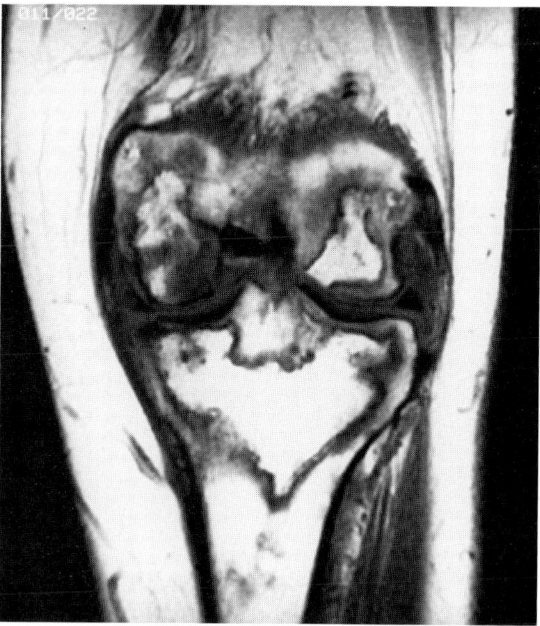

FIG. 7-64. Sagittal (**A**) and coronal (**B**) SE 500/20 images of the knee in a patient on steroids. There is avascular necrosis of both femoral condyles and a proximal tibia infarct.

TABLE 7-7. *Spontaneous osteonecrosis of the knee: radiographic and MRI features* (56)

Stage 1	Normal	Geographic area of increasing intensity T2WI[a], decreasing intensity T1WI[b]
Stage 2	Slight flattening of the femoral condyle, sclerosis of subchondral tibial bone	Geographic area with surrounding low intensity on T1WI
Stage 3	Subchondral lucency with surrounding sclerosis	Subchondral area of reduced to normal signal intensity surrounded by low intensity area on both T1 and T2WIs
Stage 4	Same but wider area of sclerosis	
Stage 5	Above changes plus degenerative joint disease	Geographic area of low intensity with joint space narrowing

[a] T2WI, T2 weighted image.
[b] T1WI, T1 weighted image.

Musculoskeletal Neoplasms and Soft Tissue Masses

A complete discussion of musculoskeletal neoplasms is included in Chapter 12. However, there are certain applications and technical aspects for evaluating the knee that are more appropriately discussed in this chapter.

Skeletal lesions are most easily characterized using routine radiography (10,11). Primary bone tumors in the knee are common (Table 7-8). About half of osteosarcomas occur in the knee. This excludes the subcategories (telangectatic OGS, parosteal OGS, etc.), which are also common in this location. Sixty percent of Ewing's sarcomas involve the pelvis or knee. Certain benign tumors are also common about the knee. Thirty-two percent of chondroblastomas and over half of giant cell tumors are located in the knee (24). Patellar tumors are rare. Patellar tumors accounted for only 0.06% of 8,542 bone tumors in the Dahlin–Unni series (24). Kransdorf et al. (50) reported a series of 42 cases. Thirty-eight were benign (chondroblastoma 16, giant cell tumor 8, simple cyst 6, hemangioma 3, osteochondroma 2, lipoma 2, and osteoblastoma 1). Three of four malignant lesions were lymphomas and there was one hemangioendotheliosarcoma. At this time, MRI is primarily reserved for staging and therapy planning of skeletal neoplasms (see Chapter 12).

Soft tissue masses about the knee are summarized in Table 7-9 (27). The MRI features of these lesions and techniques for examination are discussed in Chapter 12. Other soft tissue masses of the knee, which may mimic benign or malignant lesions, are more properly discussed here. This included popliteal cysts and ganglia. Popliteal or Baker's cysts are the most common cysts in this region. These lesions typically communicate with the joint at the junction of the medial head of the gastrocnemius and insertion of the semimembranosus (Fig. 7-69) (15,18). Cysts or bursal enlargements can also occur along the popliteus tendon and biceps femoris (66). Popliteal cysts may vary in size and they can be large and multiloculated and can contain septations. Patients usually present with knee pain, and a posterior

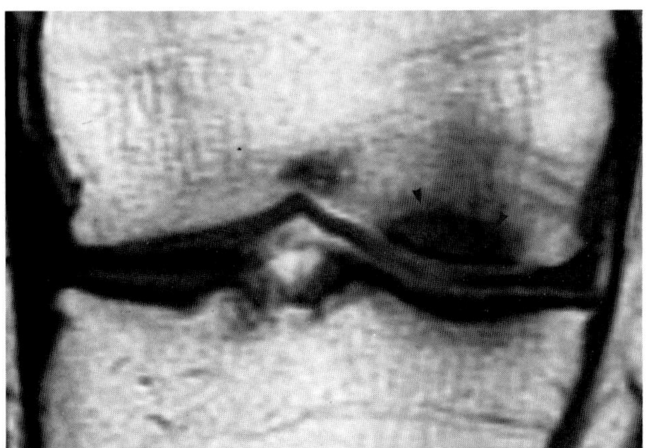

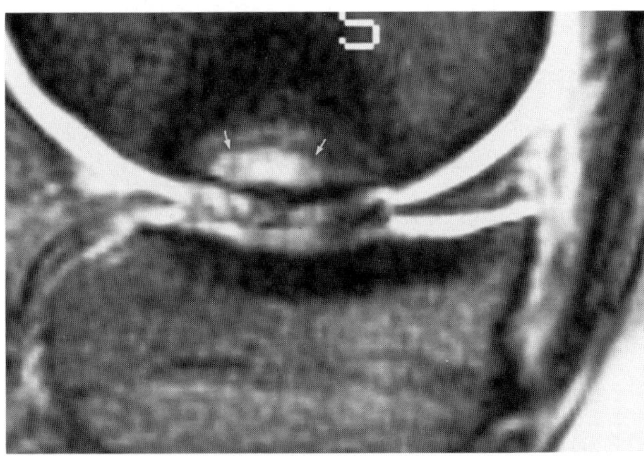

A,B

FIG. 7-65. Coronal SE 500/20 (**A**) and sagittal gradient-echo (**B**) images demonstrate spontaneous osteonecrosis of the femoral condyle (*arrows*).

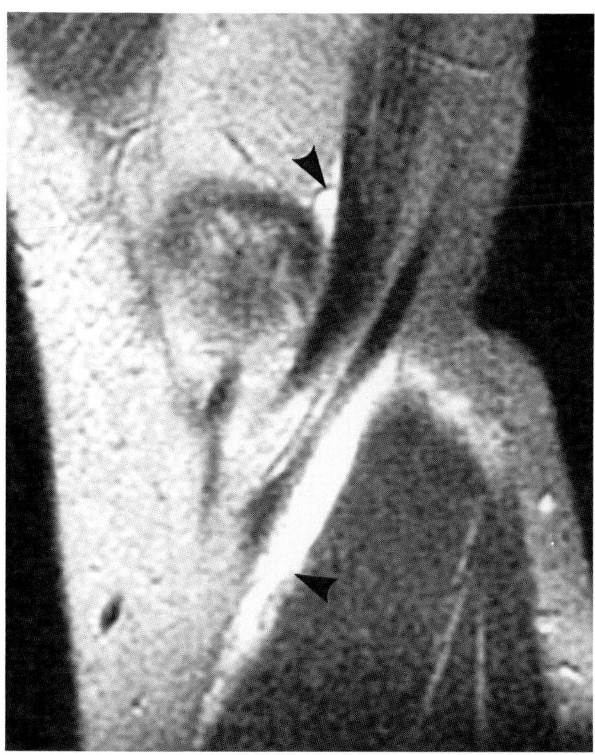

FIG. 7-66. Middle-aged female with medial joint pain. Sagittal SE 2,000/60 image shows increased signal intensity along the medial tendons (*arrowheads*) due to pes anserine bursitis.

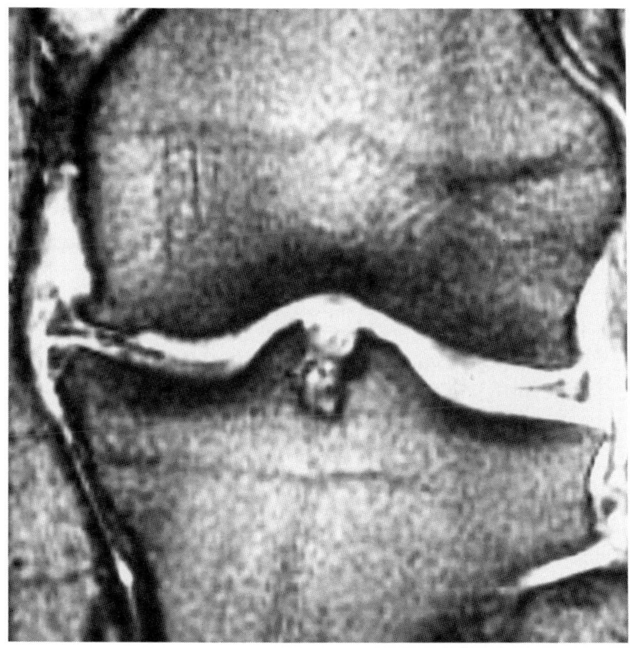

FIG. 7-67. Osteoarthritis. Coronal gradient-echo (MPGR) images show medial joint space narrowing with displacement and degeneration of the meniscus. There is also synovial herniation in the intercondylar spine region.

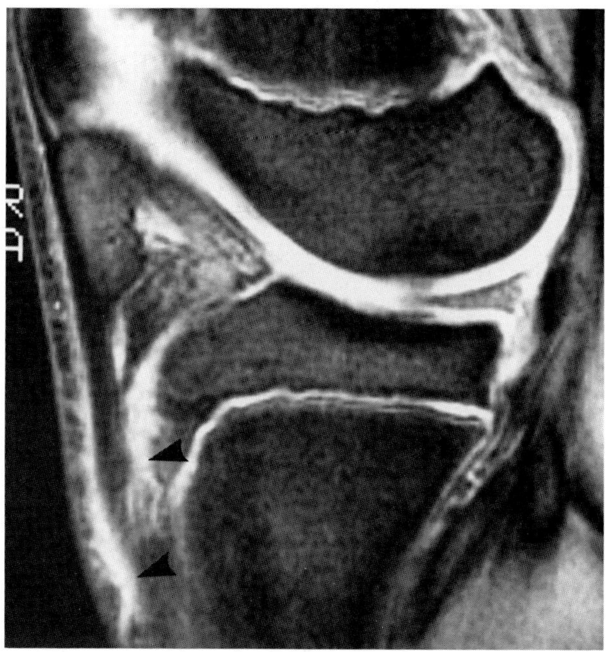

FIG. 7-68. Sagittal T2 weighted image of the knee in a 14-year-old male. There is inflammation along the distal patellar ligament (*arrowheads*) due to Osgood–Schlatter disease.

TABLE 7-8. *Primary skeletal neoplasms of the knee based on 8,542 cases* (24)

Neoplasm	Number of lesions
Malignant	
Osteosarcoma	632
Chondrosarcoma	83
Reticulum cell sarcoma	75
Fibrosarcoma	63
Ewing's sarcoma	46
Benign	
Osteochondroma	278
Giant cell tumor	223
Aneurysmal bone cysts	53
Chondroma	30
Osteoid osteoma	29
Chondroblastoma	24
Chondromyxoid fibroma	14

TABLE 7-9. *Soft tissue tumors of the knee and leg* (27)

Type of lesion	Number of cases
Liposarcoma	321
Fibrosarcoma	170
Synovial sarcoma	102
Alveolar sarcoma	63
Hemangioma	50
Rhabdomyosarcoma	40
Hemangiopericytoma	37
Epithelioid sarcoma	31
Desmoid tumor	27
Giant cell tumor of tendon sheath	15

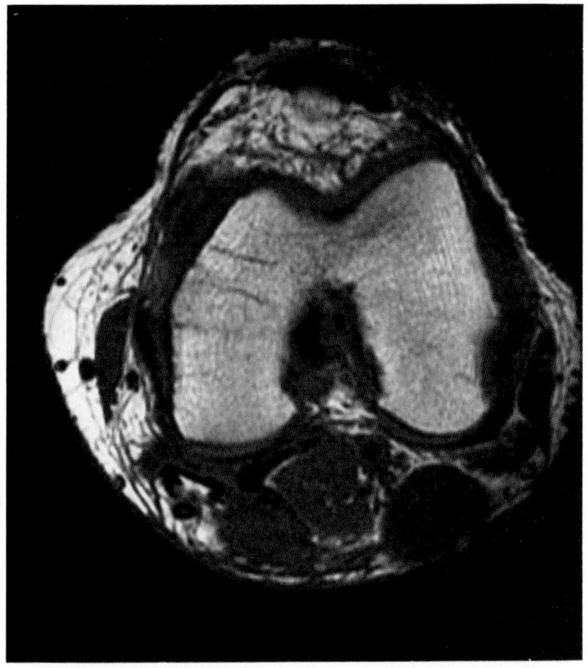

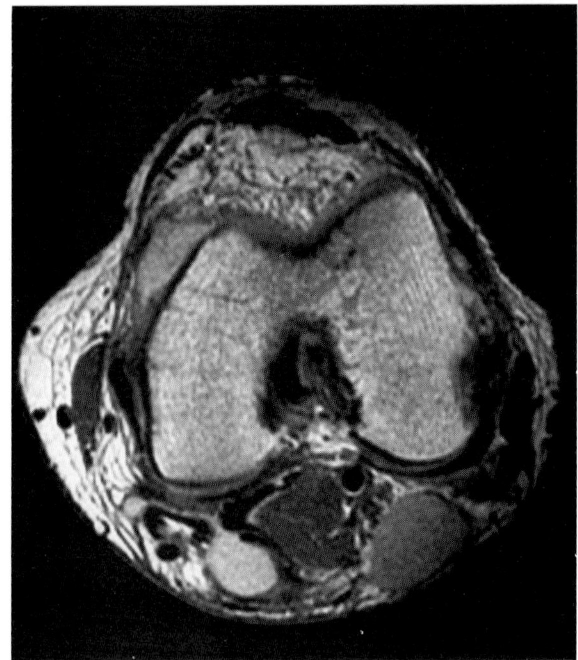

A,B

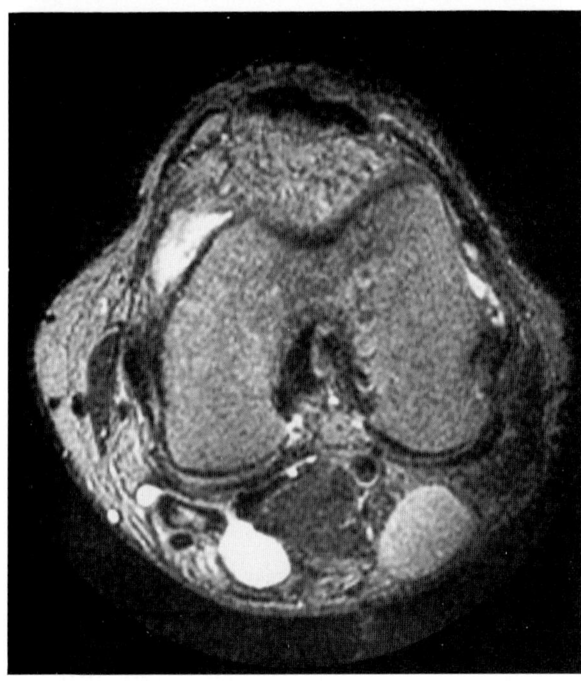

C

FIG. 7-69. Axial SE 500/20 (**A**), SE 2,000/20 (**B**), and SE 2,000/60 (**C**) images demonstrate a communicating cyst medially and a noncommunicating cyst laterally. The latter is lower signal intensity due to thick proteinaceous debris.

mass may be palpable. Meniscal tears and arthropathies (rheumatoid arthritis, osteoarthritis, etc.) are commonly associated. Rupture of these cysts may result in dissection of fluid between the soleus and gastrocnemius (3,11). Symptoms may be difficult to differentiate from deep venous thrombosis. MRI is ideally suited for diagnosis of either of these conditions. Popliteal cysts are homogeneous with high signal intensity on T2 weighted sequences and low intensity on T1 weighted sequences (Fig. 7-69). Other lesions such as distended bursae (see Table 7-2) and ganglia have similar MRI features (Fig. 7-70). Ganglia are more common along tendon sheaths and near the tibiofibular joint. Therefore, location may be somewhat useful. Both lesions can cause compression of the common peroneal nerve (100). As discussed above, meniscal cysts are located along the joint line adjacent to the menisci and are usually associated with an adjacent meniscal tear (18).

Another typically benign appearing lesion is the giant cell tumor of the tendon sheath. These lesions can appear similar to other cysts. However, often there is hemosiderin deposition, which results in reduced signal

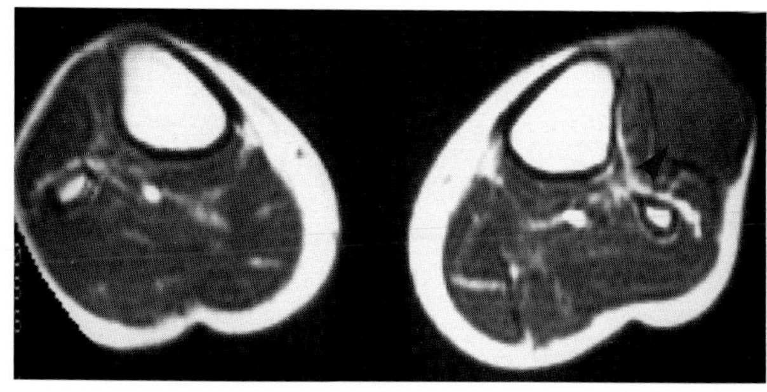
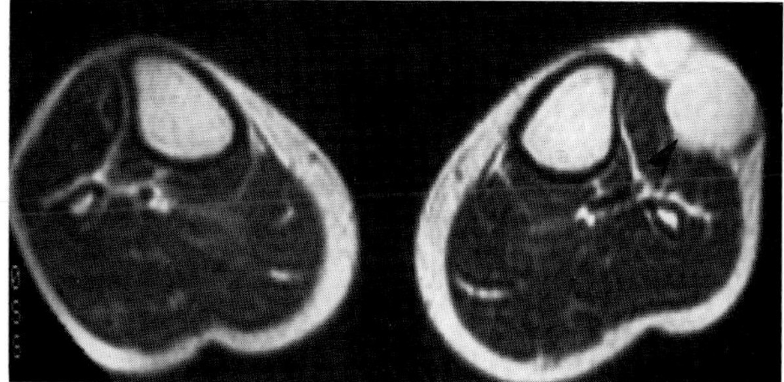

A,B

FIG. 7-70. Axial SE 500/20 (**A**) and SE 2,000/30 (**B**) images of the upper leg, demonstrating a homogeneous, well-marginated ganglion cyst (*arrowheads*).

intensity on T2 weighted sequences. This is a useful finding in characterizing the lesion.

The routine screening examination used for knee trauma is typically not used in patients referred for suspected bone or soft tissue neoplasms of the knee. Typically both T1 and T2 weighted sequences are required to properly characterize the nature of the lesions, especially in the soft tissues (11,46,63,76,106,109). We prefer to obtain images in two planes to fully evaluate the extent of lesions. The axial and sagittal or coronal planes are used. Obvious lesions can be identified and classified using two sequences and two image planes. The axial image plane is typically performed using a T2 weighted sequence and followed by either a sagittal or coronal T1 weighted sequence. This minimizes examination time without hindering diagnosis (11).

More subtle lesions, especially in the marrow, may require a STIR sequence to more easily assess the abnormalities in the marrow. Subtle soft tissue changes may dictate that the T1 and T2 weighted sequences be performed in the same image plane to more easily characterize the lesion. Vascular lesions or lesions that may encase or displace vessels may be further studied with gradient-echo sequences (GRASS) to better define the vascular anatomy (11).

Arthritis and Synovial Diseases

Early detection and characterization of arthropathies and synovial inflammatory diseases have been difficult with conventional imaging techniques. Routine radiographs may demonstrate swelling and bony erosions. Radionuclide scans can identify changes earlier but findings are not specific (48,66).

Recently, MRI has provided a new method of evaluating early articular and synovial inflammatory disease (8,32). Articular cartilage is easily identified due to the

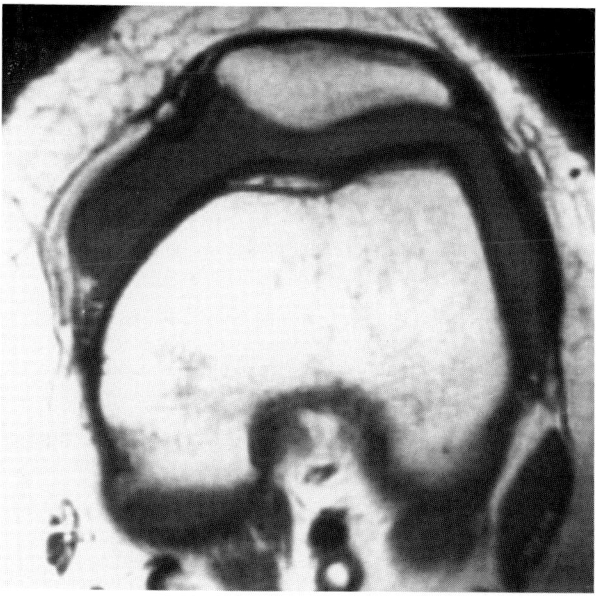
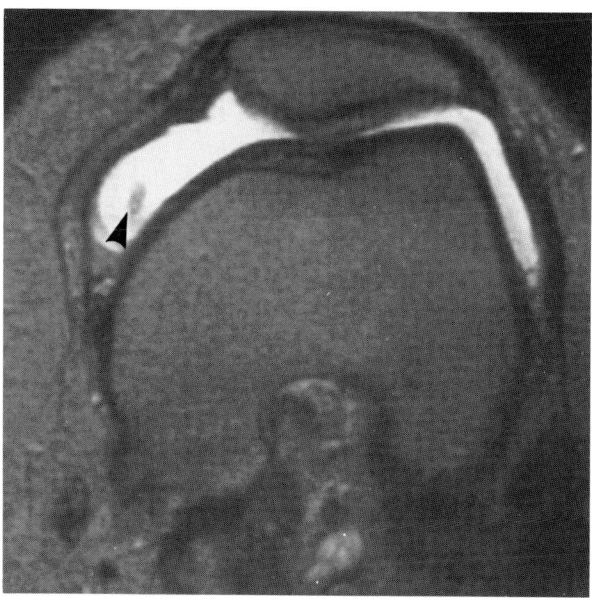

A,B

FIG. 7-71. Axial SE 500/20 (**A**) and SE 2,000/60 (**B**) images of the knee. The articular cartilage and synovial proliferation (*arrowhead* in **B**) are more easily evaluated on the T2 weighted image.

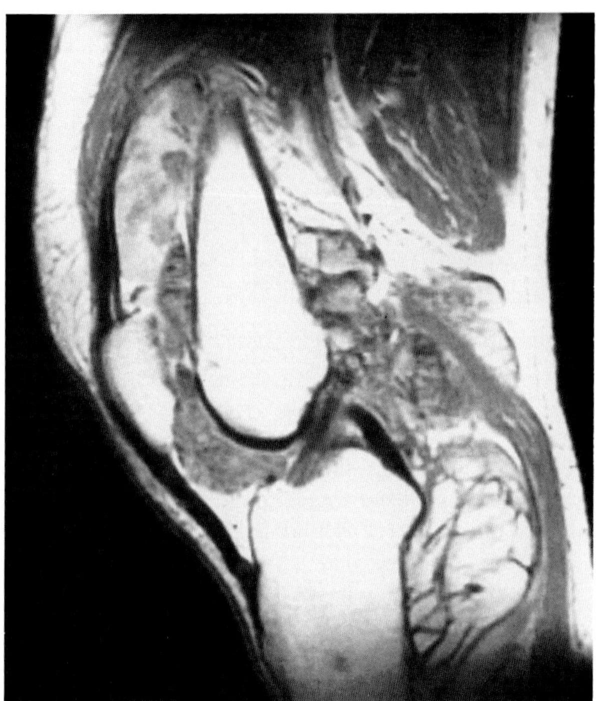

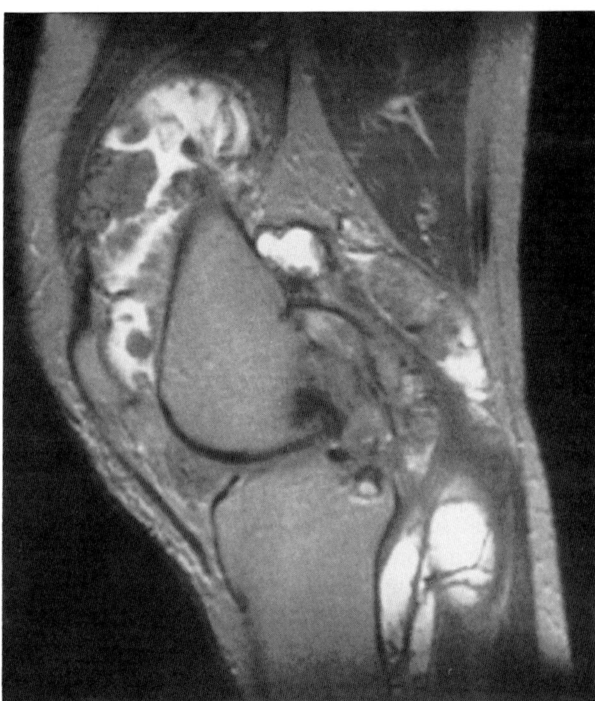

A,B

FIG. 7-72. Sagittal SE 500/20 (**A**) and SE 2,000/60 (**B**) images of the knee in a patient with pigmented villonodular synovitis. Note the multiple large areas of decreased intensity in the distended joint on the T2 weighted sequence.

contrast between cartilage and the low-intensity cortical bone. T2 or gradient-echo (TE 700; TR 12, 31, FA 25°; see Table 7-1) sequences are most useful for evaluating subtle changes in the articular cartilage. Fluid and cartilage may be difficult to clearly separate on T1 weighted sequences (Fig. 7-71). The routine screening examination is adequate for detecting early cartilage erosions. Also, changes in the growth plate and ossifying epiphysis can easily be assessed. Therefore, early changes can be detected in juvenile rheumatoid arthritis, rheumatoid arthritis, hemophilic arthropathy, and other cartilaginous disorders (6,44,45,52,72,86,96,118). The causes of synovial inflammation are numerous. Unfortunately, changes noted on MRI may not always indicate the etiology. Synovial proliferation can lead to irregular fronds that extend into the joint space. These appear as low signal intensity filling defects on T2 weighted sequences (Fig. 7-71). These changes can be identified with any chronic synovial inflammatory process. Therefore, they are not useful in separating the types of arthropathy.

Certain specific features have been noted with pigmented villonodular synovitis. This condition is a monoarticular disease that involves the knees in 80% of cases. Hemorrhagic effusions lead to histologic changes, including synovial proliferation and hemosiderin-laden macrophages (45,59,96). The latter result in focal areas of low signal intensity on T2 weighted images, presumably due to the paramagnetic effects of hemosiderin (Fig. 7-72). The areas of low intensity tend to be larger and more globular than typical synovial fronds or synovial chondromatosis (see Figs. 7-59 and 7-71).

Attempts to characterize changes in synovial fluid including T1 and T2 relaxation times, spectroscopy, and correlation of signal intensity with normal, infected, or inflammed synovial fluid have been unsuccessful (5,8,42,114). The use of contrast material has not enhanced the specificity of MRI (13,33,34,115).

REFERENCES

1. Aichroth P. Osteochondritis dissecans of the knee: a clinical survey. *J Bone Joint Surg* 1971;53:440–447.
2. Anderson JE. *Grant's atlas of anatomy,* 8th ed. Baltimore: Williams & Wilkins, 1983.
3. Anouchi YS, Parker RD, Seitz WH Jr. Posterior compartment syndrome of the calf resulting from misdiagnosis of a rupture of the medial head of the gastrocnemius. *J Trauma* 1987;27:678–680.
4. Apple JS, Martinez S, Hardaker WT, Daffner RH, Gehweiler TA. Synovial plicae of the knee. *Skeletal Radiol* 1982;7:251–254.
5. Baker DG, Schumacher HR Jr, Wolf GL. Nuclear magnetic resonance evaluation of synovial fluid and articular tissues. *J Rheumatol* 1985;12:1062–1065.
6. Beltran J, Caudill JL, Herman LA, Kantor SM, Hudson PN, Noto AM, Baran AS. Rheumatoid arthritis: MR imaging manifestations. *Radiology* 1987;165:153–157.
7. Beltran J, Noto AM, Mosure JC, Bools JC, Zuelzer W, Christoforidis AJ. Meniscal tears: MR demonstration of experimentally produced injuries. *Radiology* 1986;158:691–693.
8. Beltran J, Noto AM, Mosure JC, Weiss KL, Zuelzer W, Christoforidis AJ. The knee: surface-coil MR imaging at 1.5 T. *Radiology* 1986;159:747–751.
9. Berger PE, Ofstein RA, Jackson DW, Morrison DS, Silvino N,

Amador R. MRI demonstration of radiographically occult fractures: what have we been missing? *RadioGraphics* 1989;9:407–436.

10. Berquist TH, Ehman RL, Richardson ML. *Magnetic resonance of the musculoskeletal system.* New York: Raven Press, 1987.
11. Berquist TH. Magnetic resonance imaging of musculoskeletal neoplasms. *Clin Orthop* 1989;244:101–118.
12. Bodne D, Quinn SF, Murray WT, et al. Magnetic resonance images of chronic patellar tendinitis. *Skeletal Radiol* 1988;17:24–28.
13. Brasch RC, Bennett HF. Considerations in the choice of contrast media for MR imaging. *Radiology* 1988;166:897–899.
14. Brunner MC, Flower SP, Evancho AM, Allman FL, Apple DF, Fajman WA. MRI of the athletic knee. Findings in asymptomatic professional basketball and collegiate football players. *Invest Radiol* 1989;24:72–75.
15. Burk DL Jr, Dalinka MK, Kanal E, et al. Meniscal and ganglion cysts of the knee: MR evaluation. *AJR* 1988;150:331–336.
16. Burk DL Jr, Kanal E, Brunberg JA, Johnstone GF, Swensen HE, Wolf GL. 1.5-T surface-coil MRI of the knee. *AJR* 1986;147:293–300.
17. Clemente CD. *Gray's anatomy,* 13th ed. Philadelphia: Lea & Febiger, 1985.
18. Coral A, van Holsbeeck M, Adler RS. Imaging of meniscal cyst of the knee in three cases. *Skeletal Radiol* 1989;18:451–455.
19. Crues JV III. Magnetic resonance imaging of knee menisci. Presented at the Society of Magnetic Resonance in Medicine, Amsterdam, The Netherlands, 1989.
20. Crues JV III, Mink J, Levy TL, Lotysch M, Stoller DW. Meniscal tears of the knee: accuracy of MR imaging. *Radiology* 1987;164:445–448.
21. Crues JV III, Ryu R. MRI of the knee: Part I. *Appl Radiol* 1989;18:(7)18–23.
22. Crues JV III, Ryu R. MRI of the knee: Part II. *Appl Radiol* 1989;18:(8)12–18.
23. Daffner RH, Riemer BL, Lupetin AR, Dash N. Magnetic resonance imaging in acute tendon ruptures. *Skeletal Radiol* 1986;15:619–621.
24. Dahlin DC, Unni KK. *Bone tumors: general aspects and data on 8,542 cases,* 4th ed. Springfield, IL: CC Thomas, 1986.
25. Deutsch AL, Mink JH. Articular disorders of the knee. *Top Magn Reson Imaging* 1989;1:43–56.
26. Ehman RL. High resolution imaging of the knee: technical issues. Presented at the Society of Magnetic Resonance in Medicine, Amsterdam, The Netherlands, 1989.
27. Enzinger FM, Weiss SW. *Soft tissue tumors.* St. Louis, MO: CV Mosby, 1983.
28. Gallimore GW Jr, Harms SE. Knee injuries: high-resolution MR imaging. *Radiology* 1986;160:457–461.
29. Glashow JL, Katz R, Schneider M, Scott WN. Double-blind assessment of the value of magnetic resonance imaging in the diagnosis of anterior cruciate and meniscal lesions. *J Bone Joint Surg* 1989;71:113–119.
30. Goitz HT, Rijke AM, McCue FC III. Magnetic resonance imaging of stressed anterior cruciate ligaments. Presented at the Society of Magnetic Resonance in Medicine, Amsterdam, The Netherlands, 1989.
31. Gould ES, Taylor S, Naidich JB, Furie R, Lane L. MR appearance of bilateral, spontaneous patellar tendon rupture in systemic lupus erythematosus. *J Comput Assist Tomogr* 1987;11:1096–1097.
32. Gylys-Morin VM, Hajek PC, Sartoris DJ, Resnick D. Articular cartilage defects: detectability in cadaver knees with MRI. *AJR* 1987;148:1153–1157.
33. Hajek PC, Baker LL, Sartoris DJ, Neumann CH, Resnick D. MR arthrography: anatomic–pathologic investigation. *Radiology* 1987;163:141–147.
34. Hajek PC, Sartoris DJ, Neumann CH, Resnick D. Potential contrast agents for MR arthrography: *in vitro* evaluation and practical observations. *AJR* 1987;149:97–104.
35. Hall FJ. Arthrography of the discoid lateral meniscus. *AJR* 1977;128:993–1002.
36. Hardaker WT, Sipple TL, Bassett FH III. Diagnosis and treatment of plicae syndrome of the knee. *J Bone Joint Surg* 1980;62A:221–225.
37. Harms SE, Flamig DP, Fisher CF, Fulmer JM. 3D faster MR imaging of the knee. Presented at the Society of Magnetic Resonance in Medicine, Amsterdam, The Netherlands, 1989.
38. Harms SE, Muschler G. Three-dimensional MR imaging of the knee using surface coils. *J Comput Assist Tomogr* 1986;10:773–777.
39. Harms SE, Flamig DP, Fisher CF, Fulmer JM. New method for fast MR imaging of the knee. *Radiology* 1989;173:743–750.
40. Hartzman S, Reicher MA, Bassett LW, Duckwiler GR, Mandelbaum B, Gold RH. MR imaging of the knee. Part II. Chronic disorders. *Radiology* 1987;162:553–557.
41. Herman LJ, Beltran J. Pitfalls in MR imaging of the knee. *Radiology* 1988;167:775–781.
42. Heuck AF, Steiger P, Stoller DW, Glüer CC, Genant HK. Quantification of knee joint fluid volume by MR imaging and CT using three-dimensional data processing. *J Comput Assist Tomogr* 1989;13:287–293.
43. Hollinshead WH. *Anatomy for surgeons,* vol 3, 3rd ed. New York: Harper & Row, 1982:563–583.
44. Idy-Peretti I, Yvart J, LeBalch T. MRI of the knee: assessment and follow-up of hemophilic arthropathy. Presented at the Society of Magnetic Resonance in Medicine, Amsterdam, The Netherlands, 1989.
45. Jelinek JS, Kransdorf MJ, Utz JA, Berrey BH Jr, Thomson JD, Heekin RD, Radowich MS. Imaging of pigmented villonodular synovitis with emphasis on MR imaging. *AJR* 1989;152:337–342.
46. Kangarloo H, Dietrich RB, Taira RT, et al. MR imaging of bone marrow in children. *J Comput Assist Tomogr* 1986;10:205–209.
47. Kneeland JB, Jesmanowicz A, Hyde JS. Enhancement of parallel MR image acquisition by rotation of the plane of section. *Radiology* 1988;166:886–887.
48. König H, Sauter R, Deimling M, Vogt M. Cartilage disorders: comparison of spin-echo CHESS and FLASH sequence MR images. *Radiology* 1987;164:753–758.
49. Kornick J, Trefelner E, McCarthy S, Lynch K, Jokl P. Meniscal abnormalities in the asymptomatic population. Presented RSNA, Chicago, 1989.
50. Kransdorf MJ, Moser RP, Vinh TN, Aoki J, Callaghan JJ. Primary tumors of the patella. *Skeletal Radiol* 1989;18:365–371.
51. Kujala UM, Osterman K, Kormano M, Komu M, Schlenzka D. Patellar motion analyzed by magnetic resonance imaging. *Acta Orthop Scand* 1989;60:13–16.
52. Kulkarni MV, Droolshagen LF, Kaye JJ, Green NE, Burks DD, Janco RL, Nance EP Jr. MR imaging of hemophiliac arthropathy. *J Comput Assist Tomogr* 1986;10:445–449.
53. Lee JK, Yao L. Stress fractures: MR imaging. *Radiology* 1988;169:217–220.
54. Lee JK, Yao L, Phelps CT, Wirth CR, Czajka J, Lozman J. Anterior cruciate ligament tears: MR imaging compared with arthroscopy and clinical tests. *Radiology* 1988;166:861–864.
55. Levinsohn EM. MR imaging of extremities excels in knee evaluation. *Diagn Imag* 1989;5:100–104.
56. Lotke PA, Ecker ML. Current concepts review. Osteonecrosis of the knee. *J Bone Joint Surg* 1988;70:470–473.
57. Lynch TC, Crues JV III, Morgan FW, Sheehan WE, Harter LP, Ryu R. Bone abnormalities of the knee: prevalence and significance at MR imaging. *Radiology* 1989;171:761–766.
58. Manco LG, Berlow ME. Meniscal tears—comparison of arthrography, CT and MRI. *CRC Crit Rev Diagn Imaging* 1989; 29:151–179.
59. Mandelbaum BR, Grant TT, Hartzman S, et al. The use of MRI to assist in diagnosis of pigmented villonodular synovitis of the knee joint. *Clin Orthop* 1988;231:135–139.
60. Mesgarzadeh M, Sapega AA, Bonakdarpour A, Revesz G, Moyer RA, Maurer AH, Alburger PD. Osteochondritis dissecans: analysis of mechanical stability with radiography, scintigraphy, and MR imaging. *Radiology* 1987;165:775–780.
61. Mesgarzadeh M, Schneck CD, Bonakdarpour A. Magnetic resonance imaging of the knee and correlation with normal anatomy. *RadioGraphics* 1988;8:707–733.
62. Middleton WD, Lawson TL. *Anatomy and MRI of the joints. A multiplanar atlas.* New York: Raven Press, 1989.
63. Milgrom C, Sigal R, Robin GC, et al. MRI and CT scan com-

pared with microscopic histopathology. In osteogenic sarcoma of the proximal tibia. *Orthop Rev* 1986;15:165–169.
64. Mink JH, Deutsch AL. Occult cartilage and bone injuries of the knee: detection, classification, and assessment with MR imaging. *Radiology* 1989;170:823–829.
65. Mink JH, Levy T, Crues JV. Tears of the anterior cruciate ligament and menisci of the knee: MR imaging evaluation. *Radiology* 1988;167:769–774.
66. Mink JH, Reicher MA, Crues JV III. *Magnetic resonance imaging of the knee.* New York: Raven Press, 1987.
67. Moeser P, Bechtold RE, Clark T, Rovere G, Karstaedt N, Wolfman N. MR imaging of anterior cruciate ligament repair. *J Comput Assist Tomogr* 1989;13:105–109.
68. Munk PL, Helms CA, Genant HK, Holt RG. Magnetic resonance imaging of the knee: current status, new directions. *Skeletal Radiol* 1989;18:569–577.
69. Negendank WG, Fernandez-Madrid FR, Heilbrun LK, Teitge RA. MRI of meniscal degeneration in asymptomatic knees: evidence of a relation to clinical tears. Presented at the Society of Magnetic Resonance in Medicine, Amsterdam, The Netherlands, 1989.
70. Obletter N, Held P, Kett H, Prüll C, Breit A. Evaluation of 3D MR data sets in orthopedic cases. Presented at the Society of Magnetic Resonance in Medicine, Amsterdam, The Netherlands, 1989.
71. Patel D. Arthroscopy of the plicae—synovial folds and their significance. *Am J Sports Med* 1978;6:217–225.
72. Pettersson H, Gillespy T, Kitchens C, Kentro T, Scott KN. Magnetic resonance imaging in hemophilic arthropathy of the knee. *Acta Radiol* 1987;28:621–625.
73. Pollack MS, Dalinka MK, Kressel HY, Lotke PA, Spritzer CE. Magnetic resonance imaging in the evaluation of suspected osteonecrosis of the knee. *Skeletal Radiol* 1987;16:121–127.
74. Polly DW, Callaghan JJ, Sikes RA, McCabe JM, McMahon K, Savory CG. The accuracy of selective magnetic resonance imaging compared with the findings of arthroscopy of the knee. *J Bone Joint Surg* 1988;70:192–198.
75. Rand JA, Berquist TH. The knee. In: Berquist TH, ed. *Imaging of orthopedic trauma and surgery.* Philadelphia: Saunders, 1986:239–392.
76. Rao VM, Mitchell DG, Rifkin MD, Steiner RM, Burk DL Jr, Levy D, Ballas SK. Marrow infarction in sickle cell anemia: correlation with marrow type and distribution by MRI. *Magn Reson Imaging* 1989;7:39–44.
77. Reeder JD, Matz SO, Becker L, Andelman SM. MR imaging of the knee in the sagittal projection: comparison of three-dimensional gradient-echo and spin-echo sequences. *AJR* 1989;153: 537–540.
78. Reicher MA, Hartzman S, Bassett LW, Mandelbaum B, Duckwiler G, Gold RH. MR imaging of the knee. Part I. Traumatic disorders. *Radiology* 1987;162:547–551.
79. Reicher MA, Hartzman S, Duckwiler GR, Bassett LW, Anderson LJ, Gold RH. Meniscal injuries: detection using MR imaging. *Radiology* 1986;159:753–757.
80. Reicher MA, Lufkin RB, Smith S, et al. Multiple-angle, variable-interval, nonorthogonal MRI. *AJR* 1986;147:363–366.
81. Reiser MF, Bongartz G, Erlemann R, et al. Magnetic resonance in cartilaginous lesions of the knee joint with three-dimensional gradient-echo imaging. *Skeletal Radiol* 1988;17:465–471.
82. Resnick D, Niwayama G. *Diagnosis of bone and joint disorders,* vol 5. Philadelphia: Saunders, 1988:3289–3334.
83. Romanini L, Calvisi V, Pappalardo S, et al. Prosthetic reconstruction of the anterior cruciate ligament of the knee: the roles of CT scan and MR. *Ital J Orthop Traumatol* 1988;14:301–310.
84. Sartoris DJ, Karsunoglu S, Pineda C, Kerr R, Pate D, Resnick D. Detection of intra-articular osteochondral bodies in the knee using computed arthrotomography. *Radiology* 1985;155:447–450.
85. Seeger LL. MR imaging of the knee: acute ligamentous and osseous injury: chronic trauma. Presented at the Society of Magnetic Resonance in Medicine, Amsterdam, The Netherlands, 1989.
86. Seiler JG, Christie MJ, Homra L. Correlation of the findings of magnetic resonance imaging with those of bone biopsy in patients who have stage I or II ischemic necrosis of the femoral head. *J Bone Joint Surg* 1989;71:28–32.
87. Shahabpour M, Van Cauteren M, Handelberg F, Van Roy P, Luypaert R, Casteleyn P, Osteaux M. MRI of chondral lesions of the knee: a comparative study of 2D spin echo and 3D gradient echo imaging. Presented at the Society of Magnetic Resonance in Medicine, Amsterdam, The Netherlands, 1989.
88. Shaliriaree H. Chondromalacia. *Contemp Orthop* 1985;11:27–39.
89. Shellock FG, Mink HJ, Deutsch AL, Fox JM. Patellar tracking abnormalities: clinical experience with kinematic MR imaging in 130 patients. *Radiology* 1989;172:799–804.
90. Sick H, Burguet J. *Imaging anatomy of the knee region.* München, West Germany: Bergmann Verlag, 1988.
91. Silva I, Silver DM. Tears of the meniscus as revealed by magnetic resonance imaging. *J Bone Joint Surg* 1988;70:199–202.
92. Silverman JM, Mink JH, Deutsch AL. Discoid menisci of the knee: MR imaging appearance. *Radiology* 1989;173:351–354.
93. Smith DK, Berquist TH, An KN, Robb RA, Chai EYS. Validation of three-dimensional reconstructions of knee anatomy: CT vs. MR imaging. *J Comput Assist Tomogr* 1989;13:294–301.
94. Solomon SL, Totty WG, Lee JKT. MR imaging of the knee: comparison of three-dimensional FISP and two dimensional spin-echo sequences. *Radiology* 1989;173:739–742.
95. Soudry M, Lanir A, Angel D, Roffman M, Kaplan N, Mendes DG. Anatomy of the normal knee as seen by magnetic resonance imaging. *J Bone Joint Surg* 1986;68:117–120.
96. Spritzer CE, Dalinka MK, Kressel HY. Magnetic resonance imaging of pigmented villonodular synovitis: a report of two cases. *Skeletal Radiol* 1987;16:316–319.
97. Stafford SA, Rosenthal DI, Gebhardt MC, Brady TJ, Scott JA. MRI in stress fractures. *AJR* 1986;147:553–556.
98. Stoller DW. Fast MR improves imaging of musculoskeletal system. *Diagn Imag* 1988;2:98–103.
99. Stoller DW, Martin C, Crues JV, Kaplan L, Mink JH. Meniscal tears: pathologic correlation with MR imaging. *Radiology* 1987;163:731–735.
100. Sutro CT. Intraneural ganglion of the common peroneal nerve. *Bull Hosp Joint Dis* 1960;21:330–331.
101. Totterman S, Simon J, Szumowski J, Magagna L, Katzberg R. PEACH in the detection of musculoskeletal lesions. Presented at the Society of Magnetic Resonance in Medicine, Amsterdam, The Netherlands, 1989.
102. Totterman S, Weiss SL, Szumowski J, Katzberg RW, Hornak JP, Proskin HM, Eisen J. MR fat suppression technique in the evaluation of normal structures of the knee. *J Comput Assist Tomogr* 1989;13:473–479.
103. Tria AJ, Johnson CD, Zawadsky JP. The popliteus tendon. *J Bone Joint Surg* 1989;71:714–716.
104. Tyrrell RL, Gluckert K, Pathria M, Modic MT. Fast three-dimensional MR imaging of the knee: comparison with arthroscopy. *Radiology* 1988;166:865–872.
105. Van Heuzen EP, Golding RP, Van Zanten TEG, Patka P. Magnetic resonance imaging of meniscal lesions of the knee. *Clin Radiol* 1988;39:658–660.
106. Van Zanten TEG, Golding RP, Taets Van Amerongen AHM, Pieters R, Veerman AJP. Nuclear magnetic resonance imaging of bone marrow in childhood leukemia. *Clin Radiol* 1988;39:77–81.
107. Vellet D, Marks P, Munro T, Fowler P. MRI evaluation of subclinical, subcortical bony injuries in acute post-traumatic hemarthroses of the knee. Presented at the Society of Magnetic Resonance in Medicine, Amsterdam, The Netherlands, 1989.
108. Vellet D, Marks P, Munro T, Fowler P. Comparative evaluation of orthogonal and non-orthogonal MRI in the evaluation of acute disruption of the anterior cruciate ligament. Presented at the Society of Magnetic Resonance in Medicine, Amsterdam, The Netherlands, 1989.
109. Vogler JB, Murphy WA. Bone marrow imaging. *Radiology* 1988;168:679–693.
110. Watanabe AT, Carter BC, Teitelbaum GP, Bradley WG. Common pitfalls in magnetic resonance imaging of the knee. *J Bone Joint Surg* 1989;71A:857–862.
111. Watanabe AT, Carter BC, Teitelbaum GP, Seeger LL, Bradley

WG Jr. Normal variations in MR imaging of the knee: appearance and frequency. *AJR* 1989;153:341–344.

112. Weiss CB, Lundberg M, Hamberg P, DeHaven KE, Gillquist J. Non-operative treatment of meniscal tears. *J Bone Joint Surg* 1989;71A:811–822.
113. Wiberg G. Roentgenographic and anatomic studies of the femoropatellar joint, with special reference to chondromalacia patella. *Acta Orthop Scand* 1941;121:319–340.
114. Williamson MP, Humm G, Crisp AJ. ^{1}H nuclear magnetic resonance investigation of synovial fluid components in osteoarthritis, rheumatoid arthritis and traumatic effusions. *Br J Rheumatol* 1989;28:23–27.
115. Wolf GL. Current status of MR imaging contrast agents: special report. *Radiology* 1989;172:709–710.
116. Yao L, Lee JK. Occult intraosseous fracture: detection with MR imaging. *Radiology* 1988;167:749–751.
117. Yao L, Lee JK. Avulsion of the posteromedial tibial plateau by the semimembranosus tendon: diagnosis with MR imaging. *Radiology* 1989;172:513–514.
118. Yulish BS, Lieberman JM, Newman AJ, Bryan PJ, Muloplos GP, Modic MT. Juvenile rheumatmoid arthritis: assessment of MR imaging. *Radiology* 1987;165:149–152.
119. Yulish BS, Montanez J, Goodfellow DB, Bryan PJ, Mulopulos GP, Modic MT. Chondromalacia patellae: assessment with MR imaging. *Radiology* 1987;164:763–766.

MRI of the Musculoskeletal System, 2nd Edition, edited by T. H. Berquist. Raven Press, Ltd., New York © 1990.

CHAPTER 8

Foot, Ankle, and Calf

Thomas H. Berquist

Techniques, 253
Patient Positioning and Coil Selection, 253
Pulse Sequences and Imaging Parameters, 254
Anatomy, 273
Skeletal and Articular Anatomy, 273
Soft Tissue Anatomy, 275
Posterior Musculature, 275
Neurovascular Anatomy of the Calf, 278
Anterolateral Musculature, 278
Anterior Compartment Musculature, 279
Neurovascular Anatomy of the Anterolateral Muscles, 280
Foot Musculature, 280
Neurovascular Supply of the Foot, 284
Pitfalls and Normal Variants, 284
Clinical Applications, 285
Trauma, 285
Soft Tissue Trauma, 285
Neoplasms, 297
Arthritis/Infection, 302
Ischemic Bone and Soft Tissue Disease, 305
Miscellaneous Conditions, 309
References, 309

Proper application of imaging procedures is essential to obtain needed information for a diagnosis and therapy in patients with suspected calf, foot, and ankle pathology (9,11,12,68,107). Standard radiographic views that include AP, lateral, standing, and oblique views are essential and provide adequate screening for most skeletal abnormalities. Special views, such as fluoroscopically positioned spot films, are also useful because of the complex osseous anatomy of the foot and ankle. Conventional tomography and radionuclide studies are also valuable in detecting subtle skeletal injuries. More recently, CT has provided valuable information regarding both osseous and soft tissue pathology in the calf, foot, and ankle. Ultrasound can be used to differentiate superficial soft tissue lesions and to study abnormalities in certain tendons, especially the Achilles tendon (11). More invasive procedures, such as arthrography, tenography, and angiography, may also be required to evaluate the ligaments, tendons, and vessels (11).

Magnetic resonance imaging (MRI) is particularly suited to evaluation of the complex bone and soft tissue anatomy of the foot, ankle, and calf because of its superior soft tissue contrast and the ability to image in multiple planes. In addition, new fast-scan (gradient-echo) techniques allow pseudomotion studies with cine loop imaging (99). New software developments have also provided improved vascular studies and the potential for spectroscopic studies on clinical units.

T. H. Berquist: Mayo Medical School and Mayo Clinic, Rochester, Minnesota 55905.

TECHNIQUES

Bone and soft tissue anatomy is complex in the foot and ankle. Axial, coronal, or sagittal images adequately demonstrate the anatomy in most clinical settings. However, positioning of the foot must be carefully accomplished so the anatomy is not distorted. In some situations off-axis oblique images may be required to optimally demonstrate the anatomy.

Patient Positioning and Coil Selection

The patient should be studied with a closely coupled coil to achieve optimal signal-to-noise ratios and spatial resolution (11,70). Conventional surface coils take several configurations—flat, partial volume, or circumferential (Fig. 8-1). Different coils are suited to certain

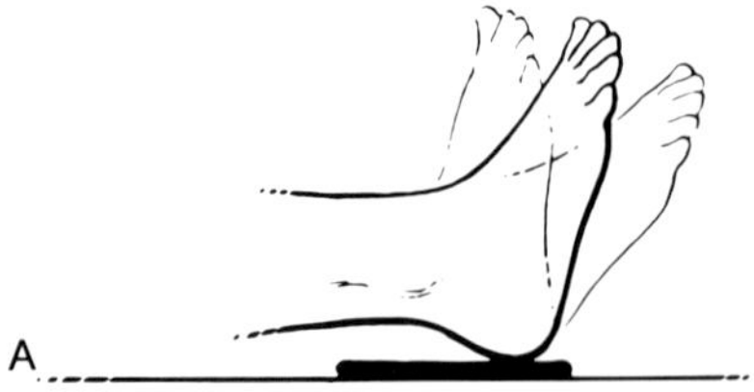

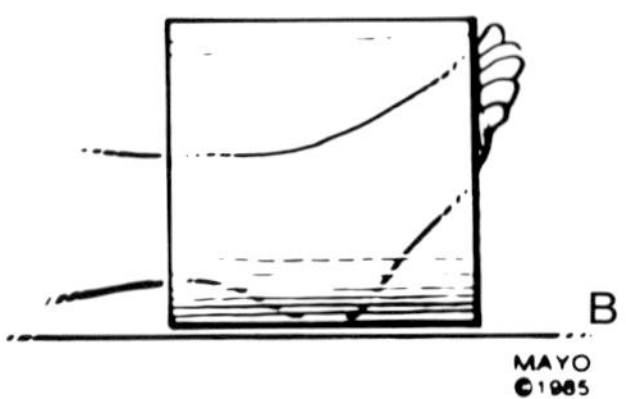

FIG. 8-1. Patient positioned for examination of the foot and ankle using flat (**A**) and circumferential (**B**) coils. The former allows more flexibility with positioning and motion studies. The circumferential coil provides more uniform signal intensity but reduces positioning options. (From ref. 10a.)

types of examination. Generally, flat circular coils, such as the 5 inch coil described in Chapter 3, or circumferential volume coils are used for examination of the foot and ankle. In certain cases, if comparison is needed, either dual coupled coils or the head coil can be used to reduce examination time (7,11,45,70,86,90). The extremity coil can be used to evaluate the calf. The head coil can be used if comparison is required.

Patients can be examined in the supine or prone position, depending on which anatomic region is being studied. The prone position is useful for examination of the forefoot and assists in reducing inadvertent motion. The prone position is also optimal for evaluating the posterior soft tissues of the calf. This avoids soft tissue compression, which can distort the anatomy. However, the hindfoot soft tissues are distorted when the patient is prone due to plantar flexion of the foot (Fig. 8-2). For example, in patients with suspected posterior or Achilles tendon pathology, it is best to have the patient supine with the foot in neutral position so that the tendons are not collapsed or buckled, which occurs when the patient is prone or the foot is in the plantar flexed position (Fig. 8-2B). The foot and ankle should be supported with foam sponges and straps to prevent motion when motion studies are not being performed. Motion studies are usually performed using the flat circular 5 inch coil.

Pulse Sequences and Imaging Parameters

Spin-echo sequences using short TE, TR (T1 weighted) and long TE, TR (T2 weighted) provide the

A,B

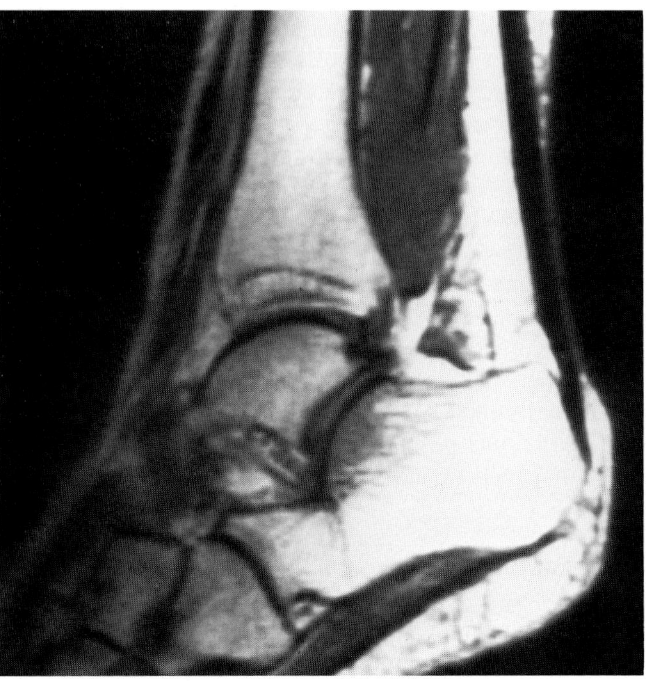

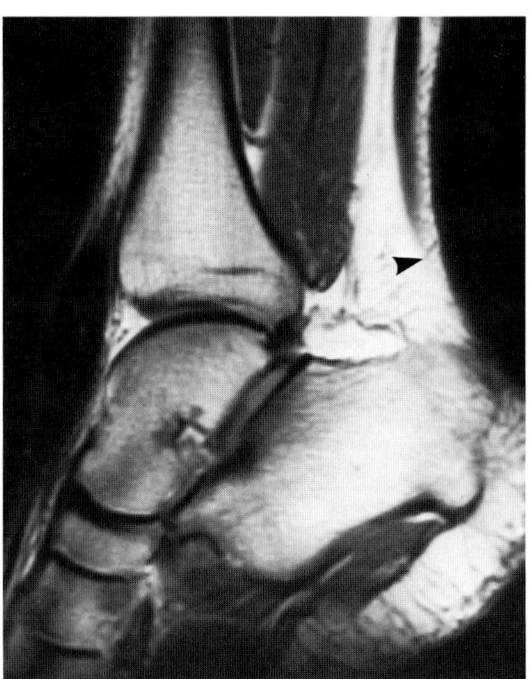

FIG. 8-2. Sagittal MR images of the ankle with the foot in neutral (**A**) and plantar flexed (prone) (**B**) positions. Note the buckling, partial volume effects on the Achilles tendon (*arrow*), and rotation of the calcaneus in (**B**).

TABLE 8-1. *MR screening examinations of the calf, foot, and ankle*

Location	Pulse sequence	Slice thickness	Matrix	Field of view (FOV)	Acquisitions (Nex)	Image time
Calf[a]						
Scout coronal	SE 200/20	Three 1 cm thick slices	128 × 256	24–32 cm	1	26 sec
Axial	SE 2,000/60,20	1 cm/skip 25 mm or 5 mm/skip 25 mm	256 × 256	24–32 cm	1	8 min 56 sec
Axial, coronal, or sagittal	SE 500/20	1 cm/skip 25 mm or 5 mm/skip 25 mm	256 × 256	24–32 cm	1	2 min 8 sec
					Total =	11 min 30 sec
Ankle						
Scout axial or sagittal	SE 200/20	Three 1 cm thick slices	128 × 256	16–20 cm	1	26 sec
Axial	SE 2,000/60,20	1 cm/skip 25 mm or 5 mm/skip 25 mm	256 × 256	16–20 cm	1	8 min 56 sec
Sagittal	SE 2,000/60,20	1 cm/skip 25 mm or 5 mm/skip 25 mm	256 × 256	16–20 cm	1	8 min 56 sec
					Total =	18 min 18 sec
Foot						
Scout sagittal	SE 200/20	Three 1 cm thick slices	128 × 256	12–16 cm	1	26 sec
Oblique axial[b]	SE 2,000/60,20	5 mm/skip 1.5–2.5 mm	256 × 256 or 192 × 256	12–16 cm	1–2	8 min 56 sec
Oblique axial or sagittal	SE 500/20	5 mm/skip 1.5–2.5 mm	256 × 256 or 192 × 256	12–16 cm	1	2 min 8 sec
					Total =	11 min 30 sec
Marrow disorders						
STIR	IR 1,500/30/100	3–5 mm/skip 1 mm	256 × 256	12–30 cm depending on area	1	6 min 40 sec
Vascular disease						
GRASS	100/12–16 flip angle 60°	5 mm/skip 2.5 mm	128 × 256	24–32 cm	2	42 sec/slice

[a] The body, extremity, or head coil can be used depending on the area to be studied.
[b] Image plane perpendicular to the sagittal to obtain true cross sections of the forefoot.

necessary information for diagnosis and evaluation of most calf, foot, and ankle disorders (7,9,11,70) (Table 8-1). We generally perform at least two pulse sequences in at least two image planes (Figs. 8-3 to 8-6). For example, in evaluation of the ankle, T2 weighted axial images along with either T1 or T2 weighted sagittal images are usually adequate to identify and characterize pathology. Similarly in the foot, these two image planes are often useful in demonstrating the pathology. In certain cases, coronal images or special oblique images are necessary to evaluate certain of the tendons and ligaments of the foot and ankle (9,11,70).

A small field of view (16–20 cm), 256 × 256 or 256 × 192 matrix, one acquisition, and 3–5 mm slice thickness with 1–2.5 mm interslice gaps appear to be most useful for defining complex foot and ankle anatomy when surface coils are used. Thicker slices may be used for screening the soft tissues in the leg (Table 8-1). We initially obtain a scout view in the plane best suited to select our initial examining sequence. The sagittal or axial plane is most often used for the scout view for the foot and ankle. A coronal scout is most often used for establishing sequences for the calf. The matrix can be reduced to 256 × 128, which allows the scout image to be obtained in approximately 26 sec using a short TE/TR sequence (see Chapter 3). Axial and sagittal T2 weighted sequences (TE 20, 80 or TE 30, 60; TR 2,000) provide an excellent screening examination for most articular and soft tissue pathology. Short TE/TR spin-echo sequences provide excellent contrast for bone marrow abnormalities and changes in fatty tissue. Short TI inversion recovery (TE 20, TI 100–150, TR 1,500) sequences are excellent for detecting subtle marrow or soft tissue pathology. Most examinations of the calf or foot and ankle can be performed in imaging times of less than 30 min (11,12,93,97).

Newer imaging techniques—specifically, gradient-echo techniques—are useful in evaluating motion and vascular anatomy (97) (Table 8-1). Specific techniques and pulse sequences are defined later as they apply to specific clinical indications.

Text continues on p. 273

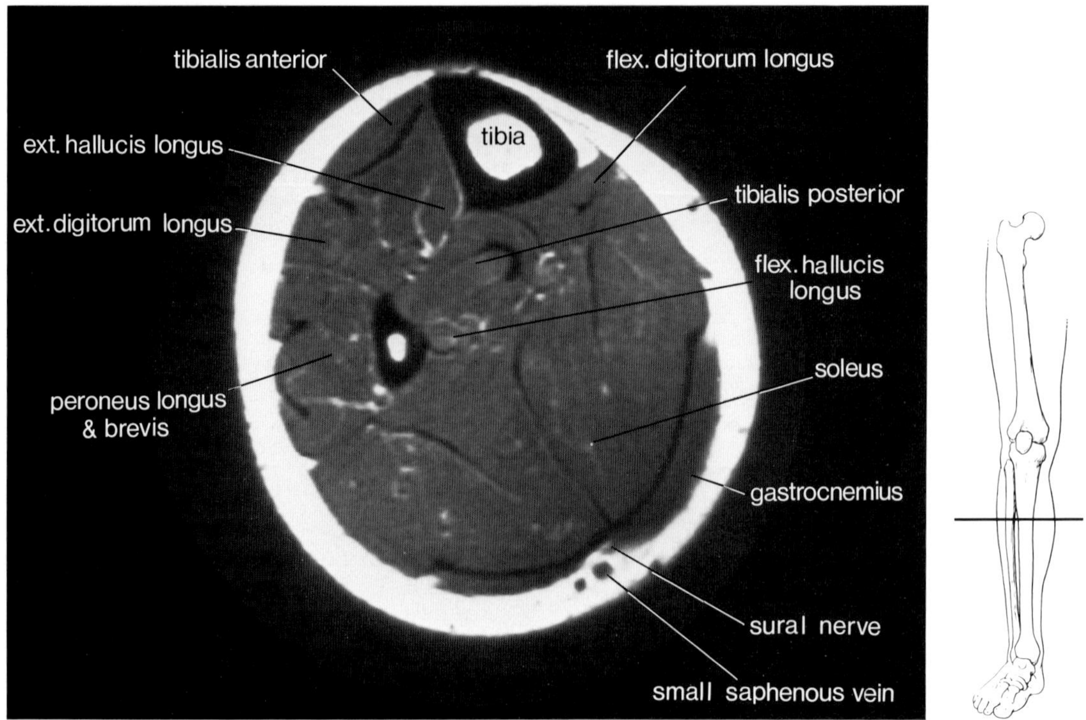

FIG. 8-3. Axial images of the calf and ankle. **A:** Axial image through the upper calf.

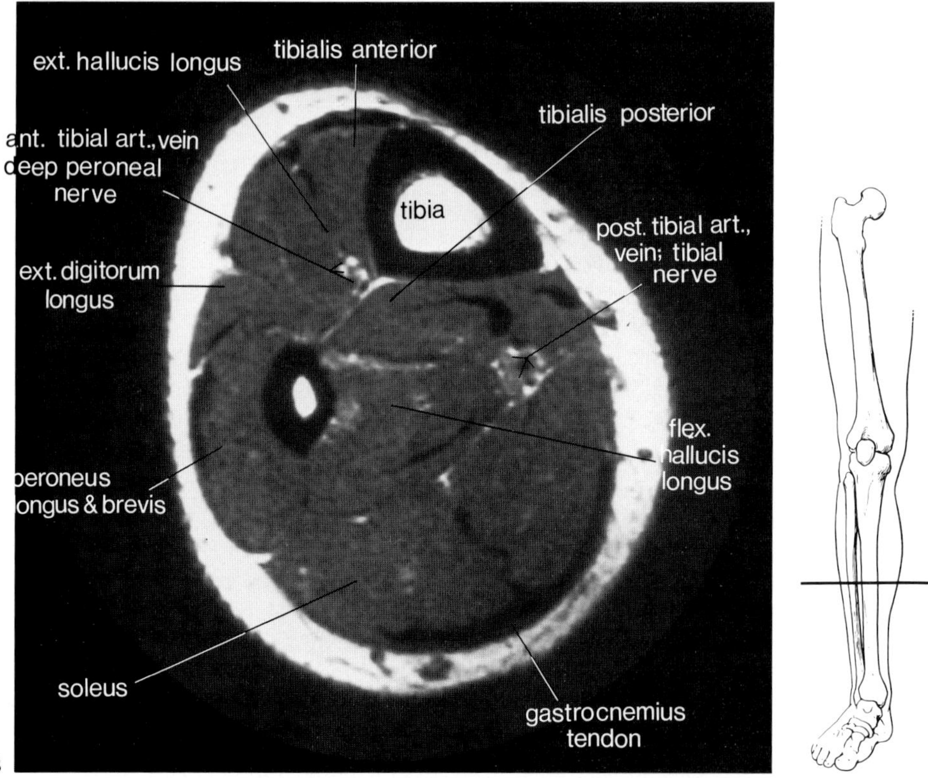

FIG. 8-3. B: Axial image through the midcalf.

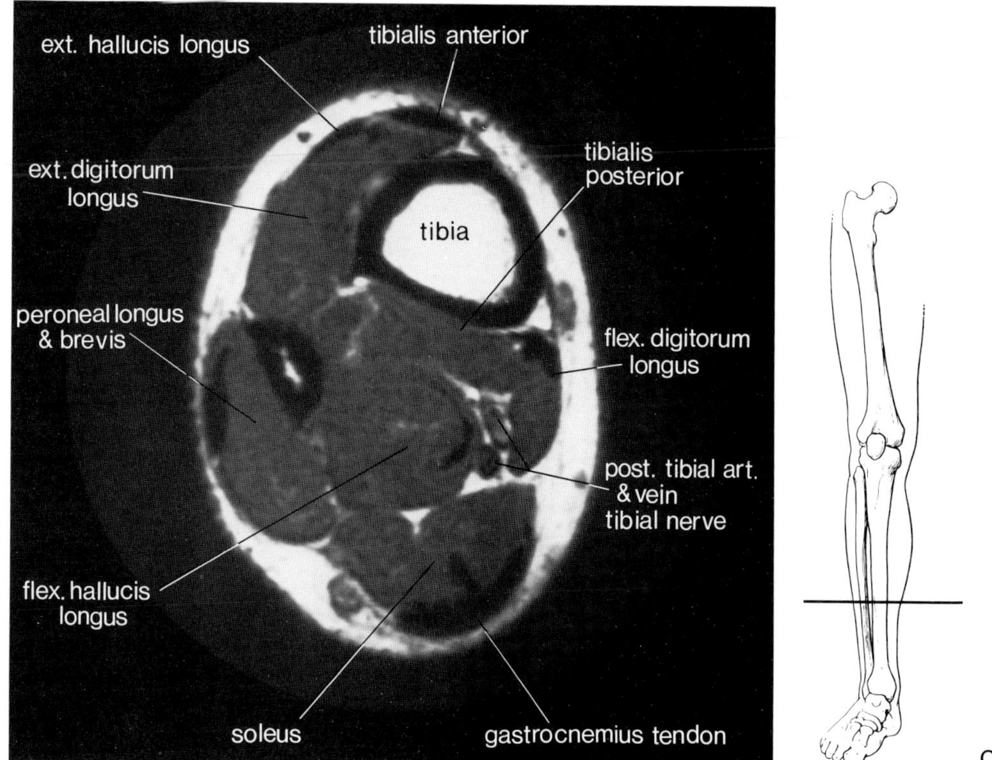

FIG. 8-3. C: Axial image through the lower calf.

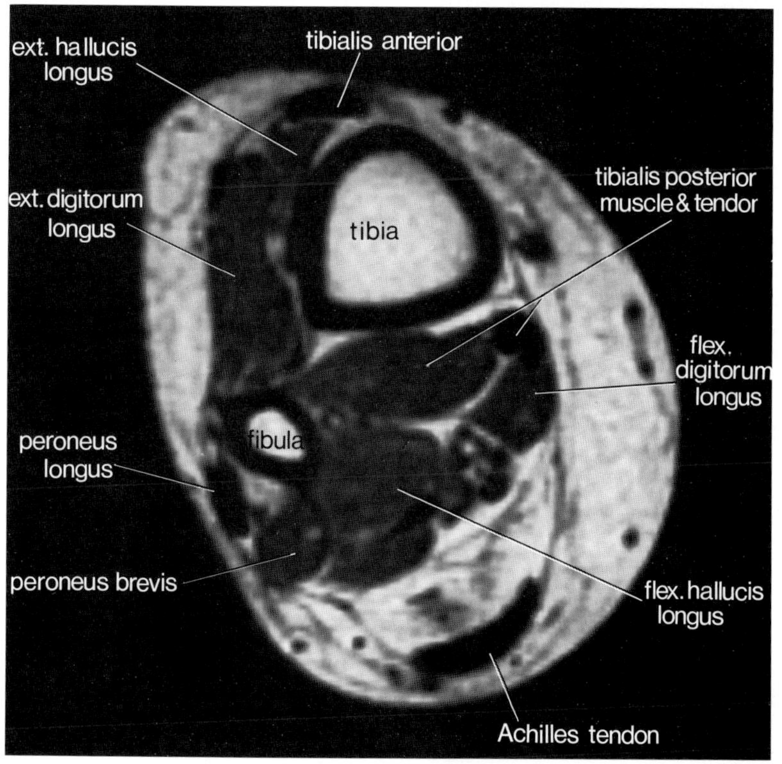

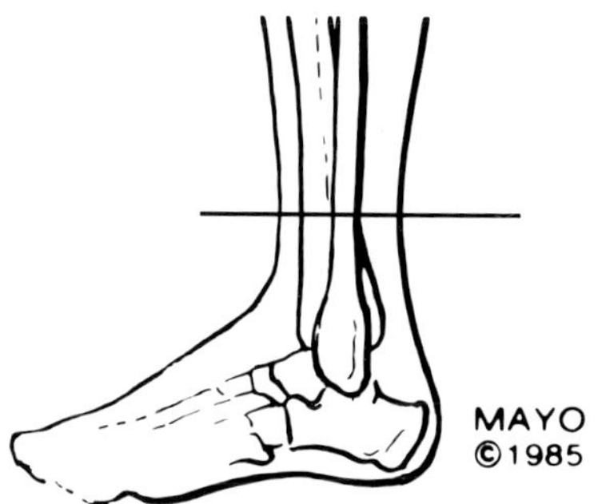

FIG. 8-3. D: Axial image through the lower calf.

E

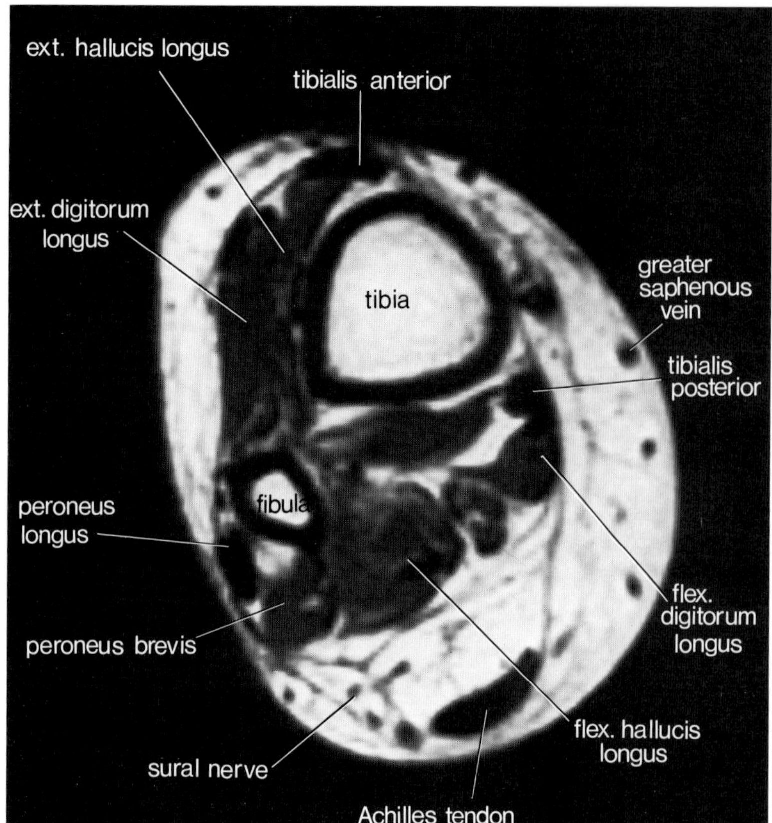

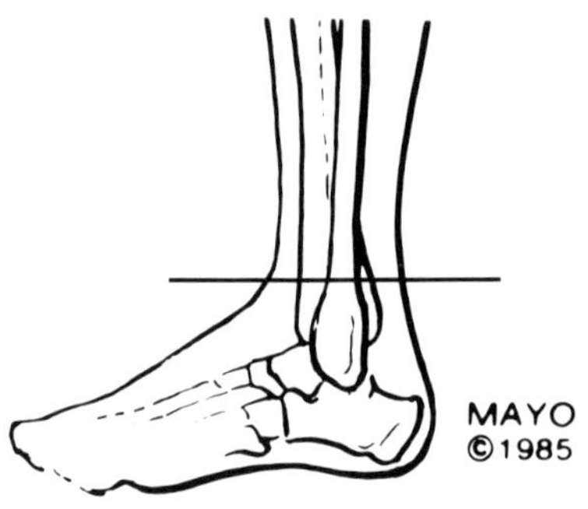

FIG. 8-3. E: Axial image through the upper ankle.

F

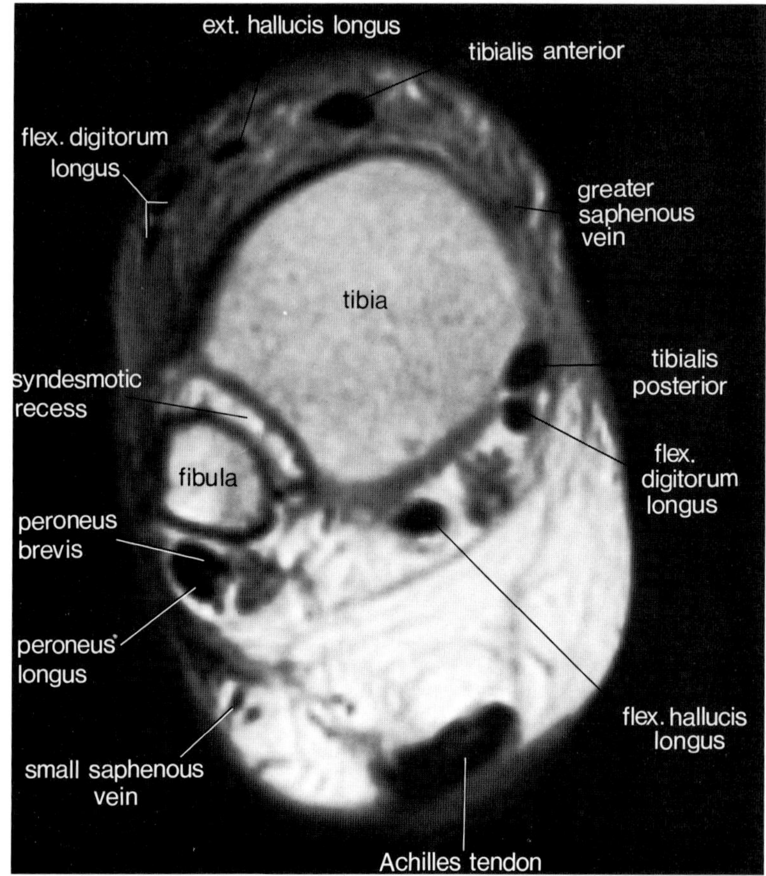

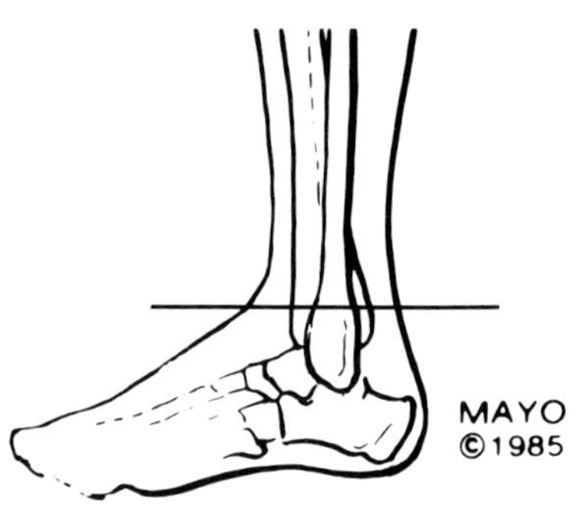

FIG. 8-3. F: Axial image through the upper syndesmosis.

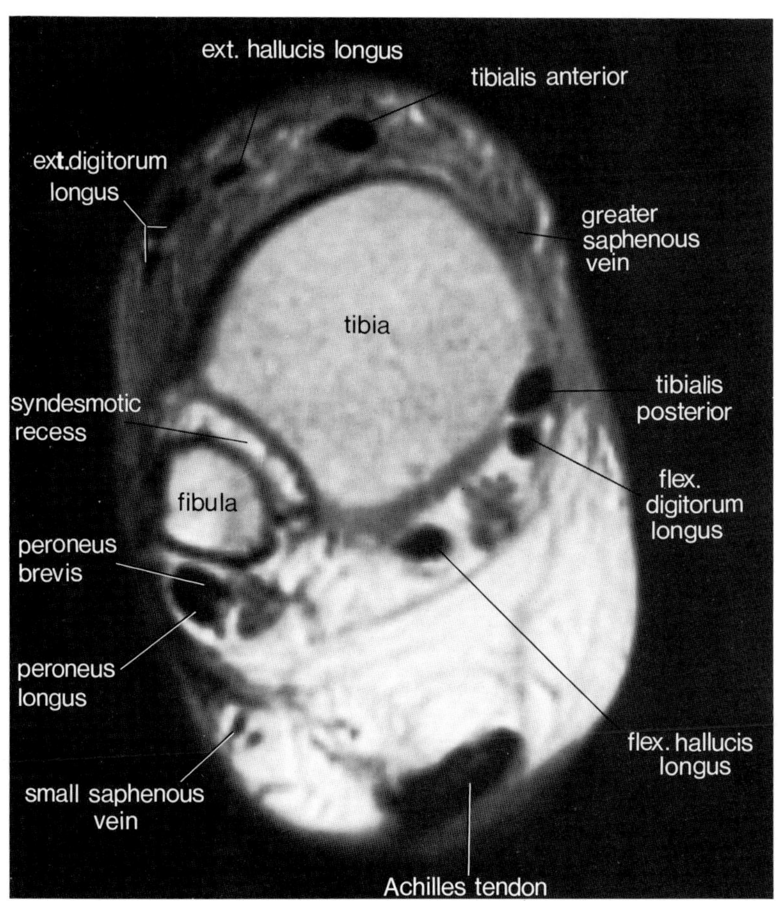

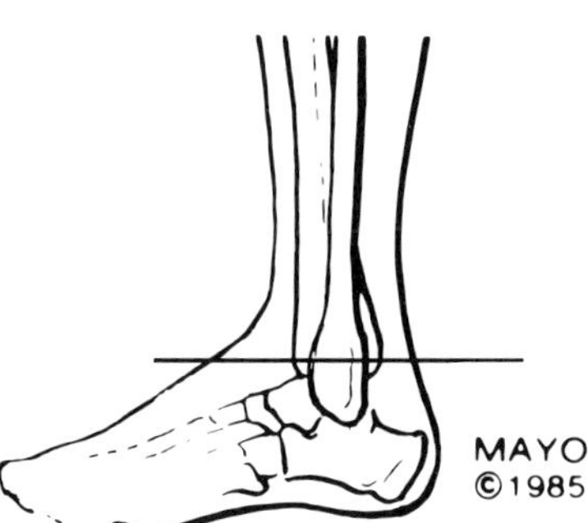

FIG. 8-3. G: Axial image through the lower syndesmosis.

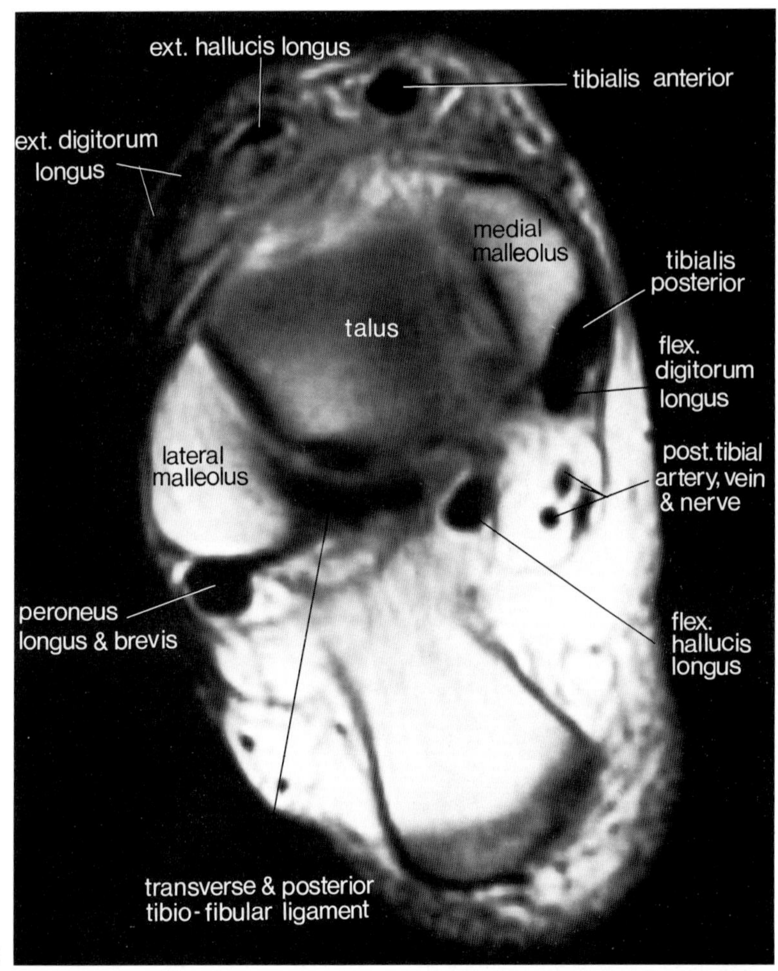

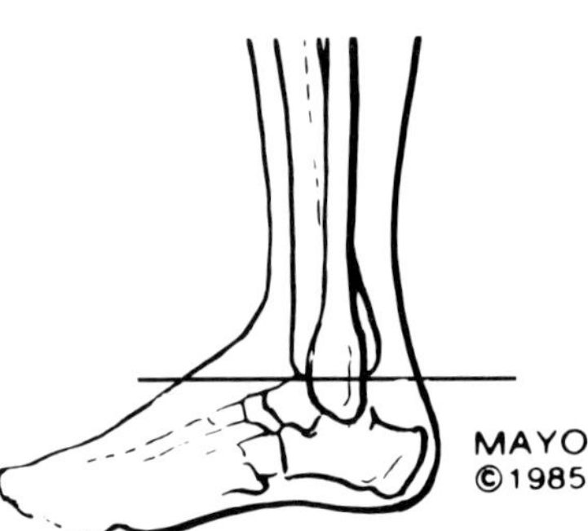

FIG. 8-3. H: Axial image through the malleoli and calcaneus.

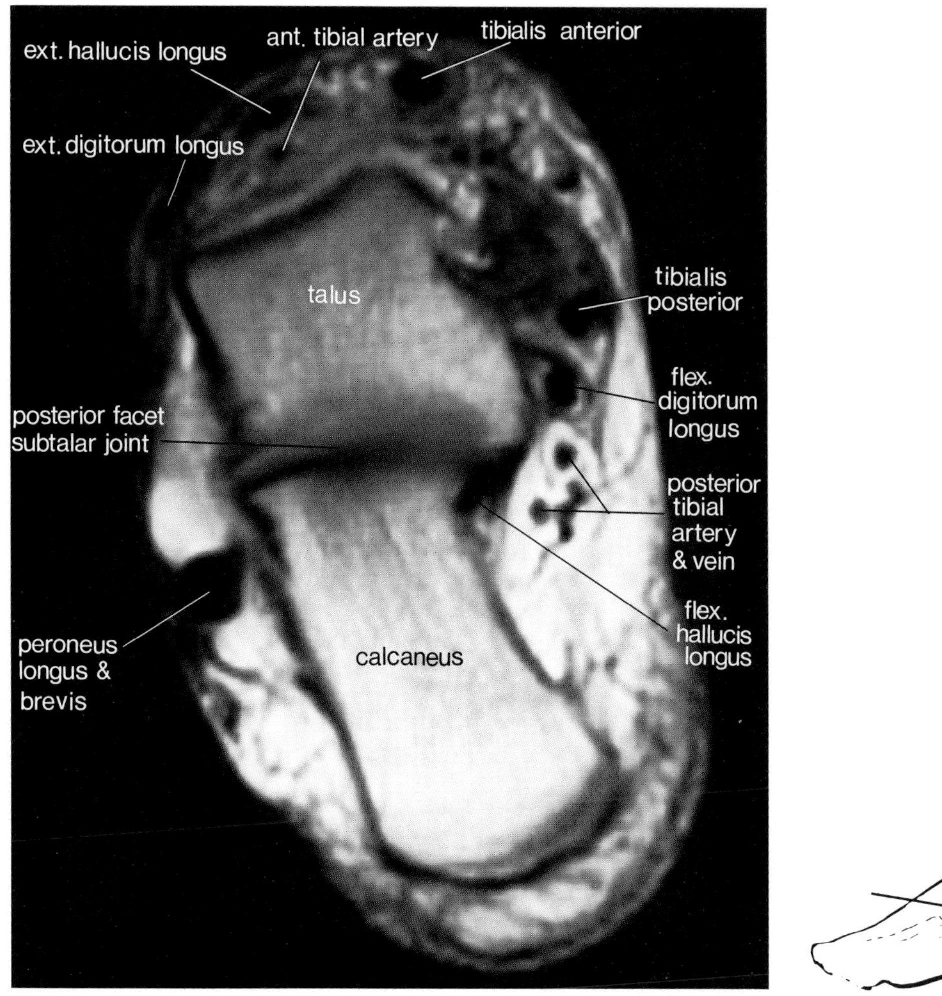

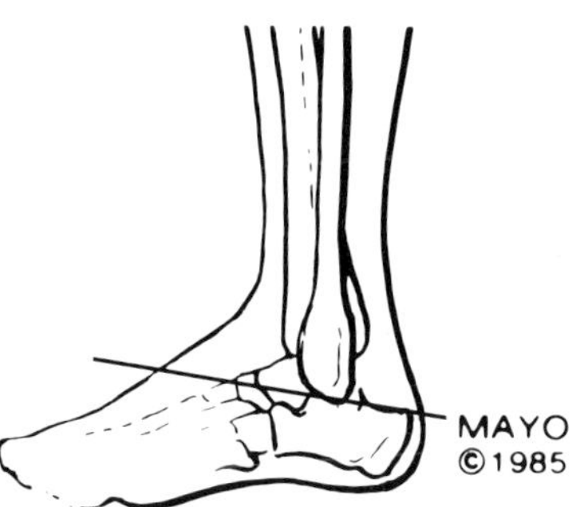

FIG. 8-3. I: Axial image through the calcaneus and posterior subtalar joint.

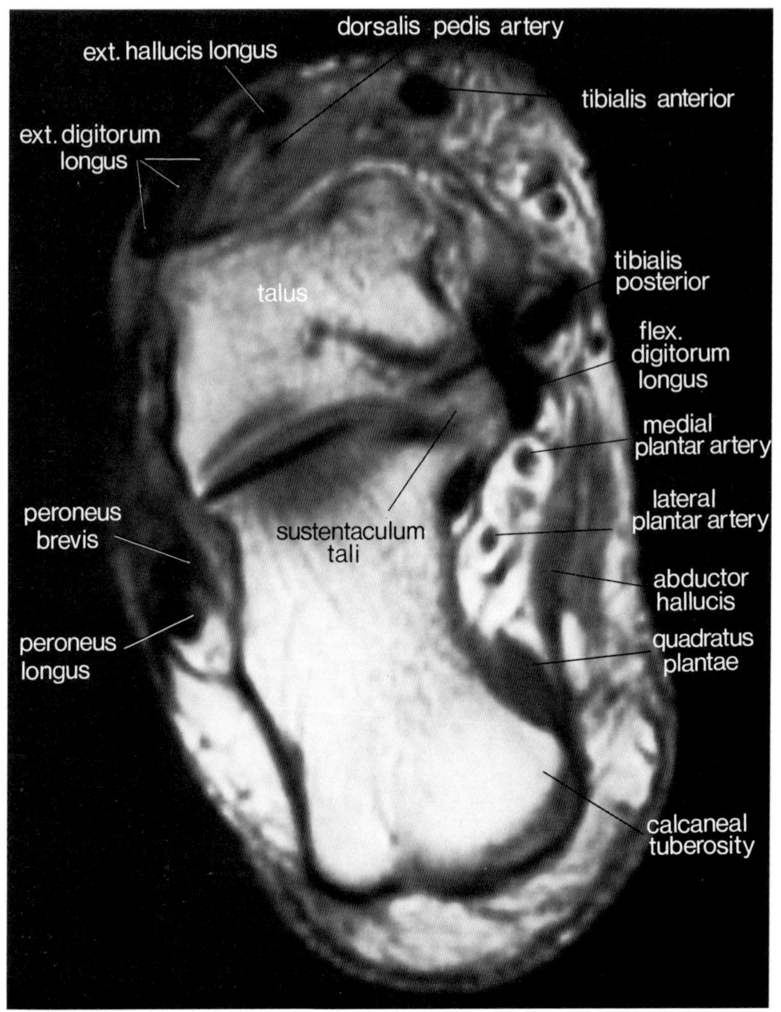

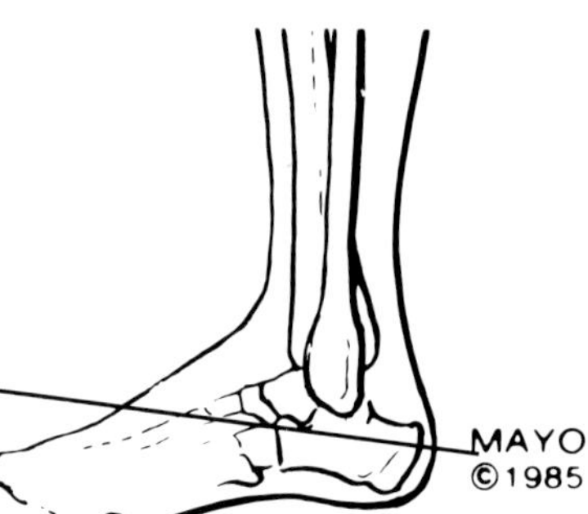

FIG. 8-3. **J:** Axial image through the sustentacular region.

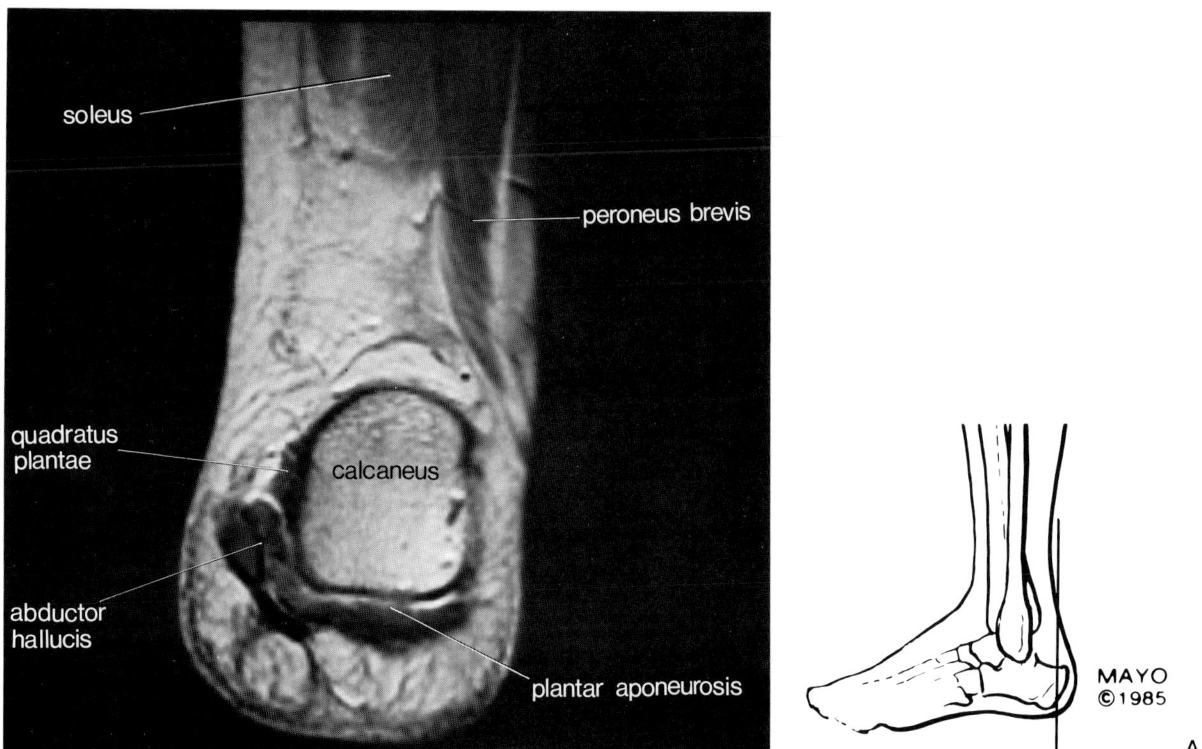

FIG. 8-4. Coronal images of the ankle and foot from posterior to anterior. **A:** Coronal image through the calcaneus.

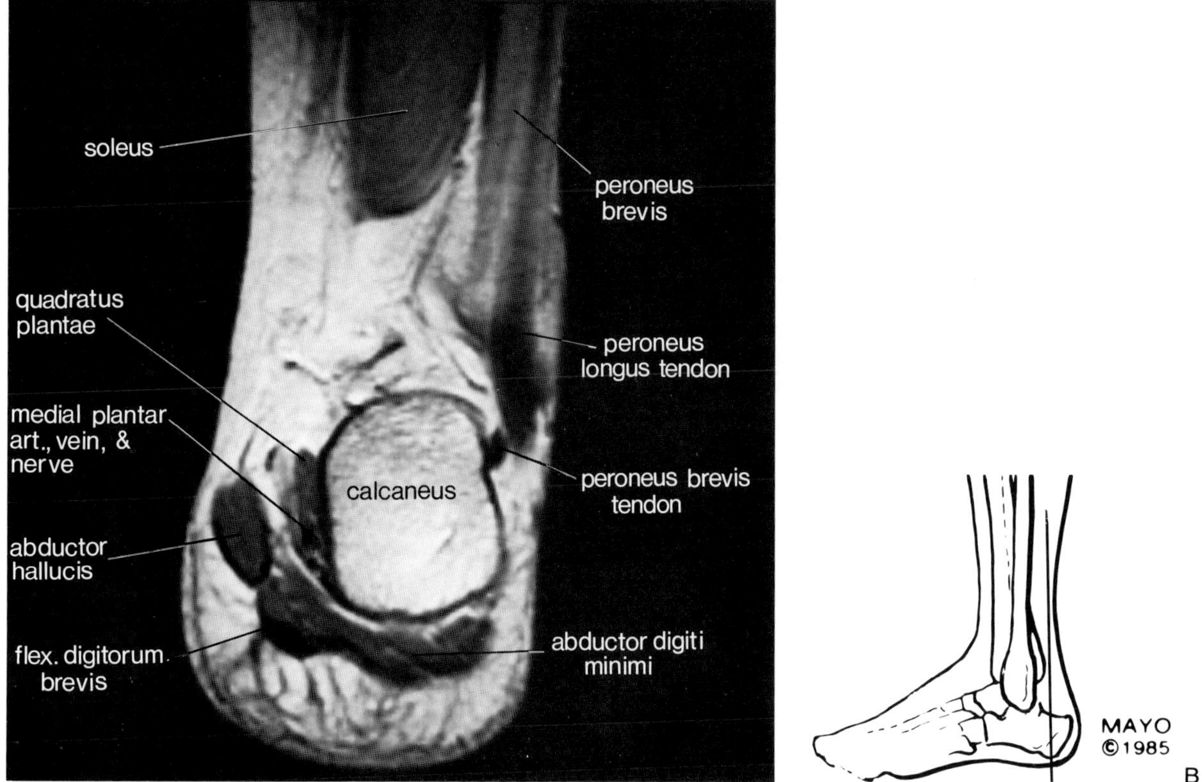

FIG. 8-4. B: Coronal image through the calcaneus in the region of the peroneal groove.

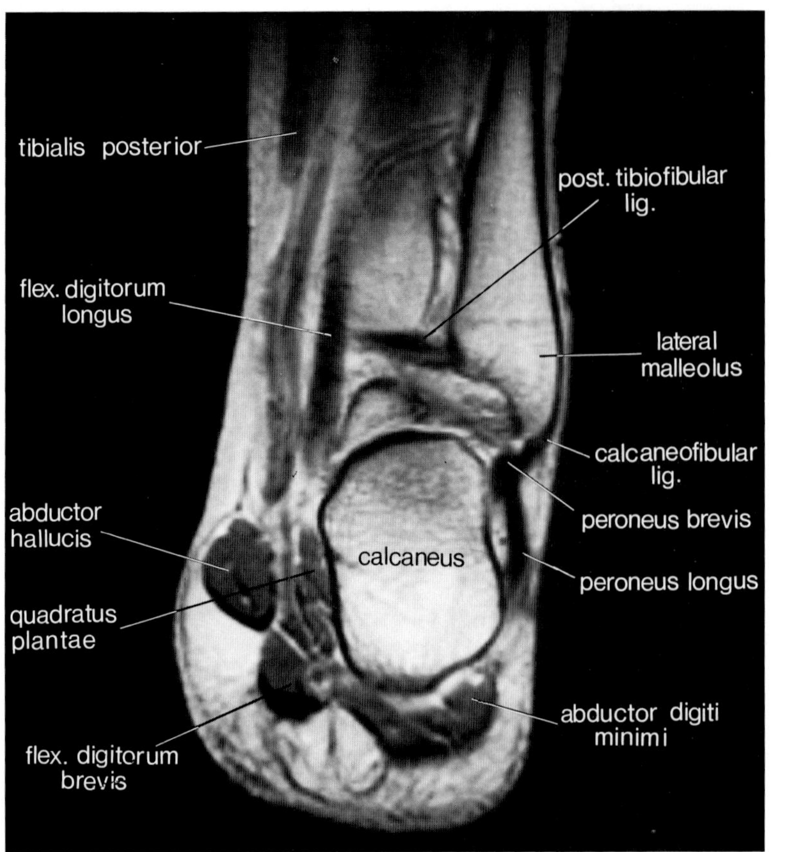

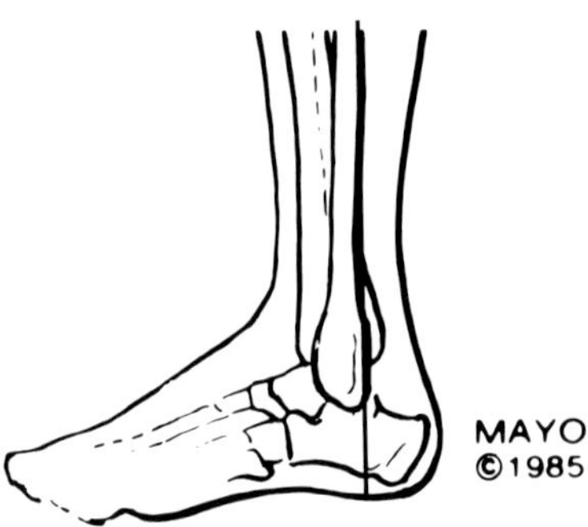

FIG. 8-4. C: Coronal image through the lateral malleolus.

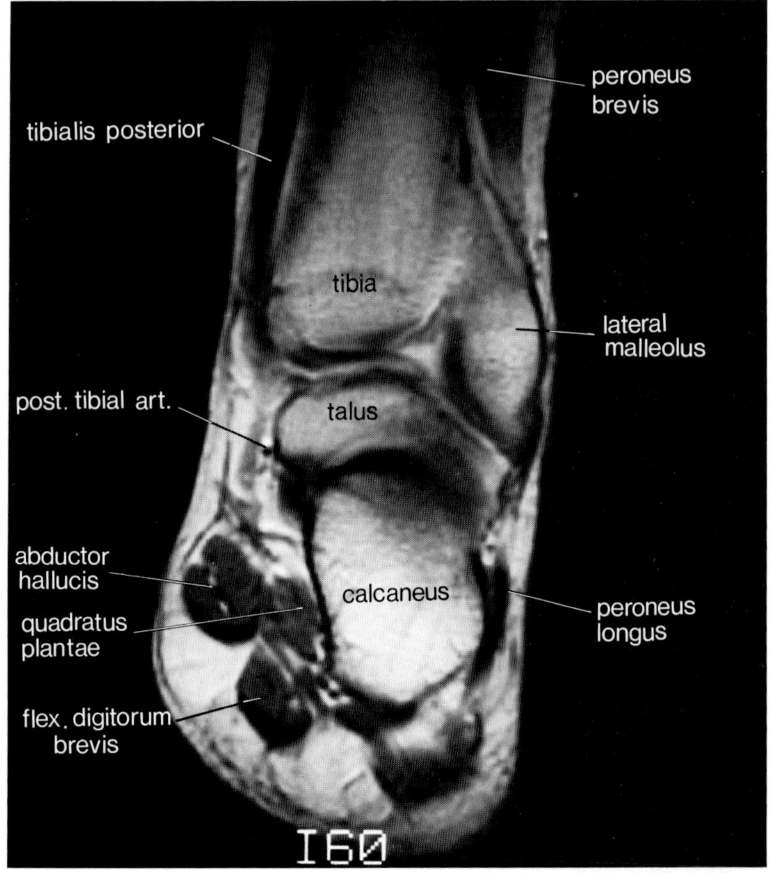

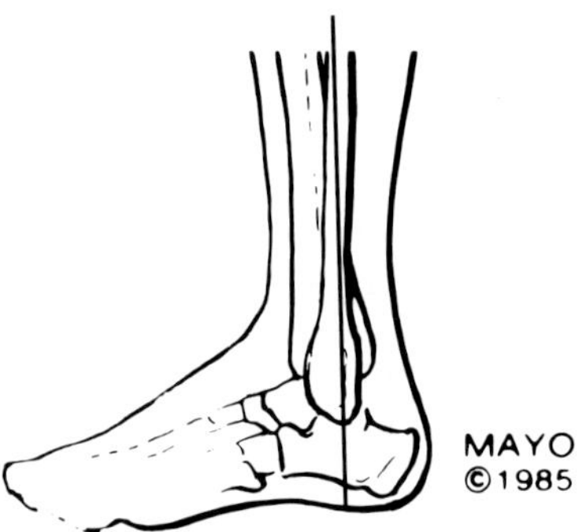

FIG. 8-4. D: Coronal image through the posterior tibiotalar joint.

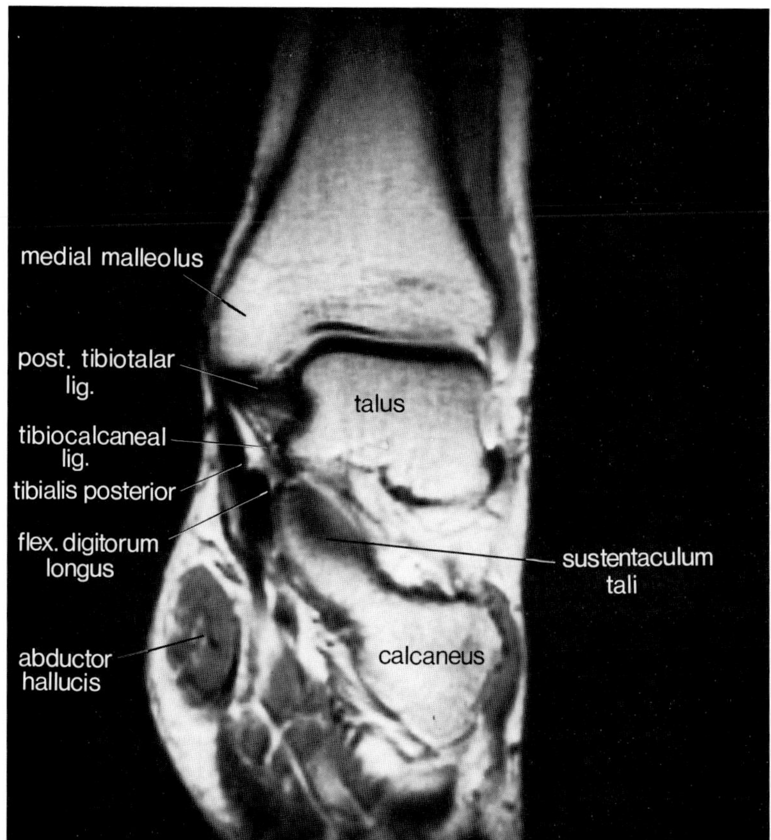

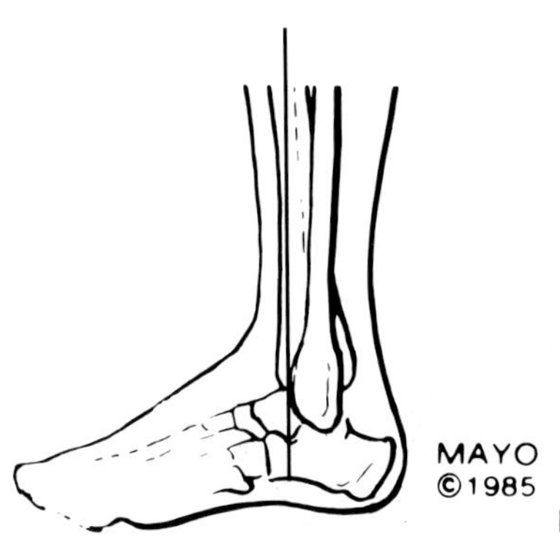

E

FIG. 8-4. E: Coronal image through the medial malleolus.

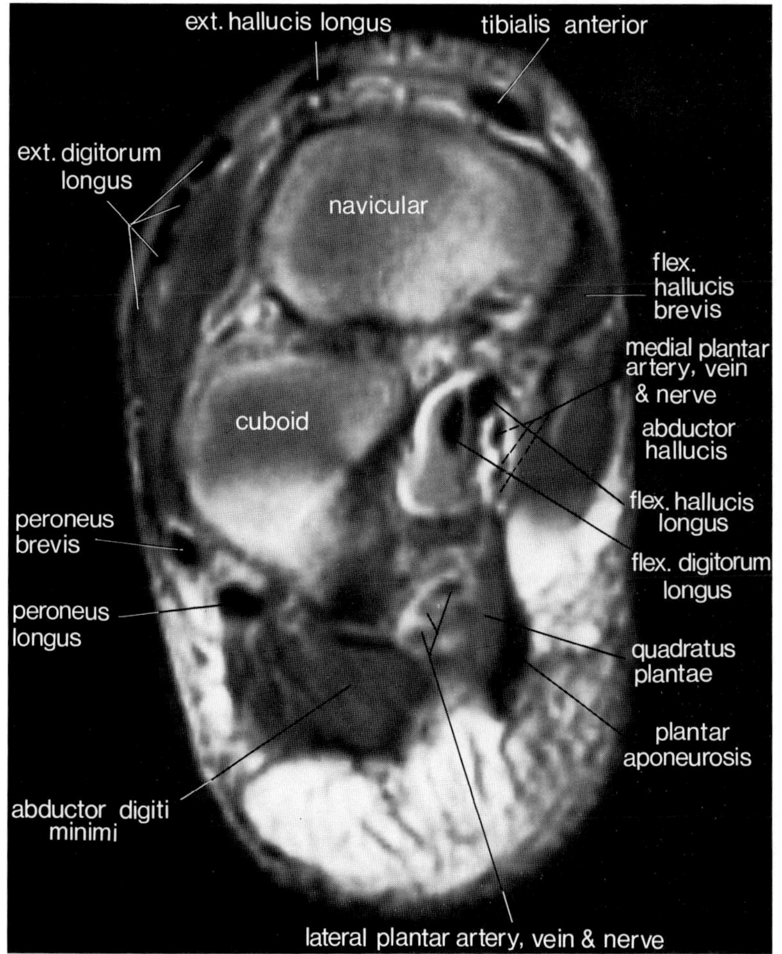

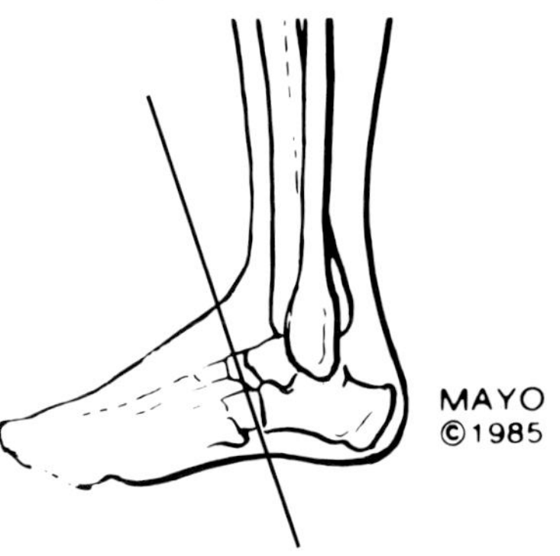

F

FIG. 8-4. F: Coronal image through the navicular.

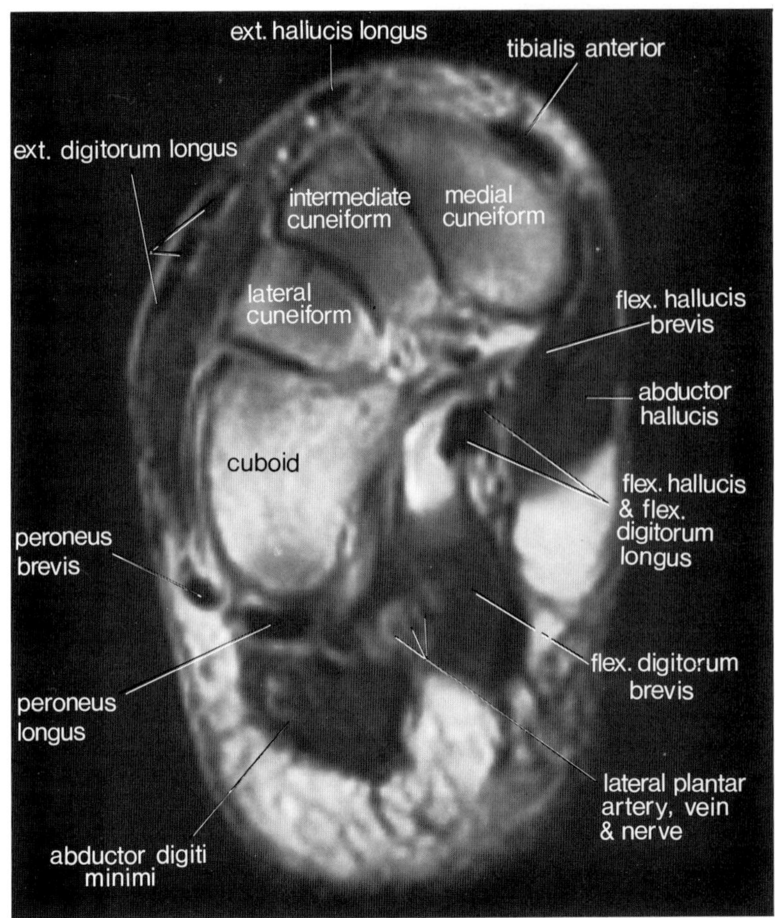

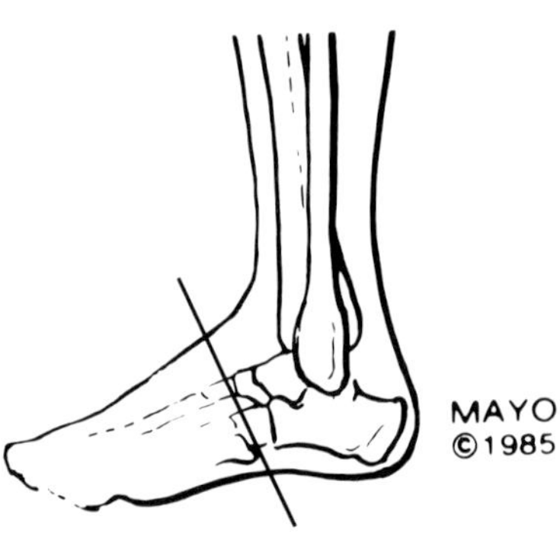

FIG. 8-4. G: Coronal image through the cuneiform.

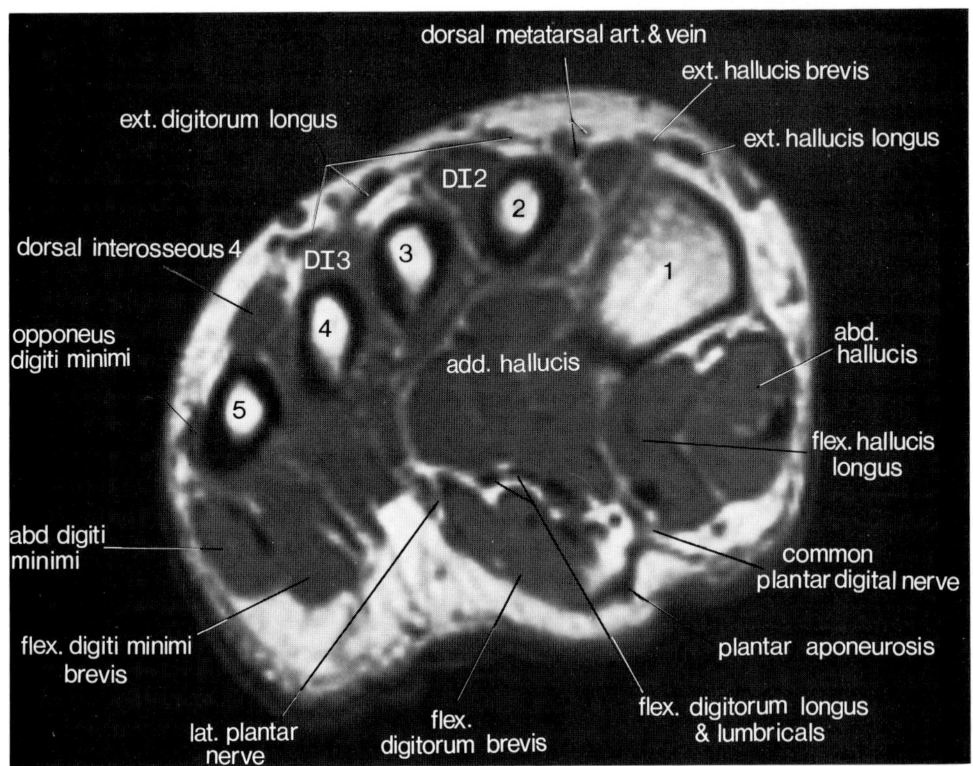

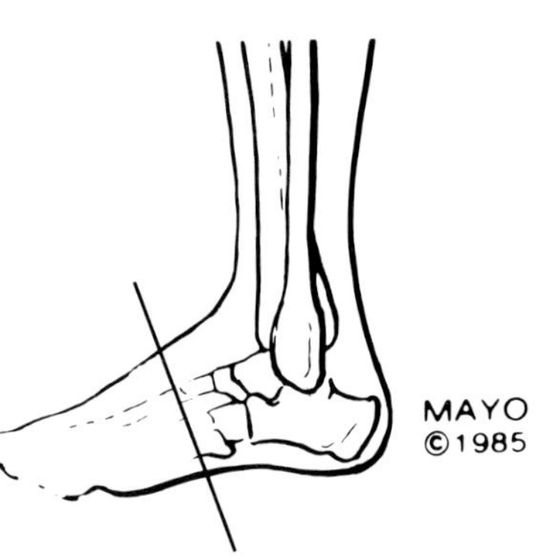

FIG. 8-4. H: Coronal image through the proximal metatarsal.

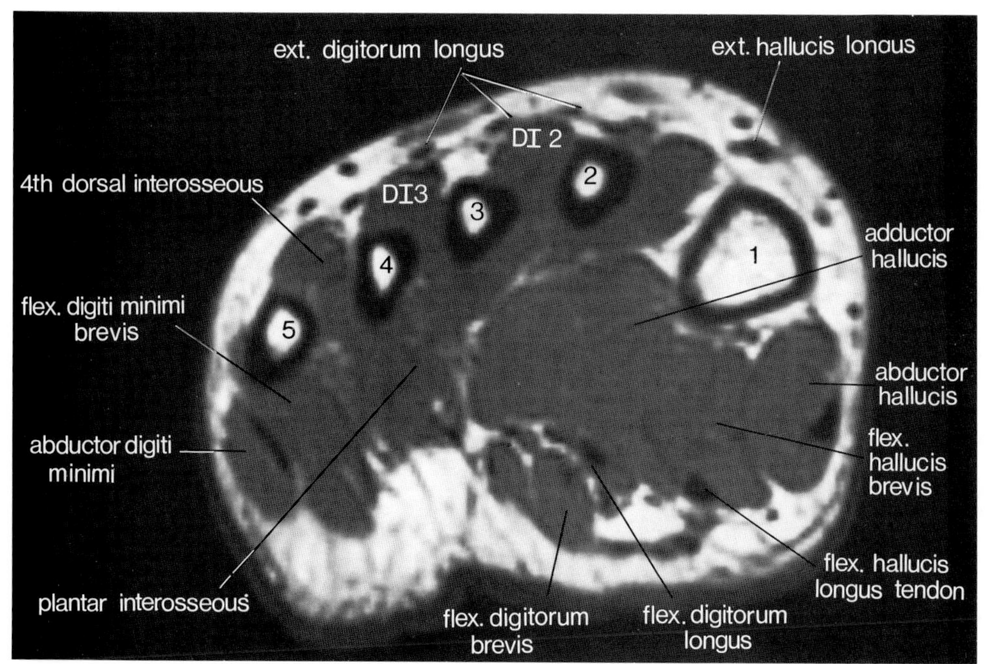

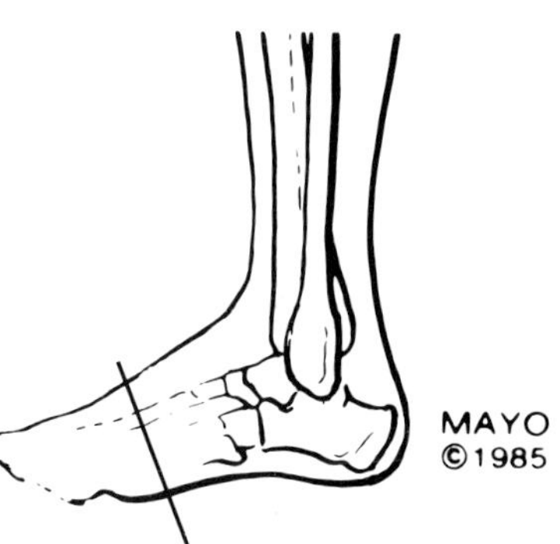

I

FIG. 8-4. I: Coronal image through the midmetatarsal region.

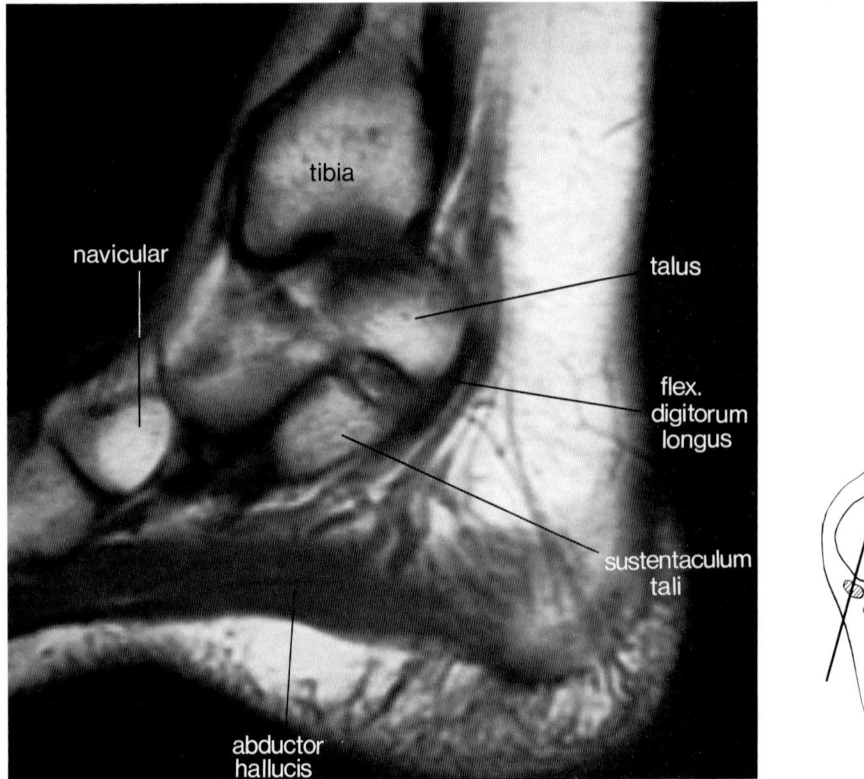

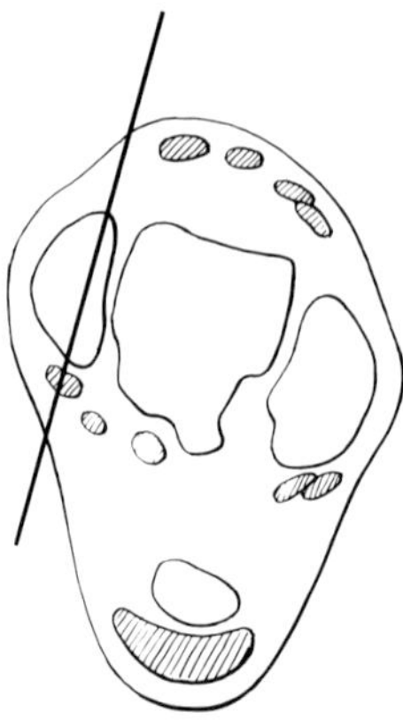

FIG. 8-5. Sagittal images of the ankle. **A:** Sagittal image through the medial malleolus.

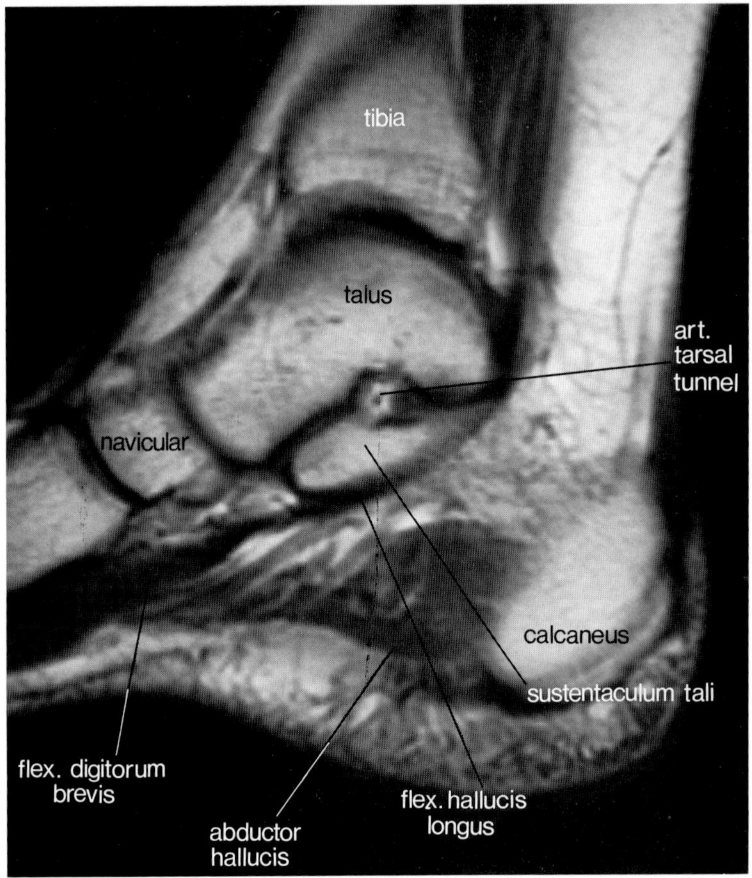

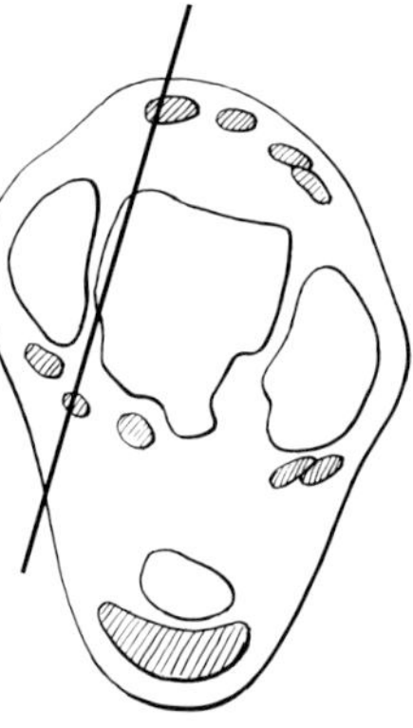

FIG. 8-5. B: Sagittal image through the sustentacular level.

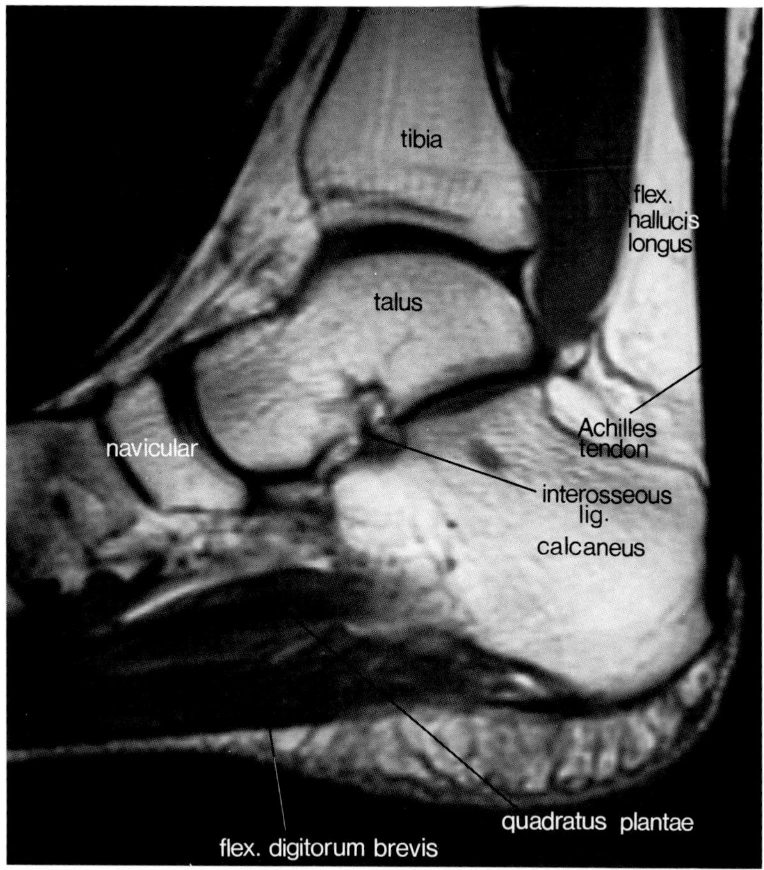

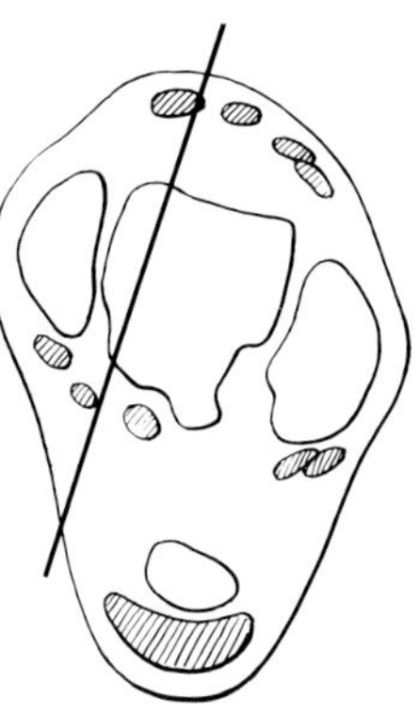

FIG. 8-5. C: Sagittal image through the medial talus.

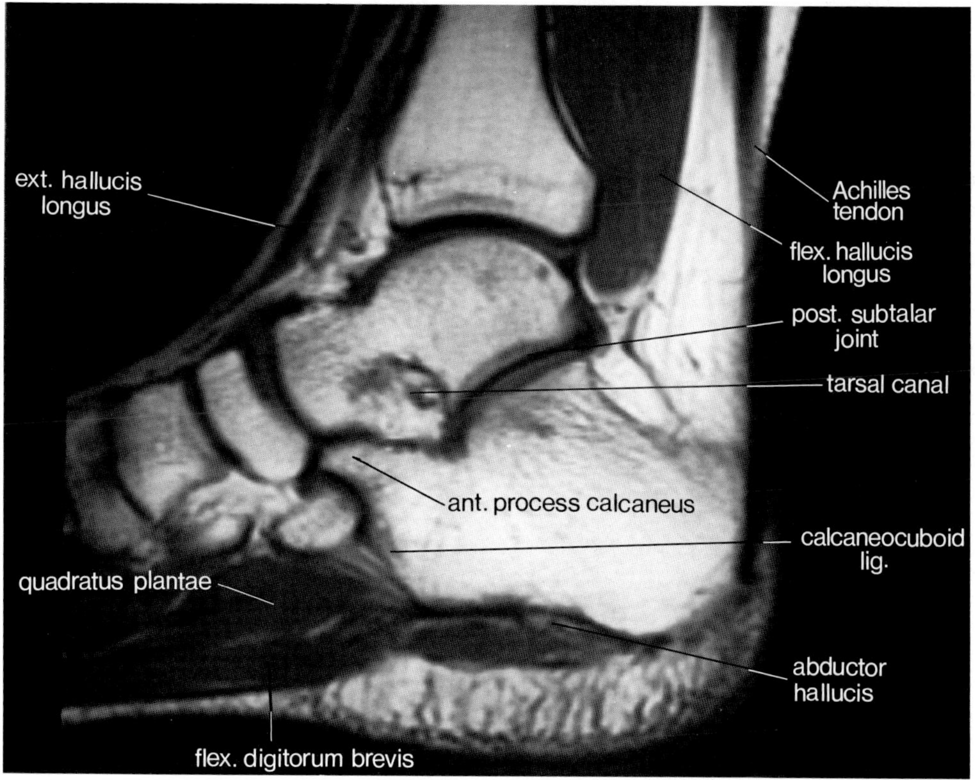

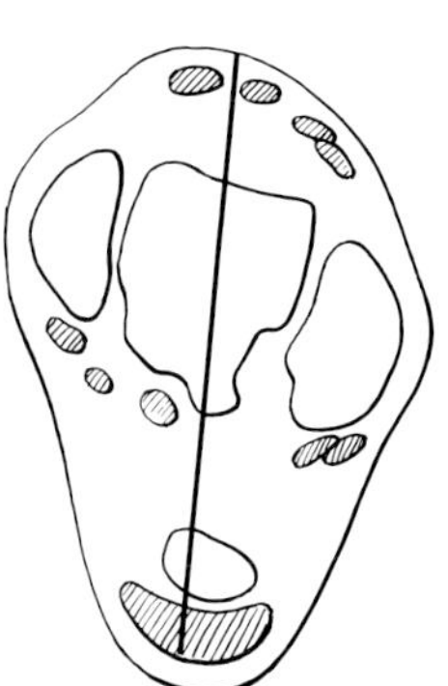

FIG. 8-5. D: Sagittal image through the midtalus.

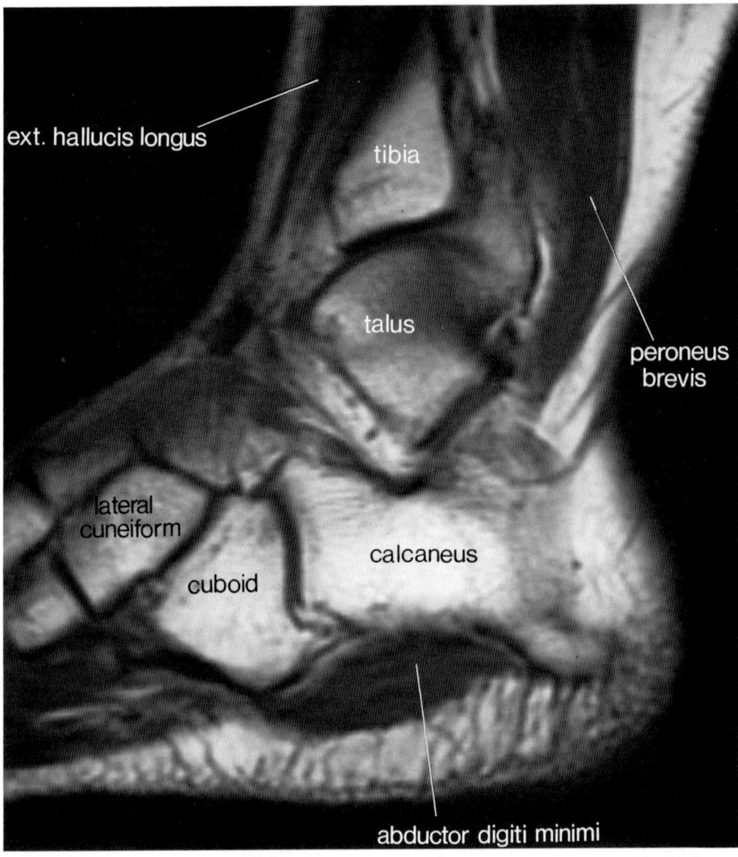

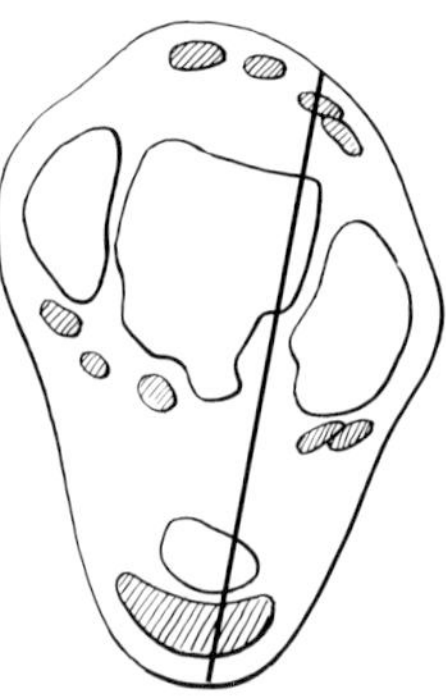

FIG. 8-5. E: Sagittal image through the lateral talus.

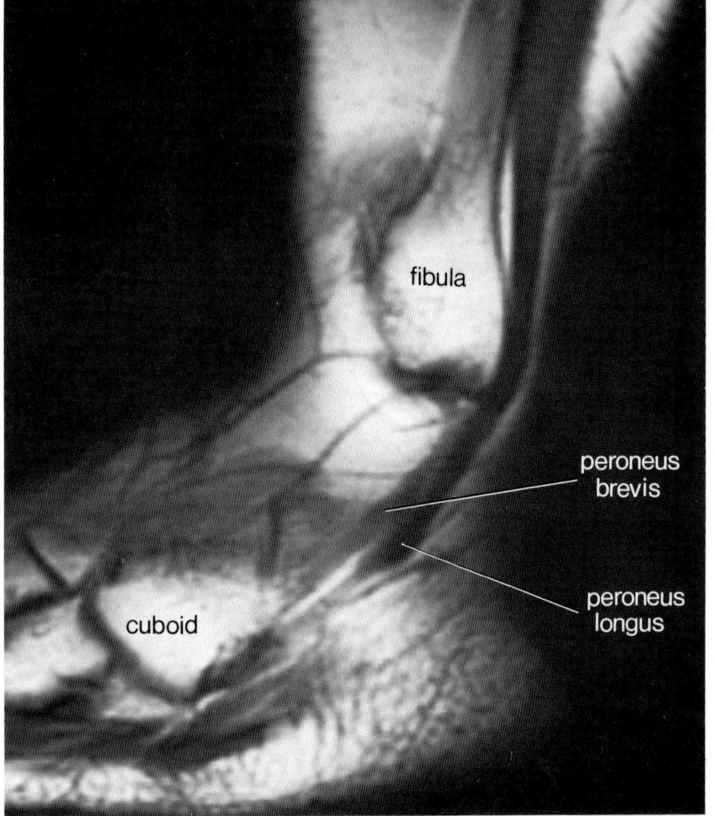

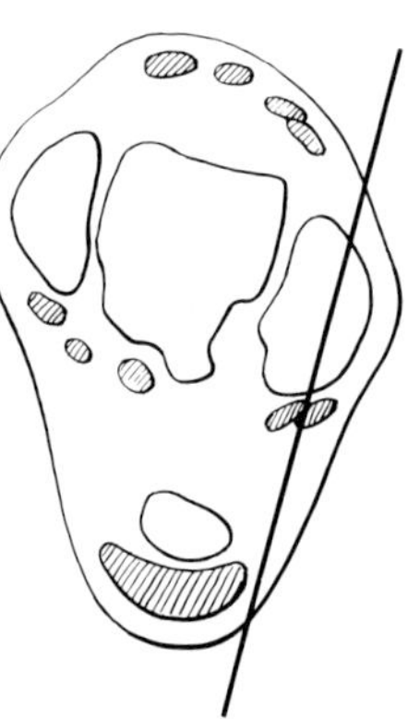

FIG. 8-5. F: Sagittal image through the lateral malleolus.

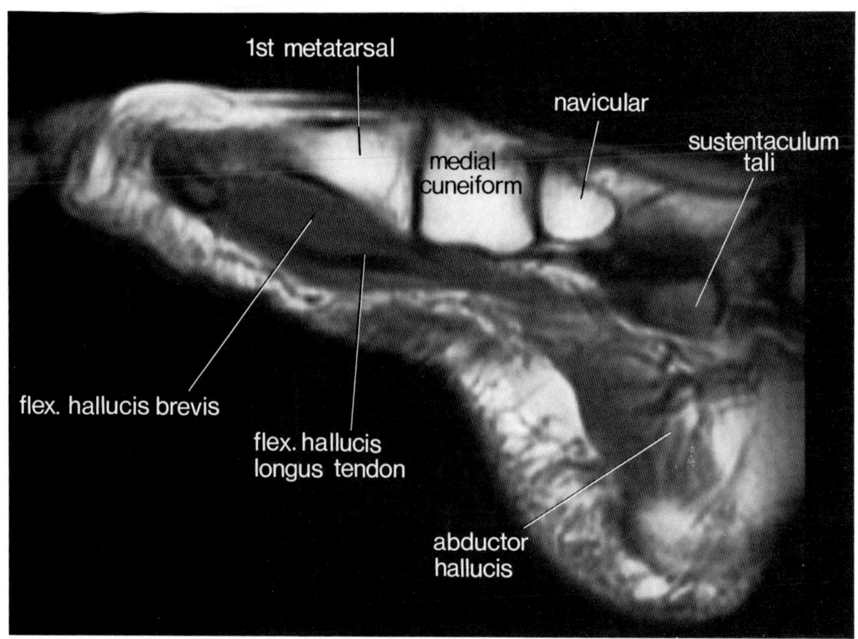

FIG. 8-6. Sagittal images of the forefoot. **A:** Sagittal image through the medial cuneiform and first metatarsal.

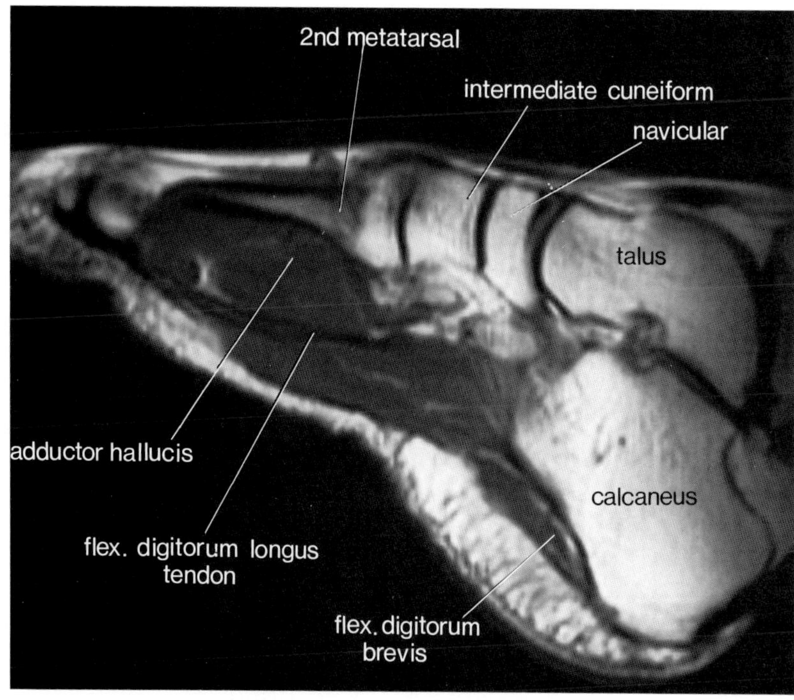

FIG. 8-6. B: Sagittal image through the second metatarsal.

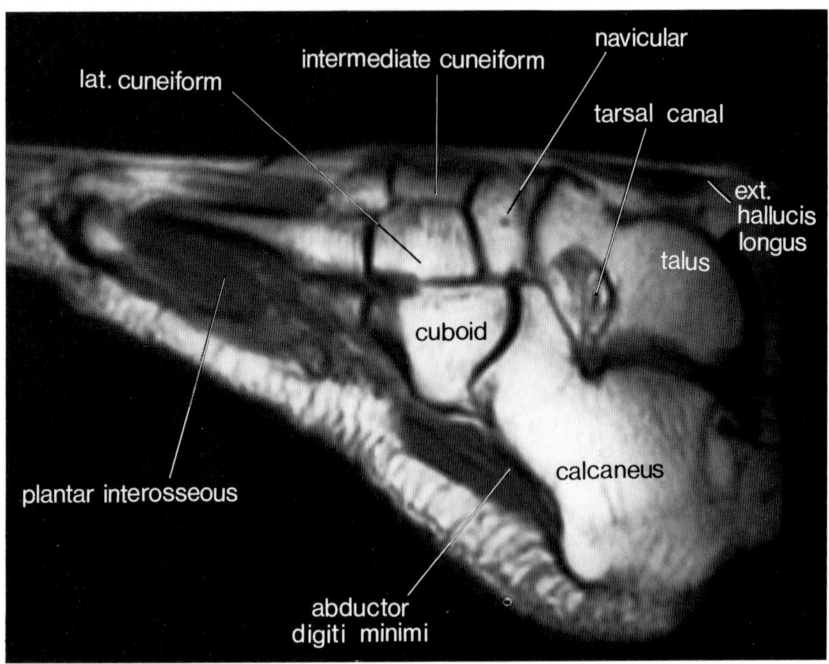

FIG. 8-6. C: Sagittal image through the intermediate cuneiform.

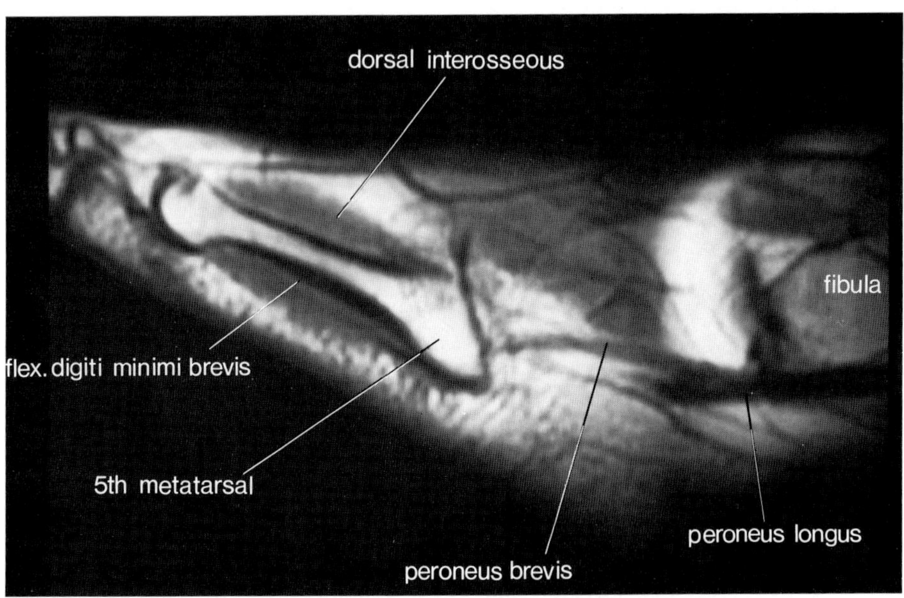

FIG. 8-6. D: Sagittal image through the fifth metatarsal.

ANATOMY

Magnetic resonance imaging (MRI) provides more diagnostic information than conventional techniques owing to improved tissue contrast and the ability to obtain multiple image planes. Therefore, a thorough knowledge of skeletal and soft tissue anatomy is even more essential than with other imaging techniques. Mastering the anatomy and biomechanics of the calf, foot, and ankle is important for evaluating MR images (Figs. 8-3 to 8-6).

Skeletal and Articular Anatomy

The ankle is composed of three osseous structures: the tibia, fibula, and talus. The triangular diaphysis of the tibia, with its three surfaces (anterior, medial, and posterior), expands at the metaphysis, forming the medial malleolus and the articular surface for the talus (Fig. 8-7). The articular surfaces are covered by hyaline cartilage, except in the most posterior aspect of the tibia. The anterior tibia is typically smooth, except for a rough anterior margin for the attachment of the anterior capsule. Posteriorly, the tibia contains grooves for the flexor hallucis longus, flexor digitorum longus, and tibialis posterior tendons (Fig. 8-3). Posterolaterally, the tibia articulates with the fibula and is bound by the interosseous membrane and anterior and posterior distal tibiofibular ligaments (Fig. 8-3) (4,12,23,47,48,82,83,90).

Supporting structures of the ankle are sometimes difficult to demonstrate with MRI, even when using off-axis oblique planes (Figs. 8-3 to 8-6). These supporting structures include the joint capsule, medial and lateral ligaments, and the interosseous ligament (Figs. 8-7 and 8-8). In addition, 13 tendons cross the ankle and there are four retinacula about the ankle (Figs. 8-3, 8-14, and 8-16). The interosseous ligament or membrane has obliquely oriented fibers and joins the tibia and fibula to its distal extent, which is just above the ankle joint. Projecting up between the distal tibia and fibula and below the interosseous ligament is the syndesmotic recess, which is seen as an area of high signal intensity extending from the joint proper on MR images (Figs. 8-3 and 8-4). Just above the tibiotalar joint, the distal anterior and distal posterior tibiofibular ligaments provide additional support as they attach to the tibia and fibula anteriorly and posteriorly (Fig. 8-8). Just anterior to the posterior tibiofibular ligament is the transverse ligament, which makes up the fourth ligament of this syndesmotic group. This ligament lies anterior to the posterior tibiofibular ligament and extends from the lateral malleolus to the posterior articular margin of the tibia just lateral to the medial malleolus (Fig. 8-9) (4,12,23,48).

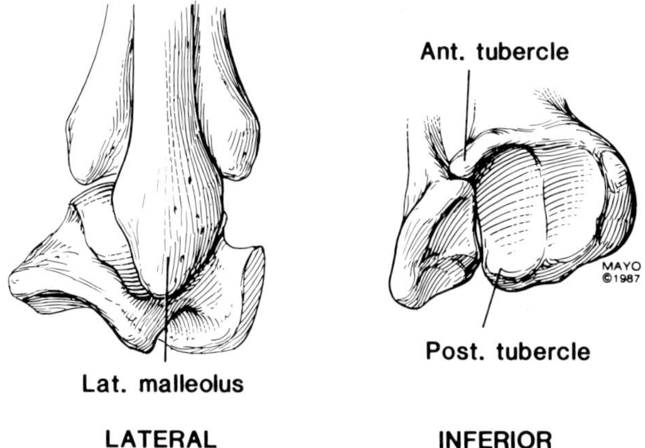

FIG. 8-7. Illustrations of the ankle seen from the lateral and infratibial surfaces. (From ref. 11, with permission.)

Medially, the deltoid ligament is a strong triangular group of fibrous tissue with its apex at the medial malleolus. As it passes caudally, the ligament fans out in a triangular fashion and divides into superficial and deep fibers. Distal insertion of this ligament is the navicular tuberosity anteriorly. The remaining fibers insert in the sustentaculum tali and talus (Fig. 8-8) (12).

There are three ligaments in the lateral complex. The anterior talofibular ligament is the weakest and most frequently injured. It passes anteriorly from the fibula to insert on the anterior to the lateral talar articular facet. The posterior ligament is much stronger than the anterior and has a nearly transverse or horizontal course from the posterior aspect of the lateral malleolus to the posterior talar tubercle. The longest of the three ligaments is the calcaneofibular ligament, which takes a nearly vertical course from the lateral malleolus to the lateral surface of the calcaneus. The peroneal tendons lie just superficial to the calcaneofibular ligament. Demonstration of all three of these ligaments is difficult on typical orthogonal MR images due to partial volume effects and the variations in the obliquity of these ligaments (Figs. 8-4 and 8-8) (4,12,23,48).

The foot is often divided into three segments: the hindfoot comprised of the talus and calcaneus, the midfoot comprised of the remaining five tarsal bones, and the forefoot comprised of the metatarsals and phalanges. The talus is the second largest of the tarsal bones and articulates with the tibia superiorly, medial and lateral malleolus and calcaneus inferiorly. The head of the talus articulates with the navicular (Figs. 8-4 and 8-5). Inferiorly, there are three articular facets. The anterior and posterior facets articulate with similarly named calcaneal facets. The middle facet is just posterior the anterior calcaneal articular facet and articulates with the sustentaculum tali (Figs. 8-3 and 8-4). The tarsal canal or sinus lies between the middle and anterior facets. The interosseous talocalcaneal ligament lies within this canal and is usually easily seen on sagittal MR images (Fig. 8-5). The tarsal canal has an oblique course between the talus and calcaneus, measuring 10–15 mm in height and 5 mm in

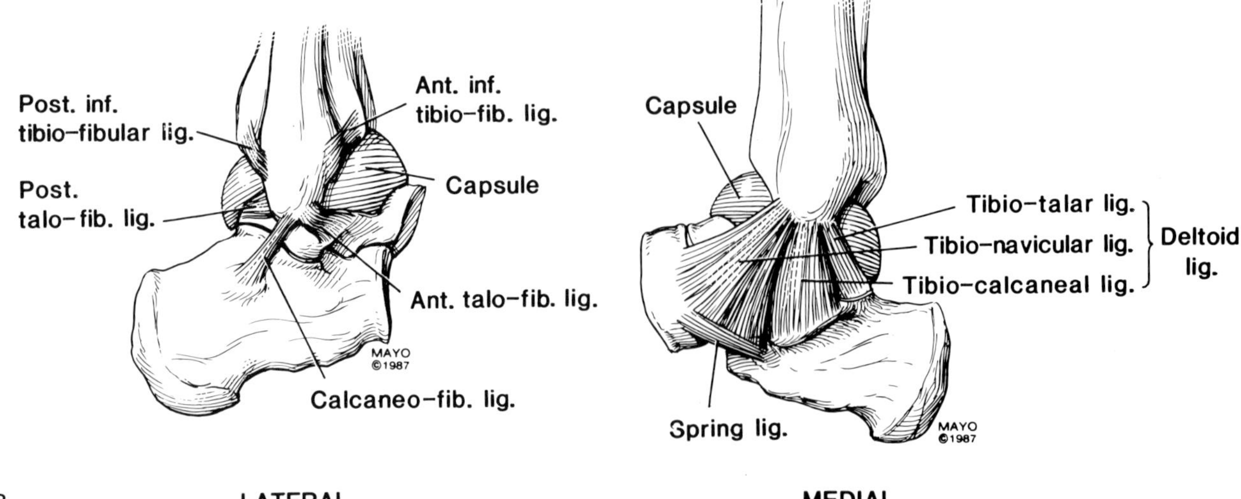

FIG. 8-8. Illustrations of the capsule, lateral (**A**) and medial (**B**) ligaments of the ankle. (From ref. 11, with permission.)

width with a length of 15–20 mm. This appearance on sagittal MR images can be confusing and can give the impression of synovitis with erosive changes in the talus (Fig. 8-5). In addition to the three superior facets, the calcaneus articulates anteriorly with the cuboid. There are two main ligaments that directly support the talocalcaneal joint. These are the interosseous talocalcaneal ligament located in the tarsal canal or sinus tarsi and the smaller lateral talocalcaneal ligaments. Ligaments of the ankle and adjacent tendons provide additional stabilization (4,12,48,82,83,90).

The remaining tarsal bones (cuboid, navicular, and three cuneiforms) make up the midfoot. The cuboid articulates with the calcaneus proximally and distally with the fourth and fifth metatarsals (Fig. 8-5). The lateral aspect of the cuboid contains a groove for the peroneus longus tendon (Fig. 8-4). The medial surface of the cuboid has an articular facet for the lateral cuneiform. Medially, the navicular articulates with the talus proximally and anteriorly with the cuneiforms and occasionally the lateral aspect of the cuboid. An additional ligamentous structure that can be seen with MRI is the spring ligament, which extends from the calcaneus to the navicular tuberosity (Figs. 8-5 and 8-8). There are other interosseous ligaments both in the dorsal and plantar surfaces of the tarsal bones.

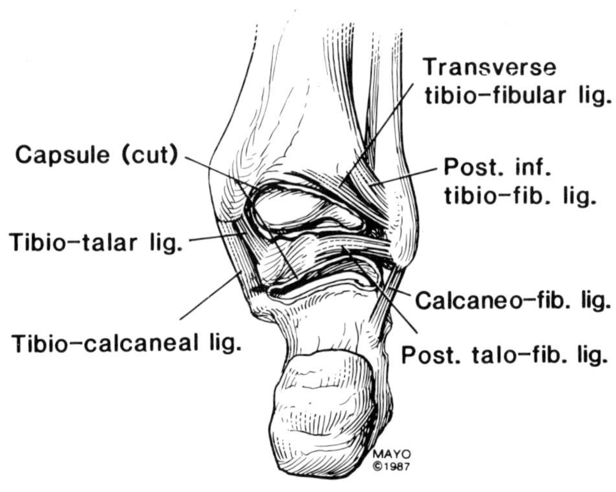

FIG. 8-9. Illustration of ligaments of the ankle seen posteriorly. (From ref. 11.)

There are three cuneiforms located distal to the navicular and medial to the cuboid. The medial cuneiform is the largest and articulates with the navicular proximally and the intermediate cuneiform laterally. Distally, it articulates with the first and second metatarsals. Lying between the medial and lateral cuneiforms is the intermediate cuneiform, which is the smallest of the three tarsal bones. It articulates with the latter and the navicular proximally and second metatarsal distally. The lateral cuneiform lies between the intermediate cuneiform and the cuboid. It articulates with both of these osseous structures plus the navicular proximally and the second through fourth metatarsals.

There are five metatarsals, which articulate with the tarsal bones. Each has three phalanges with the exception of the great toe, which typically has two. The dorsal, plantar, and interosseous ligaments support the tarsometatarsal joints and bases of the metatarsals. Distally, the transverse metatarsal ligament connects the heads of all five metatarsals. Each of the metatarsophalangeal joints is supported by collateral ligaments and plantar ligaments. Dorsally, the extensor tendons replace the

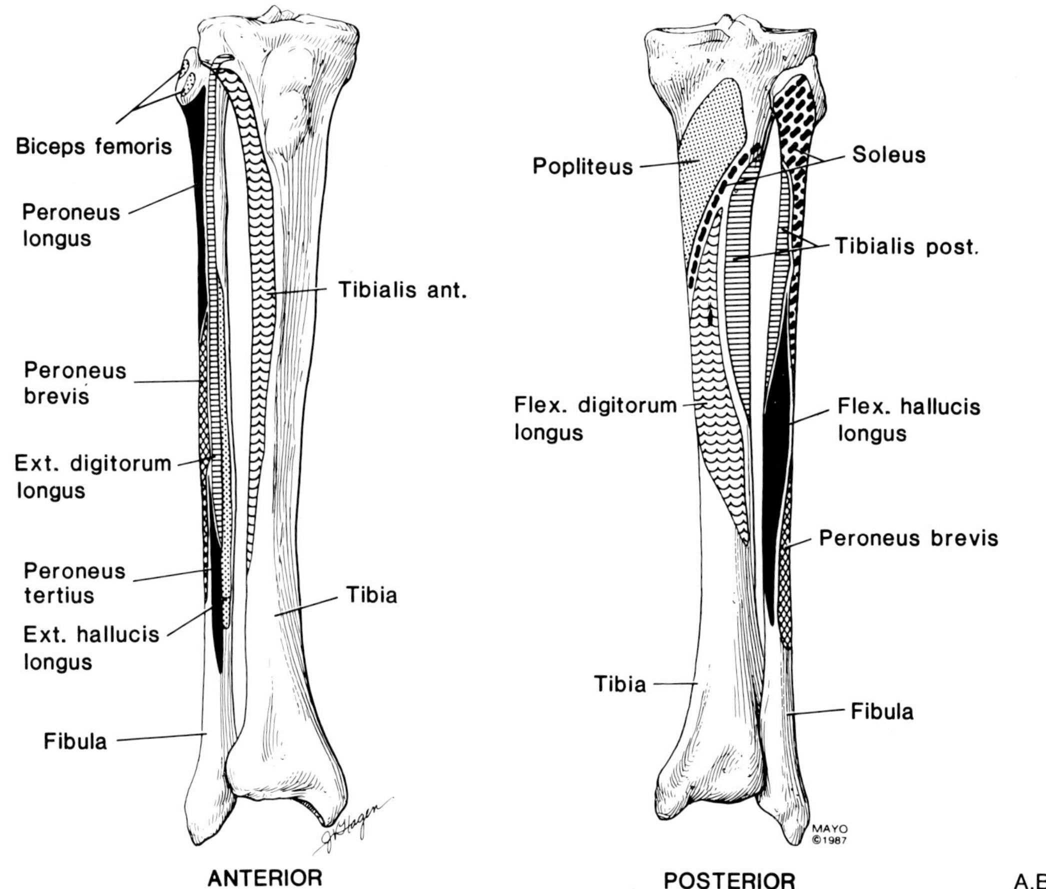

FIG. 8-10. Anterior (**A**) and posterior (**B**) illustrations of the tibia and fibula, demonstrating origins of muscles that insert on or affect the foot and ankle. (From ref. 11.)

usual dorsal ligaments seen in the midfoot (Figs. 8-4 and 8-5) (4,7,9,13,23,48,67,68).

Soft Tissue Anatomy

The lower extremity musculature develops from mesodermal tissues of the lower limb bud (12,48). Functional muscle groups are organized in fascial compartments. To simplify the muscular anatomy of the foot and ankle, we discuss compartments or functional groups of muscles, including their origins, insertions, and actions. Normal variants are also discussed.

The muscles of the leg can be divided into anterior, posterior, and lateral compartments. One of these muscles crosses only the knee; two cross the knee and ankle. The majority arise in the leg and act on both the foot and ankle (Fig. 8-10) (4,12,23,48,54,67,68).

Posterior Musculature

The superficial and deep muscles of the calf are divided into compartments by the crural fascia. The su-

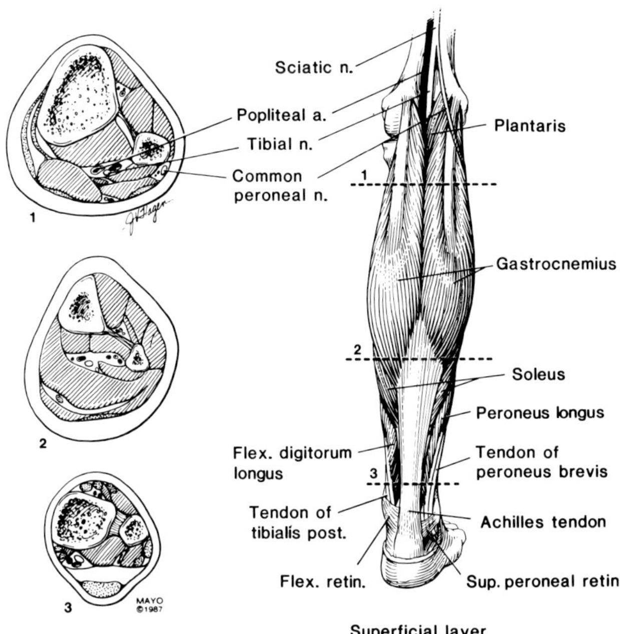

FIG. 8-11. Illustration of the superficial muscles of the calf. (From ref. 11.)

perficial muscle group includes the gastrocnemius, soleus, and plantaris (Fig. 8-11). The gastrocnemius has two heads arising from the medial and lateral femoral condyles. The two heads unite to form the bulk of the muscle in the upper calf (Fig. 8-3A). At about the midpoint of the calf, the muscle ends in a wide flat tendon. The soleus inserts into the anterior aspect of the gastrocnemius tendon. Below this level, the tendon narrows in transverse diameter and thickens, forming the Achilles tendon (tendo calcaneus), which inserts on the posterior calcaneus (Figs. 8-3, 8-5, and 8-11). The gastrocnemius plantar flexes the foot and also assists in knee flexion during nonweight bearing. Innervation is by the tibial nerve and the vascular supply is derived primarily from the posterior tibial artery (4,12,48) (Table 8-2).

The soleus lies deep to the gastrocnemius (Figs. 8-3 and 8-11) and also has two heads, one arising from the posterior superior fibula and the second from the popliteal line and posteromedial surface of the proximal tibia (Fig. 8-10). The popliteal vessels and tibial nerve pass deep to the body of the soleus. The soleus inserts in the anterior aspect of the gastrocnemius tendon, forming the thicker Achilles tendon (4,12,23,48,54).

The soleus has no effect on the knee but serves as a plantar flexor of the foot. Innervation is via the tibial nerve with vascular supply from the posterior tibial artery (Table 8-2).

The plantaris is the third muscle included in the superficial compartment (Fig. 8-12). This small muscle takes its origin from the lateral epicondyle of the femur and the oblique popliteal ligament. The belly of the muscle is only several inches long and passes between

TABLE 8-2. *Muscles of the leg, foot, and ankle* (4,23,48)

Location	Muscle	Origin	Insertion	Action	Innervation (segment)	Blood supply
Calf Superficial compartment	Gastrocnemius	Femoral condyles	Posterior calcaneus	Flexor of foot and knee	Tibial nerve (S1, S2)	Posterior tibial artery
	Soleus	Upper tibia and fibula	Gastrocnemius tendon	Plantar flexor of foot	Tibial nerve (S1, S2)	Posterior tibial artery
	Plantaris	Lateral femoral condyle and oblique popliteal ligament	Posteromedial calcaneus	Plantar flexes foot, flexes leg	Tibial nerve (L4–S1)	Posterior tibial artery
Deep compartment	Popliteus	Lateral femur and capsule of knee		Flexion and medial rotation of leg	Tibial nerve (L5, S1)	Posterior tibial artery
	Flexor hallucis longus	Posterior midfibula	Distal phalanx great toe	Flexor great toe and ankle	Tibial nerve (L5–S2)	Posterior tibial artery
	Flexor digitorum longus	Posterior tibia	Distal phalanges second to fifth toes	Flexes toes and foot and supinates ankle	Tibial nerve (L5, S1)	Posterior tibial artery
	Tibialis posterior	Posterior tibia, fibula, and interosseous membrane	Navicular, cuneiform, calcaneus, second to fourth metatarsals	Adduction of forefoot, hindfoot inversion, plantar flexion	Tibial nerve (L5, S1)	Posterior tibial artery
Lateral compartment	Peroneus longus	Lateral fibula	First metatarsal and medial cuneiform	Evertor and weak plantar flexors	Superficial and deep peroneal nerve (L4–S1)	Peroneal artery
	Peroneus brevis	Lateral fibula	Base fifth metatarsal		Superficial peroneal nerve (L4–S1)	Peroneal artery
Anterior compartment	Extensor digitorum longus	Upper tibia, fibula, and interosseous membrane	Lateral four toes	Dorsiflexes toes, everts foot	Deep peroneal nerve (L4–S1)	Anterior tibial artery
	Peroneus tertius	Distal fibula and interosseous membrane	Base fifth metatarsal	Dorsiflexes and everts foot	Deep peroneal nerve (L4–S1)	Anterior tibial artery
	Extensor hallucis longus	Distal fibula and interosseous membrane	Distal phalanx great toe	Extends great toe, weak invertor and dorsiflexion of foot	Deep peroneal nerve (L4–S1)	Anterior tibial artery
	Tibialis anterior	Lateral tibia and interosseous membrane	Medial cuneiform and first metatarsal	Strong dorsiflexion and invertor of foot	Deep peroneal nerve (L4–S1)	Anterior tibial artery

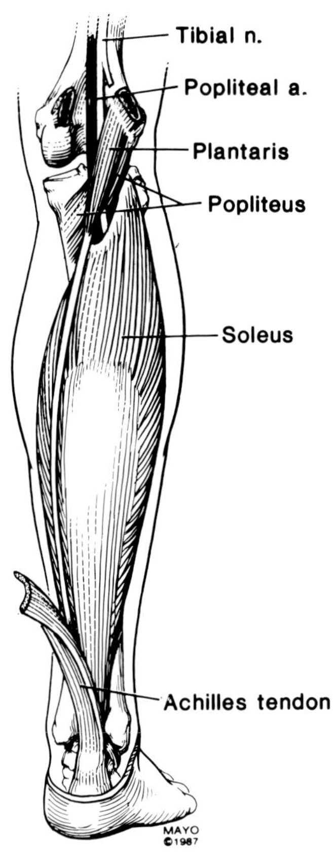

FIG. 8-12. Illustration of second layer of muscles in the calf. (From ref. 11.)

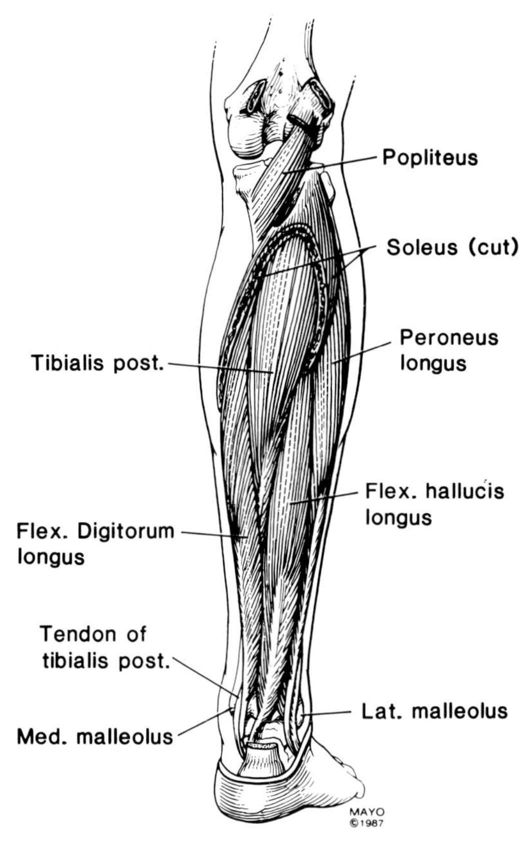

FIG. 8-13. Illustration of the deep muscles of the calf. (From ref. 11.)

the gastrocnemius and soleus in an oblique direction (Fig. 8-12). The long thin tendon passes distally along the medial margin of the Achilles to insert in the calcaneus, Achilles, or flexor retinaculum. Occasionally, the muscle is double or it may be totally absent (4,12,48). The plantaris functions as a minor flexor of the knee and plantar flexor of the foot. Innervation and blood supply are from the tibial nerve and posterior tibial artery, respectively (4,12) (Table 8-2).

The deep compartment of the calf contains the popliteus, tibialis posterior, flexor hallucis longus, and flexor digitorum longus (Figs. 8-3 to 8-5 and 8-13).

The popliteus is a small triangular muscle forming a portion of the floor of the popliteal fossa (Fig. 8-13) (4,12,48). Its origin is from the lateral femoral condyle, the arcuate popliteal ligament, and capsule of the knee. The insertion is the posterior surface of the upper tibia above the origin of the soleus (Fig. 8-13). The popliteus acts on the knee and leg as a flexor and medial rotator. Neurovascular supply is by the tibial nerve and posterior tibial artery (4,12,48) (Table 8-2).

The flexor hallucis longus is the most lateral of the three remaining deep muscles of the leg (flexor hallucis longus, flexor digitorum longus, and tibialis posterior) (Figs. 8-3 and 8-13). It arises from the lateral aspect of the middle half of the posterior fibula (Fig. 8-10) (4,12,48). Its tendon begins above the malleoli of the ankle and courses medially behind the ankle deep to the flexor retinaculum (Fig. 8-13). The tendon is posterior to the tendons of the tibialis posterior and flexor digitorum longus behind the medial malleolus (Fig. 8-3). The tendon passes along the plantar aspect of the foot to insert in the distal phalanx of the great toe (see Figs. 8-5 and 8-20). The flexor hallucis longus is a flexor of the great toe and assists in ankle flexion. The muscle is innervated by the tibial nerve and receives its blood supply from the posterior tibial artery (4,12,23,48) (Table 8-2).

The flexor digitorum longus lies medially in the deep compartment of the calf (Fig. 8-3). It arises from the upper half of the posteromedial aspect of the tibia (Fig. 8-10). Along its caudad course it passes posterior to the tibialis posterior so that at the ankle it lies between the flexor hallucis longus and tibialis posterior (Fig. 8-3). The tendon passes through the flexor retinaculum, posterior to the medial malleolus, and then divides into four slips that insert in the distal phalanges of the lateral four digits (see Figs. 8-13 and 8-20). On the plantar aspect of the foot these four tendon slips are associated with the lumbrical muscles and pass through the divided slips of the flexor digitorum brevis prior to inserting on the distal phalanges (4,12,23,48).

The flexor digitorum longus flexes the lateral four toes and also plantar flexes the foot and supinates the ankle. The muscle is innervated by branches of the tibial nerve and receives its vascular supply from posterior tibial artery branches (23,48) (Table 8-2).

The tibialis posterior is the deepest and most centrally located muscle in the deep posterior compartment (Figs. 8-3 and 8-13). It arises from the upper posterior aspects of the tibia and fibula and the interosseous membrane (Fig. 8-10). Thus, it is positioned between the flexor hallucis longus and flexor digitorum longus. The tendon passes medially deep to the flexor retinaculum and flexor digitorum longus. Therefore, it is the most anterior of the three tendons as it passes behind the medial malleolus (Fig. 8-3). The tendon flares to insert in the navicular, tarsal bones, and bases of the second to fourth metatarsals (Figs. 8-5 and 8-22) (4,12,23,48).

The tibialis posterior aids in adduction, inversion, and plantar flexion of the foot. The muscle is innervated by branches of the tibial nerve and receives its blood supply from the posterior tibial artery (48) (Table 8-1).

Table 8-2 summarizes the muscles of the calf and their functions.

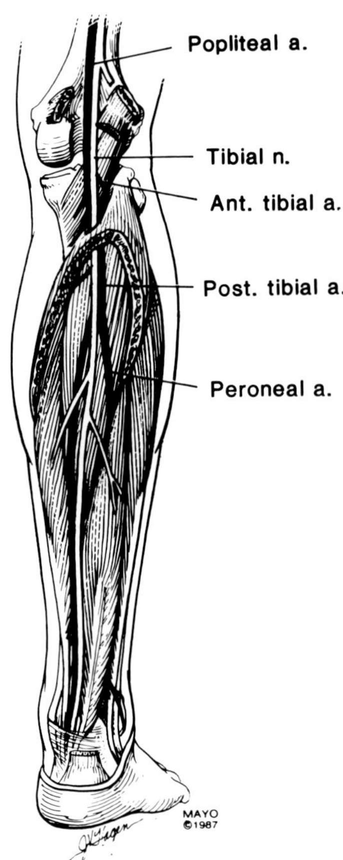

FIG. 8-14. Illustration of the major neurovascular structures in the calf. (From ref. 11.)

Neurovascular Anatomy of the Calf

The tibial nerve is a continuation of the sciatic nerve at the level of the popliteal fossa. As it passes inferiorly it enters the calf between the heads of the gastrocnemius muscle, passing deep to the soleus to lie between the soleus and tibialis posterior in the deep compartment (Figs. 8-3 and 8-14) (48). The tibial nerve sends branches to all the superficial and deep muscles of the calf (Table 8-2). At the ankle level the nerve generally lies between the flexor hallucis longus and flexor digitorum longus tendons (Fig. 8-3). Distal to the flexor retinaculum it divides, forming the medial and lateral plantar nerves (4,12,23,48).

The popliteal artery is a direct continuation of the superficial femoral artery as it passes through the adductor canal (Fig. 8-14). It divides into anterior and posterior tibial branches at the level of the popliteus muscle. The anterior tibial artery enters the anterolateral leg above the upper margin of the interosseous membrane, while the posterior tibial artery joins the tibial nerve in the deep compartment of the calf (Figs. 8-14 and 8-17). In the leg it provides muscular branches to all the calf muscles and a nutrient artery to the tibia. Its largest branch, the peroneal artery, arises high in the leg and passes deep to the flexor hallucis longus near the interosseous membrane and fibula (Figs. 8-3 and 8-14). At the ankle level, it forms anastomotic branches with the posterior tibial artery and perforates the interosseous membrane to supply the dorsal aspect of the foot. Generally, paired veins accompany the arteries. These veins are more variable and enter the popliteal vein superiorly (12,23,48).

Anterolateral Musculature

The peroneus longus and brevis are the two muscles of the lateral compartment. Both arise from the superior lateral surface of the fibula. The origin of the peroneus longus is more superior, with the muscle passing superficial to the peroneus brevis (Fig. 8-10). The muscles progress caudad in the lateral compartment with their tendons entering a common tendon sheath above the ankle (Figs. 8-3, 8-5, and 8-15). The tendons pass posterior to the lateral malleolus and deep to the superior and inferior peroneal retinacula. The tendons diverge on the lateral surface of the foot with the peroneus brevis inserting on the base of the fifth metatarsal. The peroneus longus takes an inferior course, passing under the lateral aspect of the foot where it inserts on the base of the

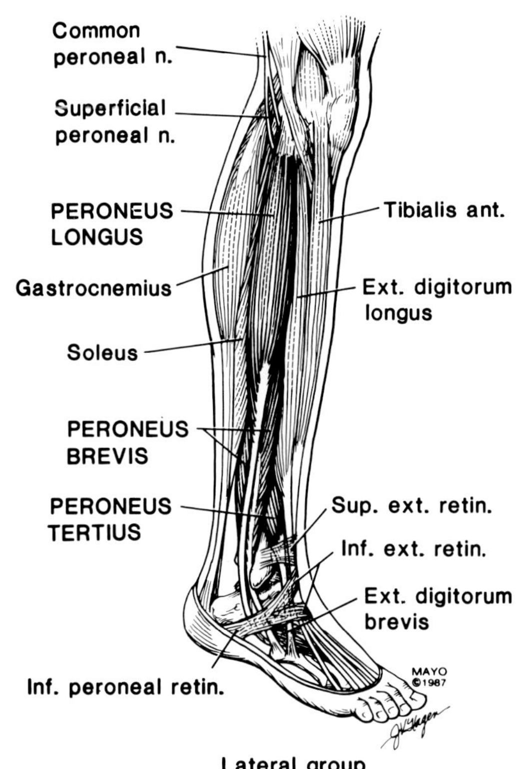

FIG. 8-15. Illustration of the lateral muscle group of the leg. (From ref. 11.)

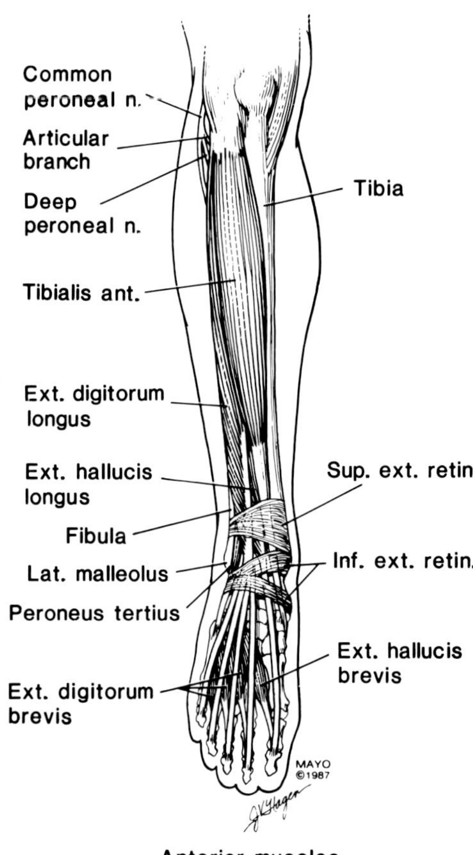

FIG. 8-16. Illustration of the anterior compartment muscles. (From ref. 11.)

first metatarsal and medial cuneiform (Fig. 8-22) (4,12,23,48).

These muscles serve as evertors of the foot and assist in plantar flexion. Innervation is from the superficial peroneal nerve with branches of the common or deep peroneal nerve supplying a portion of the peroneus longus. Vascular supply is via the peroneal artery (48) (Table 8-2).

Anterior Compartment Musculature

There are four muscles in the anterior compartment. These include the extensor digitorum longus, peroneus tertius, extensor hallucis longus, and tibialis anterior (Figs. 8-3 and 8-16) (Table 8-2).

The extensor digitorum longus is the most lateral muscle in the anterior compartment (Figs. 8-3 and 8-16). It arises from the lateral tibial condyle, anterior fibula, and interosseous membrane (Fig. 8-10). The tendon passes deep to the superior and inferior extensor retinacula prior to dividing into four slips, which insert on the dorsal aspects of the four lateral toes (Fig. 8-16). The insertions are divided such that portions insert in the middle and distal phalanges (12,23,48). This muscle dorsiflexes the toes and also assists in eversion of the foot. It is innervated by the deep peroneal nerve and receives it vascular supply from the anterior tibial artery (Table 8-2). Variations in its origin and distal insertions are not uncommon but these rarely cause confusion on MR images.

The peroneus tertius is closely associated with the extensor digitorum longus and may be considered a portion of the latter (48). It arises from the distal anterior fibula, interosseous membrane, and membrane of the peroneus brevis (Fig. 8-10). Its tendon passes deep to the extensor retinacula to insert on the dorsal aspect of the base of the fifth metatarsal (Fig. 8-16). It is supplied by the deep peroneal nerve and anterior tibial artery. This muscle varies in size and may be absent (4,12,23,48) (Table 8-2).

The extensor hallucis longus lies deep to the extensor digitorum longus and tibialis anterior (Fig. 8-3). It arises from the midfibula and interosseous membrane and becomes superficial in the lower leg (Fig. 8-10). Its tendon passes deep to the extensor retinacula to insert on the distal phalanx of the great toe (Fig. 8-16). This muscle extends the great toe and is a weak dorsiflexor and invertor of the foot. It is supplied by the deep peroneal nerve and anterior tibial artery (12,23,48) (Table 8-2).

The tibialis anterior arises from the lateral tibia surface, deep fascia, and interosseous membrane (Fig.

8-10). It passes inferiorly, becoming tendinous in the lower leg. It is the most medial tendon as it passes deep to the extensor retinacula (Fig. 8-3). It passes along the medial foot to insert in the medial cuneiform and plantar portion of the first metatarsal (Fig. 8-16) (4,12,23,48). This muscle is a strong dorsiflexor and invertor of the foot. Neurovascular supply is via the deep peroneal nerve and anterior tibial artery (48) (Table 8-2).

Neurovascular Anatomy of the Anterolateral Muscles

The common peroneal nerve is a branch of the sciatic nerve and courses laterally in the popliteal fossa. It is subcutaneous and relatively unprotected just below the fibular head (Fig. 8-17). Therefore, it is susceptible to direct trauma in this area (4,12,48). As it descends between the fibula and peroneus longus, it divides into two or three branches. These are the superficial, deep, and articular branches of the peroneal nerve. The superficial peroneal nerve lies between the peroneus longus and brevis and supplies these muscles and the subcutaneous tissues. The deep peroneal nerve courses anteriorly, deep to the peroneus longus, to supply the anterior muscles of the leg (see Table 8-2). It joins the anterior tibial artery on the anterior aspect of the interosseous membrane (4,12,48).

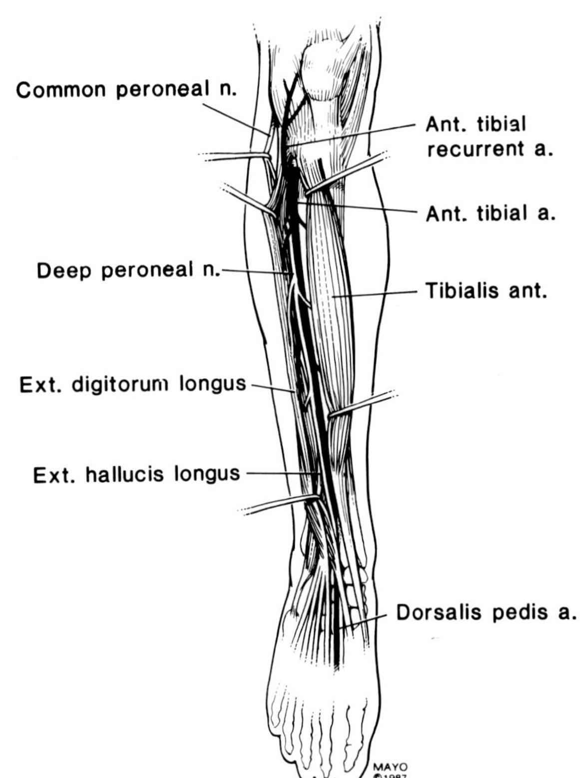

FIG. 8-17. Illustration of the anterior neurovascular anatomy. (From ref. 11.)

The anterior tibial artery passes superior to the interosseous membrane in the upper leg and then lies with the deep peroneal nerve along the anterior aspect of the interosseous membrane (Fig. 8-17). It supplies the anterior muscles and continues as the dorsalis pedis artery on the dorsum of the foot (Fig. 8-23) (4,12,23,48).

Table 8-2 summarizes the muscles of the leg, their functions, and neurovascular supply.

Foot Musculature

The muscles of the foot are generally discussed by layer rather than compartments as in the leg (Fig. 8-18) (4,11,12,23,48).

The superficial layer of plantar muscles includes the abductor hallucis, flexor digitorum brevis, and abductor digiti minimi. The abductor hallucis arises from the medial process of the calcaneal tubercle, the flexor retinaculum, and plantar aponeurosis. Its insertion is the medial side of the flexor surface of the proximal phalanx of the great toe (Figs. 8-6 and 8-19) (4,12,23,48). The medial and lateral plantar vessels and nerves pass deep to the proximal position of the muscle as they enter the foot. The muscle is supplied by branches of the medial plantar nerve and artery. The abductor hallucis functions weakly as an abductor of the metatarsophalangeal joint of the great toe (48) (Table 8-3).

The flexor digitorum brevis is the most central of the superficial plantar muscles (Figs. 8-4, 8-6, and 8-19). It arises from the medial tubercular process of the calcaneus and plantar fascia. Four tendons pass distally and divide into two slips at the level of the proximal phalanx. The tendons of the flexor digitorum longus pass through the divided brevis tendons. The divided tendon slips insert on the middle phalanx (4,48). The muscle flexes the lateral four toes. It is supplied by the medial plantar nerve and artery, with the lateral plantar nerve and artery passing deep to this muscle. It is not uncommon for the tendon to the fifth toe to be absent (38%) (23,48) (Table 8-3).

The abductor digiti minimi is the most lateral muscle in the superficial layer (Figs. 8-4 and 8-19). It arises from the lateral process of the calcaneal tubercle and the distal portion of the medial process. It inserts in the lateral aspect of the base of the proximal phalanx of the fifth toe and serves to flex and abduct the toe at the metatarsophalangeal joint. It is supplied by the lateral plantar nerve and artery (48) (Table 8-3).

The second layer of the foot is composed of the tendons of the flexor hallucis longus and flexor digitorum longus plus the quadratus plantae and lumbrical muscles (Figs. 8-4 and 8-20) (4,23,48).

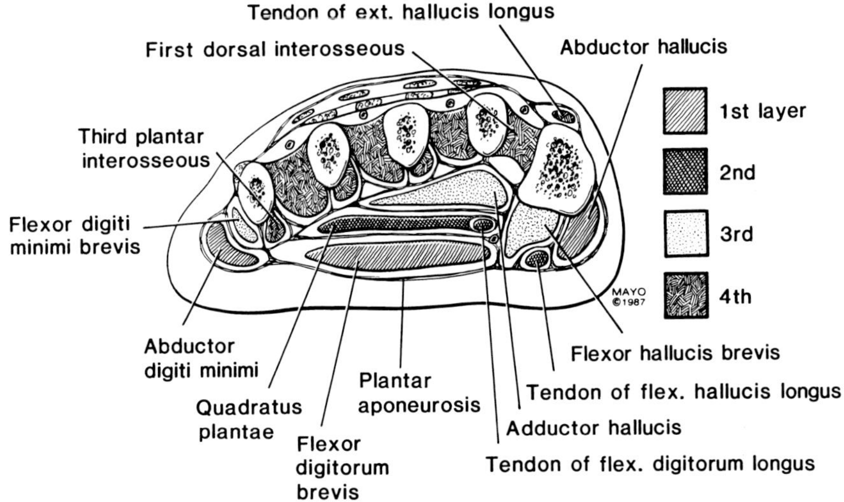

FIG. 8-18. Illustration of the muscle layers in the foot. (From ref. 11.)

The quadratus plantae has two heads, which arise from the medial and lateral plantar aspects of the calcaneal tuberosity. The muscle inserts in the lateral and posterior margin of the flexor digitorum longus just before it divides into its four tendon slips (Figs. 8-4, 8-5, and 8-20) (4,12,48). The muscle assists the flexor digitorum longus in flexing the lateral four toes. It is supplied by the lateral plantar nerve and artery. Occasionally, the lateral head or in certain cases the entire muscle may be absent (48) (Table 8-3).

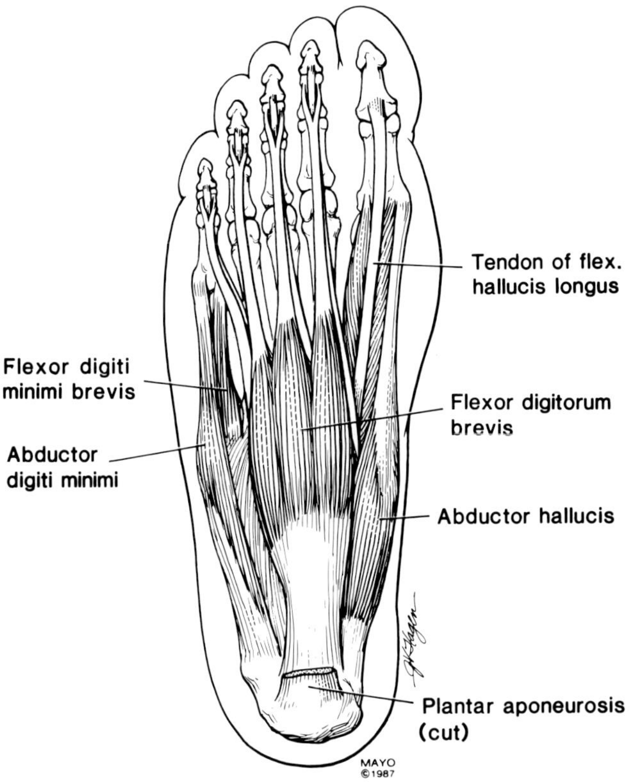

FIG. 8-19. Illustration of the superficial muscle layers of the foot. (From ref. 11.)

The four lumbrical muscles arise from the flexor digitorum longus tendon. They pass distally to insert on the medial side of metatarsophalangeal joints of the four lateral toes (Fig. 8-20). They act as flexors of the metatarsophalangeal joints. The most medial muscle is innervated by the medial plantar nerve, while the lateral plantar nerves supply the lateral three muscles. Blood supply is via the medial and lateral plantar arteries. Absence of one or more of the lumbricals has been reported. Occasionally, two muscles insert on the fourth and fifth toes (23,48) (Table 8-3).

The third layer of plantar muscles includes the flexor hallucis brevis, adductor hallucis, and flexor digiti minimi brevis (Figs. 8-4 and 8-21). The flexor hallucis brevis has two bellies arising from the plantar aspect of the cuboid and adjacent cuneiform (Fig. 8-21). The tendons insert at the sides of the base of the great toe and the sesamoids. The muscle serves as a flexor of the great toe and is supplied by the medial plantar nerve and artery (4,12,23,48).

The adductor hallucis has oblique and transverse heads (Fig. 8-21). The oblique head arises from the long plantar ligament and the second through fourth metatarsals bases (4,48). The smaller transverse head arises from the capsules of the third through fifth metatarsophalangeal joints and the deep transverse ligaments. The two heads join lateral to the great toe to insert with the lateral head of the flexor hallucis brevis. The adductor hallucis adducts and flexes the great toe. In addition, it assists in flexion of the proximal phalanx and maintaining the transverse arch (5). It is supplied by the lateral plantar arteries and nerve (48) (Table 8-3).

The flexor digiti minimi brevis arises from the cuboid and base of the fifth metatarsal and inserts in the lateral base of the proximal phalanx of the fifth toe (Fig. 8-21).

TABLE 8-3. *Muscles of the foot* (4,23,48)

Location	Muscle	Origin	Insertion	Action	Innervation (segment)	Blood supply
Plantar						
Superficial first layer	Abductor hallucis	Medial calcaneus, plantar aponeurosis, and flexor retinaculum	Proximal phalanx great toe	Flexor and abductor MTP joint great toe	Medial plantar nerve (L5, S1)	Medial plantar artery
	Flexor digitorum brevis	Medial calcaneus plantar fascia	Middle phalanges second to fifth toes	Flexor of toes	Medial plantar nerve (L5, S1)	Medial plantar artery
	Abductor digiti minimi	Lateral process calcaneal tubercle	Lateral base proximal phalanx small toe	Abductor and flexor small toe	Lateral plantar nerve (S1, S2)	Lateral plantar artery
Second layer	Quadratus plantae	Medial and lateral calcaneal tuberosity	Flexor digitorum longus tendon	Flexes terminal phalanges two to five	Lateral plantar nerve (S1, S2)	Lateral plantar artery
	Lumbricals	Flexor digitorum longus tendon	MTP joints two to five	Flexes MTP joints	Medial and lateral plantar nerve (S1, S2)	Medial and lateral plantar arteries
Third layer	Flexor hallucis brevis	Cuboid, cuneiform	Great toe	Flexor great toe	Medial plantar nerve (L5, S1)	Medial and lateral artery
	Adductor hallucis	Second to fourth metatarsal bases and third to fifth capsules transverse leg	Great toe	Adductor great toe, maintains transverse arch	Lateral plantar nerve (L5, S1)	Lateral plantar artery
	Flexor digiti minimi brevis	Cuboid and fifth metatarsal base	Proximal phalanx fifth toe	Flexes fifth toe	Lateral plantar nerve (S1, S2)	Lateral plantar artery
Fourth layer	Interossei dorsal	Metatarsal bases	Bases of second to fourth proximal phalanges	Abduct toes	Lateral plantar nerve (S1, S2)	Lateral plantar artery
	Plantar	Metatarsal bases	Bases of third to fifth proximal phalanges	Abduct toes	Lateral plantar nerve (S1, S2)	Lateral plantar artery
Dorsal	Extensor digitorum brevis	Superior calcaneus, lateral talocalcaneal ligament, extensor retinaculum	Lateral first to fourth toes	Extends toes one to four	Deep peroneal nerve (L5, S1)	Dorsalis pedis artery

The muscle serves as a flexor of the small toe and is supplied by branches of the lateral plantar nerve and artery (23,48).

The fourth and deepest layer of plantar muscles consists of seven interosseous muscles—three plantar and four dorsal (Figs. 8-4 and 8-22). The four dorsal interosseous muscles arise with two heads from the adjacent aspects of the metatarsal bases (Fig. 8-22). The tendons insert into the bases of the proximal phalanges with the two medial bellies inserting on the medial and lateral side of the second and the third and fourth inserting on the lateral sides of the third and fourth proximal phalanges. The three plantar interosseous muscles arise from the bases of the third through fifth metatarsals and insert on the medial sides of the proximal phalanges of the third, fourth, and fifth toes. Thus, the dorsal interosseous muscles are abductors and the plantar interosseous muscles are adductors. All interosseous muscles are supplied by branches of the lateral plantar artery and nerve (4,23,48) (Table 8-3).

The extensor digitorum brevis (Figs. 8-4 and 8-16) is the dorsal muscle of the foot. This broad thin muscle arises from the superior calcaneus, lateral talocalcaneal ligament, and extensor retinaculum. It takes a medial oblique course, ending in four tendons that insert in the lateral aspect of the proximal phalanx of the great toe and the lateral extensor digitorum longus tendons of the second to fourth toes. The muscle extends the great toe and second through fourth toes. It is supplied by the deep peroneal nerve and dorsalis pedis artery (4,12,23,48).

The muscles of the foot are summarized in Table 8-3.

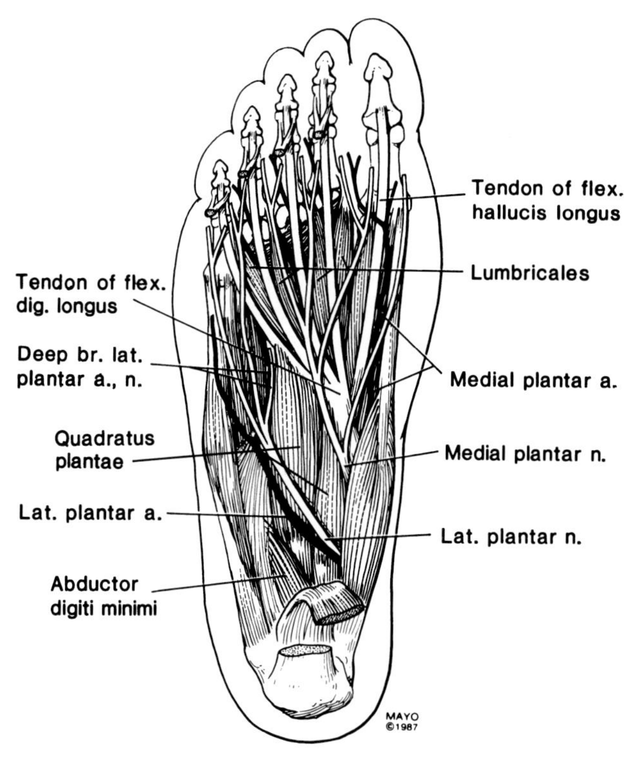

FIG. 8-20. Illustration of the second muscle layer of the foot. (From ref. 11.)

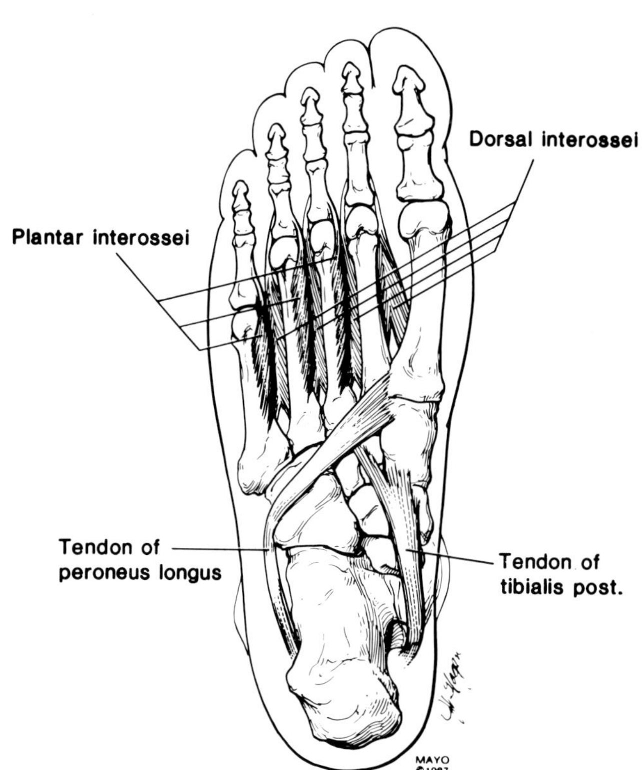

FIG. 8-22. Illustration of the deepest (fourth) layer of muscles in the foot. (From ref. 11.)

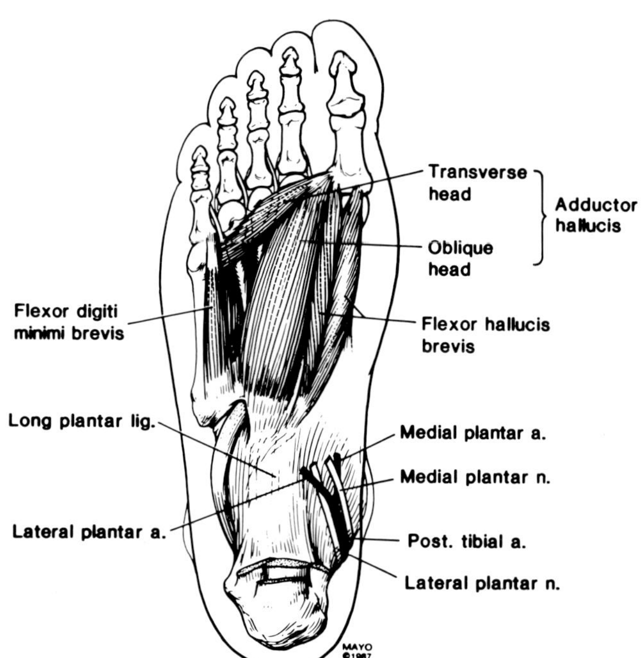

FIG. 8-21. Illustration of the third muscle layer of the foot. (From ref. 11.)

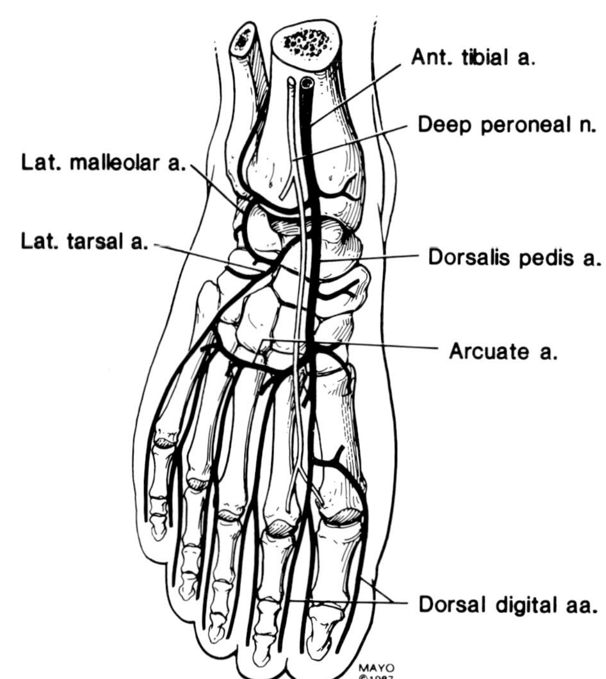

FIG. 8-23. Illustration of the dorsal neurovascular anatomy of the foot. (From ref. 11.)

Neurovascular Supply of the Foot

The anterior tibial artery continues over the midanterior aspect of the tibia, passing deep to the extensor tendons and retinacula of the ankle (Fig. 8-23). At the ankle the anterior tibial artery anastomoses with the perforating branch of the peroneal artery, both supplying the periarticular structures of the ankle. As the anterior tibial artery emerges from the extensor retinaculum, it becomes the more superficial dorsalis pedis artery. After giving off the deep plantar artery, it becomes the first dorsal metatarsal artery. This vessel courses distally, ending in digital branches of the first and second toes. Dorsal branches of the foot include medial and lateral tarsal arteries and the arcuate artery with its dorsal metatarsal branches (Fig. 8-23) (4,12,23,48).

The deep peroneal nerve accompanies the anterior tibial, dorsalis pedis, and first dorsal metatarsal arteries. It supplies the anterior muscles of the foot and leg. The superficial peroneal runs over the anterior aspect of the fibula, supplying the peroneal muscles and the lateral aspect of the foot (Fig. 8-23) (4,12,23,48).

The posterior tibial artery divides into medial and lateral plantar branches deep to the flexor retinaculum (4,48). It is accompanied by similarly named nerves and veins. The neural branches (medial and lateral plantar nerves) are branches of the tibia nerve (Fig. 8-24) (4,12,48).

The medial plantar artery is the smaller of the two branches of the posterior tibial artery and ends in digital branches to the first toe. The lateral plantar artery is larger and forms an arch at the midfoot level that gives off four metatarsal arteries with their distal digital branches (Fig. 8-24) (48). The lateral plantar artery also gives off perforating muscular branches that anastomose with the dorsal arteries. Numerous minor variations in the digital arteries have been described (4,48).

The peroneal artery passes inferior to the lateral malleolus and ends on the calcaneal surface in the lateral calcaneal artery (48).

Table 8-3 summarizes the neurovascular supply to the muscles of the foot.

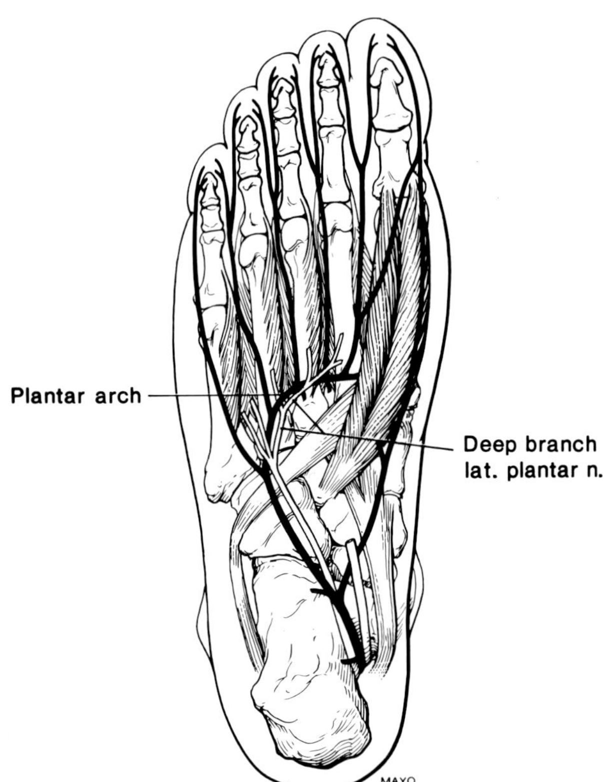

FIG. 8-24. Plantar neurovascular anatomy of the foot. (From ref. 48, with permission.)

PITFALLS AND NORMAL VARIANTS

Misinterpretation of MR images can be related to partial volume effects, flow and other artifacts, and normal anatomic variants. Recognition of these nonpathologic conditions is important to prevent misinterpretation of images and unnecessary treatment (11,105).

There are numerous soft tissue variants in the calf, foot, and ankle. Muscle variations can cause particular confusion when accessing subtle changes on MR images. For example, the gastrocnemius may have only one head, typically the medial head (48). The popliteus may originate from the inner aspect of the fibular head and insert above the oblique tibial line in 14% of cases. The normal origin and insertion are demonstrated in Fig. 8-13. A fairly common accessory flexor muscle, the accessorius longus digitorum, arises from the lower tibia, fibula, and interosseous membrane and passes anterior to the flexor retinaculum to insert with the flexor digitorum longus and quadratus plantae tendons (48).

There are several variations that may cause confusion on MR or CT images. The muscles may fuse to form one unit and occasionally the peroneus longus insertion expands to include the bases of the third to fifth metatarsals. An accessory peroneal muscle may arise from the fibula between the peroneus longus and brevis. Its tendon generally inserts in the peroneus longus tendon on the plantar aspect of the foot (12,23,48).

The peroneus quadratus is present in about 13% of patients. This arises from the posterior fibula between the longus and brevis and inserts on the peroneal trochlea of the calcaneus. The peroneus digiti minimi is rare. It arises from the lower fibula and inserts on the extensor surface of the fifth toe (12,48).

An important variant is the accessory soleus muscle. This muscle bundle extends into the pre-Achilles fat (Kager's fat) (30,33,84). This muscle may be noted incidentally or cause clinical symptoms. Patients may pre-

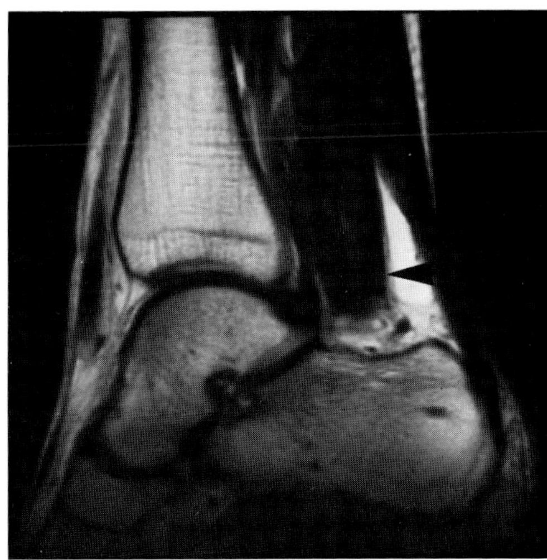

FIG. 8-25. Accessory soleus muscle. Sagittal image of the ankle in a patient with an accessory soleus muscle (*arrow*). Compare to normal sagittal images in Fig. 8-5.

sent with pain after exercise or a soft tissue mass. MRI (Fig. 8-25) can confirm the presence of this normal variant and differentiate normal muscle from a muscle tear or neoplasm (12).

One must also be familiar with accessory ossicles and variations in bony anatomy (12). However, a complete discussion of these variations is beyond the scope of this chapter.

Noto et al. (73) reviewed normal variants on MR images in 30 patients. Common variations included an irregularity of the posterior tibiotalar joint (27/30 cases), variations in signal intensity at points of tendon insertions (not to be confused with tendon rupture), and small amounts of fluid in the tendon sheath surrounding otherwise normal tendons. The latter may be particularly difficult to differentiate from early tendinitis or synovitis.

Partial volume effects can also create apparent abnormalities. Use of multiple image planes can be helpful in minimizing this problem (Fig. 8-2).

CLINICAL APPLICATIONS

The applications for MRI of the calf, foot, and ankle continue to expand (8,10,12,43,49,56,70,73,94,95). Ease of positioning, multiple image planes, and the superior contrast afforded by MRI are ideal for examination of many foot and ankle problems. In our practice (see Table 8-4), the most common applications are trauma—specifically, soft tissue trauma—neoplasms, and problem solving in patients with chronic nonspecific pain. Other indications include arthritis, both inflammatory and infectious, and osteonecrosis.

TABLE 8-4. *MRI of the foot and ankle—applications*

Indication	Patients (%)
Trauma	33
Neoplasms	19
Nonspecific pain	14
Arthritis/infection	10
Osteonecrosis	10
Problem solving	14

Trauma

Foot and ankle injuries account for 10% or more of emergency room visits (21,71). Routine radiographs and conventional techniques are still best suited for evaluation of patients with acute skeletal injuries. Chronic post-traumatic syndromes and certain soft tissue injuries may be more ideally suited to MR evaluation.

Most skeletal injuries are best evaluated with routine radiographs, tomography, and on occasion computed tomography. Although MRI is most often used to evaluate soft tissue trauma, one need not be concerned about overlooking skeletal injuries when MR examinations are performed. Subtle marrow injuries can be detected that may go undiagnosed with conventional tomography and/or CT (Fig. 8-26) (10,11,60,98,108,113). These include stress fractures and talar dome fractures (Fig. 8-27). Associated soft tissue injuries, specifically involving the tendons, can also be assessed with MRI. However, more complex fractures are better evaluated with CT (Fig. 8-28) (12).

Soft Tissue Trauma

The ligaments, capsule, and major supporting structures of the ankle have been discussed in the anatomic section of this chapter. The anatomic positions of the tendons and ligaments in the foot and ankle make it difficult to properly align all these structures in a single MR image plane. Therefore, MRI is not commonly used to identify typical ligament sprains and tears in the ankle. However, the ligaments can be demonstrated if care is taken to use the proper off-axis oblique planes. We currently still prefer arthrography and/or tenography to demonstrate partial and complete ligament tears of the medial and lateral ligament complexes of the ankle (7,14,15,17).

Computed tomography (CT) can be used to evaluate the ankle tendons, but the soft tissue contrast and limited image planes reduce its effectiveness compared to MRI (86). MRI, on the other hand, is ideally suited for evaluation of partial or complete tendon tears as well as inflammation of the tendons of the foot and ankle (7,9). There are 13 tendons that cross the ankle. These include

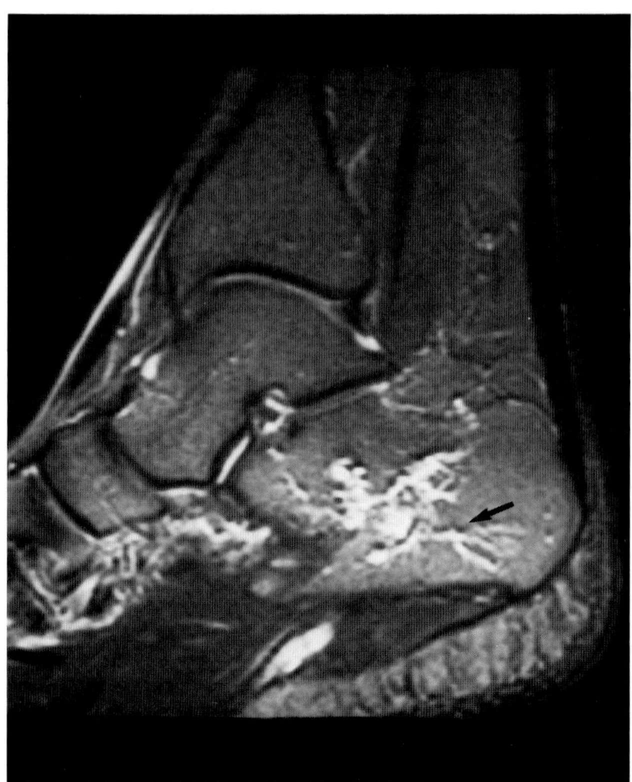

FIG. 8-26. Patient with heel pain and normal radiograph. T2 weighted (SE 2,000/60) sagittal image demonstrates a stellate area of high signal intensity (*arrow*) due to a stress fracture.

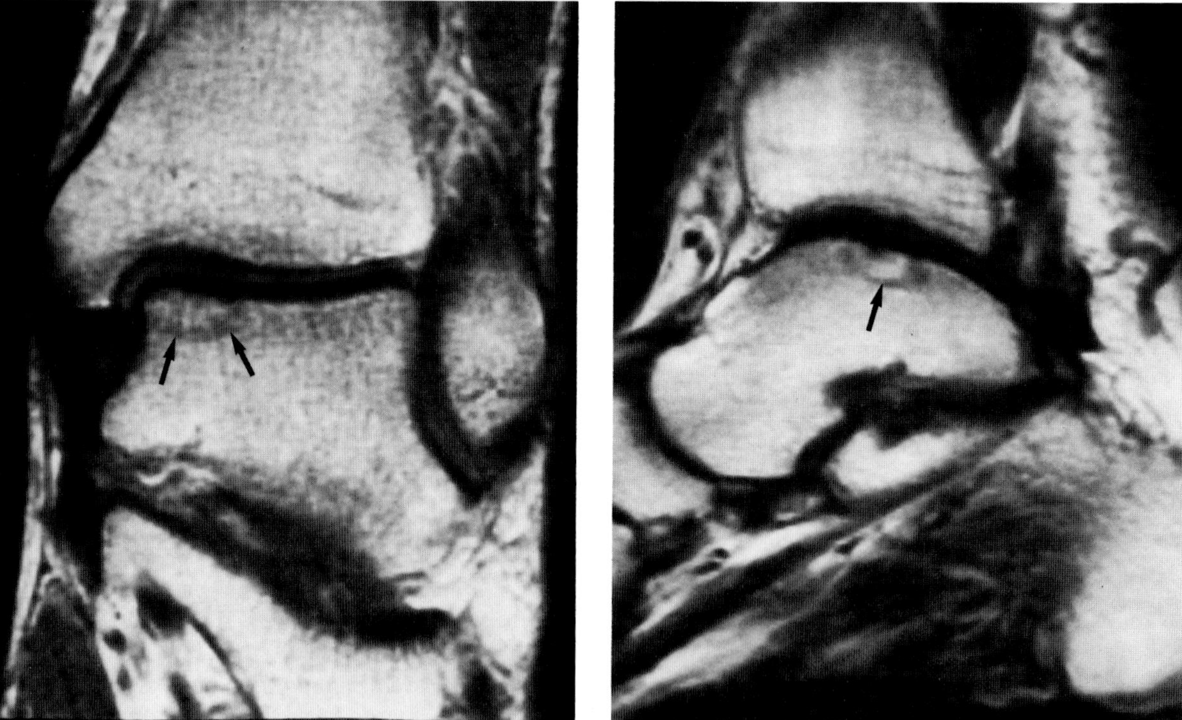

FIG. 8-27. Sagittal (**A**) and coronal (**B**) SE 500/20 images of the ankle in a patient with a suspected soft tissue injury. The talar dome fracture (*arrow*) is easily identified.

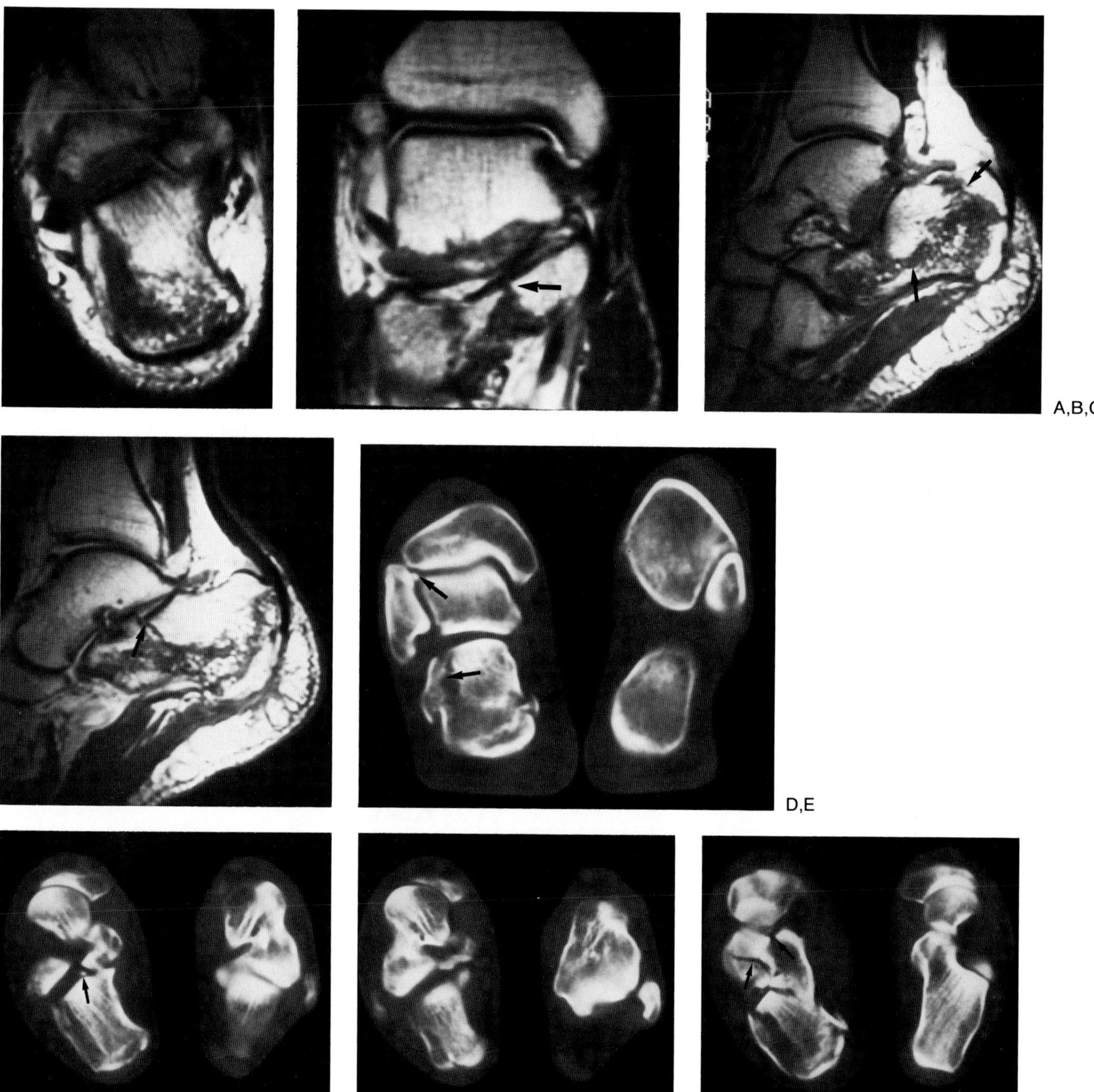

FIG. 8-28. Complex calcaneal fracture. Axial (**A**), coronal (**B**), and sagittal (**C,D**) SE 500/20 images demonstrate a complex calcaneal fracture involving the subtalar joint (*arrows*). CT images (**E–H**) more clearly demonstrate the fragments (*arrows*) and articular involvement.

the peroneus brevis and longus laterally, the Achilles tendon posteriorly, the tibialis posterior, flexor digitorum longus, and flexor hallucis longus medially, and anteriorly the tibialis anterior, extensor hallucis longus, tendons of the extensor digitorum longus, and peroneus tertius. All these tendons are enclosed within tendon sheaths, except the Achilles tendon. We typically evaluate suspected tendon pathology with spin-echo sequences in the sagittal and axial planes. The extremity coil is used with the foot in neutral position. Excessive plantar flexion buckles the tendons, which exaggerates partial volume effects. T2 weighted sequences (20/60 TE, 2,000 TR) clearly demonstrate the high signal intensity of blood or fluid in or about the normally dark tendon. Thin (3 mm) thick slices with a 1.5 mm interslice gap and a 256 × 256 matrix with one acquisition provide excellent image quality. Normally, minimal fluid is noted around these tendons on T2 weighted MR images. For purposes of discussion, it is best to consider each of the tendons in separate groups.

Peroneal Tendons

Peroneal muscles assist in pronation and eversion of the foot. The peroneus brevis tendons are anterior to the peroneus longus as they pass posterior to the lateral malleolus (see Figs. 8-5 and 8-15). In approximately 80% of patients, there is a notch in the fibula posteriorly that accommodates a portion of the peroneus brevis. In 20% this notch is either shallow or absent, which may lead to subluxation (Fig. 8-29). The two peroneal tendons are immediately adjacent to the calcaneofibular ligament between the superior and inferior retinacula through which they also pass (Fig. 8-15). Both tendons have a common sheath to the inferior margin of the superior retinaculum. At this point the sheath divides so that the peroneus longus and peroneus brevis each have their own tendon sheath. The peroneus brevis passes inferior to the lateral malleolus to insert on the base of the fifth metatarsal (Figs. 8-6 and 8-15). The peroneus longus progresses inferior to the peroneal tubercle of the calcaneus and passes to the plantar aspect of the foot, where it inserts in the base of the first metatarsal and medial cuneiform (Fig. 8-22) (11,12,23,48,87,114). This portion of the tendon can be difficult to evaluate on MRI because of its oblique position. Both peroneal tendons proximal to the base of the fifth metatarsal are easily demonstrated on the axial and sagittal planes using MRI. Therefore, diagnosis of inflammatory changes such as tendonitis, subluxation, or complete or incomplete disruption can easily be accomplished.

Patients with peroneal tendonitis generally demonstrate some thickening with increased signal intensity in the peripheral portions of the tendon and tendon sheath on T2 weighted images. A similar finding can be seen with incomplete tendon tears, except that the defect is usually more localized. T1 weighted (SE 500/20) sequences provide excellent anatomy but are not as useful for demonstrating subtle inflammatory changes and edema (11).

Diagnosis of subluxation or dislocation of the peroneal tendons is difficult. Many patients present with "ankle sprain" or recurrent "giving-way" (1,21,22). Dislocations usually occur with inversion dorsiflexion or abduction dorsiflexion injuries. Patients present with pain and swelling over the lateral malleolus, similar to an ankle sprain. Swelling can make tendon palpation difficult. Although small avulsion fractures of the lateral malleolus have been described, MRI, CT, or tenography are typically required to confirm the diagnosis (87). MRI is most useful because it can also identify other peroneal tendon pathology most effectively.

T2 weighted or gradient-echo sequences are most useful for detection of subtle subluxations or dislocations (11). Axial images with internal and external rota-

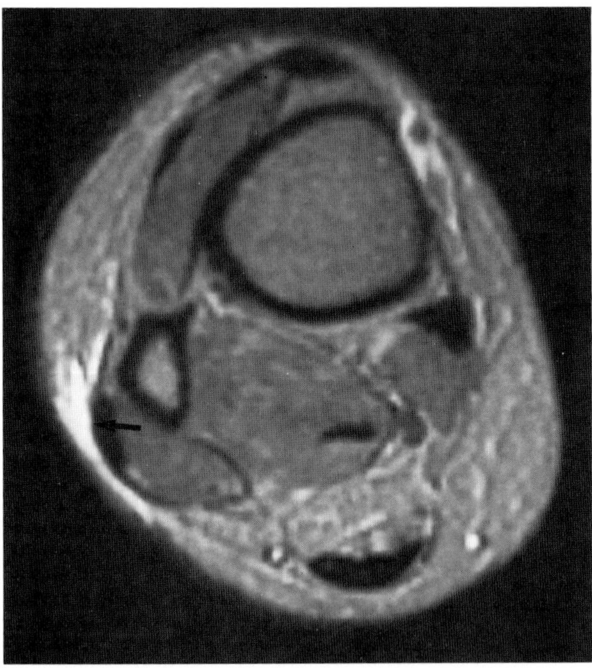

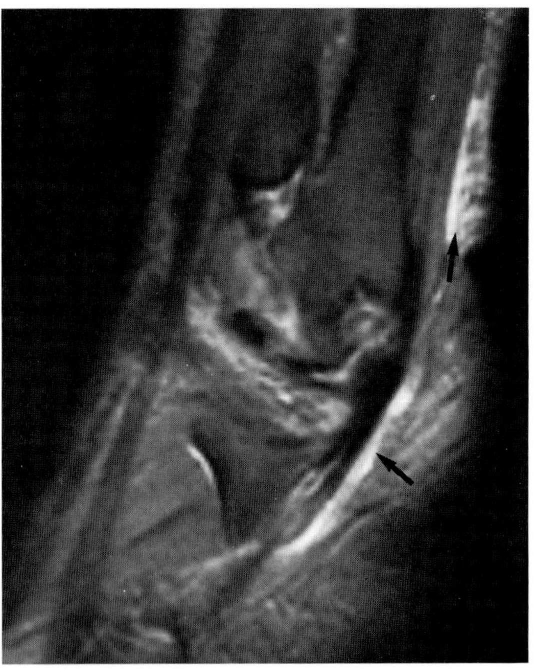

A,B

FIG. 8-29. Axial (**A**) and sagittal (**B**) T2 weighted (SE 2,000/60) images of the ankle in a patient with subluxing peroneal tendons. The only finding on static MR images may be local edema or swelling (*arrow*).

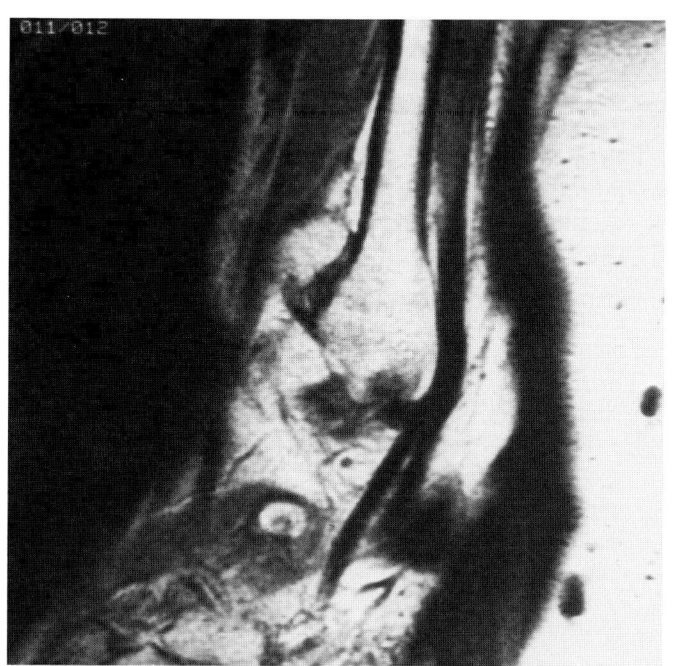

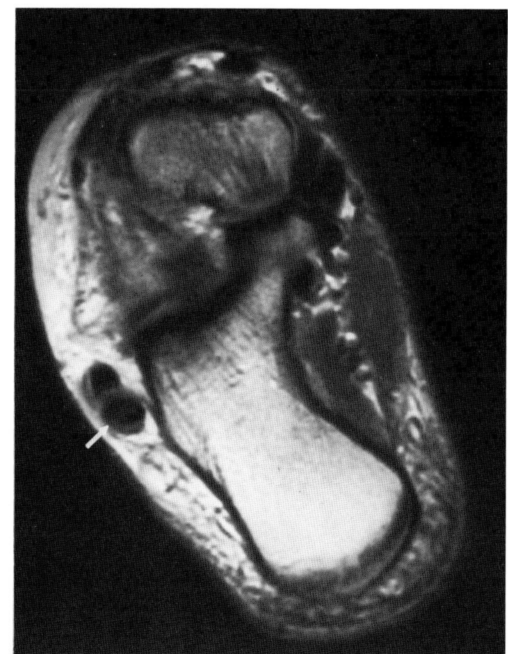

A,B

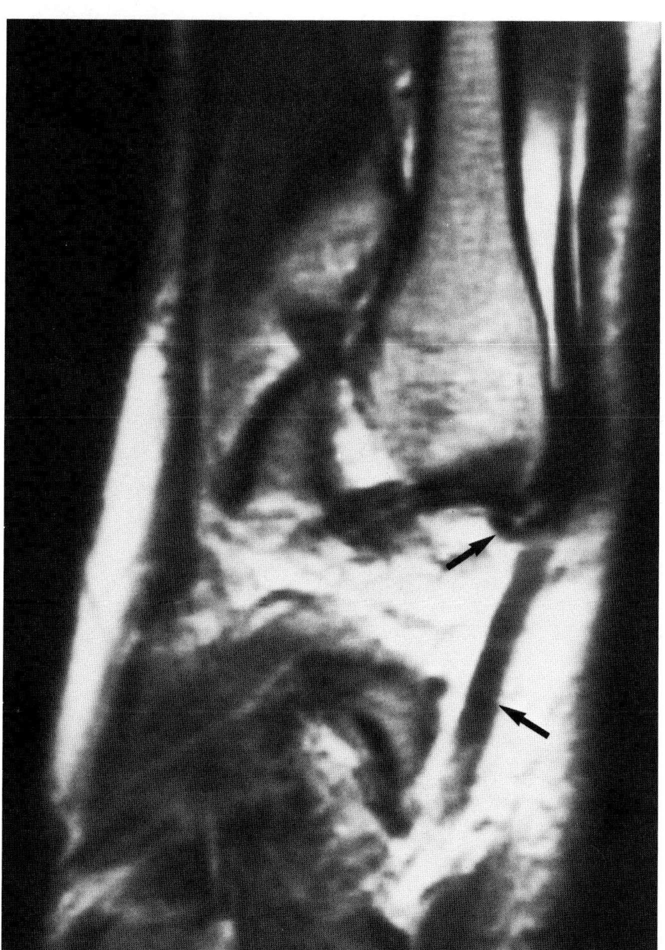

C

FIG. 8-30. Peroneus longus rupture—complete. **A:** Normal sagittal MR image showing both the peroneus brevis and longus tendons. **B:** Axial SE 2,000/60 image demonstrates thickening of the proximal end of the peroneus longus (*arrow*). **C:** Sagittal image with complete rupture of the peroneus longus shows the normal peroneus brevis (*lower arrow*) and ruptured end of the peroneus longus (*upper arrow*).

tion of the foot can be accomplished quickly with gradient-echo techniques. Cine images can be produced to simulate motion, which allows detection of subtle lesions. Tendon pathology and position changes with regard to the fibular notch are easily assessed. In some cases comparison with the opposite ankle is useful.

Ruptures of the peroneal tendon are uncommon (Fig. 8-30). However, this injury is easily overlooked so the true incidence is not known (11,21,54,87). Patients present acutely with "ankle sprain" symptoms or with chronic instability. The latter is more common in patients with arthropathy or patients on systemic steroids. Cavovarus foot deformities and compartment syndromes have also been reported with peroneal tendon rupture. When completely torn, patients are unable to evert the foot (1,54,87).

Ultrasonography, CT, MRI, and tenography can be used to evaluate peroneal tendon ruptures (11). For purposes of anatomic display and grading the injury, we find axial and sagittal T2 weighted sequences (TE 20 or 30, 60-80, TR 2,000) most useful (Fig. 8-30). Complete ruptures can be identified by absence of the tendon on the axial and sagittal images, with high signal intensity replacing the normally black tendon. Thickening and retraction of the separated tendon ends are commonly noted. Incomplete tears are demonstrated as thickening with variable degrees of increased signal intensity on T2 weighted sequences (Fig. 8-31).

Achilles Tendon

The Achilles tendon is the longest and strongest tendon in the foot and ankle. It originates where the gastrocnemius and soleus tendons join and inserts on the posterior calcaneus (Figs. 8-5, 8-11, and 8-12). In its axial presentation, the tendon thickens as it passes caudally, becoming elliptical with a slightly concave anterior and convex posterior surface (Fig. 8-3). Two to six centimeters above the ankle the fibers in the tendon cross. It is at this same level that there is some reduction in the blood supply, and therefore many tears in the Achilles tendon occur at this level (11,54).

The Achilles tendon, though one of the strongest, is commonly torn (7,11,28,52,58,72,78). Ruptures are usually the result of indirect trauma. The injury can occur during any athletic activity and at any age. Generally, ruptures occur in strenuous activities while the foot is plantar flexed or during raising up on the toes such as with pushing off or jumping with the knee extended. In nonathletes, the injury is most common in 30–50-year-old patients (11,54). Certain systemic and local conditions may predispose to tendon rupture. These include gout, systemic lupus erythematosis, rheumatoid arthritis, hyperparathyroidism, chronic renal failure, systemic or local steroids, and diabetes mellitus (11,58). Patients on systemic steroids or with systemic diseases may have simultaneous rupture of both Achilles tendons. Local

A,B
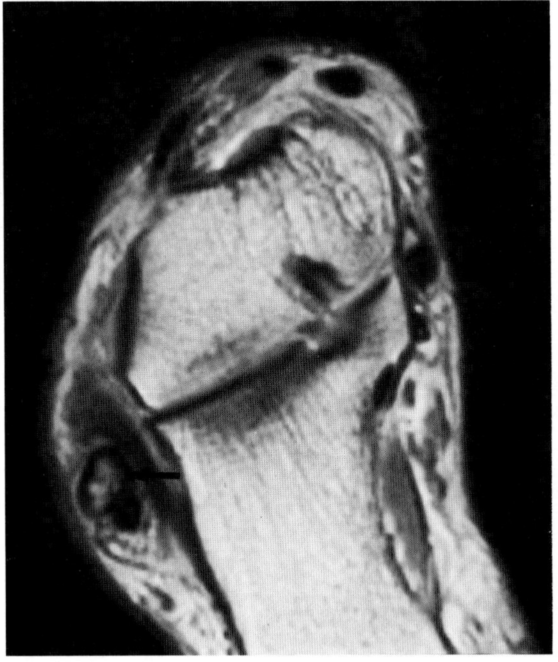
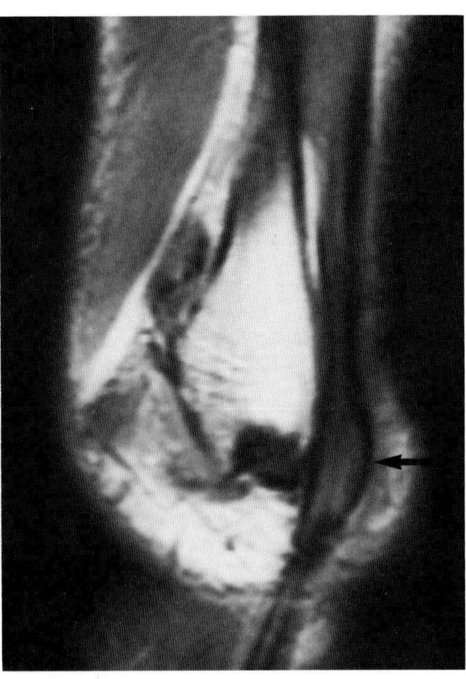

FIG. 8-31. Incomplete tear of the peroneus brevis tendon. Axial (**A**) and sagittal (**B**) SE 2,000/30 images show local thickening with increased signal intensity (*arrows*) in the tendon.

steroid injections may also lead to partial or complete disruption of the Achilles tendon (11,21,28,54,58,78).

Clinically, patients generally present with pain, local swelling, and inability to raise up on their toes on the affected side. If completely torn, a palpable defect may be noted on physical exam; however, clinical exam is not always accurate. This is because a gap in the tendon may not be palpable and patients may be able to plantar flex the foot with the toes. The exact nature of the injury can be misdiagnosed in over one-fourth of the patients (54). Differentiation from venous thrombosis, gastrocnemius, and plantaris tears may be difficult (11,54). Therefore, examination of the calf may be required when images of the Achilles tendon are normal.

Imaging of the Achilles tendon can be accomplished using several techniques, including soft tissue radiographic techniques, ultrasound, CT, and MRI (11, 81,85,86). Although all these techniques can be useful in given situations, we find MRI most useful for detection of subtle lesions and also in following the healing process in patients with partial or complete tears.

T2 weighted axial and sagittal images using a double echo (TE 20 or 30, 60; TR 2,000) provides excellent anatomy (first echo) and good contrast (fluid, hemorrhage, high intensity against normal black appearance of tendons) with normal soft tissue structures (11). Gradient-echo sequences can also be used. This reduces imaging time but the soft tissue contrast is reduced between muscle, fat, and other peritendinous tissues. We usually begin with a sagittal scout, choose the axial levels, and then use the axial images to obtain optimal sagittal images of the tendon (11).

MRI is accurate in demonstrating partial (Figs. 8-32 and 8-33) and complete (Fig. 8-34) tears, following healing (Figs. 8-35 and 8-36), and differentiating tendon tears from venous thrombosis (Fig. 8-37).

Medial Tendons

The posterior tibial, flexor digitorum longus, and flexor hallucis longus tendons make up the medial tendon group. Those tendons are located anterior to posterior in the above order (Figs. 8-3, 8-5, and 8-38). The posterior tibial tendon with its tendon sheath passes just posterior to the medial malleolus, lateral to the flexor retinaculum, and broadens at its insertion in the navicular tuberosity and base of the medial cuneiform (Fig. 8-22). The flexor digitorum longus takes a similar course proximally lying between the posterior tibial tendon and posterior tibial artery (Fig. 8-38). As it turns toward the plantar aspect of the foot, it passes superficially to the flexor hallucis longus before dividing into tendon slips that insert in the bases of the second through fifth distal phalanges (Figs. 8-4, 8-6, and 8-20). The flexor hallucis longus tendon is located more posteriorly and laterally (Fig. 8-38). It passes through a fibro-osseous tunnel be-

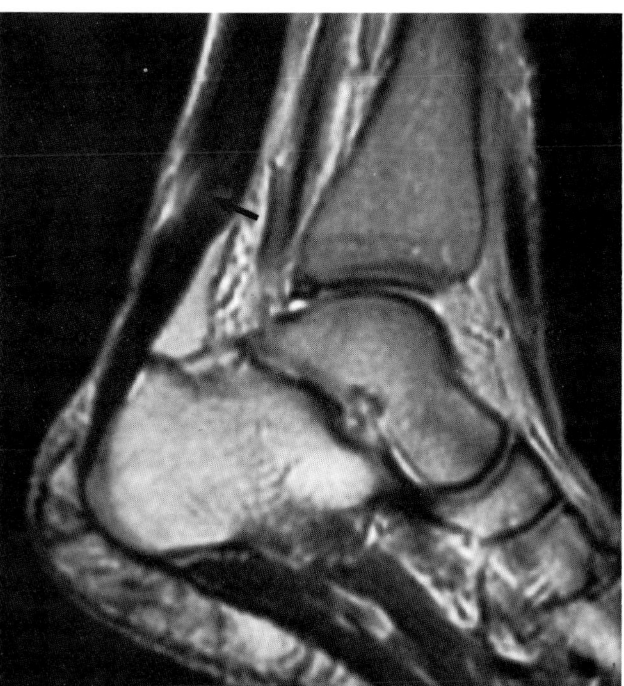
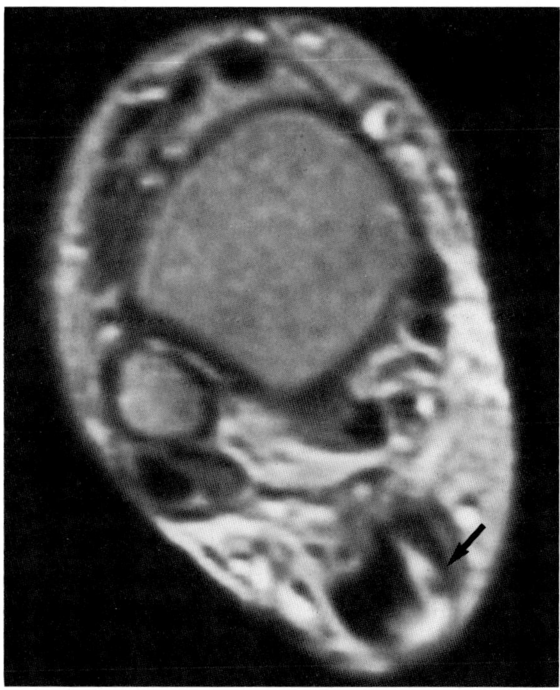

A,B

FIG. 8-32. Sagittal (**A**) and axial (**B**) SE 2,000/60 images demonstrating thickening of the Achilles tendon with a grade 1 (few fibers torn) tear (*arrow*) in the Achilles tendon.

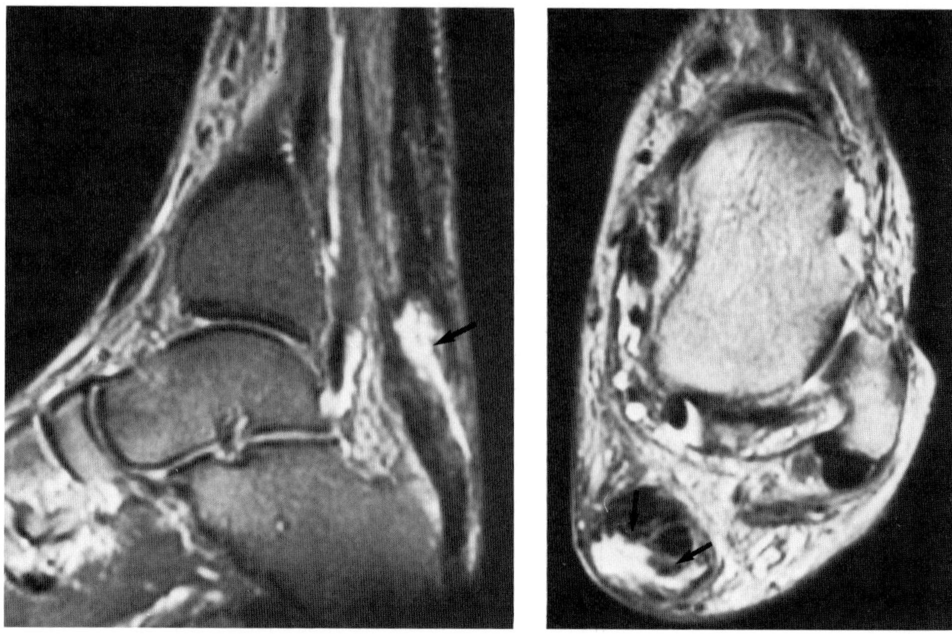

FIG. 8-33. Sagittal (**A**) and axial (**B**) images (SE 2,000/60) demonstrating a grade 2 (approximately 50% tear) tear of the Achilles tendon (*arrow*).

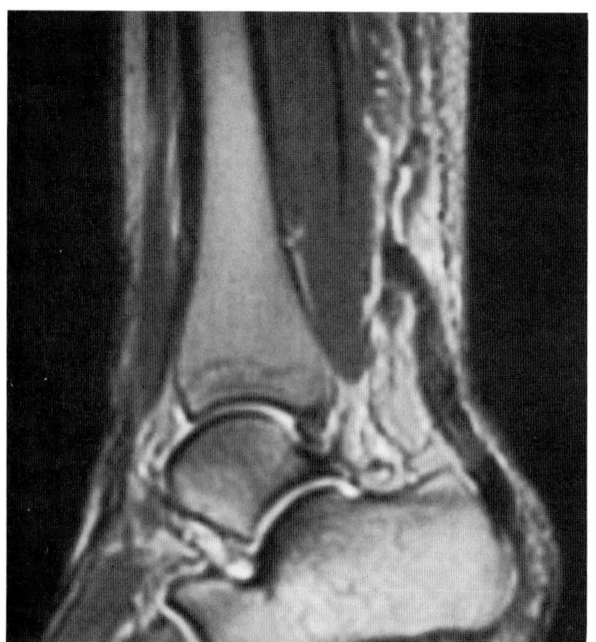

FIG. 8-34. Sagittal SE 2,000/60 image shows a "wavy" lax Achilles tendon due to a complete tear.

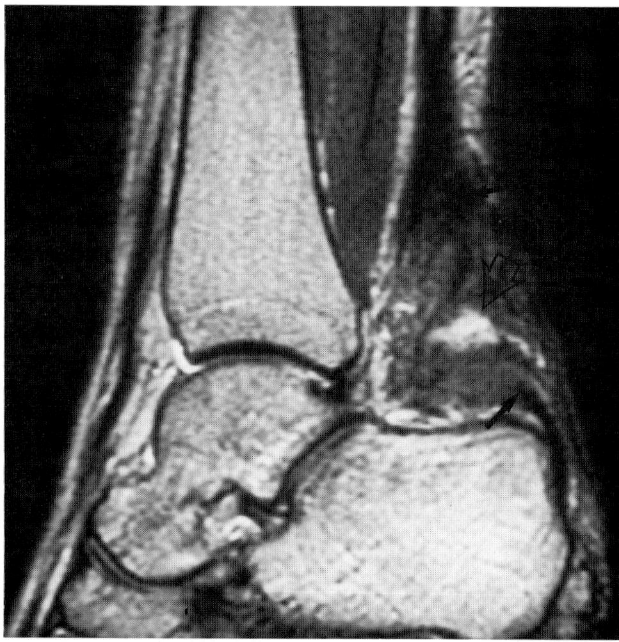

FIG. 8-35. Old complete tear of the Achilles tendon. Note the distal end (*lower arrow*), proximal end (*upper arrow*) with inflammatory changes in the fat, and active hemorrhage or edema (*open arrow*) in the tendon gap.

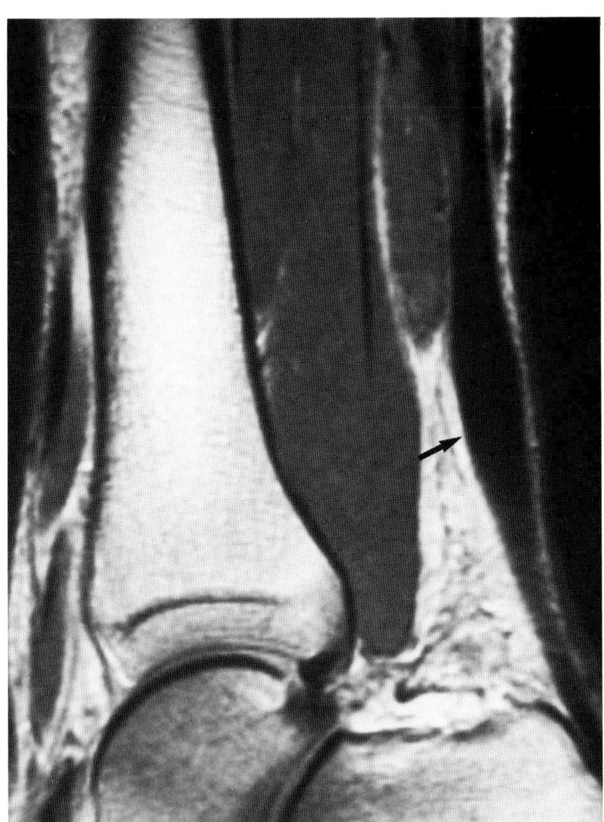

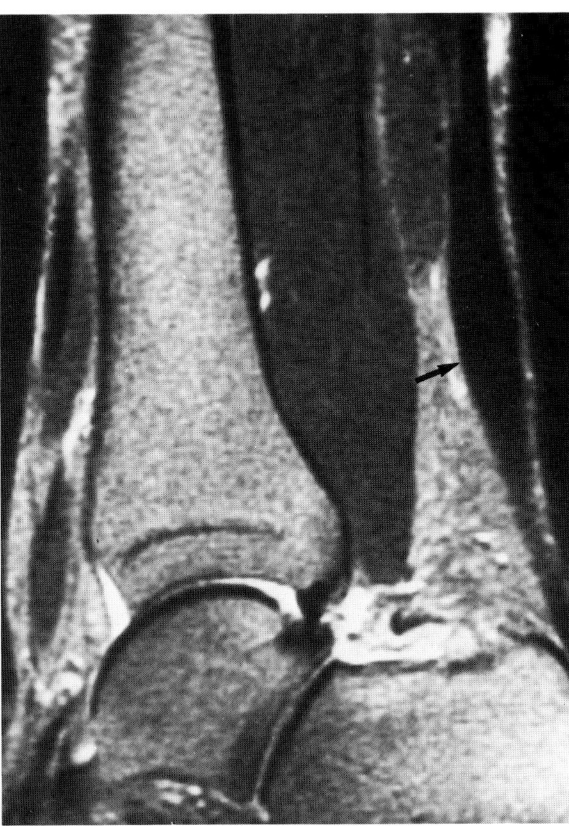

A,B

FIG. 8-36. Healed Achilles tear. T1 (SE 500/20) (**A**) and T2 (SE 2,000/60) (**B**) images show thickening (*arrow*) but no increased signal intensity in the Achilles tendon.

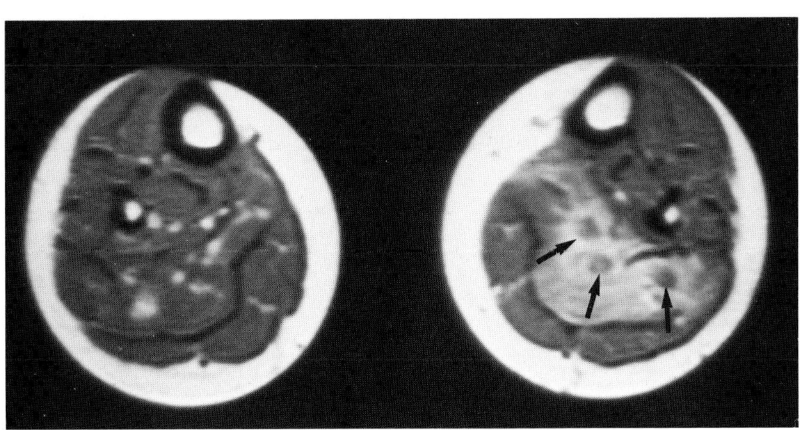

FIG. 8-37. Patient with suspected Achilles tendon tear. MRI (SE 2,000/30) shows edema in the soleus muscle with clot in three deep veins (*arrows*).

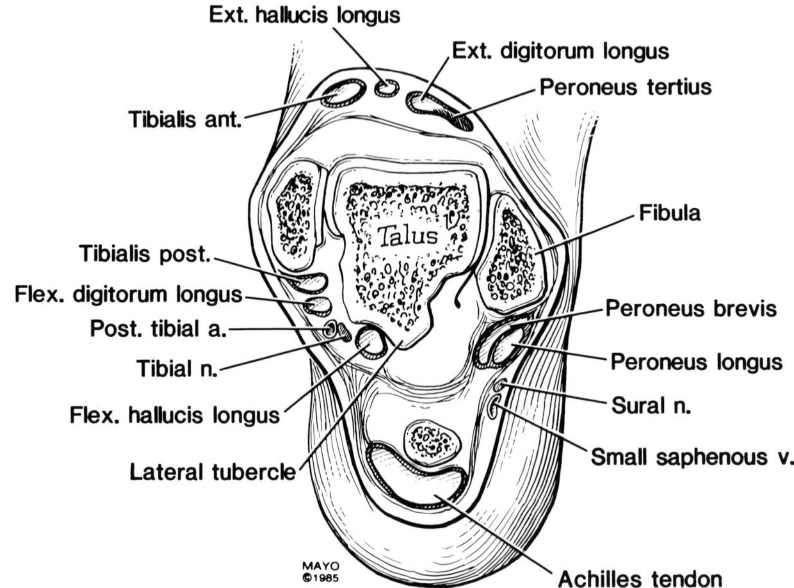

FIG. 8-38. Illustration of the tendons and neurovascular structures about the ankle. (From ref. 11.)

neath the sustentaculum tali and along the medial plantar aspect of the foot to insert in the base of the distal phalanx of the great toe (Figs. 8-3, 8-4, and 8-20) (23,48).

The posterior tibial tendon is the most commonly injured of the three medial tendons (3,11,32,54,85,86). Patients generally present with pain, local tenderness, and swelling, and physical examination may reveal a nonpalpable tendon. Rupture of the posterior tibial tendon can lead to progressive flatfoot deformity and inability to raise up on the toes, as well as weakness on inversion of the foot (11,54,85,86).

Routine radiographic techniques are usually of little value in patients with medial tendon injuries. Tenography can be accomplished, but this is difficult depending on the experience of the examiner. Evaluation of the medial tendons can be accomplished with ultrasound, CT, and MRI. As with the other tendons, in our experience, MRI has been most useful in assessing the nature and degree of tendon pathology (Fig. 8-39) (11).

Posterior tibial tendon tears have been classified by Rosenberg et al. (85) based on MRI and CT findings. Type 1 tears are incomplete with tendon thickening and vertical slits in the tendon. The tendon appears thickened with scattered areas of high signal intensity on T2 weighted images (Fig. 8-40). Type 2 injuries are partial tears with areas of attenuation in the tendon. This has the appearance of a thinned area on axial and sagittal images. When the tendon is completely torn (type 3) there is a gap in the tendon that can clearly be seen on

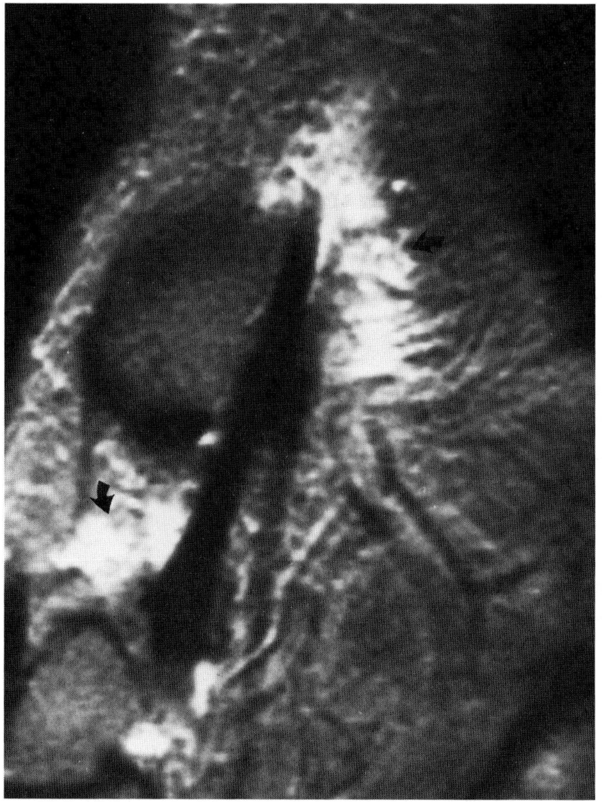

FIG. 8-39. Sagittal SE 2,000/60 image of the medial tendons in a patient with swelling and medial ankle pain. The posterior tibial tendon and flexor digitorum longus tendons are normal. There is high signal intensity in the soft tissues (*arrows*) due to edema.

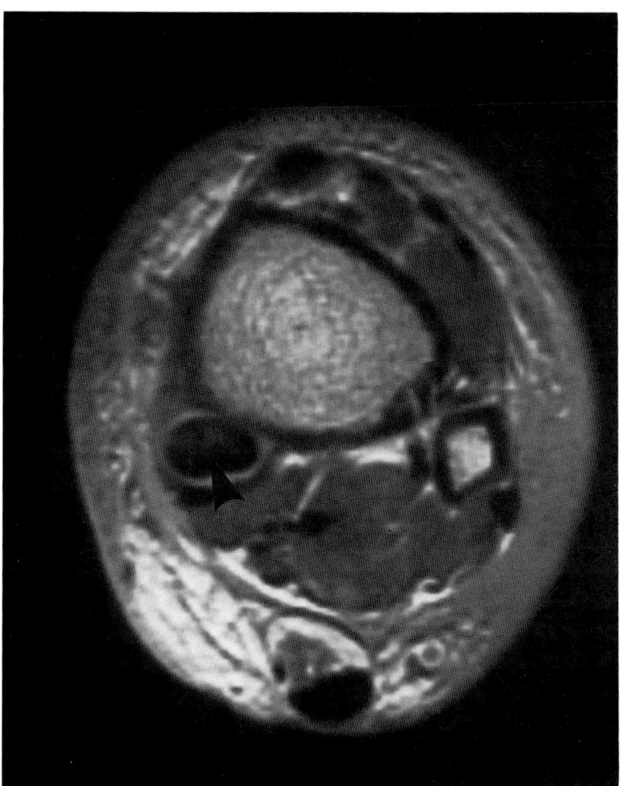

FIG. 8-40. Axial SE 2,000/60 image demonstrating an incomplete tear of the posterior tibial tendon. Note the high signal intensity in the substance of the thickened tendon (*arrowhead*) and the fluid in the tendon sheath.

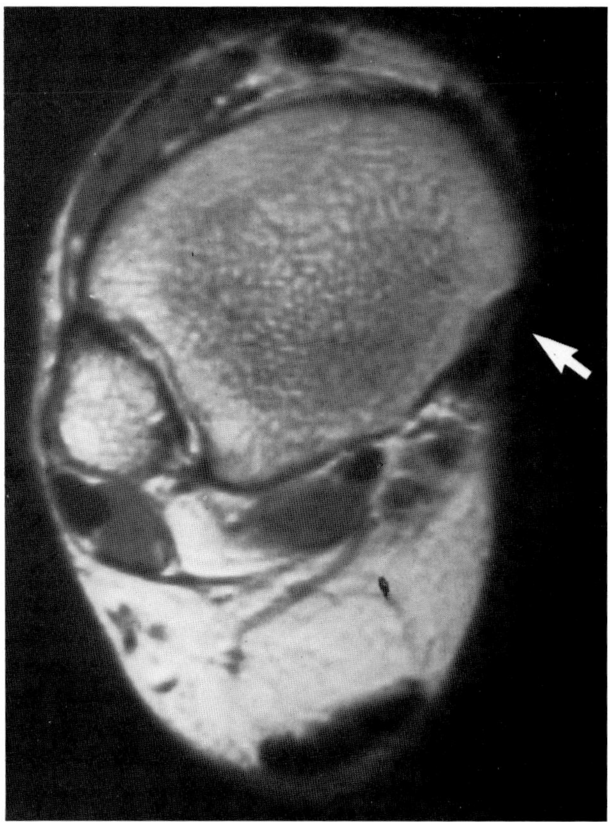

FIG. 8-41. Axial image (SE 500/20) of the ankle in a patient with a complete tear of the posterior tibial tendon. Note the complete absence (*arrow*) of the posterior tibial tendon.

sagittal images. The tendon will be absent in this section on axial images (Fig. 8-41). Older tears may have reduced signal intensity because granulation tissue begins to form about 2 weeks after injury (47). This has more intermediate signal intensity on T2 weighted sequences.

Rupture of the flexor digitorum (Fig. 8-42) and flexor hallucis longus tendons is less common. However, Garth (41) did report rupture of the flexor hallucis longus in ballet dancers and soccer players. Patients usually present with swelling, tenderness, and crepitation near the sustentaculum tali. Symptoms generally increase with flexion and extension of the great toe. Tenography, though possible for the posterior tibial tendon and flexor digitorum longus, is much more difficult for the deep and more posteriorly located flexor hallucis longus tendon. Therefore, MRI is the ideal technique for evaluation of this structure. Image features are similar regardless of which tendon is being evaluated.

Anterior Tendons

Anteriorly, the anterior tibial, extensor hallucis longus, and extensor digitorum longus tendons are all enclosed in tendon sheaths (Fig. 8-38). Acute tears are unusual but in patients with previous fractures, degen-

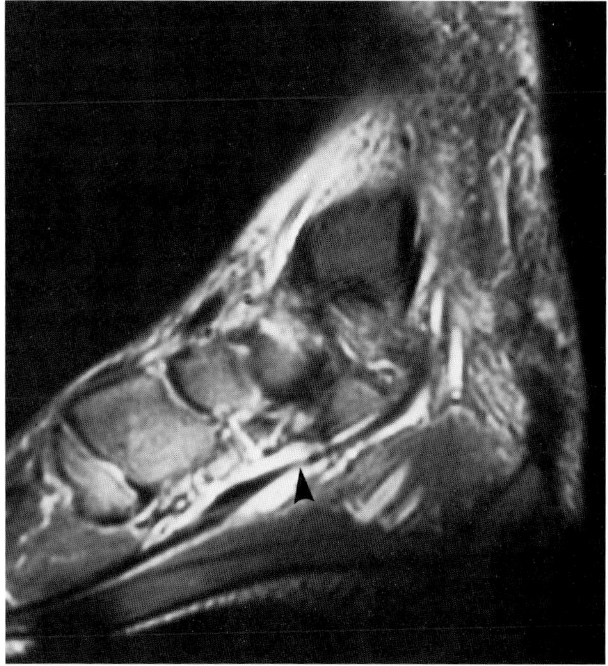

FIG. 8-42. Sagittal SE 2,000/60 image demonstrating an incomplete tear in the flexor digitorum longus tendon. There is fluid in the tendon sheath with thinning of the tendon (*arrowhead*) just distal to the sustentaculum tali.

erative arthritis, or other predisposing factors, tendon rupture can occur (54). Injury to the anterior tibial tendon is not uncommon in runners. Rupture of this tendon usually occurs as it exits the superior retinaculum. The distal segment retracts and can be palpated between the superior and inferior retinaculum (Fig. 8-43). Clinically, patients present with pain and swelling over the anterior ankle. There may also be decreased ability to dorsiflex the foot on physical examination (11,54).

Although other radiographic techniques can be used to demonstrate the anterior tendons, specifically CT, we prefer MRI to diagnose the extent of injury and also follow patients who are treated conservatively and surgically. For examination purposes, T2 weighted sequences are preferred. The increased signal intensity of the fluid and hemorrhage seen against the black or lack of signal of the tendon makes identification much easier with this technique.

Miscellaneous Soft Tissue Injuries

Other soft tissue injuries in the foot and ankle may also occur. These include compartment syndrome, plantar fasciitis, and bursitis. Inflammation of the calcaneal bursae is not uncommon (Fig. 8-44) (11,20). MRI is very useful in detection of these inflammatory changes. As noted previously, T2 weighted axial and sagittal images need to be obtained with the foot in neutral and plantar flexed positions. Normally, the pre-Achilles fat fills in the space between the tendon and calcaneus during plantar flexion (Fig. 8-45). When the anterior bursa is inflamed, this does not occur. Also, a well-defined area of high signal intensity may be seen due to a fluid-filled distended bursa (20).

Plantar fasciitis is demonstrated by the infiltrative high signal intensity in the plantar fascia on coronal and sagittal T2 weighted images. The foot should be in neutral position for the examination.

Calf Trauma

Trauma to the calf may lead to intramuscular hemorrhage or hematoma formation. Neurovascular injury and compartment syndrome may also result from direct trauma or secondary to undiagnosed muscle tears. Most ligament and tendon injuries occur about the knee or ankle (11,62,75).

Physical examination and history are important in defining the region and severity of injury. Until recently, imaging studies were usually not obtained except when venous thrombosis was suspected. It may be difficult to differentiate clinically deep venous thrombosis from dis-

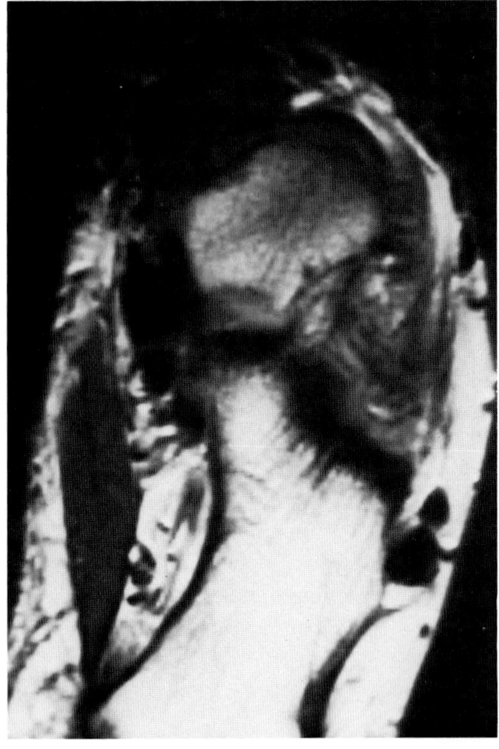
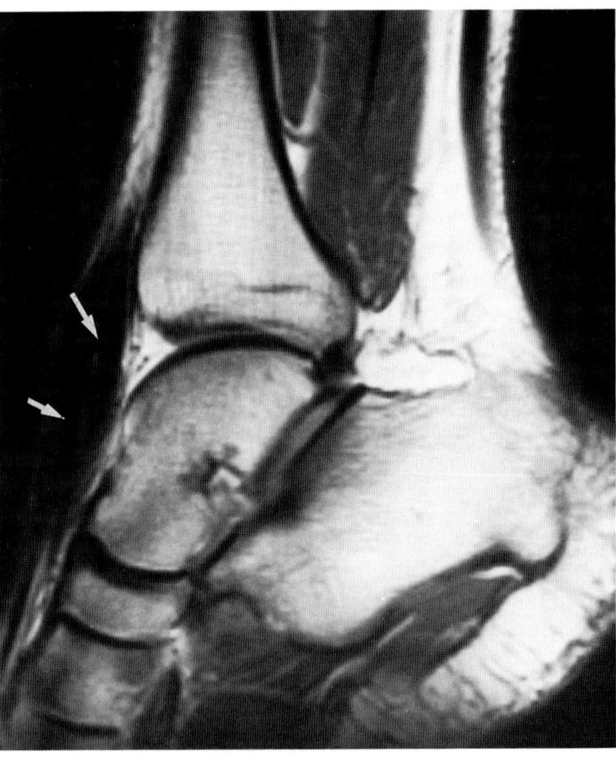

A,B

FIG. 8-43. Partial tear of the anterior tibial tendon in a jogger. Axial (**A**) and sagittal (**B**) SE 2,000/30 images show thickening and scattered areas of increased signal intensity (*arrows*) in the anterior tibial tendon.

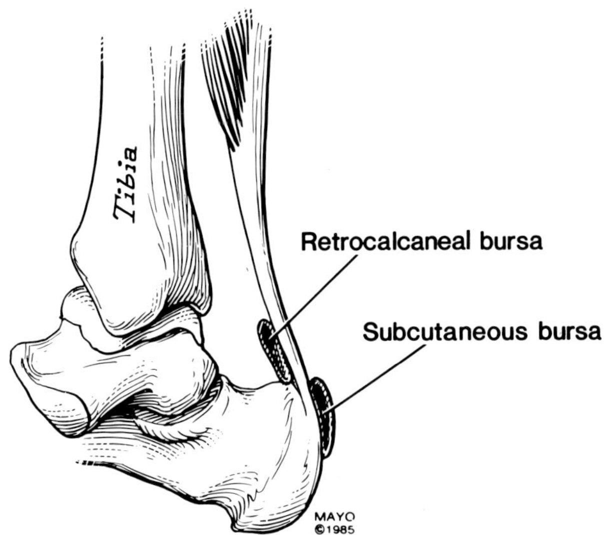

FIG. 8-44. Sagittal illustration of the calcaneal bursae. (From ref. 11.)

secting popliteal cysts, muscle tears, and Achilles tendon injuries (11,34,35,50).

MR examinations are generally performed with the patient prone to avoid compression of the soft tissues. An extremity coil or, when comparison is needed, the head coil is most often used. Axial images with 1 cm thick slices using T1 (SE 500/20) and T2 (SE 2,000/60, 20) sequences with a 256 × 256 matrix and one acquisition are usually adequate to identify the injury. On occasion, the extent of injury may be more easily appreciated with an additional T2 weighted sequence in the coronal or sagittal plane. T2 weighted sequences are most useful because acute hemorrhage or hematoma can be isointense with muscle on T1 weighted sequences (Fig. 8-46) (34,35).

Venous abnormalities can be detected with conventional spin-echo sequences (Fig. 8-47). However, flow phenomenon may cause intraluminal signal leading to false diagnosis of thromboses (35). Gradient-echo sequences (50/12–16, FA 30°) show normal flow as an area of high signal intensity. Thrombosis will be demonstrated as an area of low or reduced signal intensity (97). Inversion recovery sequences (IR 200/20/100) show thrombus as an area of high intensity and suppress fat signal (80). Either of these sequences may be added in patients with suspected thrombosis.

We have noted different responses to therapy and prolonged recovery in patients with hematomas. Patients with intramuscular hemorrhage (Fig. 8-48) tend to recover weeks to months earlier than patients with hematomas (Fig. 8-49). In addition, chronic changes (Fig. 8-50) with persistent fluid collections or scar formation (Fig. 8-51) appear to occur more frequently in patients with well-defined hematomas. This would suggest that a more aggressive approach, such as evacuation, should be considered when hematomas are identified with MRI. (See Chapter 2 for discussion of image features of blood.)

Compartment syndrome is defined as a condition in which the muscle in a fascial compartment is subjected to swelling and increased tissue, which can lead to ischemia (5,39). Clinically, patients present with pain and calf tenderness. Diminished peripheral pulses and sensory deficits may also be evident. If necrosis occurs, sequelae may include fibrosis and neurological impairment (34,35). Variations of compartment syndrome can occur. Some patients present with pain only at rest, others with pain during exercise that is relieved by rest (35). Therefore, preexercise and postexercise axial images may be required to fully evaluate these patients (39). Axial T2 weighted MR images demonstrate infiltrative high signal intensity in the muscle with bulging of the fascia (Fig. 8-52) in patients with compartment syndrome. Spectroscopy (^{31}P) may be useful in evaluating muscle ischemia and metabolism (16,65). However, to date, this has not been used frequently in the clinical setting (55).

Axial images are usually best when evaluating neurovascular injury. The course of the vessels and nerves varies so that contiguous slices can be followed to determine if hematomas or other post-traumatic changes affect the neurovascular structures. Chronic injuries can result in formation of neurofibromas.

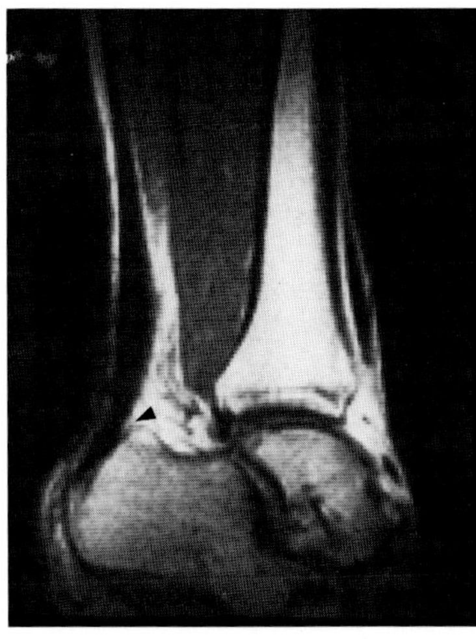

FIG. 8-45. Sagittal SE 2,000/60 image of the ankle, demonstrating extension of the fat (*arrowhead*) between the calcaneus and Achilles tendon during plantar flexion.

Neoplasms

Soft tissue neoplasms in the calf are not uncommon (see Chapter 12). Bone and soft tissue neoplasms of the

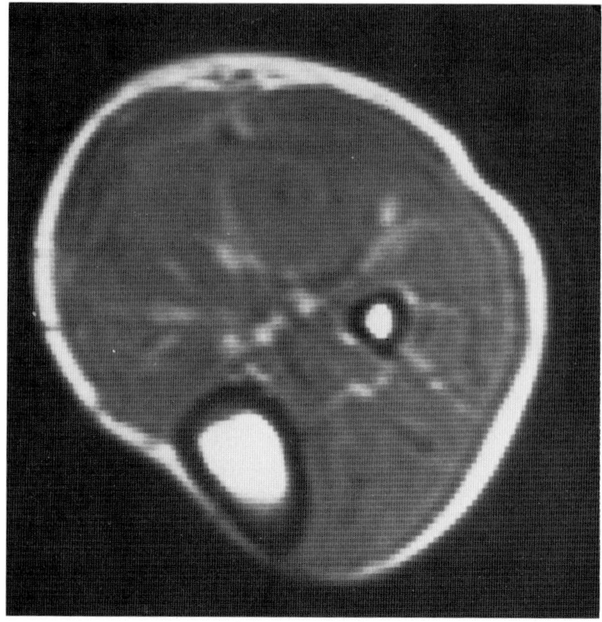

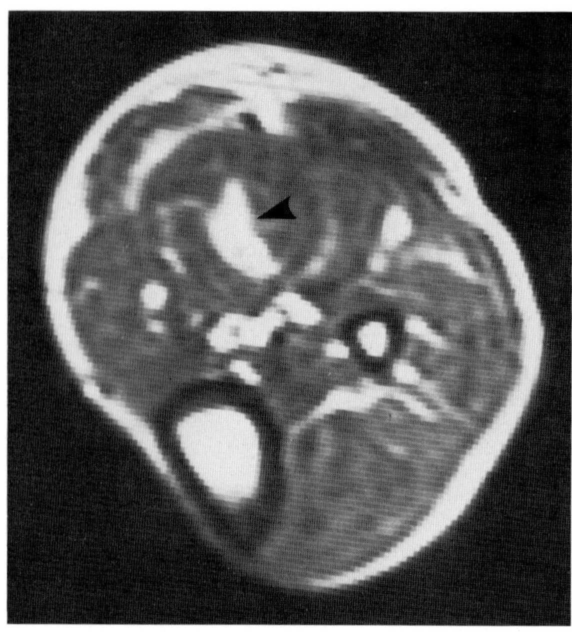

A,B

FIG. 8-46. Axial images of the calf in a patient with a tear in the medial head of the gastrocnemius. **A:** SE 500/20 image does not clearly demonstrate the muscle tear. **B:** SE 2,000/30 image clearly demonstrates the tear (*arrowhead*).

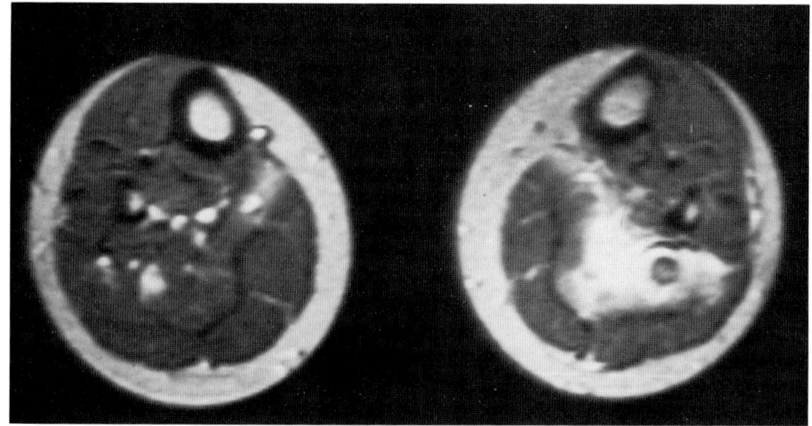

FIG. 8-47. Axial T2 weighted image of the calves. There is edema in the soleus on the right with dilatation and thrombosis in one of the deep veins.

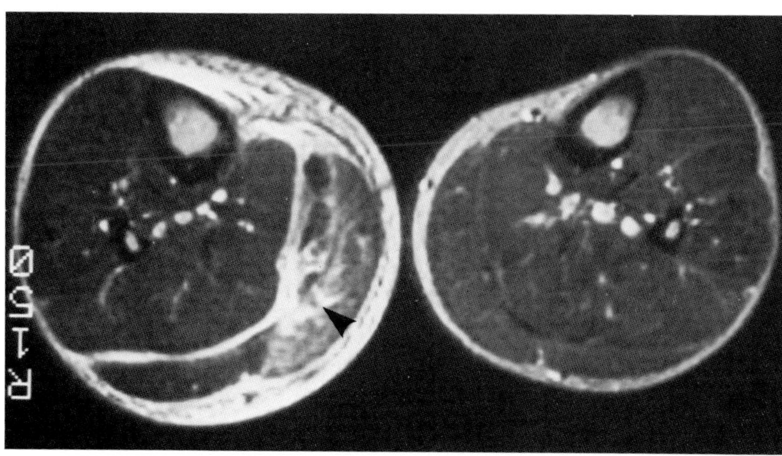

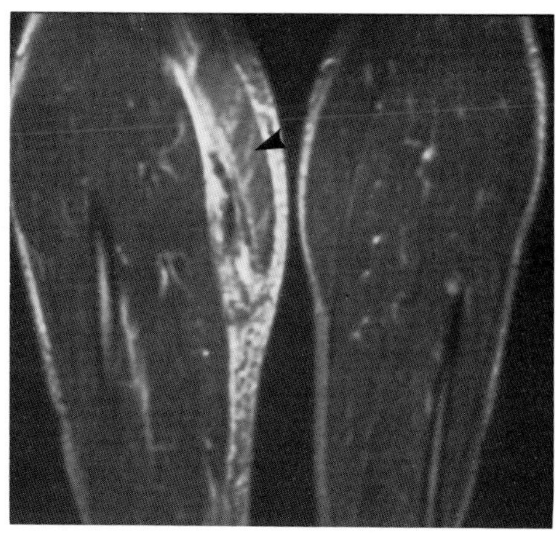

A,B

FIG. 8-48. Athlete with acute calf pain. Axial (**A**) and coronal (**B**) SE 2,000/60 images show infiltrative high signal intensity (*arrowheads*) due to hemorrhage into the medial gastrocnemius.

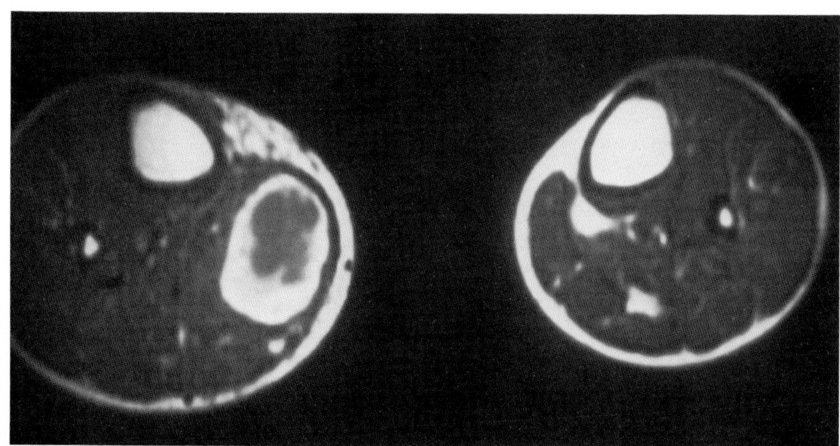

FIG. 8-49. Axial T2 weighted image of the calf in a patient with a large gastrocnemius hematoma.

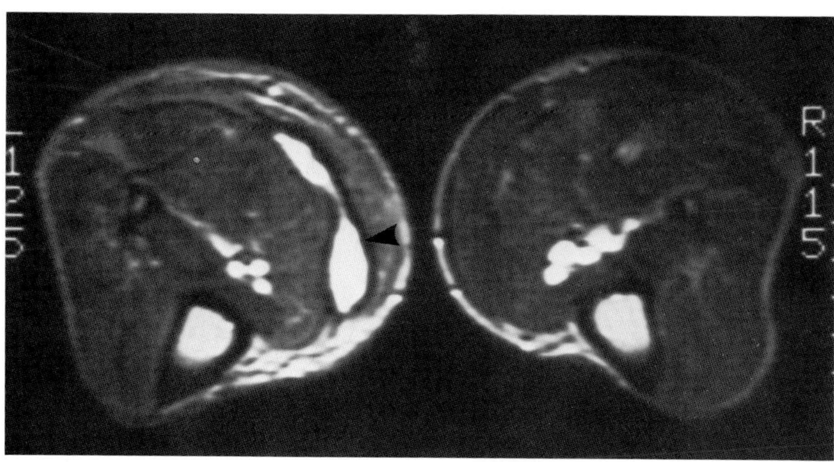

FIG. 8-50. Axial SE 2,000/60 image in a patient with a muscle tear 2 years previous. Note the fluid collection (*arrowhead*) with surrounding fibrous capsule.

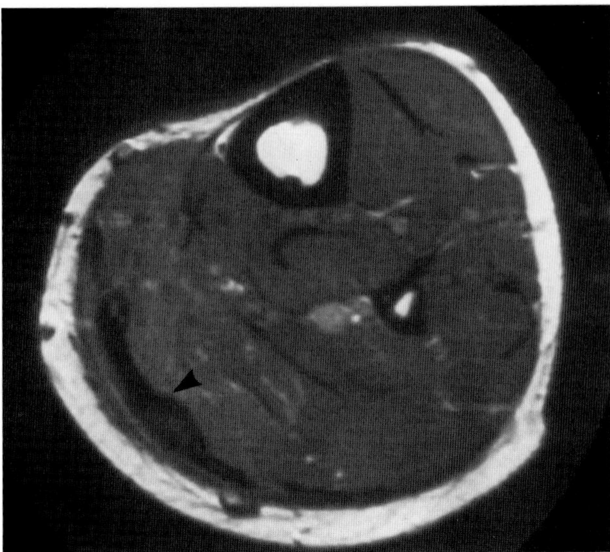

FIG. 8-51. Old gastrocnemius tear with scar tissue (*arrowhead*) replacing the muscle in the region of injury.

foot and ankle do not occur commonly. Skeletal neoplasms in the foot and ankle (see Table 8-5) account for only about 3% of all primary skeletal tumors (37,66). Skeletal metastases occur even less frequently than primary bone neoplasm. Benign lesions are slightly more common than malignant (66) (Table 8-4). All lesions summarized in Table 8-4 are more common in the ankle (tibia and fibula) than the foot (27,66). Routine radiographs are still the most useful screening technique in patients with suspected skeletal neoplasms. The features of many lesions can be characterized accurately using routine radiographic techniques (Figs. 8-53 to 8-55). Therefore, MRI is reserved mainly for those patients whose tumors are equivocal or as a staging technique for patients with suspected malignancy. MRI has essentially replaced CT as a staging technique for foot and ankle tumors (2,11,29,53,66,101,103,109).

TABLE 8-5. *Bone tumors of the foot and ankle: 8542 primary bone tumors (27,66)*

Lesion	Number of patients
Benign (202)	
Osteochondroma	34
Nonossifying fibroma	32
Osteoid osteoma	26
Giant cell tumor	26
Aneurysmal bone cyst	24
Simple bone cyst	21
Enchondroma	16
Chondromyxoid fibroma	11
Chondroblastoma	6
Osteoblastoma	4
Fibrous histiocytoma	2
Malignant (129)	
Osteogenic sarcoma	38
Ewing's sarcoma	35
Chondrosarcoma	23
Hemangioendothelial sarcoma	10
Fibrosarcoma	9
Lymphoma	8
Adimantinoma	4
Multiple myeloma	1
Desmoplastic fibroma	1

Soft tissue masses in the foot and ankle are also uncommon (24,31,36,66,88). Table 8-6 lists the soft tissue tumors of the foot and ankle in a series of 736 tumors (36). Kirby et al. (57) reviewed 83 soft tissue masses in the foot and ankle. Eighty-seven percent were benign and 13% malignant. The majority of masses are related to inflammation. Therefore, it is not surprising that most benign lesions were ganglion cysts (Fig. 8-56) and fibromatosis (Fig. 8-57) (38,92). Fibromatosis occurred most frequently in the plantar region of the midfoot. The majority of malignant lesions in this series were synovial sarcomas (57,64). Most malignant lesions were located in the heel region.

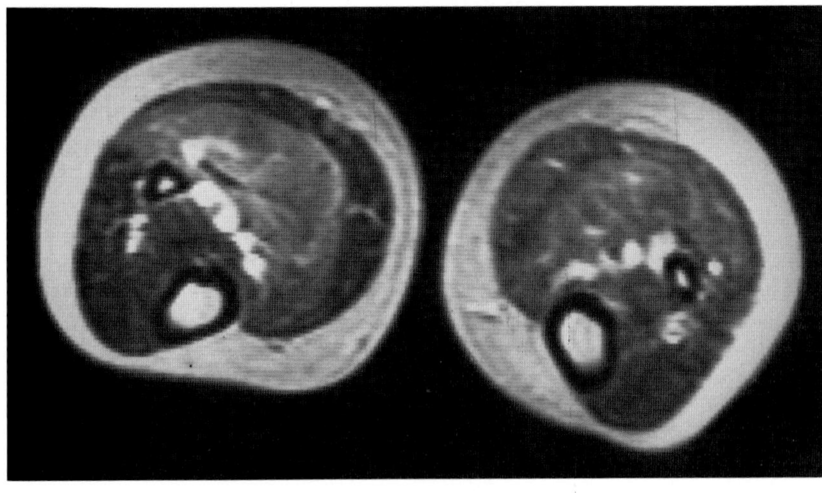

FIG. 8-52. Prone axial T2 weighted images of the calves demonstrate increased signal in the deep compartment posteriorly due to compartment syndrome.

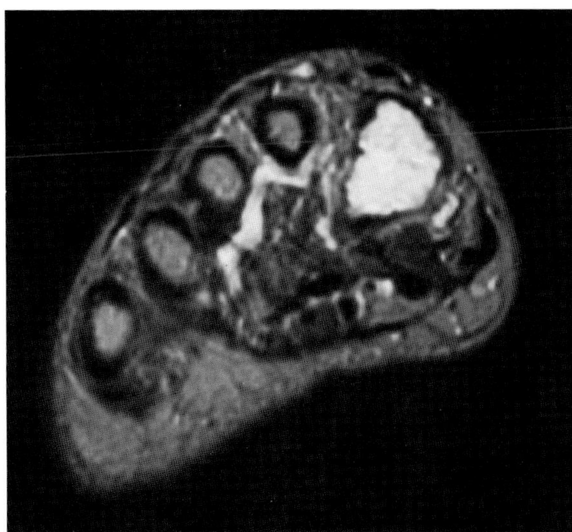

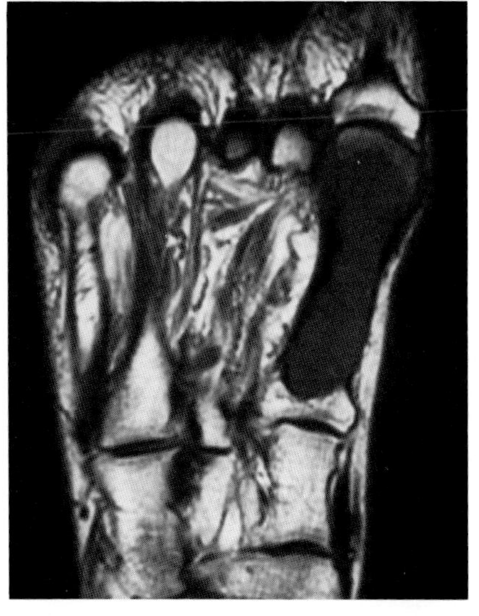

A,B

FIG. 8-53. Enchondroma. Axial (**A**) SE 2,000/60 image shows a high-intensity lesion in the first metatarsal with no soft tissue extension. Coronal (**B**) SE 500/20 image shows a low-intensity lesion involving the majority of the first metatarsal. Radiographically, an enchondroma was the more obvious diagnosis.

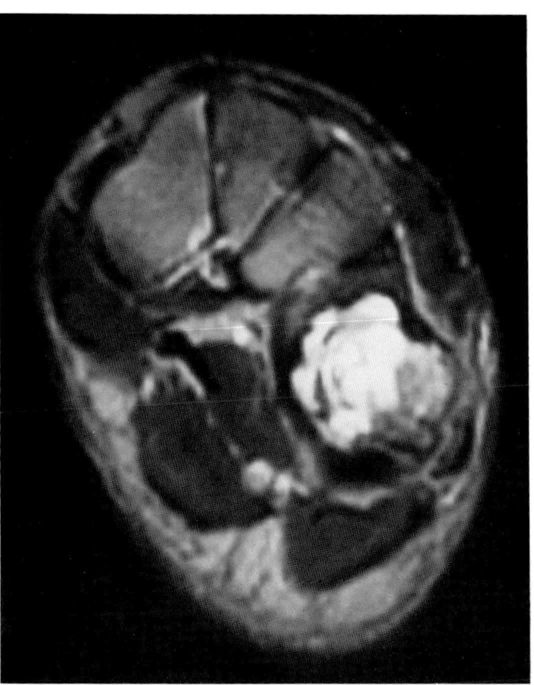

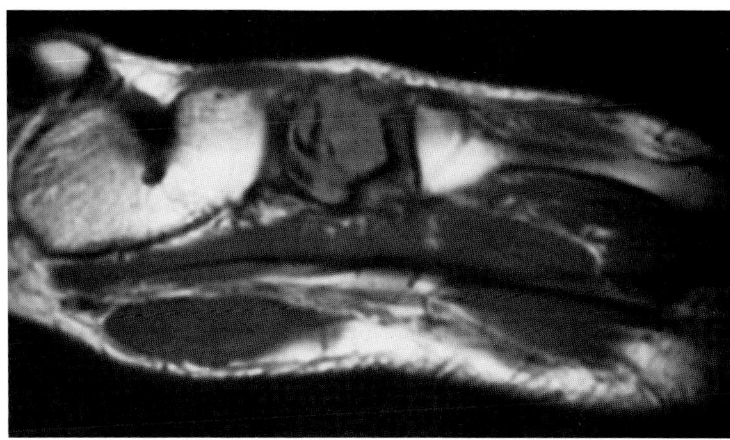

A,B

FIG. 8-54. Giant cell tumor of the cuboid. Axial (**A**) SE 2,000/60 and sagittal (**B**) SE 500/20 images show an expanding inhomogeneous lesion that could be difficult to differentiate from malignancy based on MR features. However, the soft tissues are clearly spared.

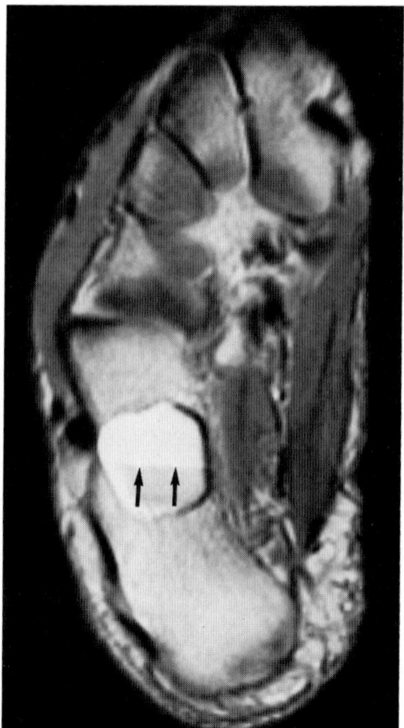

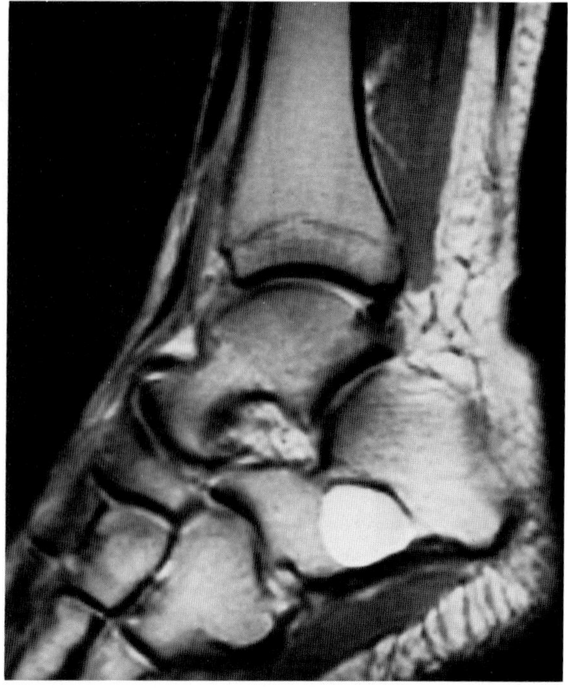

A,B

FIG. 8-55. Simple cyst. Axial (**A**) SE 2,000/30 and sagittal (**B**) SE 500/20 images demonstrate a cystic lesion in the calcaneus with a fluid–fluid level. This is nonspecific and can be noted in giant cell tumors, aneurysmal bone cysts, simple cysts, chondroblastomas, and telangiectatic osteosarcomas (51).

Neuromas are frequently responsible for foot pain. These lesions can be multiple or single. Axial MR images are most useful to identify these small lesions. Both T1 and T2 weighted images are useful to avoid confusing these lesions with the small vessels (Fig. 8-58).

Most skeletal lesions are easily detected with T1 weighted sequences due to the excellent contrast between the low intensity of pathologic tissue and high intensity of marrow fat (Fig. 8-53). Subtle lesions may be more easily detected using STIR sequences (see Table 8-1). T2 weighted sequences are ideal for identification of soft tissue extension and for evaluating soft tissue tumors (Fig. 8-58) (63). We generally perform both T1 and T2 weighted sequences in two image planes to optimally characterize and stage (extent) lesions. Gadolinium-DTPA may improve the ability of MRI to evaluate neoplasms. Early studies indicate that use of this contrast medium produces better differentiation of tumor from edema and necrotic tissue (18,37,76). A more complete discussion of musculoskeletal neoplasms can be found in Chapter 12.

TABLE 8-6. *Soft tissue tumors of the foot and ankle: 736 cases* (36)

Fibrohistiocytic tumors (inter. malignancy)	170
Glomus tumor	98
Synovial sarcoma	78
Clear cell sarcoma	54
Epithelioid sarcoma	50
Liposarcoma	49
Angiosarcoma with and without lymphedema	47
Rhabdomyosarcoma	40
Hemangiopericytoma	37
Glomangioma	29
Alveolar sarcoma (soft part)	21
Fibromatoses	18
Extraskeletal Ewing's sarcoma	18
Glomangiomyoma	14
Giant cell tumor (tendon sheath)	13

Arthritis/Infection

Imaging of inflammatory conditions in the calf and bones and joints of the foot and ankle has traditionally been accomplished using routine radiography, CT, and radionuclide studies. Recently (11,40,74,78,91,100), MRI has proved useful in early detection of synovial changes as well as changes in the articular cartilage in the small bones of the foot and ankle (6,8,11,13,77,89, 100,104,110–113). Early synovial changes and effusions can clearly be depicted, even in the small joints of the foot where they may be difficult to evaluate clinically (70,110–113). The signal intensity of joint fluid has, to date, not been useful in differentiating inflammatory arthritis such as rheumatoid arthritis from infection (Fig. 8-59). However, hemosiderin deposition and the resulting paramagnetic effects are useful in diagnosis of pigmented villonodular synovitis (11,19,25,70,96,

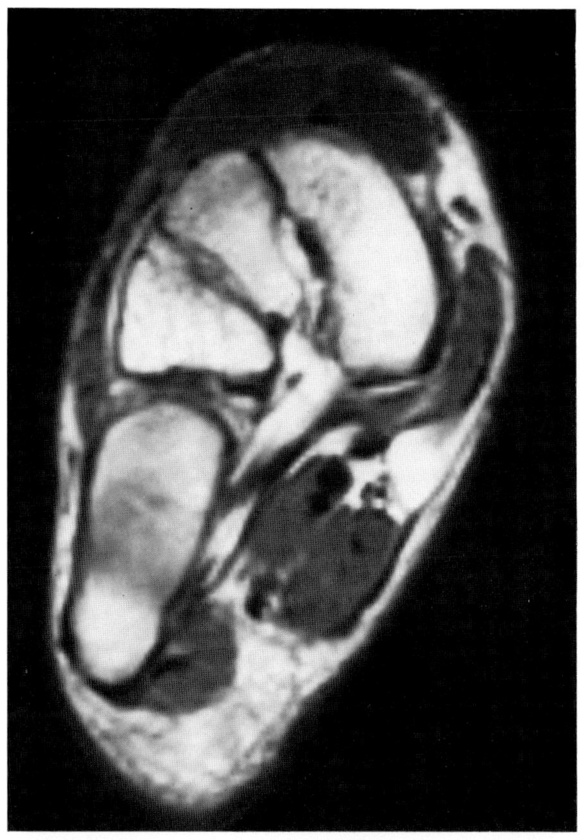

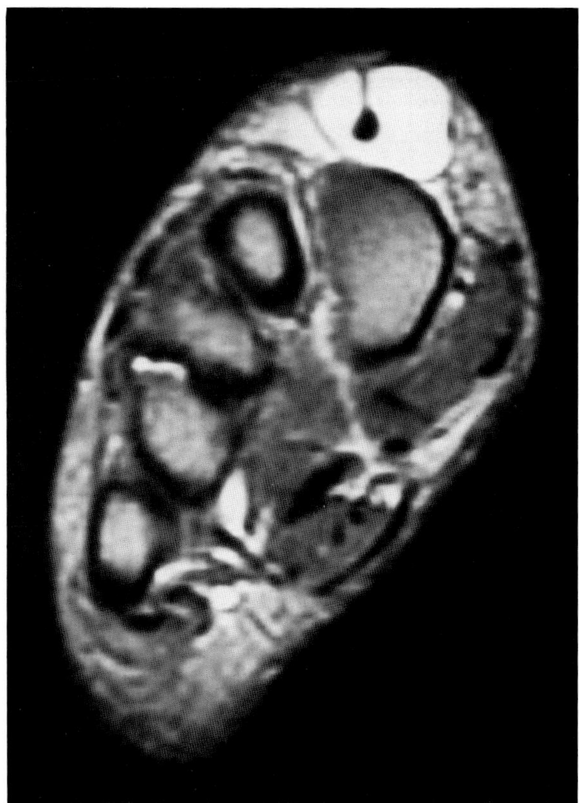

A,B

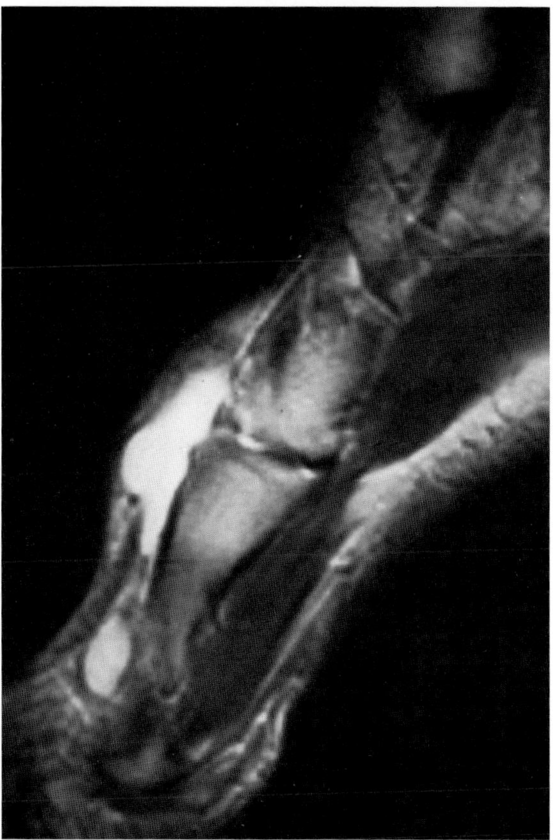

C

FIG. 8-56. Axial SE 500/20 (**A**) and 2,000/60 (**B**) and sagittal SE 2,000/60 (**C**) images of a large ganglion of the extensor hallucis longus tendon. Note the well-defined margins and homogeneity of signal intensity typical of a ganglion cyst.

A,B

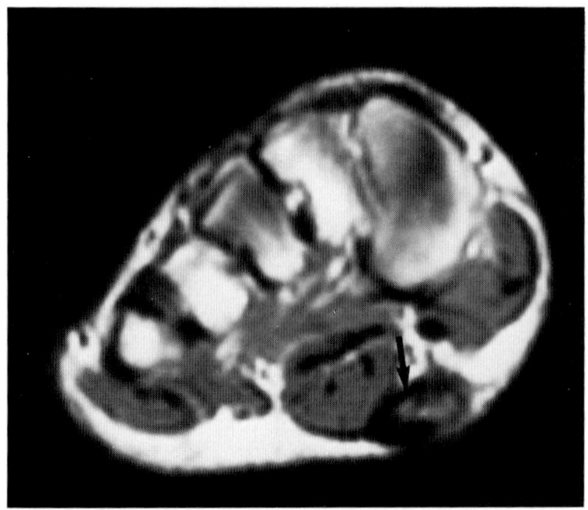

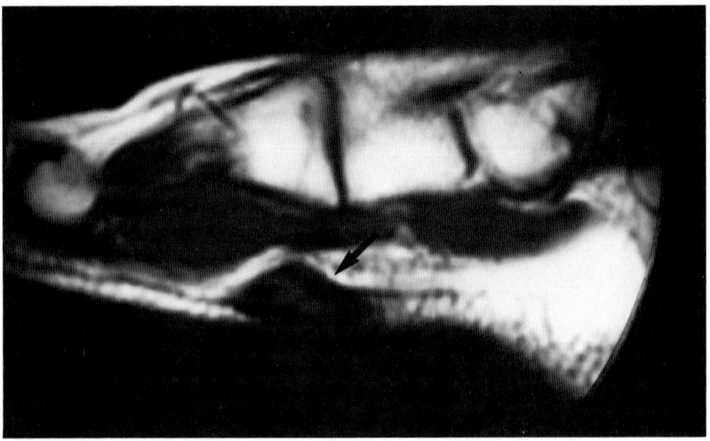

FIG. 8-57. Plantar fibromatosis. Axial (**A**) and sagittal (**B**) images show a lesion (*arrows*) with a large amount of scar or collagen (*black*) and central increased signal intensity. Findings are typical of fibromatosis or desmoid tumor.

111,112). Spectroscopy may play a role in improving specificity in the future (16).

A more thorough discussion of infection can be found in Chapter 13. However, because of the complex problem of foot infections in diabetic patients, a brief discussion is indicated here as well.

Diabetic patients have numerous problems that can make detection and categorization of lesions difficult. These patients frequently have cellulitis, ischemic and/or neurotrophic ulcers, vascular insufficiency, and neurotrophic arthritis (11,110).

Bone scanning, especially use of specific isotopes such as indium-111 labeled white blood cells and gallium-67, is highly sensitive and specific for diagnosis of acute osteomyelitis (6,11,110). However, difficulty does occur in separating osseous from soft tissue involvement with radionuclide studies. MRI is capable of distinguishing abnormalities in the marrow and soft tissues and clearly defines the anatomy and extent of the process. Osteomyelitis is demonstrated as an area of abnormally low signal intensity in the marrow on T1 weighted images and increased signal intensity on T2 weighted or short T1 inversion recovery (STIR) images (Fig. 8-60) (11,13,77,93). Detection of infection approaches 94% with MRI compared to only 71% for radionuclide studies (70,104,110).

MRI is also more useful than isotope studies in demonstrating the extent of soft tissue inflammation and

A,B

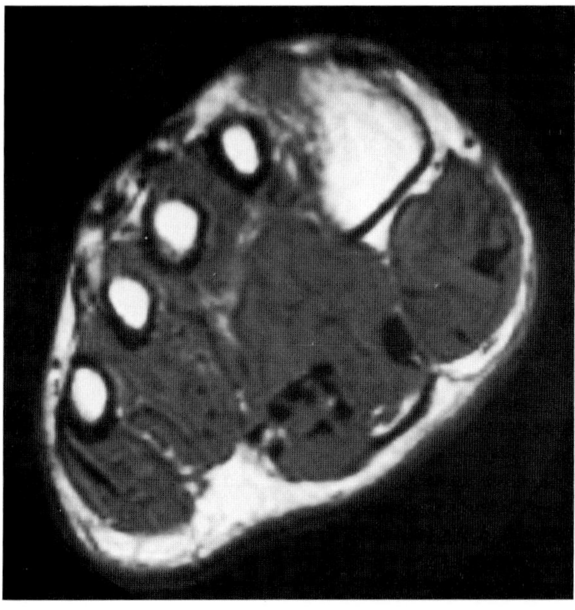

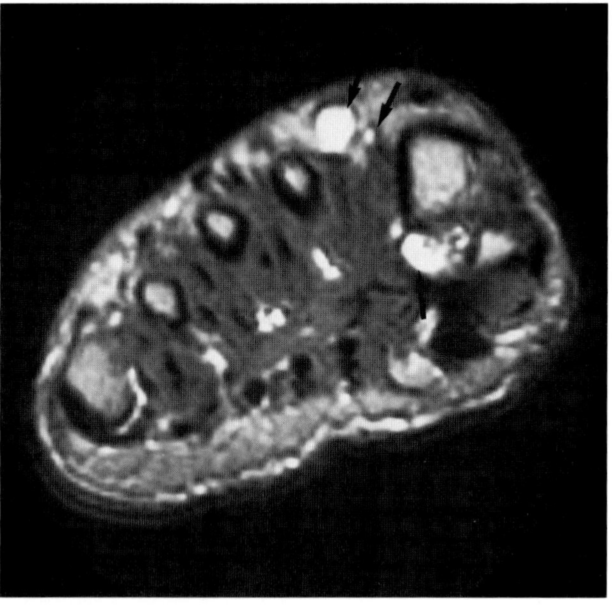

FIG. 8-58. Axial SE 500/20 (**A**) and SE 2,000/60 (**B**) images demonstrating multiple neuromas (*arrows*). The lesions are defined most easily on the T2 weighted sequence (**B**).

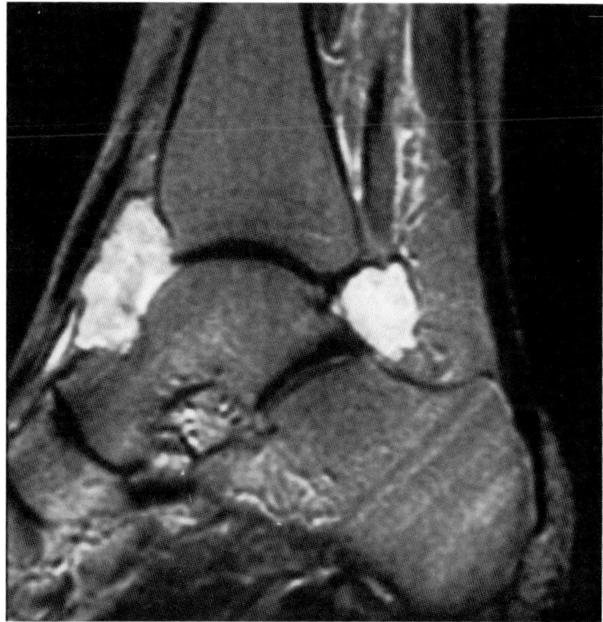

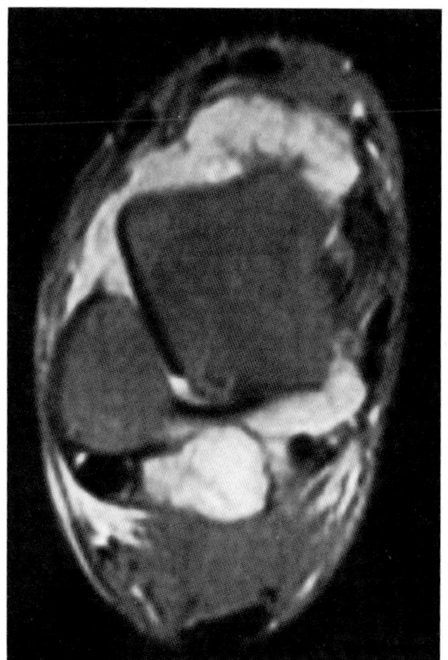

A,B

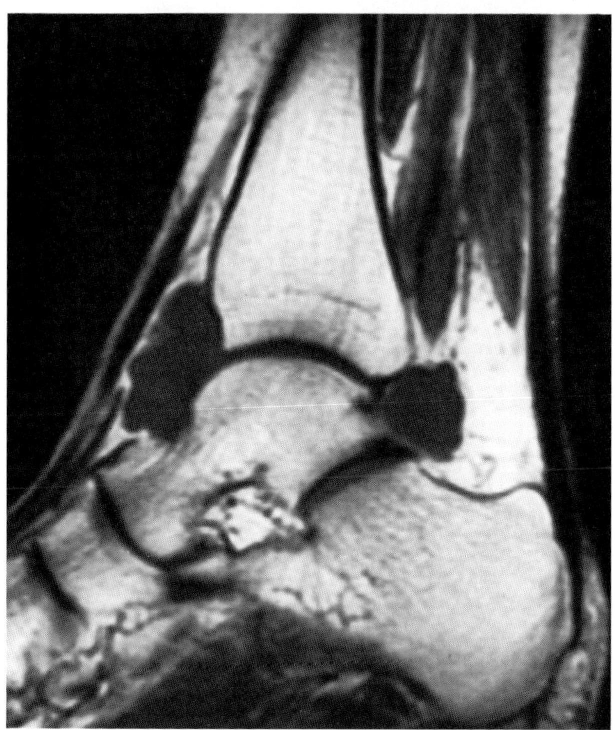

C

FIG. 8-59. SE 2,000/60 sagittal (**A**) and axial (**B**) images of the ankle demonstrate a large high signal intensity effusion in the ankle. The SE 500/20 sagittal image (**C**) shows the fluid as homogeneous low signal intensity. There are no erosions. The appearance of this fluid is nonspecific. Diagnosis post-traumatic.

abscess involvement of specific compartments in the foot (Fig. 8-61; see also Fig. 8-18). Soft tissue contrast provided by MRI is superior to CT in this regard. Delineation of the extent and compartments involved with infection is especially important if operative debridement is to be accomplished successfully.

Certain types of osteomyelitis, such as chronic osteomyelitis or Brodie's abscess, may be more difficult to evaluate with MRI than CT. Sclerotic changes with small focal areas of low attenuation, which are limited to the cortex, may be more easily demonstrated with CT.

Ischemic Bone and Soft Tissue Disease

Ischemic necrosis is a common problem in the foot and ankle, particularly in diabetics and patients with other vascular diseases (11,42,70,113). For purposes of

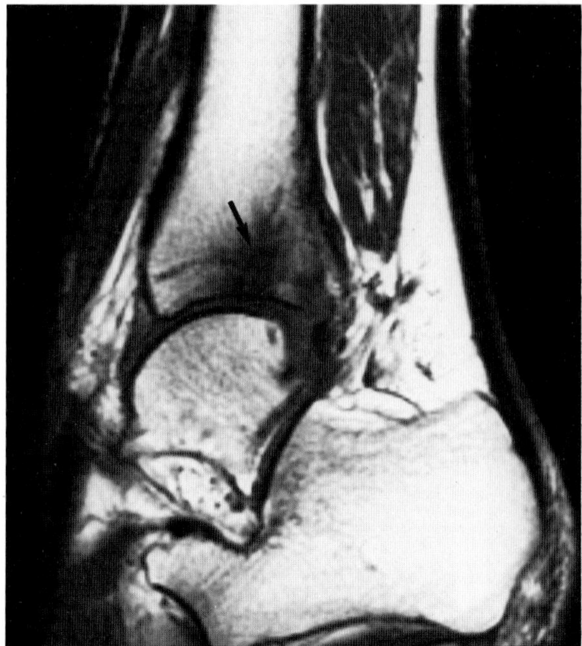
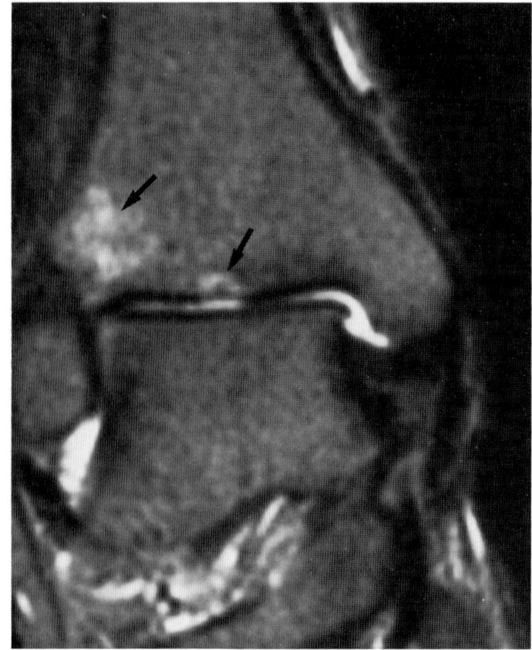

A,B

FIG. 8-60. **A:** Sagittal SE 500/20 image of the ankle demonstrates an area of low signal intensity in the distal tibia (*arrow*). **B:** Coronal SE 2,000/60 image shows fluid in the joint with a small articular defect and increased signal intensity medially (*arrows*). The joint space is narrowed. Diagnosis is osteomyelitis.

discussion, it is best to consider bone and soft tissue changes separately.

Specific areas of interest in the foot and ankle include post-traumatic avascular necrosis of the talus, which is a significant problem following fractures of this structure (11,46,94). Additional areas where avascular necrosis occurs include the metatarsal heads (Freiberg's disease) and the navicular (Köhler's disease). The MR patterns of avascular necrosis or osteonecrosis of bone in the foot and ankle are similar to those described elsewhere (see Chapter 6).

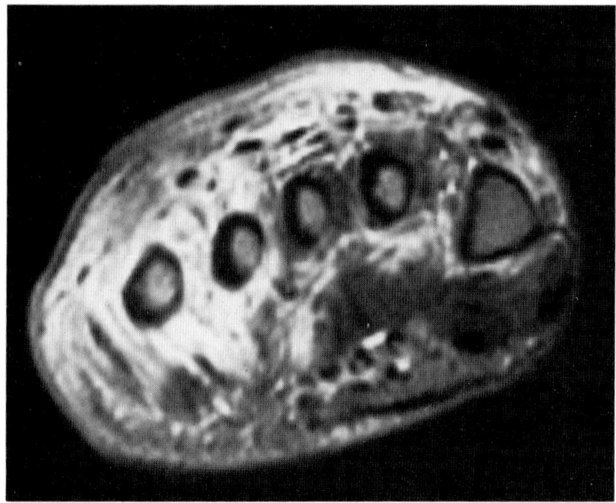

FIG. 8-61. Axial T2 weighted image of the foot showing high signal intensity in the lateral compartment primarily involving the fourth muscle layer. No abscess or osseous change. Ischemic disease in a diabetic.

Avascular necrosis in the tarsal bones, particularly the talus, is more common and generally follows significant trauma (11,46). Necrosis occurs because of the tenuous vascular supply of the tali, which have extensive articular surface area and few entrance sites for blood supply. Avascular necrosis following talar neck injury is most common after complex fracture dislocations (Hawkins type III and IV) (46). The body of the talus is more prone to osteonecrosis than the head or neck. The earliest radiographic signs do not occur for 6–8 weeks. In the presence of a fracture, radionuclide studies may not be as useful because of the increased uptake due to normal fracture healing.

MRI is a sensitive technique for early detection of avascular necrosis. Both T1 and T2 weighted sequences should be performed to assist in differentiating areas of hyperemia or revascularization (high signal intensity on T1 weighted sequences) from new bone or sclerotic areas (low signal intensity on both T1 and T2 weighted sequences) (Figs. 8-62 and 8-63) (10,113). Comparison with routine radiographs is very useful, especially when areas of bone sclerosis are present. Comparison affords more accurate interpretation of MR images.

The morphologic features may vary slightly depending on the bone (tarsals versus metatarsals) involved. Patterns of osteonecrosis in the talus may be geographic (Figs. 8-62 and 8-63), similar to those described in the femoral head (Chapter 6). Involvement of the smaller

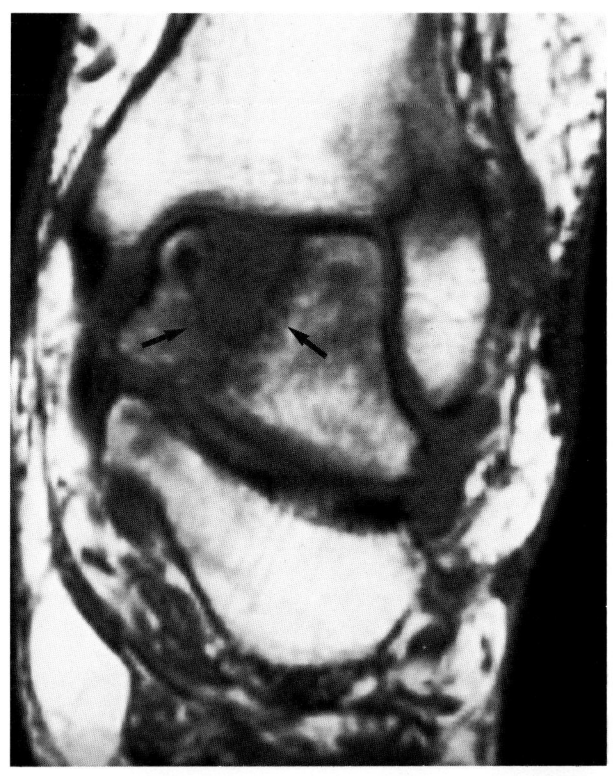

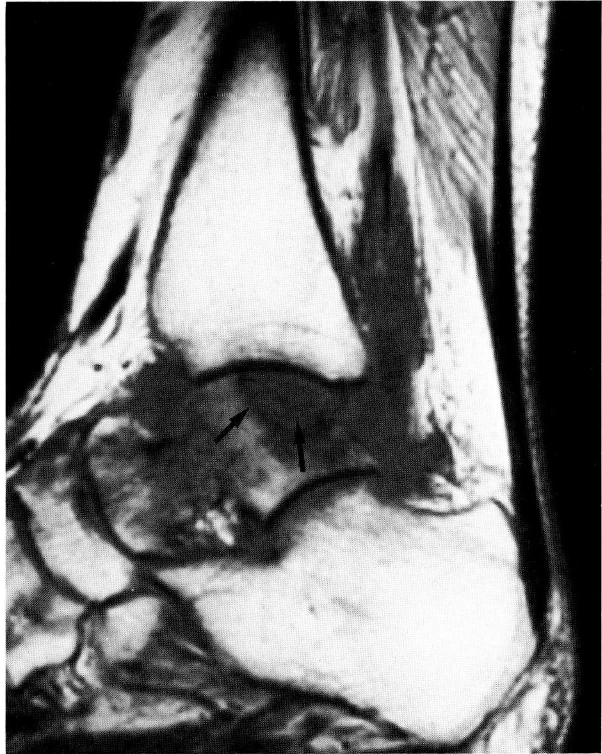

A,B

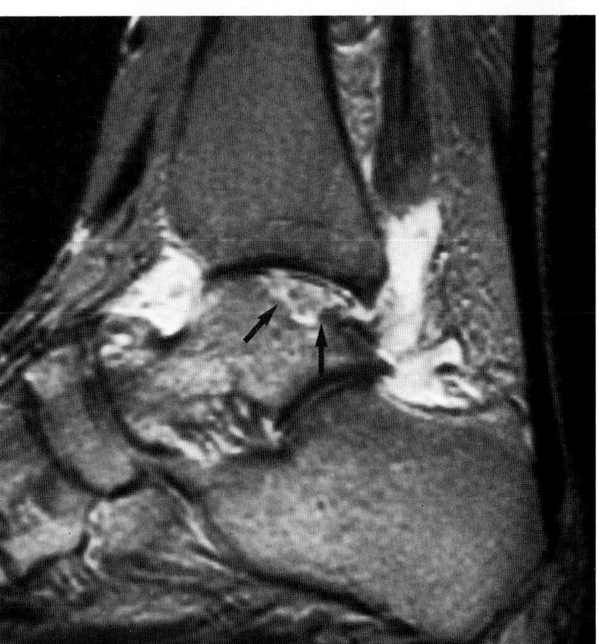

C

FIG. 8-62. Avascular necrosis of the talus. Coronal (**A**) and sagittal (**B**) SE 500/20 images demonstrate a large central area of low signal intensity (*arrows*). Its location separates this from a talar dome fracture, which occurs at the medial or lateral margin. SE 2,000/60 sagittal image (**C**) shows increased signal intensity in the avascular area. Diagnosis—healing or revascularization? Note the high signal intensity effusion in the ankle.

tarsal bones tends to be more diffuse. Uniform loss of signal intensity on T1 weighted sequences is common in Köhler's disease and spontaneous osteonecrosis of the navicular (11,44). The latter is a condition that occurs primarily in older women. Patients may have debilitating pain. Bilateral navicular involvement is common. Haller et al. (44) reported uniform low signal intensity on T1 weighted MR images with more subtle changes on T2 weighted sequences. MR features are not specific and differentiation from trauma and other inflammatory diseases may be difficult.

Osteonecrosis of the metatarsal heads (Freiberg's disease) most commonly involves the second metatarsal, but the third metatarsal and less frequently the fourth and fifth may also be involved. Females outnumber males 4:1 (11). MR images reveal changes similar to

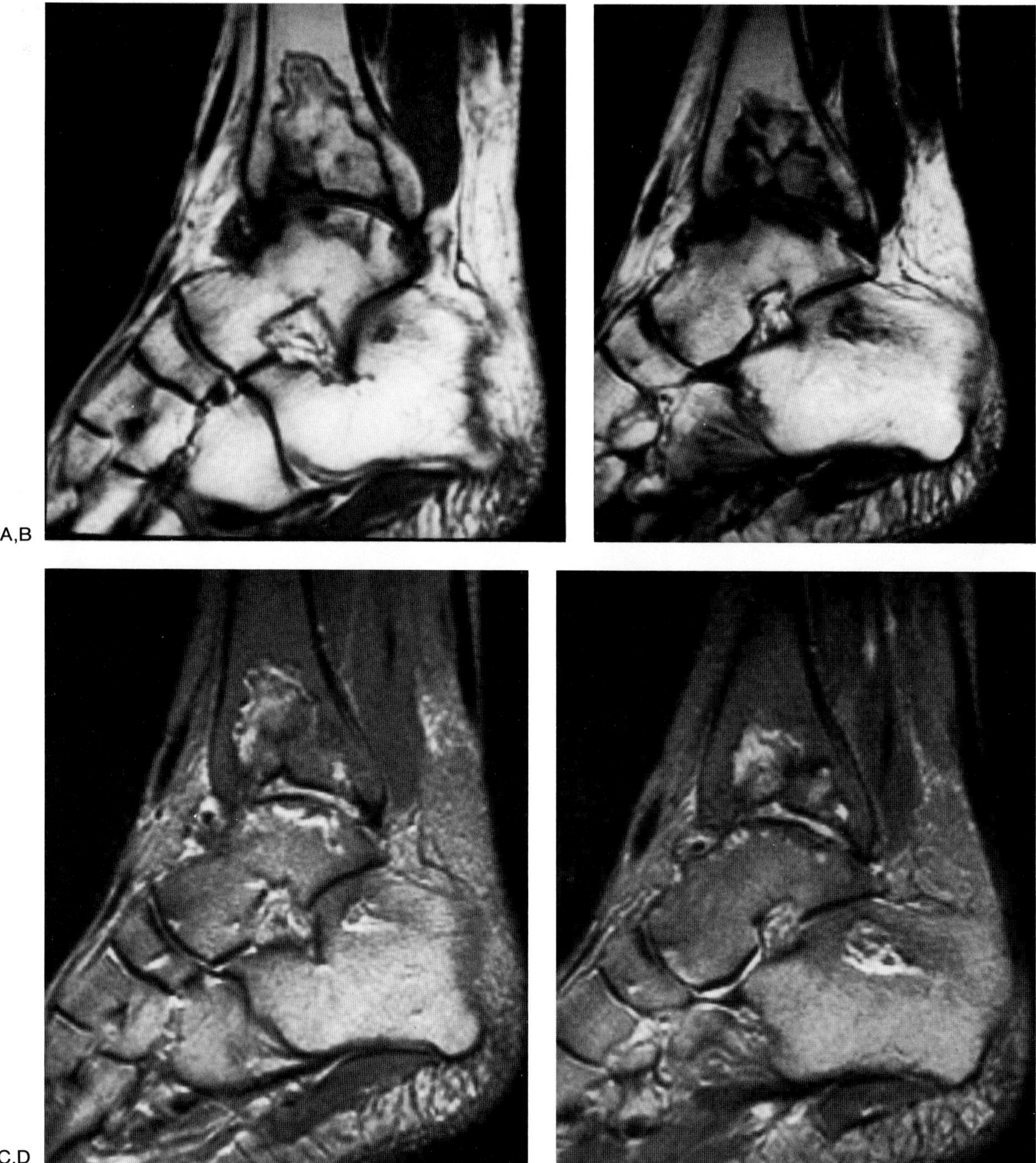

FIG. 8-63. Sagittal images of the ankle in a patient with infarcts in the tibia and calcaneus and avascular necrosis of the talus. SE 500/20 (**A, B**) and SE 2,000/60 (**C, D**) images demonstrate the classic well-marginated changes of infarction.

those described in the femoral head (Chapter 6), with a wedge-shaped area of low signal intensity on T1 weighted images. Progression to subchondral collapse and degenerative arthritis also occurs (11).

Bone infarction has a similar appearance to other areas of the skeleton (Fig. 8-63). Typically, there are well-marginated areas of low to normal signal intensity on T1 weighted sequences and areas of well-defined high signal intensity on T2 weighted sequences.

Complications of avascular necrosis in the foot and ankle do occur. The most common problems are degenerative arthritis, resulting in anatomic deformity of the articular surface. Ligament degeneration is a rare complication but has been described in bone infarcts in the distal tibia. Fibrosarcoma, osteosarcoma, and malignant fibrous histiocytoma have been reported in association with bone infarcts in the ankle (69).

Ischemic changes in the soft tissues are primarily related to vascular diseases and diabetes mellitus. The utility of MRI in determining the extent of ischemic change (Fig. 8-61) and the viability of the soft tissues has yet to be completely evaluated. Spectroscopy may play a role in the future in determining the extent of viable tissue in the leg and foot and following both surgical and medical therapy of soft tissue ischemic disorders (11).

Miscellaneous Conditions

To date, MRI has not been frequently used in diagnosis or evaluation of adult and pediatric foot deformities. There have been reports on the utility of MRI in evaluation of patients with suspected tarsal coalition (11,61). Diagnosis of this condition can be difficult prior to ossification of the tarsal bones. Also, coalitions may be only partially ossified and fibrous and cartilaginous coalitions can also occur. Prior to MRI, radionuclide studies and, more specifically, CT and conventional tomography were favored for diagnosis of this condition (61).

MRI using T1 and T2 weighted sequences is very useful in defining the type of coalition (Fig. 8-64). Bone, cartilage, and fibrous tissue can be differentiated and ossification need not be completed, which is an advantage in pediatric patients. Multiple image planes are also useful in better defining the anatomy.

There has been little utility for MRI in evaluation of many metabolic disorders (11). Hemoglobinopathies and anemias can be detected due to the changes created in the signal intensity of bone marrow on MR images (11,59). However, these changes are not specific and do not allow clear definition of the type of infiltrative process. An exception might be sickle cell anemia, where MRI could detect early changes in the marrow, such as infarction (79,91).

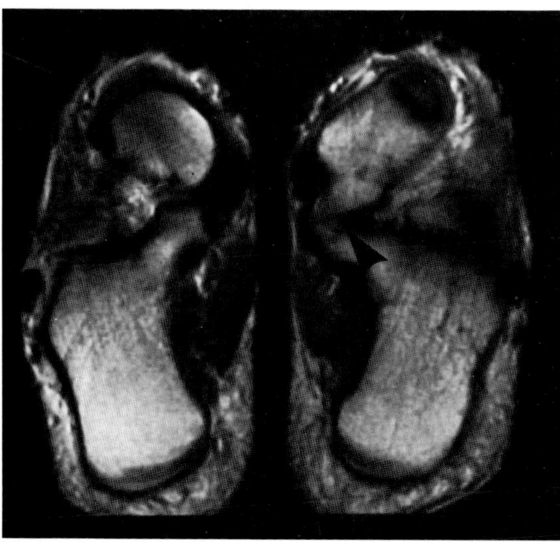

FIG. 8-64. MR image demonstrating tarsal coalition at the sustentacular articulation.

REFERENCES

1. Abraham E, Sternaman JE. Neglected rupture of the peroneal tendons causing recurrent sprains of the ankle. *J Bone Joint Surg* 1979;61A:1247–1248.
2. Aisen AM, Martel W, Braunstein EM, McMillin KI, Phillips WA, Kling TF. MRI and CT evaluation of primary bone and soft-tissue tumors. *AJR* 1986;146:749–756.
3. Alexander IJ, Johnson KA, Berquist TH. Magnetic resonance imaging in diagnosis of disruption of the posterior tibial tendon. *Foot Ankle* 1987;8:144–147.
4. Anderson JE. *Grant's atlas of anatomy,* 8th ed. Baltimore: Williams & Wilkins, 1983.
5. Anouchi YS, Parker RD, Seitz WH. Posterior compartment syndrome of the calf resulting from misdiagnosis of a rupture of the medial head of the gastrocnemius. *J Trauma* 1987;27:678–680.
6. Beltran J, McGhee RB, Shaffer PB, et al. Experimental infections of the musculoskeletal system: evaluation with MR imaging and Tc-99m MDP and Ga-67 scintigraphy. *Radiology* 1988;167:167–172.
7. Beltran J, Noto AM, Herman LJ, et al. Tendons: high-field-strength surface coil MR imaging. *Radiology* 1987;162:735–740.
8. Beltran J, Noto AM, McGhee RB, et al. Infections of the musculoskeletal system: high-field-strength MR imaging. *Radiology* 1987;164:449–454.
9. Beltran J, Noto AM, Mosure JC, et al. Ankle: surface coil MR imaging at 1.5 T. *Radiology* 1986;161:203–210.
10. Berger PE, Oftein RA, Jackson DW, Morrison DS, Silvano W, Amador R. MRI demonstration of radiographically occult fractures: what have we been missing? *RadioGraphics* 1989; 9(3):407–436.

10a. Berquist TH. *Magnetic resonance of the musculoskeletal system.* New York: Raven Press, 1987.

11. Berquist TH, ed. *Radiology of the foot and ankle.* New York: Raven Press, 1988.
12. Berquist TH, Johnson KA. *Anatomy, normal variants, and basic biomechanics.* In: Berquist TH, ed. *Radiology of the foot and ankle.* New York: Raven Press, 1988: Chap 1.
13. Berquist TH, Brown ML, Fitzgerald RH Jr, May GR. Magnetic resonance imaging: applications in musculoskeletal infection. *Magn Reson Imaging* 1985;3:219–230.
14. Black HM, Brand RL, Eichenberger MR. An improved technique for evaluation of ligamentous injury in severe ankle sprains. *Am J Sports Med* 1978;6(5):276–282.
15. Blanchard KS, Finlay DBL, Scott DJA, Ley CC, Siggens D, Allen MJ. A radiological analysis of lateral ligament injuries of the ankle. *Clin Radiol* 1986;37:247–251.
16. Blatter DD. Phosphorus-31 magnetic resonance spectroscopy of experimentally induced arthritis in rats. *Skeletal Radiol* 1987;16:183–189.
17. Bleichrodt RP, Kingma LM, Binnendijk B, Klein J. Injuries of the lateral ankle ligaments: classification with tenography and arthrography. *Radiology* 1989;173:347–349.
18. Bousquet JC, Saini S, Stark DD, Hahn PF, Nigam M, Wittenberg J, Ferrucci JT. Gd-DOTA: characterization of a new paramagnetic complex. *Radiology* 1988;166:693–698.
19. Brown JJ, vanSonnenberg E, Gerber KH, Strich G, Wittich GR, Slutsky RA. Magnetic resonance relaxation times of percutaneously obtained normal and abnormal body fluids. *Radiology* 1985;154:727–731.
20. Carroso JJ, Liu N, Traill MR, Runge VM. Physiology of the retrocalcaneal bursa. *Ann Rheum Dis* 1988;47:910–912.
21. Cass JR, Morrey BF. Ankle instability: current concepts, diagnosis and treatment. *Mayo Clin Proc* 1984;59:165–170.
22. Church CC. Radiographic diagnosis of acute peroneal tendon dislocation. *AJR* 1977;129:1065–1068.
23. Clemente CD. *Gray's anatomy,* 13th ed. Philadelphia: Lea & Febiger, 1985.

24. Cohen EK, Kressel HY, Perosio T, et al. MR imaging of soft-tissue hemangiomas: correlation with pathologic findings. *AJR* 1988;150:1079–1081.
25. Cohen JM, Weinreb JC, Maravilla KR. Fluid collections in the intraperitoneal and extraperitoneal spaces: comparison of MR and CT. *Radiology* 1985;155:705–708.
26. Cohen JM, Weinreb JC, Redman HC. Arteriovenous malformations of the extremities: MR imaging. *Radiology* 1986;158:475–479.
27. Dahlin DC, Unni KK. *Bone tumors: general aspects and data on 8,542 cases,* 4th ed. Springfield, IL: CC Thomas, 1986.
28. Daffner RH, Reimer BL, Lupetin ARE, et al. Magnetic resonance imaging in acute tendon ruptures. *Skeletal Radiol* 1986;15:619–621.
29. Demas BE, Heelan RT, Lane J, Marcove R, Hajdu S, Brennan MF. Soft-tissue sarcomas of the extremities: comparison of MR and CT in determining the extent of disease. *AJR* 1988;150:615–620.
30. Dokter G, Linclau LA. The accessory soleus muscle: symptomatic soft tissue tumor or accidental finding. *Neth J Surg* 1981;33(3):146–149.
31. Dooms GC, Hricak H, Sollitto RA, Higgins CB. Lipomatous tumors and tumors with fatty component: MR imaging potential and comparison of MR and CT results. *Radiology* 1985; 157:479–483.
32. Downey DJ, Simkin DA, Mack LA, Richardson ML, Kilcoyne RF, Hansen ST. Tibialis posterior tendon rupture. *Arthritis Rheum* 1988;31:441–446.
33. Dunn AW. Anomalous muscle simulating soft tissue tumors in the lower extremities. *J Bone Joint Surg* [Am] 1965;47A:1397–1400.
34. Ehman RL, Berquist TH. Magnetic resonance imaging of trauma. *Radiol Clin North Am* 1986;24:291–319.
35. Ehman RL, Berquist TH, McLeod RA. MR imaging of the musculoskeletal system: a 5-year appraisal. *Radiology* 1988;166: 313–320.
36. Enzinger FM, Weiss SW. *Soft tissue tumors.* St. Louis, MO: CV Mosby, 1983.
37. Erlemann R, Reiser MF, Peters PE, et al. Musculoskeletal neoplasms: static and dynamic Gd-DTPA-enhanced MR imaging. *Radiology* 1989;171:767–773.
38. Fischer HJ, Lois JF, Gomes AS, et al: Radiology and pathology of malignant fibrous histocytomes of soft tissues. *Shel. Radiol.* 1985;13:202–206.
39. Fleckenstein JL, Canby RC, Parkey RW, Peshock RM. Acute effects of exercise on MR imaging of skeletal muscle in normal volunteers. *AJR* 1988;151:231–237.
40. Fletcher BD, Scoles PV, Nelson AD. Osteomyelitis in children: detection by magnetic resonance—work in progress. *Pediatr Radiol* 1984;150:57–60.
41. Garth WP. Flexor hallucis tendonitis in a ballet dancer. *J Bone Joint Surg* 1981;63A:1489.
42. Goergen TG, Danzig LA, Resnick D, Owen CA. Roentgen evaluation of the tibiotalar joint. *J Bone Joint Surg* [Am] 1977;59A:874–877.
43. Hajek PC, Baker LL, Bjorkengren A, Sartoris DJ, Neumann CH, Resnick D. High-resolution magnetic resonance imaging of the ankle: normal anatomy. *Skeletal Radiol* 1986;15:536–540.
44. Haller J, Sartoris DJ, Resnick D, Pathria MN, Berthoty D, Howard B, Nordstrom D. Spontaneous osteonecrosis of the tarsal navicular in adults: imaging findings. *AJR* 1988;151:355–358.
45. Hardy CJ, Katzberg RW, Frey RL, Szinowski J, Totterman S, Mueller OM. Switched surface coil system for bilateral MR imaging. *Radiology* 1988;167:835–838.
46. Hawkins LG. Fractures of the neck of the talus. *J Bone Joint Surg* 1970;52A:991–1002.
47. Helal B, Wilson D. *The foot.* New York: Churchill Livingston, 1988.
48. Hollinshead WH. *Anatomy for surgeons,* vol 3, 3rd ed. New York: Harper & Row, 1982: 563–583.
49. Jacobs AM, O'Leary RJ, Totty WG, Hardy DC. Magnetic resonance imaging of the foot and ankle. *Clin Podiatr Med Surg* 1987;4:903–924.
50. Jung M, Kletter K, Dudczak R, et al. Deep venous thrombosus: scintigraphic diagnosis with In-111 labeled monoclonal antifibrin antibodies. *Radiology* 1989;173:469–475.
51. Kaplan PA, Murphey M, Greenway G, Resnick D, Sartoris DJ, Harms S. Fluid levels in giant cell tumors of bone: report of two cases. *J Comput Tomogr* 1987;11:151–155.
52. Keene JS, Lash EG, Fisher DR, DeSmet AA. Magnetic resonance imaging of Achilles tendon rupture. *Am J Sports Med* 1989;17:333–337.
53. Keigley BA, Haggar AM, Gaba A, Ellis BI, Froelich JW, Wu KK. Primary tumors of the foot: MR imaging. *Radiology* 1989;171:755–759.
54. Kelikian H, Kelikian AS. *Disorders of the ankle.* Philadelphia: Saunders, 1985.
55. Keller U, Oberhansli R, Huber P, et al. Phosphocreatine content and intracellular pH of calf muscle measured by phosphorus NMR spectroscopy in occlusive arterial disease of the legs. *Eur J Clin Invest* 1985;15:382–388.
56. Kingston S. Magnetic resonance imaging of the ankle and foot. *Clin Sports Med* 1988;7:15–28.
57. Kirby EJ, Shereff MJ, Lewis MM. Soft-tissue tumors and tumor-like lesions of the foot. An analysis of eighty-three cases. *J Bone Joint Surg* 1989;71:621–626.
58. Kleinman M, Grass AE. Achilles tendon rupture following steroid injection. *J Bone Joint Surg* 1983;65A:1345–1347.
59. Lanir AM, Hadar H, Cohen I, Tal Y, Benmair J, Schreiber R, Clouse ME. Gaucher disease: assessment with MR imaging. *Radiology* 1986;161:239–244.
60. Lee JK, Yao L. Stress fracture: MR imaging. *Radiology* 1988;169:217–220.
61. Lee MS, Harcke HT, Kumer SJ, Bassett GS. Subtalar joint coalition in children: new observations. *Radiology* 1989;172:635–639.
62. Logigan EL, Berger AR, Bhagwan TS. Injury to the tibial and peroneal nerves due to hemorrhage in the popliteal fossa. *J Bone Joint Surg* 1989;71A:768–770.
63. Mahajan H, Kim EE, Wallace S, Abello R, Benjamin R, Evans HL. Magnetic resonance imaging of malignant fibrous histiocytoma. *Magn Reson Imaging* 1989;7:283–288.
64. Mahajan H, Lorigan JG, Shirkhoda A. Synovial sarcoma: MR imaging. *Magn Reson Imaging* 1989;7:211–216.
65. Mancini DM, Ferraro N, Tuchler M, Chance B, Wilson JR. Detection of abnormal calf muscle metabolism in patients with heart failure using phosphorus-31 NMR. *Am J Cardiol* 1988;62:1234–1240.
66. McLeod RA. Bone and soft tissue neoplasms. In: Berquist TH, ed. *Radiology of the foot and ankle.* New York: Raven Press, 1988.
67. Middleton WD, Macrander S, Lawson TL, et al. High resolution surface coil magnetic resonance imaging of the joints: anatomic correlation. *RadioGraphics* 1987;7:645–683.
68. Middleton WD, Lawson TL. *Anatomy and MRI of the joints: a multiplanar atlas.* New York: Raven Press, 1988.
69. Mirra JM, Bullough PG, Marcove RC, Jacobs B, Huvos AG. Malignant fibrous histiocytoma and osteosarcoma in association with bone infarcts. *J Bone Joint Surg* 1979;56A:932–940.
70. Mitchell MJ, Sartoris DJ, Resnick D. The foot and ankle. *Top Magn Reson Imaging* 1989;1:57–73.
71. Morrey BF, Cass JR, Johnson KA, Berquist TH. Foot and ankle. In: Berquist TH, ed. *Imaging of orthopedic trauma and surgery.* Philadelphia: Saunders, 1986:407–498.
72. Newmark H, Olken SM, Mellon WS, Malhotra AK, Halls J. A new finding in radiographic diagnosis of Achilles tendon rupture. *Skeletal Radiol* 1982;8:223–224.
73. Noto AM, Cheung Y, Rosenberg ZS, Norman A, Leeds NE. MR imaging of the ankle: normal variants. *Radiology* 1989;170:121–124.
74. Oloff-Soloman J, Soloman MA. Special techniques in the evaluation of arthritic disease. *Clin Podiatr Med Surg* 1988;5:25–36.
75. Pakter RL, Fishman EK, Zerhouni EA. Calf hematoma—computed tomographic and magnetic resonance findings. *Skeletal Radiol* 1987;16:393–396.
76. Pettersson H, Slone RM, Spanier S, Gillespy T, Fitzsimmons JR,

Scott KN. Musculoskeletal tumors: T1 and T2 relaxation times. *Radiology* 1988;167:783–785.

77. Quinn SF, Murray W, Clark RA, Cochran C. MR imaging of chronic osteomyelitis. *J Comput Assist Tomogr* 1988;12:113–117.
78. Quinn SF, Murray WT, Clark RA, et al. Achilles tendon: MR imaging at 1.5 T. *Radiology* 1987;164:767–770.
79. Rao VM, Fishman M, Mitchell DG, et al. Painful sickle cell crisis: bone marrow patterns observed with MR imaging. *Radiology* 1986;161:211–215.
80. Rapoport S, Sostman HD, Dope C, Camputaro CM, Holcomb W, Gore JC. Venous clots: evaluation with MR imaging. *Radiology* 1987;162:527–530.
81. Reinig JW, Dorwart RH, Roden WC. MRI of a ruptured achilles tendon. *J Comput Assist Tomogr* 1985;9:1131–1134.
82. Resnick D. Radiology of the talocalcaneal articulations. *Radiology* 1974;111:581–586.
83. Rhea JT, Salvatore DA, Sheahan J. Radiographic anatomy of the tarsal bones. *Med Radiogr Photogr* 1983;59:2–8.
84. Romanus B, Lindahl S, Stener B. Accessory soleus muscle: a clinical and radiographic presentation of 11 cases. *J Bone Joint Surg* 1986;68A:731–734.
85. Rosenberg ZS, Cheung Y, Jahss MH, Noto AM, Norman A, Leeds NE. Rupture of posterior tibial tendon: CT and MR imaging with surgical correlation. *Radiology* 1988;169:229–235.
86. Rosenberg ZS, Cheung Y, Jahss MH. Computed tomography scan and magnetic resonance imaging of the ankle tendons. An overview. *Foot Ankle* 1988;8:297–307.
87. Rosenberg ZS, Feldman F, Singson RD. Peroneal tendon ruptures: CT analysis. *Radiology* 1986;161:743–748.
88. Russell WO, Cohen J, Enzinger F, et al. A clinical and pathologic staging system for soft tissue sarcomas. *Cancer* 1977;40:1562–1570.
89. Santoro JP, Cachia VV, Sartoris DJ, Resnick D. Nonspecific inflammation in the foot demonstrated by magnetic resonance imaging. *J Foot Surg* 1988;27:478–483.
90. Sartoris DJ, Resnick D. Cross-sectional imaging of the foot: text of anatomic knowledge. *J Foot Surg* 1988;27:374–383.
91. Sebes JI. Diagnostic imaging of bone and joint abnormalities associated with sickle cell hemoglobinopathies. *AJR* 1989;152:1153–1159.
92. Sherry CS, Harms SE. MR evaluation of giant cell tumors of the tendon sheath. *Magn Reson Imaging* 1989;7:195–201.
93. Shuman WP, Baron RL, Peters MJ, Tazioli PK. Comparison of STIR and spin echo MR imaging at 1.5T in 90 lesions of the chest, liver, and pelvis. *AJR* 1989;152:853–859.
94. Sierra A, Potchen EJ, Moore J, Smith HG. High field magnetic resonance imaging of asceptic necrosis of the talus. *J Bone Joint Surg* 1986;68A:927–928.
95. Solomon MA, Oloff-Solomon J. Magnetic resonance imaging in the foot and ankle. *Clin Podiatr Med Surg* 1988;5:945–965.
96. Spritzer CE, Dalinka MK, Kressel HY. Magnetic resonance imaging of pigmented villonodular synovitis. *Skeletal Radiol* 1987;16:316–319.
97. Spritzer CE, Sussman SK, Blunder RA, Saeed M, Herfkens RJ. Deep venous thrombosis evaluation with limited flip-angle, gradient refocused MR imaging: preliminary experience. *Radiology* 1988;166:371–375.
98. Stafford SA, Rosenthal DI, Gebhardt MC, Brady TJ, Scott JA. Case report—MRI in stress fracture. *AJR* 1986;147:553–556.
99. Stoller DW, Genant HK, Goumas CG, et al. Fast MR improves imaging of musculoskeletal system. *Diagn Imag* 1988;10:98–103.
100. Tang JSH, Gold RH, Bassett LW, et al. Musculoskeletal infection of the extremities: evaluation with MR imaging. *Radiology* 1988;166:205–209.
101. Tehranzadeh J, Mnaymneh W, Ghavam C, Morillo G, Murphy BJ. Comparison of CT and MR imaging in musculoskeletal neoplasms. *J Comput Assist Tomogr* 1989;13:466–472.
102. Terrier F, Hricak H, Revel D, Alpers CE, Reinhold CE, Levine J, Genant HK. *Invest Radiol* 1985;20:813–823.
103. Totty WG, Murphy WA, Lee JKT. Soft-tissue tumors: MR imaging. *Radiology* 1986;160:135–141.
104. Unger E, Moldofsky P, Gatenby R, et al. Diagnosis of osteomyelitis by MR imaging. *AJR* 1988;1509:605–610.
105. Vogler JB, Helmes CA, Callan PW. *Normal variants and pitfalls in imaging.* Philadelphia: Saunders, 1986.
106. Weekes RG, Berquist TH, McLeod RA, Zimmer WD. Magnetic resonance imaging of soft-tissue tumors: comparison with computed tomography. *Magn Reson Imaging* 1985;3:345–352.
107. Weissman SD. *Radiology of the foot.* Baltimore: Williams & Wilkins, 1983.
108. Yao L, Lee JK. Occult intraosseous fracture: detection with MR imaging. *Radiology* 1988;167:749–751.
109. Yeager BA, Schiebler ML, Wertheim SB, et al. Case report—MR imaging of osteoid osteoma of the talus. *J Comput Assist Tomogr* 1987;11:916–917.
110. Yuh WTC, Corson JD, Baraniewski HM, et al. Osteomyelitis of the foot in diabetic patients: evaluation with plain film, ^{99m}Tc-MDP bone scintigraphy, and MR imaging. *Am. J. Roent.* 152:795–800, 1989.
111. Yulish BS, Lieberman JM, Newman AJ, et al. Juvenile rheumatoid arthritis: assessment with MR imaging. *Radiology* 1987;165:149–152.
112. Yulish BS, Lieberman JM, Strandjord SE, Bryan PJ, Mulopulos GP, Modic MT. Hemophilic arthropathy: assessment with MR imaging. *Radiology* 1987;164:759–762.
113. Yulish BS, Mulopulos GP, Goodfellow DB, Bryan PJ, Modic MT, Dollinger BM. MR imaging of osteochondral lesions of the talus. *J Comput Assist Tomogr* 1987;11:296–301.
114. Zeiss J, Saddemi SR, Ebraheim NA. MR imaging of the peroneal tunnel. *J Comput Assist Tomogr* 1989;13(5):840–844.

MRI of the Musculoskeletal System, 2nd Edition, edited by T. H. Berquist.
Raven Press, Ltd., New York © 1990.

CHAPTER 9

Shoulder and Arm

Thomas H. Berquist

Techniques, 314
Glenohumeral Joint, 314
Arm, 316
Brachial Plexus, 316
Anatomy, 334
Osseous Anatomy, 334
Muscular Anatomy, 337
Bursae, 341
Neurovascular Anatomy, 341
Applications, 343
Shoulder and Arm, 343
Trauma, 343
Postoperative Changes, 348
Capsular Abnormalities, 349
Infection and Inflammatory Diseases, 351
Osteonecrosis, 351
Neoplasms, 353
Brachial Plexus Lesions, 354
References, 355

There are numerous clinical problems relating to the shoulder, arm, and brachial plexus. The last has been partially discussed in Chapter 5; however, a more detailed discussion of brachial plexus lesions is given in this chapter. There is some overlap in clinical syndromes relating to the shoulder, upper extremity, and brachial plexus, but for purposes of discussion each area is considered separately.

Most patients with shoulder pathology present with pain and/or pain with reduced range of motion. To date, shoulder evaluation has been based on clinical data as well as findings from routine radiographs (3,14,27). Routine radiographs are still an important part of the workup of patients with shoulder pain because subtle changes in both the bone and soft tissue can lead to proper selection of additional imaging techniques (3). In many patients, this may mean arthrography, CT, or arthrotomography (3,27,66,68,70). In recent years, magnetic resonance imaging (MRI) has begun to replace these techniques since the information obtained is significantly greater and MRI is a noninvasive technique. Similarly, soft tissue problems involving the upper arm are easily assessed with MRI. An additional benefit of MRI is the ability to image the shoulder and arm in any orthogonal or off-axis oblique plane (6,90–92).

The brachial plexus can be evaluated with myelography and CT. However, the complex anatomy, along with inability to clearly demonstrate all neurovascular structures, has hindered these techniques to some degree (8,69). Myelography only demonstrates the spinal canal and nerve root sheaths, while CT, though it demonstrates soft tissue pathology to some degree, has difficulty in clearly differentiating all neurovascular structures. In addition, there is significant artifact in the shoulder region on many CT scanners, which makes examination of this area somewhat suboptimal. Examination of the brachial plexus using MRI can be accomplished in the axial, sagittal, and coronal planes, which allows more complete evaluation of neurovascular structures as they exit the paraspinal tissues and extend into the axillary and shoulder regions (8,69).

This chapter discusses the techniques, anatomy, and applications for evaluating the shoulder, brachial plexus,

T. H. Berquist: Mayo Medical School and Mayo Clinic, Rochester, Minnesota 55905.

and upper arm. Variations in techniques depend on the clinical setting. Anatomy in sagittal, coronal, and axial planes, especially with regard to the course of the neural structures, is stressed.

TECHNIQUES

Technique in MRI examination of the shoulder or brachial plexus region varies depending on the clinical symptoms. For purposes of discussion, it is best to consider the shoulder, arm, and brachial plexus region separately because there are significant differences in the methods for MRI examination (Table 9-1).

Glenohumeral Joint

New software and coil techniques have greatly enhanced the ability of MRI examinations to properly evaluate patients with shoulder symptoms. A particularly important development is the ability to perform off-axis small field of view images in the shoulder region. This allows the patient to be examined in a more comfortable position with the arm at the side. Larger patients may need to be rotated slightly with the uninvolved arm above the head in order to properly position the patient in the gantry (Fig. 9-1). Off-axis small field of view with the surface coil is still the most optimal technique in these patients. In some cases, the body coil with a smaller field of view can be used but image quality is usually suboptimal.

In most situations, the patient is placed supine in the magnet with a single or dual circular 5 inch surface coil placed over the shoulder to be examined (Figs. 9-1 and 9-2). When using dual coils, one coil is above and the other below the shoulder with a connector between the two coils. An advantage of this configuration is the additive signal created by the two coils (21,35,36,44). New

TABLE 9-1. *MR examinations of the shoulder, arm, and brachial plexus*

	Pulse sequence	Slice thickness/gap	Field of view (FOV) (cm)	Matrix	Excitations (Nex)	Image time
Shoulder						
Coronal scout	SE 200/20	Three 1 cm/no skip	30–48	128 × 256	1	26 sec
Axial	SE 2,000/60,20	3 mm/skip 1.5 mm	16–20	192 × 256	2	12 min 48 sec
Oblique coronal (in plane of glenohumeral joint)	SE 2,000/60,20	2 mm/skip 1.5 mm	16–20	192 × 256	2	12 min 48 sec
Sagittal (perpendicular to glenohumeral joint)	SE 500/20	5 mm/no skip	16–20	256 × 256 or 192 × 256	1 2	2 min 8 sec 3 min 12 sec
					Total	28 min 10 sec to 19 min 14 sec
Arm						
Coronal scout	SE 200/20	Three 1 cm/no skip	30–48	128 × 256	1	26 sec
Axial	SE 2,000/60,20	0.5–1 cm/skip 2.5–5 mm	~24	192 × 256	2	12 min 48 sec
Axial, coronal, or sagittal	SE 500/20	0.5–1 cm/skip 2.5–5 mm for axial; 3–5 mm/no skip for coronal or sagittal of humerus	~24	256 × 256	1	2 min 8 sec
STIR	TR 1,500, TE 30 TI 150	3–5 mm	~24	192 × 256	2	9 min 36 sec
					Total	15 min 14 sec to 24 min 50 sec
Brachial plexus						
Coronal scout	SE 200/20	Three 1 cm/no skip	30–48	128 × 256	1	26 sec
Axial	SE 2,000/60,20	5 mm/skip 2.5 mm	24–30	192 × 256	2	12 min 48 sec
Sagittal	SE 500/20	5 mm/no skip	24–30	256 × 256	1	2 min 8 sec
					Total	15 min 22 sec

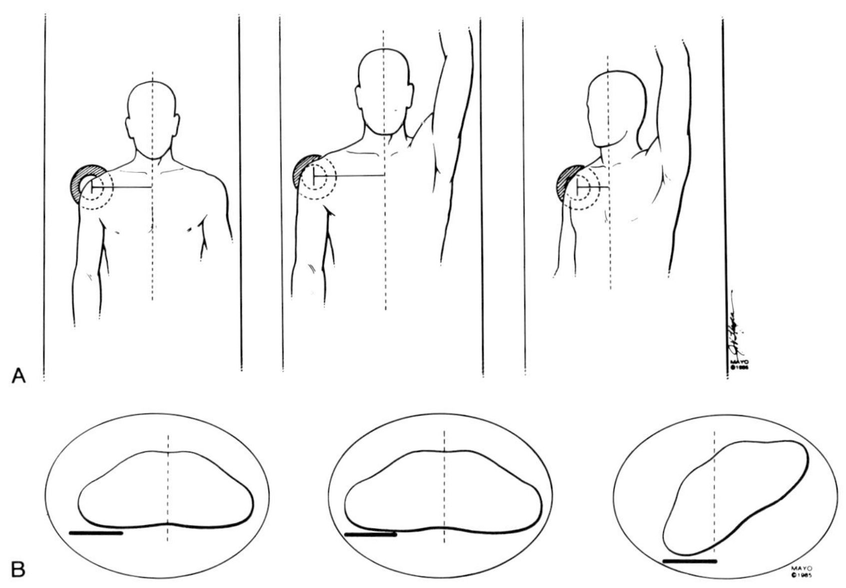

FIG. 9-1. Illustrations of patient positioned for shoulder examination using a circular coil. Changes in patient position are demonstrated in the frontal (**A**) and axial (**B**) planes to indicate the relationship of the shoulder to the gantry center. The position on the left in (**A**) is most comfortable but can only be used successfully with off-axis small field of view capabilities.

shoulder coils are being configured to improve image quality in the shoulder.

In most situations, the patient is being examined for suspected tear of the rotator cuff, the glenoid labrum, or other soft tissue abnormalities involving the periarticular soft tissues of the shoulder (37). Our routine examination (Table 9-1) consists of three image planes using T2 and T1 weighted spin-echo sequences (Figs. 9-3 to 9-6). A coronal scout film is obtained initially using 128 × 256 matrix, a 30–48 cm field of view, and three 1 cm thick sections. This sequence takes approximately 26 sec. The scout image is used to select the image locations for the axial T2 weighted (SE 2,000/60,20) sequence (Fig. 9-4). A 16–20 cm field of view is usually optimal, depending on patient size, and 3 mm thick slices with 1.5 mm interslice gaps are used to study the area from the axillary region through the superior aspect of the acromioclavicular joint. Following this portion of the examination, coronal sections are obtained in the same plane as the scapula or perpendicular to the glenohumeral articulation (Figs. 9-3B and 9-5) (23,90–92). These images are obtained using the same field of view with either 256 × 256 or 192 × 256 matrix and 3 mm slices with a 1.5 mm skip between slices (90–92). The same pulse sequence is used in the coronal plane. This provides optimal anatomic detail and also demonstrates synovial fluid as high signal intensity, allowing subtle changes in the rotator cuff and glenoid labrum to be more easily appreciated. These two sequences are usually adequate to evaluate rotator cuff tears and glenolabrum pathology. However, we generally also perform sagittal images (Fig. 9-6) parallel to the glenohumeral joint (Fig. 9-3C). This is useful for evaluating the undersurface of the AC joint and supraspinatus muscle for impingement (90–92). This sequence is performed using the same field of view with a spin-echo sequence (500/20) and 5 mm thick contiguous slices (Table 9-1). In patients with significant discomfort or claustrophobia, gradient-echo sequences can be used to reduce image time.

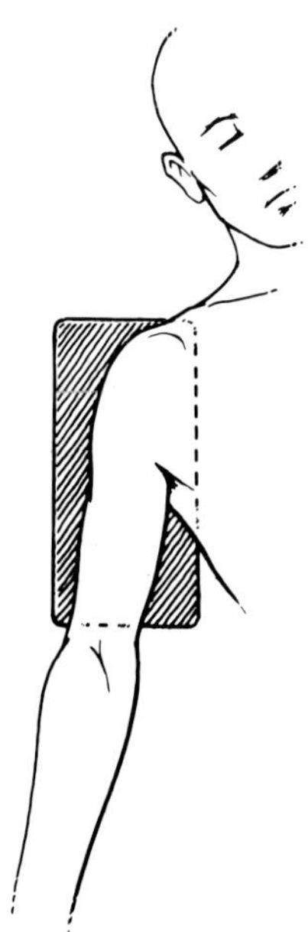

FIG. 9-2. Illustration of patient positioned for examination of the arm using the rectangular-shaped "license plate" coil.

In some situations, additional sequences or image planes may be indicated but the above technique is gen-

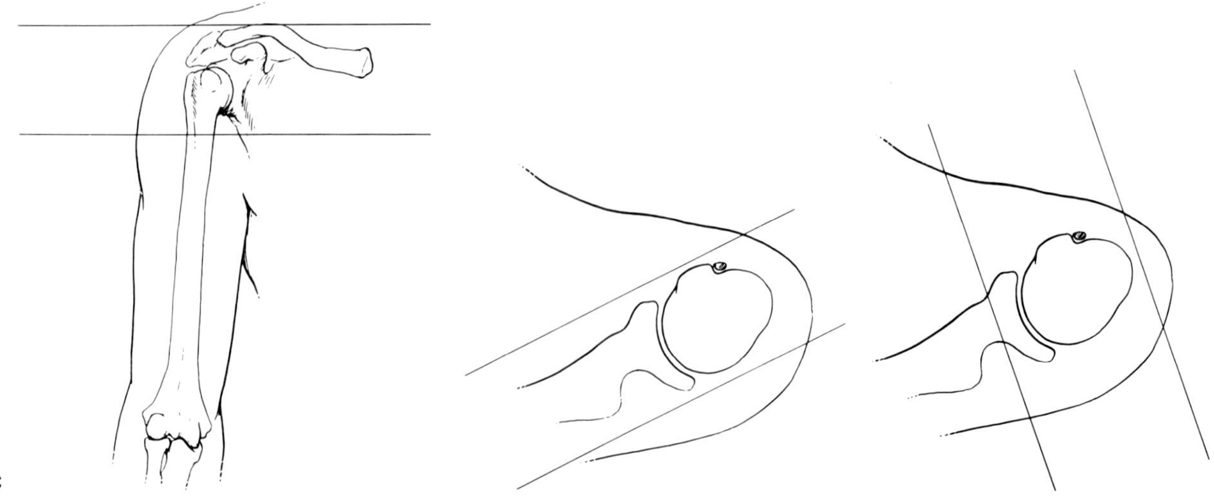

A,B,C

FIG. 9-3. Illustration of imaging regions for evaluation of the shoulder. **A:** Coronal illustration demonstrating the region studied (between lines) with axial images. **B:** Axial illustration demonstrating the region studied by coronal images. **C:** Axial illustration demonstrating the region and angle of sagittal images.

erally appropriate for most shoulder or glenohumeral joint pathology. In certain cases, subtle marrow abnormalities may be detected more easily using short TI inversion recovery sequences (STIR); or when the glenoid labrum is not optimally noted with the routine examination, radial GRILL images may be used to further define this anatomy (59).

Arm

MR evaluation of the arm may be included as a portion of the shoulder examination or performed separately. The patient should be supine. The license plate coil or body coil can be used depending on patient size (Fig. 9-2). Patients with suspected bone or soft tissue pathology in the arm are usually examined with axial T2 weighted images with either 1 cm or 5 mm slice thicknesses depending on the area of interest. Axial double-echo T2 weighted sequences (SE 2,000/60,20) provide an excellent screening examination. This sequence can be followed by T1 weighted axial images if soft tissue pathology is suspected; or if marrow pathology is suspected, sagittal or coronal images should be selected along the plane of the humerus using either T1 weighted spin-echo sequences or, in some cases, STIR or chemical shift images to evaluate subtle changes in the marrow or the humerus. Table 9-1 lists the different examinations for the shoulder and arm as well as the parameters and examination times.

Brachial Plexus

Examination of the brachial plexus requires a different approach. The cervical spine is frequently examined as part of the study (see Chapter 5). Routine cervical spine examination may be done first to exclude any spinal canal or proximal nerve root abnormalities. These techniques are fully discussed in Chapter 5 (see Figs. 5-4 to 5-6). The area to be examined when evaluating the brachial plexus (cervical spine to humerus) is large, so the body coil is usually used. When symptoms are unilateral, a small off-center field of view is used (Fig. 9-7). When both sides are being examined, a larger field of view is required. Examination of the more peripheral aspect of the brachial plexus is usually accomplished with T2 weighted axial (Fig. 9-8) and T1 weighted sagittal (Fig. 9-9) images. The axial images are obtained using cardiac and respiratory gaiting to minimize the artifact from respiratory and cardiac motion. Slice thickness of 5 mm with 2.5 mm skip and a 24–32 cm field of view will usually allow the side of interest to be completely evaluated (Fig. 9-7A). Axial images are usually obtained from the midcervical level (C3–C4) to the midhumerus, which allows the lower neck, shoulder, and upper arm to be completely included in the field of view (Fig. 9-7A).

There is considerable fat along the course of the neurovascular bundle of the brachial plexus. Therefore, sagittal T1 weighted images provide optimal evaluation of the nerve roots as they exit the spinal foramina and extend into the soft tissues of the neck and arm (8,69). The nerve roots appear as small low signal intensity structures with this sequence and are accompanied by the larger arteries and veins as they extend peripherally. Soft tissue masses in the brachial plexus region are seen as low-intensity areas and are clearly separated from the fat around the neurovascular bundle. In most situations, the axial and sagittal images provide an adequate

Text continues on p. 334.

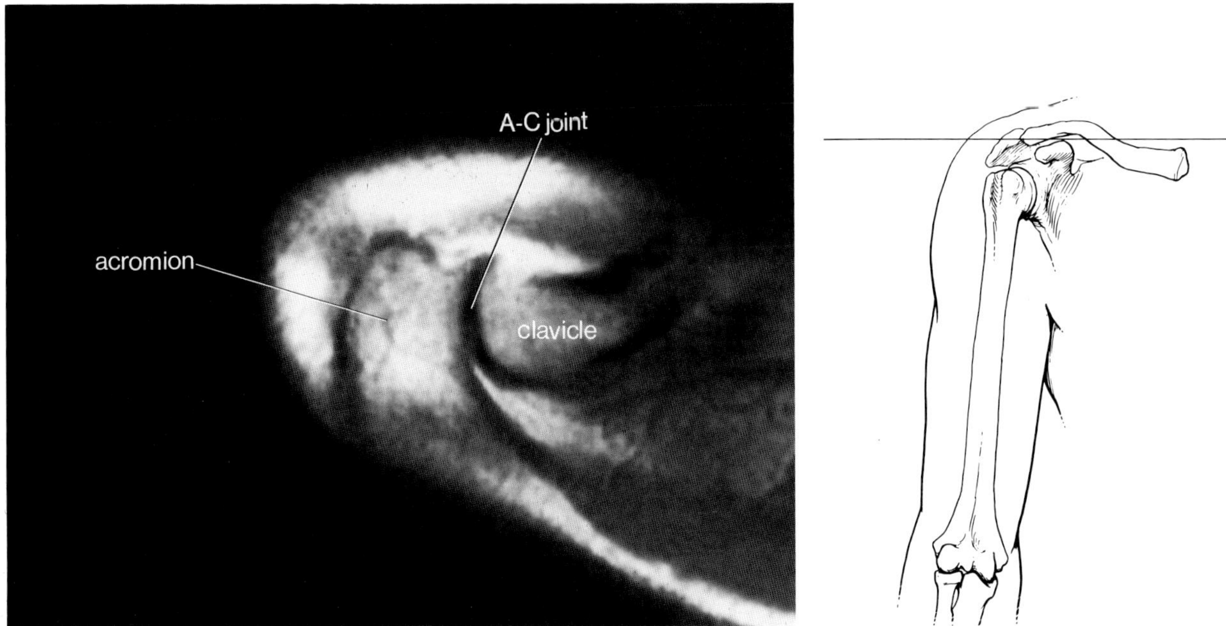

FIG. 9-4. Axial MR images of the shoulder with illustration of anatomic levels. **A:** Axial image through the acromioclavicular joint.

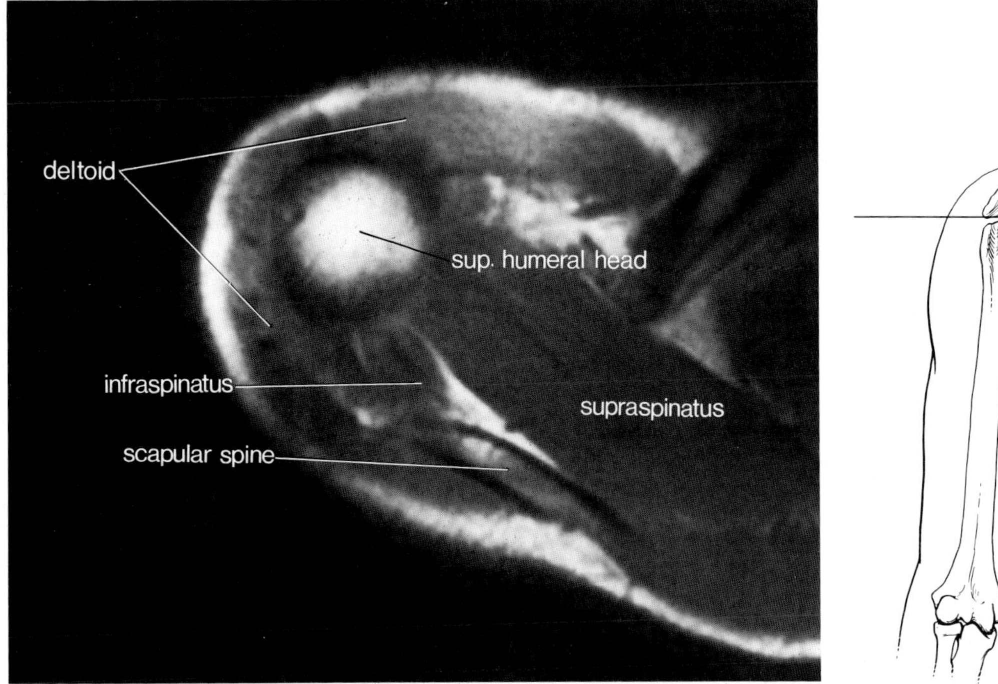

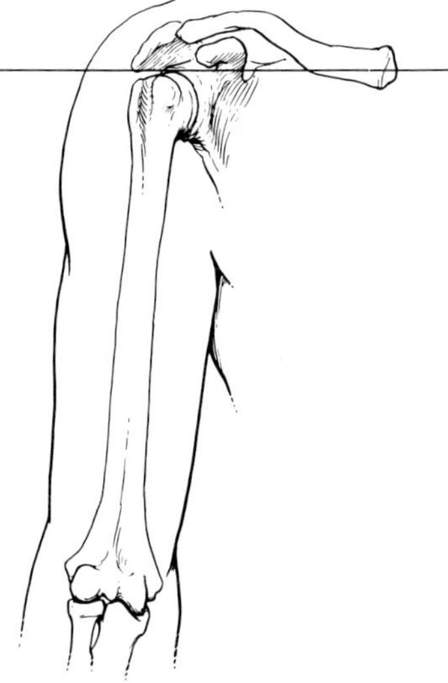

FIG. 9-4. B: Axial image through the supraspinatus.

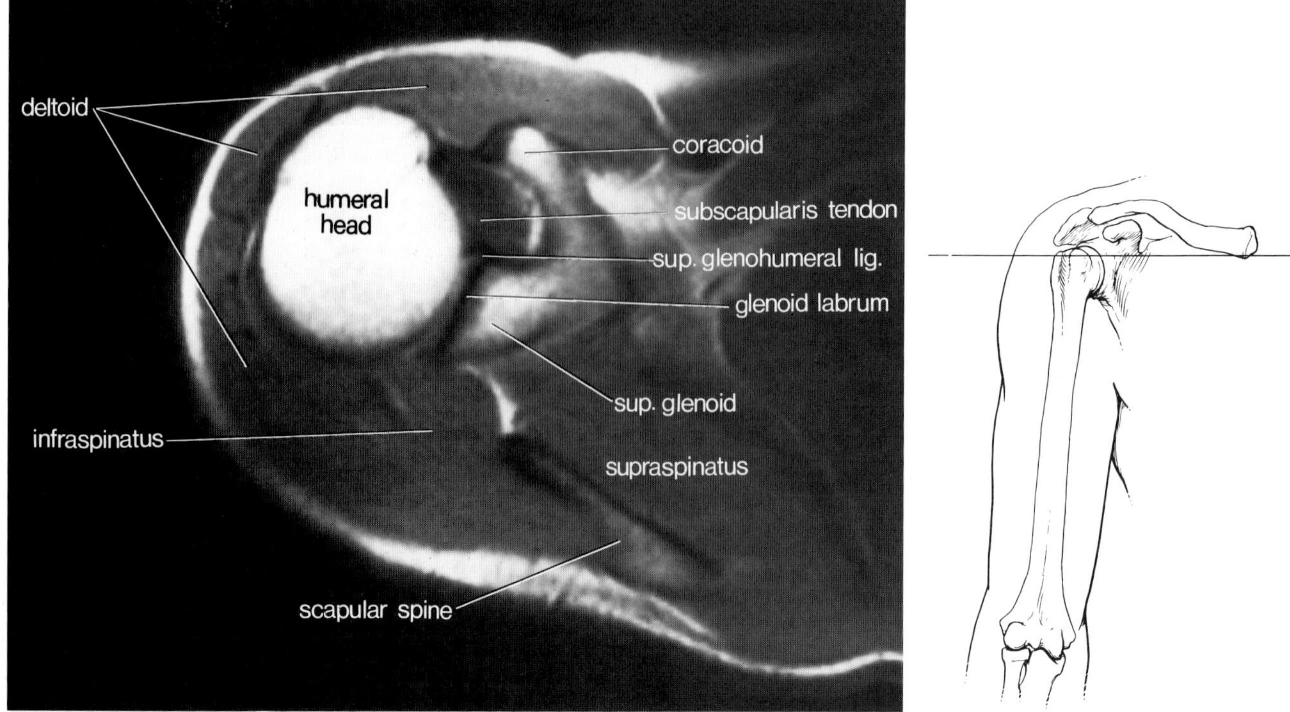

FIG. 9-4. C: Axial image through the upper glenoid and coracoid.

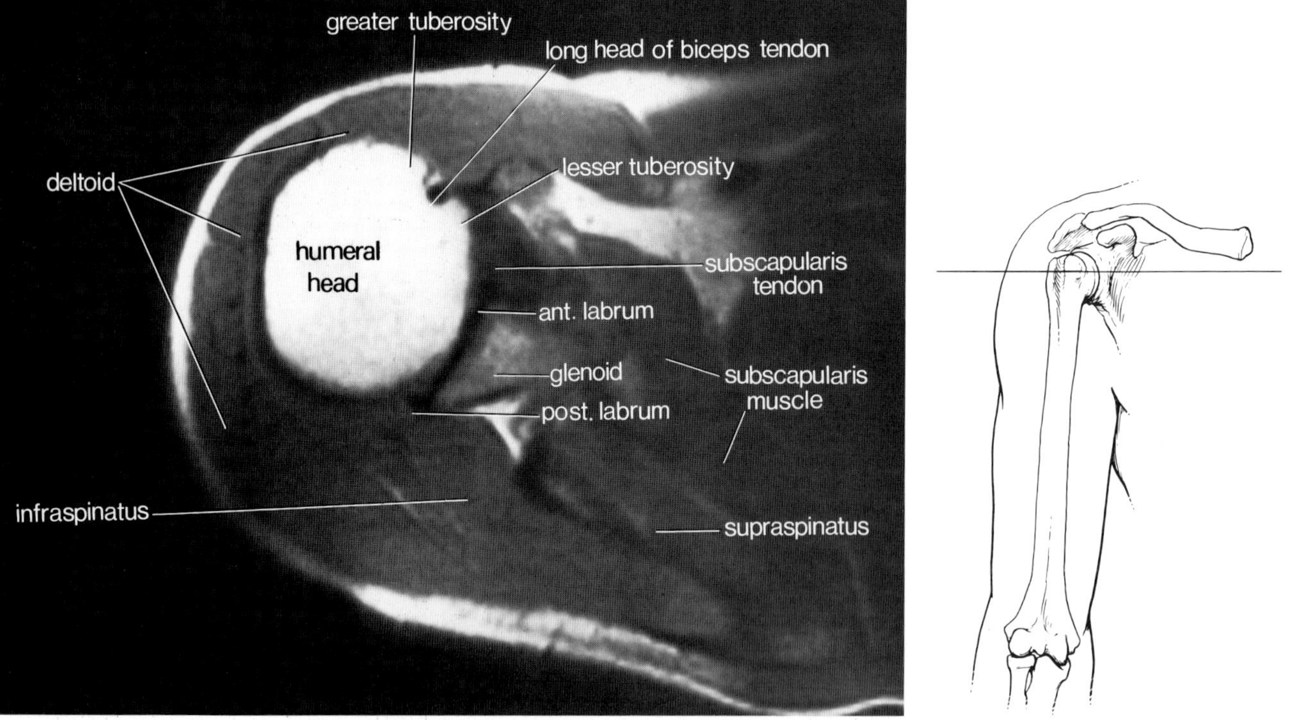

FIG. 9-4. D: Axial image through the humeral head and glenoid demonstrating the normal labrum.

E

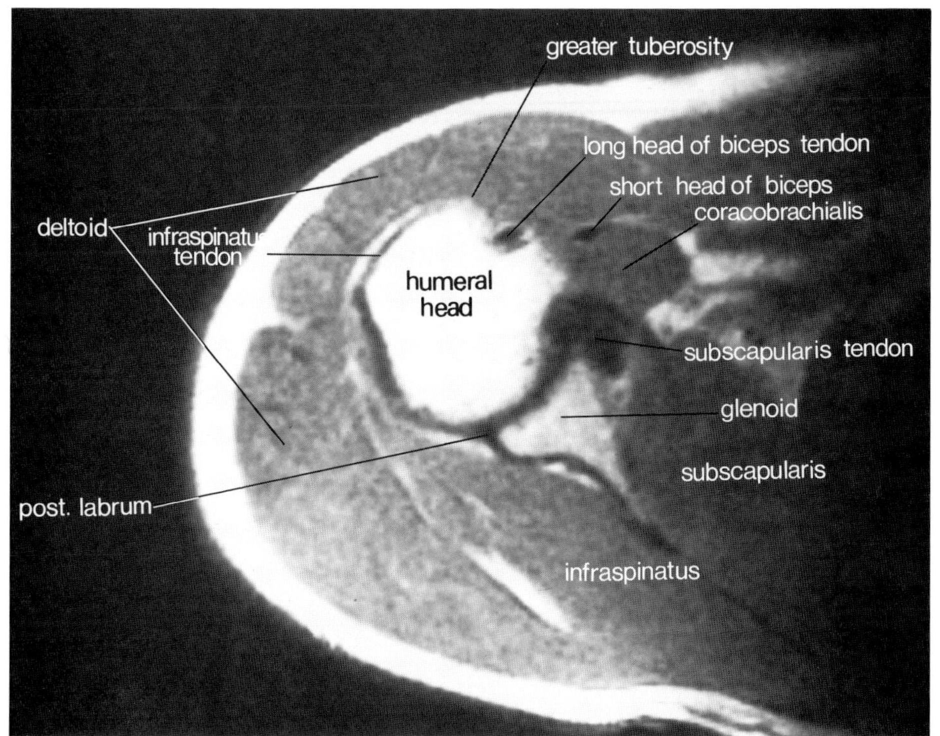

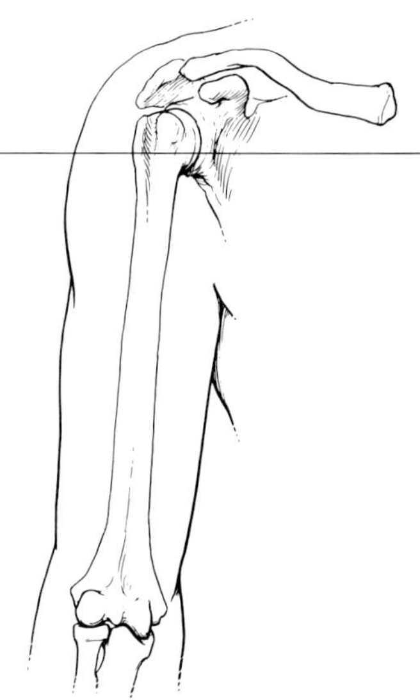

FIG. 9-4. E: Axial image through the lower humeral head.

F

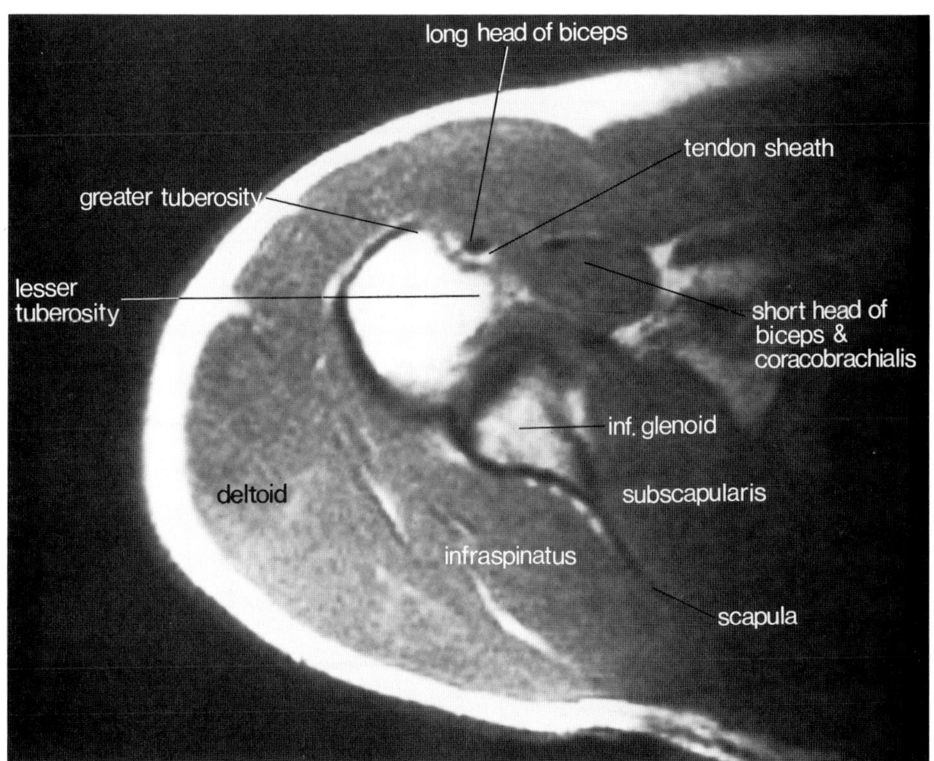

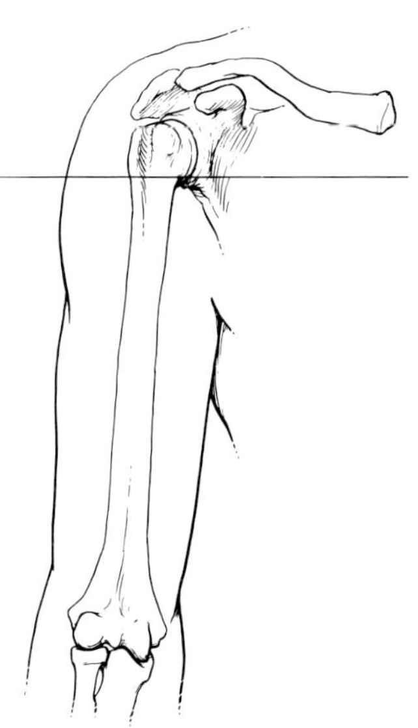

FIG. 9-4. F: Axial image through the lower glenoid.

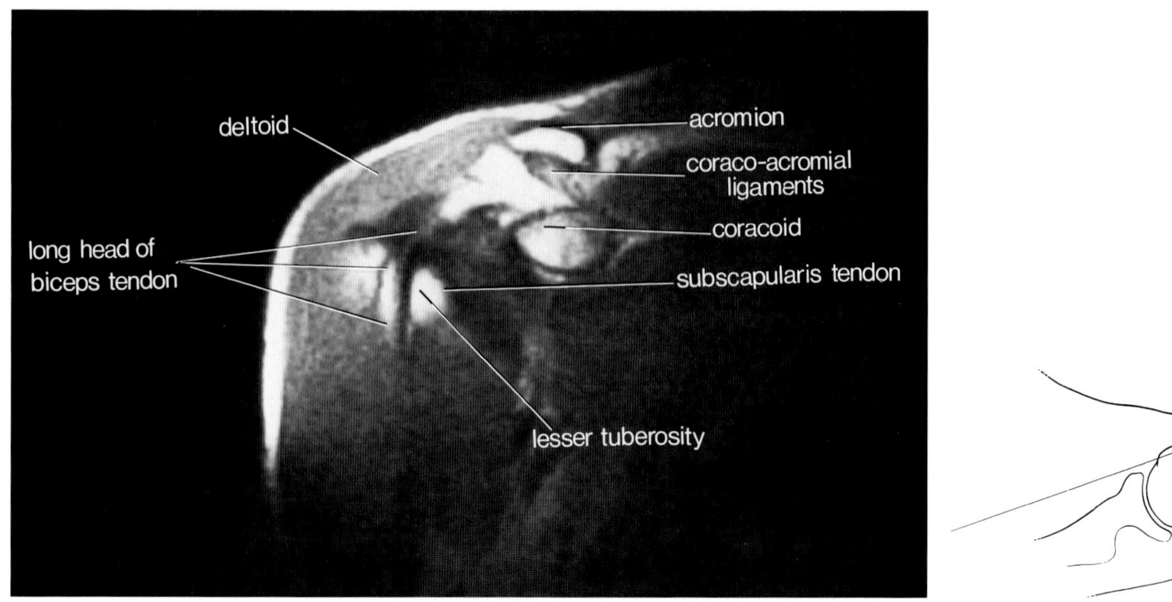

FIG. 9-5. Coronal MR images of the shoulder with illustration of levels. **A:** Coronal image through the anterior shoulder at the biceps tendon and coracoid level.

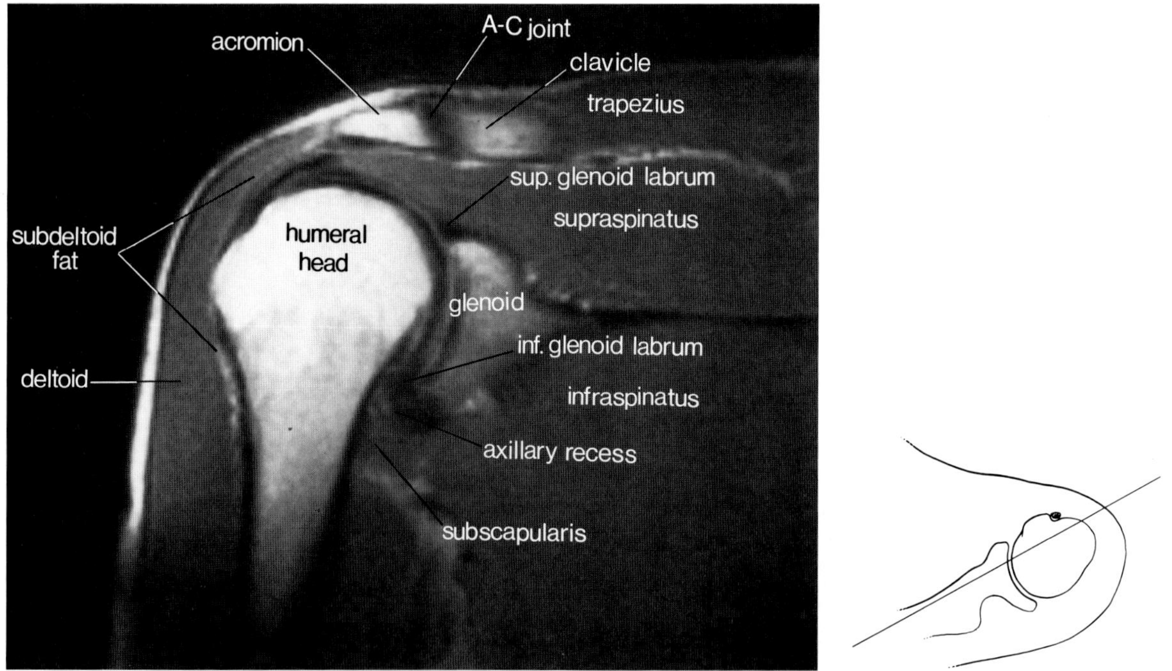

FIG. 9-5. **B:** Coronal image through the humeral head and acromioclavicular joint.

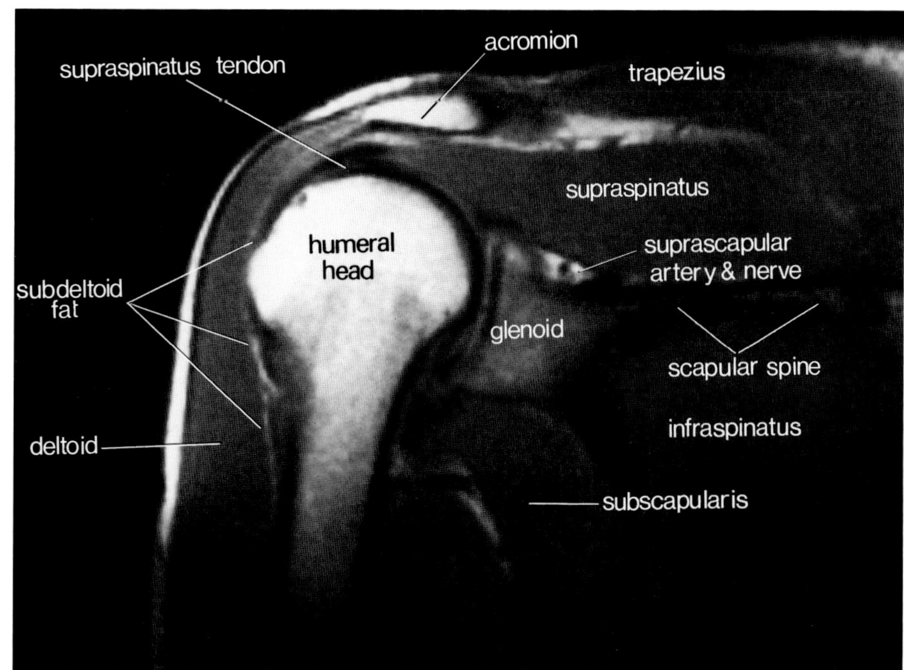

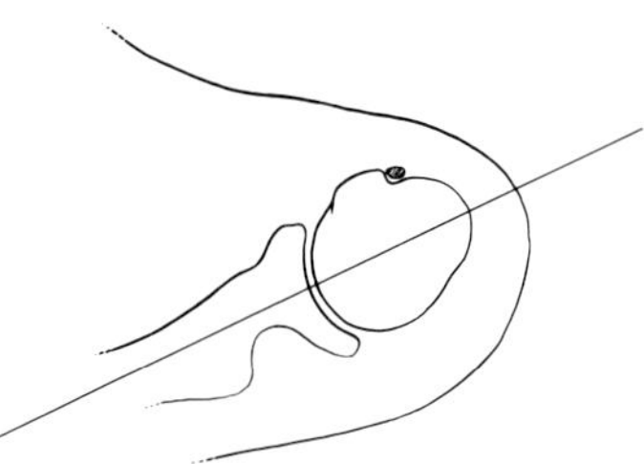

FIG. 9-5. C: Coronal image through the glenohumeral joint.

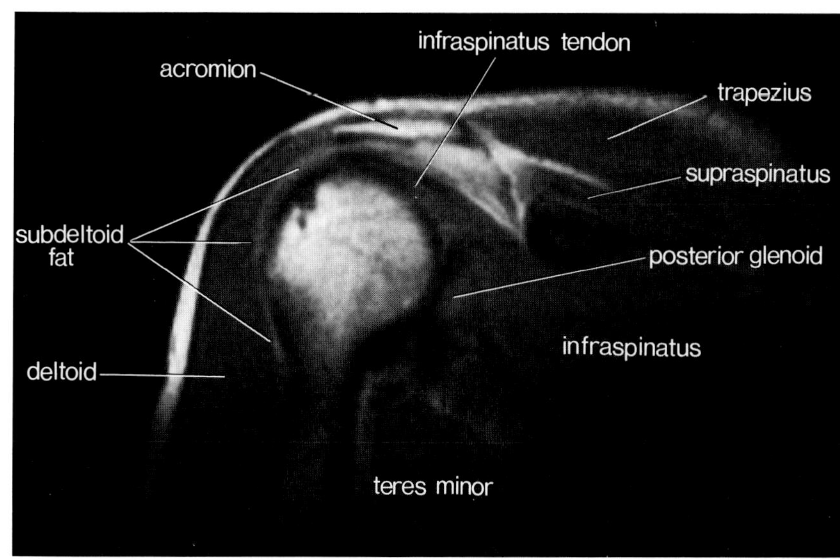

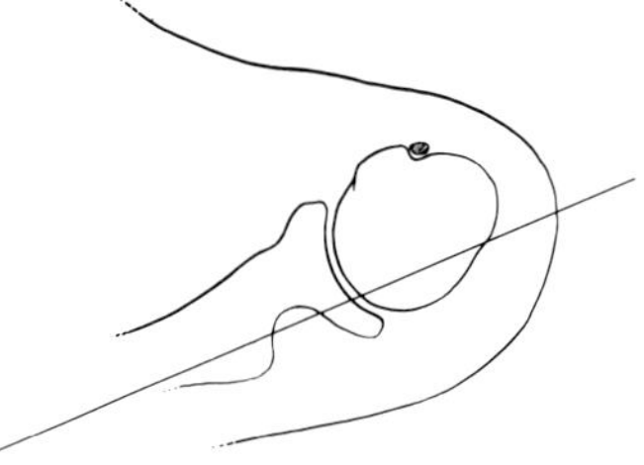

FIG. 9-5. D: Coronal image through the posterior glenoid.

E

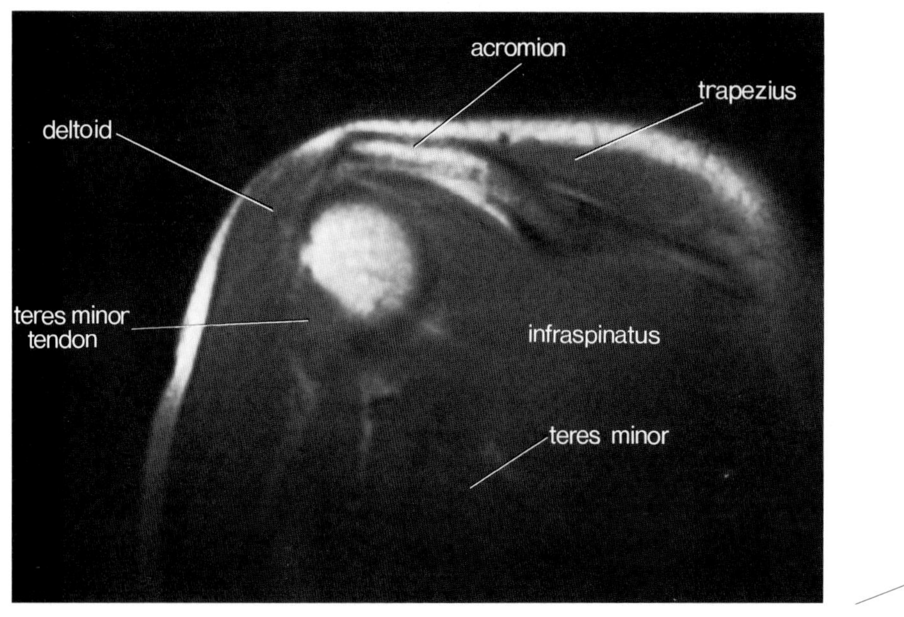

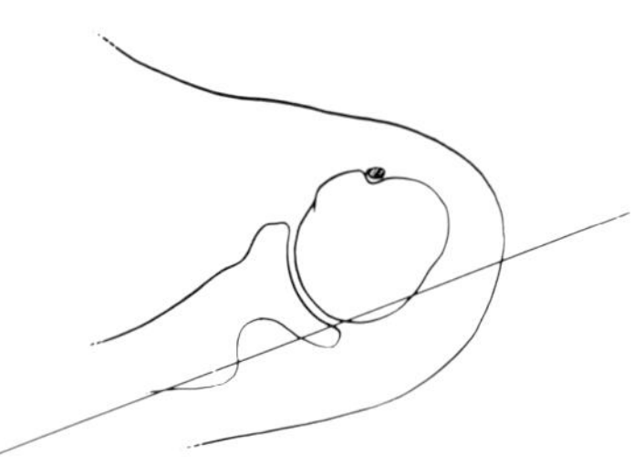

FIG. 9-5. E: Coronal image through the acromion and posterior head.

A

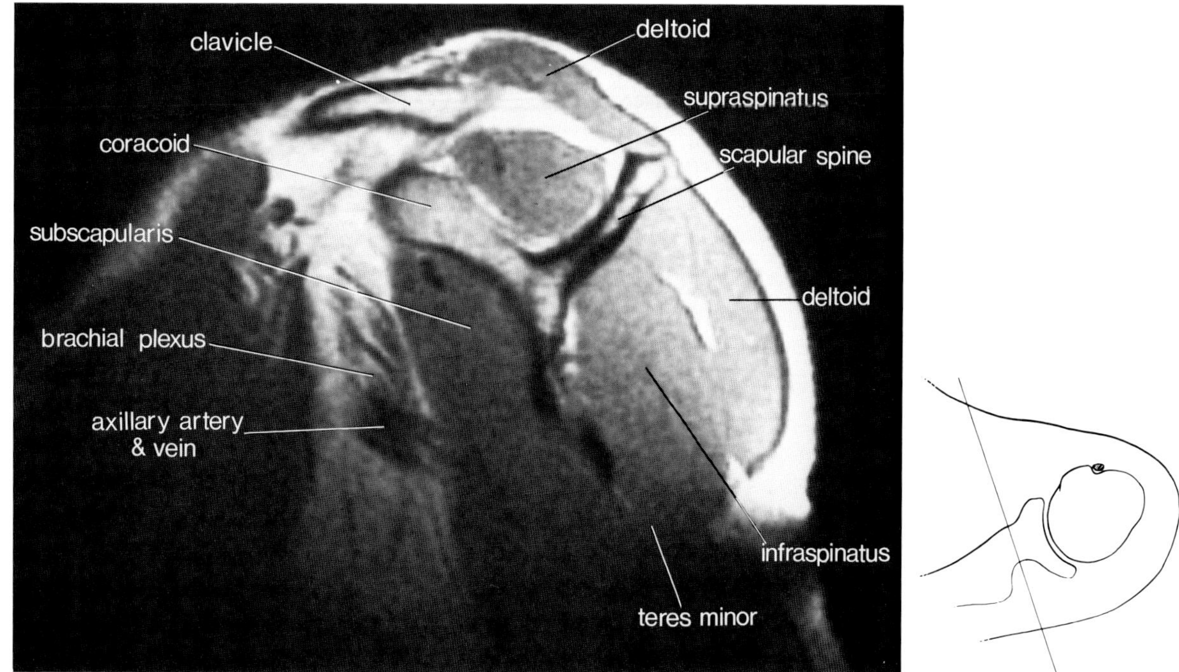

FIG. 9-6. Sagittal images of the shoulder with illustrations for level of section. **A:** Sagittal image through the coracoid and scapular spine.

B

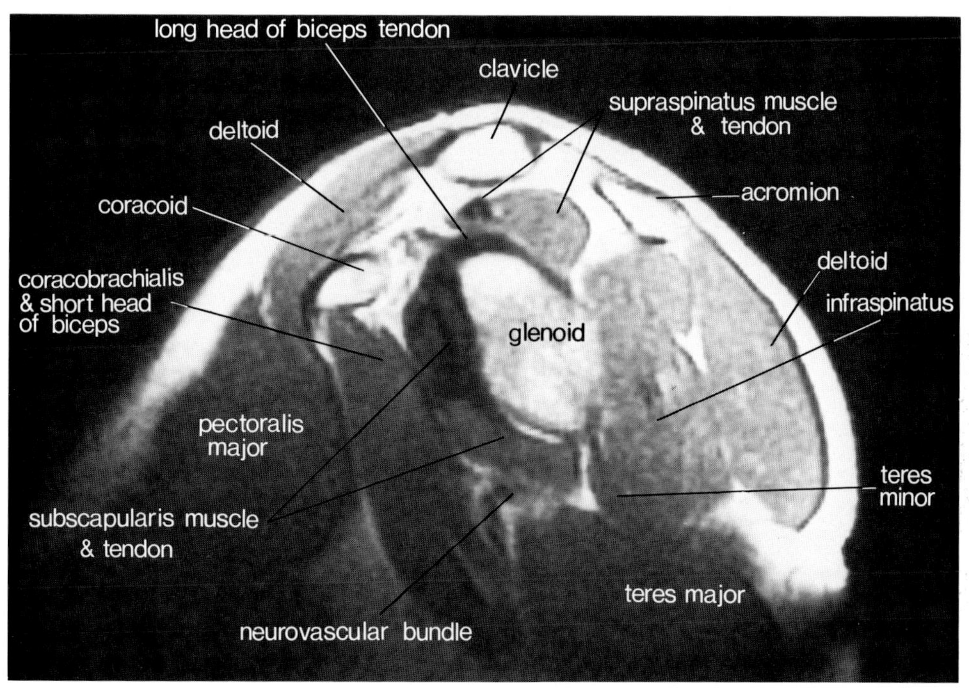

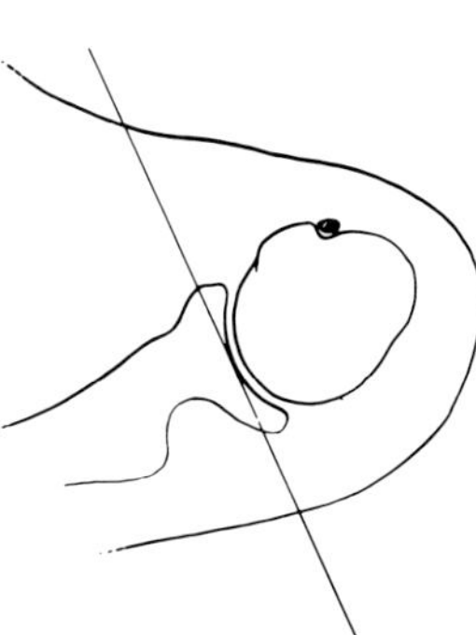

FIG. 9-6. B: Sagittal image through the glenoid.

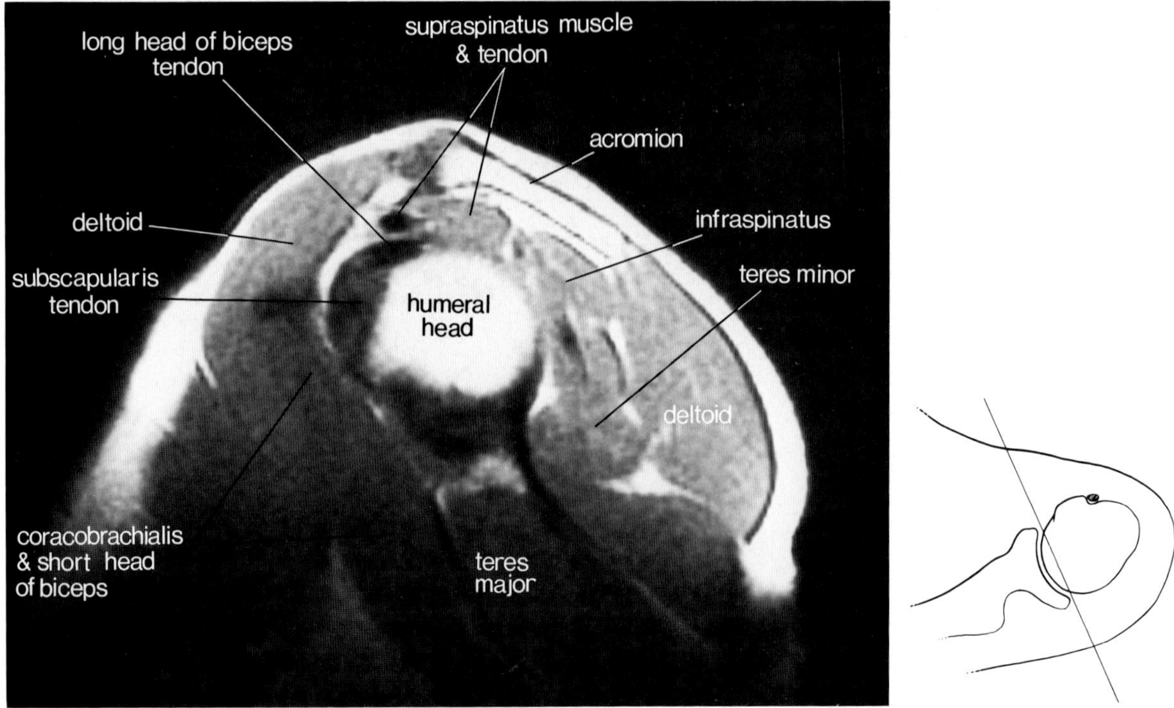

FIG. 9-6. C: Sagittal image through the acromioclavicular joint.

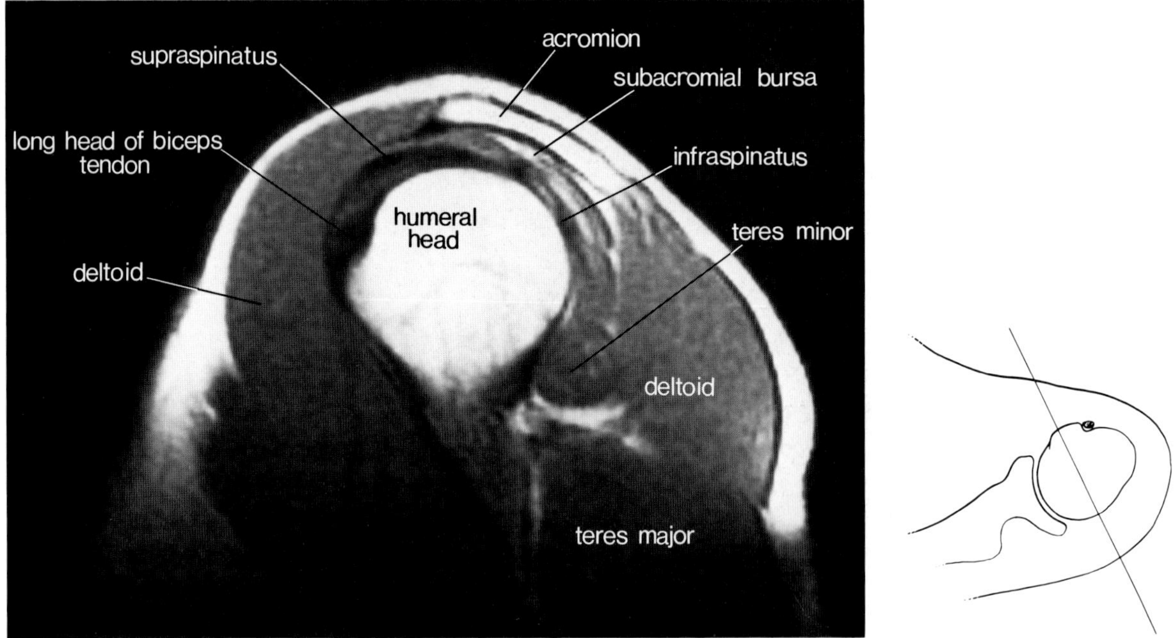

FIG. 9-6. D: Sagittal image through the humeral head and acromion.

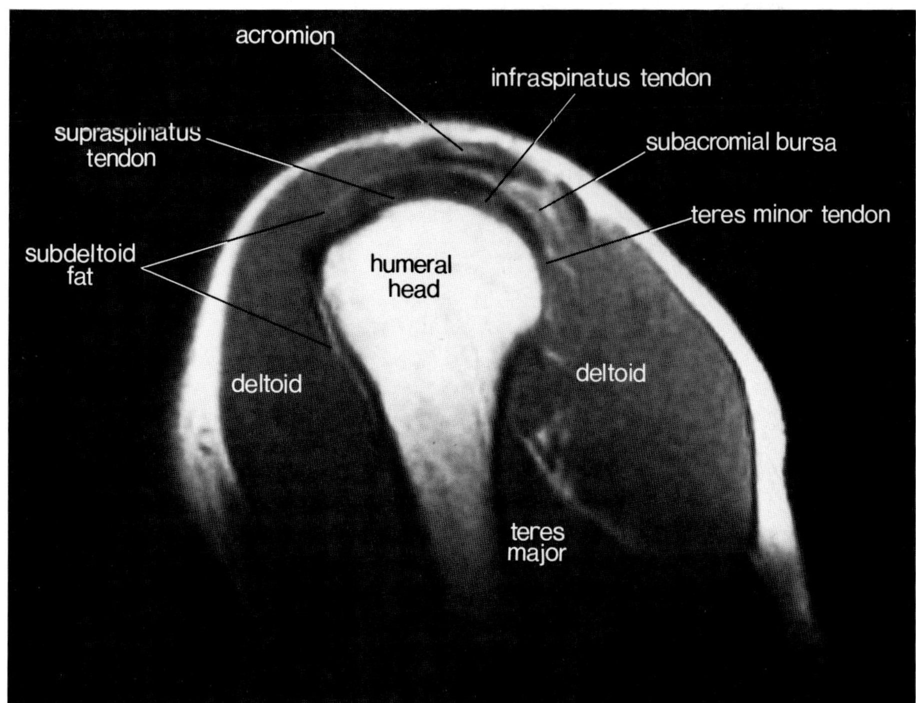

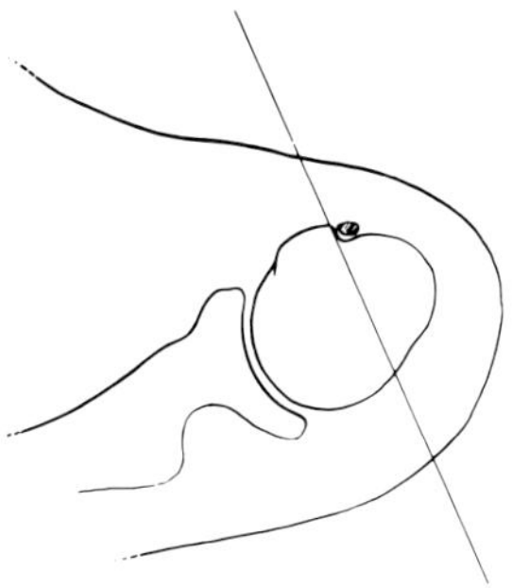

E

FIG. 9-6. E: Sagittal image through the lateral humeral head.

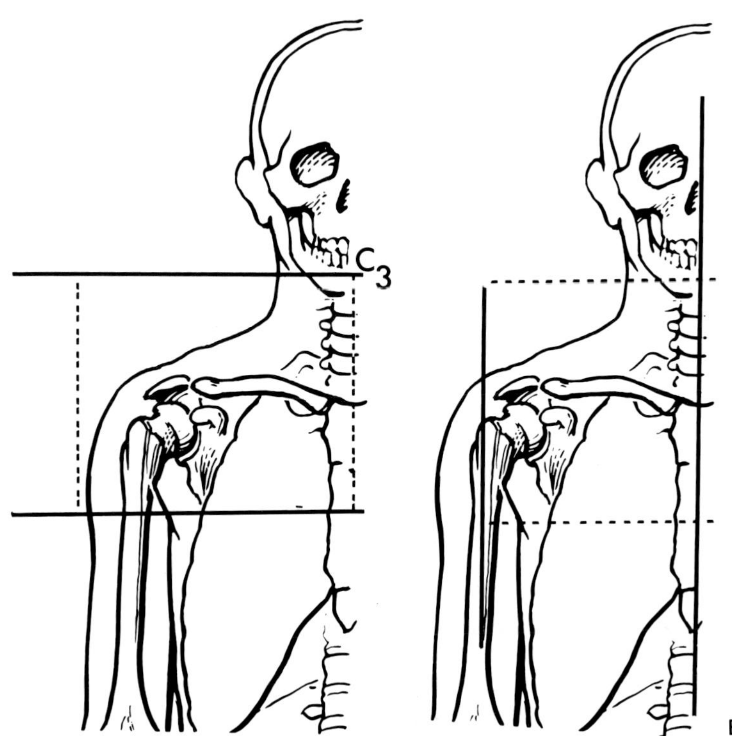

FIG. 9-7. Illustration of area studied with axial (**A**) and sagittal (**B**) imaging of the brachial plexus.

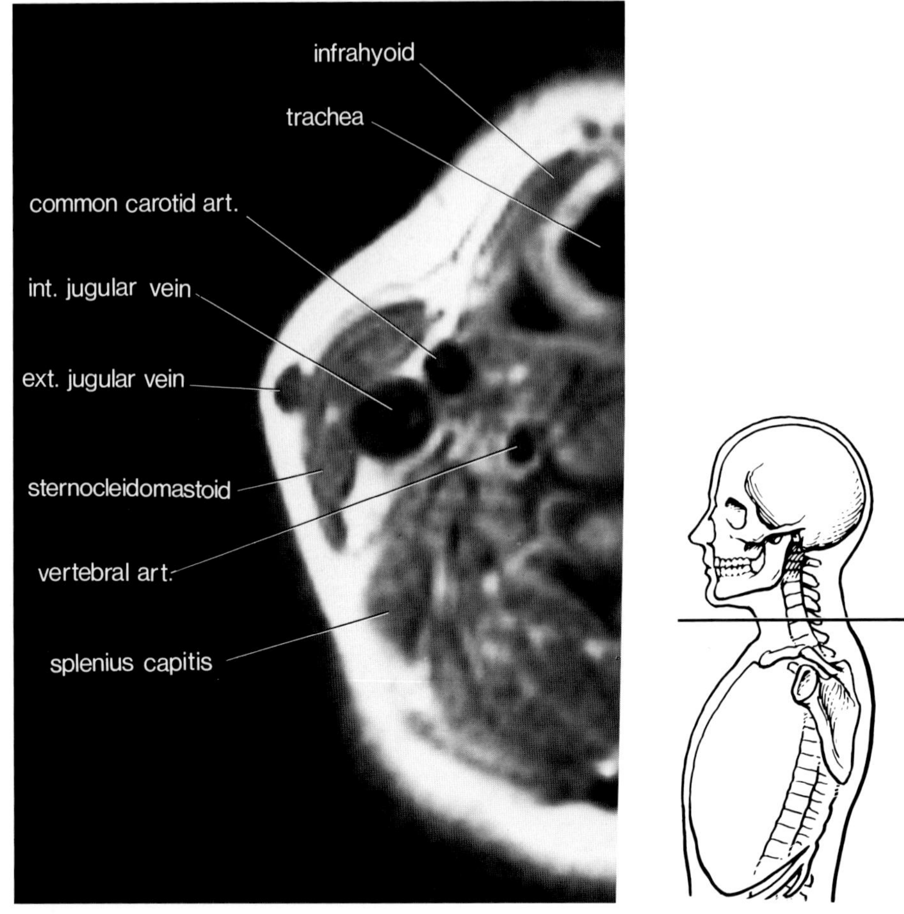

FIG. 9-8. Axial images of the brachial plexus region with illustrations for level. **A:** Axial image through the lower cervical region.

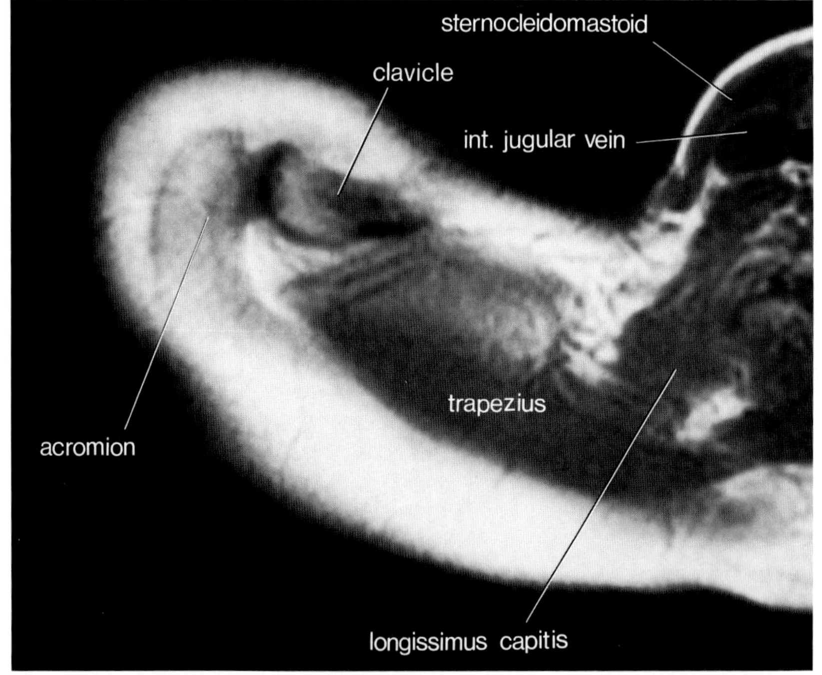

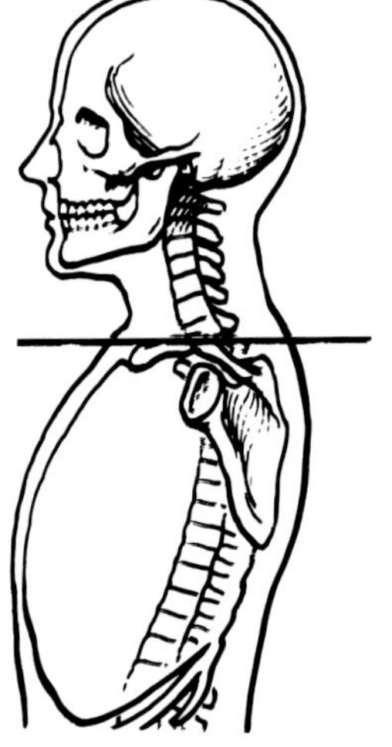

FIG. 9-8. B: Axial image at the base of the neck.

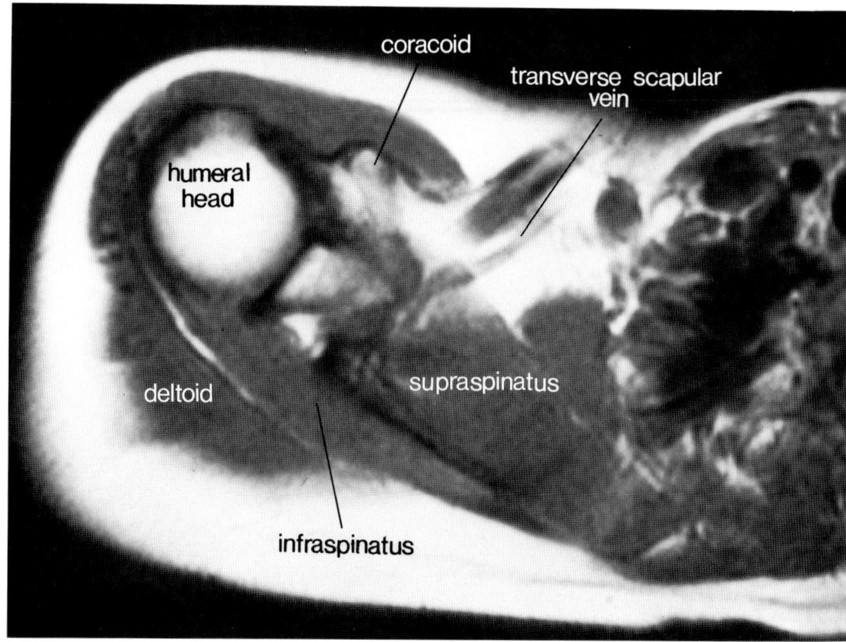

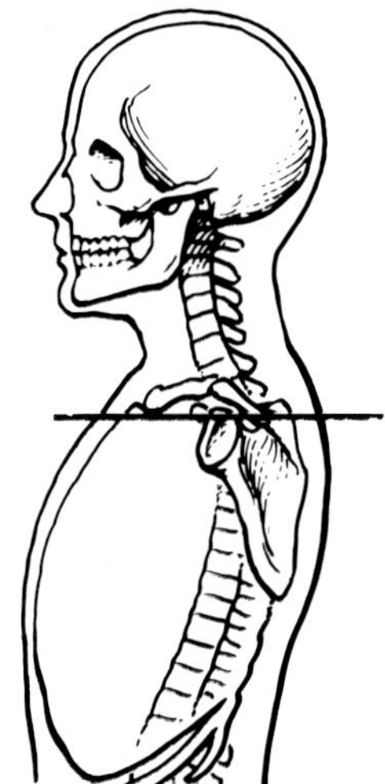

FIG. 9-8. C: Axial image through the upper humeral head.

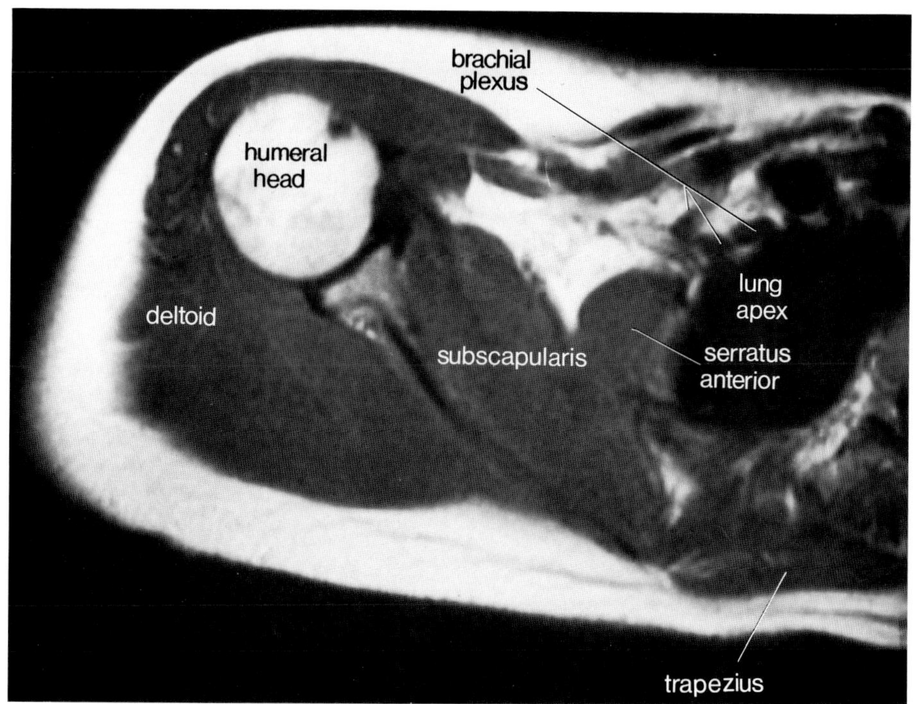

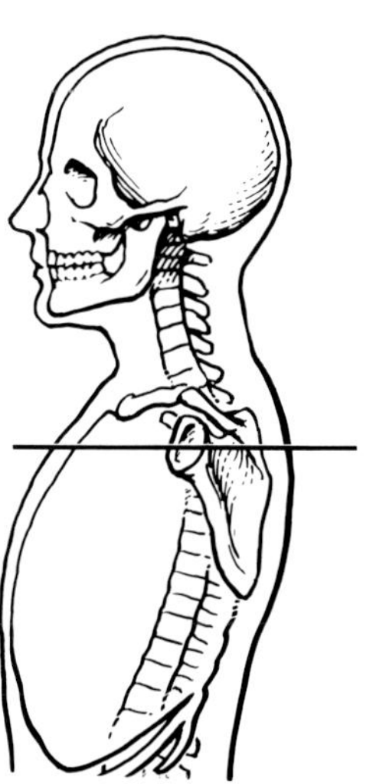

FIG. 9-8. D: Axial image through the glenohumeral level.

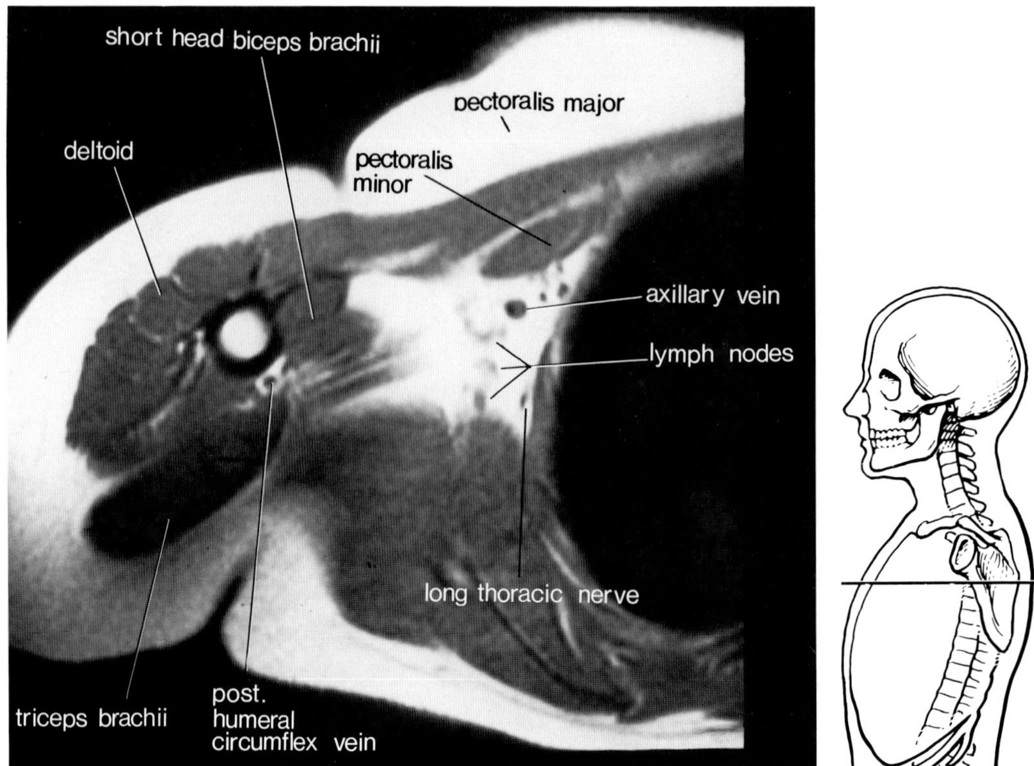

FIG. 9-8. E: Axial image through the upper arm and axilla.

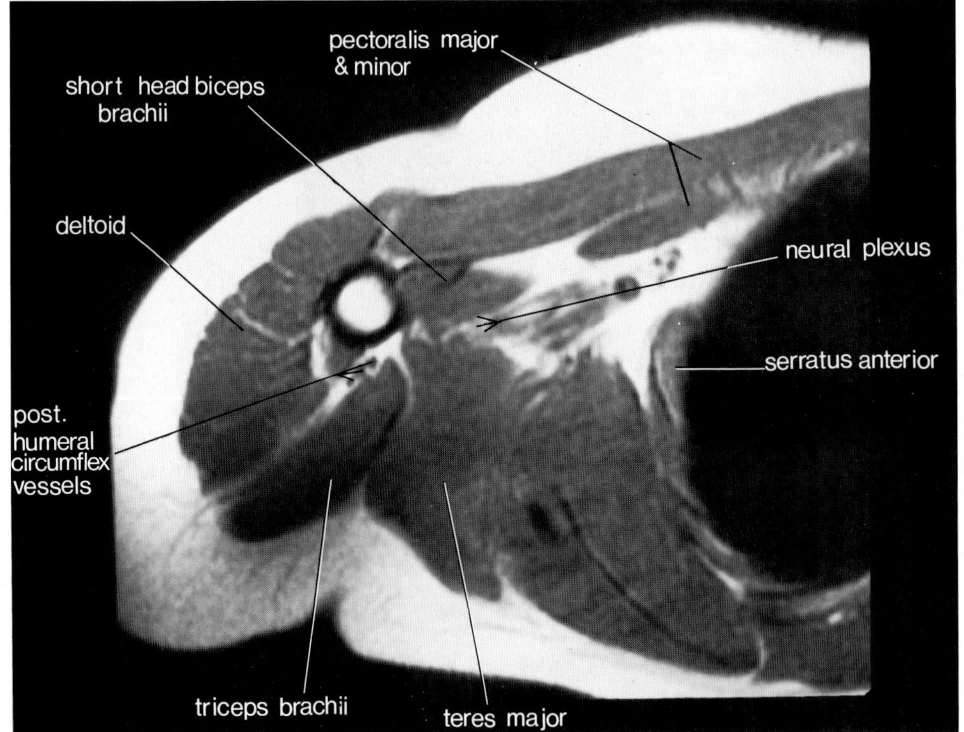

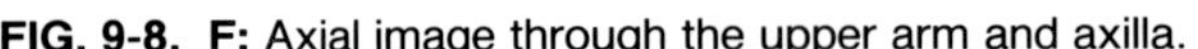

FIG. 9-8. F: Axial image through the upper arm and axilla.

G

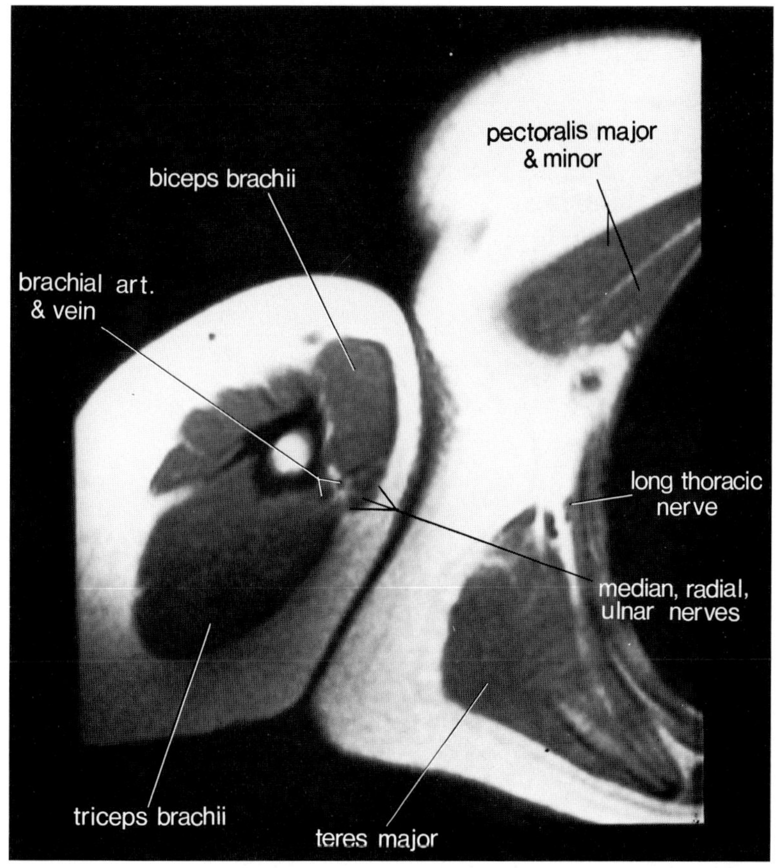

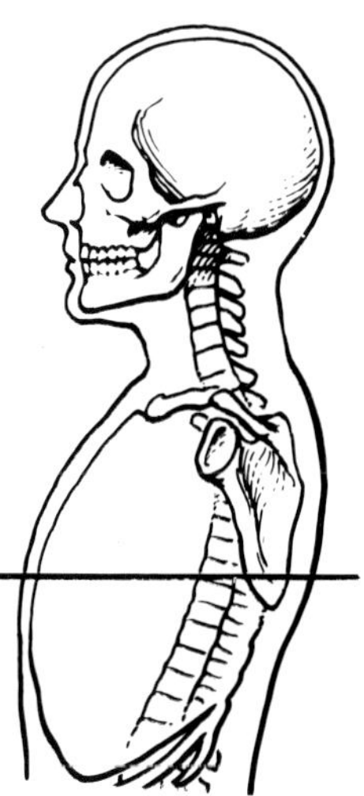

FIG. 9-8. G: Axial image through the upper humerus.

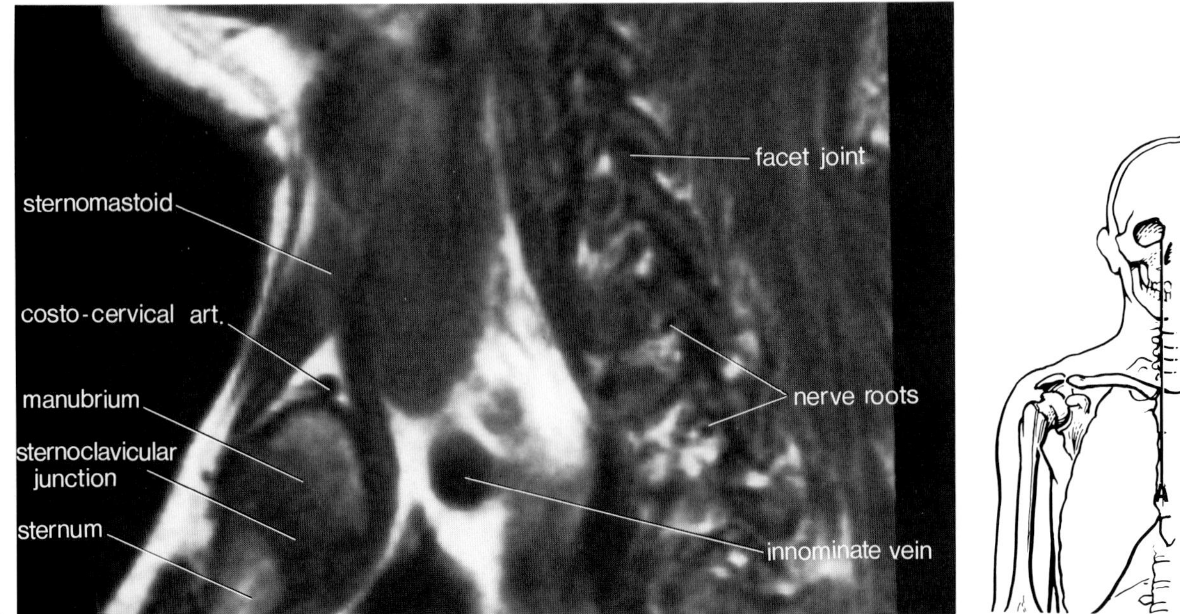

FIG. 9-9. Sagittal images of the brachial plexus region with illustration for level of section. **A:** Sagittal image through the facets and intervertebral foramina.

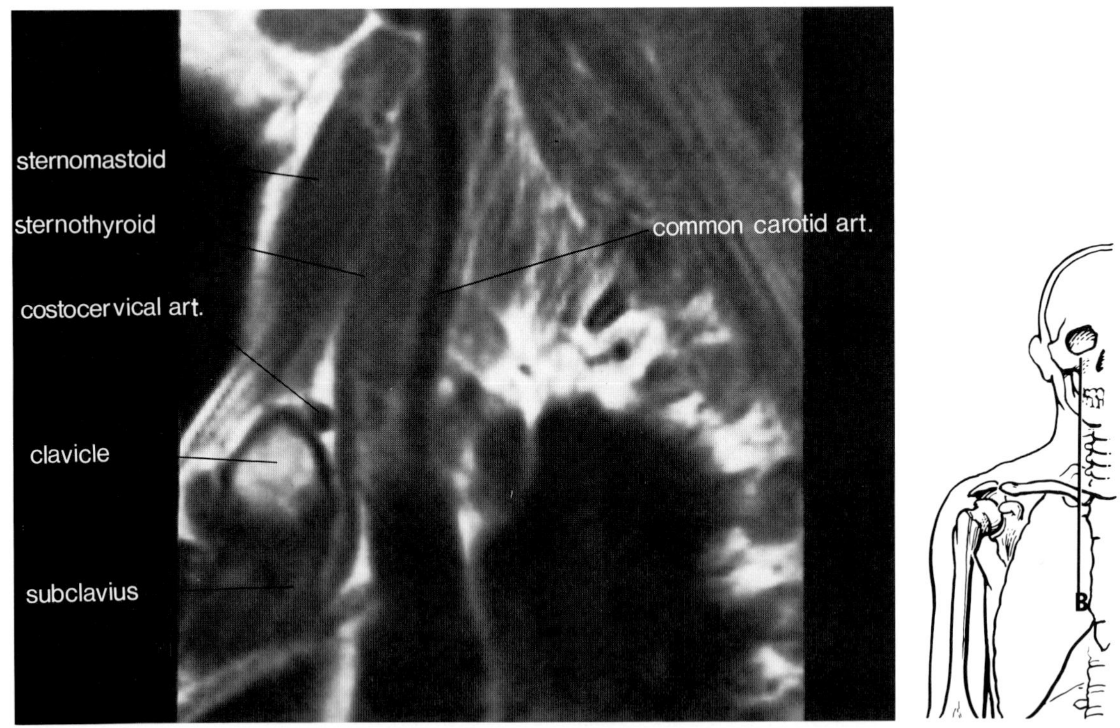

FIG. 9-9. B: Sagittal image through the carotid artery.

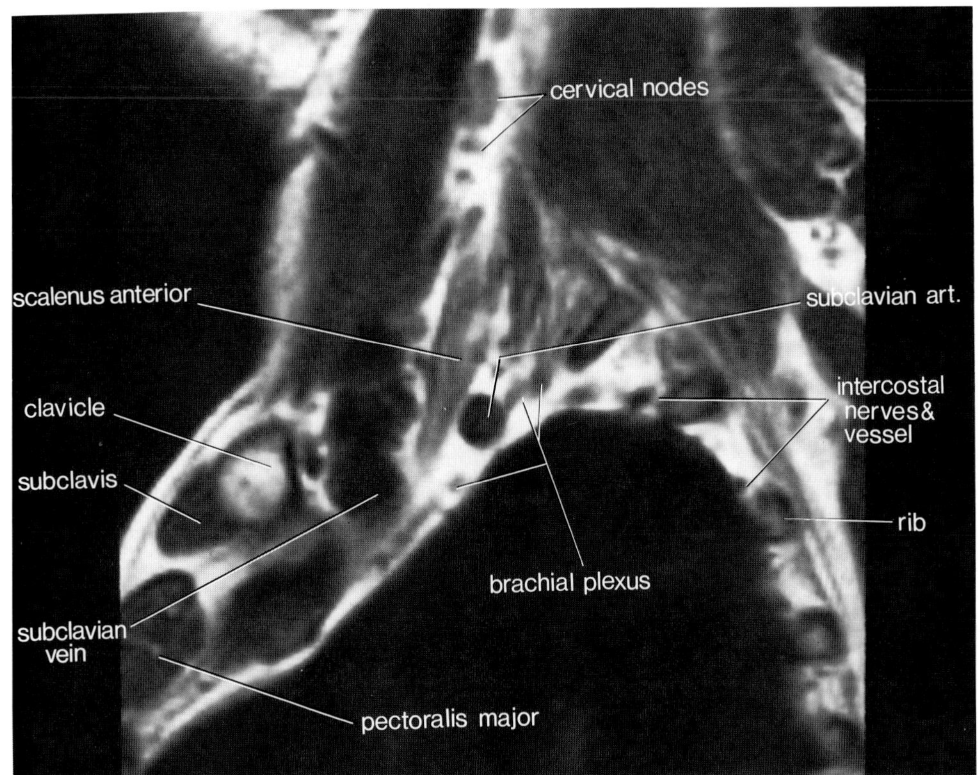

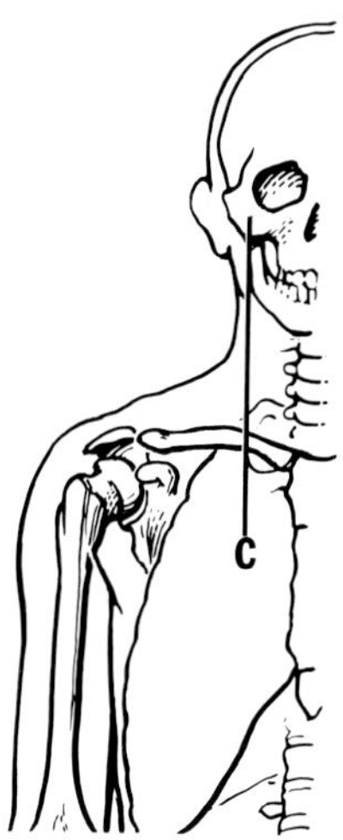

FIG. 9-9. C: Sagittal image through the lateral neck.

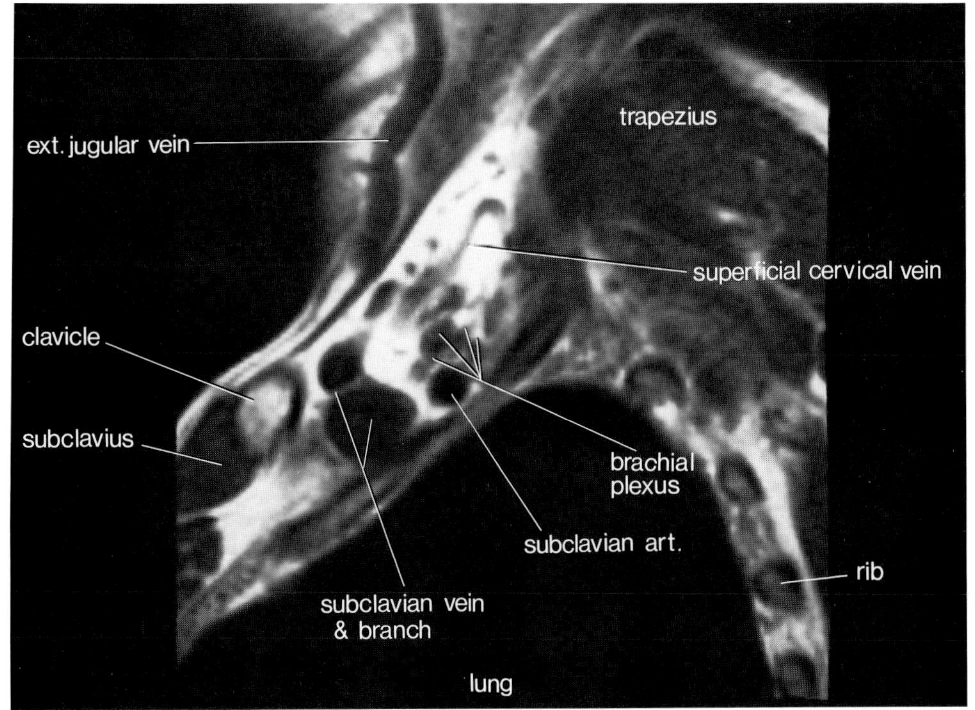

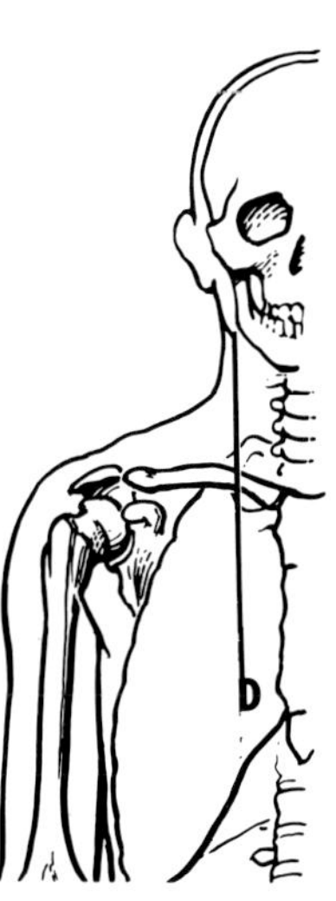

FIG. 9-9. D: Sagittal image through the external jugular vein region.

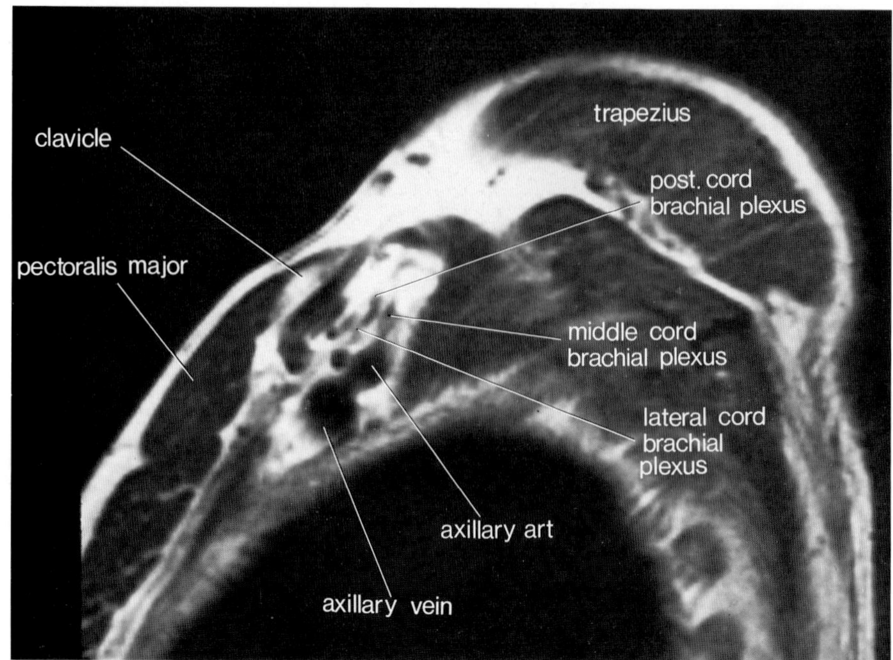

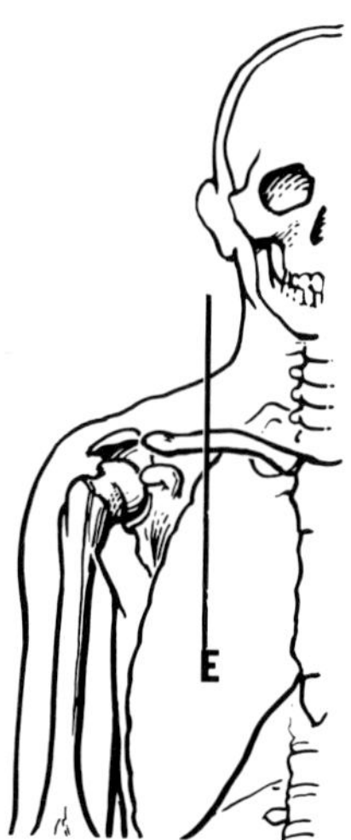

FIG. 9-9. E: Sagittal image through the lateral chest.

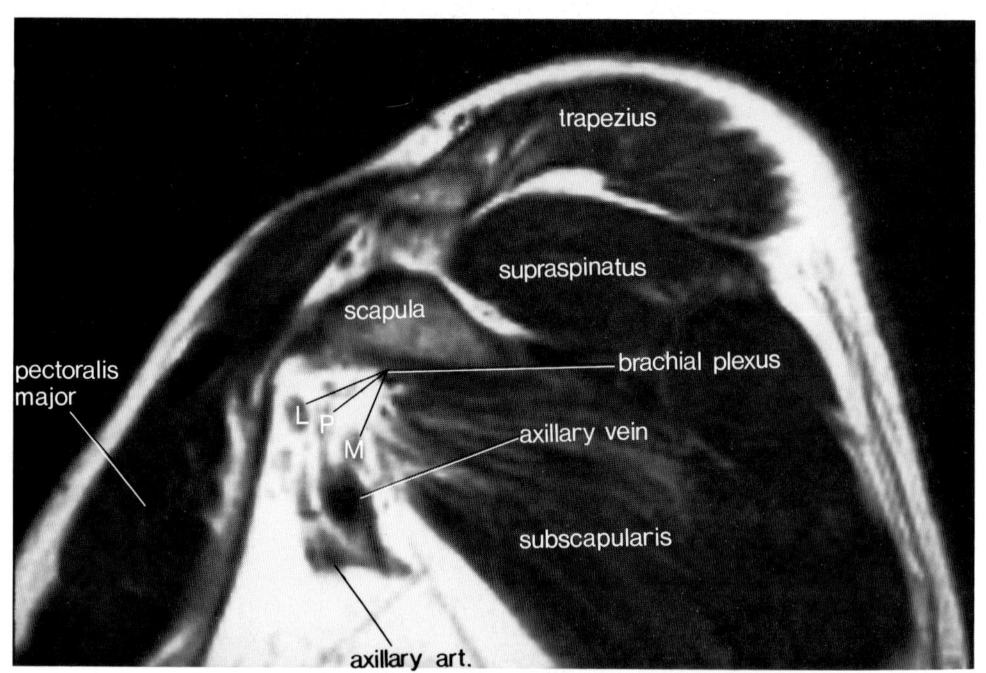

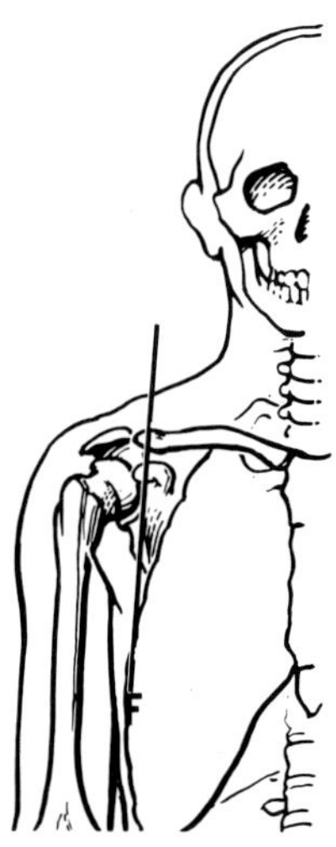

FIG. 9-9. F: Sagittal image through the lateral scapula.

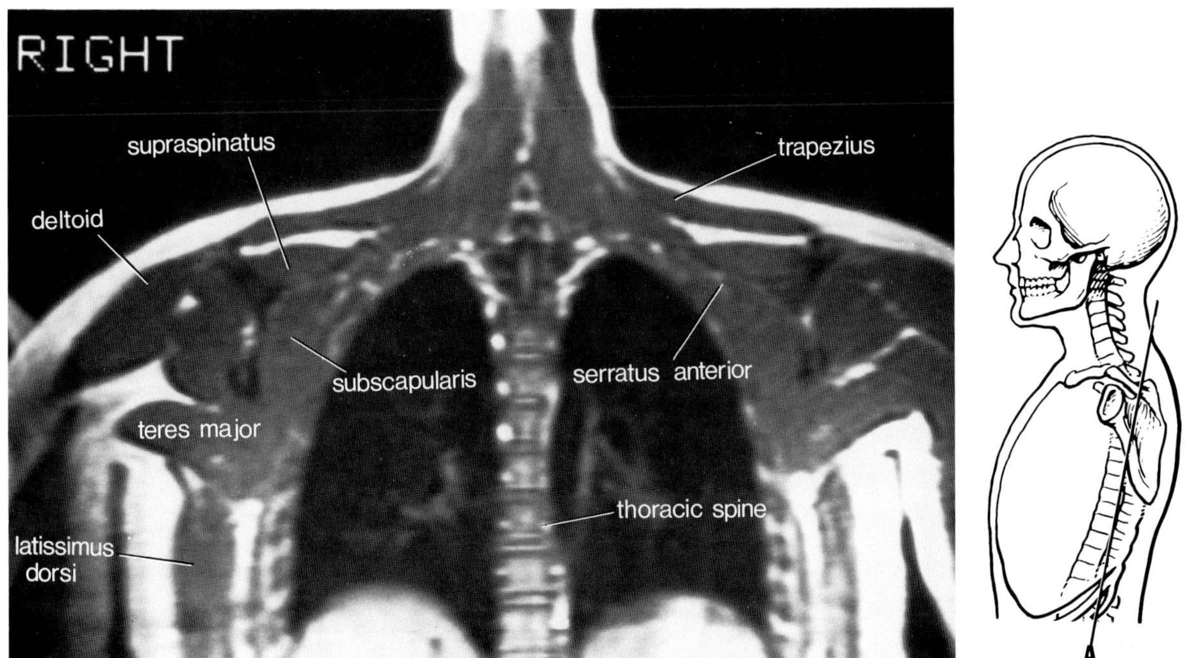

FIG. 9-10. Coronal images of neck and shoulders with illustrations for level of section. **A:** Coronal image through the thoracic spine.

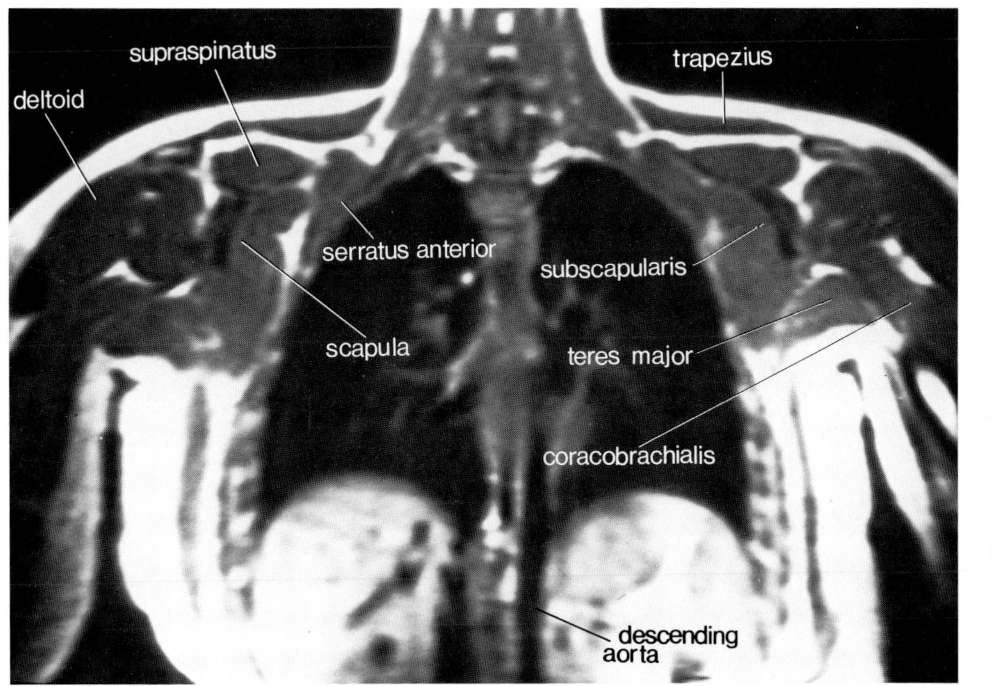

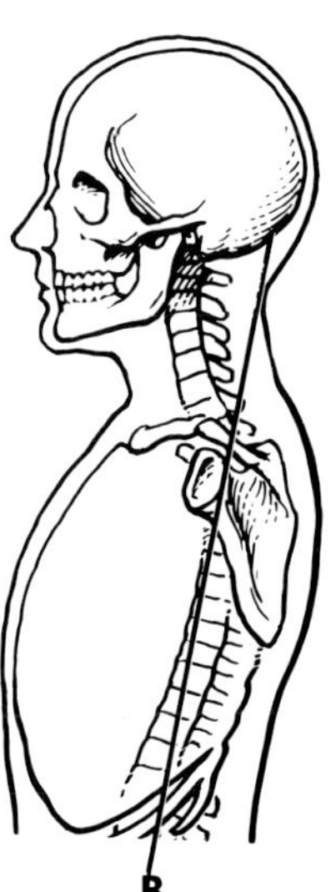

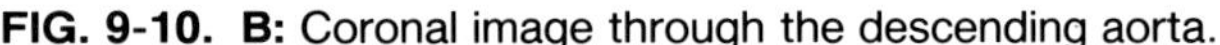
FIG. 9-10. B: Coronal image through the descending aorta.

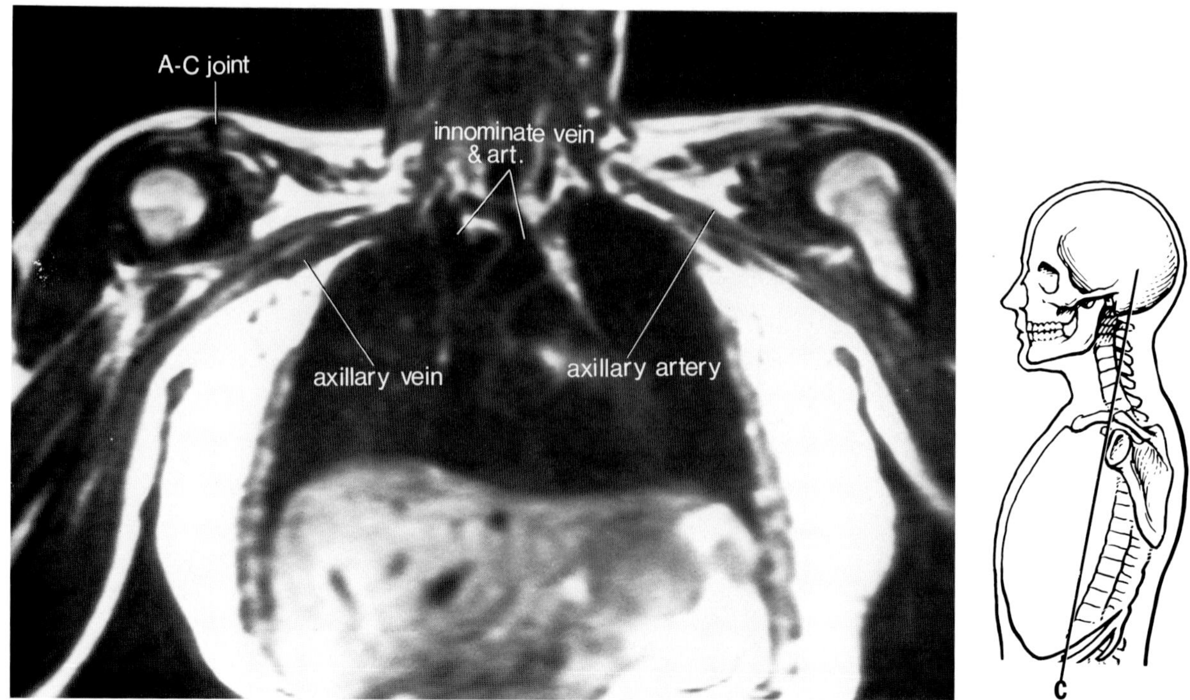

FIG. 9-10. C: Coronal image through the neurovascular region.

screening examination for brachial plexus pathology. In certain cases, coronal images (Fig. 9-10) or additional sequences may be needed. This is discussed more completely in the clinical applications section of this chapter.

ANATOMY

Osseous Anatomy

The shoulder is comprised of three bony structures—the clavicle, scapula, and humerus. The glenohumeral joint is a ball-and-socket joint. The humeral head is four times larger than the glenoid fossa of the scapula. This permits significant range of motion but also results in an increased susceptibility to instability. The majority of the muscles acting on the humerus are for adduction. Therefore, the clavicle and the sternoclavicular articulation provide important support in maintaining the muscular efficiency of the shoulder (3,34).

There are two main articulations in the shoulder region—the acromioclavicular joint and the glenohumeral joint (Fig. 9-11). The acromioclavicular joint is formed by the capsule about the clavicle and acromion and is lined with synovial fluid. In some cases the joint is divided by a small articular disk. Motion at this articulation is limited to slight gliding movements between the scapula and clavicle. Supporting structures between the acromion of the scapula and the distal clavicle include the acromioclavicular ligament and the coracoacromial ligament, which extends from the coracoid process to the undersurface of the acromion just distal to the acromioclavicular joint. The coracoclavicular ligament is divided into the conoid and trapezoid bands (Fig. 9-12).

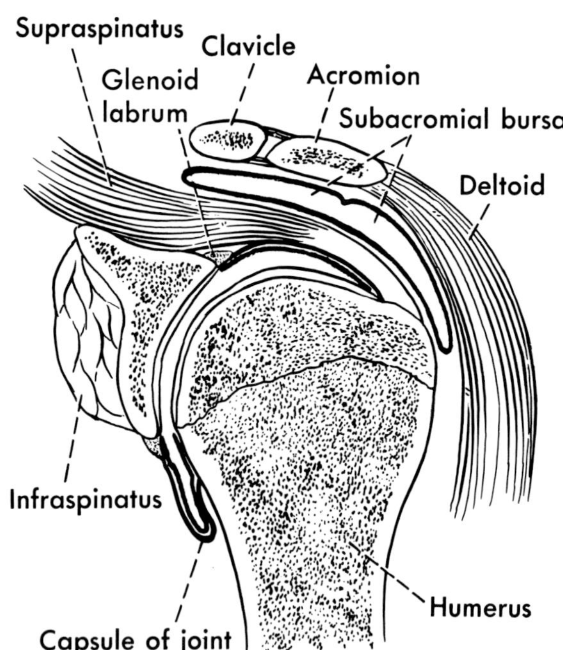

FIG. 9-11. Illustration of the shoulder, demonstrating the glenohumeral and acromioclavicular joints and surrounding structures. (From ref. 34, with permission.)

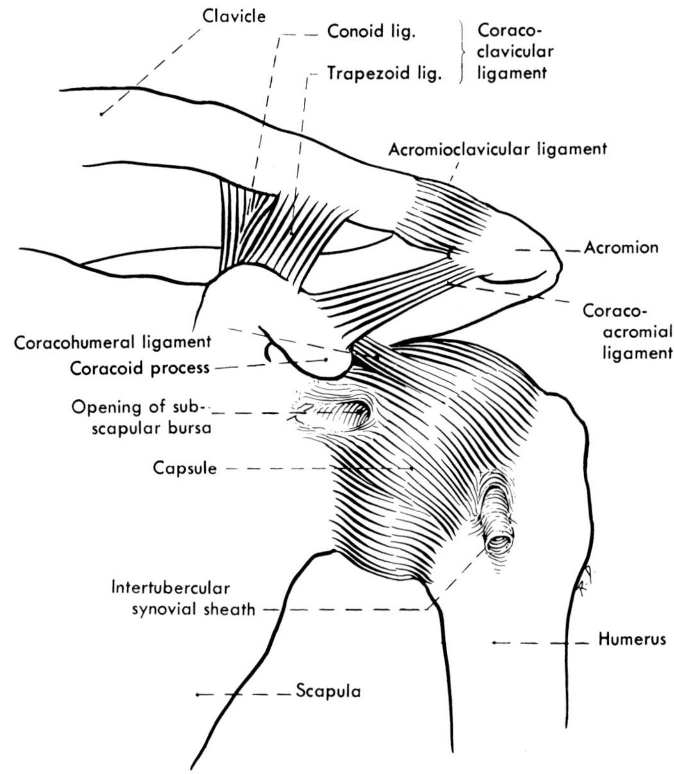

FIG. 9-12. Illustration of the ligaments of the shoulder. (From ref. 34, with permission.)

These ligaments prevent upper displacement of the clavicle by the muscle forces of the trapezius and sternocleidomastoid muscles (2,34,39).

The glenohumeral articulation is formed by the shallow glenoid cavity, which is surrounded by a cartilaginous labrum or lip (Fig. 9-13). This labrum is composed of fibrocartilage similar to the meniscus in the knee and is therefore seen as a triangular dark or low-intensity structure on MR images (Figs. 9-4 to 9-6). The labrum is somewhat blunted or rounded posteriorly and generally more triangular and sharper appearing anteriorly (89). The capsule of the shoulder is lined with synovial membrane, which arises from the margin of the glenoid labrum and extends around the head of the humerus anteriorly and posteriorly where it attaches at about the level of the physeal line or anatomic neck. The capsule therefore usually closely approximates the margins of the articular cartilage of the humeral head (Fig. 9-14). There are variations in the anterior capsular attachment that may play a role in recurrent dislocations. Type I attaches in or near the labrum (Fig. 9-15). Types II and III attach to the scapula more proximally. Capsules that attach more medially (type IV) either predispose or are the result of recurrent dislocations (93). The synovial membrane continues between the greater and lesser tuberosities, forming a sheath for the long head of the biceps tendon. This sheath extends for variable lengths into the upper arm. Extension of the tendon sheath distal to the groove should not be confused with disruption (3). The synovium also extends through a small defect in the capsule anteriorly to form the subscapular or subcoracoid bursa (Fig. 9-14) (2,3,34,93).

The capsule of the shoulder is supported by several areas of thickening or fibrous capsular ligaments (Figs.

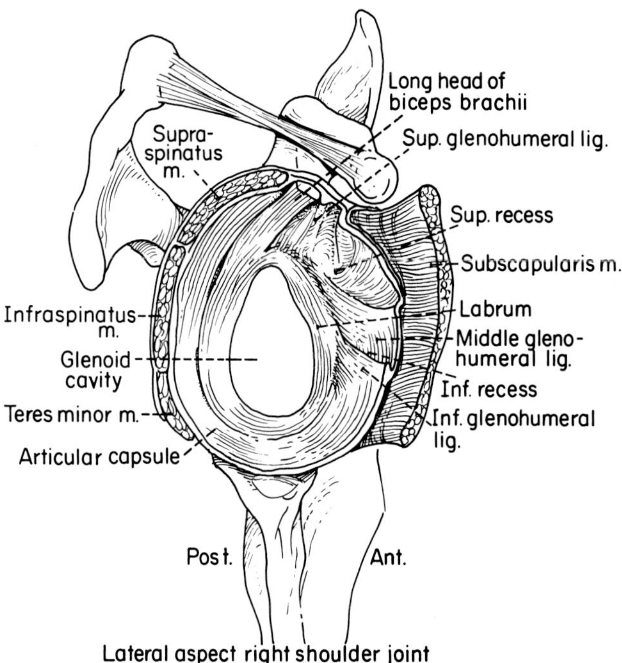

FIG. 9-13. Illustration of the shoulder, demonstrating the glenoid articular surface, labrum, and supporting structures. (From ref. 57a, with permission.)

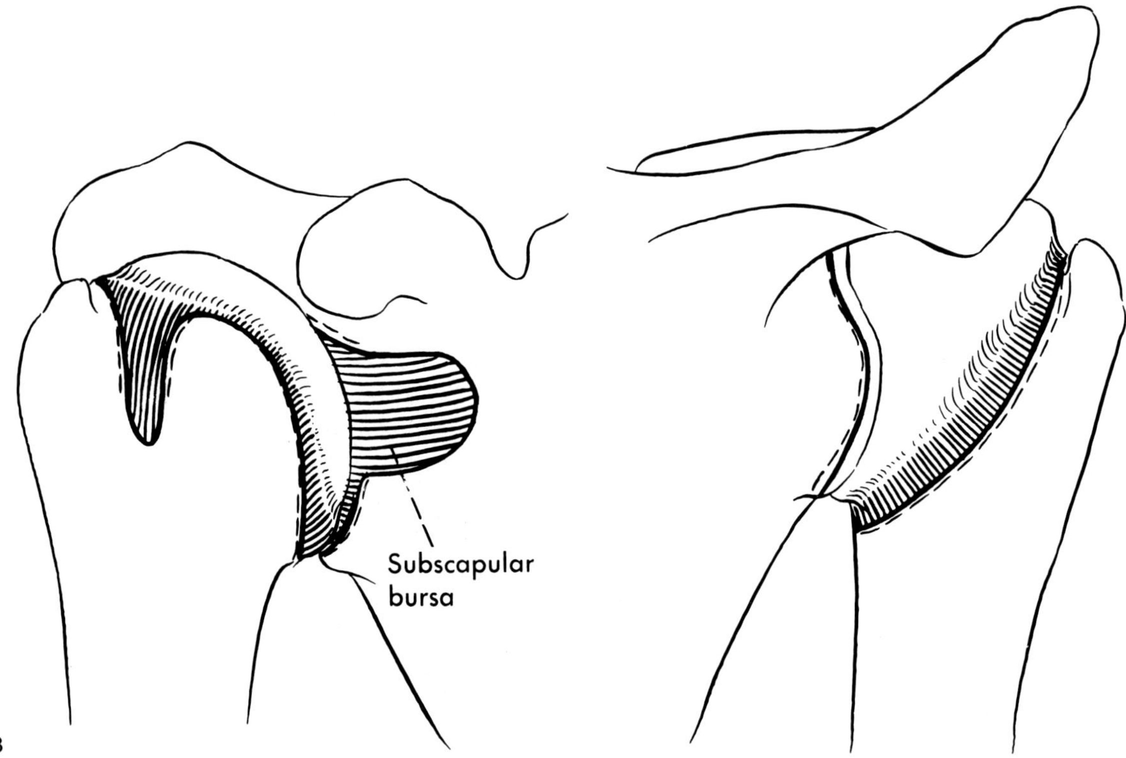

FIG. 9-14. Illustration of capsular attachments of the shoulder as seen anteriorly (**A**) and posteriorly (**B**). (From ref. 34, with permission.)

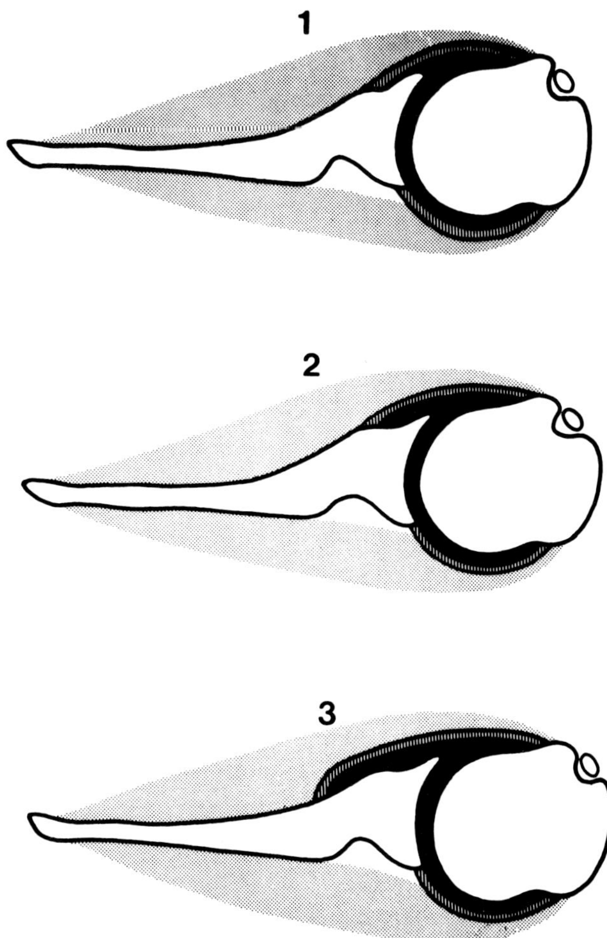

FIG. 9-15. Illustration of variations in the anterior capsular attachments. Type I, in or near anterior glenoid labrum; type II, along scapular neck; type III, medial to glenoid neck. (From ref. 93, with permission.)

9-12 and 9-13). The most consistent of these ligaments is the coracohumeral ligament (Fig. 9-12), which is a strong band arising from the most lateral edge of the coracoid process and extending over the superior aspect of the shoulder to attach to the greater tuberosity. The glenohumeral ligaments vary in thickness and may be difficult to appreciate on MR images (Figs. 9-4 and 9-13). The inferior glenohumeral ligament is usually the most obvious. It extends from the middle anterior margin of the glenoid labrum to the lower medial aspect of the humeral neck. The middle glenohumeral ligament is attached somewhat superior to this, extending from both the labrum and the coracoid and attaching to the anterior aspect of the lesser tuberosity (Fig. 9-13). The superior glenohumeral ligament arises at the same level as the middle glenohumeral ligament and extends in a parallel manner to the middle glenohumeral ligament (Fig. 9-13). The transverse ligament extends across the greater and lesser tuberosities, enclosing the synovial sheath and long head of the biceps tendon (2,15,34).

Muscular Anatomy

There are numerous muscles that act on the scapula, shoulder, and glenohumeral articulation. The most important of these, from a clinical standpoint, are the intrinsic muscles of the shoulder comprised of the deltoid and rotator cuff group. The deltoid is a large muscle covering the shoulder superficially, which arises from the lateral third of the clavicle, the acromion, and the spine of the scapula (Figs. 9-4 to 9-6 and 9-16). The fibers of the deltoid all converge distally and laterally to insert on the deltoid tuberosity on the lateral aspect of the upper humerus (Fig. 9-16). The deltoid serves as a powerful abductor of the humerus (2,34) (Table 9-2).

The supraspinatus muscle (Figs. 9-4 to 9-6 and 9-16B) is a critical muscle and tendon unit in evaluating patients with rotator cuff tears (3,90–92). The supraspinatus muscle arises from the supraspinous fossa of the scapula and is covered by the trapezius in its proximal portion. As the muscle extends peripherally, it passes under the acromion, coracoclavicular ligament, and AC joint (Fig. 9-6) to insert on the most superior of the three facets of the greater tuberosity. The tendon of the supraspinatus is broad, covering the top of the shoulder and blending with the capsule superiorly. The primary function of the supraspinatus is to assist the deltoid in abduction of the humerus (2,34,54,72,75) (Table 9-2).

The infraspinatus arises from the infraspinous fossa of the scapula (Fig. 9-16B). As it passes laterally, it is often separated from the scapula by a bursa that sometimes communicates with the shoulder joint (Table 9-3). The infraspinatus is separated from the supraspinatus by the scapular spine (Fig. 9-16B). Its tendon forms the upper posterior portion of the rotator cuff and inserts in the greater tuberosity posterior and inferior to the supraspinatus tendon (2,34,40,43).

The teres minor arises from the middle half of the lateral scapular border and extends in an oblique upward direction to insert as a large flat tendon on the most posterior and inferior of the three facets of the greater tuberosity (Fig. 9-16B). Like the infraspinatus, the teres minor is primarily an external rotator of the humerus (2,34).

Along with the supraspinatus, infraspinatus, and teres minor, the subscapularis makes up the fourth of the rotator cuff muscles (3,34). The subscapularis arises from the anterior subscapular surface of the scapula with its fibers converging and extending laterally to insert in a broad tendon or band along with the capsule on the lesser tuberosity of the humerus and the crest below

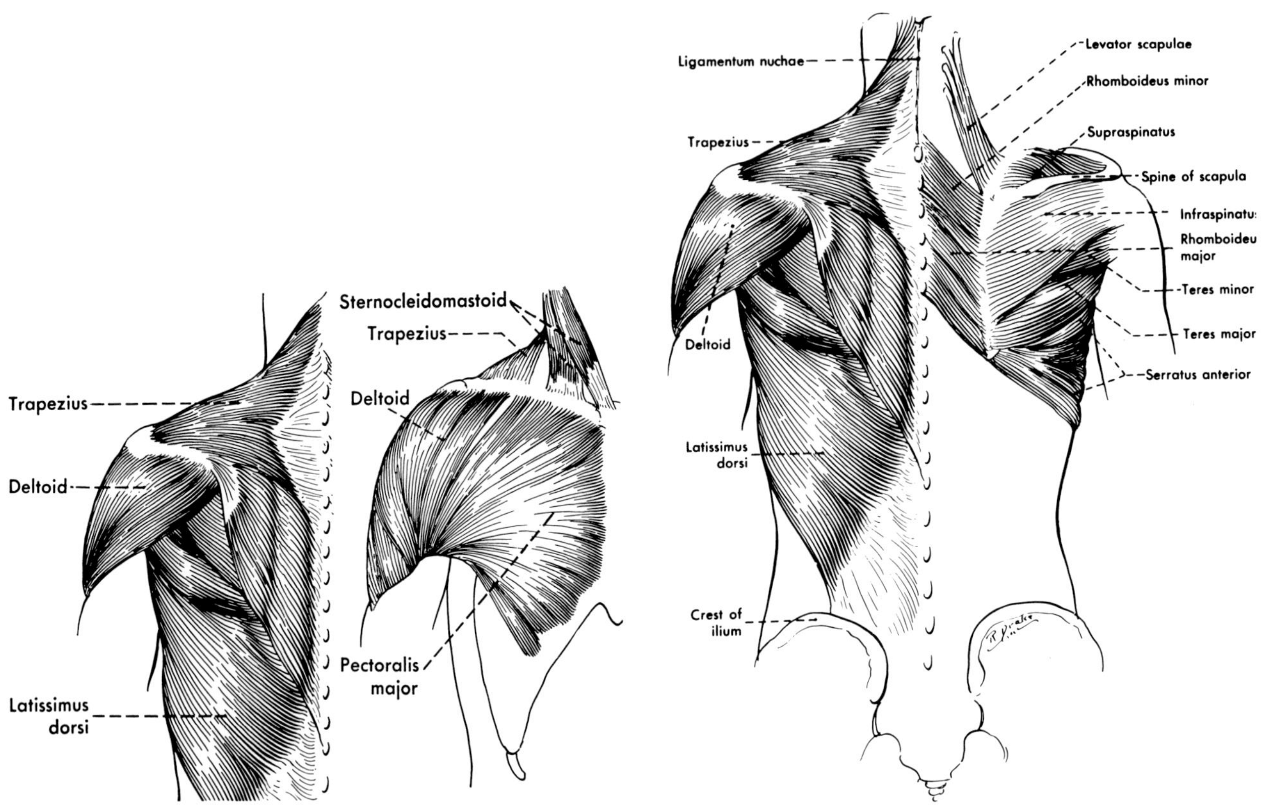

FIG. 9-16. Illustration of the extrinsic shoulder muscles from anterior (**A**) and posterior (**B**). (From ref. 34, with permission.)

TABLE 9-2. *Muscles of the shoulder and upper arm* (2,34)

Muscles	Origin	Insertion	Action	Innervation
Intrinsic				
Deltoid	Lateral clavicle, acromion, scapular spine	Deltoid tuberosity humerus	Abductor of humerus	Axillary nerve (C5,C6)
Supraspinatus	Supraspinous fossa of scapula	Greater tuberosity superiorly	Abductor of humerus	Suprascapular nerve (C5,C6)
Infraspinatus	Infraspinous fossa of scapula	Posterior inferior greater tuberosity	Lateral rotation of humerus	Suprascapular nerve (C5,C6)
Teres minor	Lateral midscapular border	Lateral inferior facet, greater tuberosity	External rotator of humerus	Axillary nerve (C5,C6)
Subscapularis	Suprascapular fossa	Lesser tuberosity	Internal rotator of humerus	Subscapular nerves (C5–C7)
Teres major	Inferior lateral scapula	Medial intertubercular groove	Internal rotation, adduction, extensor of humerus	Subscapular nerve (C5–C6)
Extrinsic				
Trapezius	Ligamentum nuchae, thoracic spinous processes	Distal clavicle, acromion, scapular spine	Retractor and elevator of scapula	Spinal accessory and C2,C3
Latissimus dorsi	Spinous processes T6–T12, lumbar, upper sacrum	Medial intertubercular groove	Adductor, internal rotator and extensor of humerus	Thoracodorsal nerve (C6–C8)
Levator scapulae	Posterior tubercles, C1–C4 transverse processes	Upper medial scapula	Elevates medial scapula	Cervical plexus (C3–C4)
Rhomboideus major	C2–T5 spinous processes	Posterior medial scapula	Retractor of scapula	Dorsal scapular nerve (C5)
Rhombodeus minor	Ligamentum nuchae C7 and T1 spinous processes	Posterior medial scapula at base of scapular spine		
Serratus anterior	Anterior ribs 1–9	Anterior medial scapula	Protractor, anterior drawing of scapula	Long thoracic nerve (C5–C7)
Pectoral region				
Pectoralis major	Inferomedial clavicle, sternum and costochondral junctions	Lateral intertubercular groove	Adductor of humerus	Medial and lateral anterior thoracic nerves (C5–T1)
Pectoralis minor	Anterior ribs 2–5	Coracoid of scapula	Depresses angle of scapula	Medial pectoral nerve (C8–T1)
Subclavius	Anteromedial first rib	Midinferior clavicle	Stabilizes sternoclavicular joint	Subclavian nerve

TABLE 9-3. *Shoulder bursae* (2,3,34)

Bursa	Location	Normal joint communication
Subscapular	Between subscapulosus tendon and capsule	Yes
Infraspinatus	Between capsule and infraspinatus tendon	Inconsistent
Subdeltoid	Between deltoid and rotator cuff	No
Subacromial	Between acromion and rotator cuff (usually contiguous with subdeltoid)	No
Subcoracoid	Between coracoid and subscapularis (may be contiguous with subacromial)	No
Coracobrachialis	Between coracobrachialis and subscapularis	No
Latissimus dorsi	Between latissimus and teres major	No
Teres major	Between teres and humeral insertion	No
Pectoralis major	Between pectoralis and humeral insertion	No

From ref. 3, with permission.

this tuberosity (Figs. 9-4 to 9-6 and 9-13). This large triangular-shaped muscle forms the posterior wall of the axilla with the axillary vessels and brachial plexus passing across and anterior to the muscle. The subscapularis bursa or recess lies between the muscle and the neck of the scapula and can communicate with the shoulder joint (Fig. 9-14A) (Table 9-3). The primary function of the subscapularis is internal rotation of the humerus (2,34) (Table 9-2).

The teres major (Fig. 9-16B) arises on the dorsal aspect of the scapula from its lower lateral border and extends anteriorly to insert below the subscapularis on the medial aspect of the intertubercular groove. The teres major is an additional internal rotator of the humerus and when acting with the latissimus dorsi also serves as an extensor and adductor of the humerus. The muscle is innervated by the subscapular nerve, which receives its branches from the C5–C6 levels (34).

The extrinsic muscles of the shoulder arise from the vertebral column or thoracic cage and attach to the scapula or humerus (Fig. 9-16). Two of these muscles—the trapezius and latissimus dorsi—completely cover the deep musculature of the back as they course to insert in the shoulder region (Fig. 9-16). The trapezius has a long broad origin from the upper superior nuchal line of the occipital bone, ligamentum nuchae, and upper thoracic spinous processes (Fig. 9-16). The upper fibers insert on the posterior superior aspect of the distal clavicle, while the middle fibers insert more inferiorly on the border of the acromion and spine of the scapula. The lower fibers insert on a more clearly defined tendon at the base of the scapular spine. There is commonly a small bursa between the tendon of the lower fibers and the spine of the scapula (Fig. 9-3). The trapezius serves as a retractor of the scapula and an elevator of the scapula. It is innervated by the accessory spinal nerve and roots from C3 and C4 (2,34).

The latissimus dorsi is a second very broad-based muscle taking its origin from the lower six thoracic spinous processes and the spinous processes of the lumbar and upper sacral vertebrae (Figs. 9-10 and 9-16). Superiorly, the muscle's origin is covered by the lower fibers of the trapezius. This broad triangular muscle extends superiorly to its insertion along the medial wall of the intertubercular or bicipital groove. There is a bursa between the tendons of latissimus dorsi and the teres major that, when inflamed, can be seen as an area of well-defined high intensity on MR images. The chief actions of the latissimus dorsi are adduction, internal rotation, and extension of the humerus. The muscle is supplied by the thoracodorsal nerve with roots from C6 through C8 (2,34) (Table 9-2).

The levator scapulae (Fig. 9-16) arises from the posterior tubercles of the upper first through fourth transverse processes of the cervical spine. The muscle then passes in an oblique posteroinferior direction to insert on the superior angle of the medial scapular border. It is deep to the sternocleidomastoid superiorly and trapezius inferiorly. The main function of this muscle is to elevate the scapular border. The muscle is innervated by the deep cervical plexus from the third and fourth roots (2,34) (Table 9-2).

The rhomboid muscles (Fig. 9-16) are often divided into minor and major groups; however, in reality, especially on MR images, the muscle is difficult to separate into two groups. The muscles take a broad origin from the ligamentum nuchae and spinous processes of C2 through T5 to pass laterally and insert on the posterior medial aspect of the scapula near the base of the scapular spine. The chief functions of these muscles are to retract the scapula, and they are innervated by the dorsoscapular nerve, which is primarily derived from the C5 root (2,34) (Table 9-2).

The serratus anterior (Figs. 9-8 and 9-10) is a large flat muscle that covers the thoracic cage laterally and acts primarily on the scapula. It arises from the outer surfaces of the proximal eight or nine ribs and extends around the lateral aspect of the thoracic cage to insert on the anterior medial aspect of the scapula. The chief function of this muscle is to protract or draw the scapula anteriorly. The muscle is supplied by the long thoracic nerve, which typically arises from cervical nerves (2,34) (Table 9-2).

Three muscles constitute the musculature of the pectoral region. These include the pectoralis major, pectoralis minor, and subclavius muscles (Figs. 9-8 and 9-9). The pectoralis major is a large triangular- or fan-shaped muscle covering much of the upper thorax. The pectoralis major has an extensive origin from the medial inferior aspect of the clavicle, the lateral margin of the sternum, and the chondral junctions of the upper ribs. The fibers of this muscle converge to form a broad tendon that passes just anterior to coracobrachialis and biceps brachii. The muscle then passes deep to the anterior margin of the deltoid to insert on the crest of the greater tubercle or lateral aspect of the intertubercular groove. The pectoralis major is a strong adductor of the humerus and is innervated by two nerves, the lateral and medial (anterior thoracic) nerves (2,34) (Table 9-2).

The pectoralis minor is deep to the pectoralis major and arises from the anterior aspects of the second through fifth ribs. The muscle passes in a superior and oblique direction to insert on the coracoid process of the scapula. Its chief action is to depress the angle of the scapula. Nerve supply is via the medial pectoral nerve (C8–T1) (2,34) (Table 9-2).

The subclavius (Fig. 9-9) is a small muscle that takes its origin from the junction of the first rib and its articular cartilage and passes upward and laterally to insert on the inferior aspect of the midclavicle. This muscle is covered by the pectoralis major and is innervated by a small branch of the subclavian nerve. It is often seen as a small intermediate-density structure beneath the clavicle on the sagittal images and should not be confused with a soft tissue mass (2,34) (Table 9-2).

Bursae

There are numerous bursae about the shoulder that are of importance in identification and excluding significant pathology. Table 9-3 summarizes these bursae and their locations. It is important to note that the subscapular bursa normally communicates with the shoulder joint. The infraspinatus bursa inconsistently communicates with the shoulder joint, and the remaining bursa should not, in normal patients, communicate with the glenohumeral joint (3). The most important of these bursae are the subdeltoid and subacromial bursae (Fig. 9-11), which are normally contiguous, do not communicate with the shoulder joint, but can be inflamed. Inflammation does not generally occur in the absence of impingement and rotator cuff tear (3,40,54, 72,75,90–92).

Neurovascular Anatomy

Because of its complexity and significant clinical implications, the brachial plexus is discussed separately from the arterial and venous anatomy of the shoulder and upper arm. The brachial plexus (Figs. 9-9 and 9-17) arises from the anterior rami of the fifth, sixth, seventh, and eighth cervical and first thoracic nerves. In some

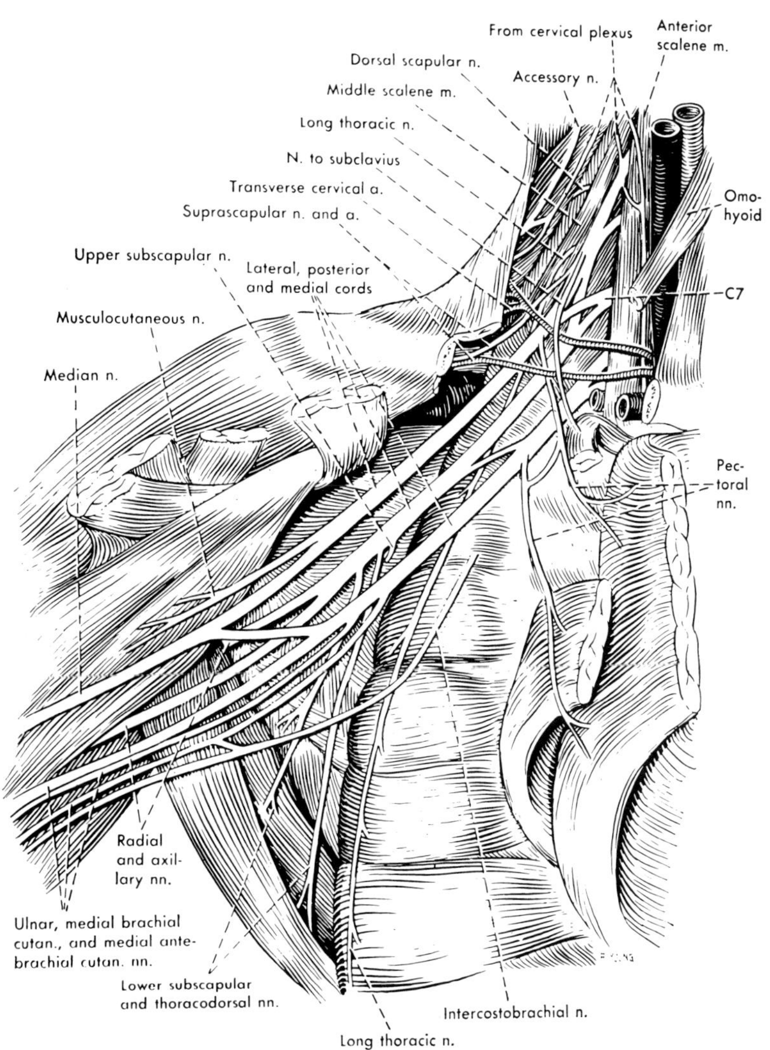

FIG. 9-17. Illustration of the brachial plexus and branches. (From ref. 34, with permission.)

situations C4 also forms a portion of the brachial plexus. In most situations the C5 and C6 roots form the upper, C7 the middle, and C8 and T1 the lower trunks of the brachial plexus. Each trunk then divides to form anterior and posterior divisions. The anterior divisions of the upper and middle trunks form the lateral cord (Figs. 9-9 and 9-17). The anterior division of the lower trunk continues as the medial cord (Figs. 9-9 and 9-17). The posterior divisions of the upper, middle, and lower trunks unite to form the posterior cord (Figs. 9-9 and 9-17). The branches arising from these cords are demonstrated in Fig. 9-17. Sagittal MR images usually clearly define the nerve roots as they exit the intervertebral foramen (Fig. 9-9). As one passes peripherally, it is more difficult to identify the individual cords and branches of the brachial plexus. However, there are certain relationships that can easily be identified and followed on contiguous MR sections (2,8,34,69).

In the lower neck, the brachial plexus lies above the subclavian artery, except for the lower trunk, which lies posterior to this vessel. This relationship is maintained as the brachial plexus crosses the first rib and enters the axilla. Upon entering the axillary region, the brachial plexus is more closely grouped to the axillary artery and vein (Fig. 9-18). At this level the lateral cord and a major portion of the posterior cord lie lateral and superior to the axillary artery. The lower trunk of the medial cord is posterior to the artery with the major continuation of the other groups closely approximated to the vessel (Figs. 9-9 and 9-18). On sagittal images this forms a closely approximated group of low-intensity structures (Fig. 9-9) (2,8,34,69).

Figure 9-19 demonstrates the major vascular supply of the shoulder. The subclavian artery along with the transverse cervical and subscapular arteries is generally clearly demonstrated on MR images. These are most easily demonstrated in the coronal plane (Fig. 9-10C). The smaller branch vessels are more difficult to identify on conventional spin-echo sequences. However, new reconstruction techniques using GRASS images clearly define the major branch vessels including the circumflex vessels, thoracodorsal artery, and other branch vessels around the glenohumeral articulation. The nerve branches of the brachial plexus generally closely follow the courses of the subclavian and axillary artery branches (Fig. 9-18) (2,15,34).

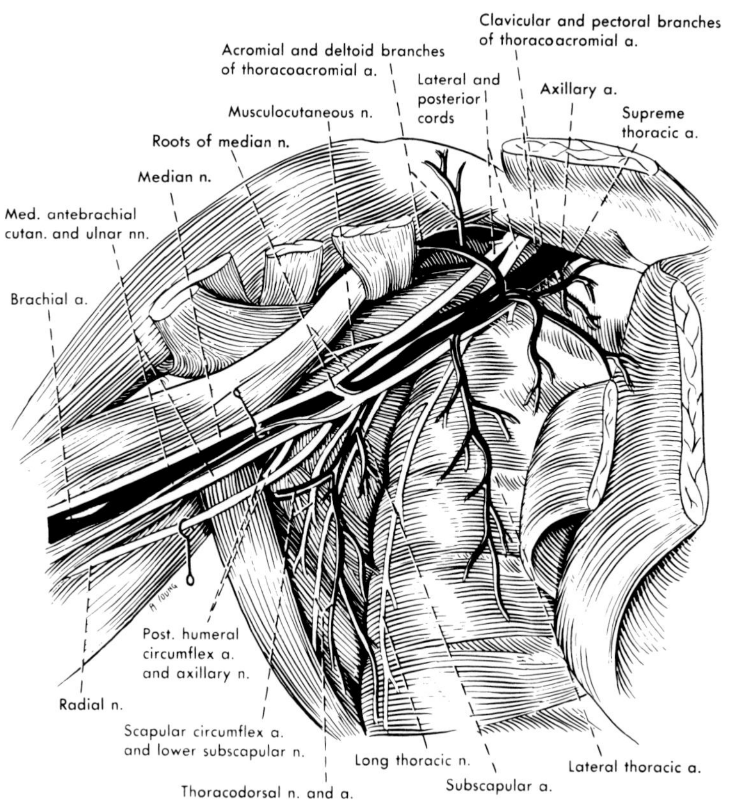

FIG. 9-18. Illustration of the vascular and neural anatomy in the axillary region. (From ref. 34, with permission.)

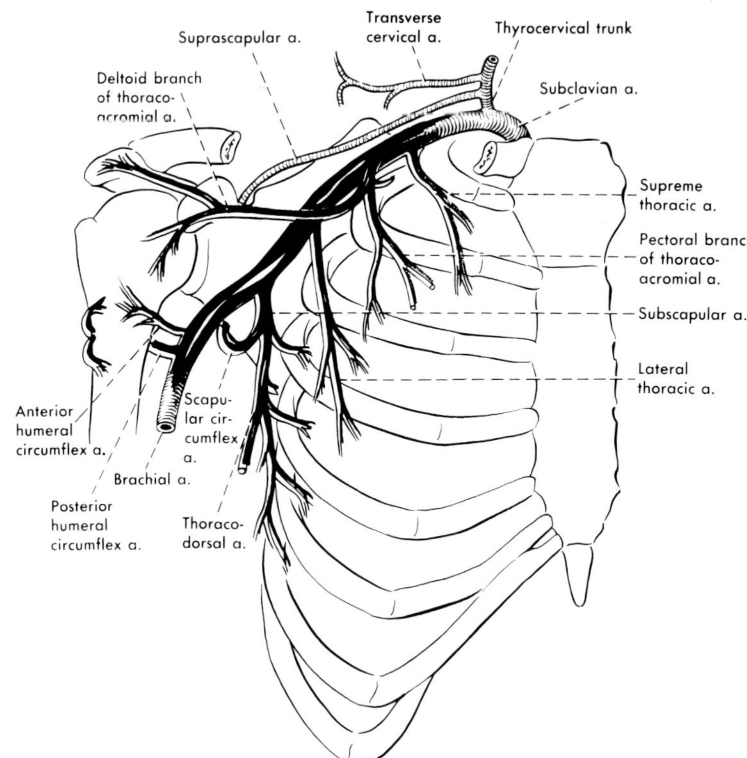

FIG. 9-19. Illustration of the major vascular anatomy of the shoulder. (From ref. 34, with permission.)

APPLICATIONS

Routine radiography is an important initial examination for screening patients with shoulder, arm, and suspected brachial plexus lesions (3,28). Other techniques including radionuclide studies, CT, and arthrography also have an important role in evaluating these patients (1,6,7,11,22,53,67). In recent years ultrasound has become a useful tool in some institutions for screening patients with suspected rotator cuff tears, but this technique is limited in its ability to identify other abnormalities in the shoulder region (14,31,33,48,55,77). Because of the clinical presentations and anatomic and examination differences, we discuss the shoulder and arm separately from brachial plexus examinations.

Shoulder and Arm

The majority of patients who are referred for MRI of the shoulder or arm present with pain or restricted range of motion in the shoulder. The most common clinical indications for MRI are patients referred with suspected rotator cuff tears or impingement, defects in the glenolabrum, osteonecrosis, suspected soft tissue or bony neoplasms, and infectious or inflammatory disorders (90–93).

Trauma

Routine radiography and radionuclide studies are usually sufficient for identifying subtle and/or complete fractures in the shoulder and humerus. Occasionally, conventional tomography or, in the shoulder region, computed tomography is needed to clearly identify the position of the fracture fragments (3,19,22). MRI, to date, has not played a significant role in evaluating osseous trauma. However, subtle fractures can easily be identified with MRI and certainly, if they are present, one should not be concerned that they will be overlooked (Fig. 9-20) (13,21).

The primary application of MRI for shoulder and upper arm trauma is evaluation of soft tissue injuries. Most of these injuries are chronic in nature. MRI is less commonly used to evaluate acute injuries.

The most common application for MRI is evaluation of patients with suspected rotator cuff tear or impingement syndrome (6,25,26). The majority (95%) of rotator cuff lesions are the result of chronic impingement of the supraspinatus tendon against the acromial arch (9,61,92). Neer (61) divided rotator cuff disease into three stages. The initial stage (stage I) consists of edema or hemorrhage in the rotator cuff, specifically the supraspinatus tendon. During stage II there is progression of the inflammatory stage to a more fibrotic process. The

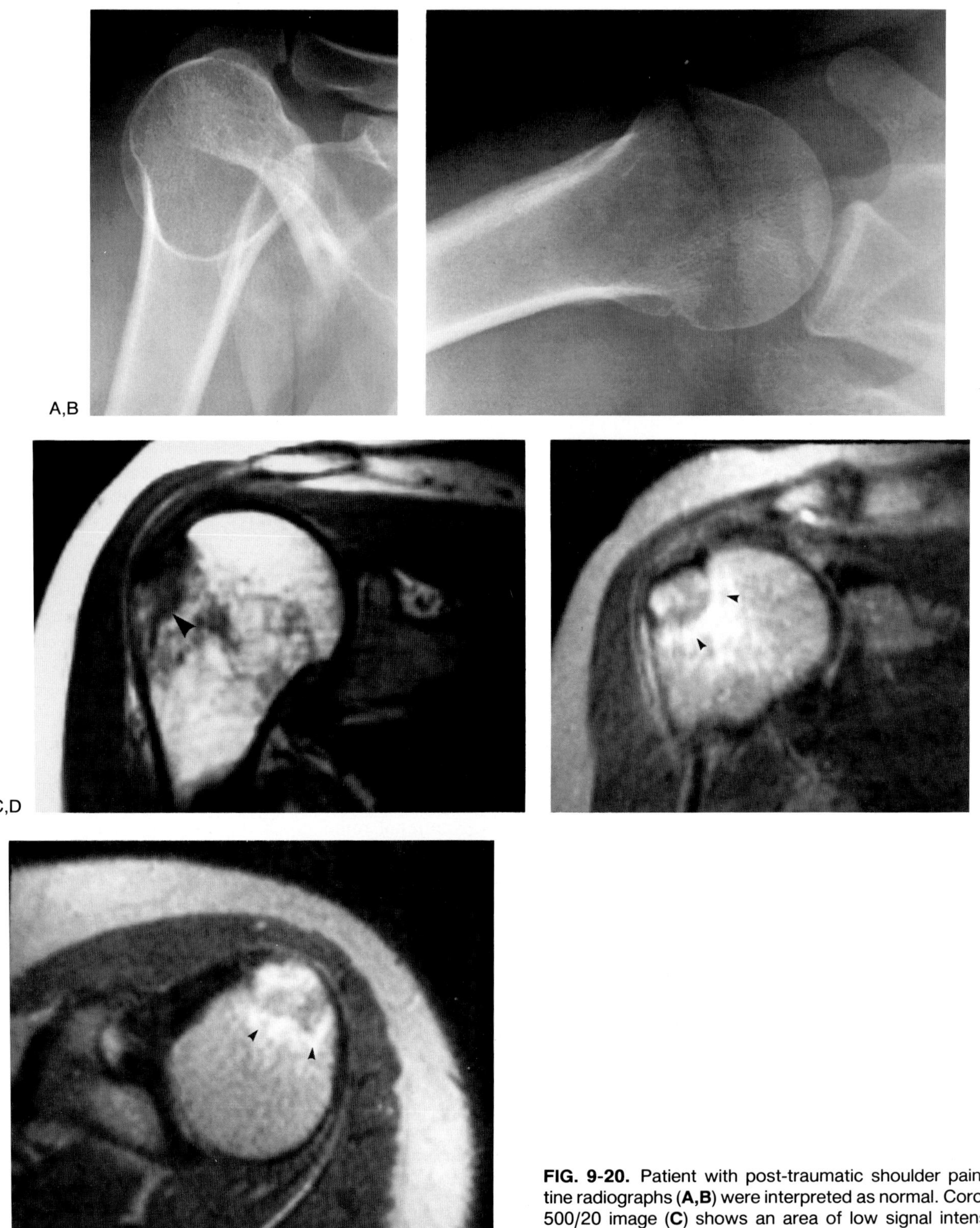

FIG. 9-20. Patient with post-traumatic shoulder pain. Routine radiographs (**A,B**) were interpreted as normal. Coronal SE 500/20 image (**C**) shows an area of low signal intensity involving the greater tuberosity with a fracture line (*arrowhead*) medially. Coronal (**D**) and axial (**E**) SE 2,000/60 images show the fracture line with reactive hyperemia (*arrowheads*) around the fracture.

final stage, stage III, results in a tear of the rotator cuff. The most susceptible area in the cuff is approximately 1 cm from the insertion of the supraspinatus tendon into the greater tuberosity. This critical zone is where the majority of tendon ruptures occur. Chronic impingement of this avascular area leads to tendinitis or inflammation during the first stage of the degeneration period (50). This abnormality is identifiable on MR images, which is important since inflammatory changes may be reversible. As the degenerative process continues to stage II and then stage III, progressive change in the supraspinatus tendon and AC joint region occur (20,61,62). Therefore, in evaluating MRI of the shoulder, it is important to compare the routine radiographs to obtain some predictive value from the secondary osseous changes, especially in the AC joint as well as the position of the humeral head in relation to the AC joint (3). On the normal AP radiograph in external rotation, the distance between the undersurface of the acromion and humeral head should measure 1 cm. When this space is reduced to 7 mm or less, the presence of a rotator cuff tear is almost certain (3).

MRI is particularly suited for evaluation of the shoulder because it is capable of detecting lesions in the rotator cuff as well as other abnormalities in the glenohumeral joint, acromioclavicular joint, and the associated periarticular soft tissues (41,42,73,74,91).

The technique described in this chapter consisting of axial, coronal, and sagittal T2 and T1 weighted sequences is well suited for evaluating patients with suspected rotator cuff tears. Patients with stage I disease (Fig. 9-21) or tendinitis have an intact rotator cuff. However, there is increased signal intensity within the supraspinatus tendon. This is generally most obvious on T2 weighted sequences but can be seen as an area of intermediate signal intensity (gray) on T1 weighted sequences. This increased signal intensity is most likely due to edema, inflammation, and hemorrhage in the tendon. During this stage of rotator cuff disease, the subacromial bursa is generally not fluid distended and the normal fat plane between the rotator cuff and deltoid is clearly demonstrated. In contrast to MRI, arthrograms would be normal during this stage of rotator cuff disease. Histologic changes during this phase of rotator cuff disease show inflammation and mucoid degenerative changes within the tendon (42,61,91–93).

Additional osseous and articular changes in the AC joint may also be evident in patients at this time. These are easily demonstrated on the coronal and sagittal images, which usually demonstrate expansion, either fibrocartilaginous or osseous, of the subacromial joint with deformity of the adjacent supraspinatus muscle (Fig. 9-22) (42,91).

The ability to demonstrate early changes in the rotator cuff is important in treatment planning, specifically developing surgical criteria for management of patients with impingement syndrome. Patients who fail to respond to conservative therapy in this setting may require acromioplasty and excision of the coracoacromial ligament to prevent stage II and III disease (20,61,62).

In patients with complete rotatory cuff tears, it is important to identify the ends of the tendons and calculate as closely as possible the size of the tear (3,27,29). Coronal and sagittal images are usually sufficient in this re-

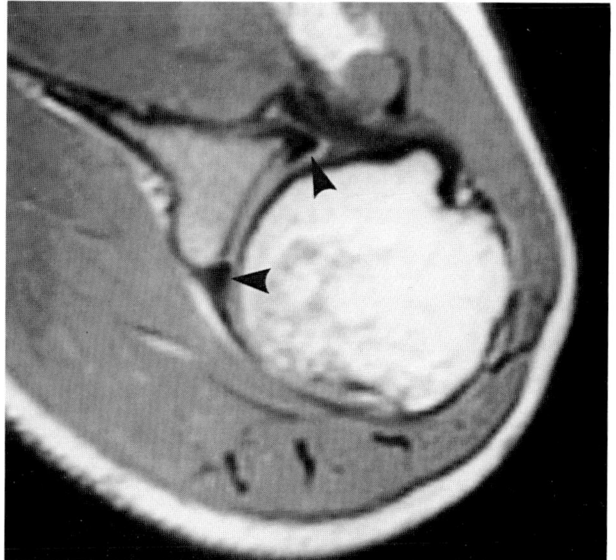
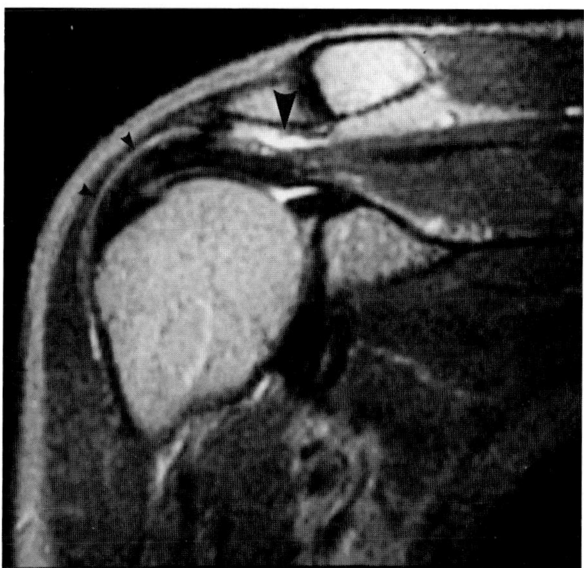

A,B

FIG. 9-21. Stage I cuff disease: **A:** Axial SE 2,000/20 image shows normal anterior and posterior labrum (*arrowheads*). **B:** Coronal SE 2,000/60 shows slight increased signal in the rotator cuff with a normal deltoid fat stripe (*small arrowheads*). There is increased signal intensity in the subacromial bursa (*large arrowhead*) due to bursitis.

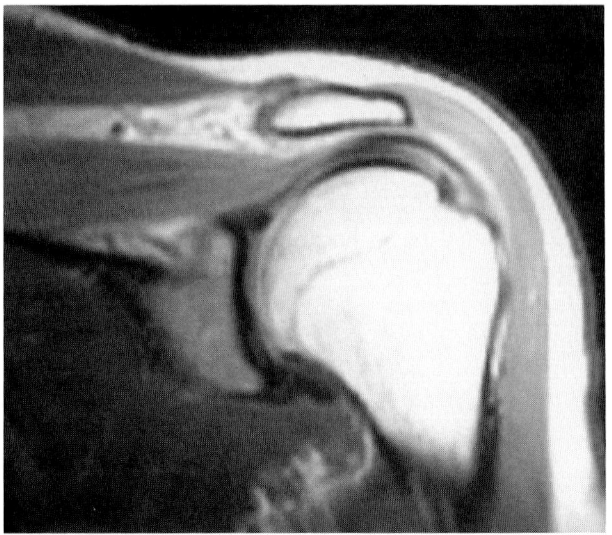
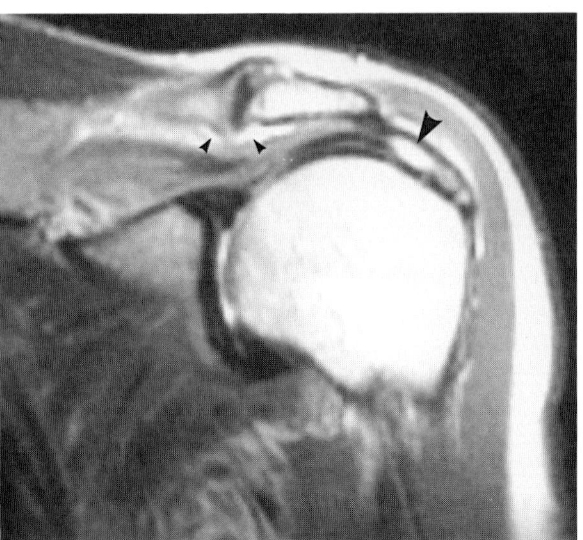

A,B

FIG. 9-22. Coronal SE 2,000/20 images demonstrating increased signal in the cuff (**A**) and focal cystic change (*large arrowhead*) and hypertrophy of the AC joint (*small arrowheads*) causing impingement (**B**).

gard and, again, T2 weighted sequences provide the best contrast distinction between the dark tendon and the high-intensity signal of the fluid between the ends of the torn tendon (Fig. 9-23). In addition to demonstrating the tear, the tendon thickness is also important. In chronic disease the tendon is often significantly thinned. Additional findings include fluid in the subacromial and subdeltoid bursae and disruption of the normal subdeltoid fat stripe. It is not unusual in advanced disease to see communication from the glenohumeral joint through a tear into the subacromial bursa with continued extension into the acromioclavicular joint. In addition, cystic or ganglion-like lesions may appear on the dorsal aspect of the AC joint in patients with advanced chronic rotator cuff tears (Fig. 9-24). These patients may also demonstrate atrophy and retraction of the supraspinatus muscle along with the secondary osseous changes previously described (3,90–93).

MR experience is more limited with incomplete rotator cuff tears (42,45,93). Incomplete tears may occur superiorly or inferiorly and are demonstrated as areas of increased signal intensity involving only a partial thickness of the tendon, usually in a linear fashion perpendicular to the course of the tendon (Fig. 9-25). These findings may be difficult to differentiate from tendinitis. In this setting, double-contrast arthrography with weight-bearing views may still be the most effective in identifying subtle tears of the inferior surface of the tendon (3,27). However, superior defects would require bursography, which is a more difficult technique to perform

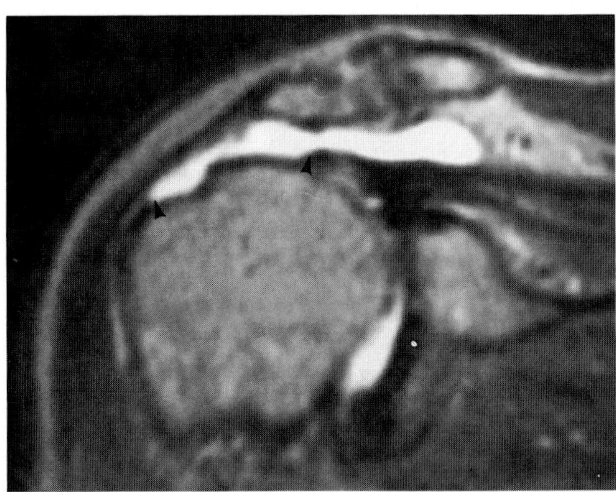
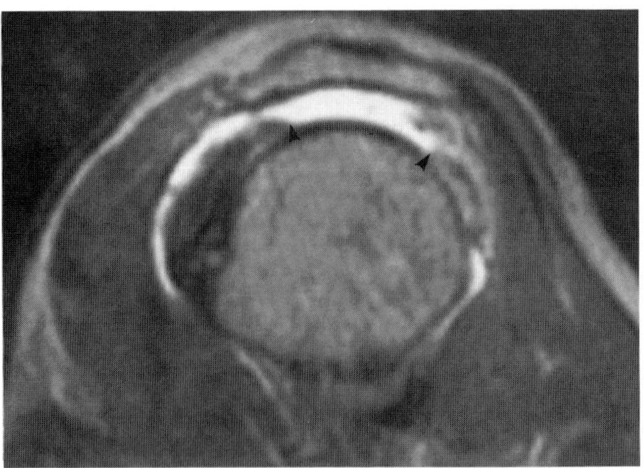

A,B

FIG. 9-23. Stage III or complete rotator cuff tear. **A:** Coronal image (SE 2,000/60) shows a large fluid collection and degenerative disease in the AC joint. The size of the cuff tear (*arrowheads*) can be identified on this view and the coronal (**B**) view (*arrowheads*).

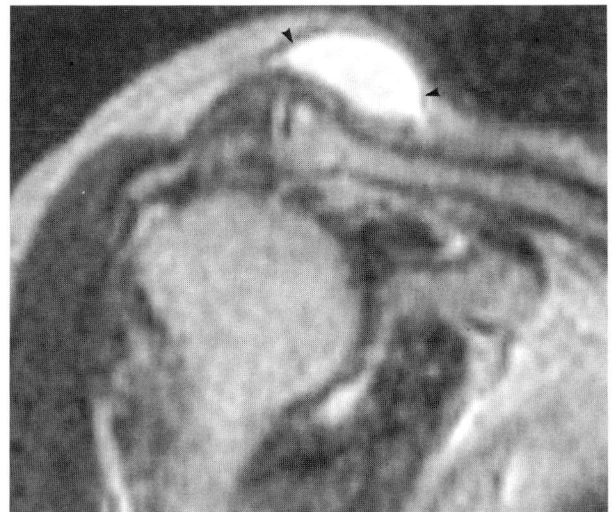

FIG. 9-24. Chronic rotator cuff tear. Image quality is degraded by motion due to patient discomfort. Note the humeral head lies immediately below the AC joint. There is a high signal intensity cyst (*arrowheads*) due to degeneration of the AC joint and a chronic rotator cuff tear.

(47,79). Therefore, it is apparent that, at some point, MRI will also be the technique of choice in this regard.

Based on the work of Kneeland et al. (45) and Zlatkin et al. (90,92), diagnostic criteria for MRI have been developed. Criteria are based on changes involving the rotator cuff, as well as secondary signs involving the subacromial and subdeltoid fat planes and bursae. The grading system is as follows: A normal tendon with normal signal intensity and morphology is considered grade 0 (Fig. 9-5). Grade 1 tendons have increased signal but normal width and morphology (Fig. 9-21). A grade 2 tendon shows increased signal intensity with change in morphology such as tendon thinning or irregularity (Fig. 9-26). Grade 3 tendons have discontinuity, with increased signal in the region of tendinous disruption best appreciated on T2 weighted images (Fig. 9-23) (36,93).

Zlatkin et al. (90,92) reported the accuracy of shoulder MRI using these criteria. Sensitivity, specificity, and accuracies of 91%, 88%, and 89%, respectively, for all tears, partial and complete, were demonstrated. MRI was also noted to be more sensitive than arthrog-

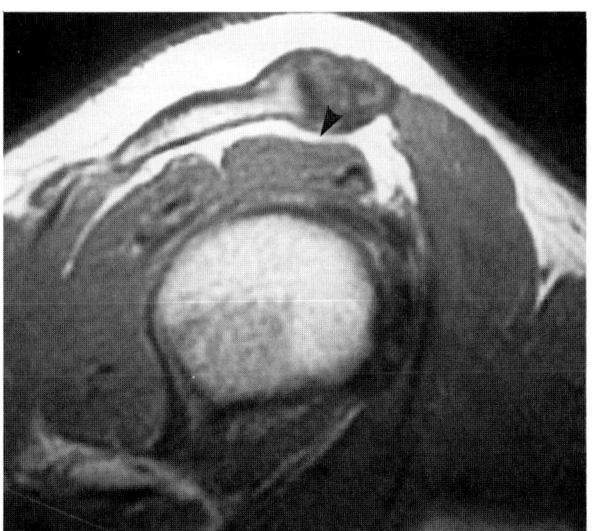

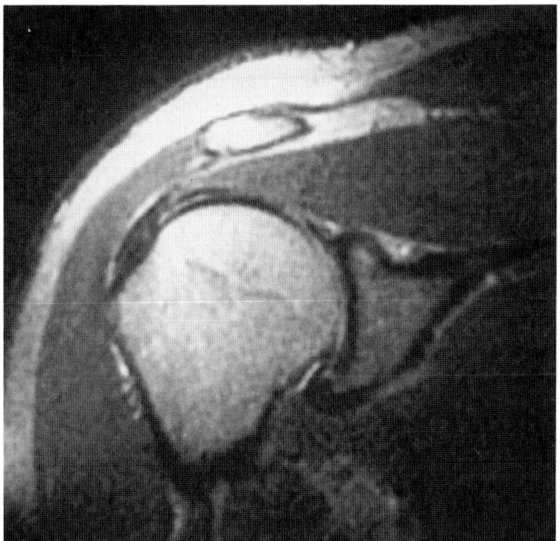

A,B

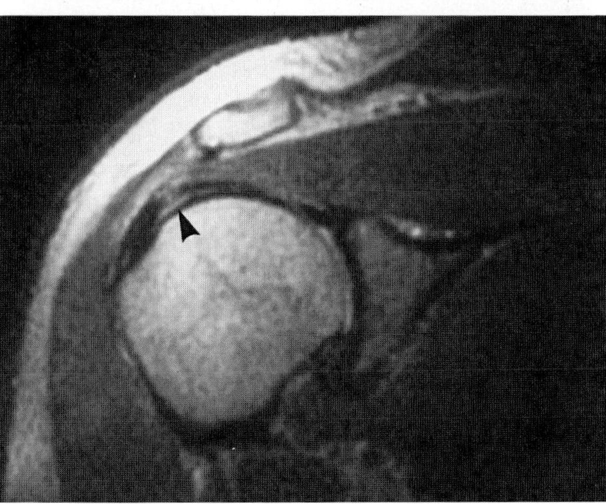

C

FIG. 9-25. Patient with an acute injury and shoulder pain. Sagittal SE 500/20 image (**A**) shows mild impingement with hypertrophy of the AC joint and indentation (*arrowhead*) of the supraspinatus. Coronal SE 2,000/60 images show increased signal in the rotator cuff on the first section (**B**) and a focal defect (*arrowhead*) with some irregularity of the fat plane in the adjacent section (**C**). Partial or focal complete tear?

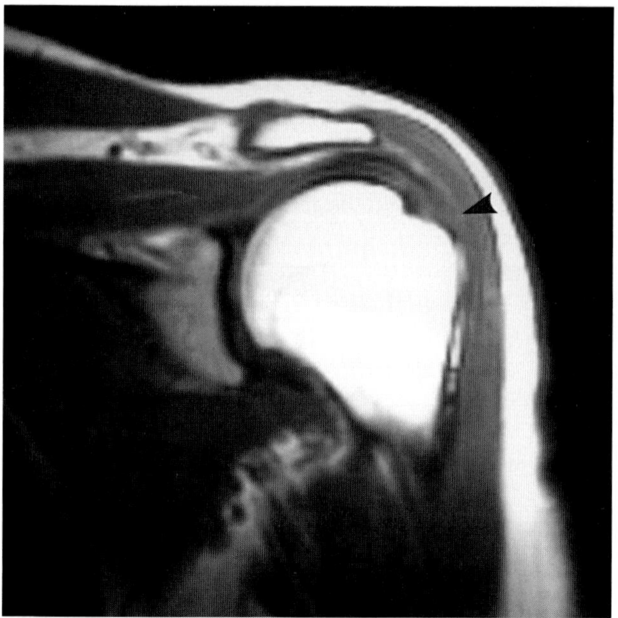

FIG. 9-26. Grade 2 tendon changes. T1 weighted (SE 500/20) image shows increased signal in the cuff with irregularity (*arrowhead*) near the insertion.

raphy in the diagnosis of small anterior supraspinatus tendon tears.

Evancho et al. (25) correlated MR findings with surgery and arthroscopy. MRI demonstrated a sensitivity of 80%, a specificity of 94%, and an accuracy of 89% for complete tears. When partial and complete tears were evaluated as a group, the sensitivity and accuracy were reduced to 69% and 84%, respectively.

It is important to compare the results of MRI with other accepted imaging techniques, specifically arthrography, bursography, and ultrasonography (19,86). Both single- and double-contrast arthrography have been accurate in detection of rotator cuff tears. However, unless combined with bursography, partial superior tears and impingement are difficult to diagnose (27,30,47,79). Bursography is invasive and difficult to perform unless the procedure is performed by an experienced examiner (3,92).

Burk et al. (6) compared the results of arthrography, MRI, and ultrasound in a group of 38 patients referred for suspected rotator cuff tears. Both MRI and double-contrast arthrography demonstrated sensitivities of 92% and specificities of 100% for normal cuffs. Diagnosis of cuff tears was equal with both techniques. Ultrasound was 63% sensitive for diagnosis of cuff tears and demonstrated a specificity of only 50% for intact rotator cuffs. Others report ultrasound to have accuracy of 87–94% for diagnosis of rotator cuff tears (48,55). Soble et al. (77) compared arthrography with ultrasonography and found that 92% of cuff tears were detected. Importantly, the negative predictive value of ultrasonography was 95%. However, in the operated group the specificity of ultrasound was only 73% compared to 100% for arthrography.

Arthrography is an accurate (98%) but invasive technique for diagnosis of rotator cuff tears but is of little value in evaluating impingement (6,56). Ultrasound is accurate in some physicians' hands but has not achieved the wide acceptance of MRI or arthrography due to the experience required by examiners and the difficulty in achieving acceptance in the orthopedic community. Physicians not involved in performing and interpreting ultrasound find the image difficult to evaluate (14,77). MRI is noninvasive and provides a method of screening for many osseous and soft tissue abnormalities. Though refinements are still in progress, it appears to be the noninvasive technique of choice for evaluating impingement and rotator cuff pathology (6,92,93).

Postoperative Changes

Surgical procedures to correct or repair rotator cuff tears and impingement may be directed at direct repair of the rotator cuff defect and/or resection of portions of the acromion and distal clavicle (20,32,60–63). Though results are usually satisfactory, up to 26% of patients may have recurrent symptoms. Inadequate acromial resection or recurrent cuff tear should be considered (49,87). Adhesive capsulitis may also occur (3). Arthrography is the most valuable technique for diagnosis of adhesive capsulitis. However, the more common problems with regard to the cuff and adequacy of the acromioplasty are difficult to answer accurately. Calvert et al. (7) reported postoperative leaks that mimic rotator cuff tears in 18 of 20 patients after rotator cuff repair. Changes in the subacromial bursa or resection of this structure can also cause confusion in interpreting arthrographic findings.

Ultrasonography has been useful in evaluating patients following rotator cuff repair. Though experience is limited, accuracies up to 98% for diagnosing postoperative recurrent tears have been reported (49).

MRI has the potential to evaluate the rotator cuff and osseous structures (Fig. 9-27). Coronal and sagittal images are ideal for following patients after acromioplasty. T1 weighted sequences are sufficient for evaluating the adequacy of acromial and clavicular resection. The sagittal plane is most useful in this regard. Double-echo (SE 2,000/60,20) T2 weighted sequences in the coronal plane are more ideally suited for evaluating the integrity of the rotator cuff (Fig. 9-28). This is more difficult due to the postoperative changes in the subacromial region, which lead to obliteration of the subdeltoid fat that is an important secondary structure for diagnosis of rotator cuff tears (92).

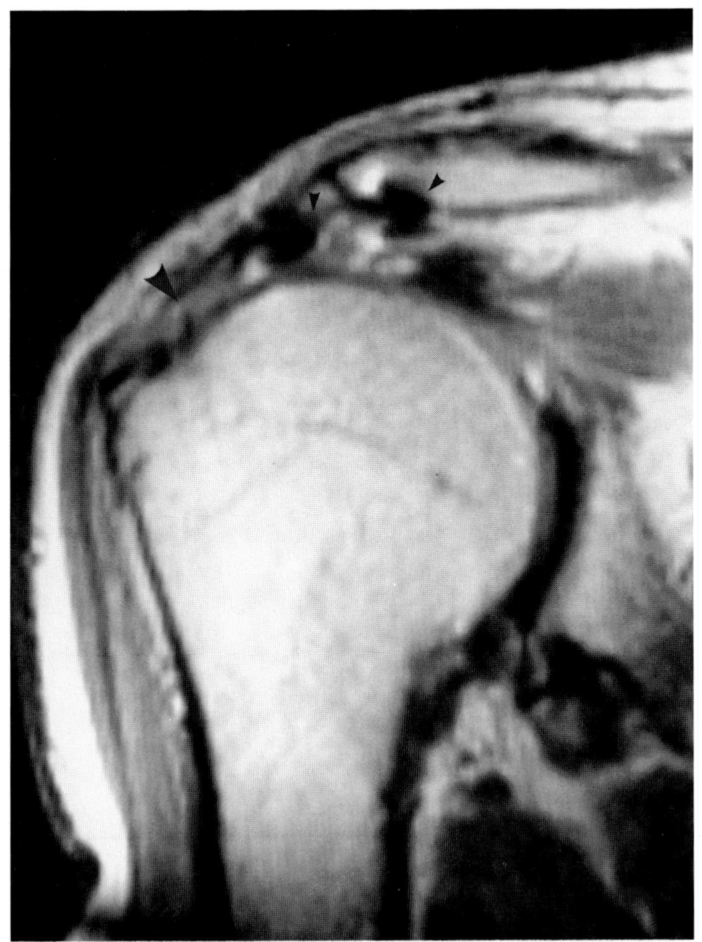
A

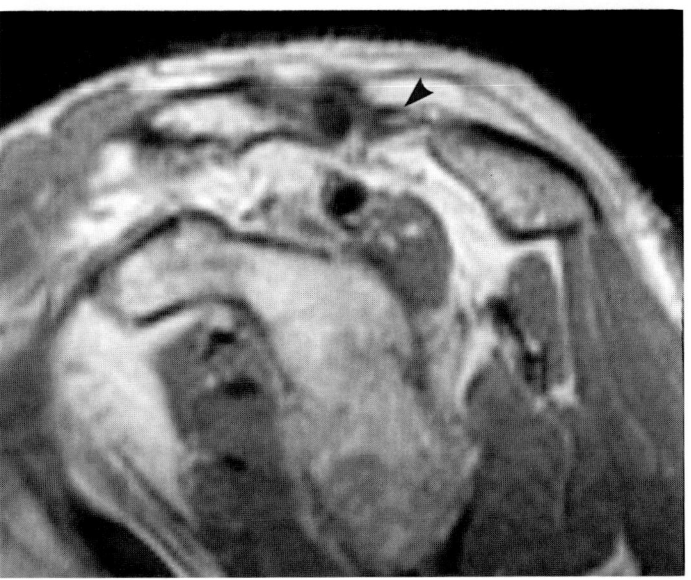
B

FIG. 9-27. Postoperative cuff repair and acromioplasty. **A:** Coronal SE 2,000/20 image shows postoperative artifacts (*small arrowheads*) with intermediate signal intensity in the rotator cuff (*large arrowhead*). There is no subdeltoid fat plane to assist in evaluation of the cuff. **B:** Sagittal SE 500/20 image shows adequate osseous resection (*arrowhead*) with a normal supraspinatus.

Capsular Abnormalities

As noted in the anatomy section, the capsular structures of the shoulder consist of the synovial membrane, the capsule, the associated glenohumeral ligaments, glenoid labrum, and associated bursae and recesses (2,34,84,85). Subscapularis muscle and tendon are also closely applied to the anterior capsule (2,3,34). Imaging of the shoulder capsule has conventionally been accomplished using either conventional or CT or arthroto-

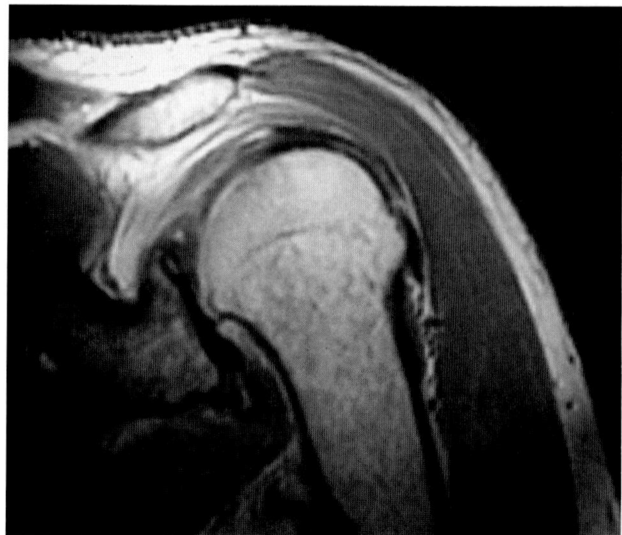
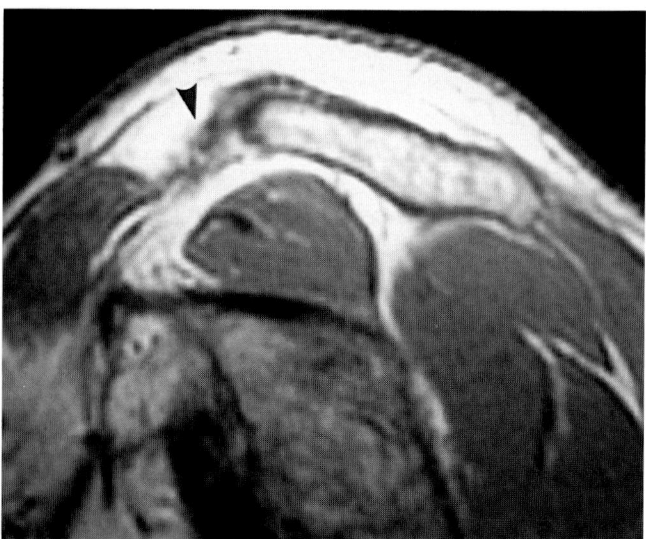

A,B

FIG. 9-28. Postoperative cuff repair and acromioplasty. **A:** Coronal image shows superior subluxation of the humeral head. There is increased signal intensity in the rotator cuff but it is intact. **B:** Sagittal image demonstrates adequate resection (*arrowhead*) with no impingement.

mography (53,89). Contrast arthrography provides valuable information regarding the size and integrity of the capsule and also allows intra-articular injections of anesthetic and/or a combination of anesthetic and steroidal compounds to treat and diagnose certain shoulder disorders (3).

Capsular volume is difficult to evaluate with MRI since the degree of distention of the capsule cannot be evaluated unless contrast material of some type is injected. Recently, gadolinium-DTPA has been advocated as an MR arthrography contrast agent. However, to date there has not been significant experience to clearly understand its implications in MRI of the shoulder (89). Certainly, fluoroscopically monitored injections of contrast material are much more efficacious than MR arthrography at this point. Therefore, patients who are being evaluated for subtle changes in the synovial lining or for changes in capsular volume such as adhesive capsulitis are still studied to better advantage with conventional arthrography or arthrography combined with CT or tomography (3,53).

Disruption of the shoulder capsule can be detectable by arthrography or MRI. Loss of integrity of the capsule or its adjacent or associated ligaments can be identified on MRI as poorly defined areas of increased signal intensity adjacent to the capsule on T2 weighted sequences. Capsular lesions are most easily evaluated in the axial and coronal planes.

Recurrent shoulder dislocations are a common problem in orthopedic practice (9,20). Originally, it was felt that the Bankhart lesion (glenoid labral tear or osteochondral fracture of the inferior labrum) was the main lesion resulting in recurrent anterior dislocation (58,64,65,71,85). More recently the entire anterior capsule mechanism has been implicated (see Fig. 9-15) (58,71,84). Type II and type III capsular insertions are more often associated with instability (93).

Until recently, arthrography with CT has been the technique of choice for evaluating the glenoid labrum (41,53). T2 weighted or gradient-echo sequences can be used to evaluate the glenoid labrum as well. Conventional axial and coronal images (Fig. 9-29) will demonstrate the entire labrum; however, it might be optimal to

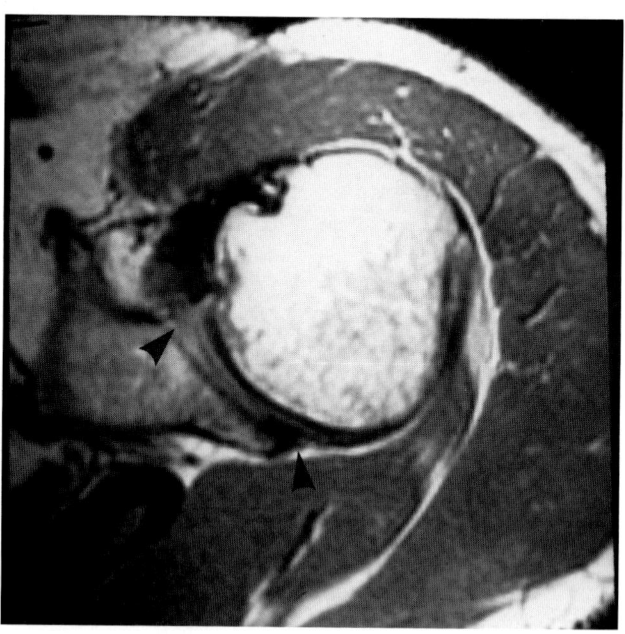

FIG. 9-29. Axial SE 2,000/20 image showing a normal posterior labrum (*arrowhead*) and complete tear with absence of the anterior labrum (*arrowhead*).

use radial GRIL sequences, similar to those described for the knee, to optimally look at the labrum tangentially (59). Currently, most software does not provide the capability to select multiple off-axis radial GRIL images.

Normally, the glenoid labrum has a triangular shape and appears black or low intensity on spin-echo and gradient-echo sequences. There are some variations in the appearance of the labrum as it is generally sharper anteriorly and slightly more rounded posteriorly (Fig. 9-30) (53,89). Disruptions of the labrum are seen as linear areas of high signal intensity on MR images. Complete avulsion or total absence of the labrum is easily identified (Fig. 9-29). Degenerative changes within the labrum that do not communicate with the articular surface, similar to those changes described in the knee, may also be evident. The clinical significance of these is probably similar to changes in the knee meniscus, and therefore a glenoid labrum tear should not be suggested unless there is a clear linear defect that articulates with the articular surface of the labrum or a labral detachment. Tears are most commonly identified anteriorly, and therefore if GRIL techniques are not available, the axial plane is usually best suited to identify these lesions (59,89).

Infection and Inflammatory Diseases

The shoulder, specifically the glenohumeral joint, is frequently involved in osteoarthritis and other types of inflammatory arthropathies. Soft tissue changes as well as early changes in the articular and osseous structures of the shoulder are more easily defined using MRI than conventional radiography. Chronic synovial changes such as proliferative synovitis can also be demonstrated without the use of contrast material. These changes are, however, not specific and do not preclude the need for aspiration to obtain fluid for more specific analysis, especially infection (76,92).

Osteomyelitis and infectious arthritis involving the shoulder can also be detected early (82). The extent of bone and soft tissue involvement can be more clearly defined using MRI than conventional radiographs or radionuclide scans (4). Certain other inflammatory diseases such as pigmented villonodular synovitis (78) and giant cell tumors of the tendon sheath can be somewhat more specifically identified due to hemosiderin deposition in the proliferative synovium (46). The paramagnetic effects of hemosiderin result in shortening of the T2 relaxation time, which causes areas of low signal intensity in the normally high-intensity synovial fluid (46). A more complete discussion of infection and arthropathies can be found in Chapters 13 and 15.

Osteonecrosis

Detection of early avascular necrosis or osteonecrosis of the humeral head can be difficult with routine radiographs and radionuclide studies (4,10). Later, once these

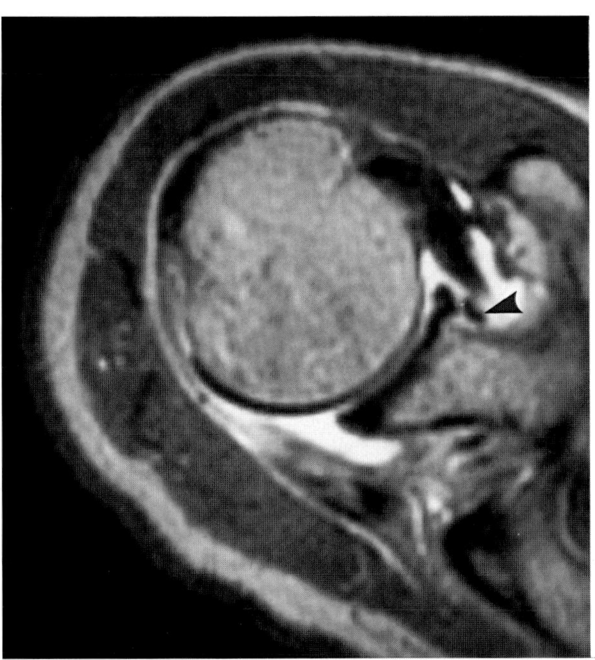

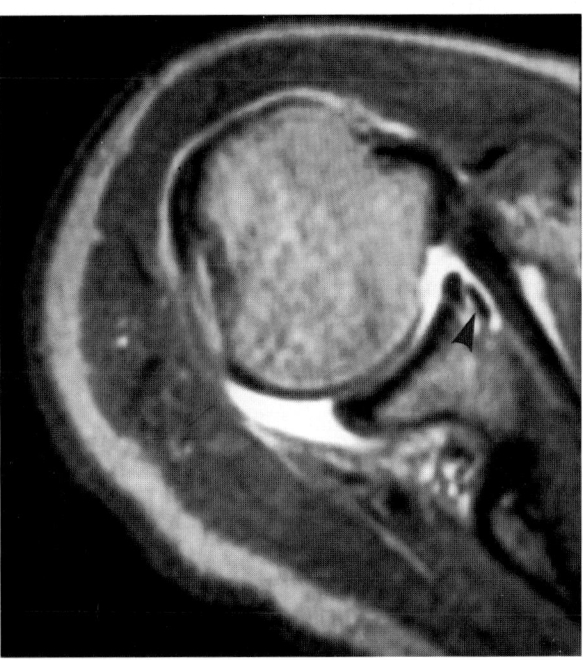

A,B

FIG. 9-30. Normal glenoid labrum. Axial SE 2,000/60 images (**A,B**) show fluid in the joint with normal anterior and posterior labra. The capsular insertion (*arrowhead*) should not be mistaken for anterior labral abnormalities.

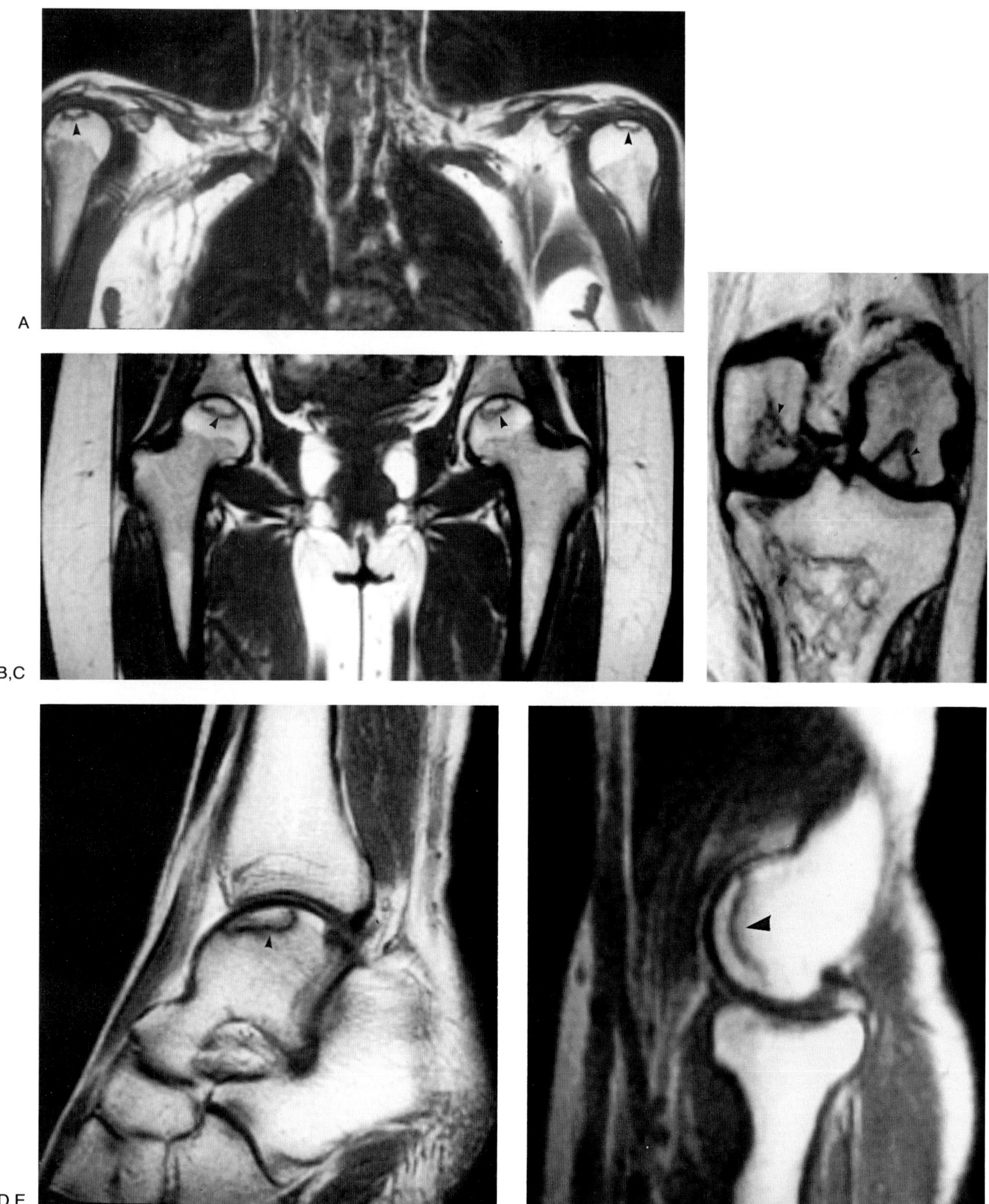

FIG. 9-31. Renal transplant patient on systemic steroid therapy. Screening SE 500/20 coronal images of the shoulders (**A**), hips (**B**), and knees (**C**) and sagittal images of the ankle (**D**) and elbow (**E**) show classic MR images of avascular necrosis (*arrowheads*). There are also bone infarcts in the tibia.

TABLE 9-4. *Skeletal neoplasms of the shoulder (18)*

Lesion	Number of shoulder/total lesions	Percentage of total
Benign		
Osteochondroma	136/727	19
Chondroma	31/245	13
Chondroblastoma	20/79	25
Giant cell tumor	16/425	4
Osteoid osteoma	10/245	4
Hemangioma	3/80	4
Osteoblastoma	1/63	2
Malignant		
Myeloma	37/556	7
Lymphoma	54/469	12
Chondrosarcoma	99/634	16
Dedifferentiated chondrosarcoma	18/79	23
Osteosarcoma	137/1,274	11
Ewings sarcoma	60/402	15
Fibrosarcoma	22/207	11

changes have become obvious, the radiographic appearance is typical and MRI is not usually indicated.

The appearance of osteonecrosis in the humeral head does not differ significantly from the hip (51,57). A complete discussion of the etiology and pathophysiology of osteonecrosis is included in Chapter 6 and is not repeated here.

Screening for avascular necrosis in the shoulder can be accomplished with coronal SE 500/20 images using a large field of view (include both shoulders), the body coil, 256 × 256 matrix, and 1 Nex (Fig. 9-31). This examination can be performed in less than 5 min. Early or subtle changes may require surface coils to more clearly delineate the changes in one or both shoulders. In this setting, coronal and sagittal images are useful to evaluate the articular cartilage and the area of involvement.

Neoplasms

MRI has become the technique of choice for staging of musculoskeletal neoplasms, whether they are primary or metastatic (1,4,88). Soft tissue and bony lesions in the shoulder are no exception.

Characterization of bony lesions is still most easily accomplished using routine radiographs (4,88). However, T1 weighted sequences or, in certain situations, STIR sequences provide valuable information regarding the extent of bony involvement in primary, metastatic, and infiltrative lesions such as lymphoma or leukemia (12,17,38,52,80,81). Table 9-4 lists the incidence of benign and malignant osseous lesions in the shoulder and upper humerus (18).

Data on locations of soft tissue tumors is less readily available than on osseous neoplasms (18,24). There are not many soft tissue lesions that more commonly occur in the shoulder region except subcutaneous or superficial lipomas and extra-abdominal desmoid tumors. Subcutaneous lipomas are most common in the shoulder, upper arm, and back. Desmoids (Fig. 9-32) occur most frequently in the shoulder (81/367 or 22.2%) (24). Malignant lesions that can more commonly involve the shoulder include epithelioid sarcoma (9%) and alveolar soft tissue sarcomas (17%) (24).

Soft tissue involvement is generally best demonstrated with T2 weighted sequences. Generally, both T1 and

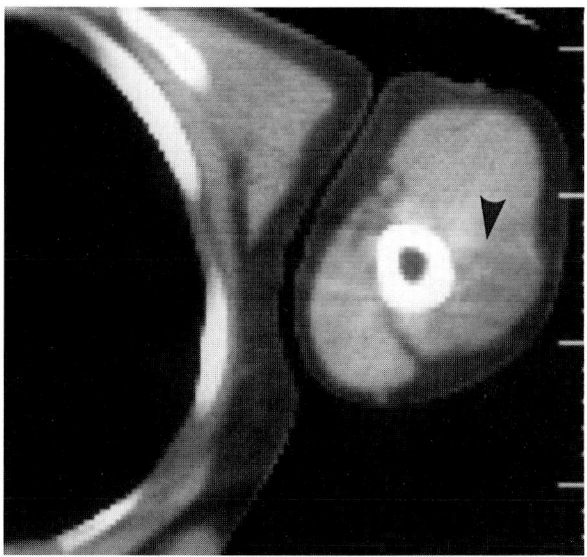

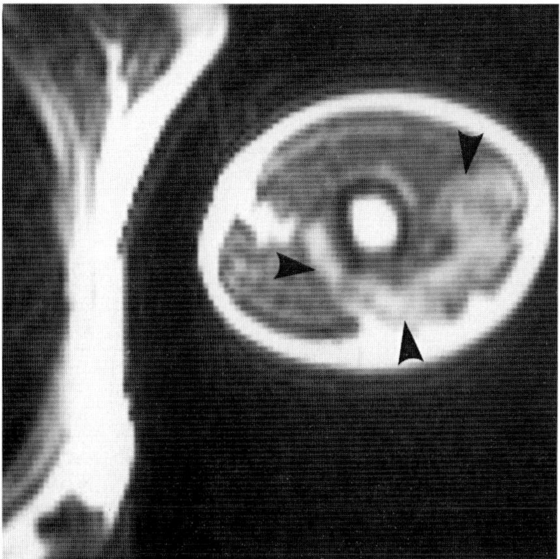

A,B

FIG. 9-32. Desmoid tumor CT scan (**A**) was interpreted as normal. The beam hardening artifact obscures the subtle low-intensity area (*arrowhead*) in the soft tissues. The 0.15 T MR image (**B**) (SE 2,000/30) demonstrates the lesion and its extent (*arrowheads*) more clearly.

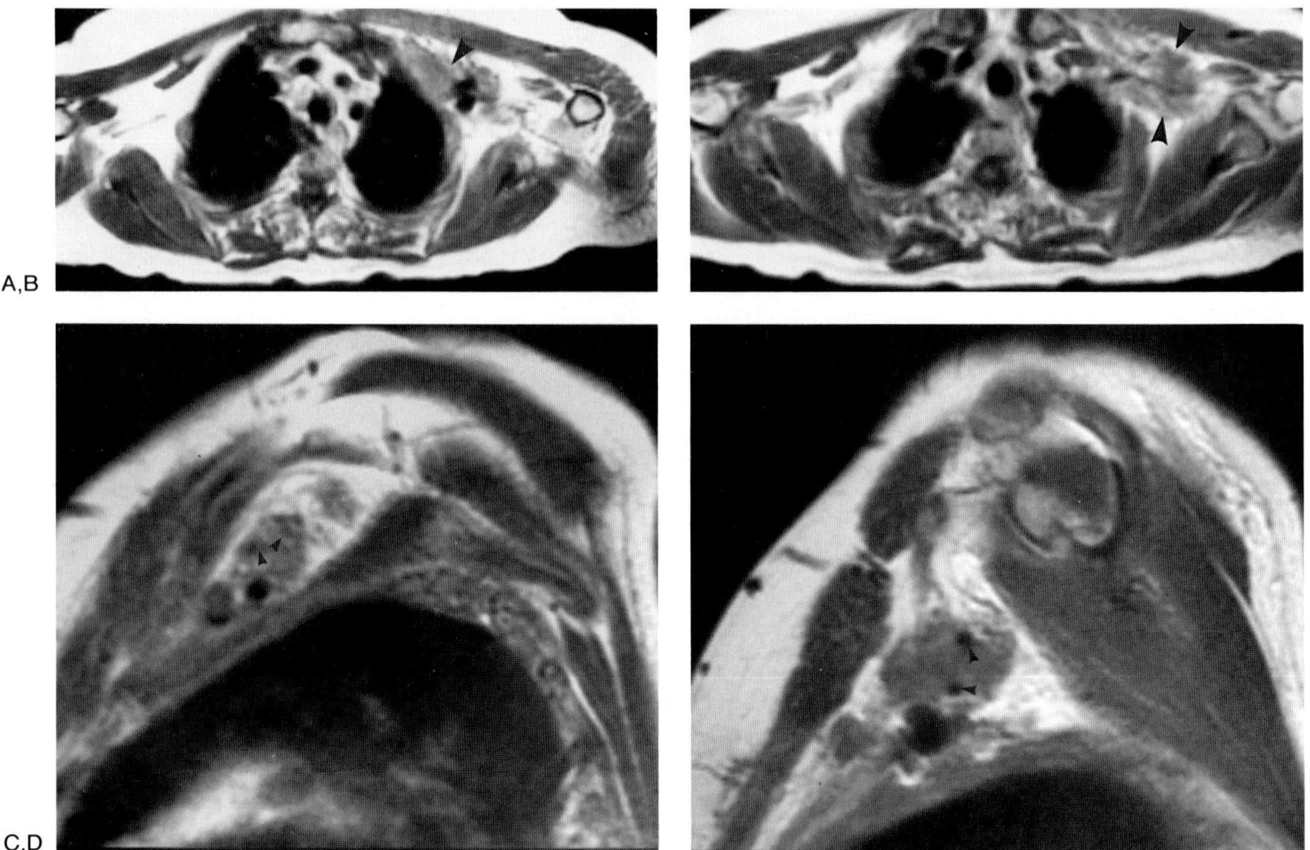

FIG. 9-33. Metastasis involving the brachial plexus. Axial SE 2,000/20 images show metastasis (*arrowhead*) involving the chest wall (**A**) and along the neurovascular bundle (**B**). Sagittal images (SE 500/20) show encasement of the nerve roots (*arrowheads*) (**C,D**).

T2 weighted sequences are indicated to characterize the type of lesion (4,12). Specific soft tissue lesions, especially those that are benign, are more often histologically predictable than malignant lesions; however, image characteristics that are discussed more fully in Chapter 12 are very useful in identifying the nature of the lesion (4).

BRACHIAL PLEXUS LESIONS

As noted above, the brachial plexus is a difficult area to image with most radiographic techniques. CT has significant limitations, including restriction of imaging planes and artifacts from the shoulder (69). In addition, it is more difficult to distinguish neurovascular structures from nodes in the brachial plexus region using conventional CT techniques. The superior soft tissue contrast and multiple image planes available with MRI provide significant advantages in this regard (5,8,69).

Early experience with MRI suggests that it may be useful for evaluating neoplasms (primary neural, metastatic, or adjacent soft tissue masses), differentiating neoplasm from postradiation changes, and evaluating trauma to the neural plexus (8,69).

The technique for examination was discussed earlier in this chapter. We typically use T2 weighted (SE 2,000/60,20) axial and T1 weighted (SE 500/20) sagittal images (Fig. 9-33). The double-echo sequence provides an excellent anatomic and pathologic screening technique. Neoplasms and active pathologic processes demonstrate increased signal intensity on the second echo (2,000/60), and fat signal is suppressed. This is particularly useful in separating radiation fibrosis from neoplasm. This can be a significant clinical problem (83). Fibrosis has low signal intensity on T1 and T2 weighted sequences. Edema (of the nerves or surrounding tissues) and tumors show increased intensity on T2 weighted sequences.

Saggital T1 weighted sequences provide a method of following the neural structures for the intervertebral foramina laterally to the brachial plexus and into the axillary region (40). The low signal intensity of the nerves in the high signal intensity fatty tissue provides excellent contrast.

In certain cases gradient-echo sequences or T1 weighted sequences are used. These sequences are particularly useful in following the nerve roots as they exit the cord and enter their sheaths (16).

Although more experience is needed, it would appear that MRI is the imaging technique of choice for evaluating the brachial plexus (8,69).

REFERENCES

1. Aisen AM, Martel W, Braunstein EM, McMillin KI, Phillips WA, King TF. MRI and CT evaluation of primary bone and soft tissue tumors. *AJR* 1986;146:749–756.
2. Anderson JE. *Grant's atlas of anatomy,* 8th ed. Baltimore: Williams & Wilkins, 1983.
3. Berquist TH. *Imaging of orthopedic trauma and surgery.* Philadelphia: Saunders, 1986.
4. Berquist TH, Ehman RL, Richardson ML. *Magnetic resonance of the musculoskeletal system.* New York: Raven Press, 1987.
5. Blair DN, Rapoport S, Sostman HD, Blair OC. Normal brachial plexus: MR imaging. *Radiology* 1987;165:763–767.
6. Burk LD, Karasick D, Kurtz AB, et al. Rotator cuff tears: prospective comparison of MR imaging with arthrography, sonography, and surgery. *AJR* 1989;153:87–92.
7. Calvert PT, Pacher NP, Stoker DJ, Bayley JI, Kessell L. Arthrography of the shoulder after operative repair of the torn rotator cuff. *J Bone Joint Surg* 1986;68:147–150.
8. Castagno AA, Shuman WP. MR imaging in clinically suspected brachial plexus. *AJR* 1987;149:1219–1222.
9. Cofield RH. Rotator cuff disease of the shoulder. *J Bone Joint Surg* 1985;67:974–979.
10. Coleman BG, Kressel HY, Dalinka MK, Scheibler ML, Burk DL, Cohen EK. Radiographically negative avascular necrosis: detection with MR imaging. *Radiology* 1988;168:525–528.
11. Beltran J, Gray LA, Bools JC, Zuelzer W, Weis LD, Unverferth LF. Rotator cuff lesions of the shoulder: evaluation by direct sagittal CT arthrography. *Radiology* 1986;160:161–165.
12. Beltran J, Simon DC, Katz W, Weis LD. Increased MR signal intensity in skeletal muscle adjacent to malignant tumors: pathologic correlation and clinical relevance. *Radiology* 1987;162:251–255.
13. Berger PE, Ofstein RA, Jackson DW, Morrison DS, Silvino N, Amador R. MRI demonstration of radiographic occult fractures: what have we been missing? *Radiographics* 1989;9:407–436.
14. Brandt TD, Cardone BW, Grant TH, Post M, Weiss CA. Rotator cuff sonography: a reassessment. *Radiology* 1989;173:323–327.
15. Carter BL, Morehead J, Walpert JM, Hammerschlag SB, Griffiths HJ, Kahn PC. *Cross-sectional anatomy: computed tomography and ultrasound correlation.* New York: Appleton-Century Crofts, 1977.
16. Czervionki LF, Daniels DL, Ho PSP, et al. Cervical neural foramina: correlative anatomic and MR imaging study. *Radiology* 1988;169:753–759.
17. Daffner RH, Lupetin AR, Dash N, Deeb ZL, Sefczek RJ, Schapiro RL. MRI in the detection of malignant infiltration of bone marrow. *AJR* 1986;146:353–358.
18. Dahlin DC, Unni KK. *Bone tumors: general aspects and data on 8,542 cases.* Springfield, IL: CC Thomas, 1986.
19. Dalinka MK, Kricun ME, Zlatkin MB, Hibbard CA. Modern diagnostic imaging in joint disease. *AJR* 1989;152:229–240.
20. Depalma AF. *Surgery of the shoulder.* Philadelphia: Lippincott, 1983.
21. Deutsch AL, Mink JH. Musculoskeletal trauma. *Top Magn Reson Imaging* 1989;1(4):53–66.
22. Deutsch AZ, Resnick D, Mink JH, et al. Computed and conventional arthrotomography of the glenohumeral joint: normal anatomy and clinical experience. *Radiology* 1984;153:603–609.
23. Edelman RR, Stark DD, Sairi S, et al. Oblique planes of section in MR imaging. *Radiology* 1986;159:807–810.
24. Enzinger FM, Weiss SW. *Soft tissue tumors.* St. Louis: CV Mosby, 1983.
25. Evancho AM, Stiles RG, Fajman WA, Flower SP, Macha T, Brunner MC, Fleming L. MR imaging diagnosis of rotator cuff tears. *AJR* 1988;151:751–754.
26. Fritts HM, Craig E, Kyle R, Strefling M, Miller D, Heithoff H, Schellhas K. MR imaging of the shoulder: clinical experience and surgical correlation. Read before the 73rd Scientific Assembly and Annual Meeting of the Radiologic Society of North America, Chicago, 1988.
27. Goldman AB, Ghelman B. The double contrast shoulder arthrogram: a review of 158 studies. *Radiology* 1978;127:655–663.
28. Goldman AB. Calcific tendonitis of the long head of the biceps brachii distal to the glenohumeral joint: plain film radiographic findings. *AJR* 1989;153:1011–1016.
29. Greenway GD, Danzig LA, Resnik D, Haghighi P. The painful shoulder. *Med Radiogr Photogr* 1982;58:22–67.
30. Hall FM, Rosenthal DI, Goldberg RP, Wyshak G. Morbidity from shoulder arthrography: etiology, incidence and prevention. *AJR* 1981;136:56–62.
31. Harcke AT, Grissom LE, Finkelstein MS. Evaluation of the musculoskeletal system with sonography. *AJR* 1988;150:1253–1261.
32. Hawkins RJ. The rotator cuff and biceps tendon. In: Evarts CM, ed. *Surgery of the musculoskeletal system.* New York: Churchill Livingstone, 1983.
33. Hodler J, Fretz CJ, Terrier F, Gerber C. Rotator cuff tears: correlation of sonographic and surgical findings. *Radiology* 1988;169:791–794.
34. Hollinshead WH. *Anatomy for surgeons, Volume 3. The trunk and extremities.* Philadelphia: Lippincott, 1982:259–436.
35. Hoult D. The NMR receiver: a description and analysis of design. *Prog Nucl Magn Reson Spectrosc* 1978;12:41–47.
36. Huber DJ, Mueller E, Heribes A. Oblique magnetic resonance imaging of normal structures. *AJR* 1985;145:843–846.
37. Huber DJ, Sauter R, Mueller E, Requardt H, Weber H. MR imaging of the normal shoulder. *Radiology* 1986;158:405–408.
38. Imhof H, Hajek PC, Kramer J, Ritschl P. Gd-DTPA: help in diagnosis of malignant bone lesions? Read before the 73rd Scientific Assembly and Annual Meeting of the Radiological Society of North America, Chicago, 1988.
39. Kellman GM, Kneeland JB, Middleton WD, et al. MR imaging of the supraclavicular region: normal anatomy. *AJR* 1987;148:77–82.
40. Kieft GJ, Bloem JH, Obermann WR, Verbout AJ, Rozing PM, Doornbos J. Normal shoulder: MR imaging. *Radiology* 1986;159:741–745.
41. Kieft GJ, Bloem JL, Rozing PM, Obermann WR. MR imaging of recurrent anterior dislocation of the shoulder: comparison with CT arthrography. *AJR* 1988;150:1083–1087.
42. Kieft GJ, Bloem JL, Rozing PM, Obermann WR. Rotator cuff impingement syndrome: MR imaging. *Radiology* 1988;166:211–214.
43. Kieft GH, Sartoris DJ, Bloem JL, et al. Magnetic resonance imaging of glenohumeral joint disease. *Skeletal Radiol* 1987;16:285–290.
44. Kneeland JB, Carrera GF, Middleton WD, et al. Rotator cuff tears: preliminary application of high-resolution MR imaging with counter rotating current loop-gap resonators. *Radiology* 1986;160:695–699.
45. Kneeland JB, Middleton WD, Carrera GF, et al. MR imaging of the shoulder: diagnosis of rotator cuff tears. *AJR* 1987;149:333–337.
46. Kottal RA, Vogler JB III, Matamoros A, Alexander AH, Cookson JL. Pigmented villonodular synovitis: a report of MR imaging in two cases. *Radiology* 1987;163:551–553.
47. Lie S, Mast WA. Subacromial bursography: techniques and clinical application. *Radiology* 1982;144:626–630.
48. Mack LA, Matsen FA III, Kilcoyne RF, Davies PK, Sickler ME. US evaluation of the rotator cuff. *Radiology* 1985;157:205–209.
49. Mack LA, Nyberg DA, Matsen FR III, Kilcoyne RF, Harvey D. Sonography of the postoperative shoulder. *AJR* 1988;150:1089–1093.
50. MacNab I, Hastings D. Rotator cuff tendinitis. *Can Med Assoc J* 1968;99:91–98.
51. Markisz JA, Knowles JR, Altchek DW, Schneider R, Whalen JP, Cahill PT. Segmental patterns of avascular necrosis of the femoral heads: early detection with MR imaging. *Radiology* 1987;162:717–720.
52. McKinstry CS, Steiner RE, Young AT, Jones L, Swirsky D, Aber V. Bone marrow in leukemia and aplastic anemia: MR imaging before, during, and after treatment. *Radiology* 1987;162:701–707.

53. McNiesch LM, Callaghan JJ. CT arthrography of the shoulder; variations of the glenoid labrum. *AJR* 1987;149:963–966.
54. Middleton WD, Kneeland JB, Carrera GF, et al. High-resolution MR imaging of the normal rotator cuff. *AJR* 1987;148:559–564.
55. Middleton WD, Edelstein G, Reinus WR, Melson GL, Totty WG, Murphy WA. Sonography detection of rotator cuff tears. *AJR* 1985;144:349–353.
56. Mink JH, Harris E, Rappaport M. Rotator cuff tears: evaluation using double-contrast shoulder arthrography. *Radiology* 1985;157:621–623.
57. Mitchell DG, Kundel JL, Steinberg ME, Kressel HY. Avascular necrosis of the hip: comparison of MR, CT and scintigraphy. *AJR* 1986;147:67–71.
57a. Morrey BF, Chao EY. Recurrent anterior dislocation of the shoulder. In: Black J, Dumpleton JH, eds. *Clinical biomechanics: a case history approach.* New York: Churchill Livingstone, 1981.
58. Moseley HG, Overgaard B. The anterior capsular mechanism in recurrent anterior dislocation of the shoulder: morphological and clinical studies with special reference to the glenoid labrum and the glenohumeral ligaments. *J Bone Joint Surg* 1962;44:913–927.
59. Munk PL, Holt RG, Helms CA, Genant HK. Glenoid labrum: preliminary work with use of radial sequence MR imaging. *Radiology* 1989;173:751–753.
60. Neer CS III. Anterior acromioplasty for the chronic impingement syndrome of the shoulder: a preliminary report. *J Bone Joint Surg* 1972;54:41–50.
61. Neer CS III. Impingement lesions. *Clin Orthop* 1983;173:70–77.
62. Neviaser RJ. Tears of the rotator cuff. *Orthop Clin North Am* 1980;11:295–303.
63. Nixon JE, Distefano V. Ruptures of the rotator cuff. *Orthop Clin North Am* 1975;6:423–447.
64. Oveson J, Sojbjerg JO. Lesions in different types of anterior glenohumeral joint dislocations. *Arch Orthop Trauma Surg* 1986;105:216–218.
65. Pappas AM, Goss TP, Kleiman PK. Symptomatic shoulder instability due to lesions of the glenoid labrum. *Am J Sports Med* 1983;11:279–288.
66. Pennes DR, Jonsson K, Buckwalter K, Braunstein E, Blasier R, Wojty SE. Computed arthrotomography of the shoulder: comparison of examinations made with internal and external rotation of the humerus. *AJR* 1989;153:1017–1019.
67. Rafii M, Firooznia H, Bonamo JJ, Minkoff J, Golimbu C. Athlete shoulder injuries: CT arthrographic findings. *Radiology* 1987;162:559–564.
68. Rafii M, Firooznia H, Golimbu C, Minkoff J, Bonamo J. CT arthrography of the capsular structures of the shoulder. *AJR* 1986;146:361–367.
69. Rapoport S, Blair DN, McCarthy SM, Desser TS, Hammers LW, Sostman HD. Brachial plexus: correlation of MR imaging with CT and pathologic findings. *Radiology* 1988;167:161–165.
70. Resnick DR. Shoulder arthrography. *Radiol Clin North Am* 1981;19:243–255.
71. Rose CO, Patel D, Southnayd WW. The Bankart procedure. *J Bone Joint Surg* 1978;60:1–16.
72. Rothman RH, Marvel JP, Heppenstall RB. Anatomic considerations in the glenohumeral joint. *Orthop Clin North Am* 1975;6:341–352.
73. Seeger LL, Gold RH, Bassett LW. Shoulder instability: evaluation with MR imaging. *Radiology* 1988;168:695–697.
74. Seeger LL, Gold RH, Bassett LW, Ellman H. Shoulder impingement syndrome: MR findings in 53 shoulders. *AJR* 1988;150: 343–347.
75. Seeger LL, Ruszkowski JT, Bassett LW, Kay SP, Kahmann RD, Ellman H. MR imaging of the normal shoulder: anatomic correlation. *AJR* 1987;148:83–91.
76. Sims RE, Genant HK. Magnetic resonance imaging of joint disease. *Radiol Clin North Am* 1986;24:179–188.
77. Soble MG, Kaye AD, Guay RC. Rotator cuff tear: clinical experience with sonographic detection. *Radiology* 1989;173:319–321.
78. Spritzer CE, Dalinka MK, Kressel HY, Alavi A, Axel L. Magnetic resonance imaging of pigmented villonodular synovitis: a report of two cases. *AJR* 1986;147:67–71.
79. Strizak AM, Danzig L, Jackson DW, Greenway G, Resnick D, Staple T. Subacromial bursography. *J Bone Joint Surg* 1982;64:196–201.
80. Sundaram M, McGuire MH, Fletcher J, Wolverson MK, Heiberg E, Shields JB. Magnetic resonance imaging of lesions of synovial origin. *Skeletal Radiol* 1986;15:110–116.
81. Sundaram M, McDonald DJ. The solitary tumor or tumor like lesion of bone. *Top Magn Reson Imaging* 1989;1(4):17–29.
82. Tang JS, Gold RH, Bassett LW, Seeger LL. Musculoskeletal infection of the extremities: evaluation with MR imaging. *Radiology* 1988;166:205–209.
83. Thomas J, Colby M. Radiation-induced or metastatic brachial plexopathy. *JAMA* 1971;222:1392–1395.
84. Townley CO. The capsular mechanism in recurrent dislocation of the shoulder. *J Bone Joint Surg* 1950;32:370–380.
85. Turkel SJ, Panio MW, Marshall JL, Girgis FG. Stabilizing mechanisms prevent anterior dislocation of the glenohumeral joint. *J Bone Joint Surg* 1981;63:1208–1217.
86. Wilson AJ, Totty WG, Murphy WA, Hardy DC. Shoulder joint: arthrographic CT and long term follow-up with surgical correlation. *Radiology* 1989;173:329–333.
87. Wolfgang GL. Surgical repair of tears of the rotator cuff of the shoulder. *J Bone Joint Surg* 1974;56A:14–26.
88. Zimmer WD, Berquist TH, McLeod RA, et al. Bone tumors: magnetic resonance imaging versus computed tomography. *Radiology* 1985;155:709–718.
89. Zlatkin MB, Bjorkengren AG, Gylys-Morin V, Resnik D, Sartoris DJ. Cross-sectional imaging of the capsular mechanism of the glenohumeral joint. *AJR* 1988;150:151–158.
90. Zlatkin MB, Iannotti JP, Roberts MC, Esterhai JC, Dalinka MK, Kressel HY, Lenkinski RE. Rotator cuff disease. Diagnostic performance of MR imaging. *Radiology* 1989;172:223–229.
91. Zlatkin MB, Reicher MA, Kellerhouse LE, McDade W, Vetter L, Resnick D. The painful shoulder: MR imaging of the glenohumeral joint. *J Comput Assist Tomogr* 1988;12:995–1001.
92. Zlatkin MB, Dalinka MK. The glenohumeral joint. *Top Magn Reson Imaging* 1989;1(3):1–13.
93. Zlatkin MB, Dalinka MK, Kressel HY. Magnetic resonance imaging of the shoulder. *Magn Reson Q* 1989;5(1):3–22.

MRI of the Musculoskeletal System, 2nd Edition, edited by T. H. Berquist.
Raven Press, Ltd., New York © 1990.

CHAPTER 10

Elbow and Forearm

Thomas H. Berquist

Techniques, 357
Patient Positioning and Coil Selection, 357
Pulse Sequences and Image Planes, 358
Anatomy, 370
Articular Structures, 370
Bursae, 371
Muscles of the Elbow and Forearm, 371
Extensors, 377
Deep Extensors, 379
Neurovascular Anatomy, 380
Pitfalls, 382
Applications, 382
Trauma, 382
Neoplasms, 384
Avascular Necrosis (Osteonecrosis), 388
Infection/Inflammatory Arthropathies, 390
Miscellaneous Conditions, 390
References, 393

Magnetic resonance imaging (MRI) of the elbow and forearm can clearly define normal bone and soft tissue anatomy and pathology (8,16). Clinical information (symptomatic region, the relationship of symptoms to flexion, extension, pronation, and supination) and the type of pathology suspected are important in planning the MRI examination. In order to solve a given clinical problem, the patient must be comfortable, properly positioned, and the best image planes and pulse sequences selected to optimize lesion identification and characterization.

TECHNIQUES

Patient Positioning and Coil Selection

Patient positioning is as important with MRI as with other radiographic techniques (see Chapter 3). The types of coil available, gantry limitations, patient size, and clinical status may lead to suboptimal examinations, particularly in the upper extremity. The confining nature of the MR gantry reduces positioning options, especially for larger patients. Patients are usually most comfortable when supine with the elbow extended and arm at their side (Fig. 10-1). The circular or license plate shaped flat coils can be used in this position. The circular coil is optimal for localized evaluation of the elbow, while the larger license plate coil is preferred for examination of larger areas such as the forearm or elbow and forearm (Fig. 10-2). Partial volume and circumferential coils for the upper extremity are also available. Positioning the patient with the arm at the side can only be accomplished when software allows the use of off-axis small field of view (8,9).

Different positions and coils may be required when software does not permit off-center placement of surface coils (off-axis small field of view) or when patients are too large. The elbow can be moved closer to the center of the magnet by rotating the patient and/or placing the elbow above the head (Fig. 10-3 and middle of Fig. 10-1). In the latter position a volume (circumferential) coil can be used. A volume or circumferential coil provides more uniform signal intensity, avoiding the problem of signal drop-off seen with flat surface coils (36,40). Unfortunately, patient discomfort can be significant when the arm is above the head. As a result, images may be degraded by motion artifact. In our initial review of 200 upper extremity cases, we found image degradation due to motion in 25%. Motion artifact is usually not a

T. H. Berquist: Mayo Medical School and Mayo Clinic, Rochester, Minnesota 55905.

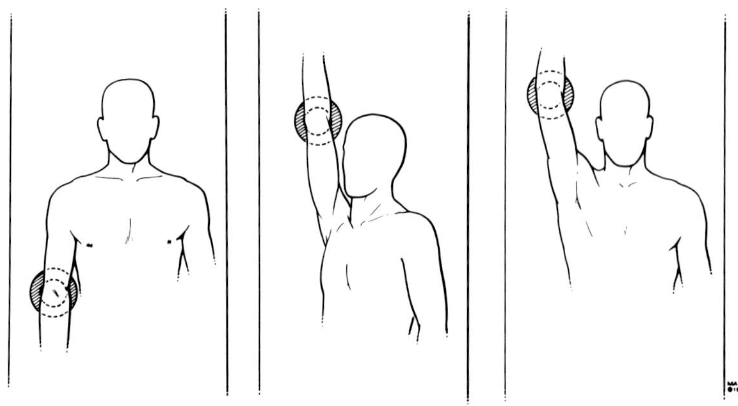

FIG. 10-1. Illustration of positions for imaging the elbow. The most easily tolerated is the arm at the side (**left**). When the arm is positioned above the head (**middle** and **right**), the patient has more difficulty tolerating the examination.

problem when the patient is supine with the arm at the side (8,9).

In certain situations, such as biceps insertion pathology, positioning the patient with the elbow flexed displays anatomy to better advantage (Fig. 10-4). This may be impossible with large patients. Smaller patients can be rotated into the oblique position with the elbow flexed at the side. Axial examinations during pronation and supination are also useful for evaluating the biceps tendon and subtle abnormalities in the radioulnar joint. Both axial and sagittal images should be obtained. When motion studies are required, it is usually best to use gradient-echo sequences (see below) and cine studies. Videotapes of the examination can easily be produced. This technique provides more information than static images in areas where motion is important to analyze (8).

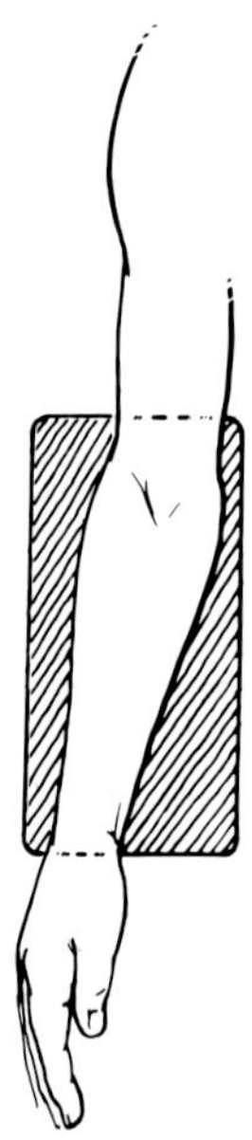

FIG. 10-2. Illustration of license plate coil for examining the elbow and forearm. (From ref. 8, with permission.)

Comparison of both extremities is useful in patients with subtle pathology. This doubles the examination time with conventional coils and software. Dual coils are being developed that allow simultaneous examinations of both upper extremities. This will reduce image time significantly without reduction in image quality (28,53).

Pulse Sequences and Image Planes

Many examinations of the elbow and forearm can be performed in the axial plane using T1 (SE 500/20) and T2 (SE 2,000/20–30, 60–80) weighted sequences. This will generally provide sufficient information to screen for most suspected abnormalities (9).

In most situations a coronal scout is obtained (Fig. 10-5, Table 10-1). Three 1 cm thick slices are obtained using a spin-echo sequence (200/20), large field of view (FOV) (32–40 cm), 256 × 128 matrix, and one excitation or average. This can be accomplished in approximately 26 sec with a 128 × 256 matrix or 52 sec with a 256 × 256 matrix and one excitation. The first axial images are usually performed using a T2 (SE 2,000/30, 60 or 2,000/20, 80) sequence. Soft tissue contrast is superior with this pulse sequence so the likelihood of overlooking an abnormality is remote (Table 10-1). Initial axial slice thicknesses vary depending on the region of interest and size of the suspected or palpable lesion (Fig. 10-6). Larger, palpable lesions can be evaluated with 1 cm thick slices and 0.25–0.5 cm interslice gaps. Thinner (3–5 mm/skip 1.5–2.5 mm) slices are used when more subtle pathology is suspected. We typically use a 16–24 cm FOV, 192 × 256 matrix, and two excitations, which provides excellent image quality. The axial T2 weighted sequence takes 12.8 min using these parameters (Table 10-1). The second sequence is a T1 weighted scan using SE 500/20 sequence in either the axial, coronal, or sagittal plane (Figs. 10-7 and 10-8) depending on the clinical symptoms and findings on the

Text continues on p. 370

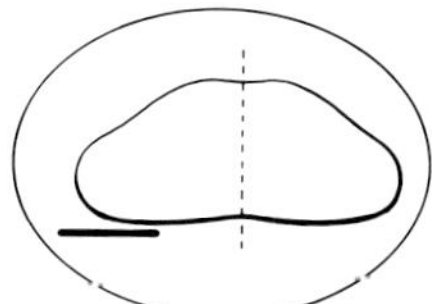
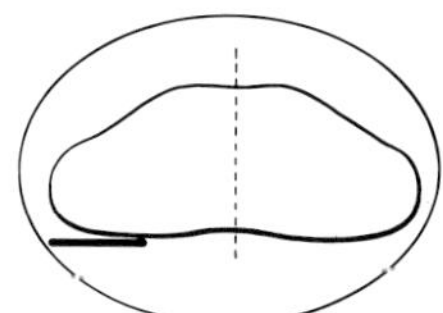
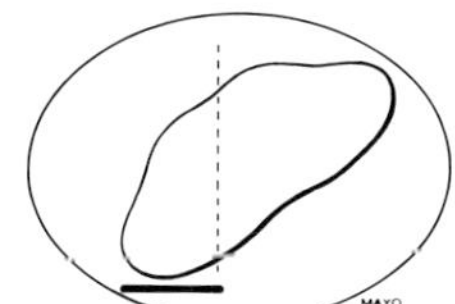

FIG. 10-3. Illustration of the effect of rotating the patient to bring the upper extremity closer to the midline. **Left:** Average patient size. **Middle:** Larger patient with extremities closer to gantry. **Right:** Rotated patient with upper extremity nearer midline.

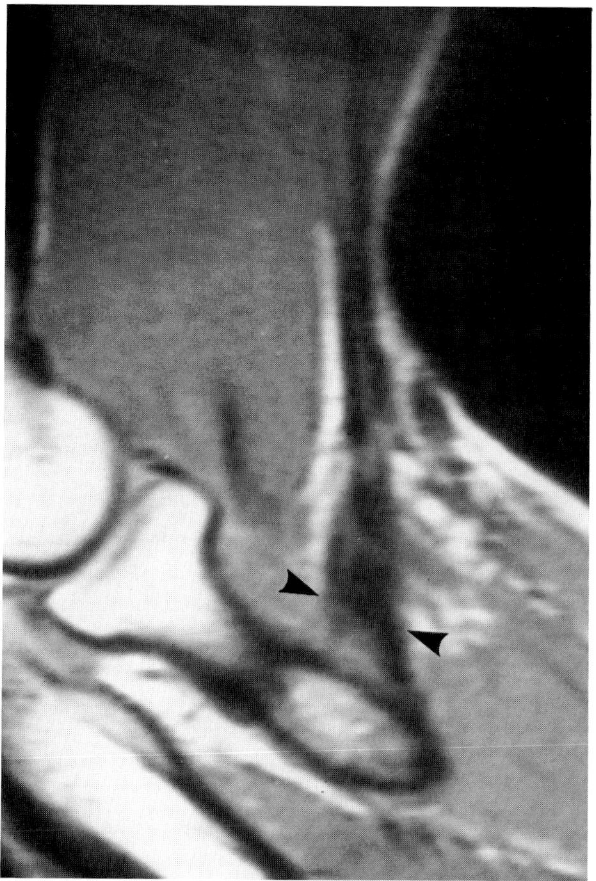

FIG. 10-4. Sagittal (SE 500/20) image of the elbow, demonstrating the biceps tendon as it expands (*arrowheads*) near its attachment on the tuberosity of the radius.

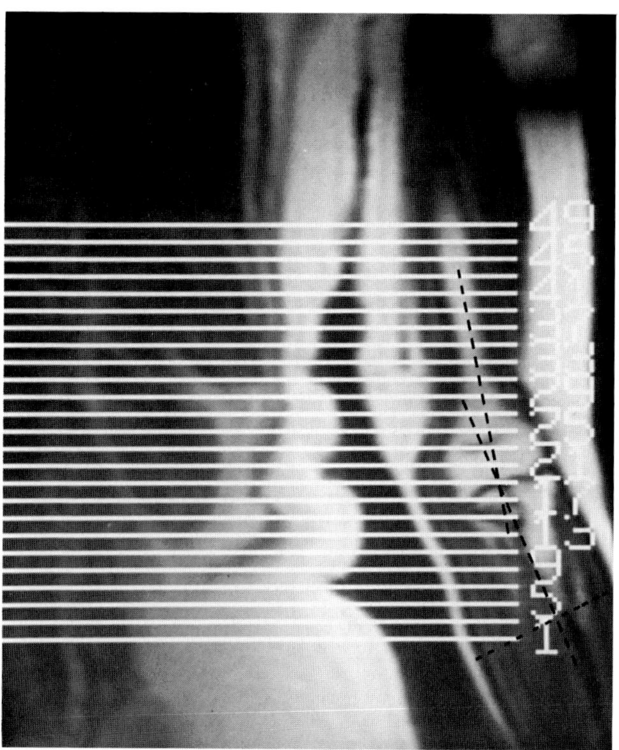

FIG. 10-5. Coronal scout image of the elbow with axial image planes selected. The left side of the trunk is also seen due to the large (40 cm) field of view. The axis of the humerus and forearm (*dark lines*) must be considered to obtain true axial images. The normal carrying angle of the elbow is 3–29°. Therefore, axial images of the forearm need to be angled (*transverse line*).

TABLE 10-1. *Routine MR examination of the elbow and forearm*

	Pulse sequence	Slice thickness	FOV (cm)	Matrix	Excitations	Image time
Scout (coronal)	SE 200/20	1 cm	32–40	256 × 128	1	26 sec
				256 × 256		52 sec
Axial	SE 2,000/20–30, 60–80	5 mm/skip 2.5 mm	16–24	256 × 256	1	8.53 min
		1 cm/skip 2.5 mm		256 × 192	2[a]	12.8 min
Axial, coronal, or sagittal	SE 500/20	5 mm/skip 2.5 mm	16–24	256 × 256	1	2.13 min
		1 cm/skip 2.5 mm		or		
				256 × 256	2[a]	4.26 min
				Total image time		11.26–17.91 min

[a] Best for small patients and children to improve image quality.

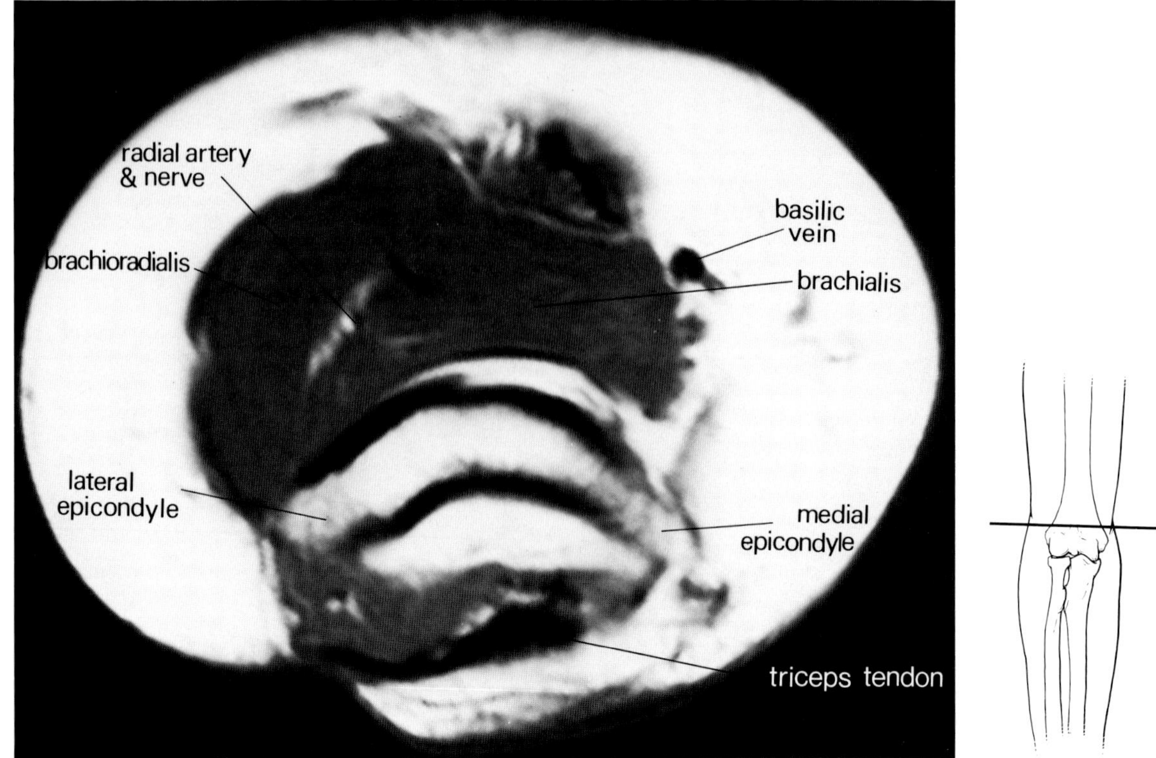

FIG. 10-6. Axial MR images (SE 500/20) of the elbow and forearm with anatomy labeled. **A:** Axial image through the supracondylar region.

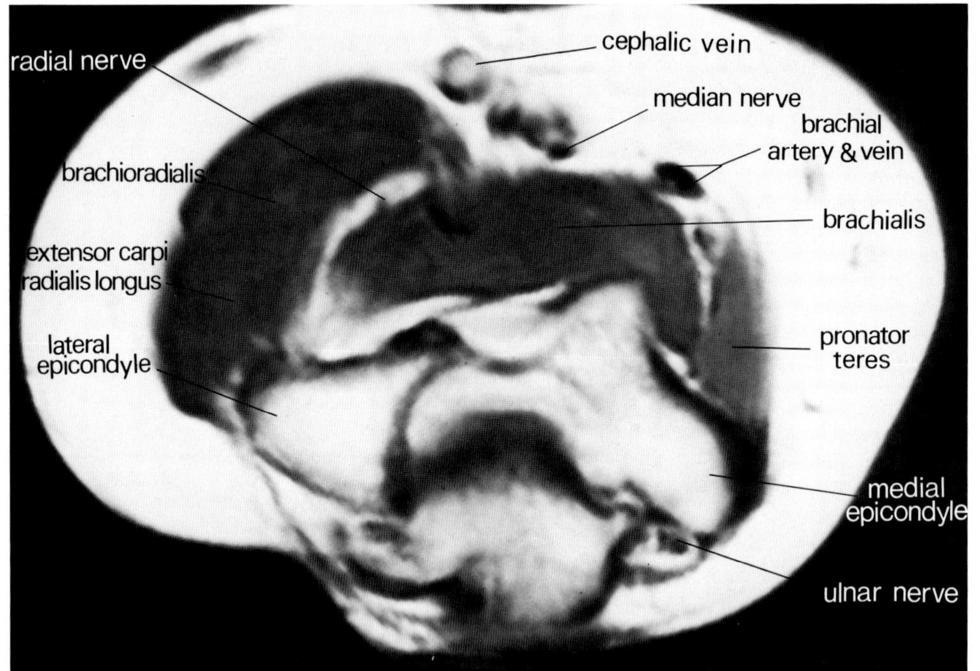

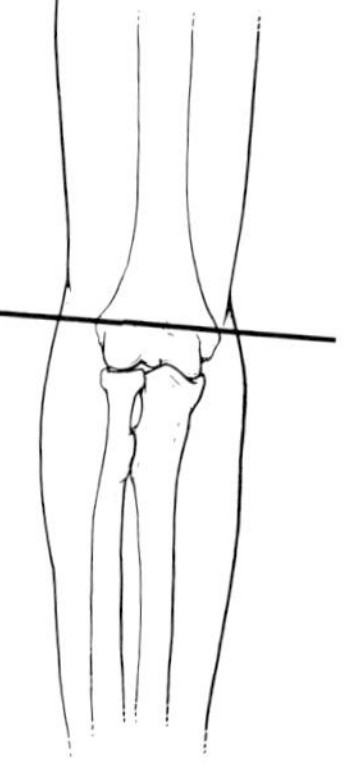

FIG. 10-6. B: Axial image through the medial and lateral epicondyle.

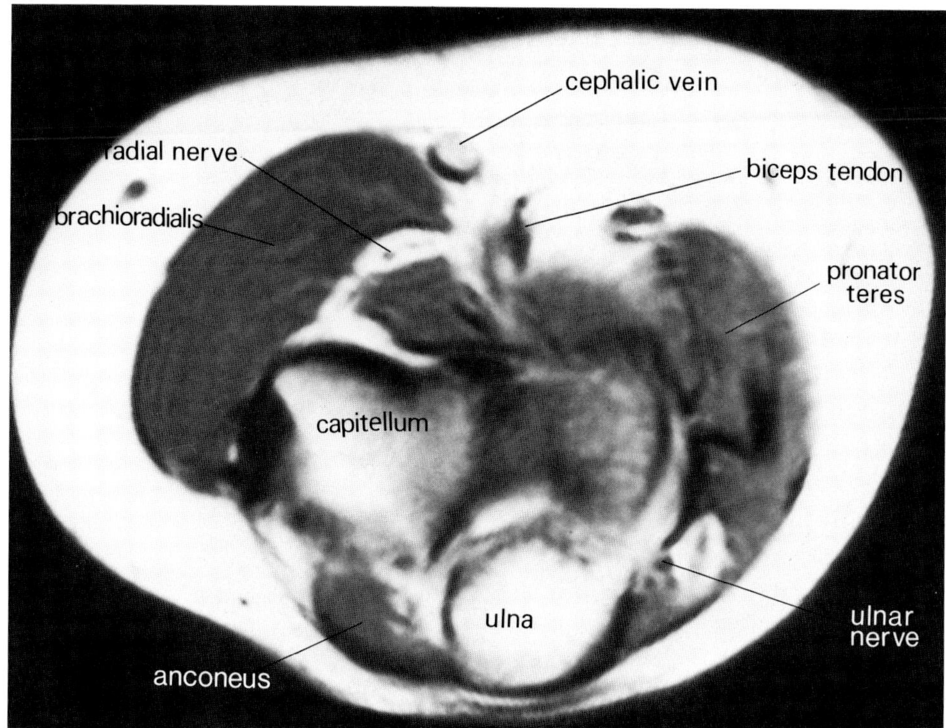

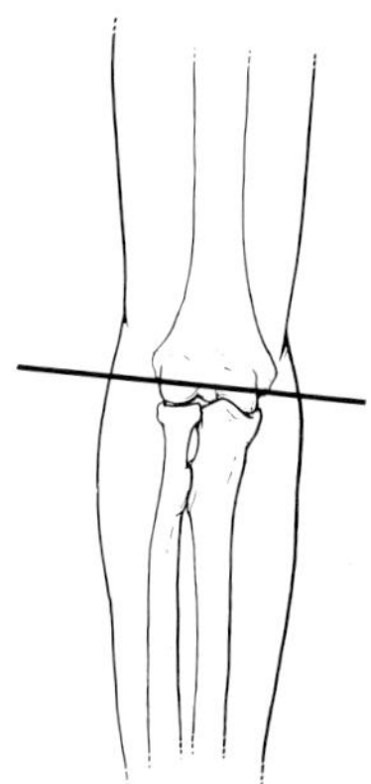

FIG. 10-6. C: Axial image through the capitellum.

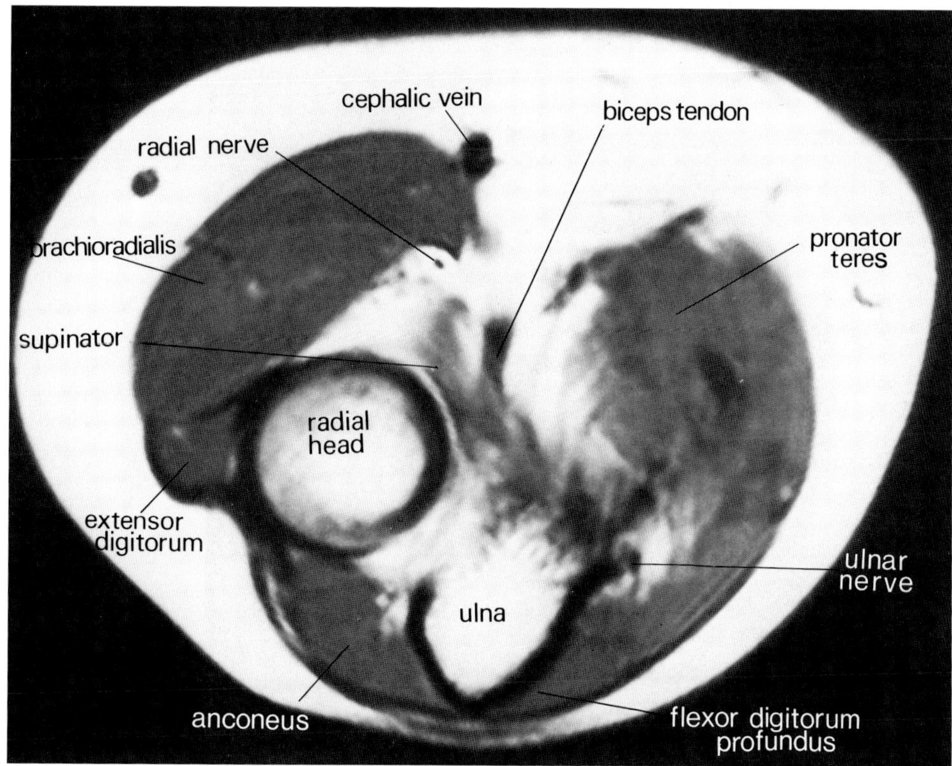

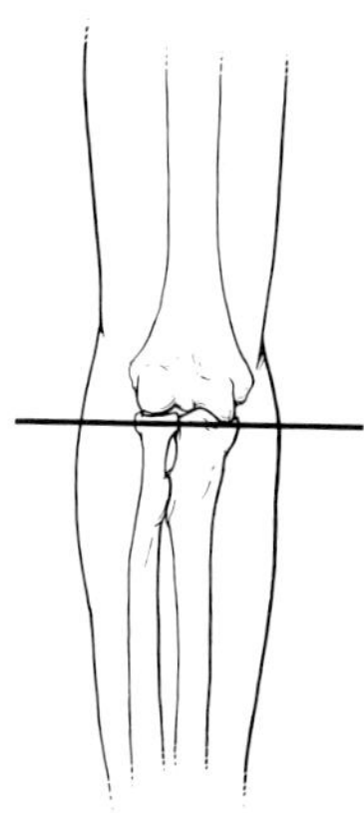

FIG. 10-6. D: Axial image through the radial head.

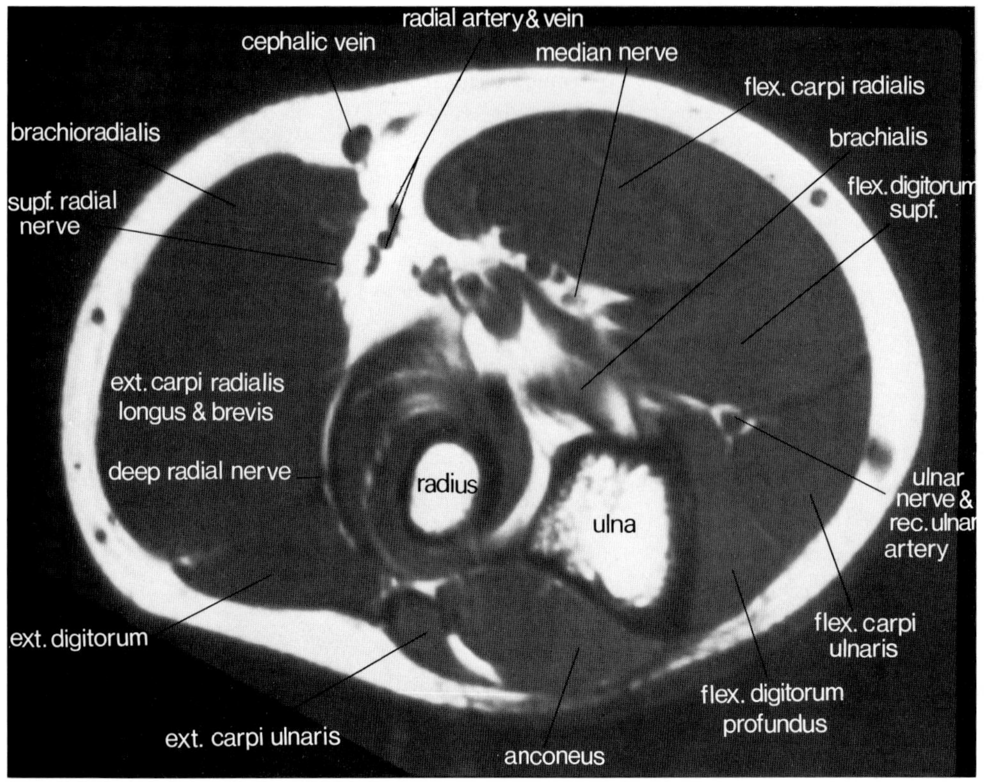

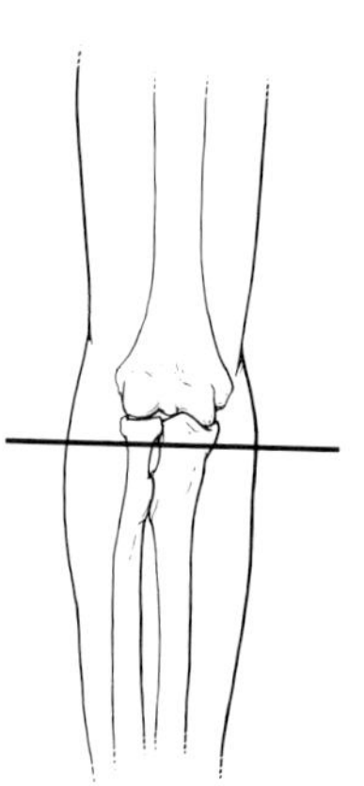

FIG. 10-6. E: Axial image at a level just distal to the radial head.

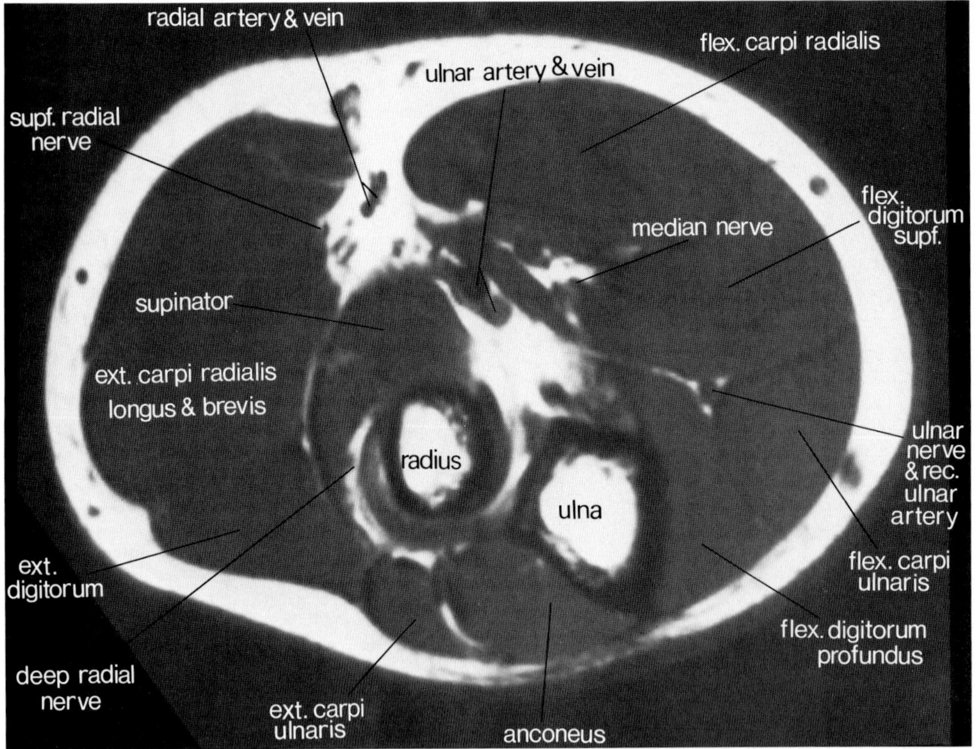

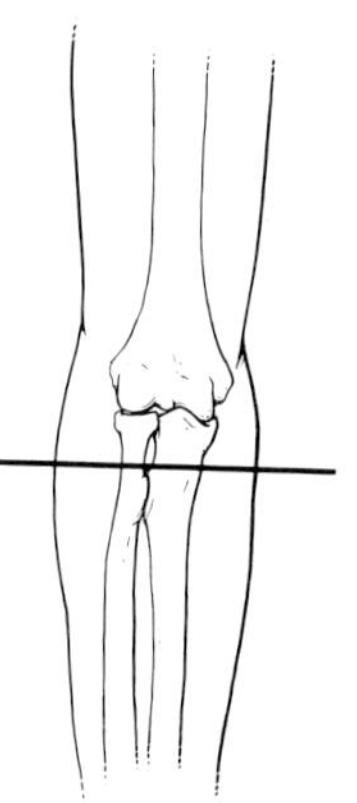

FIG. 10-6. F: Axial image through the radial neck.

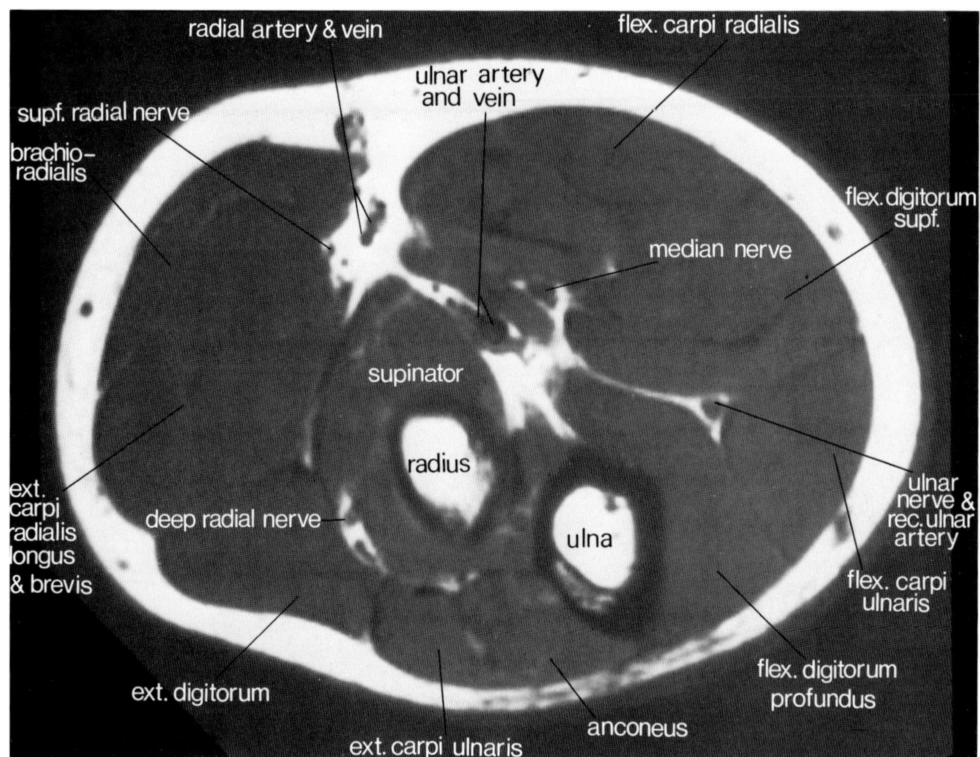

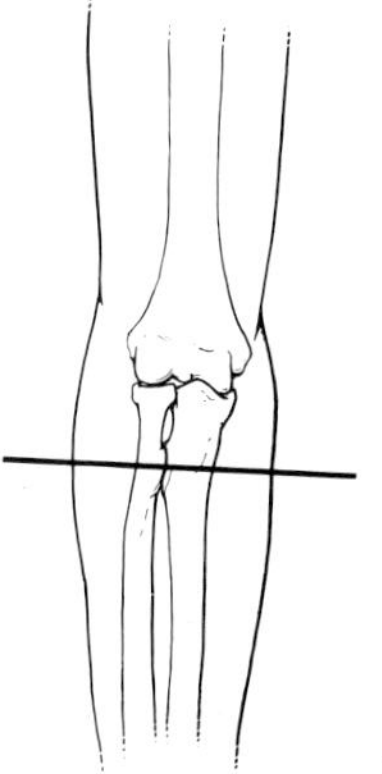

FIG. 10-6. G: Axial image at the level of the radial tuberosity.

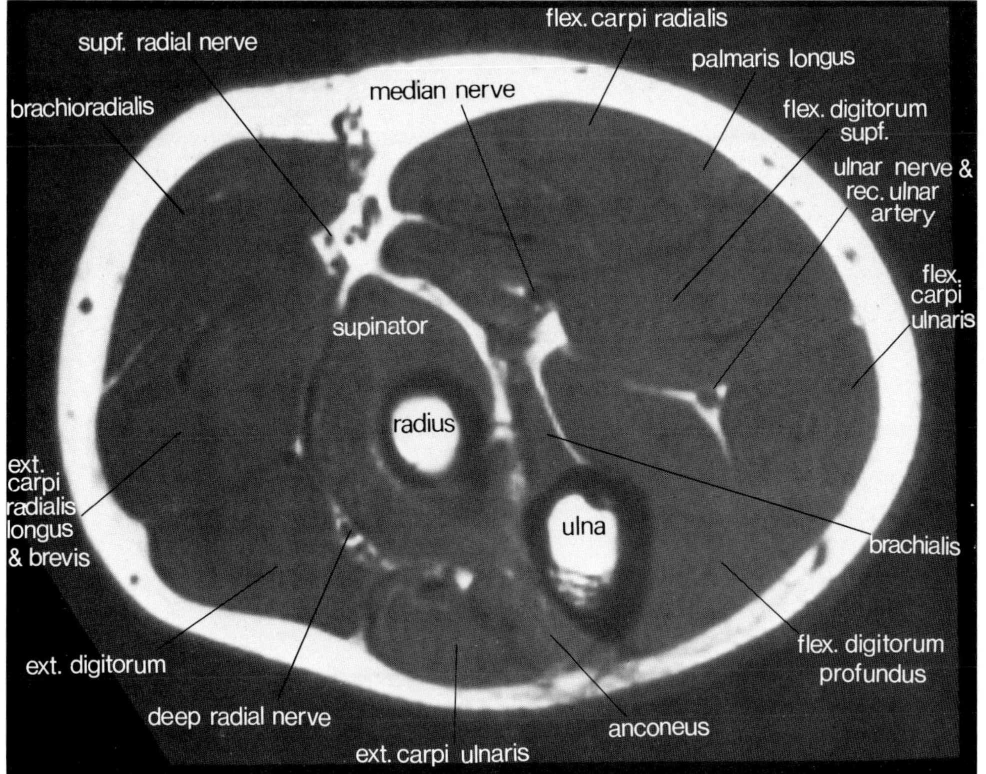

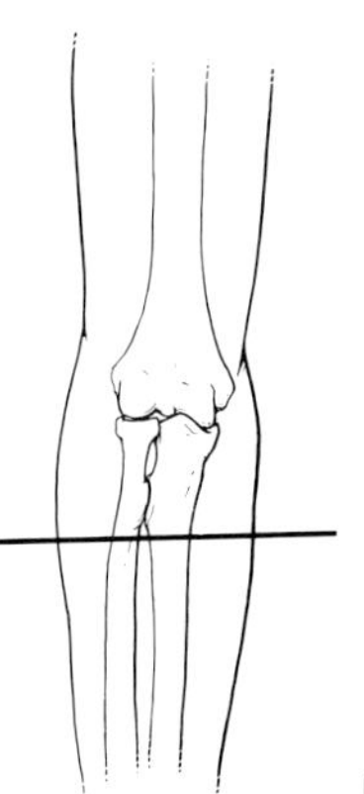

FIG. 10-6. H: Axial image below the tuberosity level.

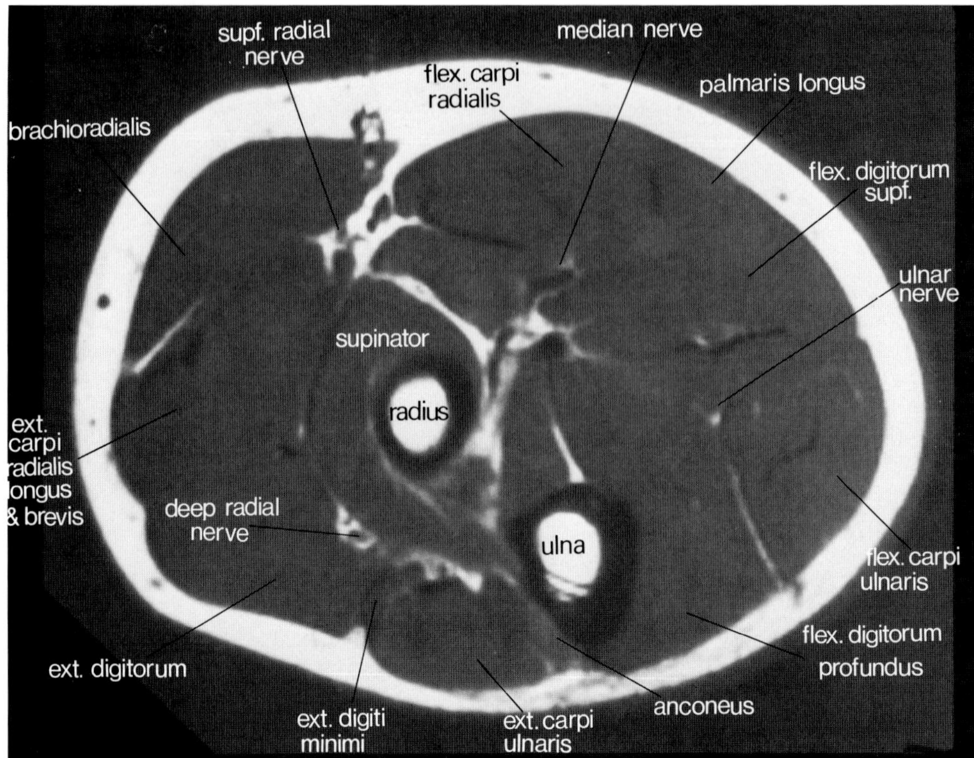

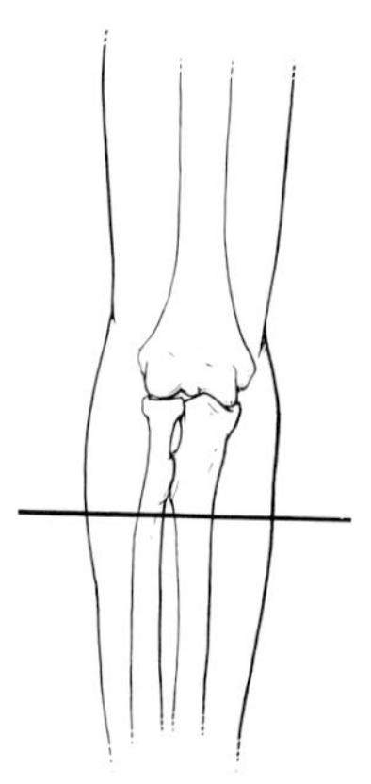

FIG. 10-6. I: Axial image proximal forearm.

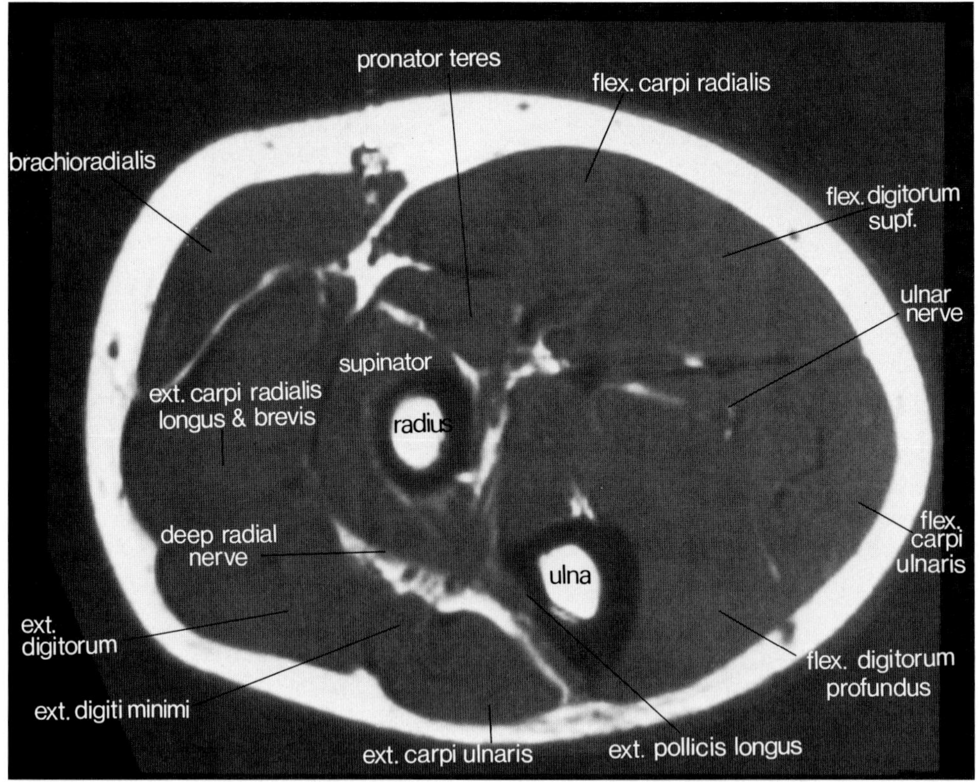

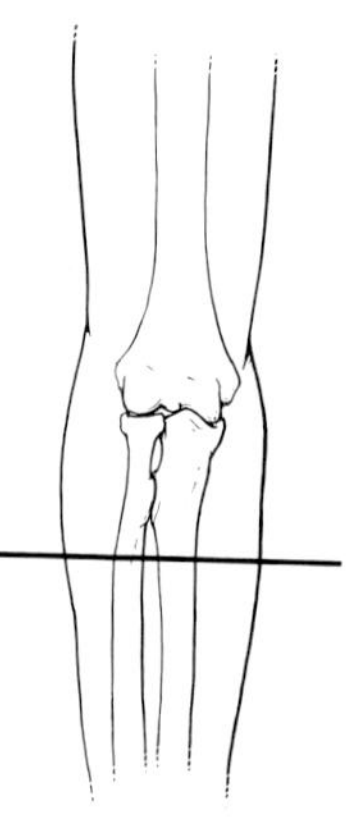

FIG. 10-6. J: Axial image proximal forearm.

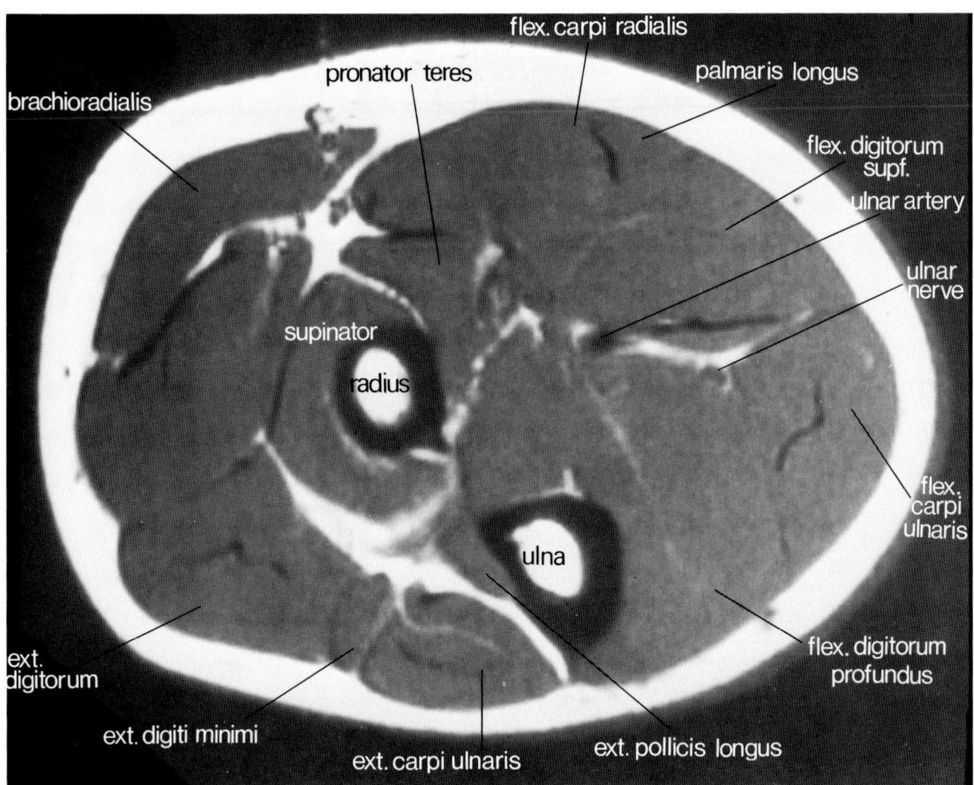

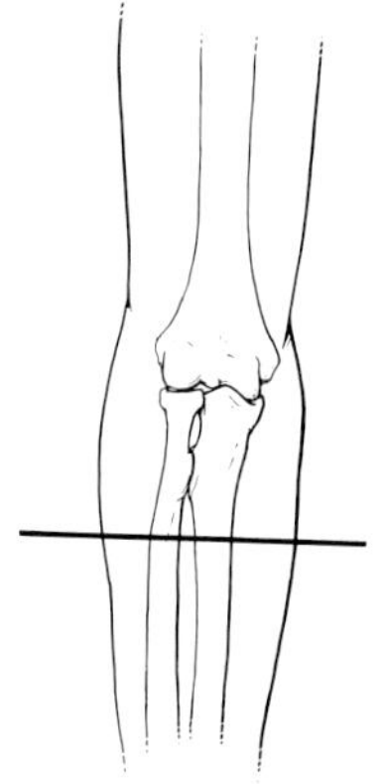

FIG. 10-6. K: Axial image proximal forearm.

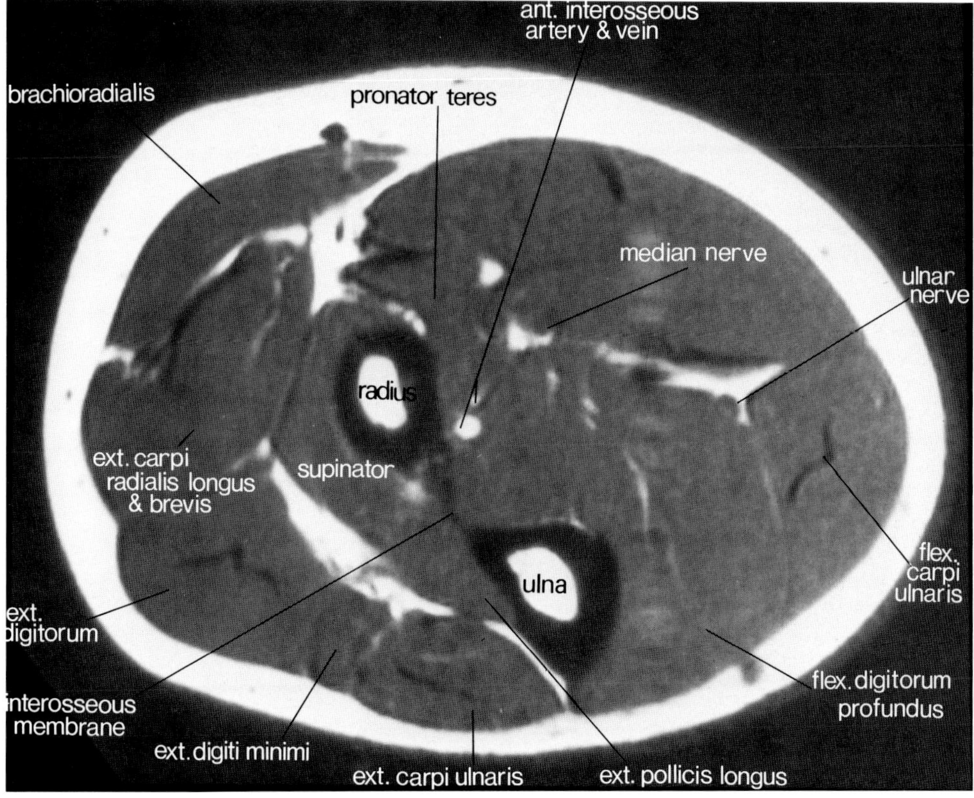

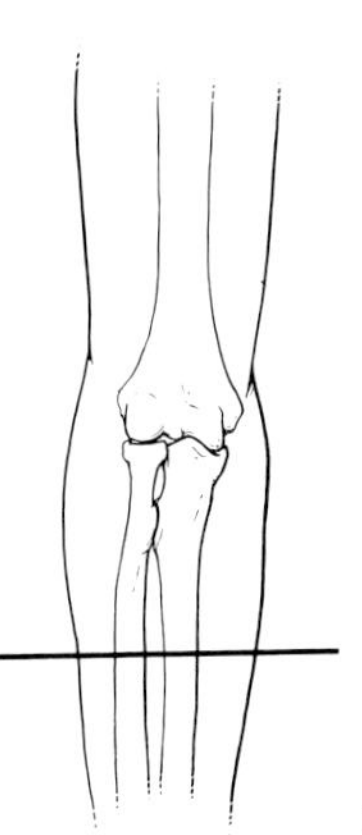

FIG. 10-6. L: Axial image proximal forearm.

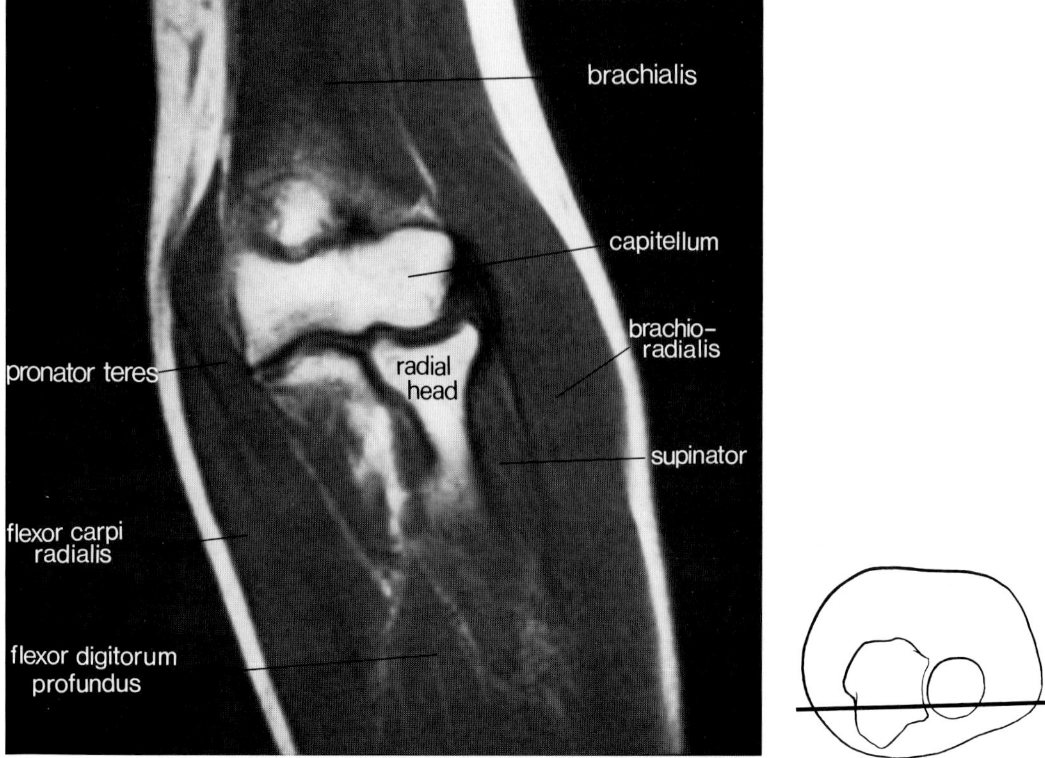

FIG. 10-7. Coronal images of the elbow and forearm with anatomy labeled. **A:** Coronal image through posterior elbow and forearm.

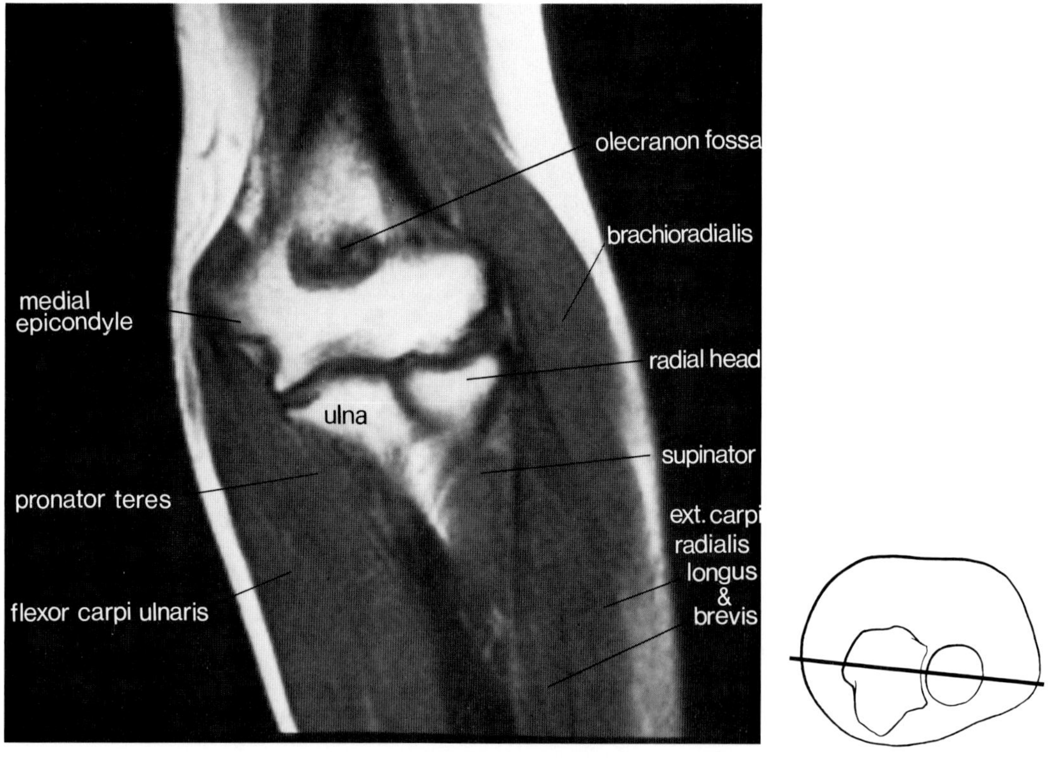

FIG. 10-7. B: Coronal image through midelbow and forearm.

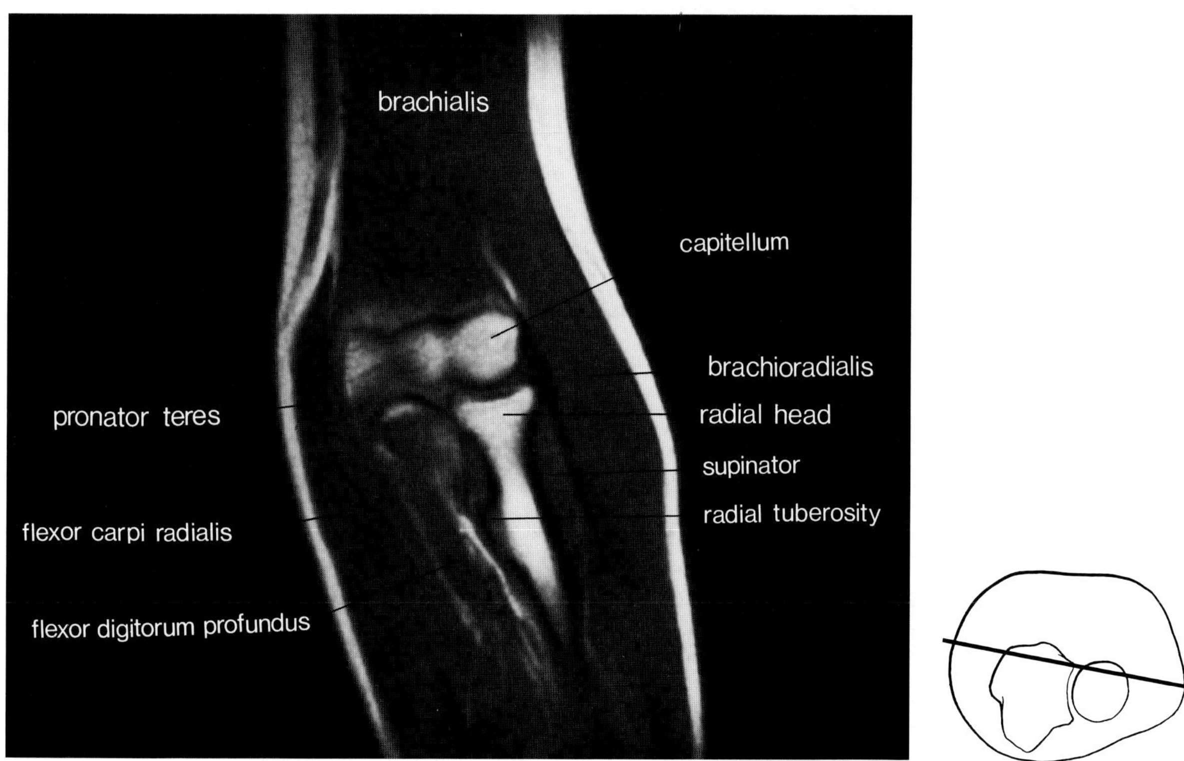

FIG. 10-7. C: Coronal image through anterior elbow and forearm.

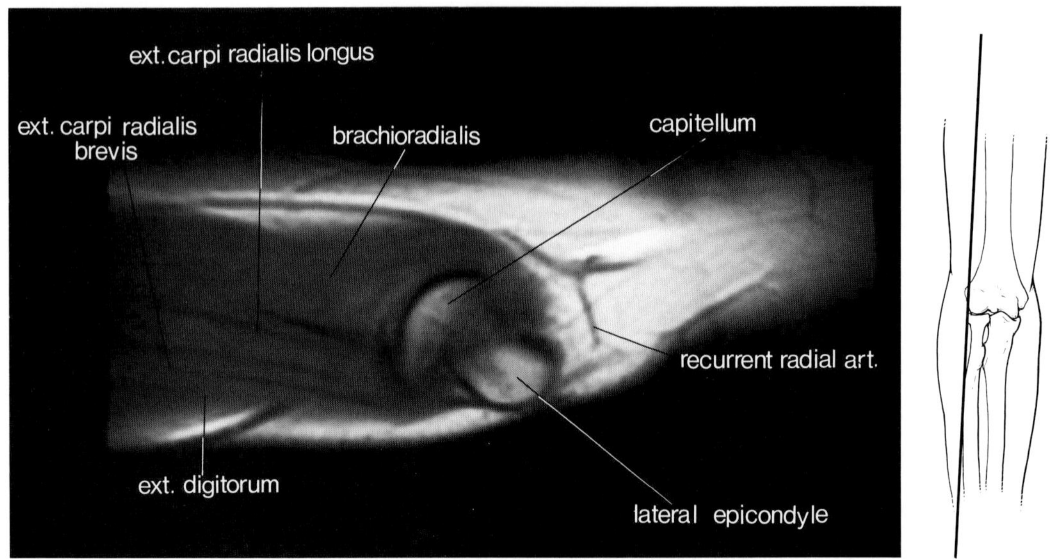

FIG. 10-8. Sagittal images of the elbow and forearm with anatomy labeled. **A:** Sagittal image through lateral epicondyle.

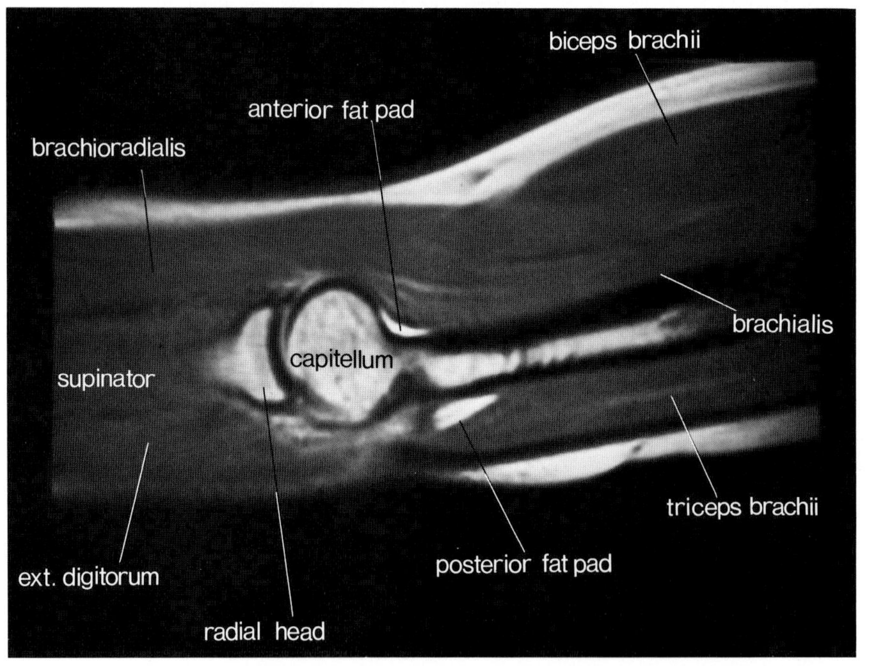

FIG. 10-8. B: Sagittal image through lateral radiocapitellar joint.

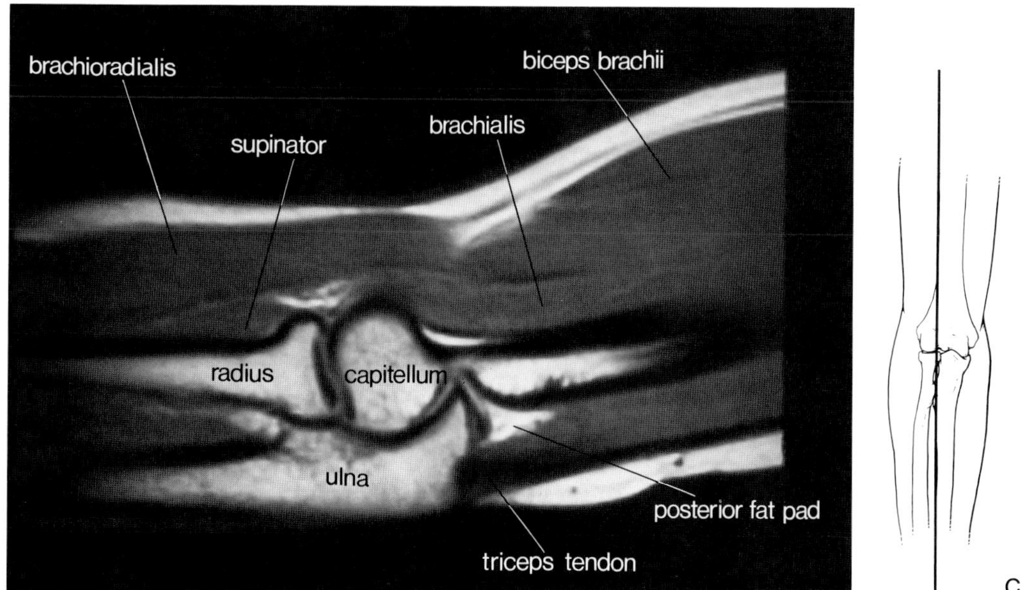

FIG. 10-8. C: Sagittal image through ulnar aspect of radiocapitellar joint.

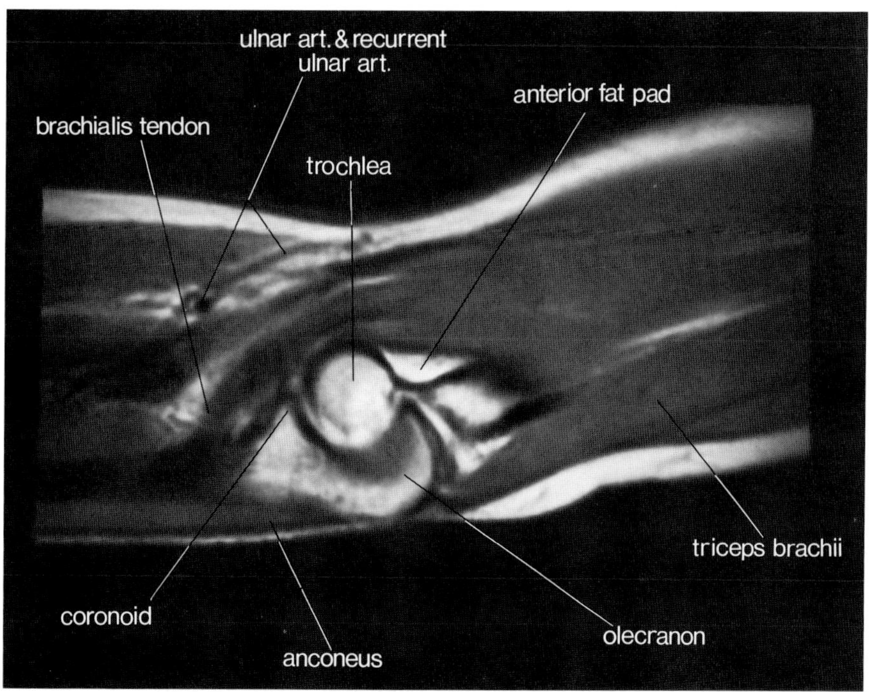

FIG. 10-8. D: Sagittal image through ulnar–trochlear articulation.

axial images. The FOV, matrix size, and excitations are the same as described with the T2 weighted sequence. This sequence takes 2.13–4.26 min (Table 10-1). No further studies may be needed if the examination is normal or if the lesion is clearly identified and characterized. If the nature or extent of the lesion is unclear, further image planes and sequences may be needed.

Inversion recovery, short T1 inversion recovery (STIR), gradient-echo sequences (GRASS, GRIL, FLASH, etc.), and chemical shift sequences may be indicated in certain situations. Inversion recovery sequences provide more purely T1 weighted images than spin-echo sequences with short TR/TE (500/20) (see Chapter 2). These sequences are not commonly used in musculoskeletal imaging. However, short T1 inversion recovery sequences can be very useful for evaluating subtle lesions, specifically in bone marrow. This pulse sequence (TE 30, TR 1,500, TI 100–150) can be performed in 75% of the time required for a typical T2 weighted spin-echo sequence (SE 2,000/60–80). In addition, STIR sequences provide superior contrast by adding the effects of prolonged T1 and T2 and by suppressing fat signal. This provides contrast ratios of up to 18:1 for pathologic lesions to fat and 12:1 for pathology compared to muscle (23,49).

Gradient-echo sequences with reduced flip angles and short TRs provide excellent flexibility for rapid imaging in different positions (48). These techniques are especially useful when evaluating articular problems that require evaluating anatomic changes during flexion, extension, supination, and pronation (minimum TR/TE, flip angle 30–70°, 2–4 Nex). Static GRASS images are particularly useful for evaluating vascular anatomy and pathology (3,12–15,26).

Chemical shift imaging can be used in marrow to separate fat and water signal intensity. Marrow is normally 30% fat and 70% H_2O (blood cells) in adults. Spin-echo sequences may not provide the necessary contrast to separate fat and water (47). Chemical shift techniques are not commonly used in the elbow and forearm. Additional technical data are discussed later as they apply to specific clinical applications.

ANATOMY

Anatomy of the elbow and forearm is complex but effectively demonstrated by MRI (9,16,33,34) (Figs. 10-6 to 10-8).

Articular Structures

The elbow articulations are formed by three osseous structures. The lower end of the humerus, consisting of the capitellum and the trochlea, articulates with the radial head and ulna, respectively (Fig. 10-7). The radial head also articulates with the adjacent radial notch of the ulna (1,17,29). All articular surfaces are covered with hyaline cartilage, which is seen as an area of intermediate signal intensity on spin-echo MR images (16,33,34). The articular capsule of the elbow is thin anteriorly and posteriorly with additional support provided anteriorly by the brachialis muscle and posteriorly by the triceps muscle (Fig. 10-8). Supplementary support medially and laterally is provided by the radial and ulnar collateral ligament complexes (29,35) (Fig. 10-9). These ligaments can be identified on the axial images and coronal MR images (9,16) (Fig. 10-10). The anterior capsule attaches to the humerus just above the radial and coronoid fossae and extends beyond the coronoid process of the ulna to the anterior portion of the annular ligament (Fig. 10-11A). The posterior capsule is closely related to the triceps tendon and attaches to the humerus above the olecranon fossa, attaching inferiorly to the upper and lateral margins of the trochlear notch of the ulna, the roughened area on the lateral side of the ulna, and the annular ligament of the radius (Fig. 10-11B). Medially and laterally the capsule blends with the medial and lateral collateral ligaments. The capsule is not usually clearly demonstrated on MR images unless there is an effusion. In this setting it is often best appreciated on axial and sagittal images (Figs. 10-6 and 10-8). It may be difficult to separate the capsule from the brachialis muscle anteriorly and triceps tendon posteriorly (2,29,35).

Varus and valgus injuries to the elbow can result in disruption of either the radial or ulnar collateral ligaments and capsule (9,35). Therefore, these structures need to be further defined (Fig. 10-9). The medial (ulnar) collateral ligament attaches above the anterior inferior aspect of the medial epicondyle, becoming triangular as it progresses distally. The ligament commonly forms three bands, which are continuous with each other. The anterior band runs anteriorly from the epicondyle to attach on the medial edge of the coronoid process. The middle band also extends from the epicondyle, expanding to attach along the ridge between the coronoid and olecranon process, and blends with the transverse band, which stretches between the olecranon and coronoid processes (Fig. 10-9A). The posterior portion of the ligament extends from behind the medial epicondyle, running slightly posteriorly to attach on the medial aspect of the olecranon (Fig. 10-9A). The lateral (radial) collateral ligament is attached to the anterior inferior aspects of the lateral epicondyle, deep to the common extensor tendon. It extends distally to insert in the annular ligament of the radius and fibers of the supinator muscle (Fig. 10-9B). There is an additional ligament that extends between the radial neck and ulna, termed the quadrate ligament. The annular ligament is a well-defined structure that attaches anteriorly and posteriorly to the radial notch of the ulna (Fig. 10-9B). This

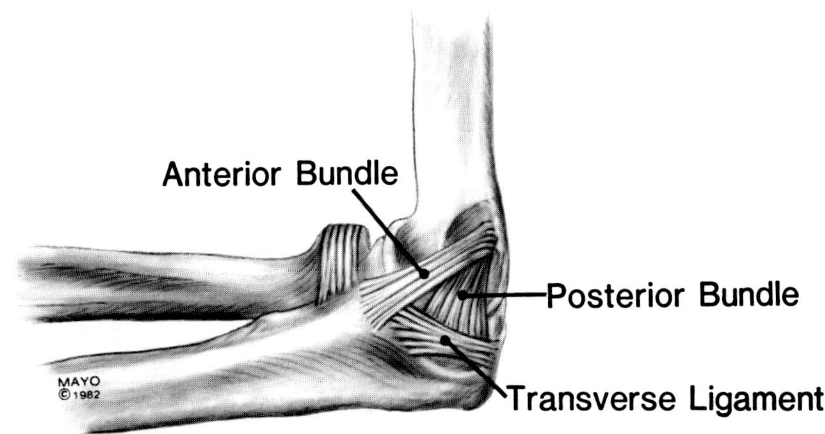

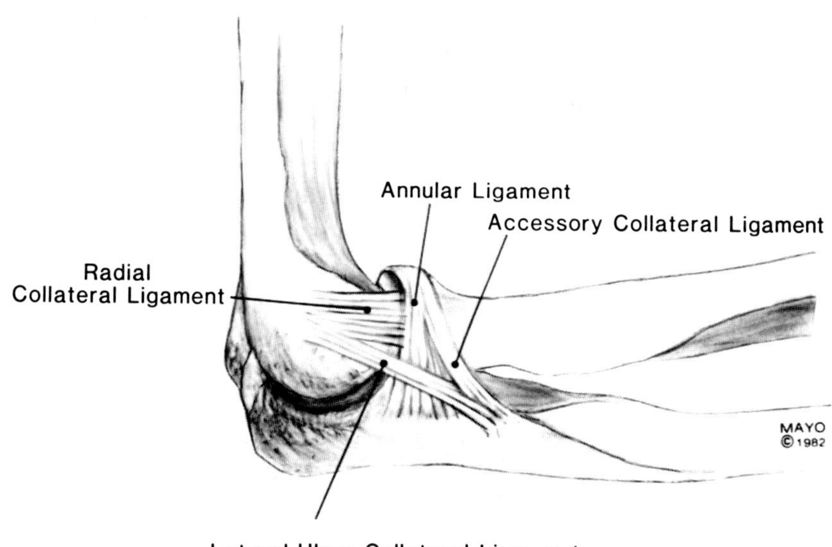

FIG. 10-9. Lateral illustrations of the ligaments of the elbow from the medial (**A**) and lateral (**B**) sides. (From ref. 35, with permission.)

somewhat thin ligament is best seen on axial MR images (2,29,35) (Fig. 10-6).

The capsule of the elbow joint is lined with synovial membrane (Fig. 10-11) with two prominent anterior and posterior fat pads that are intracapsular but extrasynovial. These have commonly been used in evaluating routine radiographs but can also be useful in MR evaluations (Fig. 10-8).

Bursae

There are several important superficial and deep bursae about the elbow that should be emphasized because of the potential for confusion with cysts or other pathology on MR images. Superficial bursae include the olecranon and the medial and lateral epicondylar bursae. There are three potential olecranon bursae locations. The most common is the subcutaneous olecranon bursa. There are also intratendinous and subtendinous bursae in the olecranon region (29,35) (Fig. 10-12, Table 10-2). The subtendinous bursa is best seen on axial and sagittal MR images and should not be confused with an elbow effusion. An inflamed bursa can be differentiated from a simple effusion by the lack of fluid in the anterior compartment of the elbow. The other two superficial bursae, the medial epicondylar and lateral epicondylar, should not be confused with disruptions or tears in the medial and lateral collateral ligaments. Figure 10-13 demonstrates the location of the other superficial and deep bursae in the elbow region. The relationship of these bursae to branches of the radial and ulnar nerves (Fig. 10-13) is important (29,35). These bursae are normally not identified but when inflamed and fluid-filled, they can be demonstrated on T2 weighted MR images. In this setting the bursae will appear as homogeneous high-intensity structures with clearly defined margins.

Muscles of the Elbow and Forearm

The muscular anatomy of the elbow and forearm is complex (Tables 10-3 and 10-4). Generally, there are four basic movements in the elbow and forearm. The

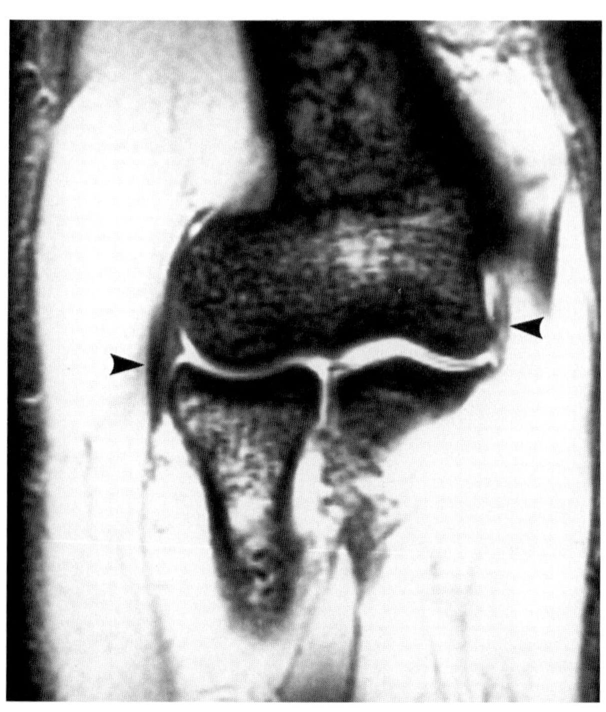

FIG. 10-10. Coronal GRASS image of the elbow, demonstrating the radial and ulnar collateral ligaments (*arrowheads*).

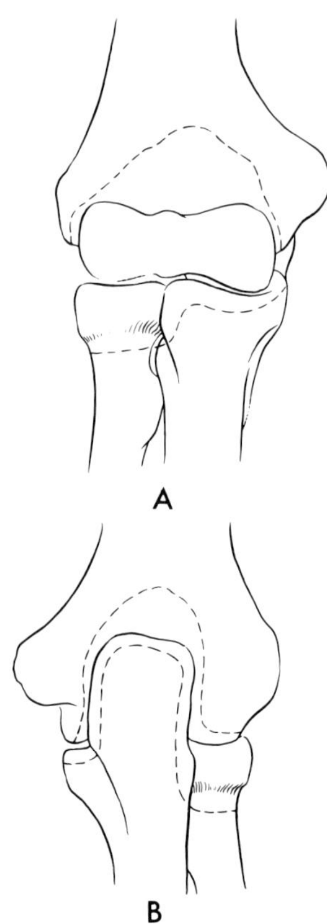

FIG. 10-11. Illustrations of the capsule of the elbow (*broken lines*) seen in a cut coronal anterior (**A**) and posterior (**B**) display. (From ref. 29, with permission.)

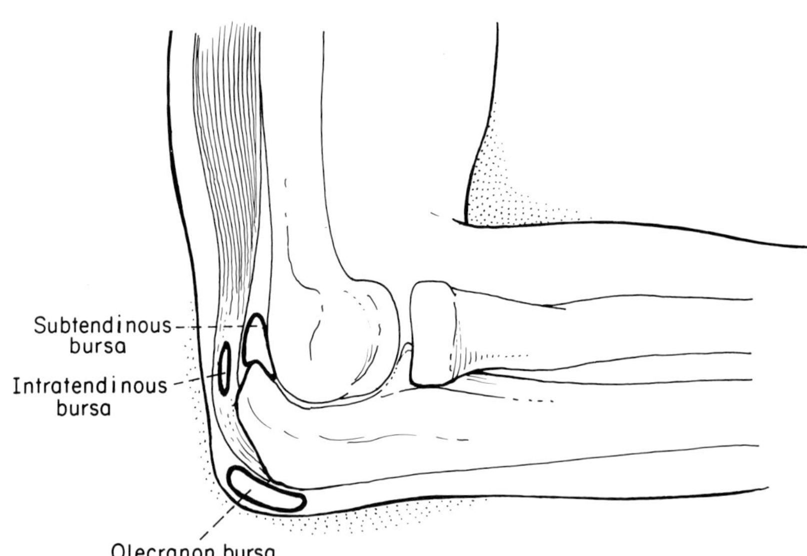

FIG. 10-12. Illustration of the olecranon bursae. The superficial subcutaneous bursa is most commonly seen. The intratendinous and subtendinous bursae are less frequently identified. (From ref. 35, with permission.)

TABLE 10-2. *Elbow bursae (35)*

Superficial
Olecranon (subcutaneous, intratendinous, subtendinous)
Medial epicondylar
Lateral epicondylar
Deep
Radiohumeral bursa
Supinator bursa
Bicipital bursa
Subextensor carpi radialis brevis bursa
Ulnar nerve bursa

elbow is limited to flexion and extension. Pronation and supination occur between the radius and ulna. It should be kept in mind that in the extended position the normal carrying angle of the elbow ranges from 3° to 29° (see Fig. 10-5). When discussing the muscles of the elbow and forearm, it is simplest to discuss them based on their functions (Tables 10-3 and 10-4) (2,17,29,35).

There are two major categories as described above: namely, flexors and extensors, and pronators and supinators. The chief flexors of the elbow are the biceps, brachialis, and brachioradialis (Figs. 10-6, 10-8, and 10-14 and Table 10-3). The biceps brachii crosses the elbow anteriorly to insert on the radial tubercle and serves as a supinator in addition to a flexor (29) (Figs. 10-4, 10-6, 10-14). The brachialis is a large muscle that arises from the anterior humerus and passes anterior to the elbow before inserting on the proximal ulna near the coronoid process (Figs. 10-6, 10-7, and 10-14). The brachioradialis arises from the radial side of the distal hu-

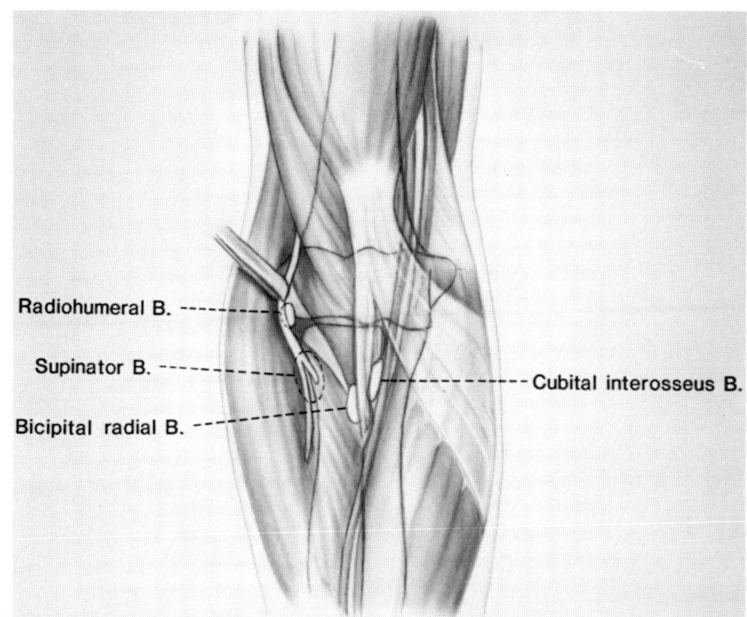

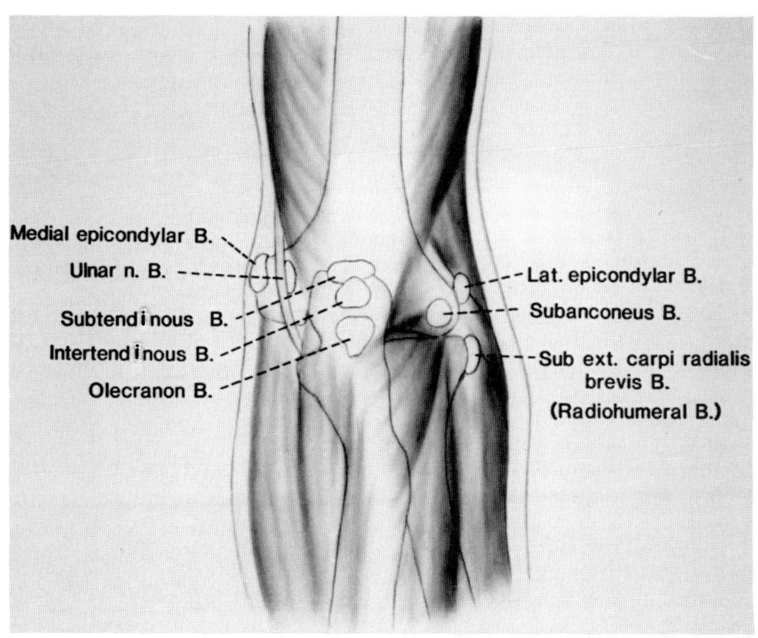

FIG. 10-13. Illustrations of the bursae of the elbow seen anteriorly (**A**) and posteriorly (**B**). Note the relationship of the bursae to the ulnar nerve and neural branches anteriorly (**A**). (From ref. 35, with permission.)

TABLE 10-3. *Muscles of the elbow*

Muscle	Origin	Insertion	Action	Blood supply	Innervation
Biceps brachii	Two heads: (1) supraglenoid tubercle and (2) coracoid	(1) Radial tuberosity (bursa separates tendon from tuberosity) and (2) aponeurosis to forearm flexors	Elbow flexor, supinator	Brachial branches	Musculocutaneous C5–C6
Brachialis	Lower two-thirds of anterior humerus	Coronoid and ulnar tuberosity	Elbow flexor	Brachial branches	Musculocutaneous C5–C6
Brachioradialis	Supracondylar ridge of lateral humerus	Distal lateral radius	Elbow flexor	Radial and radial recurrent arteries	Radial C5–C6
Pronator teres	Two heads: (1) medial supracondylar ridge and interosseous membrane and (2) coronoid of ulna	Midlateral radius	Pronation, accessory elbow flexor	Ulnar and recurrent ulnar arteries	Median C5–C7
Triceps brachii	Three heads: (1) infraglenoid tubercle, (2) posterior humerus above radial groove, and (3) lower two-thirds of posterior humerus	Olecranon	Elbow extensor	Profunda brachii	Radial
Anconeus	Posterolateral epicondyle	Lateral olecranon and proximal ulna	Elbow extensor	Recurrent radial artery	Radial
Supinator	Lateral epicondyle, radial ligament, annular ligament, ulna	Upper lateral radius	Supination	Radial artery	Median

merus (Fig. 10-14), crossing the lateral epicondyle and extending distally to insert just proximal to the metaphysis of the radius (Figs. 10-6 to 10-8). This muscle in its activity as a flexor is aided by the adjacent muscles of the extensor group, especially the extensor carpi radialis longus (29,35). A fourth and less important flexor of the elbow is the pronator teres, which functions optimally only when the forearm is pronated. The pronator teres arises from the supercondylar portion of the humerus, extending obliquely across the medial aspect of the elbow to insert on the upper third of the radius (29,35) (Figs. 10-6 to 10-8 and 10-14) (29).

Extension of the elbow (Table 10-3) is accomplished primarily by the triceps, especially the medial head, and the anconeus (1,29) (Figs. 10-6, 10-8, and 10-15). The triceps takes its origin (three heads) from the infraglenoid tubercle of the scapula, posterior humerus above the radial groove, and the lower posterior humerus (1,29,35) (Fig. 10-15). It inserts on the olecranon. The anconeus (Figs. 10-6, 10-8, and 10-15) arises from the posterior lateral epicondyle and extends distally and medially to insert on the lateral ulna (Fig. 10-15) (29,35).

The main pronators of the radius and ulna are the pronator teres proximally and the pronator quadratus distally (Tables 10-3 and 10-4, Fig. 10-16). The pronator teres (Figs. 10-6, 10-8, and 10-16) originates from the medial supracondylar ridge and coronoid of the ulna. It passes distally and laterally to insert on the lateral aspect of the midradius (1,29). The origins and insertions of the pronator quadratus are discussed in Chapter 11.

Supination is accomplished by the supinator and biceps brachii muscle with some supination resulting from contraction of the extensor pollicis longus, abductor pollicis longus, and to a lesser extent the extensor carpi radialis longus and brachioradialis (29,35) (Fig. 10-17). The supinator (Figs. 10-6 to 10-8 and 10-17) originates from the lateral epicondyle, lateral ligament complex, and adjacent ulna. The muscle passes distally to insert on the upper lateral radius (1,29). Pronation is almost exclusively innervated by the median nerve, while supination is innervated by the musculocutaneous and radial nerves (29) (Table 10-3).

The majority of the forearm muscles arise from the humerus and cross the elbow prior to inserting distally (12,19,24). The flexor group arises from the medial humerus and/or ulna. This muscle group is supplied by both the median and ulnar nerve but the median nerve is the major contributor (Table 10-4). The extensors arise from the lateral aspect of the humerus and radius

TABLE 10-4. *Muscles of the forearm*

Muscles	Origin	Insertion	Action	Innervation
Flexors				
Superficial group				
Pronator teres	Two heads: (1) medial supracondylar ridge and interosseous membrane and (2) coronoid of ulna	Midlateral radius	Pronator elbow flexor	Median C5–C7
Flexor carpi radialis	Common flexor tendon (medial epicondyle)	Second metacarpal base	Wrist flexor	Median
Palmaris longus	Common flexor tendon (medial epicondyle)	Palmar aponeurosis	Wrist flexor	Median
Flexor carpi ulnaris	Two heads: (1) common flexor tendon and (2) medial olecranon and upper posterior two-thirds of ulna	Hamate hook and fifth metacarpal base	Wrist flexor	Ulnar
Intermediate group				
Flexor digitorum superficialis	Two heads: (1) common flexor tendon and (2) upper radius and distal tubercle	Bases of middle phalanges two to five	Flexion PIP joints	Median
Deep group				
Flexor digitorum profundus	Anterior two-thirds of ulna and interosseous membrane	Distal phalanges two to five	Flexion of fingers	Median and ulnar
Flexor pollicis longus	Middle one-third of radius and interosseous membrane	Distal phalanx thumb	Thumb flexor	Median
Pronator quadratus	Distal one-quarter of anterior ulna	Distal one-quarter of anterior radius	Pronation	Median
Extensors				
Superficial group				
Brachioradialis	Lower two-thirds of anterior humerus	Coronoid and ulnar tuberosity	Elbow flexor	Radial C5–C6
Extensor carpi radialis longus	Lower one-third of supracondylar ridge humerus	Radial dorsal base second metacarpal	Extend wrist	Radial
Extensor carpi radialis brevis	Common extensor tendon lateral epicondyle	Base third metacarpal	Extend wrist	Radial
Extensor digitorum	Common extensor tendon lateral epicondyle	Distal phalanges two to five	Common extensor fingers	Radial
Extensor digiti minimi	Extensor digitorum	Distal small finger	Extensor fifth finger	Radial
Extensor carpi ulnaris	Two heads: (1) common extensor tendon and (2) posterior ulnar border	Medial side base fifth metacarpal	Wrist extensor, ulnar abduction	Radial
Deep group				
Abductor pollicis longus	Posterior ulna, interosseous membrane, middle posterior radius	Lateral base first metacarpal	Long abduction thumb	Radial
Extensor pollicis brevis	Midposterior radius	Base proximal phalanx of thumb	Extensor thumb	Radial
Extensor pollicis longus	Middle one-third of posterior radius	Base distal phalanx of thumb	Extends phalanges of thumb	Radial
Extensor indicis	Posterior radius and interosseous membrane	Proximal phalanx index finger	Extensor index finger	Radial

and are supplied predominantly by the radial nerve (29) (Table 10-4).

The flexor group is divided into three layers: superficial, intermediate, and deep (1,29). The superficial layer originates predominantly from the common flexor tendon at the medial epicondyle (Fig. 10-18). Muscles in the superficial group include the pronator teres, flexor carpi radialis, palmaris longus, and flexor carpi ulnaris (Fig. 10-18, Table 10-4). The pronator teres originates with two heads from the common flexor tendon and also a small head from the coronoid process of the elbow. It extends to insert under the brachialis at the lateral aspect of the midradius. The flexor carpi radialis also originates from the common flexor tendon at the

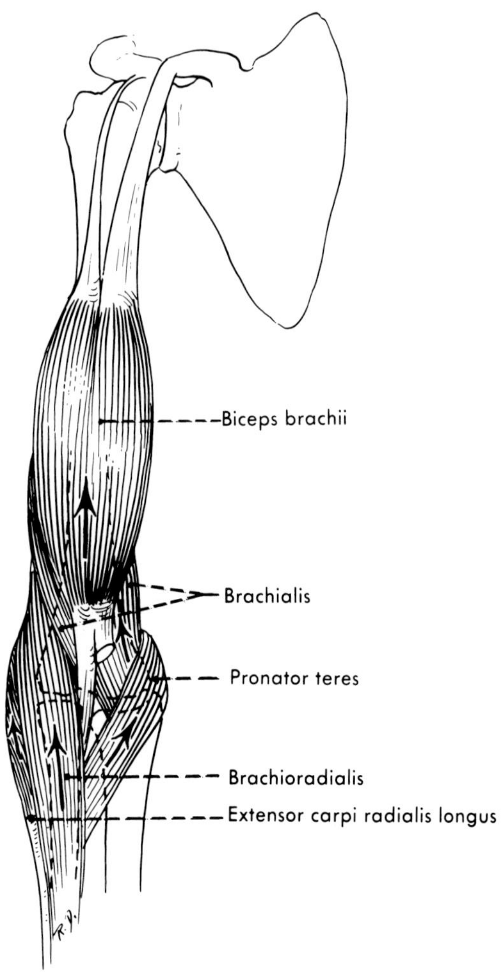

FIG. 10-14. Illustration of the superficial flexor muscles of the elbow. (From ref. 29, with permission.)

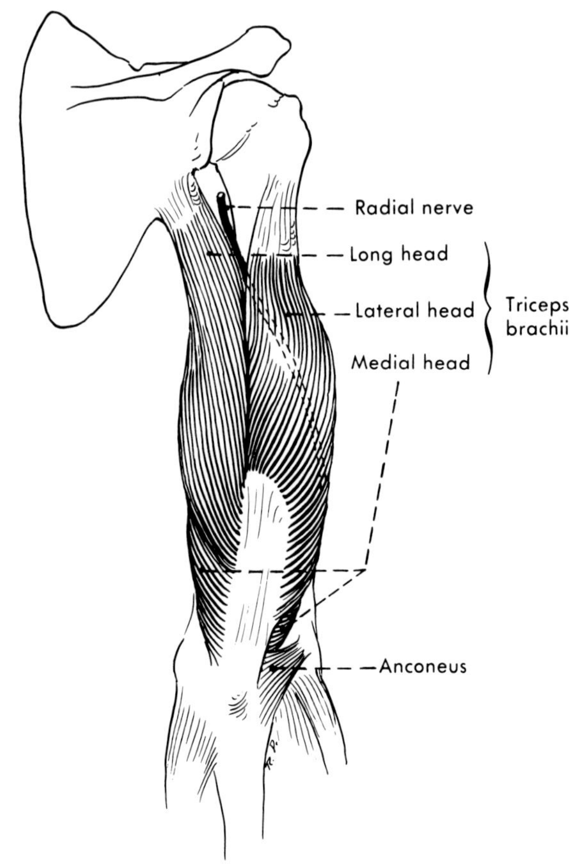

FIG. 10-15. Illustration of the extensors of the elbow. (From ref. 29, with permission.)

medial epicondyle and extends distally, crossing the flexor retinaculum along the groove of the trapezium to insert in the second metacarpal base. The flexor carpi radialis along its course covers part of the flexor digitorum superficialis (Fig. 10-6). Palmaris longus arises from the common flexor tendon medially and extends for only about one-third the length of the forearm. Distally, the tendinous portion crosses the wrist superficial to the flexor retinaculum (Figs. 10-6 and 10-18) and continues to become a part of the palmar aponeurosis in the hand. The flexor carpi ulnaris, the last of the superficial group, also has two heads, the first arising from the common flexor tendon, the second from the olecranon and posterior upper two-thirds of the ulna. This muscle covers the ulnar nerve and vessels along much of its course in the forearm (Fig. 10-6) and crosses the wrist through the pisohamate and pisometacarpal ligaments to insert on the hamate hook and fifth metacarpal base (1,16,29,35).

The flexor digitorum superficialis (sublimis) forms the intermediate layer of the flexor group (Fig. 10-19). This muscle also arises from the medial common flexor tendon and has a second head from the upper radius distal to the tubercle. This large flat muscle covers the median nerve and ulnar nerve and artery as it courses distally in the forearm (17,29) (Figs. 10-6 and 10-19). Prior to traversing the flexor retinaculum, the muscle gives off four tendons that, after passing through the flexor retinaculum and carpal tunnel, have common sheaths with the flexor digitorum profundus. The four tendons split distally to insert on either side of the bases of the second through fifth middle phalanges (1,29).

The deep flexor group includes the flexor digitorum profundus, flexor pollicis longus, and pronator quadratus (Fig. 10-20, Table 10-4). The flexor digitorum profundus arises from the anterior two-thirds of the ulna in its midportion and the interosseous membrane. This muscle also divides into four tendons, which join the flexor digitorum superficialis in a common tendon sheath as they pass beneath the flexor retinaculum and carpal tunnel. The tendons insert in the bases of the distal phalanges two through five (1,17,29). The flexor pollicis longus arises from the middle one-third of the radius and interosseous membrane and has an independent tendon sheath distally as it passes through the car-

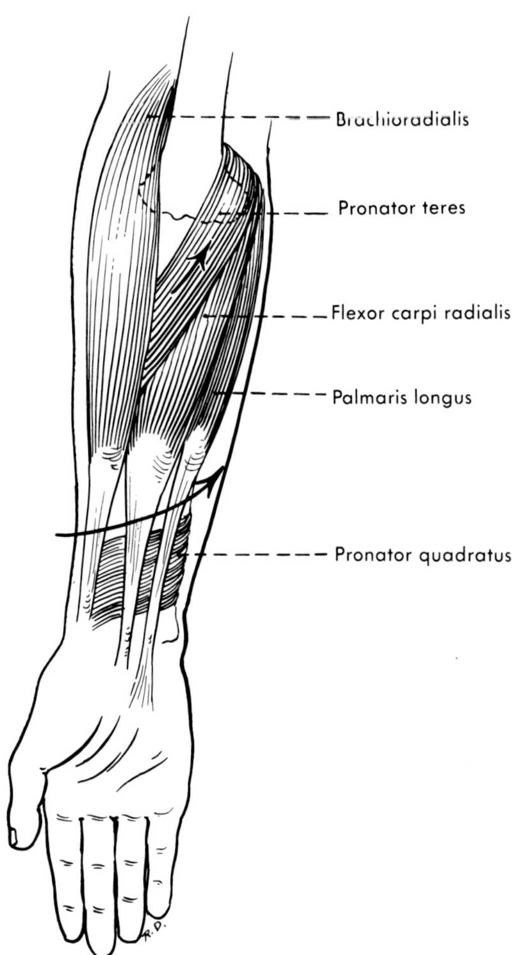

FIG. 10-16. Illustration of the pronators of the forearm. (From ref. 29, with permission.)

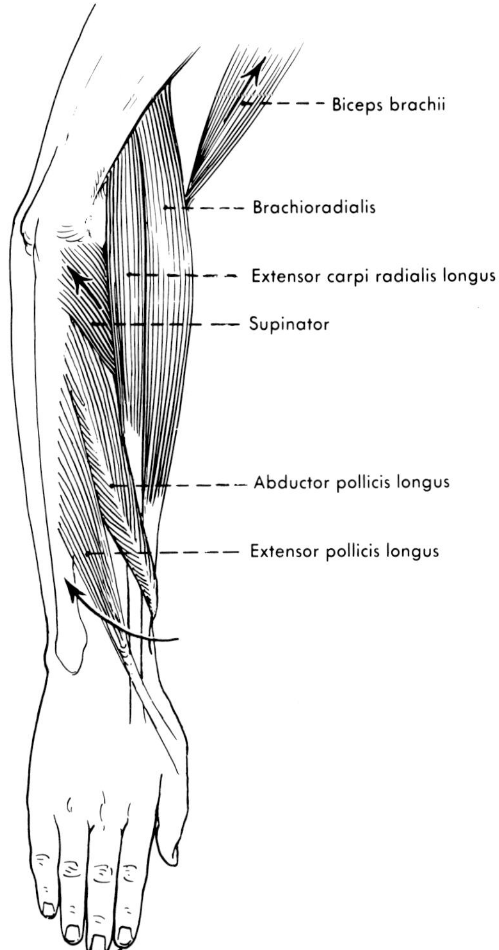

FIG. 10-17. Illustration of the supinators of the forearm. (From ref. 29, with permission.)

pal tunnel. Thus, it is located more radially and separate from the flexor digitorum profundus and flexor digitorum superficialis tendons (Fig. 10-6; see Figs. 11-17 and 11-23). Upon leaving the carpal tunnel, the flexor pollicis longus passes to the thenar muscle region to insert in the distal phalanx of the thumb. The third and final muscle of the deep group is the pronator quadratus, which is a flat quadrangular muscle lying behind the flexor digitorum longus and flexor pollicis longus. This muscle arises from the distal ulna to insert in the distal radius in a near transverse direction (Fig. 10-20; see Fig. 11-4 and Chapter 11) (1,17,29,35).

Extensors

The extensor muscles of the forearm are actually flexors of the elbow as noted above. All the extensor muscles are supplied by the radial nerve (29). The extensor muscles, like the flexors, are divided into superficial and deep compartments. The superficial group includes the brachioradialis, extensor carpi radialis longus, extensor digitorum, extensor digiti minimi, and extensor carpi ulnaris (1,29) (Fig. 10-21). The brachioradialis, as described above, has a long origin above the supercondylar ridge, where it lies between the brachialis and triceps muscle. The radial nerve lies between it and the brachialis (Fig. 10-6). Superiorly, the brachioradialis partially covers the extensor carpi radialis longus as it passes distally to insert on the lateral side of the distal radius. The extensor carpi radialis longus, arising from the lower third of the anterior supercondylar ridge, is covered superiorly by the brachialis. The extensor carpi radialis longus overlaps the extensor carpi radialis brevis and gives rise to a flat tendon at the level of the midforearm. It then accompanies its companion, the extensor carpi radialis brevis, distally. The extensor carpi radialis longus extends along the posterior radial surface deep to the abductor pollicis longus and extensor pollicis longus, passing under the extensor retinaculum where it shares a common tendon sheath with the extensor carpi radialis brevis to insert on the radial dorsal aspect of the base of the second metacarpal (Figs. 10-6 to 10-8). At this loca-

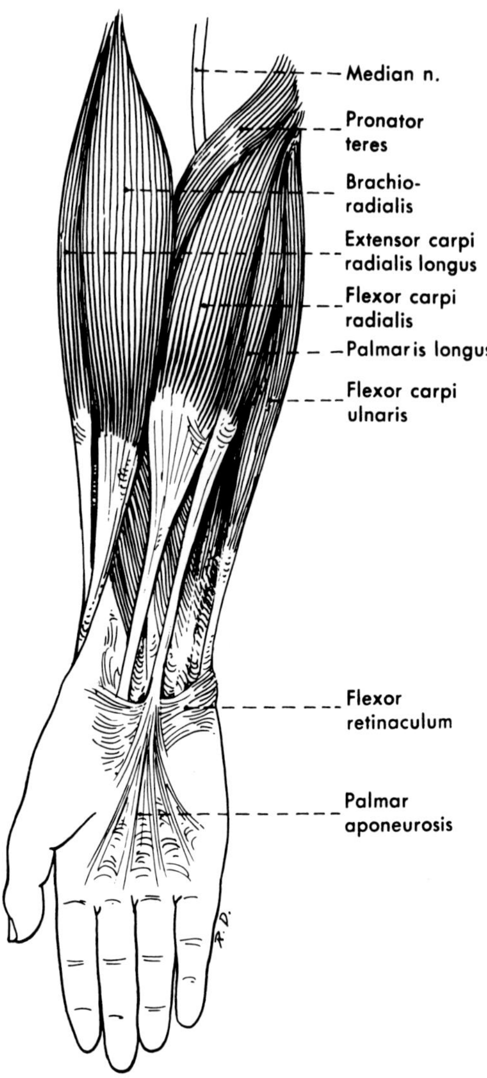

FIG. 10-18. Illustration of the superficial flexor and extensor muscles of the forearm. (From ref. 29, with permission.)

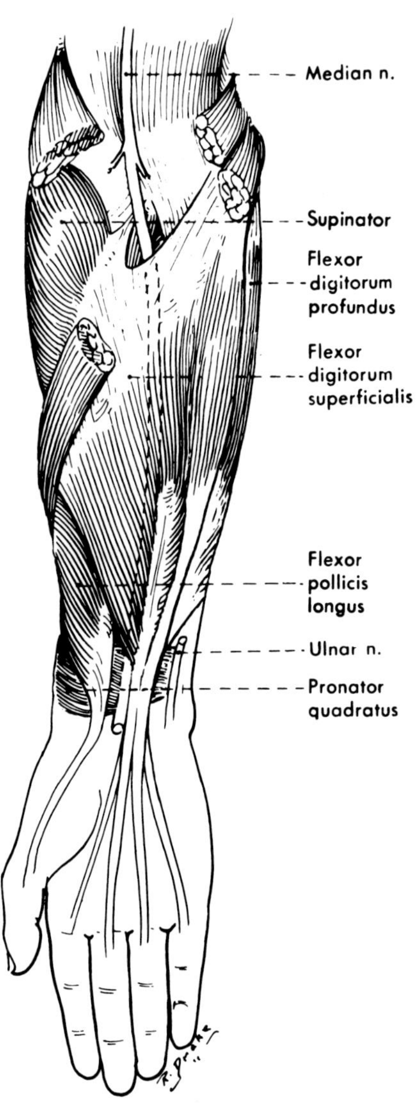

FIG. 10-19. Illustration of the intermediate flexor compartment of the forearm. Note the relationship of the muscles to the median nerve. (From ref. 29, with permission.)

tion there may be a small bursa between the second metacarpal base and the tendon. This bursa is usually not visible on MR images unless it is inflamed and distended with fluid. The extensor carpi radialis brevis is the most lateral of the extensor muscles and arises from the common extensor tendon at the lateral epicondyle and also has a small head that arises from the radial collateral ligament. This muscle is largely covered by the extensor carpi radialis longus in its proximal portion (Figs. 10-6 and 10-21). The extensor digitorum is located adjacent to it on the ulnar side. In the distal forearm, the muscle is separated from the extensor digitorum by the abductor pollicis longus and extensor pollicis brevis (Figs. 10-6 and 10-21). At the wrist, the tendon of the extensor carpi radialis brevis lies immediately adjacent to the ulnar side of the extensor carpi radialis longus and both tendons share a common sheath as they pass under the extensor retinaculum. The extensor carpi radialis longus inserts in the base of the third metacarpal. Its chief function is to extend the wrist, but it also assists in elbow flexion. The extensor digitorum (extensor digitorum communis) is the common extensor of the fingers. This muscle occupies the central portion of the dorsal forearm. It arises in the common extensor tendon and shares an origin with the belly of the extensor digiti minimi. Distally, three to four tendons are present with a common sheath within the extensor retinaculum. The sheath is shared with the extensor digiti indicis. The tendons pass under the extensor retinaculum and receive slips from the lumbricalis and interosseous muscles in the hand, thereafter dividing into central and lateral bands (also see Chapter 11). The central bands insert on the middle and lateral bands on the sides of the distal phalanges. The primary

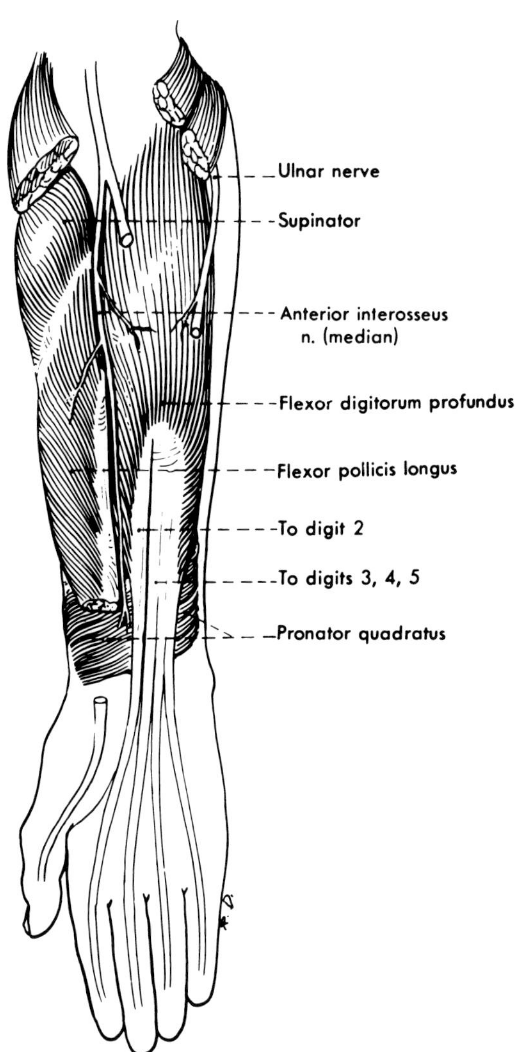

FIG. 10-20. Illustration of deep flexors of the forearm. Note the relationships to the radial and ulnar nerves. (From ref. 29, with permission.)

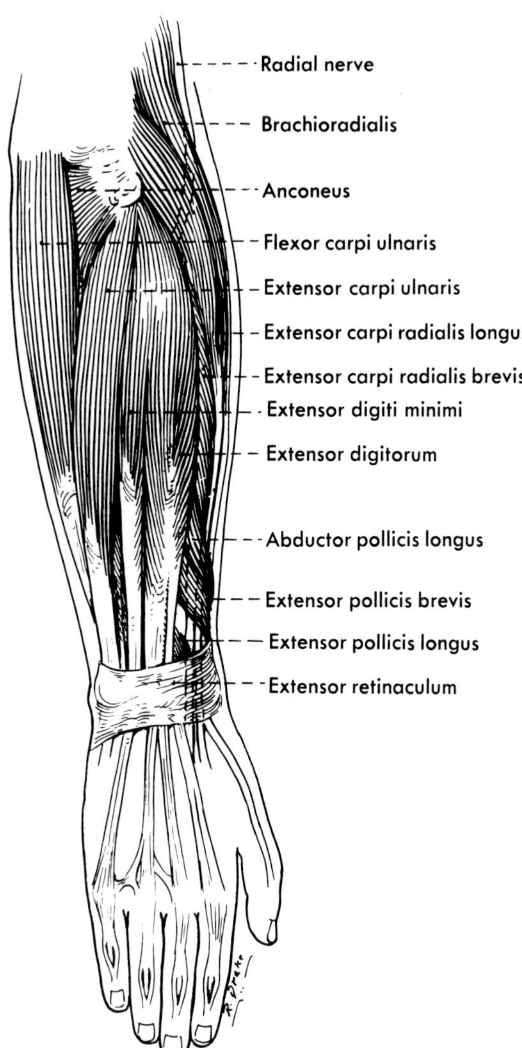

FIG. 10-21. Illustration of the extensor muscles of the forearm. (From ref. 29, with permission.)

function of the extensor digitorum is to serve as an extender and abductor of the fingers. The extensor digiti minimi arises largely from a septum adjacent to the extensor digitorum and occupies a superficial position on the dorsal forearm between the extensor digitorum and extensor carpi ulnaris. The slendor tendon of this muscle continues in a separate compartment under the extensor retinaculum to insert on the dorsal aspect of the small finger in a similar fashion to the extensor digitorum. The extensor carpi ulnaris is the most medial of the superficial muscles. It has two heads, the first arising from a lateral epicondyle via the common extensor tendon, the second from the posterior border of the ulna. The tendon of this muscle passes through a special compartment in the extensor retinaculum and also through the ulnar groove. The insertion is the medial side of the base of the fifth metacarpal. Its primary functions are wrist extension and ulnar abduction (1,17,29,35).

Deep Extensors

The deep extensors of the forearm include the abductor pollicis longus, extensor pollicis brevis, extensor pollicis longus, and extensor indicis (Fig. 10-22). The supinator is included in this group because of its position in the deep compartment (Fig. 10-6). The abductor pollicis longus is the long abductor of the thumb and arises from the posterior ulna distal to the supinator and also from the interosseous membrane and the middle third of the posterior radius. The muscle passes obliquely to emerge between the extensor carpi radialis brevis and extensor digitorum with the extensor pollicis brevis me-

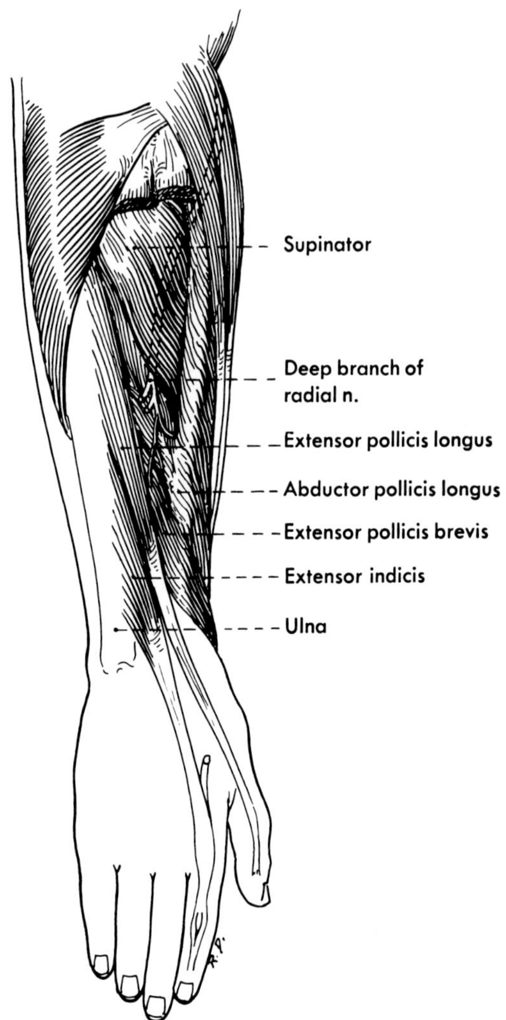

FIG. 10-22. Illustration of the deep extensor muscles of the forearm. (From ref. 29, with permission.)

dial and inferior to it (Figs. 10-6 and 10-22). The abductor pollicis longus and extensor pollicis brevis pass superficial to the radial extensor tendons and both share a common sheath at the wrist. At this level it lies superior to the radial artery and passes to the dorsum of the hand, where it inserts in the base of the first metacarpal on its lateral side (also see Chapter 11). The abductor pollicis longus serves as a radial abductor of the wrist and also a radial extender of the thumb. The extensor pollicis brevis is the short extensor of the thumb and arises from the midportion of the posterior radius distal to the abductor pollicis longus and also from the interosseous membrane. It passes between the extensor digitorum and abductor pollicis longus and crosses the wrist superficial to the radial extensors. This tendon forms the anterior boundary of the anatomic snuff box. The radial artery is deep to this tendon and the tendon of the abductor pollicis longus. The extensor pollicis brevis inserts in the base of the proximal phalanx of the thumb, where it serves as an extensor of the thumb and radial abductor of the wrist. The extensor pollicis longus arises from the middle posterior third of the radius and interosseous membrane, in contact with the abductor pollicis longus, and partially overlaps the extensor pollicis brevis superiorly. At the wrist, it lies on the radial side of the extensor digitorum. The tendon runs obliquely across the wrist in a separate compartment under the extensor retinaculum and in a groove just medial to the radial tubercle. It emerges to form the dorsal margin of the anatomic snuff box. Its tendon covers or is dorsal to the extensor pollicis brevis and inserts in the base of the distal phalanx of the thumb. This muscle serves as an extender of both phalanges of the thumb. The final muscle of the deep compartment is the extensor indicis or extensor indicis proprius, which is the extensor of the index finger. It arises distal to the extensor pollicis longus on the posterior radius and interosseous membrane and is largely covered by the superficial muscle group along its course. The tendon passes deep to the extensor digiti minimi and deep to the extensor digitorum with which it shares a common sheath in the dorsum of the hand. Along the dorsal aspect of the hand it lies on the ulnar side of the extensor digitorum and inserts with an expansion on the dorsal aspect of the proximal phalanx (1,17,29,35) (see also Fig. 11-17).

Neurovascular Anatomy

Knowledge of the neurovascular anatomy and the relationship of the neurovascular structures to the various muscles and compartments of the elbow and forearm is critical for evaluating MR images (Fig. 10-23). Soft tissue masses and traumatic conditions including nerve compression syndromes involving these structures can cause significant clinical symptoms (9,17,35,45). Therefore, it is important that the relationships of the arteries, veins, and nerves to the various compartments and muscle groups are appreciated. Following the nerves and vessels is most easily accomplished with contiguous axial images (Fig. 10-6). Because of the variation in the course of these structures, they are rarely included in their entirety in the coronal or sagittal planes. New three-dimensional volume imaging and angiographic techniques will provide excellent visualization of the major vascular structures; however, following the course of nerves and identifying lesions in or adjacent to nerves will likely still be most easily accomplished on axial images (16,17,33,34).

At the level of the distal humerus (Fig. 10-6A), the brachial artery is located anteromedially adjacent to its accompanying vein. The median nerve usually lies along the medial aspect at the junction of the biceps and brachialis muscles. The ulnar nerve is positioned more posteriorly along the medial aspect of the triceps (Figs. 10-6 and 10-23). At this same level, the radial nerve is

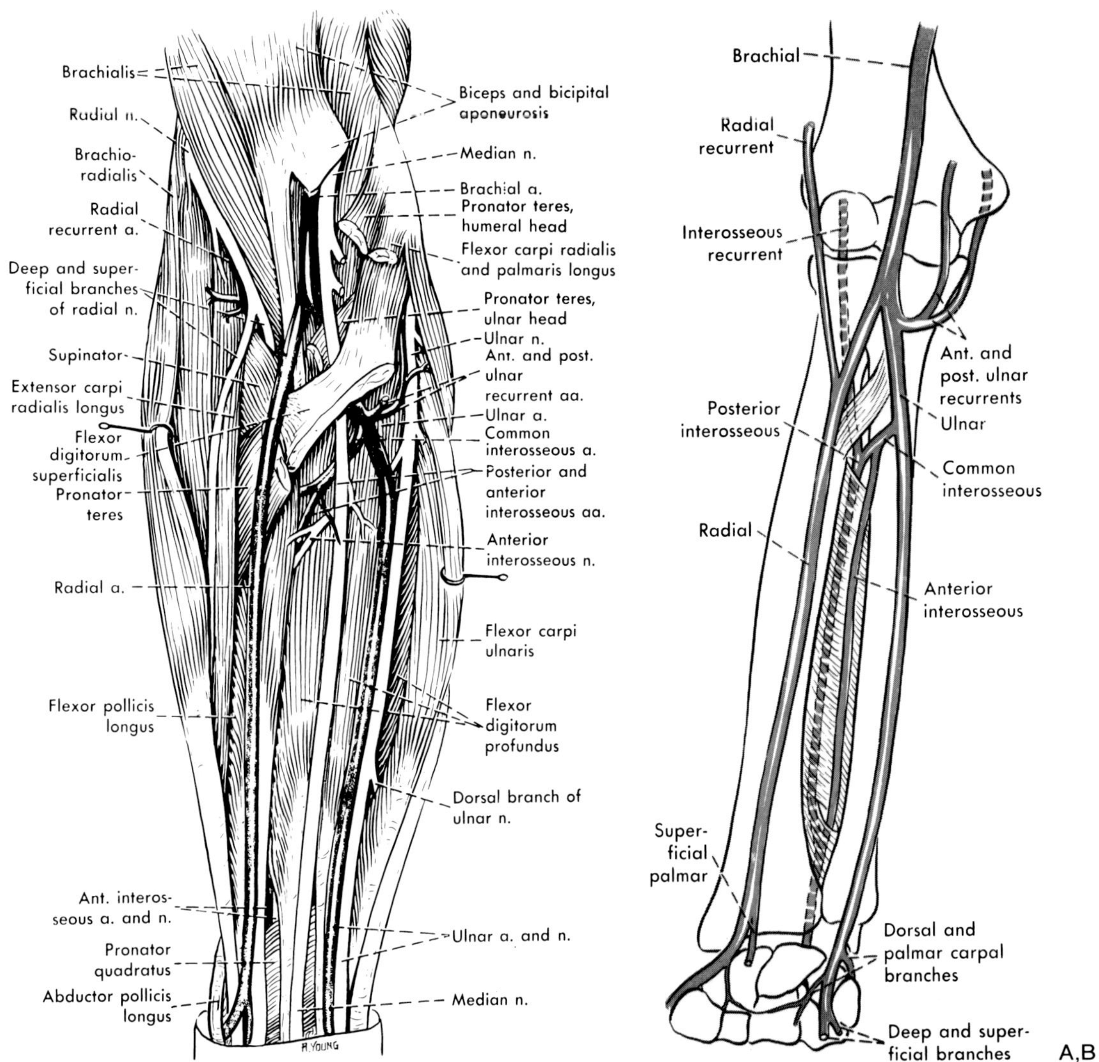

FIG. 10-23. Illustrations of the neurovascular (**A**) and major arterial (**B**) anatomy of the elbow and forearm. (From ref. 29, with permission.)

most commonly seen between the brachialis muscle and brachioradialis just anterior to the lateral aspect of the supracondylar portion of the humerus. Near the elbow the radial nerve courses anteriorly along the margin of the brachialis muscle and medial to the brachioradialis (Fig. 10-23) to a point just above the supinator, where it divides into the deep and superficial branches. Once this division has occurred, the nerve as seen on MR images (small low-intensity structure) is more difficult to follow into the forearm (Fig. 10-6). However, at this point the superficial branch of the nerve lies anterior to the extensor carpi radialis longus and the deep branch is generally seen either within or between the supinator and extensor digitorum posterior to the radius (Figs. 10-6 and 10-23). The median nerve courses along the anterior aspect of the antecubital fossa, passing beneath the flexor digitorum superficialis to lie between this muscle and the flexor digitorum profundus as it passes distally into the forearm (Figs. 10-19 and 10-23). The median nerve is a larger structure and usually can easily be identified on axial MR images (Fig. 10-6). The ulnar nerve passes posterior to the medial epicondyle and is clearly identified on most images at this level (Fig. 10-6). More distally, the ulnar nerve is usually located between the flexor digitorum profundus and the flexor carpi ulnaris (Figs. 10-6 and 10-23).

The major vessels in the elbow and forearm are more easily identified than the smaller, low signal intensity nerves. The brachial artery courses with the median nerve in the antecubital fossa prior to dividing into the radial and ulnar arteries. The radial artery continues distally superficial to the flexor pollicis longus as it extends into the forearm. The ulnar artery usually accompanies the median nerve along its course superficial to the flexor digitorum profundus. Figure 10-23 demonstrates the major neurovascular anatomy of the forearm and elbow.

PITFALLS

Pitfalls in MRI of the elbow and forearm are usually related to normal anatomic variants (20), technical errors, improper coil selection, or flow and other imaging artifacts (8,9,39).

The list of normal anatomic variants involving the elbow and forearm is potentially long. A frequent osseous variant is the supracondylar process. This "hook-like" bony projection is usually noted 1–2 inches above the medial epicondyle. This structure is almost always asymptomatic. However, compression of the median nerve or brachial artery can occur (29,35). Identification of this process is easily accomplished with routine radiography. However, the process with the ligamentous band to the medial epicondyle and relationship to neurovascular structures may most easily be viewed with coronal and axial MR images (9).

Soft tissue anomalies, including combination of muscle bellies, accessory origins or absence of one of the heads when multiple origins are present, and total absence (palmaris longus 12.9%), are not unusual. These changes are not usually clinically significant (29). Readers are referred to anatomic references for a more complete discussion of normal anatomic variants (1,29,35).

Other errors in interpretation of MR images are due to improper choice of pulse sequences, image planes, coils, and patient position (see Chapter 3). Many mistakes can be avoided by careful review of clinical history and physical findings.

Image artifacts are more fully discussed in Chapters 1 and 3. Most artifacts in the upper extremity are due to motion and/or flow. Flow artifacts can be useful. For example, if a small ganglion cyst is suspected, the flow artifact can be used to differentiate vessels from the cysts. Flow artifact can cause signal enhancement in vessel lumina, which may mimic a cyst. Flow artifacts may also create problems in image interpretation. Flow artifact suppression techniques (see Chapter 3) can reduce artifacts; however, it is still useful to change the phase-encoding direction in order to prevent artifacts from degrading important areas on the image (8,9,26) (Fig. 10-24).

APPLICATIONS

The most common clinical applications for MRI of the elbow and forearm are trauma, neoplasms and other mass lesions, avascular necrosis (osteonecrosis), infection, and problem solving. The latter category includes patients with complex symptoms who have had normal conventional studies including CT, ultrasonography, and arthrography (8,9).

Trauma

Routine radiographs, radionuclide studies, and conventional tomography or computed tomography (CT) are generally sufficient for detection and classification of skeletal injuries. However, it is not uncommon to detect subtle skeletal injuries with MRI that were overlooked or not identifiable with conventional techniques (8,9). Occult fractures in the marrow and stress fractures can be identified early with MRI (31,52). In the case of stress

A,B

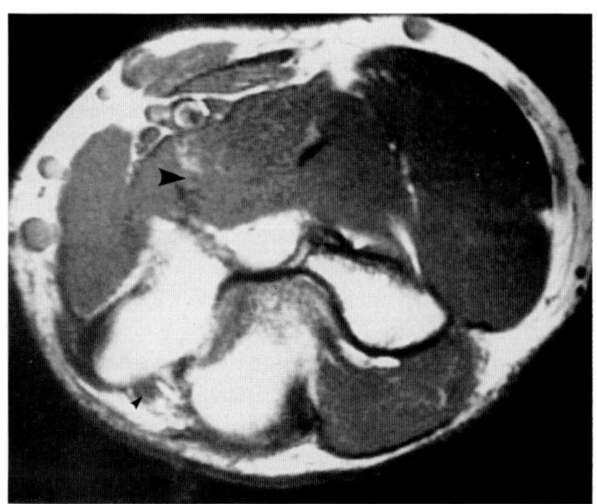

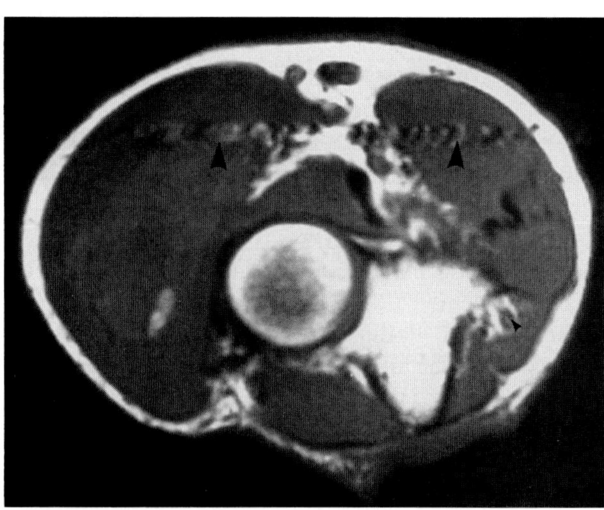

FIG. 10-24. Axial images of the elbow showing flow artifact in the vertical Y axis (**A**) and transverse (**B**) or X axis. The ulnar nerve region (*small arrowheads*) is distorted by flow artifact in (**A**), which could interfere with diagnosis of pathology in this region.

fractures we still prefer radionuclide imaging. However, if findings (clinical and radionuclide scan) are atypical, MRI is an excellent technique for clarifying the nature of the lesion. Cortical changes are most obvious on T2 weighted images. Fractures have high signal intensity compared with the dark cortical bone. Marrow fat is suppressed with the use of these sequences (SE 2,000/60–80), so a stellate area of high or low signal intensity may be noted. The former occurs with medullary edema or fluid and blood at the fracture site (8,9,52). When signal intensity is decreased on T2 weighted sequences, it usually is due to trabecular compression. Marrow trauma is seen as an area of low signal intensity on T1 weighted images. MRI also can be useful in monitoring the healing process and for differentiating between fibrous union and nonunion (see Fig. 11-27). In patients with fibrous union, the signal intensity is decreased on both T1 and T2 weighted sequences. If nonunion is present, the signal intensity is increased due to fluid along the fracture line (8).

Articular or joint-related injuries are typically evaluated with arthrography or tenography in combination with motion studies, stress views, and, in certain cases, CT or arthrotomography. An additional advantage of these invasive techniques is the ability to perform simultaneous diagnostic and therapeutic injections. Ultrasonography may be useful for evaluating the superficial tendons. The primary applications for MRI of articular trauma include detection of capsular disruptions and subtle articular defects or early osteonecrosis, as well as evaluation of pericapsular tendons, muscles, and nerves (9,11,25,27,37,38,51).

Defects in the articular cartilage can easily be defined with MRI. Usually more than one image plane should be used so the size of the defect and its position can clearly be defined. Defects in the capsule are usually easily defined, but in some cases distention of the joint with fluid or contrast material (Gd-DTPA) may be necessary (27).

Tendon injuries are more common in the upper extremity than the lower extremity (1). Inflammation or partial tearing in the medial and lateral complexes is a common problem in athletes. Isolated ruptures of these tendons, the biceps and triceps tendons, occur less frequently (35).

Ruptures of the biceps tendon at the insertion into the radial tuberosity account for only 3–10% of biceps tendon injuries (1). Patients usually present with acute onset of pain in the antecubital region following lifting a heavy object (2,35). Routine radiographs may show avulsion of the radial tuberosity and/or swelling with obliteration of the supinator fat stripe. However, MRI is probably best suited to define the tendon and extent of injury. Axial and sagittal image planes provide the best information (Fig. 10-25). The forearm must be properly positioned for sagittal images to optimize visualization

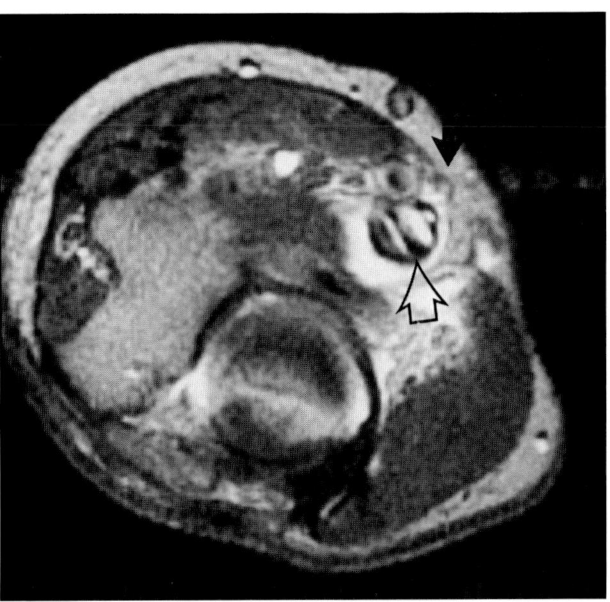

FIG. 10-25. Axial SE 2,000/60 image of the elbow showing a grade 2 tear in the biceps tendon (*open arrow*). Note the flow artifact (*closed arrow*) that obscures a portion of the lesion. Switching phase direction would prevent this problem.

of the tendon (Fig. 10-4). This requires palpation of this region prior to patient positioning. Operative treatment is indicated for both complete ruptures and incomplete ruptures with significant function loss (35). MRI is also useful in following the healing process and in patients with continued symptoms after therapy (Fig. 10-26).

Rupture of the triceps tendon is rare. Anzel et al. (2) reported eight triceps ruptures in 856 cases of upper extremity tendon disruption. Disruption usually occurs with a deceleration force to the arm while the triceps is contracted. The injury has also been reported in patients with systemic diseases or patients on steroid therapy (35). Routine radiography is more useful in triceps injury as up to 80% of patients will have avulsion fractures of the olecranon (25). MRI in the axial and sagittal planes is useful in defining the extent of injury.

Snapping triceps tendon is an uncommon disorder. This condition occurs most commonly in young adults (22). The snapping is typically noted medially and posteriorly. The sensation of snapping may be due to anomalous triceps insertions or subluxation of the ulnar nerve. Most commonly, the problem is due to subluxation of the medial head of the triceps over the medial epicondyle. MRI is ideal for identification of the ulnar nerve (Fig. 10-6) and the associated local inflammation that accompanies this disorder (Fig. 10-27). Axial T2 weighted images in pronation and supination or varying degrees of elbow flexion are useful in detecting subluxation. Patient size may be a limiting factor because the elbow must be at the patient's side and the patient in the oblique position to accomplish this maneuver. The flat 5

A,B

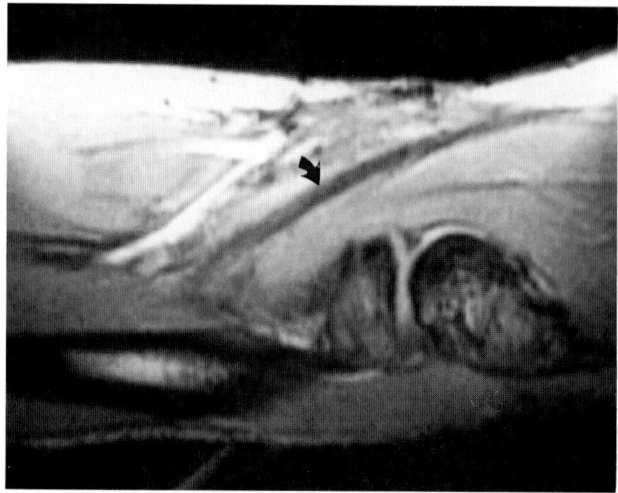

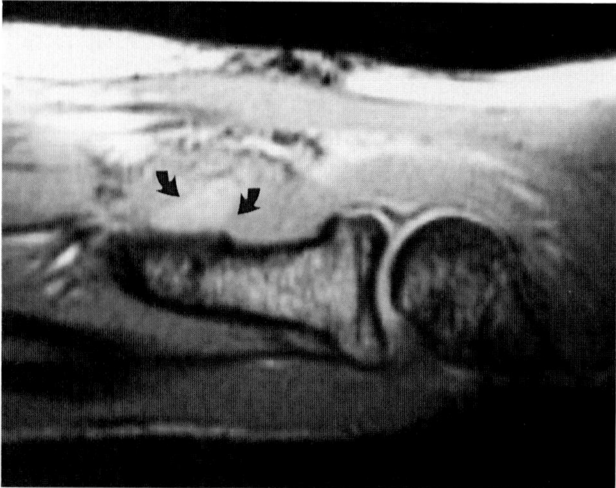

FIG. 10-26. GRASS images in the sagittal plane taken in varying degrees of pronation and supination. The first position (**A**) shows the biceps tendon (*arrow*). The second position does not demonstrate the tendon but clearly shows a recurrent ganglion (*arrows*) below the tendon which caused snapping with motion.

inch circular coil is optimal when motion studies are indicated (Fig. 10-1).

Patients with medial and lateral epicondylitis can be evaluated with MRI to determine the extent of inflammation and whether an actual tear is present. However, the majority of these patients are treated symptomatically and imaging studies are not performed. Lateral tendonitis typically involves the origin of the extensor carpi radialis brevis, while medial involvement occurs at the origins of the flexors and pronator teres (29,35). Inflammation medially may result in ulnar nerve compression (35). In advanced cases surgical intervention with ulnar nerve transfer may be indicated (37). In this setting MRI may be useful to evaluate the position of the ulnar nerve in relation to the medial epicondyle and

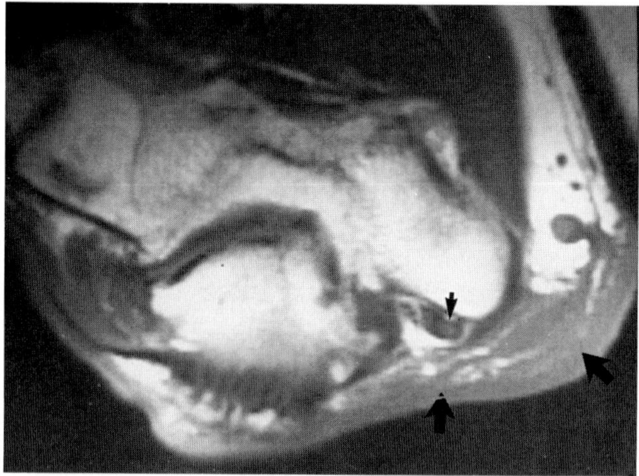

FIG. 10-27. Axial T1 weighted image of the elbow showing chronic inflammatory changes in the subcutaneous fat (*arrows*) adjacent to the ulnar nerve (*small arrow*).

adjacent soft tissues (Fig. 10-27). Other nerve and muscle injuries in the elbow and forearm can also be demonstrated using MRI.

The above injuries are detected most easily with T2 weighted sequences. Spin-echo (2,000/30–60 or 2,000/20–80) sequences provide anatomic (SE 2,000/20–30) and T2 weighted (SE 2,000/60–80) information. The latter provides the best contrast between joint fluid, edema, or hemorrhage (high signal intensity) and muscle, tendons, ligaments, and articular cartilage (Fig. 10-25). Similar data can be obtained with fast-scan techniques such as GRASS or GRIL (Fig. 10-26). Although these pulse sequences are somewhat noisier than SE sequences, the information can be obtained quickly, and cine studies are possible. Cine studies are particularly useful when motion studies are indicated: for example, radioulnar motion in the elbow during supination and pronation (8,9). More recently, some authors have suggested that intra-articular injection of Gd-DTPA may improve the accuracy of MRI in evaluating joint pathology (27). This work is not conclusive at this time.

Neoplasms

Bone and Soft Tissue Neoplasms

The majority of patients (54% at the Mayo Clinic) are referred for evaluation of the elbow and forearm because of suspected soft tissue masses or to exclude postoperative residual or recurrent neoplasm (8–10). MRI is the technique of choice for evaluating soft tissue neoplasms in the extremities. The paucity of fat and the beam hardening artifact from cortical bone greatly reduce the

TABLE 10-5. *Skeletal neoplasms of the elbow and upper forearm* (19)

Neoplasm	Number of elbow and forearm/total
Benign	
Osteoid osteoma	16/245
Osteochondroma	10/640
Giant cell tumor	8/425
Chondroma	1/245
Chondromyxoid fibroma	1/39
Chondroblastoma	0/79
	36/1,673
Malignant	
Lymphoma	17/469
Osteosarcoma	13/1274
Ewing's sarcoma	12/402
Myeloma	11/556
Chondrosarcoma	4/634
Fibrosarcoma	3/207
	60/3,512

utility of computed tomography (CT) in these regions. Lesions are identified more easily with MRI because of its superior soft tissue contrast. MRI is especially useful for demonstrating neurovascular, soft tissue, and articular involvement. In addition, the image features are often useful, although not specific, in predicting the nature of the lesion (8–10).

Bone Tumors

Osseous neoplasms in the elbow are rare and are not commonly evaluated with MRI (19) (Table 10-5). Routine radiographs usually are sufficient for detection of skeletal neoplasms (Fig. 10-28). Characterization of the lesion is also usually possible with radiographs, so that only indeterminate or obviously malignant lesions require staging with MRI. The latter are rare in the elbow and forearm (Table 10-5). When MR examination is required, it is usually to determine the extent of bone and soft tissue involvement. This is accomplished most easily with the use of the circular or license plate coil. The larger license plate coil allows a larger field of view, so that skip areas in the humerus or forearm are not overlooked when a lesion in the elbow is being studied (8–10) (Figs. 10-1 and 10-2).

MRI examinations for musculoskeletal neoplasms usually begin with a coronal scout image. Axial T2 weighted (SE 2,000/30–60 or 2,000/20–80) images are used to evaluate the extent of cortical and soft tissue involvement. If the nature of the lesion is obvious, a second sagittal or coronal T1 weighted image is obtained, with care being taken to select an image plane that includes the entire osseous or soft tissue region in the image slices. This usually requires an oblique adjustment in the sagittal or coronal images. Slice thicknesses of 5–10 mm with 1.5–2.5 mm skip, a field of view to include the entire area of suspected involvement (usually less than 24 cm), a 256 × 256 matrix, and 1 excitation (NSA) are usually adequate. As noted above, the coil selected should include the region of interest plus potential skip areas. With these parameters the image time for this examination is approximately 15 min (see Chapter 12, where technical aspects are discussed more completely).

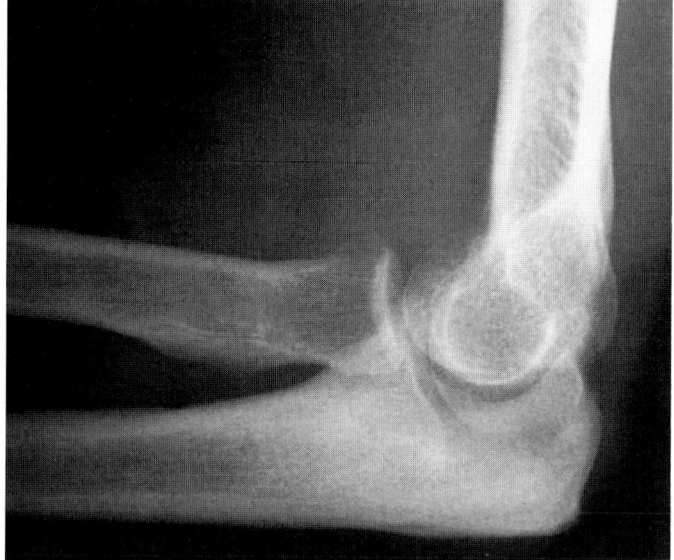

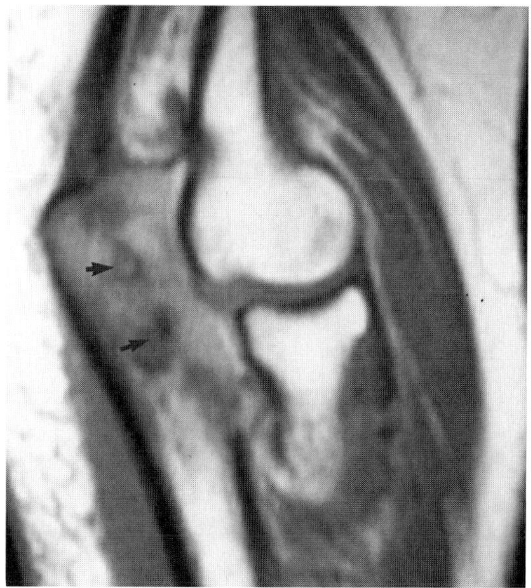

A,B

FIG. 10-28. Lateral view of the elbow (**A**) shows sclerosis in the olecranon region. T1 weighted (SE 500/20) sagittal image (**B**) shows reduced signal intensity in the same region with two small areas (*arrows*) of no signal with central areas of intermediate intensity. Diagnosis is osteoid osteomas.

Soft Tissue Tumors

Benign soft tissue tumors usually are well marginated, have homogeneous signal intensity, and do not encase neurovascular structures or invade bone (10,24). Edema is common with malignant lesions but less frequent with benign tumors (6). The T1 and T2 relaxation times of benign lesions overlap considerably with those of malignant lesions and thus are not useful in characterizing or predicting the histologic appearance of tumors. The appearance of certain lesions, however, has been accurately defined with the use of the previously described criteria and the increased experience with MRI (10).

Lipomas are common benign soft tissue lesions that maintain a homogeneous high signal intensity (as observed for subcutaneous fat) on both T1 and T2 weighted sequences (Fig. 10-29). The lesions are well marginated but may contain fibrous septations (10,21). Liposarcoma should be considered when areas of inhomogeneity or shaggy margins are noted in a fatty tumor (10).

Benign cysts have high signal intensity on T2 weighted sequences and homogeneous low signal intensity on T1 weighted images. These lesions are very distinct and well marginated, even when complicated by hemorrhage or infection. The signal intensity of these complicated cysts may be lower on T2 and higher on T1 weighted sequences (9,10).

Other than lipomas, most benign lesions are well marginated, homogeneous, and have a high signal intensity on T2 weighted sequences and a low signal intensity on T1 weighted sequences. The exception to this general rule occurs with two lesions: hemangiomas and desmoid tumors (9,10). Hemangiomas and other vascular malformations often are irregular, have mixed signal intensity, and may be extensive. The numerous vessels are usually obvious, and, when MRI data are combined with clinical data, the diagnosis usually is obvious (Fig. 10-30). Differentiation of veins, arteries, and dilated lymphatic vessels is not always possible. Selective angiography may still be necessary to identify the feeding arteries and draining veins in arteriovenous malformations (9,10,18).

Desmoid tumors are aggressive, often hypocellular fibrous lesions. The margins are frequently irregular (80% in the Mayo Clinic experience), and the masses have inhomogeneous signal intensity or a malignant appearance (Fig. 10-31). Resection of these lesions often requires extensive surgery, and recurrence is common (9,10) (see Chapter 12).

Most malignant soft tissue neoplasms are irregular, at least at some point along their margins. Irregular margins may also be due to local inflammation rather than malignant extension. Beltran et al. (6) described increased signal intensity around masses on T2 weighted sequences. This finding was more common with malignant lesions but also was seen in some patients with infection and hemorrhage. The sensitivity of this finding

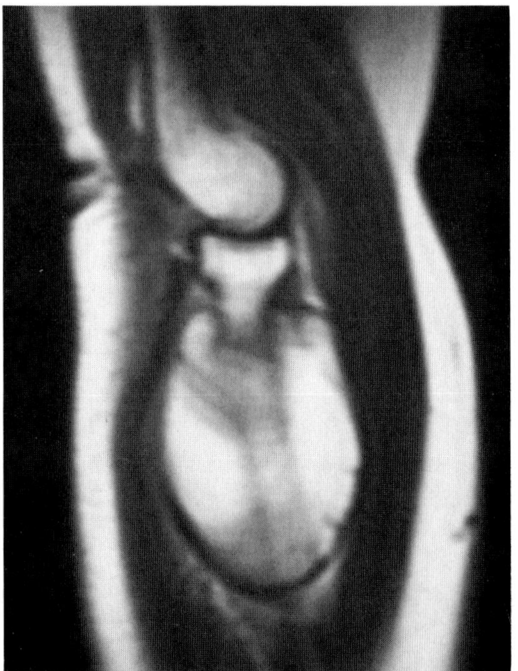
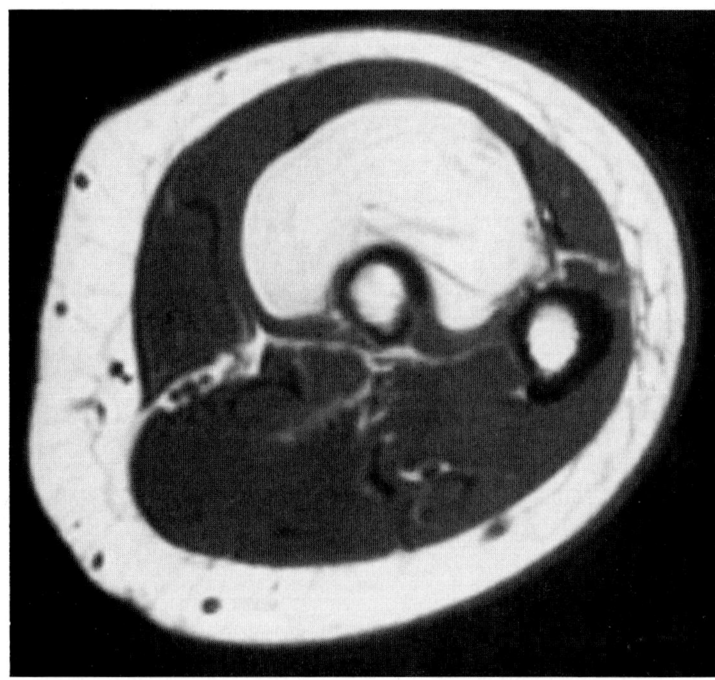

A,B

FIG. 10-29. Sagittal (**A**) and axial (**B**) images of a benign lipoma. The lesion is homogeneous and has the same signal intensity as subcutaneous fat.

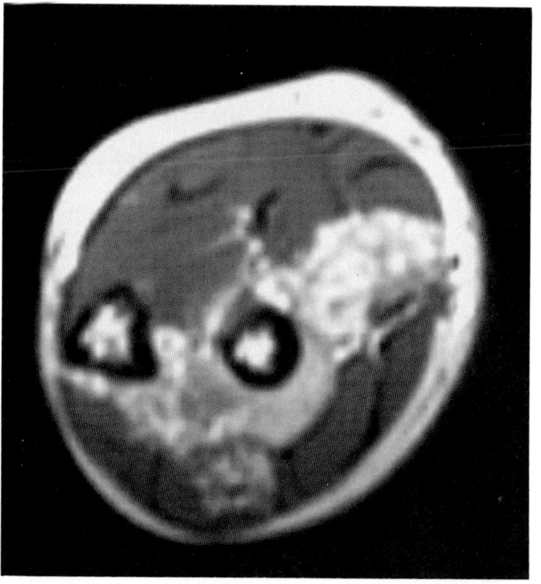

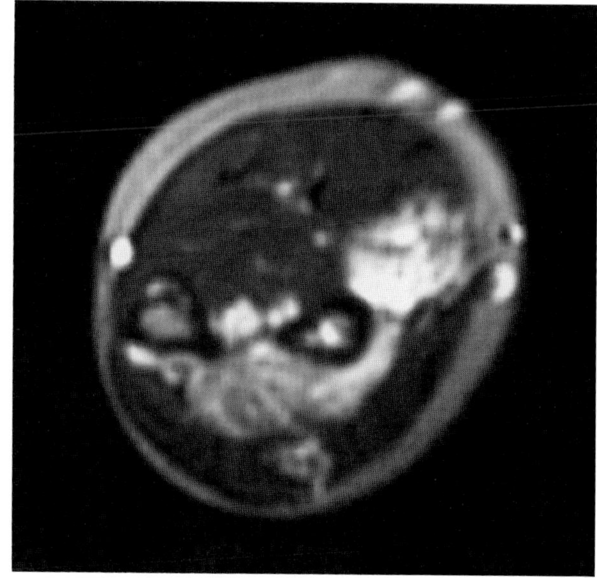

A,B

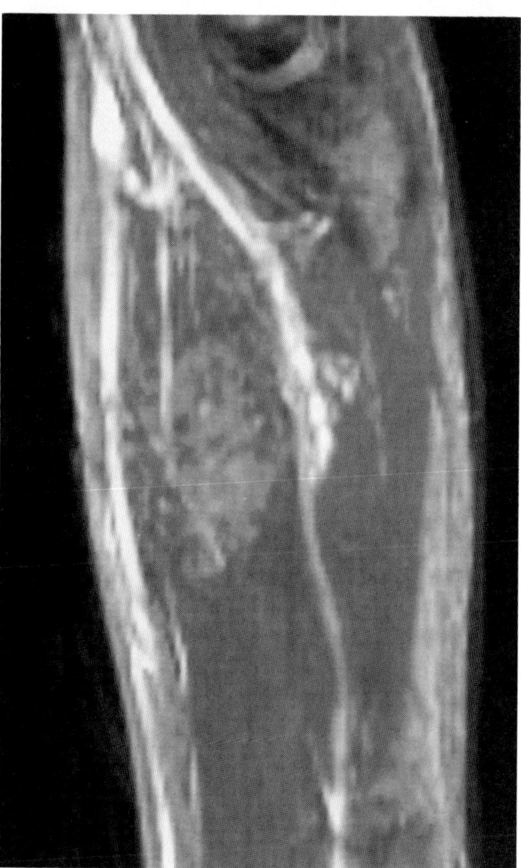

C

FIG. 10-30. Axial SE 500/20 (**A**), SE 2,000/60 (**B**), and sagittal GRASS (**C**) images of a hemangioma. The vascular anatomy is well demonstrated using GRASS imaging.

in predicting malignancy was 80%, specificity 50%, and accuracy 64%. Some malignant lesions are well marginated. Therefore, inhomogeneous signal intensity, which is noted in most malignancies, may be a more useful sign for distinguishing benign from malignant disorders. Generally, the signal intensity is inhomogeneous on both T1 and T2 weighted sequences. Inhomogeneity, however, usually is most obvious on T2 weighted sequences (Fig. 10-32). Neurovascular encasement and bone involvement also occur more frequently with malignant lesions.

The above image criteria are less useful in patients

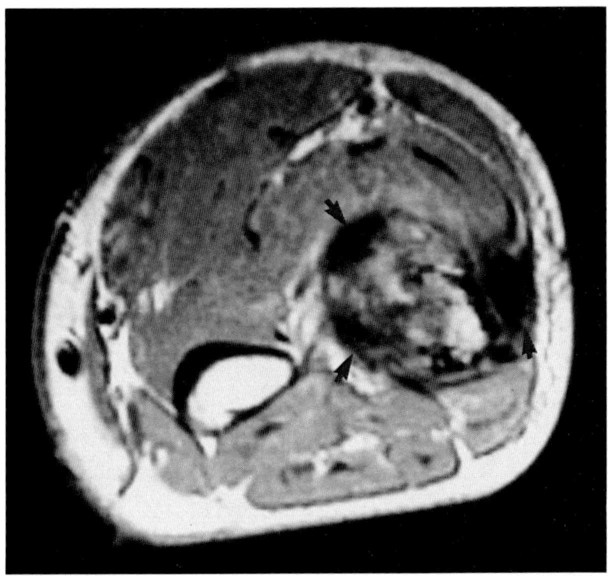

FIG. 10-31. Axial image of the forearm with a desmoid tumor. Note the numerous areas of low-intensity fibrous tissue (*arrows*).

who have recently undergone surgery or a diagnostic needle biopsy. Inflammatory changes and hemorrhage or hematoma from the procedure can create inhomogeneity in the signal intensity, which makes classification of lesions difficult.

A more complete discussion of musculoskeletal neoplasms, postoperative changes, metastasis, and MRI specificity is given in Chapter 12.

Avascular Necrosis (Osteonecrosis)

Osteonecrosis or avascular necrosis occurs less frequently in the elbow than other anatomic sites. However, patients with systemic disease or on steroid therapy can develop osteonecrosis in this region. Most often, osteonecrosis or osteochondrosis in the elbow occurs in young adults or teenagers and typically involves the capitellum (11). Patients present with dull pain in the elbow. Symptoms frequently increase with exercise. Local swelling and reduced extension of the elbow are common findings. The condition is frequently seen in young males (age 7–12) during ossification of the capitellar epiphysis. The local lesion of osteochondrosis is most common in the anterior central capitellum at the point of maximum contact with the radial head (11,38,51). Though the etiology is somewhat controversial, the condition is generally considered to be related to ischemia and/or trauma (11,51).

Since treatment is dictated by the imaging appearance of these lesions, it is important to accurately define the bone and cartilage changes. Type I lesions are undisplaced fragments with intact articular cartilage. Type II lesions have defects in the articular cartilage and may be partially displaced. Type III lesions are completely detached (11,51). Operative treatment is indicated for type II and type III lesions.

Imaging of osteochondritis dissecans or osteonecrosis (adults) should begin with routine radiography. In certain cases radionuclide scans are important for early detection. However, if one considers the importance of classifying this lesion and evaluating unossified cartilage it becomes apparent that MRI is ideally suited to evaluate these patients (Fig. 10-33).

Prior to MRI, arthrography was frequently required to evaluate the articular cartilage. However, T2 weighted sequences in two image planes provide excellent visualization of the size and position of the osseous or cartilaginous lesion and the articular cartilage. In general, sagittal and coronal images are most useful. The MRI features of osteonecrosis in the elbow are similar to the changes described in the hip. On T1 weighted images

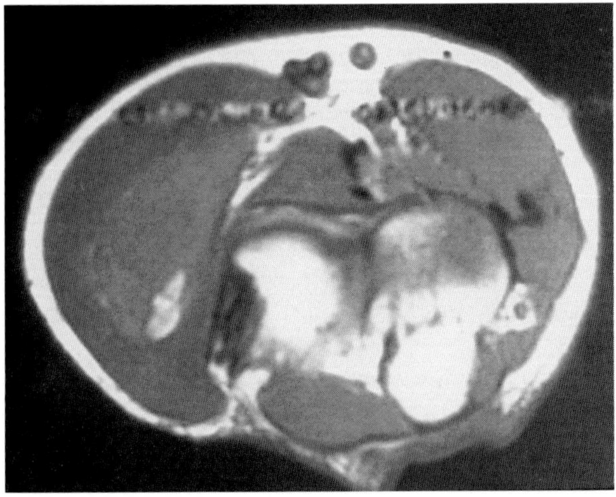

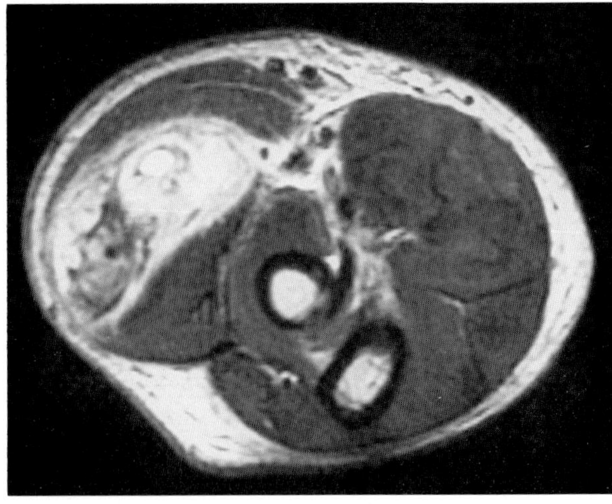

A,B

FIG. 10-32. Axial SE 500/20 (**A**) and SE 2,000/60 (**B**) images of a forearm sarcoma. The characteristics of the lesion are better demonstrated on the T2 weighted sequence (**B**).

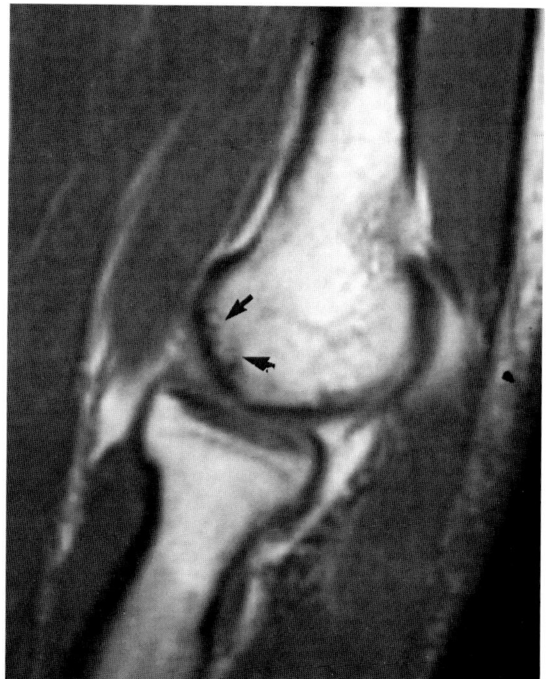

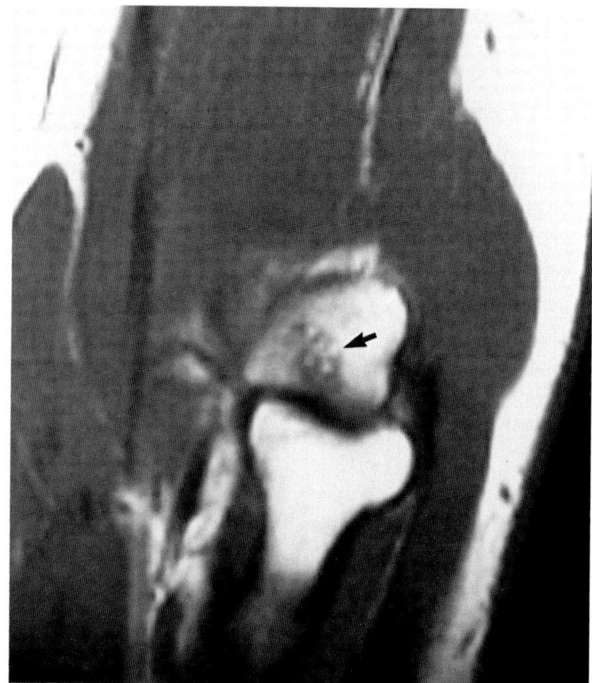

A,B

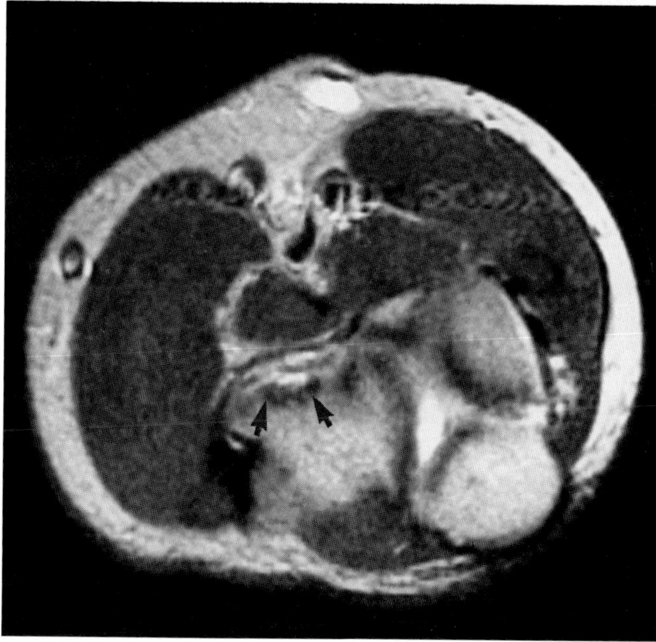

C

FIG. 10-33. Osteonecrosis of the capitellum. SE 500/20 sagittal (**A**) and coronal (**B**) images show a small defect (*arrows*) with intact articular cartilage. The axial SE 2,000/60 image (**C**) shows increased intensity with a low-intensity margin (*arrows*).

the area of necrosis is usually isointense with normal marrow and is surrounded by a low-intensity margin. In the early stages the low-intensity margin is due to hyperemia. On T2 weighted images high signal intensity is noted in this hyperemic zone. When new bone formation occurs around the infarcted region, the signal intensity is reduced on both T1 and T2 weighted sequences. Variable signal intensity at the necrotic margin is due to mixed resorption and new bone deposition. Articular cartilage (intermediate signal intensity) can clearly be defined on either T1 or T2 weighted sequences. However, subtle fissures or linear defects may be identified more easily on T2 weighted sequences (Fig. 10-33).

Early experience with MRI of the hip and wrist suggests that the technique is also useful for following patients with low-grade lesions who are considered for conservative therapy. Return of normal signal intensity has been correlated with improvement in patient symptoms (8,9).

Infection/Inflammatory Arthropathies

Musculoskeletal infections may present with an acute, rapidly progressing course or may be insidious. Determination of the extent of involvement is important in planning proper medical or surgical management. Routine radiographs and CT are useful for this purpose (7,9,50). Radioisotope studies are particularly sensitive in the early stages of infection. Technetium-99m, gallium-67, and indium-111 labeled leukocytes provide sensitive and fairly specific methods for diagnosis of infection. The anatomic extent, however, may be inaccurate, especially in the articular regions, and differentiation of cellulitis or soft tissue infection from bone involvement is not always possible (7,9,32).

Skeletal infections typically begin in medullary bone. The resulting hyperemia and inflammation cause alterations in the intensity of medullary bone on MR images. The excellent tissue contrast and multiplanar imaging provided by MRI may allow earlier and more accurate assessment than is possible with current imaging techniques. Therefore, acute osteomyelitis may be evident on MR images when radiographic findings are negative (9,41,46,49).

As with other musculoskeletal abnormalities, the examination generally requires both T1 and T2 weighted sequences to provide the necessary contrast between normal and abnormal tissue and to detect and characterize subtle abnormalities. Short TR/TE SE sequences (SE 500/20) can be performed quickly and provide high spatial resolution. Infection is seen as an area of decreased signal intensity compared with the high signal intensity of normal marrow. Changes in cortical bone, periosteum, and muscle are often less obvious. T2 weighted sequences (SE 2,000/60 or 2,000/80) demonstrate infection as areas of high signal intensity, which is ideal for identifying abnormal areas in cortical bone and soft tissues. Normal signal from fat in marrow is suppressed with this sequence, so when compared with normal marrow infected areas are seen as areas of higher signal intensity (7,9,47). In certain situations, more than two sequences may be required to improve tissue characterization. For example, chemical shift imaging may provide valuable information about fat, water (cellular elements), or inflammatory changes in bone marrow. More recently, short inversion time (TI) IR (STIR) sequences have proved useful in skeletal diseases including infection. A TI of 100–150 msec, a TE of 30 msec, and a TR of 1,500 msec will suppress fat signal, so that areas of inflammation are clearly seen by their marked increase in signal (23).

The specificity of MRI in diagnosing osteomyelitis needs to be defined more clearly. In marrow, cortical bone, periosteum, and soft tissue, increased signal intensity is noted on T2 weighted sequences, and decreased signal intensity is evident on T1 weighted sequences. Similar findings have been noted with neoplasms. The only reliable image feature noted to date has been increased signal intensity in medullary bone with a well-defined low-intensity margin. This observation has been noted with both infection and benign tumors (9). Infection must be present for several weeks to produce the reactive region in the medullary bone that is responsible for this finding.

Infectious arthritis generally is monoarticular and, like osteomyelitis, usually involves the lower extremities. Joint space changes and soft tissue swelling may be noted on radiographs, but early bone changes are not appreciated for 1–2 weeks in a pyogenic infection and may take months to develop with tuberculous arthritis. Isotope studies with the use of ^{99m}Tc are sensitive in detecting early changes but are nonspecific. ^{67}Ga and ^{111}In leukocyte scans are more specific in this regard (5,7,32).

The role of MRI in joint space infection is unclear. Early bone and soft tissue changes and effusions are easily detected (4,5,42). Findings, however, are nonspecific and could be noted with many other arthritides (44,54). Characterization of the type of fluid present in the joint would be useful. Generally, the T1 and T2 relaxation times of transudates are longer than those of exudates. Infected fluid and blood in the joint tend to have an intermediate signal intensity and may be inhomogeneous on T2 weighted images. Normal synovial fluid has a uniformly high signal intensity with this sequence. This information is not sufficient to obviate joint aspiration to identify the offending organism. In addition, effusions and capsular distention may be evident in any inflammatory arthritis. Pigmented villonodular synovitis is the exception to the rule. The lipid-laden macrophages and hemosiderin deposition create fairly specific MRI changes (44) (Fig. 10-34).

Miscellaneous Conditions

There are numerous evolving applications for MRI. Also, special "problem solving" situations continue to develop in patients where other imaging techniques have not defined the problem. In these settings the data to state that MRI is the technique of choice may not be complete. However, the early findings clearly indicate MRI may be superior in certain clinical settings. Certain problems in the elbow and forearm fall into these categories.

Nerve Entrapment Syndromes

Chronic pain with or without localized neurologic disease is a common indication for MRI of the elbow and forearm. Generally, patients are referred to exclude soft tissue masses or primary peripheral nerve tumors.

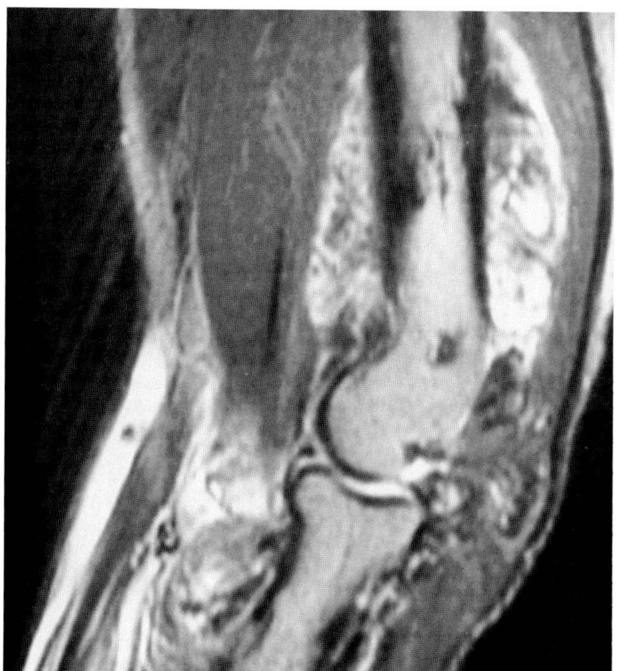

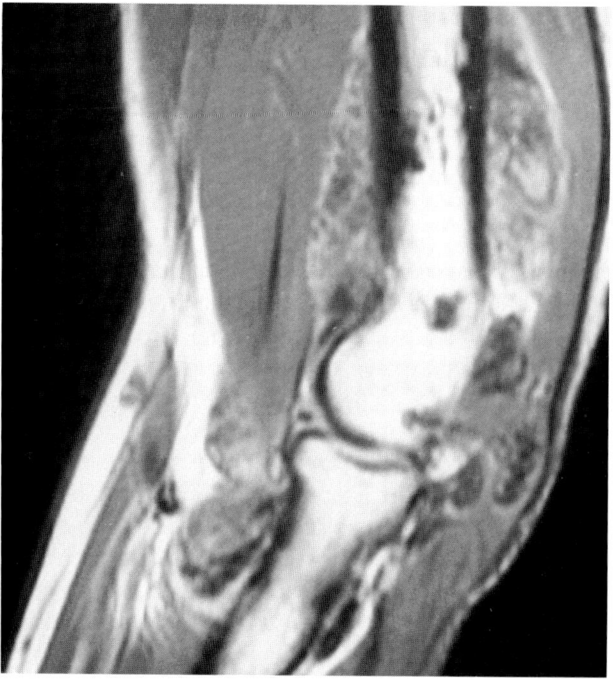

A,B

FIG. 10-34. Sagittal T1 (**A**) and T2 (**B**) weighted images demonstrate extensive synovitis with multiple areas of low signal intensity due to pigmented villonodular synovitis.

There is no question that MRI is ideally suited for detection of these lesions (8,9) (Fig. 10-35). However, subtle changes along the nerves of the elbow and forearm may also be evaluated by MRI (Fig. 10-6). This requires careful evaluation of the nerves and adjacent anatomy (Fig. 10-23).

Nerve compression or entrapment syndromes have been categorized into four different lesions (35,43,45). A first degree lesion (neuraproctic) shows conduction defects, but there are no structural changes in the nerve. This type of lesion may be due to blunt trauma, ischemia, or compression, and return to function can be expected with proper treatment. Second degree lesions (axonometric) have disruption of the sheath and nerve fibers, but connective tissue is intact and regeneration can occur. More advanced third degree and fourth degree lesions (neurometric) usually result in complete motor and sensory loss and typically occur when compression has been present for more than $1\frac{1}{2}$ years (43). Third and fourth degree injuries are more common in

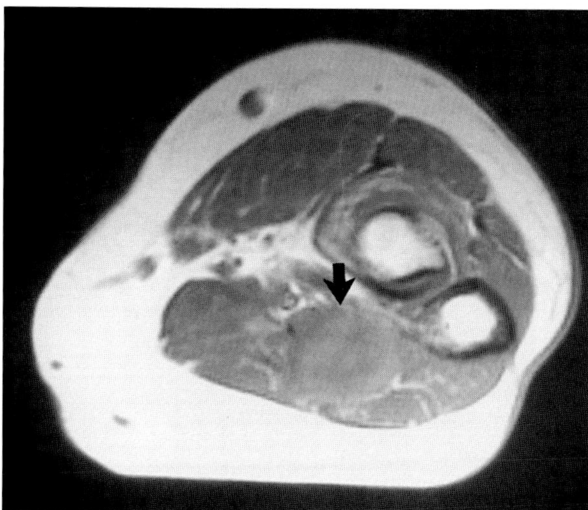

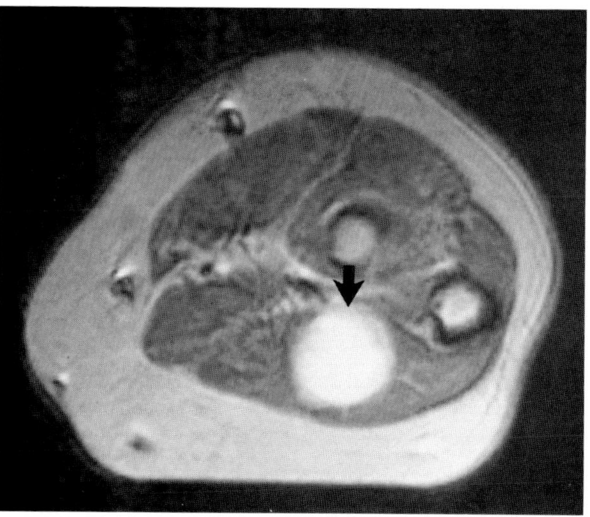

A,B

FIG. 10-35. Axial SE 500/20 (**A**) and SE 2,000/60 (**B**) images of the forearm in a patient with a benign neuroma (*arrow*).

regions where motion or friction occur in addition to compression (35,43,45).

The causes of nerve compression are numerous and summarized in Table 10-6. However, from an imaging standpoint it is important to be familiar with the common locations and anatomy where nerve compression syndromes typically occur (Table 10-7). This information is essential when planning the MR examination. The radial nerve and its posterior interosseous and superficial branches are susceptible to compression in several areas. Compression can occur from the lateral margin of the triceps to the distal forearm. Therefore, an extensive thin slice (≤5 mm) MR examination is required. Localization of the problem to the posterior interosseous or superficial branches can assist in planning the MR examination (Table 10-7). For example, the most common site of compression of the posterior interosseous branch is at the upper margin of or in the region of the supinator (43) (Fig. 10-23). Motor paralysis to the extensor muscles is common with compression of the posterior interosseous branch of the radial nerve (see Table 10-4). Some patients present with minor symptoms resembling tennis elbow. Compression of the superficial branch (Fig. 10-23) typically occurs in the proximal forearm or elbow region (43,45).

The ulnar nerve passes posterior to the medial epicondyle and then enters the anterior compartment several centimeters distal to the elbow (2) (Figs. 10-6 and 10-23). These areas are the most common locations for nerve compression syndromes. Compression in the forearms is rare (43,45). The etiology of ulnar nerve compression does not differ significantly from the radial nerve (Table 10-6). Several exceptions, primarily anatomic, include bone changes in the medial epicondyle and the anomalous muscle, anconeus epitrochlaris (29,43). The ulnar nerve can also be compressed between the ulnar and humeral heads of the flexor carpi ulnaris during flexion (29). Patients generally present with parasthesias on the fourth and fifth fingers. Later, sensory loss or flexion deformities due to motor loss can occur. Prior to performing localized MRI of the elbow and upper forearm, we must exclude the cervical spine or thoracic outlet as the source of ulnar neuropathy.

TABLE 10-6. *Etiology of nerve compression in the forearm and elbow*

Fibrous adhesions
Muscle anomalies
Vascular anomalies
Bursal enlargement
Ganglia
Musculotendinous inflammation
Bone and soft tissue trauma
Neoplasms
Vascular occlusion

TABLE 10-7. *Nerve compression syndromes of the elbow and forearm (43)*

Nerve	Location of compression
Radial nerve	Distal arm to distal forearm
Posterior interosseous branch	Proximal supinator (arcade of Frohse)
Superficial branch	Proximal forearm, elbow
Ulnar nerve[a]	Medial epicondyle
Medial nerve[b]	Distal humerus (supracondylar process), pronator teres origin

[a] Cervical spine and thoracic outlet pathology may also cause ulnar nerve symptoms.
[b] May be confused with carpal tunnel syndrome.

The median nerve rests on the brachialis muscle near the brachial artery, vein, and biceps tendon in the medial aspect of the distal arm (1,29). At the elbow it passes along the humeral head of the pronator teres (Figs. 10-6

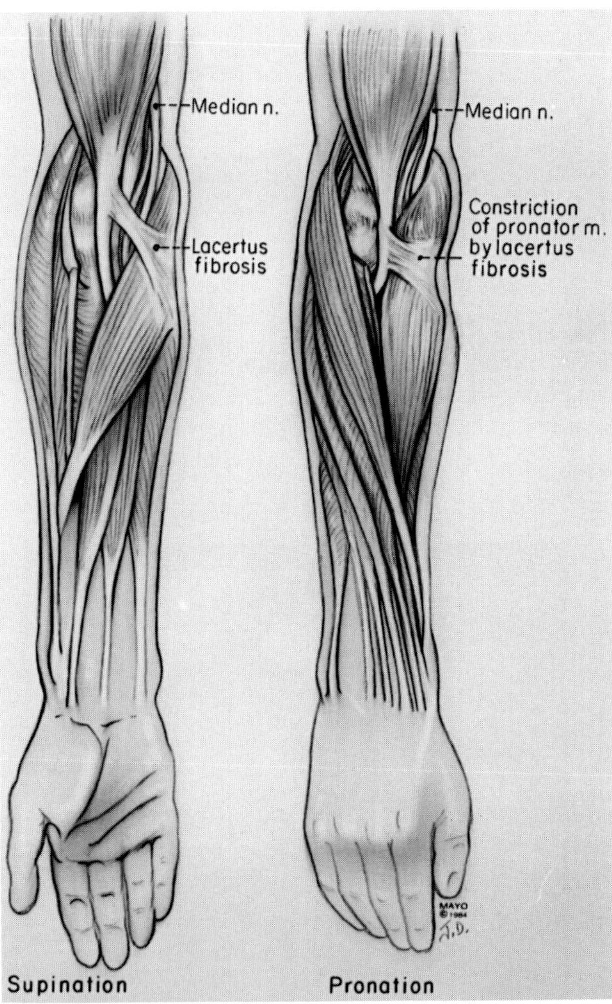

FIG. 10-36. Illustration of the median nerve and its relationship to the lacertus fibrosis and pronator teres. Compression can occur during pronation and supination at this level. (From ref. 35, with permission.)

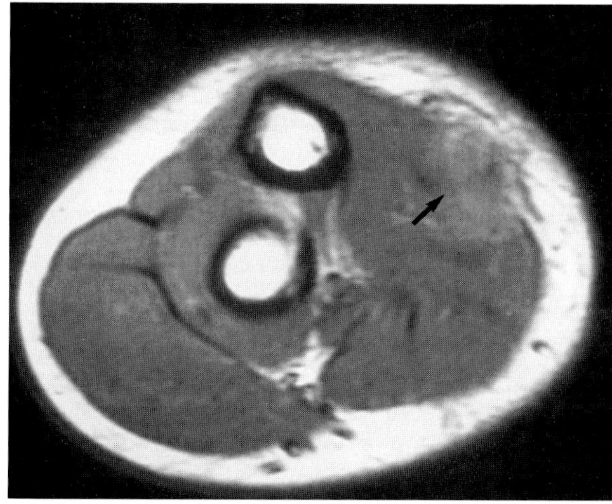

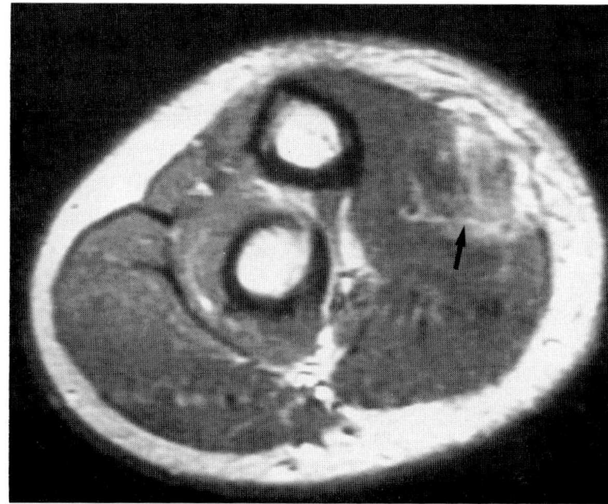

A,B

FIG. 10-37. Axial SE 500/20 (**A**) and SE 2,000/60 (**B**) images in a patient with radial nerve symptoms caused by a local granulomatous infection (*arrows*).

and 10-23) and then beneath it to lie between the flexor digitorum profundus and superficialis in the forearm (1,29,35).

Compression typically occurs at the supracondylar process or near the origin of the pronator teres (Fig. 10-36). The etiology may vary (Table 10-7) but, particularly in the pronator teres syndrome, may be related to repetitive strenuous activity, usually industrial professions (30). Patients present with vague discomfort or numbness in the median nerve distribution of the hand. Thus, one must consider carpal tunnel syndrome in the differential diagnosis. Therefore, if MRI of the elbow and upper forearm is normal, one should also evaluate the wrist.

Compression syndromes involving the anterior interosseous and musculocutaneous nerves (Fig. 10-23) have also been described but are uncommon (30). MR evaluation of patients with suspected nerve compression syndromes can be complex. The course of the nerves and their size (especially branches of the median, ulnar, and radial nerves) make them difficult to follow unless thin (≤5 mm) axial images are obtained. A scout coronal image is obtained to select the necessary FOV. T2 weighted axial images (SE 2,000/20–30, 60–80) provide excellent anatomic detail and allow easy detection of soft tissue inflammation and masses along the nerves (Fig. 10-37). One must consider evaluation of the cervical spine and thoracic outlet and use flexion and extension GRASS images if the axial images are normal in a patient with suspected nerve compression (Table 10-7). The carpal tunnel region should be evaluated when the median nerve is normal at the elbow and upper forearm.

The data obtained from MRI and EMG studies can be extremely valuable in determining the proper management of patients with nerve compression syndromes.

MRI applications for the elbow and forearm will continue to expand. Chapter 15 discusses evolving MR applications in the musculoskeletal system.

REFERENCES

1. Anderson JE. *Grant's atlas of anatomy,* 8th ed. Baltimore: Williams & Wilkins, 1983.
2. Anzel SH, Covey KW, Weiner AD, Lipscomb DR. Disruption of muscles and tendons: analysis of 1,014 cases. *Surgery* 1959;45:406–414.
3. Axel L. Blood flow effects in magnetic resonance imaging. *AJR* 1984;143:1157–1166.
4. Beltran J, Caudell JL, Herman LA, Kantor SM, Hudson PN, Noto AM, Baran AS. Rheumatoid arthritis: MR imaging manifestations. *Radiology* 1987;165:153–157.
5. Beltran J, Noto AM, Herman LJ, Mosure JC, Burk JM, Christoforidis AJ. Joint effusions: MR imaging. *Radiology* 1986; 158:133–137.
6. Beltran J, Simon DC, Katz W, Weis LD. Increased MR signal intensity in skeletal muscle adjacent to malignant tumors. *Radiology* 1987;162:251–255.
7. Berquist TH, Brown ML, Fitzgerald RH, May GR. Magnetic resonance imaging: application in musculoskeletal infection. *Magn Reson Imaging* 1985;3:219–230.
8. Berquist TH. MR imaging of the elbow and wrist. *Top Magn Reson Imaging* 1989;1:15–27.
9. Berquist TH. *Magnetic resonance of the musculoskeletal system.* New York: Raven Press, 1987.
10. Berquist TH. Magnetic resonance imaging of musculoskeletal neoplasms. *Clin Orthop* 1989;244:101–118.
11. Bianco AJ. Osteochondritis dissecans. In: Morrey BF, ed. *The elbow and its disorders.* Philadelphia: Saunders, 1985:254–259.
12. Bradley WG. When should GRASS be used. *Radiology* 1988;169:574–575.
13. Bradley WG Jr, Waluch V. Blood flow: magnetic resonance imaging. *Radiology* 1985;154:443–450.
14. Bradley WG Jr, Waluch V, Lai KS, Fernandez E, Spaler C. Appearance of rapidly flowing blood on magnetic resonance images. *AJR* 1984;143:1167–1174.
15. Bradley WG Jr. Flow phenomena in MR imaging. *AJR* 1988;150:983–994.
16. Bunnell DH, Fisher DA, Bassett LA, Gold RH, Ellman H. Elbow joint: normal anatomy on MR images. *Radiology* 1987;165:527–531.
17. Carter BL, Morehead J, Walpert SM, Hammerschlag SB, Griffiths HJ, Kahn PC. *Cross-sectional anatomy: computed tomography*

and ultrasound correlation. New York: Appleton-Century-Crofts, 1977.
18. Cohen JM, Weinreb JC, Redman HC. Arteriovenous malformations of the extremities. MR imaging. *Radiology* 1986;158:475–479.
19. Dahlin DC, Unni KK. *Bone tumors: general aspects and data on 8,542 cases.* Springfield, IL: CC Thomas, 1986.
20. Dobyns JH. Congenital abnormalities of the elbow. In: Morrey BF, ed. *The elbow and its disorders.* Philadelphia: Saunders, 1985:161–181.
21. Dooms GC, Hricak H, Sollitto RA, Higgins CB. Lipomatous tumors and tumors with fatty component: MR imaging potential and comparison of MR and CT results. *Radiology* 1985;157:479–483.
22. Dreyfuss U. Snapping elbow due to dislocation of the medial head of the triceps. *J Bone Joint Surg* 1978;60B:56–57.
23. Dwyer AM, Frank JA, Sank VJ, Reenig JW, Hickey AM, Doppman JL. Short-TI inversion-recovery pulse sequence: analysis and initial experience in cancer imaging. *Radiology* 1988;168:827–836.
24. Enzinger FM, Weiss SW. *Soft tissue tumors.* St. Louis: CV Mosby, 1983.
25. Farrar EL III, Lippert FG III. Avulsion of the triceps tendon. *Clin Orthop* 1981;161:242–246.
26. Felmlee JP, Ehman RL. Spatial presaturation: a method for suppressing flow artifacts and improving depiction of vascular anatomy in MR imaging. *J Comput Assist Tomogr* 1987;11:369–377.
27. Hajek PC, Sartoris DJ, Neumann CH, Resnick D. Potential contrast agents for MR arthrography: *in vitro* evaluation and practical observations. *AJR* 1987;149:97–104.
28. Hardy CJ, Katzberg RW, Frey RL, Szumowski J, Totterman S, Mueller OM. Switched surface coil system for bilateral MR imaging. *Radiology* 1988;167:835–838.
29. Hollinshead HW. *Anatomy for surgeons. Volume 3, The back and limbs,* 3rd ed. New York: Harper & Row, 1982.
30. Kopell HP, Thompson WAL. The pronator syndrome. *N Engl J Med* 1958;259:713–715.
31. Lee JK, Yao L. Stress fractures: MR imaging. *Radiology* 1988;169:217–220.
32. Lewin JS, Rosenfield NS, Hoffner PB, Downing D. Acute osteomyelitis in children: combined Tc-99m and Ga-67 imaging. *Radiology* 1986;158:795–804.
33. Middleton WD, Lawson TL. *Anatomy and MRI of the joints.* New York: Raven Press, 1989.
34. Middleton WD, Macrander S, Lawson TL, et al. High resolution surface coil magnetic resonance imaging of the joints: anatomic correlation. *Radiographics* 1987;7:645–683.
35. Morrey BF, ed. *The elbow and its disorders.* Philadelphia: Saunders, 1985.
36. Narayama PA, Brey WW, Kulkarni MV, Sievenpiper CL. Compensation for surface coil sensitivity variation in magnetic resonance imaging. *Magn Reson Imaging* 1988;6:271–274.
37. Nirschl RP. Muscle and tendon trauma: tennis elbow. In: Morrey BF, ed. *The elbow and its disorders.* Philadelphia: Saunders, 1985:481–496.
38. Omer GEJ. Primary articular osteochondrosis. *Clin Orthop* 1981;158:33–40.
39. Pusey E, Lofkin RB, Brown RK, Solomon MA, Stark DD, Tarr RW, Hanafee WN. Magnetic resonance imaging artifacts: mechanism and clinical significance. *Radiographics* 1986;6(5):891–911.
40. Reiman TH, Heiken JP, Totty WG, Lee JKT. Clinical MR imaging with a Helmholtz-type surface coil. *Radiology* 1988;169:564–566.
41. Rosen BR, Flemings DM, Kushner DC, et al. Hematologic bone marrow disorders: quantitative chemical shift MR imaging. *Radiology* 1988;169:799–804.
42. Sims RE, Genant HK. Magnetic resonance imaging of joint disease. *Radiol Clin North Am* 1986;24:179–188.
43. Spinner M, Linscheid RL. Nerve entrapment syndromes. In: Morrey BF, ed. *The elbow and its disorders.* Philadelphia: Saunders, 1985.
44. Spritzer CE, Dalinka MK, Kressel HY. Magnetic resonance imaging of pigmented villonodular synovitis: a report of two cases. *Skeletal Radiol* 1987;16:316–319.
45. Sutherland S. *Nerves and nerve injuries.* Baltimore: Williams & Wilkins, 1978.
46. Tang JSH, Gold RH, Bassett LW, Seeger LL. Musculoskeletal infection of the extremities: evaluation with MR imaging. *Radiology* 1988;166:205–209.
47. Unger E, Moldofsky P, Gatenby R, Hartz W, Broder G. Diagnosis of osteomyelitis by MR imaging. *AJR* 1988;150:605–610.
48. VanderMeuler P, Groen JP, Tinus AMC, Brantink G. Fast field echo imaging: an overview and contrast calculations. *Magn Reson Imaging* 1988;6:355–368.
49. Vogler JB III, Murphy WA. Bone marrow imaging. *Radiology* 1988;168:679–693.
50. Wing VW, Jeffrey RB, Federle MP, Helms CA, Trofton P. Chronic osteomyelitis examined by CT. *Radiology* 1985; 154:171–174.
51. Woodward AH, Bianco AJ. Osteochondritis dissecans of the elbow. *Clin Orthop* 1975;110:35–44.
52. Yao L, Lee JK. Occult intraosseous fracture: detection with MR imaging. *Radiology* 1988;167:749–751.
53. Wright SM, Wright RM. Bilateral MR imaging with switched mutually coupled receiver coils. *Radiology* 1989;170:249–255.
54. Yulish BS, Lieberman JM, Newman AJ, Bryan PJ, Mulopulos GP, Modic MT. Juvenile rheumatoid arthritis: assessment with MR imaging. *Radiology* 1987;165:149–152.

MRI of the Musculoskeletal System, 2nd Edition, edited by T. H. Berquist. Raven Press, Ltd., New York © 1990.

CHAPTER 11

Hand and Wrist

Thomas H. Berquist

Techniques, 395
Anatomy, 410
Osteology, 411
Ligamentous and Articular Anatomy, 411
Muscular Anatomy, 413
Neurovascular Anatomy, 418
Pitfalls, 419
Clinical Applications, 420
Trauma, 421
Musculoskeletal Neoplasms, 422
Infection, 425
Arthritis, 425
Avascular Necrosis, 426
Carpal Tunnel Syndrome, 429
Ulnar Nerve Compression, 431
Miscellaneous Conditions, 433
References, 433

Imaging of the hand and wrist can be difficult due to the complex bone and soft tissue anatomy. Routine radiographs and fluoroscopically positioned spot films are usually adequate for identification of fractures. Subtle changes may require radionuclide studies followed by tomography to clearly define the nature of bone lesions. Invasive techniques such as arthrography and tenography have been used to identify ligament and tendon injuries. Ultrasonography has been used to evaluate tendons and computed tomography (CT) is the technique of choice for evaluating subluxations of the distal radioulnar joint (9). MRI has become increasingly useful in defining soft tissue abnormalities, subtle bone lesions, and ischemic changes in the hand and wrist. When properly performed, MRI may replace more conventional techniques in diagnosing certain disorders of the hand and wrist (10,12,14,29–31,40,49).

TECHNIQUES

MRI examinations of the hand and wrist can be difficult to perform due to limitations in positioning and coil selection (10,11). Patient comfort is an essential part of the examination. If the position is difficult to tolerate, one can expect significant problems with motion artifact. In our initial review of upper extremity MRI studies, we noted motion artifacts or incomplete studies due to patient discomfort in 25% of cases.

Positioning depends on patient size, information required (i.e., motion studies), software, and coil availability. Uniform signal intensity is most easily obtained using a wrap-around, partial volume, or Helmholtz coil system (Fig. 11-1) (3,10,31,32,49). The small flat coils (3 and 5 inches) are also adequate for hand and wrist imaging (Fig. 11-2). Flat coils allow more flexibility for positioning and motion studies. When patient size allows, it is best to position the arm at the side. Dual coils are now available which allow simultaneous evaluation of both hands and wrists (23). The wrist can also be positioned over the abdomen with the elbow flexed. However, the coil must be supported and separated from the abdominal wall or motion artifact becomes a problem. Larger patients may need to be rotated with the arm above the head (Fig. 11-1). This position is difficult to tolerate due to shoulder discomfort (11).

Optimal image quality in hand and wrist imaging requires a small field of view (FOV) (Fig. 11-3). We typically use an 8–12 cm FOV for examinations with both flat and volume coils. Off-axis, small field of view is needed if the coil is positioned away from the central axis of the magnet (see Chapter 3). Therefore, if this software is not available, one must position the arm above the head to achieve the proper FOV (Fig. 11-1).

Text continues on p. 407

T. H. Berquist: Mayo Medical School and Mayo Clinic, Rochester, Minnesota 55905.

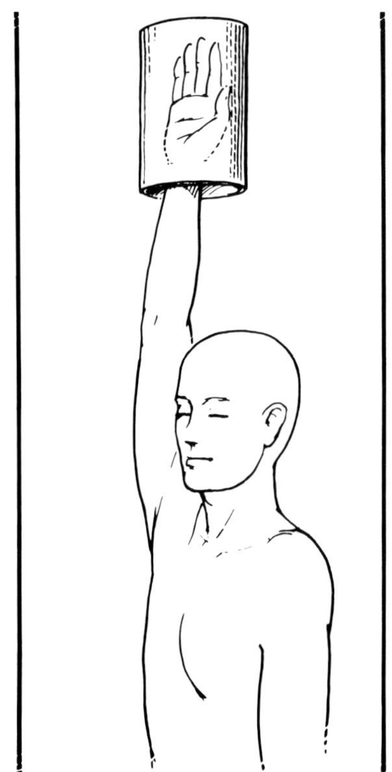

FIG. 11-1. Illustration of a patient positioned for evaluation of the hand and wrist using a circumferential (volume) coil. The arm is above the head. This position is not easily tolerated and motion artifacts are likely to occur. (From ref. 10, with permission.)

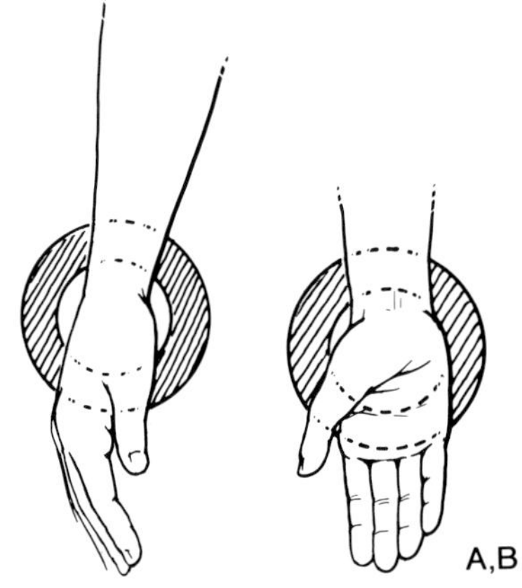

FIG. 11-2. Illustration of patient positioned with arm at the side and the wrist in the lateral (**A**) and supine (**B**) positions. A flat 5 inch coil is used. (From ref. 10, with permission.)

A,B

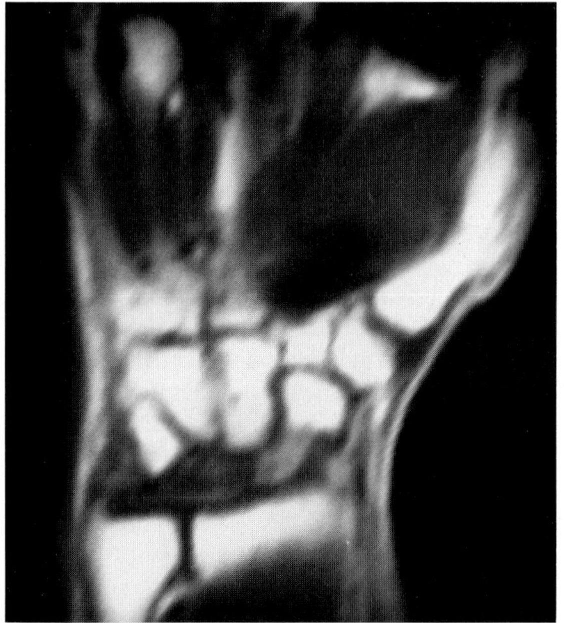

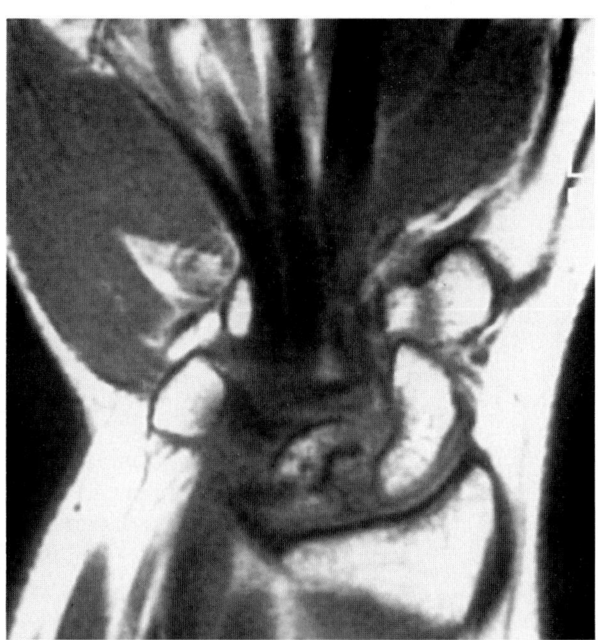

FIG. 11-3. Coronal images of the wrist (SE 500/20) with a 24 cm (**A**) and 12 cm (**B**) field of view (FOV). Note the marked improvement in image quality with small FOV.

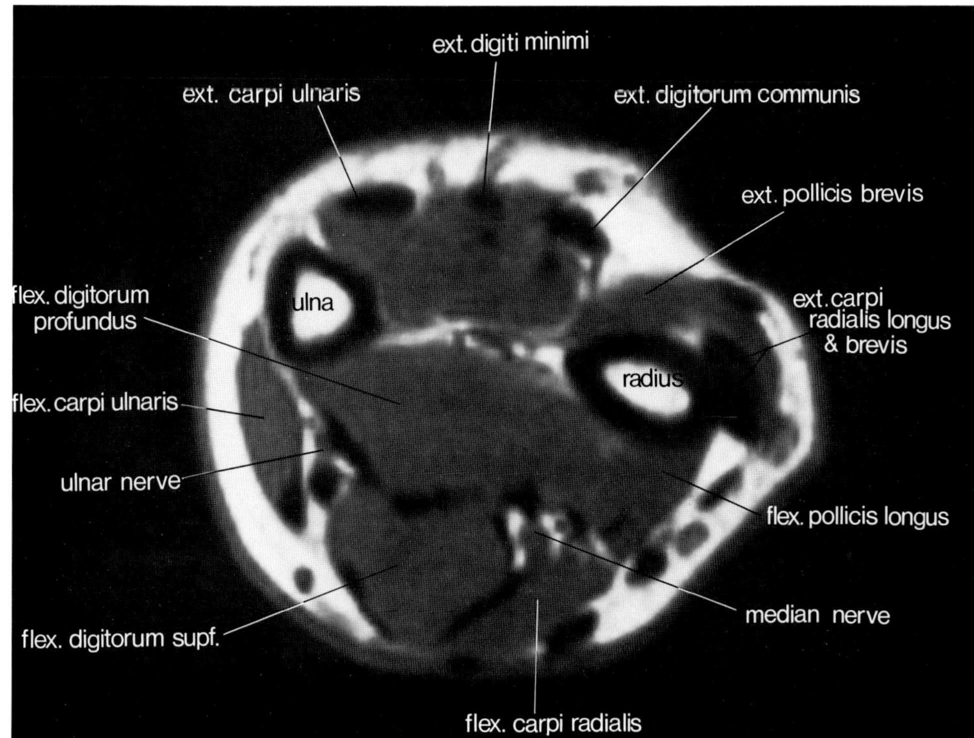

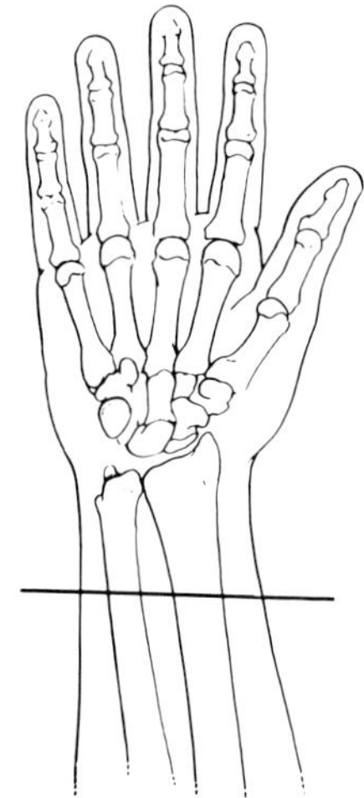

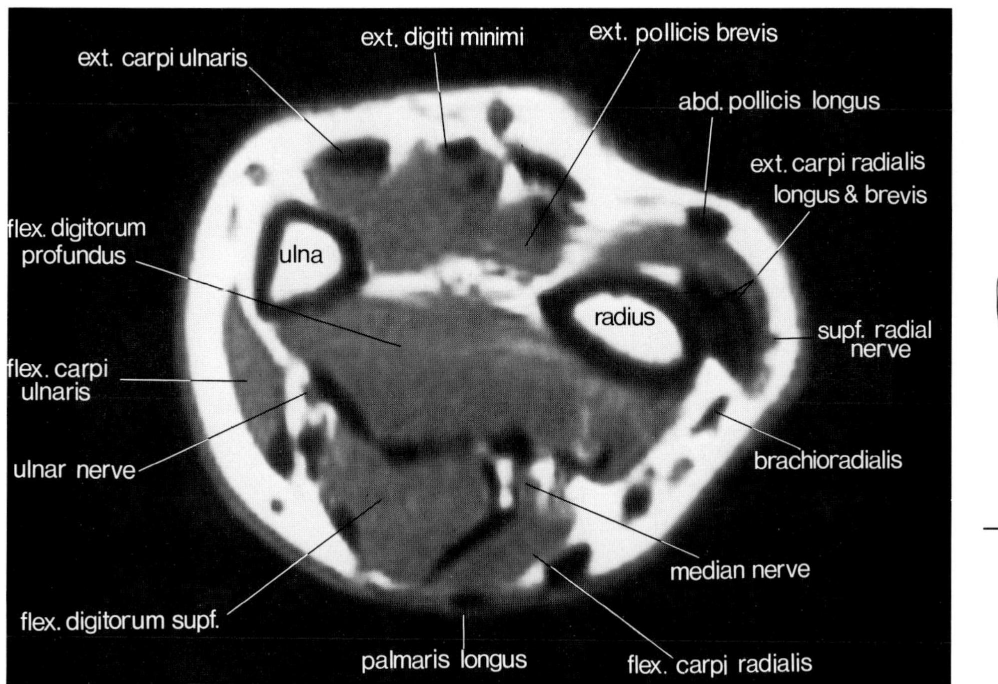

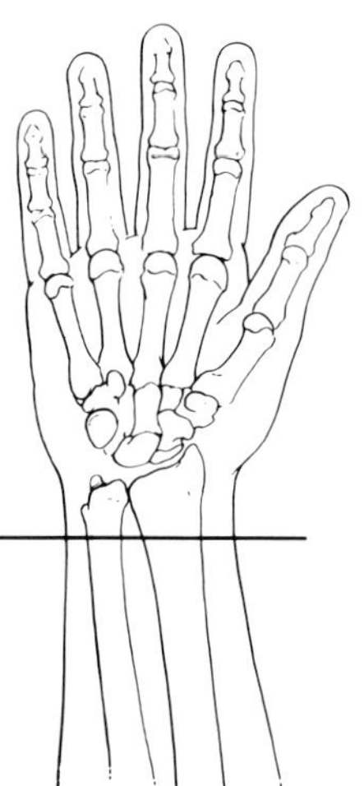

FIG. 11-4. Axial images of the distal forearm, wrist, and hand with illustration for plane of section (DI, dorsal interosseous; PI, palmar interosseous). **A,B:** Axial images distal forearm.

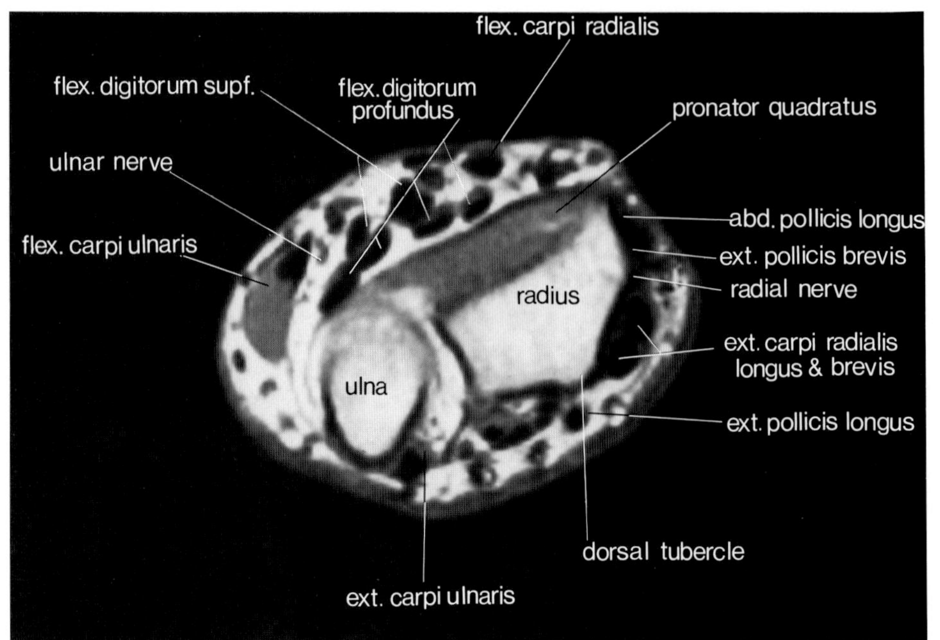

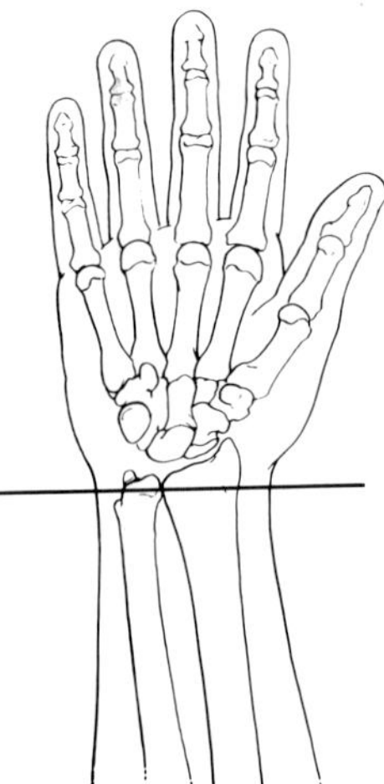

FIG. 11-4. C: Axial image through the radioulnar joint (prone).

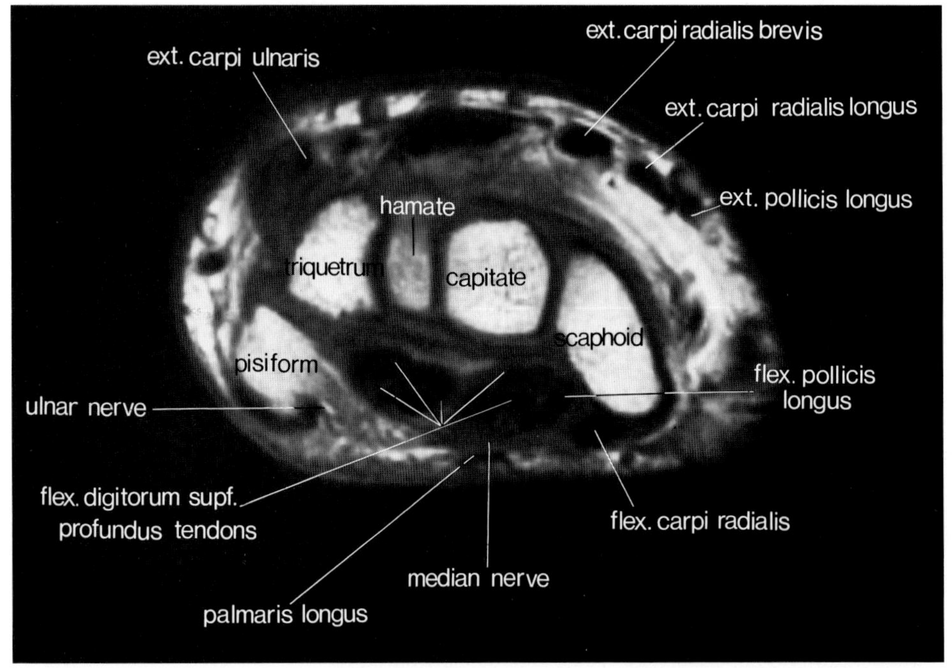

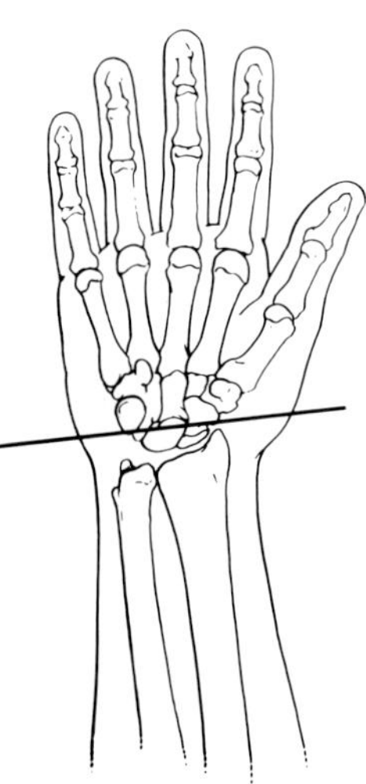

FIG. 11-4. D: Axial image through the scaphoid (supine).

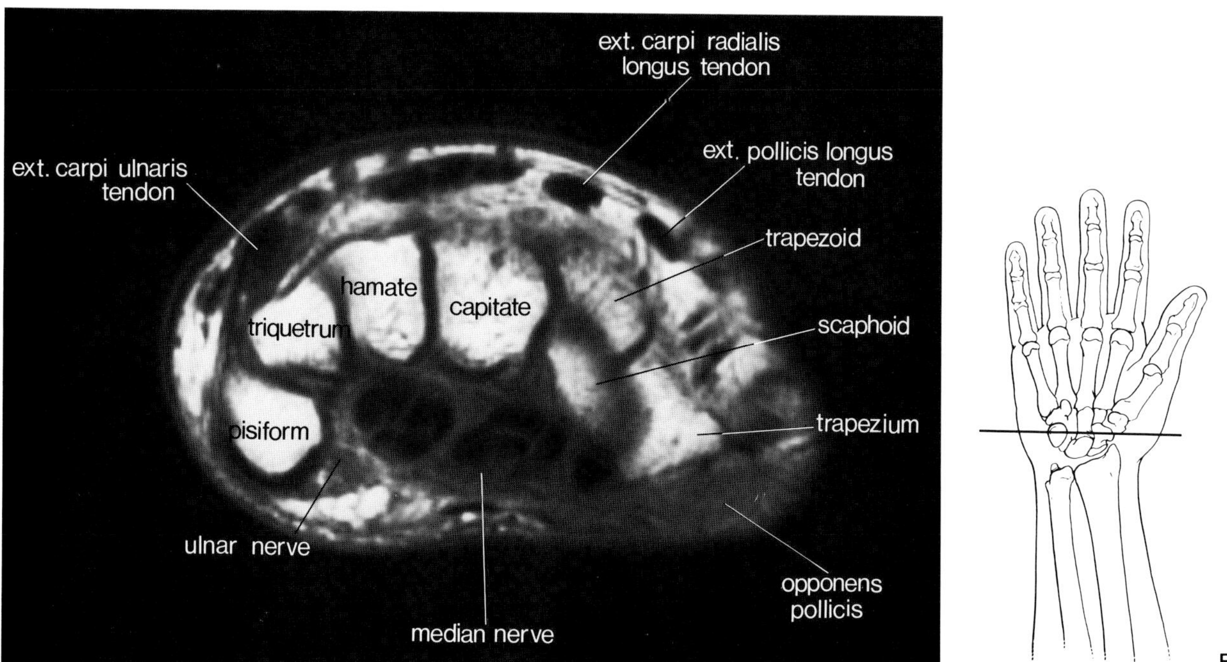

FIG. 11-4. E: Axial image through pisotriquetral articulation and Guyon's canal.

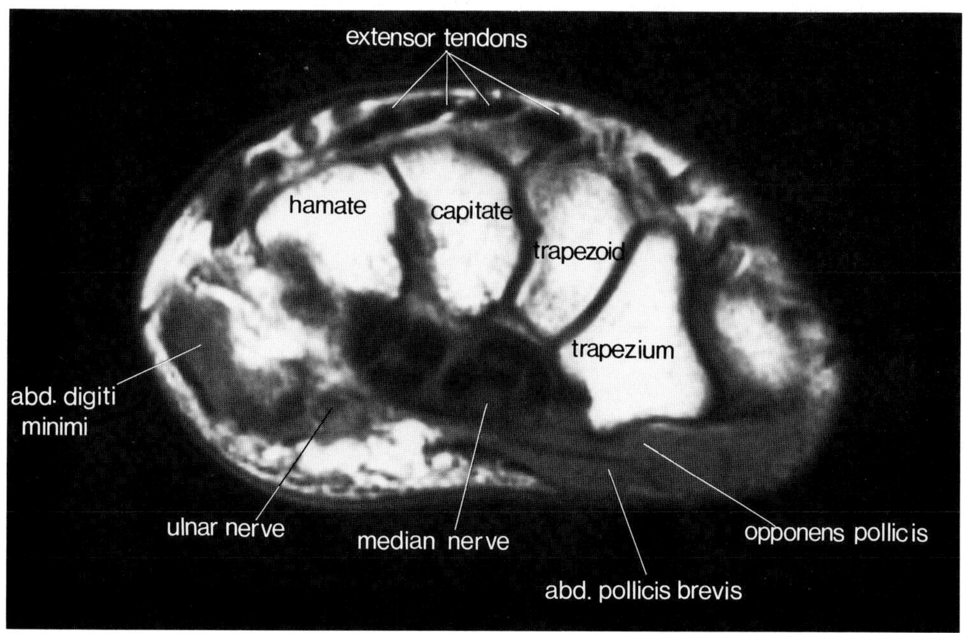

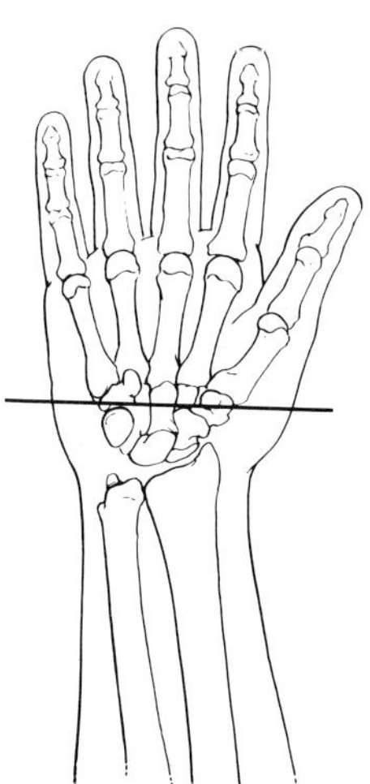

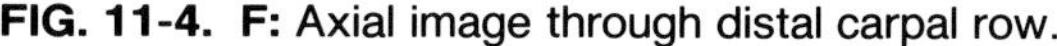
FIG. 11-4. F: Axial image through distal carpal row.

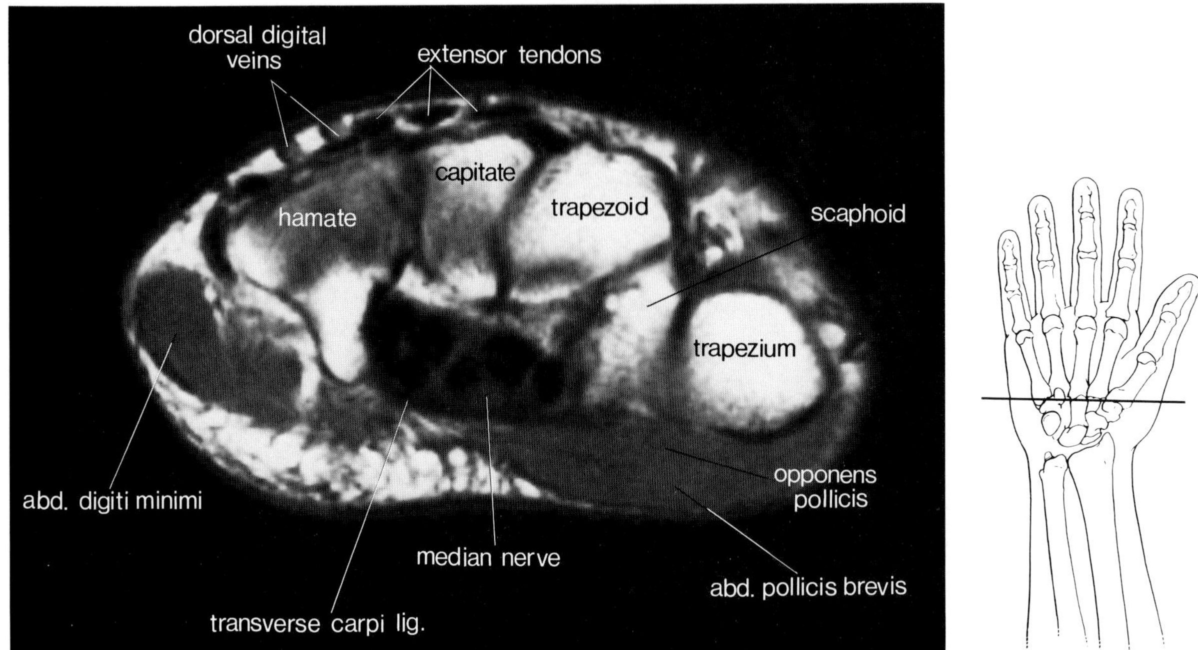

FIG. 11-4. G: Axial image through distal carpal row at the hook of the hamate.

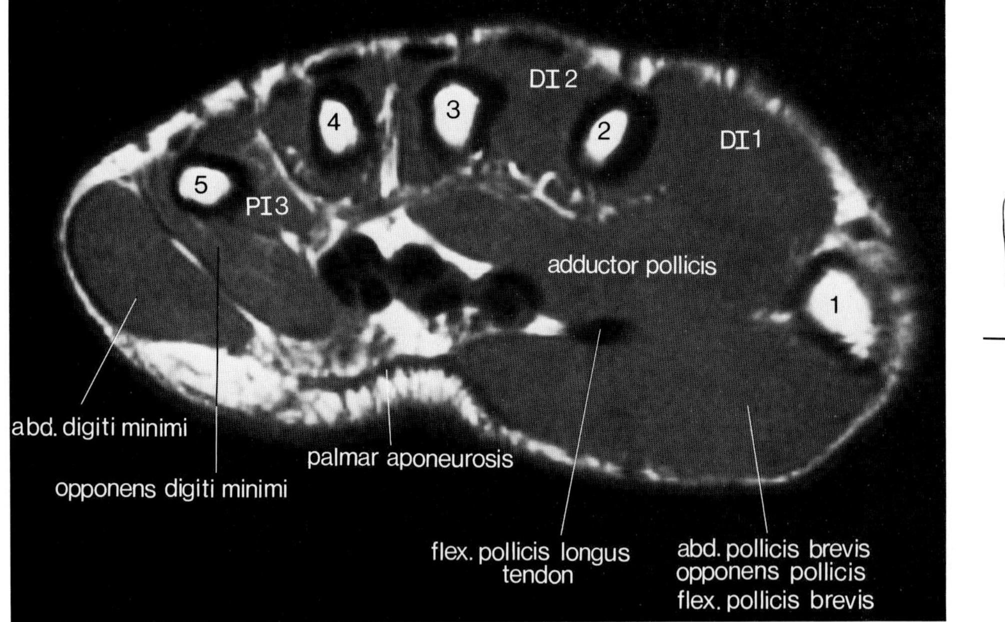

FIG. 11-4. H: Axial image through thenar region.

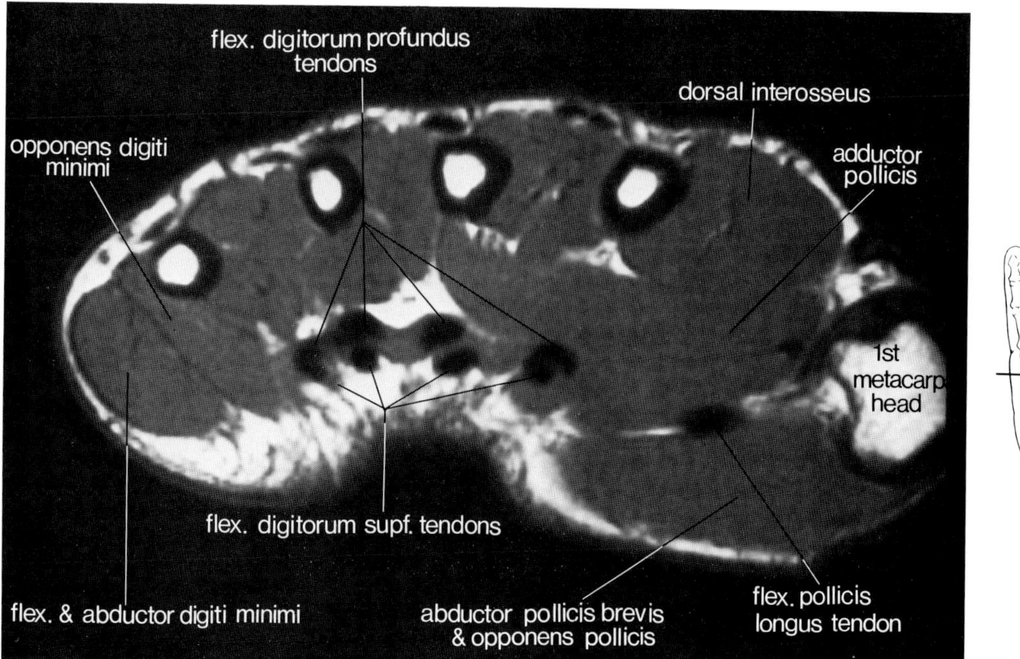

FIG. 11-4. I: Axial image through first metacarpal head.

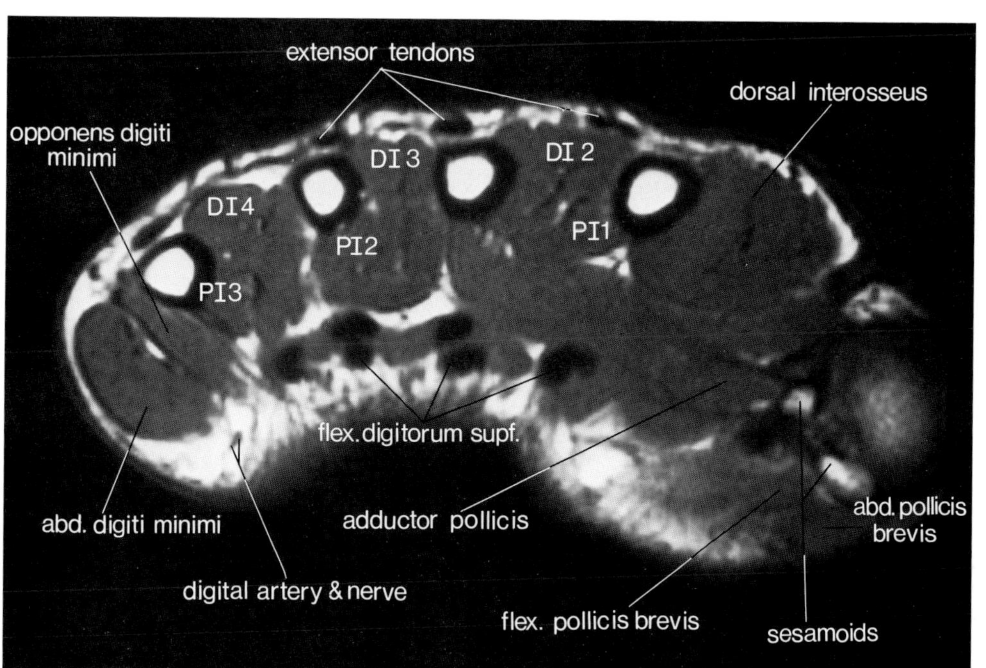

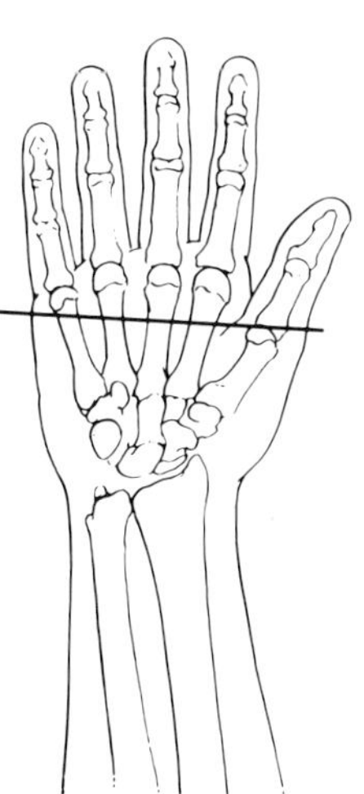

FIG. 11-4. J: Axial image through the first MCP joint level.

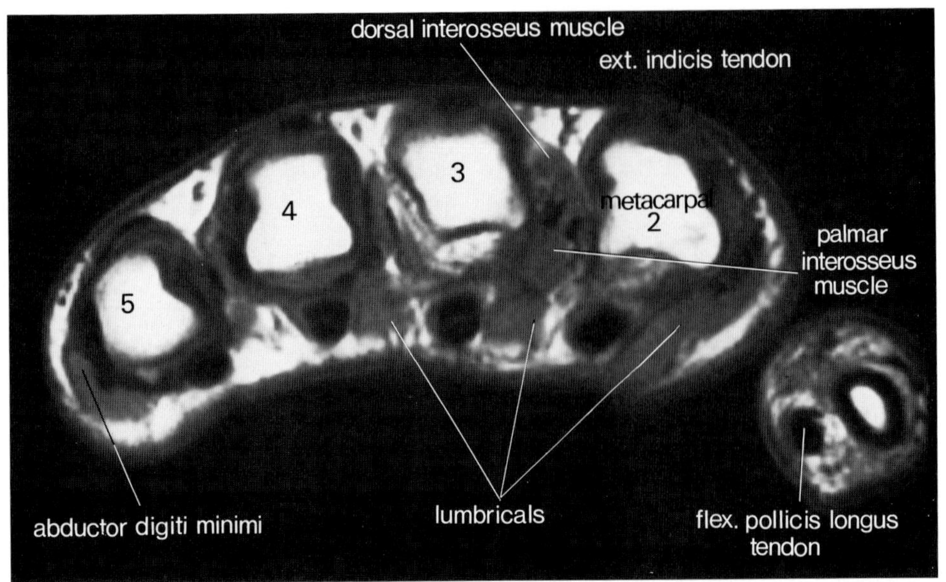

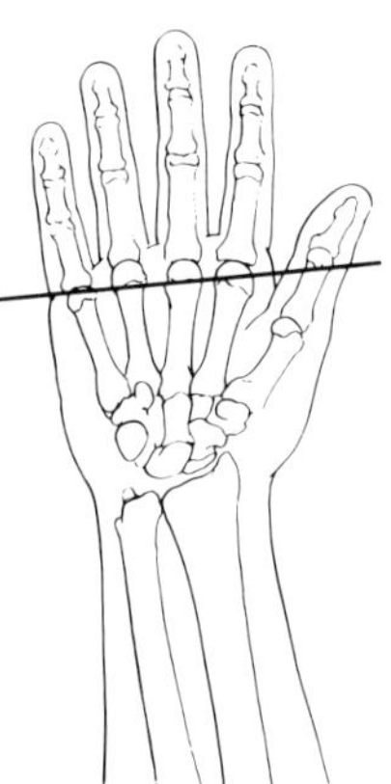

FIG. 11-4. K: Axial image through metacarpal heads two to five.

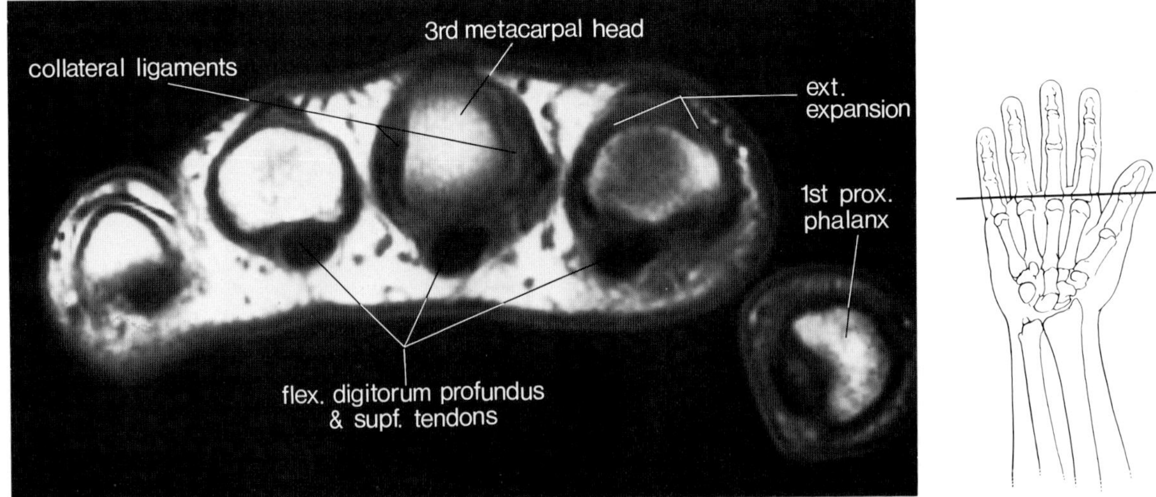

FIG. 11-4. L: Axial image through proximal phalangeal bases and third metacarpal head.

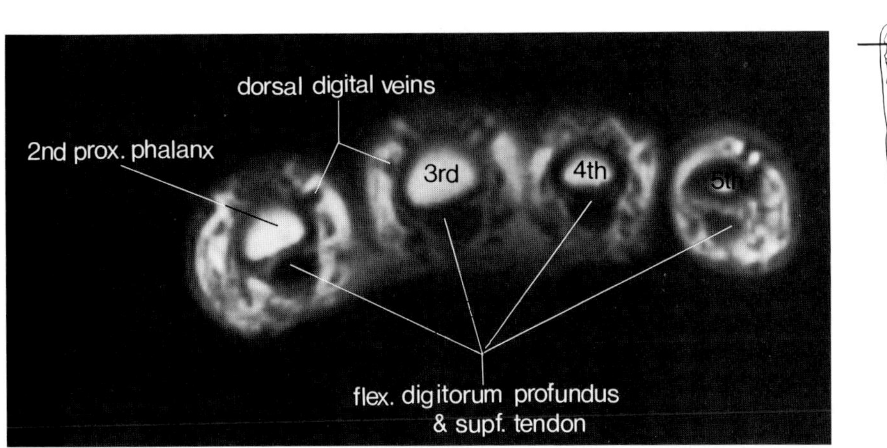

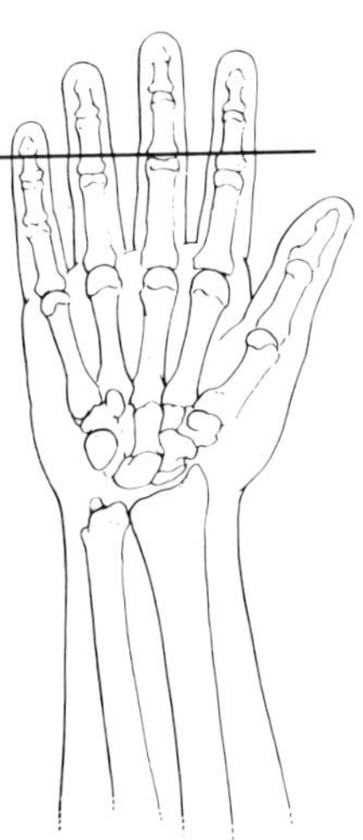

FIG. 11-4. M: Axial image through the second to fourth phalanges.

A

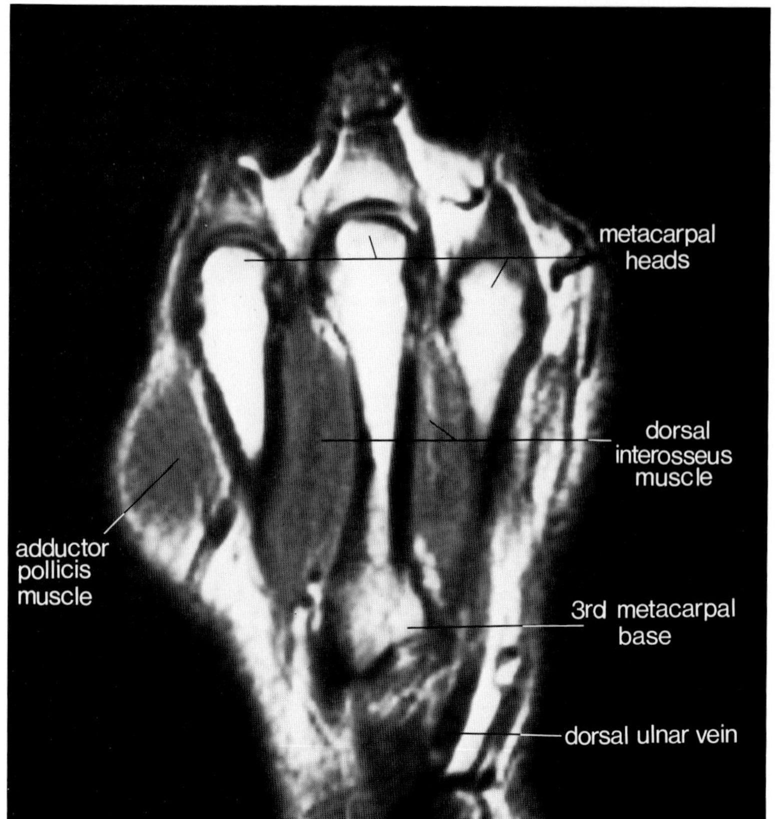

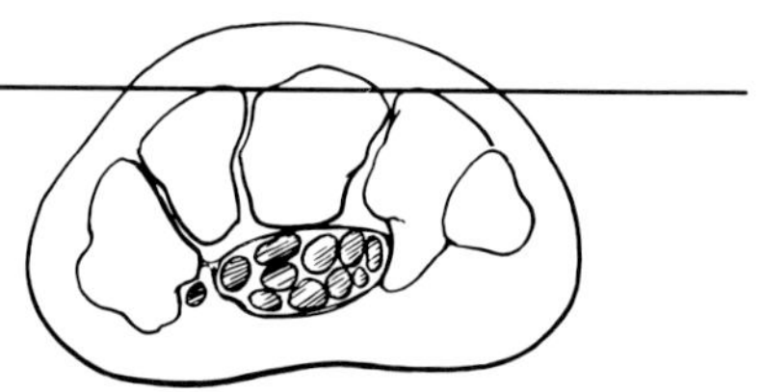

FIG. 11-5. Coronal images of the hand and wrist with illustrations of plane section. **A:** Dorsal image of the hand.

B

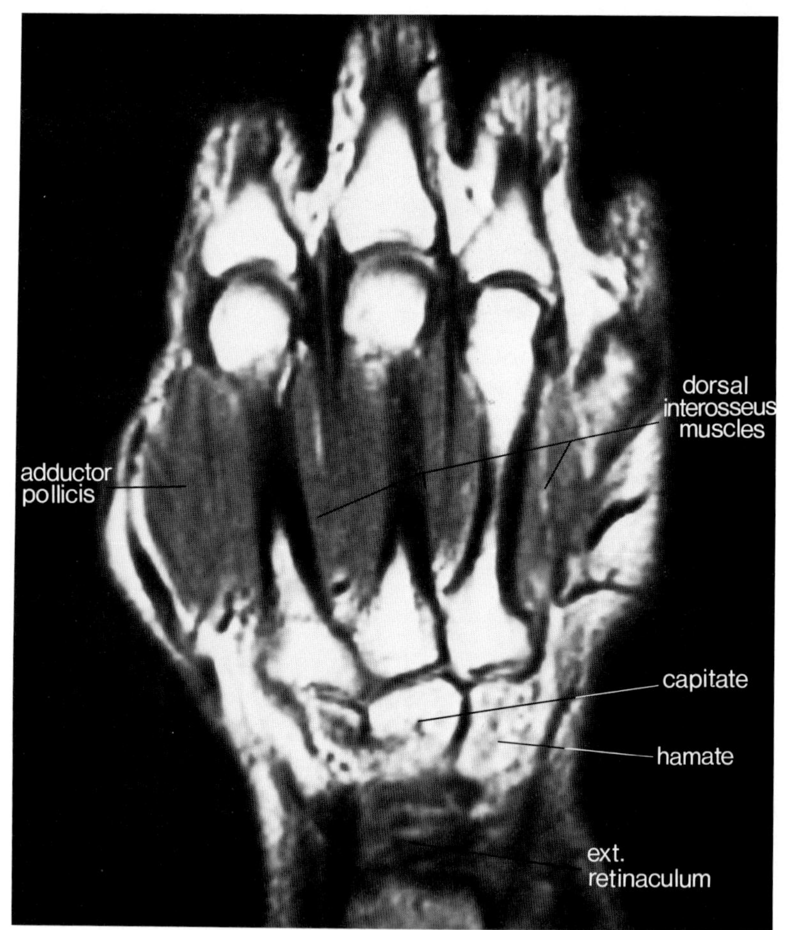

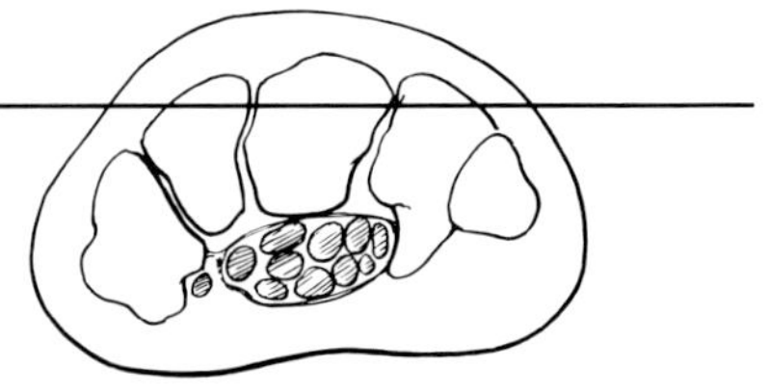

FIG. 11-5. B: Dorsal image of the hand and wrist.

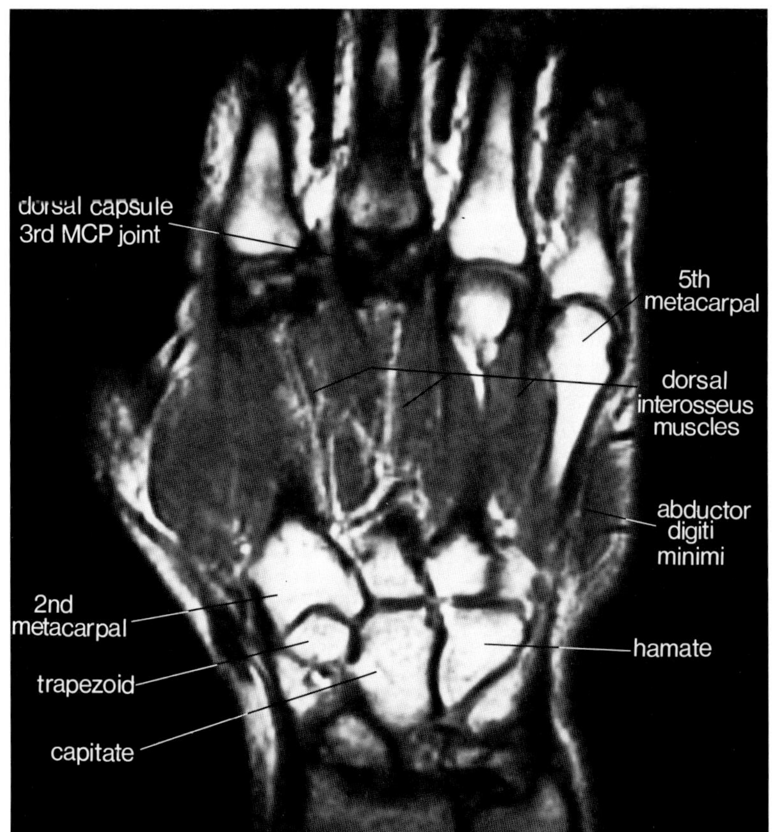

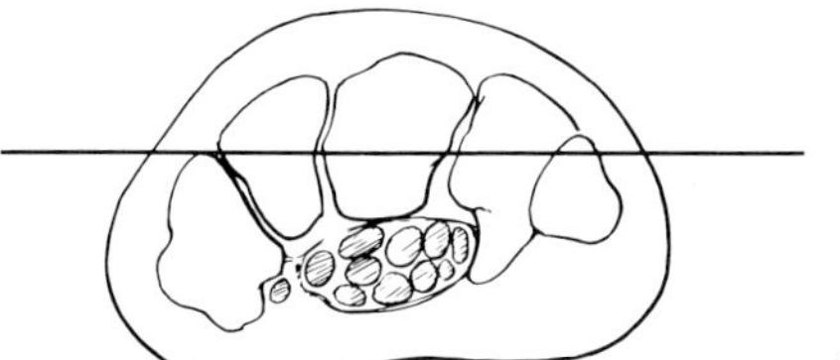

FIG. 11-5. C: Image through dorsal carpal bones and muscles of the hand.

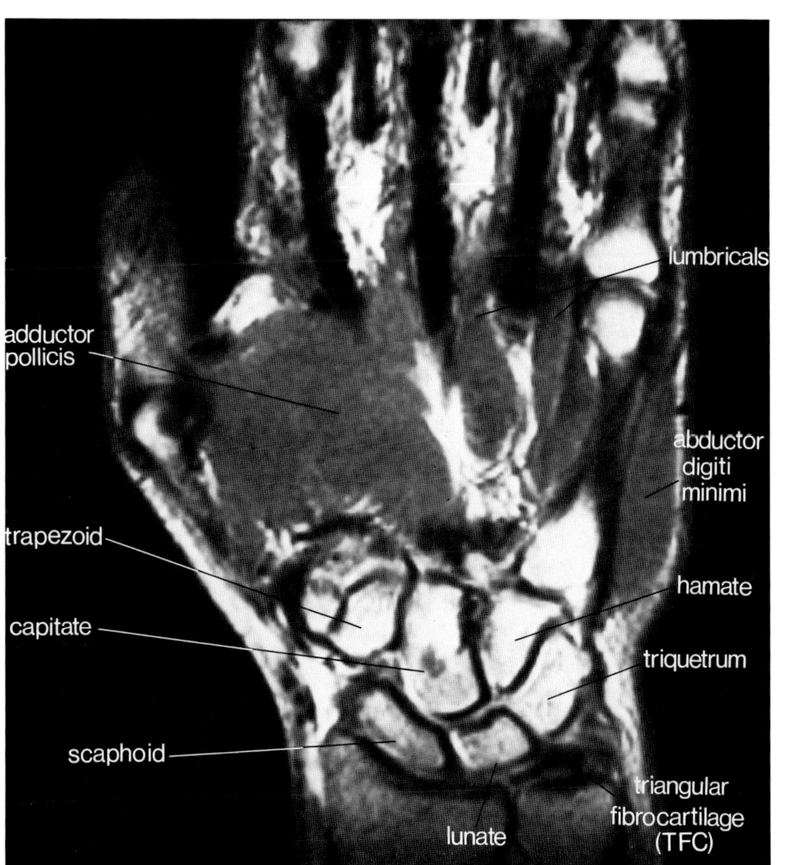

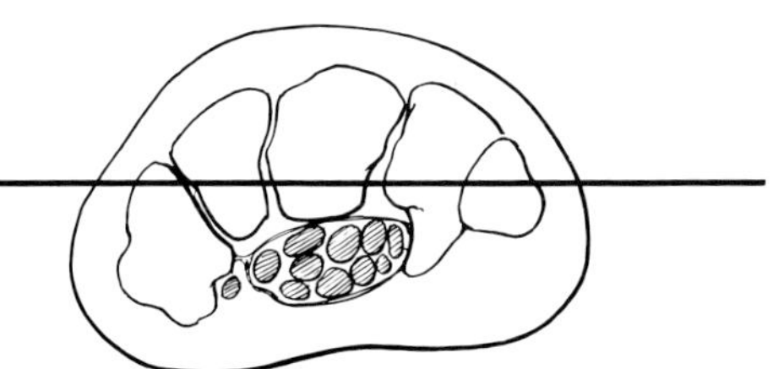

FIG. 11-5. D: Image through carpal bones and thenar muscles.

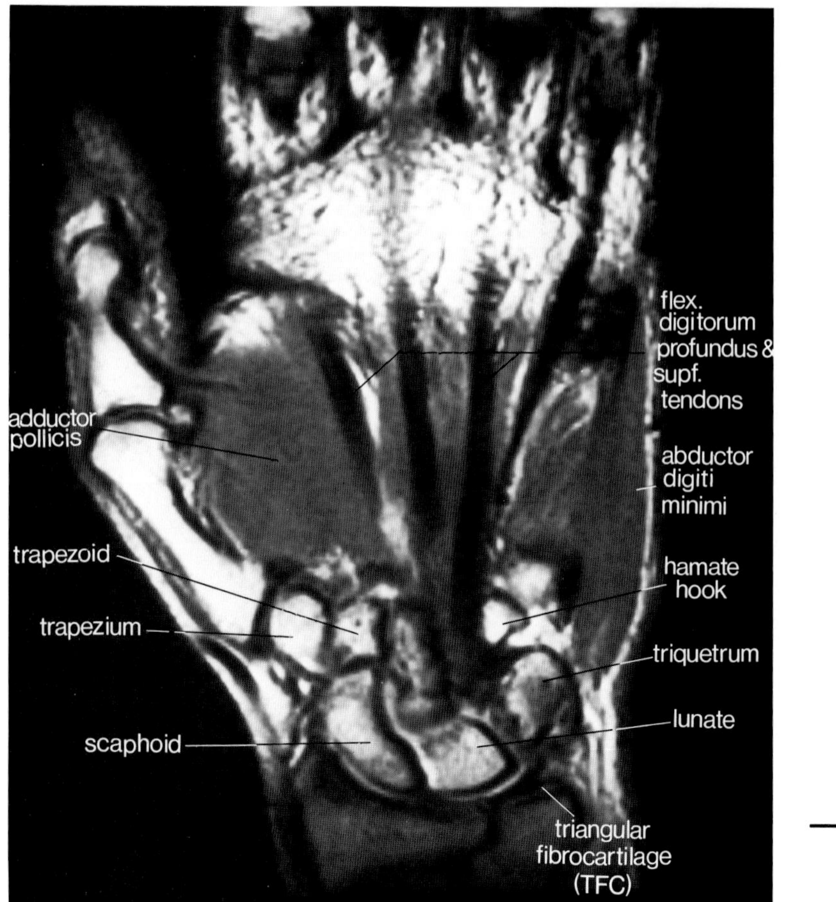

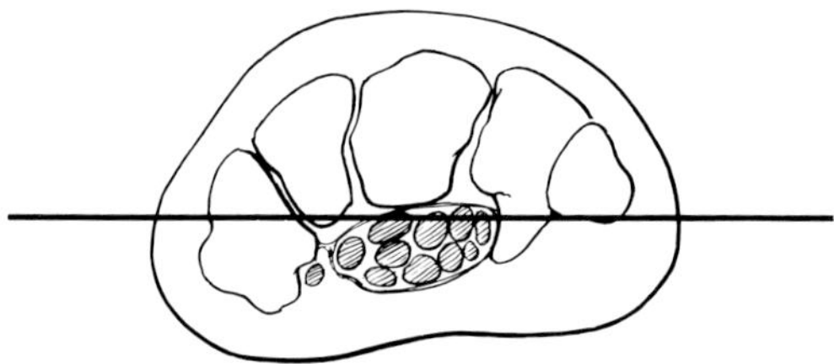

FIG. 11-5. E: Image through carpal bones and flexor tendons of the hand.

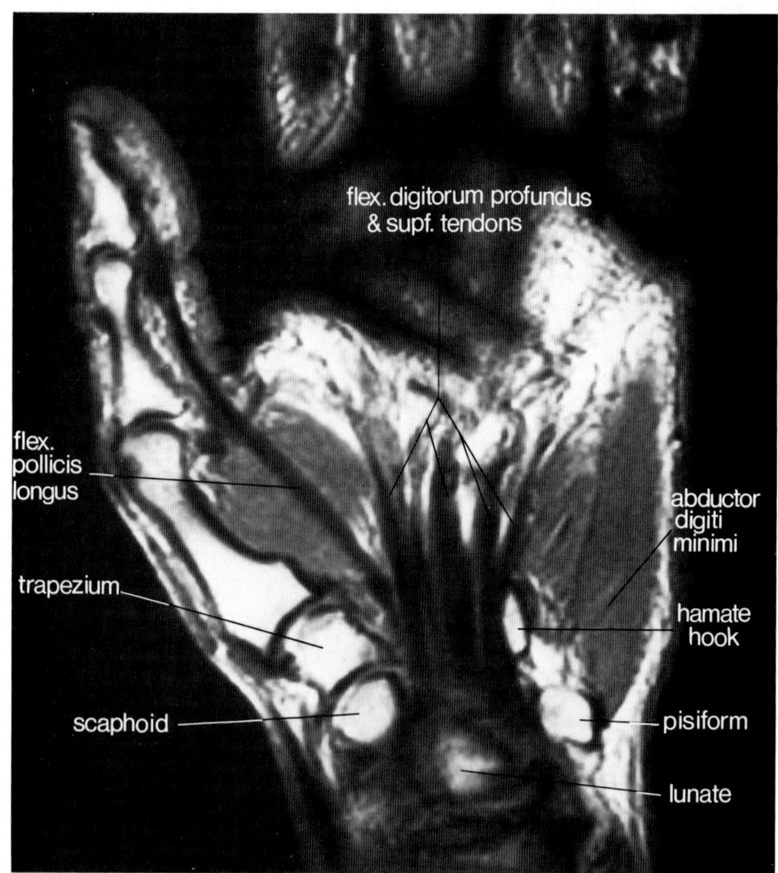

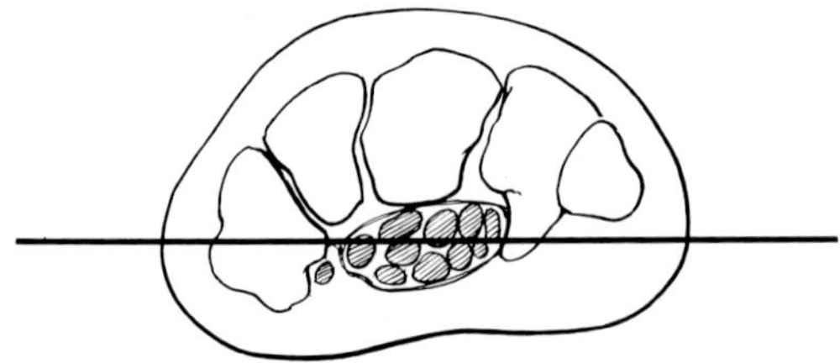

FIG. 11-5. F: Image through volar aspect of wrist.

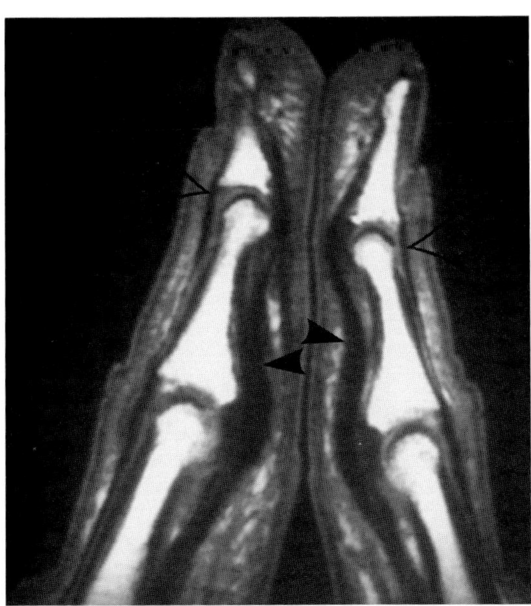

FIG. 11-6. Sagittal images of both index fingers using the flat 3 cm coil. Extensor (*open arrows*) and flexor (*closed arrowheads*) tendons are well demonstrated.

Once the patient has been positioned, the proper pulse sequences and image planes must be selected to demonstrate the anatomy and pathology (Table 11-1). An effective screening examination can be accomplished by beginning with either a coronal or sagittal scout (SE 150–400/20). This should include the full area of the hand and wrist to be examined. We typically follow this sequence with an axial T2 weighted sequence (SE 2,000/20–30, 60–80) using 5 mm thick slices, minimal interslice gap, 256 × 256 matrix with 1 excitation (8 min 56 sec) or 256 × 192 matrix with 2 excitations (13 min). A small field of view (8–12 cm), no phase, no frequency wrap, and presaturation techniques are used to reduce flow artifacts and maximize image quality (Fig. 11-4). The second sequence chosen varies, depending on the findings of the first sequence or clinical indication for the examination (Table 11-1). A coronal T1 weighted sequence (SE 500/20) with 3–5 mm slice thicknesses, no skip, and other setup data above is usually adequate as a second sequence to provide a good screening technique for bone and soft tissue pathology (Fig. 11-5) (3,10,12,13).

Additional sequences may be indicated in specific clinical situations or when abnormalities are evident on the initial sequences which dictate further sequences are required to characterize the lesion. For example, if an abnormality is suspected in a specific phalangeal segment, sagittal T2 (SE 2,000/30, 60) or gradient-echo sequences (TE 13, TR 100–400, flip angle 30°–70°) will define the structures, including vasculature, to better advantage. The sagittal sequence should be performed with thin slices (3 mm) and aligned with the tendon or osseous structure (Fig. 11-6) (10,20).

Specific anatomic areas can be examined with the 3 inch coil, an 8 cm field of view, and sequences that may differ from the screening examination described above. Specifically, the scaphoid is demonstrated most completely using the coronal and sagittal planes (Figs. 11-5 and 11-7). T1 and T2 weighted sequences should be performed to fully evaluate the bone and articular anatomy. Evaluation of the distal radioulnar joint often requires pronation, supination, and neutral T2 weighted axial images. This allows functional anatomic information and evaluation of subtle soft tissue abnormalities. Cine motion studies can be performed quickly using GRASS or GRIL sequences (Fig. 11-8). Soft tissue abnormalities in the carpal tunnel can be studied using axial SE 2,000/30,60 and SE 500/20 sequences. These

TABLE 11-1. *MR imaging[a] of the hand and wrist*

Anatomic structures	Image planes	Pulse sequences
Distal radius and ulna	Axial, coronal	SE 2,000/30,60, SE 500/20
Distal radial ulnar joint	Axial—pronation and supination, coronal	SE 2,000/30,60 or GRIL (GRASS interleaved)
Soft tissue proximal	Axial	SE 2,000/30,60 or 20,80
Wrist	Sagittal[b]	SE 2,000/30,60 or 20,80
Carpal tunnel	Axial	SE 2,000/30,60 or 20,80 and SE 500/20
Carpal bones		SE 500/20
Scaphoid, hamate	Coronal, sagittal	SE 500/20, SE 500/20 and 2,000/30,60 in one plane
Other carpal bones	Axial, coronal	SE 500/20, SE 500/20
Metacarpals and phalanges	Axial, oblique sagittal	SE 2,000/30,60 or 20,80 and SE 500/20
Soft tissues of hand	Axial	SE 500/20 and SE 2,000/30,60 or 20,80
Tendons	Axial, sagittal	SE 2,000/30,60 or 20,80 and GRASS[c] (FA 25°–70°, minimum TE, TR)
Vascular anatomy	Axial, coronal	GRASS

[a] FOV, 8–12 cm; matrix, 256 × 256 or 192 × 256; 1–2 Nex.
[b] Best for soft tissue ganglia.
[c] For motion studies.

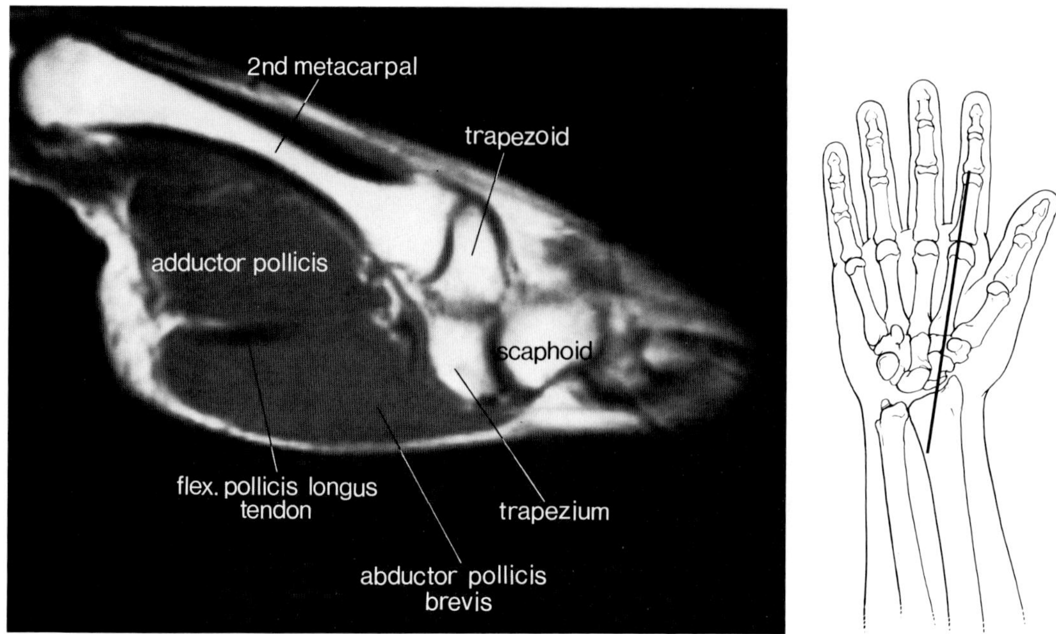

FIG. 11-7. Sagittal images of the hand and wrist with illustrations for plane of section. **A:** Radial aspect of the wrist through the scaphotrapezial articulation.

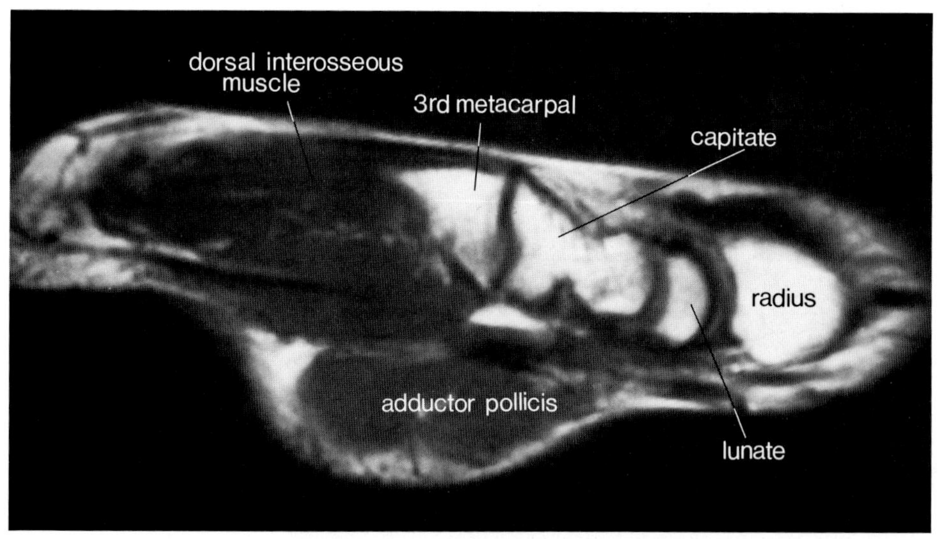

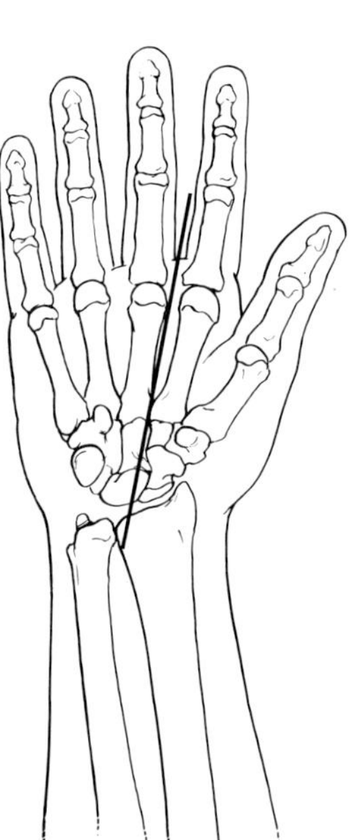

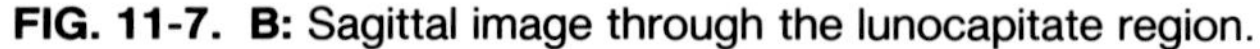

FIG. 11-7. B: Sagittal image through the lunocapitate region.

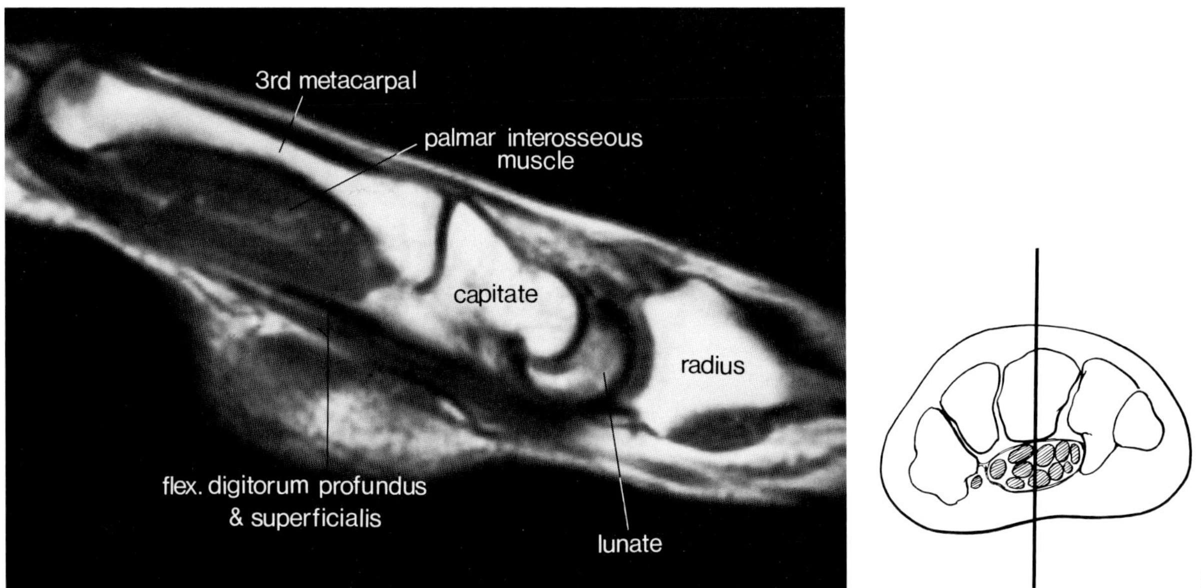

FIG. 11-7. C: Sagittal image through the third metacarpal.

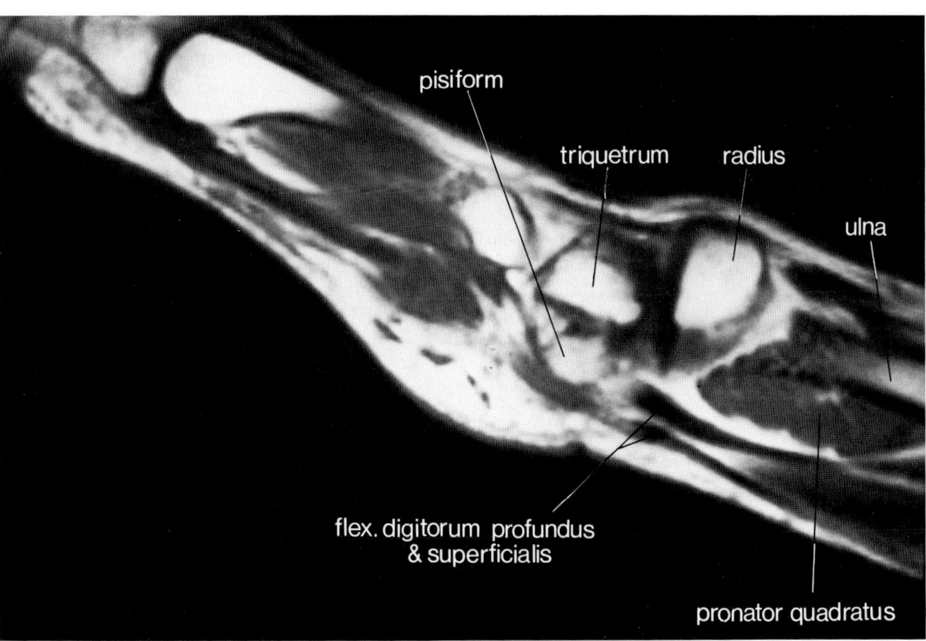

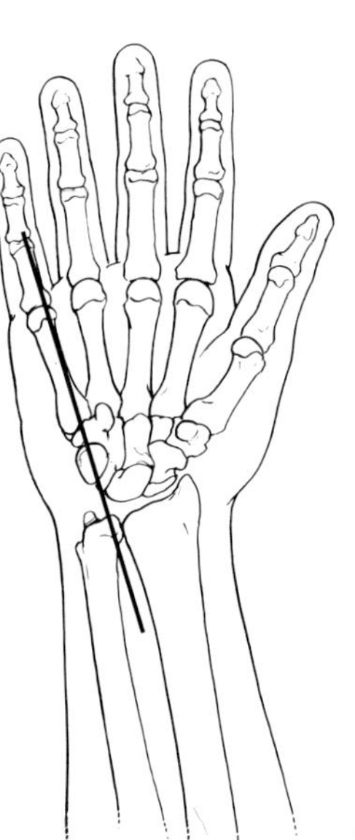

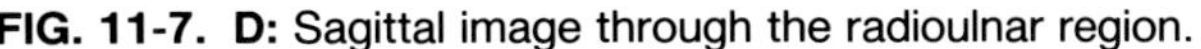

FIG. 11-7. D: Sagittal image through the radioulnar region.

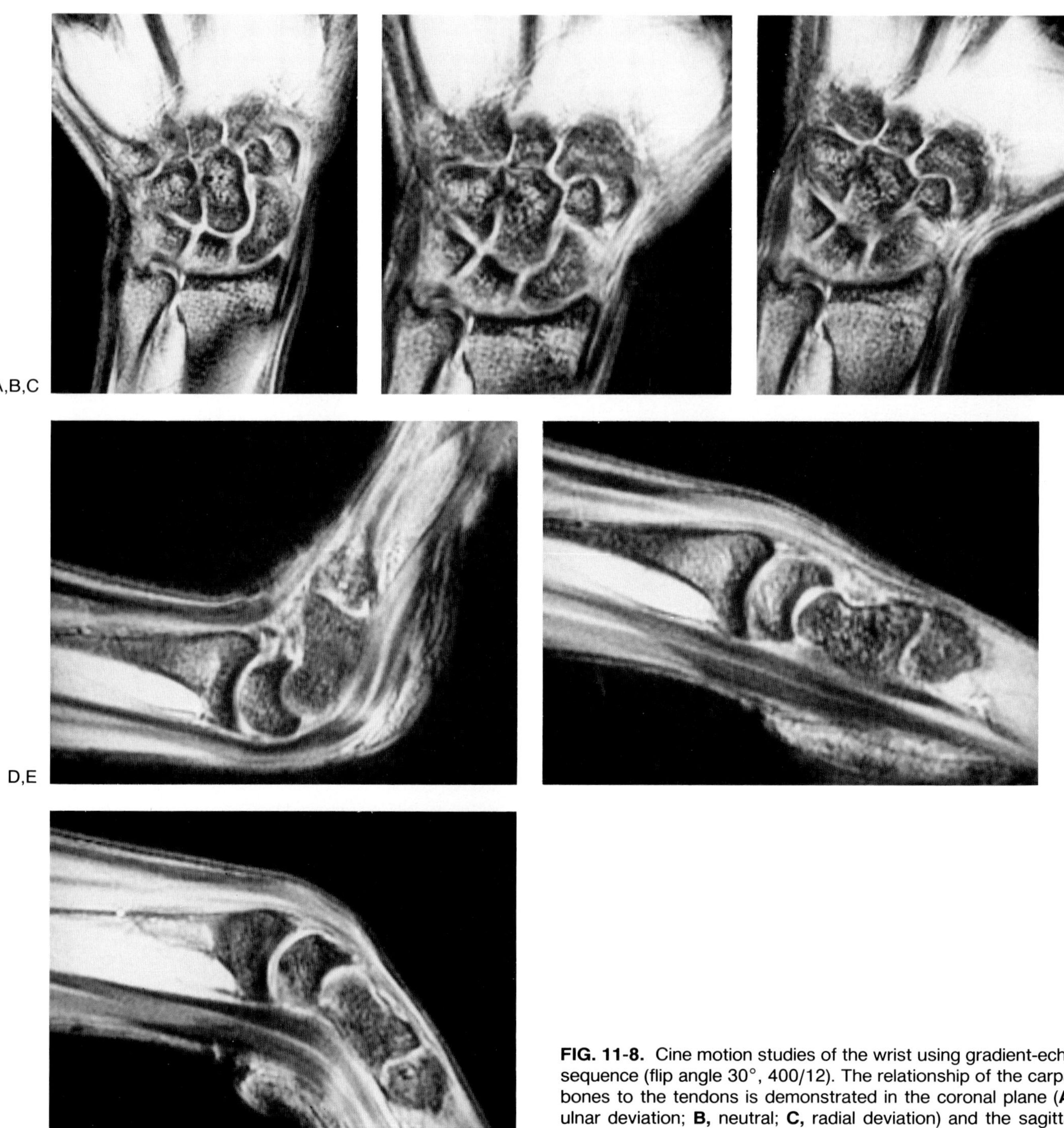

FIG. 11-8. Cine motion studies of the wrist using gradient-echo sequence (flip angle 30°, 400/12). The relationship of the carpal bones to the tendons is demonstrated in the coronal plane (**A,** ulnar deviation; **B,** neutral; **C,** radial deviation) and the sagittal plane (**D,** extension; **E,** neutral; **F,** flexion). (From ref. 10, with permission.)

images provide more than adequate evaluation of the median nerve and surrounding structures (12,29–31). Vascular anatomy is demonstrated most completely using GRASS or volume reconstruction techniques (Table 11-1). More specific techniques will be discussed with specific clinical applications.

ANATOMY

The osseous and soft tissue anatomy of the hand and wrist is complex. Therefore, in the past, numerous imaging techniques have been required for thorough evaluation. MRI is an additional technique that can provide valuable information regarding subtle soft tissue and bone pathology (3,9–11).

Osteology

There are eight carpal bones in the wrist and five metacarpal bones and 14 phalanges in the hand. Bones of the wrist form three major articular groups composed of the distal radioulnar joint, the radiocarpal joint, and the midcarpal articulation. The distal radial metaphysis and epiphysis is a largely cancellous bone with only a thin cortical shell, which makes this region ideally suited for MRI. The distal radius is elongated on its radial side, forming the radial styloid (Fig. 11-5). Distally, the radius has two articular fossae for the scaphoid and lunate. Distal articular surface normally angles 14° toward the ulna in the frontal plane and 12°–15° volarly in the lateral or sagittal plane (Figs. 11-5 and 11-7). There is a notch in the ulnar side of the radius, termed the sigmoid notch, which articulates with the distal ulna. Of importance, on the dorsal surface of the radius are the sulci and palpable dorsal protuberance termed Lister's tubercle. These osseous changes assist in forming the dorsal compartments for the extensor tendons of the wrist (Figs. 11-4 and 11-9) (52). The cortex in the distal ulna is somewhat thicker than the radius and it also has a spikelike projection on the most ulnar aspect termed the ulnar styloid. The head of the ulna articulates with the distal radius via the sigmoid notch and the lunate and triquetrum distally. It is separated from the latter two structures by a triangular fibrocartilage complex (Fig. 11-10). This is discussed more completely later. The carpal bones are composed of three anatomic groups (Fig. 11-11). The proximal row consists of the scaphoid, lunate, triquetrum, and overlapping pisiform. The proximal surfaces of these bones should form a smooth unbroken arch in the coronal plane. In the sagittal plane the angle formed by the scaphoid and lunate should be between 30° and 60° (see Fig. 11-7). A second osseous anatomic group, the distal carpal row, consists of the trapezoid, capitate, and hamate. The third compartment is composed of the trapezium and five metacarpals (2,9,24,52).

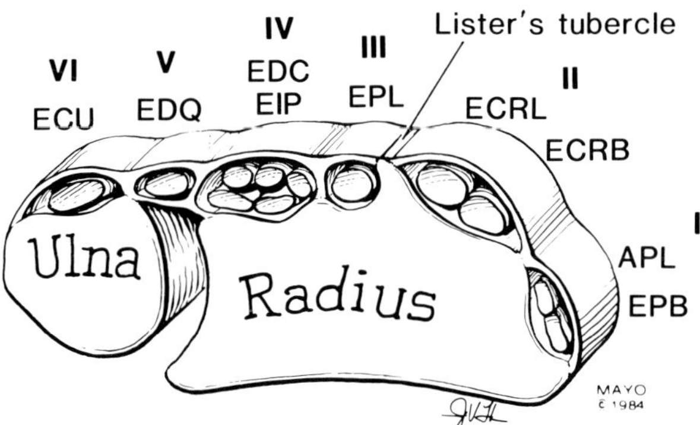

FIG. 11-9. Axial illustration of the first through sixth compartments of the wrist. I, abductor pollicis longus (APL) and extensor pollicis brevis (EPB); II, extensor carpi radialis longus and brevis (ECRL, ECRB); III, extensor pollicis longus (EPL); IV, extensor digitorum communis (EDC) and extensor indicis proprius (EPI); V, extensor digiti quinti (EDQ); VI, extensor carpi ulnaris (ECU). (From ref. 52, with permission.)

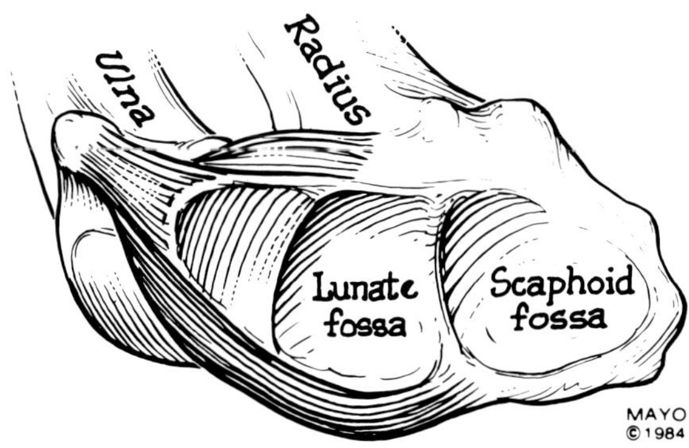

FIG. 11-10. Illustration of the triangular fibrocartilage complex. (From ref. 52, with permission.)

The proximal and middle phalanges of the fingers are similar in structure with proximal and distal flaring. The osseous composition of these structures is primarily cancellous. There are two phalanges on the thumb because it lacks a middle phalanx. The remaining digits have three phalanges (2,24,52).

Ligamentous and Articular Anatomy

The ligamentous anatomy of the wrist is complex due to the stabilization required for the numerous carpal bones and extensive motion. The orientation of the ligaments about the wrist is also complex, making it difficult to include all the dorsal or volar ligaments in any one orthogonal MR image plane (9,10,12).

The distal radioulnar joint is stabilized primarily by the triangular fibrocartilage complex. This complex consists of several components that blend with one another and include the triangular fibrocartilage, the ulnocarpal meniscus, the ulnar collateral ligament, and the volar and dorsal distal radioulnar ligaments (Fig. 11-10). The triangular fibrocartilage is most easily identified on coronal images (Fig. 11-5), with the dorsal and volar ligaments most easily seen on axial images (Fig. 11-4). Additional support of the distal radioulnar joint is provided by the interosseous membrane between the radius and ulna, the extensor carpi ulnaris tendon, and the concavity of the sigmoid notch of the radius (Fig. 11-4) (24,52).

Stability of the wrist is largely provided by the palmar and dorsal ligaments (Fig. 11-11). As can be noted from

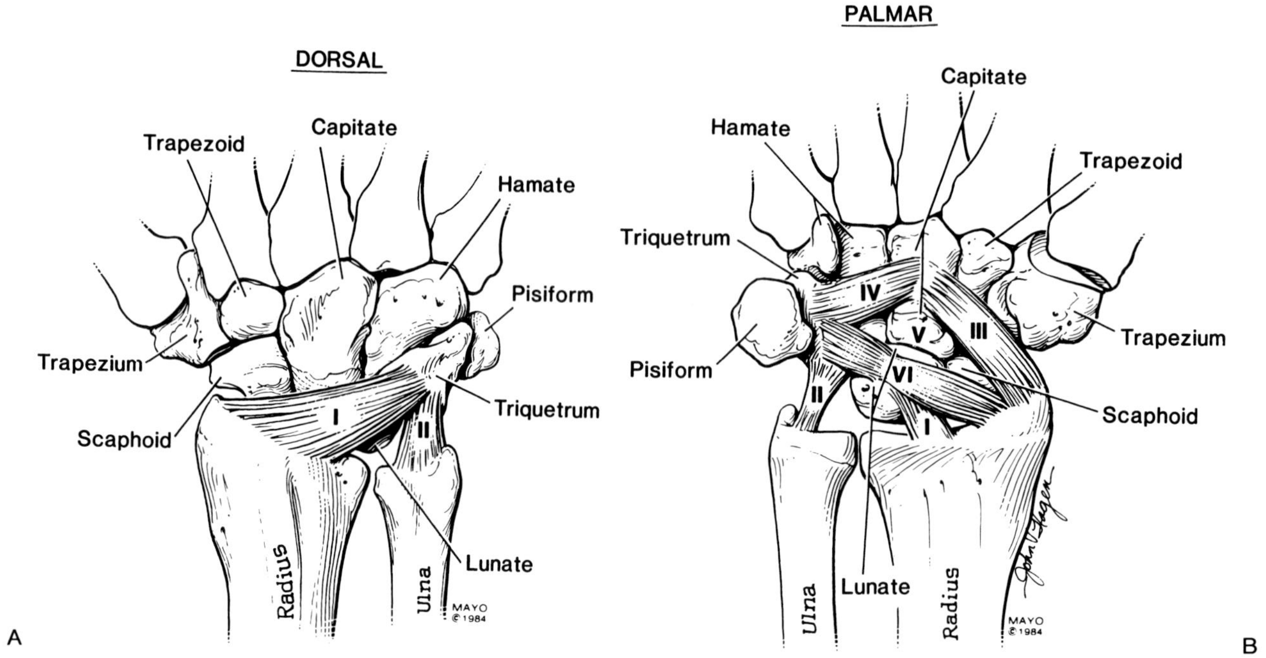

FIG. 11-11. Illustrations of the dorsal (A) and volar (B) ligaments of the wrist. I, radiolunotriquetral ligament; II, ulnotriquetral ligament; III, radiocapitate ligament; IV, capitotriquetral ligament; V, space of Poirier; VI, radioscapholunate ligament. (From ref. 52, with permission.)

the illustrations defining the anatomy of these structures (Fig. 11-11), it is difficult to define them in their entirety on any given axial or coronal MR image. The palmar ligaments consist of two concentric arches originating from the volar margin of the radius and inserting into the triquetrum and triangular fibrocartilage complex (Figs. 11-10 and 11-11A). The first group is composed of the radiolunotriquetral ligament, which crosses obliquely and distally from the distal radius to insert in the lunate and volar aspect of the triquetrum. The ulnotriquetral ligament extends in a nearly direct sagittal plane from the distal ulna to insert adjacent to the radiolunotriquetral ligament in the volar aspect of the triquetrum. The more distal or second arch is composed of the radiocapitate ligament, which originates more laterally near the radial styloid and extends obliquely to insert in the volar aspect of the capitate. The ulnar aspect of this arch is completed by the capitotriquetral ligament, which extends obliquely and proximally from the capitate to insert in the volar aspect of the triquetrum. Between the two arches is an area of thinning in the capsule termed the space of Poirier. In addition to these two arches, there is a short ligament extending from the radius to the lunate, termed the ligament of Testut or the radioscapholunate ligament. Dorsally, there are two main ligaments, the radiolunotriquetral and the ulnotriquetral (Fig. 11-11B). The ligamentous support of the metacarpophalangeal and interphalangeal joints is similar, composed primarily of a capsule as well as volar and collateral ligaments (Fig. 11-12) (2,24,52).

Within the ligamentous and capsular anatomy of the wrist there are numerous compartments (Fig. 11-13). Using T2 weighted sequences, the synovial fluid in these compartments can easily be identified with MRI. However, defects in the interosseous ligaments are difficult to identify and the compartments more difficult to separate than when conventional arthrography is used. The compartments as demonstrated in Fig. 11-13 include the radiocarpal joint, distal radioulnar joint, intercarpal joint, carpometacarpal joints, first carpometacarpal joint, outer carpometacarpal joint, and pisotriquetral joint (2,9,24,52).

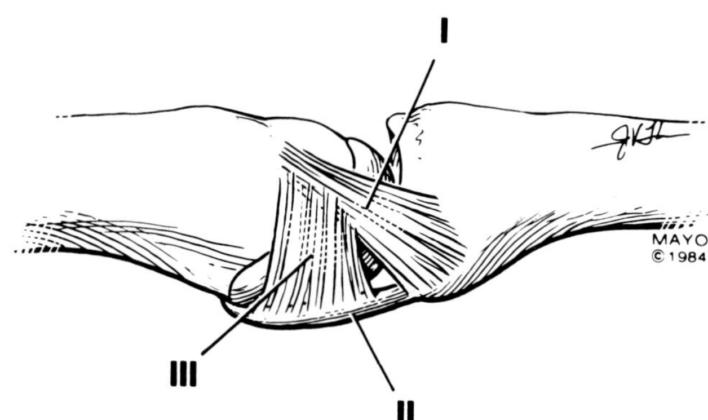

FIG. 11-12. Illustration of the supporting ligaments of the metacarpophalangeal joints. I, collateral ligaments; II, volar plate; III, accessory collateral ligaments. (From ref. 52, with permission.)

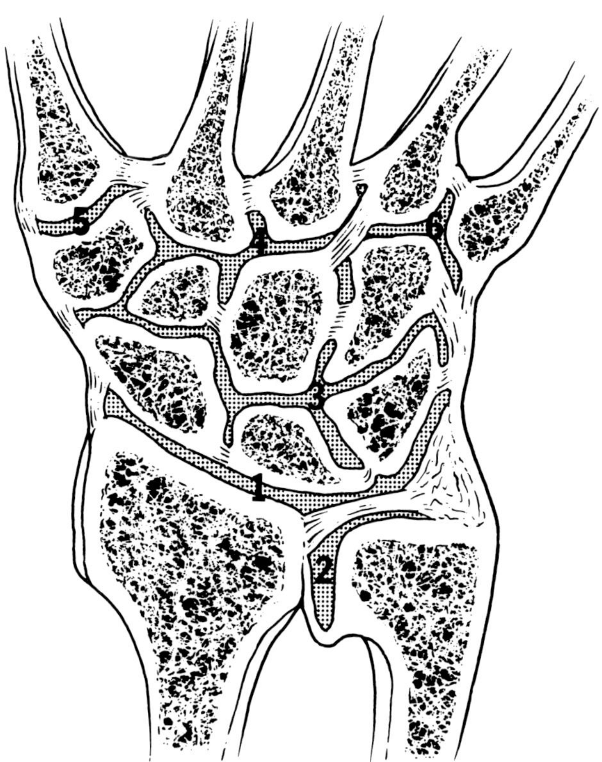

FIG. 11-13. Illustration of the compartments in the wrist. 1, radiocarpal; 2, distal radioulnar; 3, intercarpal; 4, common carpometacarpal; 5, first carpometacarpal; 6, outer carpometacarpal. (From ref. 52, with permission.)

Muscular Anatomy

Many of the muscles and tendons that cross the wrist originate at the elbow or proximal forearm and have been discussed previously in Chapter 10. The muscles of the forearm, which are largely responsible for flexion and extension of the wrist, have been thoroughly discussed in Chapter 10 and, except for some essential anatomy, are not reviewed here. This section primarily deals with those muscles directly related to the bones of the hand and wrist with regard to their origins and insertions (Table 11-2).

The chief flexors of the wrist are the flexor carpi radialis and flexor carpi ulnaris. The palmaris longus is a minor flexor of the wrist (Fig. 11-14) (2,24). Extension of the wrist is largely due to the extensor carpi radialis longus and brevis and the extensor carpi ulnaris (Fig. 11-15). During radial deviation of the wrist, the primary muscles involved are the abductor pollicis longus and extensor pollicis brevis. Ulnar deviation of the wrist is accomplished primarily by the extensor carpi ulnaris (Fig. 11-16) (24).

There are typically four lumbrical muscles, which arise from the flexor digitorum profundus tendons and extend along the radial aspects of the second through fifth metacarpals to insert in the extensor aponeurosis of the proximal phalanx on the radial side. The muscles can be identified in the axial and coronal planes (Figs.

TABLE 11-2. *Muscles of the hand* (2,24)

Muscles	Origin	Insertion	Action	Innervation
Lumbricals (four)	Tendons of flexor digitorum profundus	Extensor aponeurosis	Extensors of interphalangeal joints	Radial or first and second lumbricals—median nerve, third and fourth —ulnar nerve
Flexor pollicis longus	Anterior middle third of radius and interosseous membrane	Distal phalanx thumb	Flexor of thumb	Median nerve (anterior interosseous branch)
Interossei				
Palmar (three)	First, fourth, and fifth metacarpal diaphysis	Extensor aponeurosis	Abduction and adduction of fingers	Deep branch of ulnar nerve
Dorsal (four)	First through fifth metacarpal diaphyses	Proximal phalanges		
Abductor pollicis brevis	Flexor retinaculum, trapezium	Radial side proximal phalanx thumb	Abductor of thumb	Median nerve
Flexor pollicis brevis	Flexor retinaculum, trapezium, and trapezoid	Radial flexor aspect proximal phalanx thumb	Flexes and rotates thumb	Median nerve
Opponens pollicis	Flexor retinaculum, trapezium	Radial diaphysis first metacarpal	Stabilize and opposition of thumb	Median nerve
Adductor pollicis	Third metacarpal, trapezium, trapezoid, capitate	Base proximal phalanx thumb		Median nerve
Palmaris brevis	Palmar aponeurosis (ulnar side)	Medial skin palm	Draws skin laterally	Deep branch of ulnar nerve
Abductor digiti minimi	Pisiform	Ulnar base fifth proximal phalanx	Abductor of fifth finger	Deep branch of ulnar nerve
Flexor digiti minimi brevis	Hamate hook, flexor retinaculum	Ulnar base fifth proximal phalanx	Flexor of fifth MCP joint	Deep branch of ulnar nerve
Opponens digiti minimi	Flexor retinaculum, distal hamate hook	Fifth metacarpal diaphysis	Draws fifth metacarpal anteriorly	Deep branch of ulnar nerve

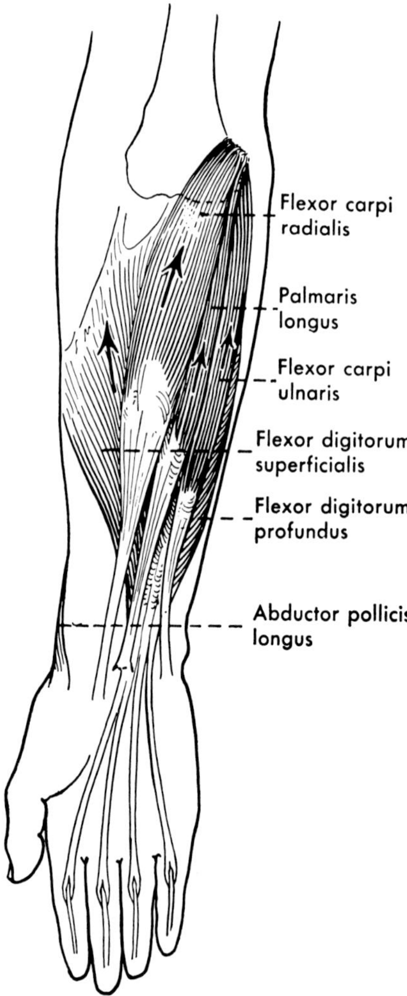

FIG. 11-14. Illustration of the flexor muscles of the wrist. (From ref. 24, with permission.)

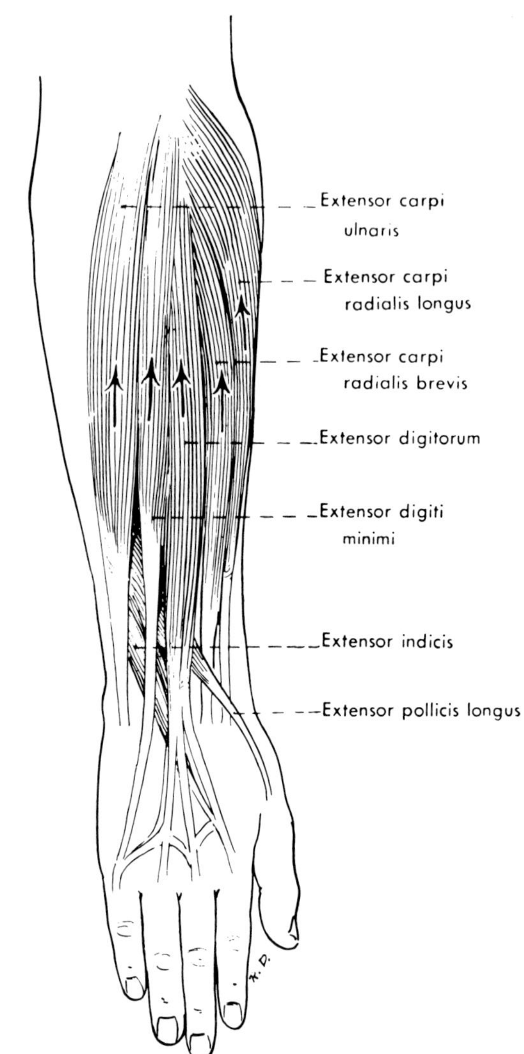

FIG. 11-15. Illustration of the extensor muscles of the wrist. (From ref. 24, with permission.)

11-4 and 11-5) and are seen as tissue of muscle signal intensity between the flexor digitorum profundus tendons proximally and along the radial aspect of the metacarpals adjacent to the interosseous muscles more distally (2,24). Insertions are not usually clearly defined on MR images. The flexor pollicis longus has been discussed in Chapter 10; however, its function is important in the hand and wrist, so certain aspects need to be repeated. As noted in Table 11-2, the muscle originates from the anterior aspect of the middle third of the radius. The tendon passes through the radial side of the carpal tunnel (Fig. 11-17) radial to the superficial and deep flexor tendons (Figs. 11-4, 11-5, and 11-7). A synovial sheath of the flexor pollicis longus tendon begins just proximal to the flexor retinaculum and extends distally to near the insertion of the tendon on the distal phalanx of the thumb (2,24,52) (Table 11-2).

The interosseous muscles form the deepest layer of the muscles in the hand and are divided into palmar and dorsal groups (Fig. 11-4). The palmar group consists of three muscles that take their origin on the radial aspect of the fifth and fourth metacarpals and the ulnar aspect of the second metacarpal. The muscles pass distally between the metacarpophalangeal joints to insert on the extensor aponeurosis. The dorsal interossei originate from adjacent metacarpals, the first from the first and second metacarpal, the second from the second and third, the third from the third and fourth, and the fourth from the fourth and fifth metacarpal diaphyses. The muscles pass dorsally and distally to insert with a palmar and dorsal slip into the bases of the proximal phalanges. The interosseous muscles, both palmar and dorsal, are innervated by the deep branch of the ulnar nerve and function in abduction and adduction of the fingers of the hand (2,24) (Table 11-2).

The thenar eminence or muscle group is comprised of the abductor pollicis brevis and superficial head of the flexor pollicis brevis, which overlie the opponens pollicis

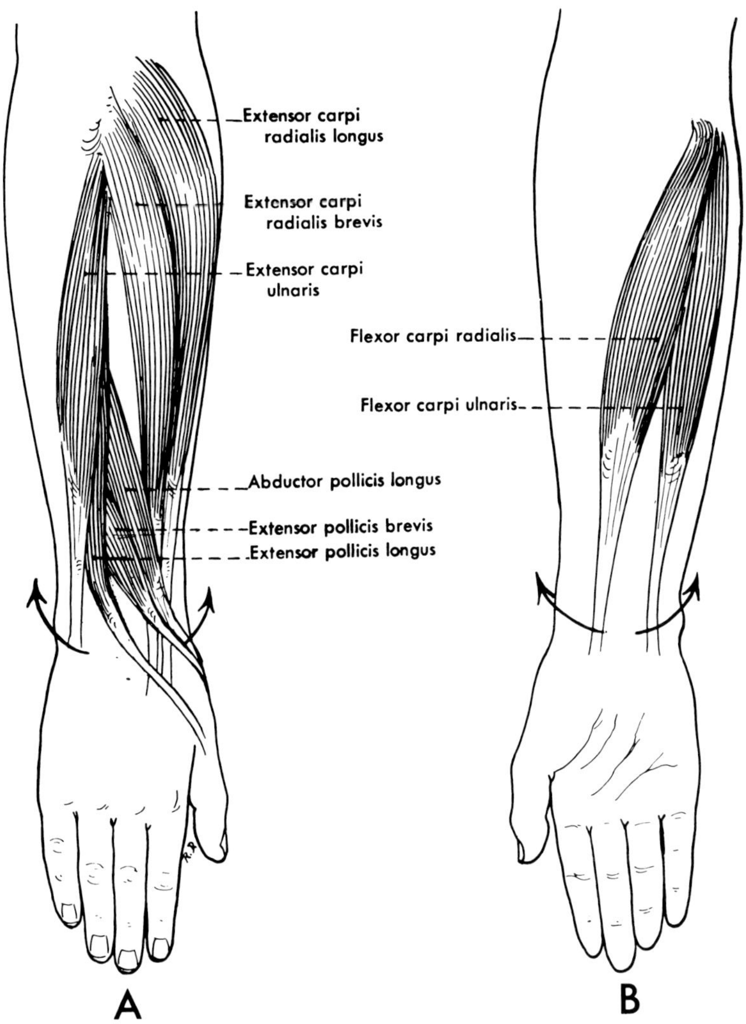

FIG. 11-16. Illustration of muscles for ulnar and radial deviation of the wrist seen from the dorsal (**A**) and volar (**B**) aspects of the forearm and wrist. (From ref. 24, with permission.)

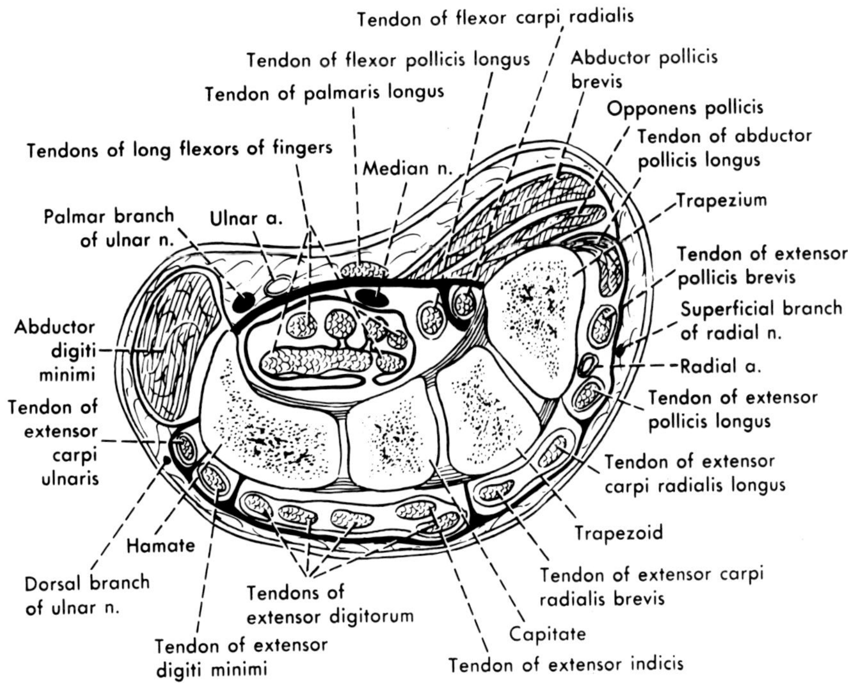

FIG. 11-17. Axial illustration of the carpal tunnel region. (From ref. 24, with permission.)

(Fig. 11-4). The abductor pollicis brevis arises from the flexor retinaculum and has deeper origins from the trapezium and trapezoid. This somewhat triangular muscle extends distally to insert in the radial aspect of the proximal phalanx of the thumb. It serves as the primary abductor of the thumb. The flexor pollicis brevis has two heads, one superficial and the other deep. The superficial head arises from the trapezium and flexor retinaculum and the deep head from the trapezoid. The muscle extends distally to form a tendon that inserts on the radial flexor side of the base of the proximal phalanx of the thumb. The primary function is flexion and rotation of the thumb. The opponens pollicis is partially covered by the abductors and flexors of the thumb and arises from the flexor retinaculum and trapezium to insert on the radial surface of the diaphysis of the first metacarpal. The adductor pollicis arises with both oblique and transverse heads. The transverse head arises from the ulnar surface of the third metacarpal diaphysis and the oblique head from the base of the third metacarpal and flexor aspects of the trapezium, trapezoid, and capitate. The triangular muscle extends to insert at the base of the proximal phalanx of the thumb. This muscle serves to adduct the metacarpal and flex the metacarpophalangeal joint of the thumb (2,24,52) (Table 11-2).

The hypothenar muscle group consists of one superficial and three deep muscles. The superficial muscle is the palmaris brevis, which arises from the ulnar side of the palmar aponeurosis and extends medially to attach into the skin along the medial border of the palm. This muscle is superficial to the ulnar nerve and artery (24). The deep muscles include the abductor digiti minimi, flexor digiti minimi brevis, and opponens digiti minimi (Fig. 11-4). The abductor digiti minimi is the most superficial of the three deep muscles. It arises from the distal surface of the pisiform and passes distally along the medial aspect of the hand to insert along the ulnar side of the base of the fifth proximal phalanx. This muscle abducts the little finger at the metacarpophalangeal joint. It acts along with the dorsal interosseous muscle in

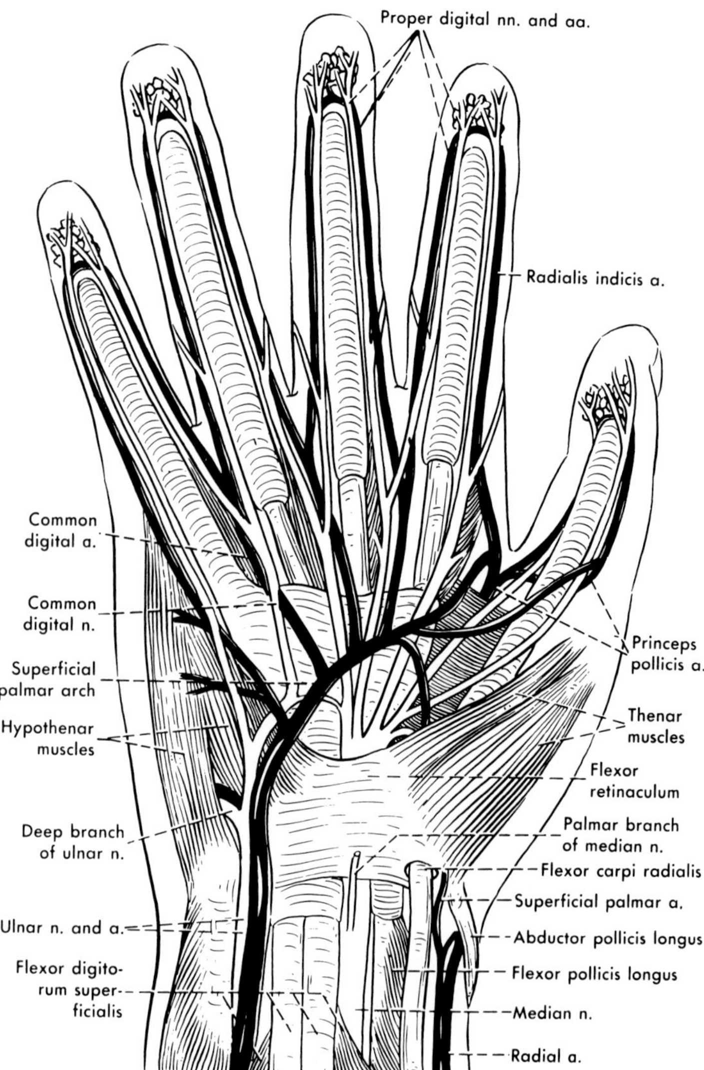

FIG. 11-18. Illustration of the neurovascular anatomy on the volar aspect of the hand and wrist. (From ref. 24, with permission.)

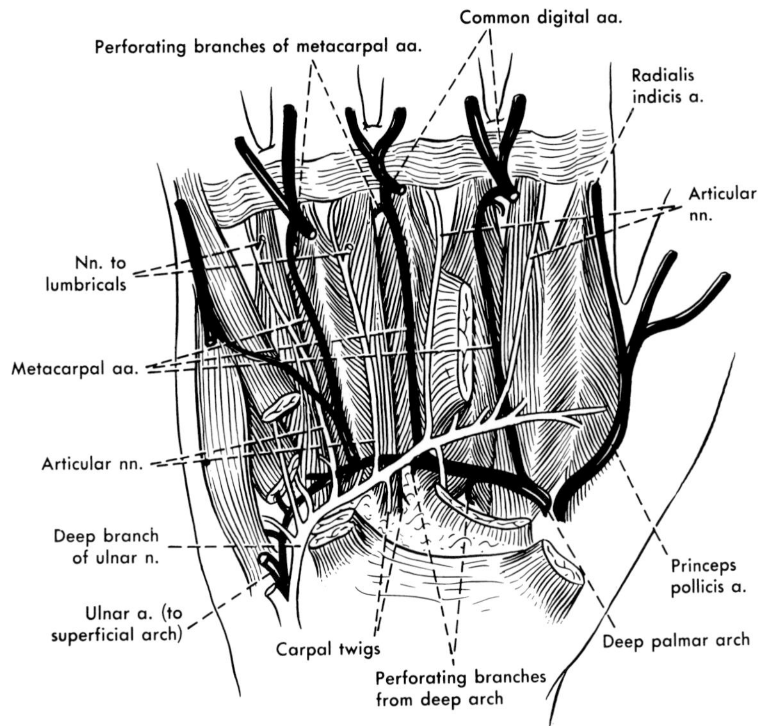

FIG. 11-19. Illustration of the deep palmar arch and deep branch of the ulnar nerve. (From ref. 24, with permission.)

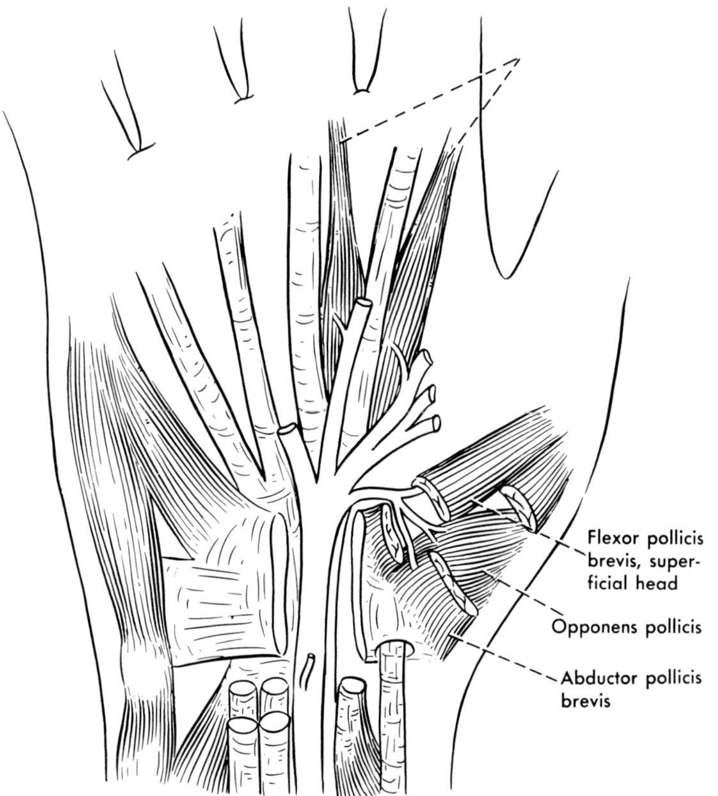

FIG. 11-20. Illustration of the median nerve and branches. (From ref. 24, with permission.)

assisting in abduction or spreading of the fingers. The flexor digiti minimi brevis arises more distally than the abductor digiti minimi and takes its origin from the hook of the hamate and flexor retinaculum. This muscle passes more obliquely and medially and inserts in the same position as the abductor. The main function of this muscle is a flexor of the fifth metacarpophalangeal joint. The third and final muscle of the deep hypothenar group is the opponens digiti minimi. This muscle is the deepest and arises deep to the abductor and flexor from the flexor retinaculum and distal hook of the hamate, taking an oblique course to insert along the ulnar aspect of the fifth metacarpal diaphysis. This muscle draws the fifth metacarpal anteriorly. All muscles of the hypothenar group are supplied by the deep branch of the ulnar nerve (2,24,52) (Table 11-2).

Neurovascular Anatomy

The neurovascular anatomy of the hand and wrist is complex. Since there are numerous causes of nerve compression in this region, it is especially essential to understand the anatomy and relationship of these structures in the hand and wrist (12,24,29–31,55). MR evaluation of neurovascular anatomy is most easily accomplished by following the major nerve branches proximal to distal on axial images (Fig. 11-4). On the ulnar side of the distal forearm proximal to the carpal tunnel, the ulnar artery, nerve, and their accompanying veins lie deep to the flexor carpi ulnaris (Fig. 11-4). The nerve is generally medial to the artery at this level (Fig. 11-18). At the level of the pisiform, these structures pass along the lateral or radial side of the pisiform, passing deep to the volar carpal ligament and then distally into the palm of the hand anterior to the flexor retinaculum but deep to the palmaris brevis muscle (Fig. 11-4) (12,24, 29,30,55). At the level of the pisiform, the ulnar nerve typically divides into superficial and deep branches (Fig. 11-19). Also at the pisiform level the nerve and accompanying vascular structures lie between the volar carpal ligament and flexor retinaculum in a space commonly known as Guyon's canal. Lesions proximal to or within

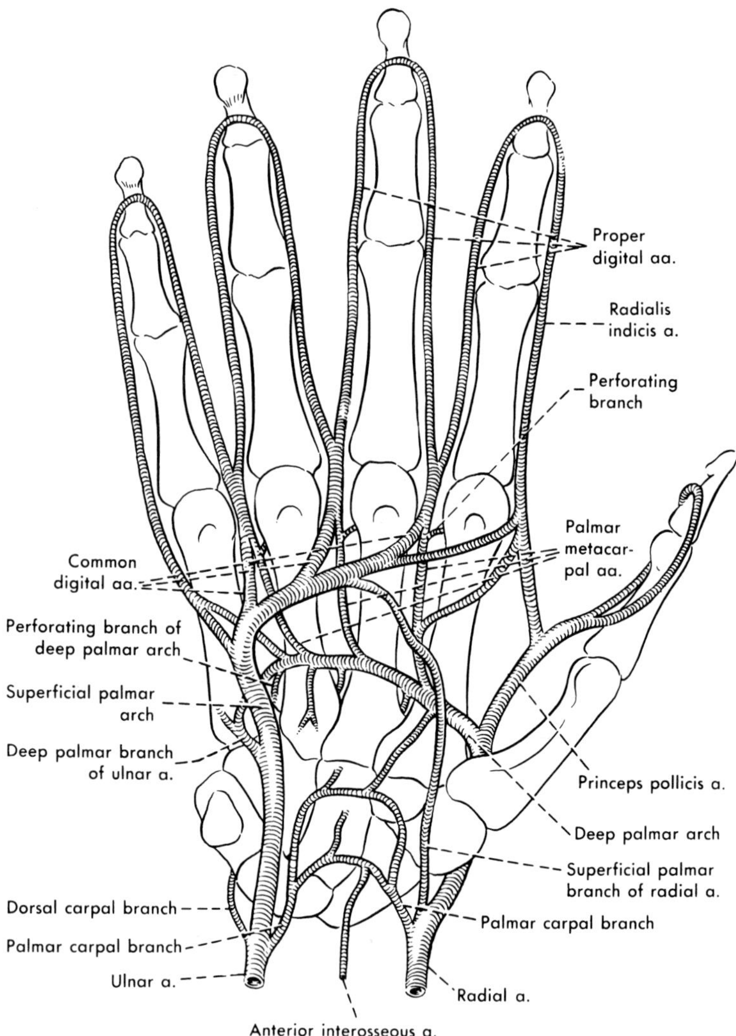

FIG. 11-21. Illustration of the vascular anatomy of the hand and wrist. (From ref. 24, with permission.)

the canal can produce both sensory and motor abnormalities in the ulnar nerve distribution (Fig. 11-4E) (24,29,30).

The two flexor digitorum muscles (superficial and profundus) are lateral to the ulnar nerve and vessels at the level of the wrist (Fig. 11-18). The tendon of the palmaris longus lies superficially. These structures are most easily identified on axial MR images (Fig. 11-4). The midline volar structures of the wrist, as they enter the carpal tunnel, tend to form three layers. The most superficial or anterior layer is formed by the flexor digitorum superficialis. The middle layer is formed by the superficial flexor of the index and middle fingers, and the most posterior or deepest layer is formed by the flexor digitorum profundus tendons. All tendons have a common sheath just before they pass under the flexor retinaculum. The palmaris longus tendon is the most superficial and midline structure at the wrist level (Figs. 11-4 and 11-7) (2,24,55).

The median nerve lies deep to the flexor digitorum superficialis through much of the forearm (Figs. 11-4 and 11-20). Just proximal to the wrist, it emerges on the radial side of the superficial flexor and passes forward and medially to lie in front of the flexor tendons in the carpal tunnel (Figs. 11-4 and 11-20). At the distal margin of the flexor retinaculum, the median nerve divides into five or six branches. These small branches are difficult to identify, even when thin slice axial MR images are obtained (10,12,55).

The muscle planes and fascial compartments of the palm basically divide the palm into three compartments —the thenar, hypothenar, and central compartments (Fig. 11-17). These compartments, along with the tendon sheaths of the flexor tendons, are anatomically important in the spread of inflammatory and infectious diseases (24).

The complex vascular anatomy of the hand and wrist is demonstrated in Figs. 11-18, 11-19, and 11-21. The major vessels can be demonstrated to better advantage on coronal and axial MR images (Figs. 11-4 and 11-5). More peripheral digital branches and an overview of vascular anatomy is most easily accomplished by using thin gradient-echo (GRASS) sequences, either in the axial or coronal plane, and reformatting the images with special software that demonstrates only the vascular anatomy.

PITFALLS

Pitfalls of MRI of the hand and wrist may be caused by anatomic variants, improper techniques, and artifacts created by software and hardware problems.

There are numerous anatomic variants in the hand and wrist. A complete discussion of bone and soft tissue variants is beyond the scope of this chapter. However, certain variants deserve mention as they may be encountered more commonly on MR images.

The carpal bones generally develop from a single ossification center. Therefore, anomalous conditions such as bipartate or tripartate carpal bones are not common. Unfortunately, when bipartate and tripartate carpal bones do occur, they involve the most commonly fractured carpal bone, the scaphoid (24,34). The most common appearance is two separate ossicles separated at the wrist, a common site of scaphoid fractures. The capitate and hook of the hamate may also develop from multiple ossification centers. When this occurs, differentiation from fracture may be difficult with MRI (9,34). Fusion of carpal bones, typically the lunate and triquetrum, is unusual but is reported in up to 6% of the black population (Fig. 11-22) (34).

Soft tissue variants are common. Neurovascular variations in the dorsal and palmar arches may be noted in up to one-third of patients (24). Fortunately, this is not usually a significant problem when interpreting MR images. Anomalous muscles may cause problems clinically because patients present with soft tissue masses or asymmetry when compared with the opposite extremity. Though the exact variation may not be apparent on MR images, the demonstration of a muscle density structure can be confirmed by MRI. Thus, a neoplasm can be excluded.

Variations in the flexor tendon sheaths are more significant. Anomalies may lead to changes in patterns of spread of infection. Also, confusion of tenosynovitis with a ganglion can occur. Most often the common

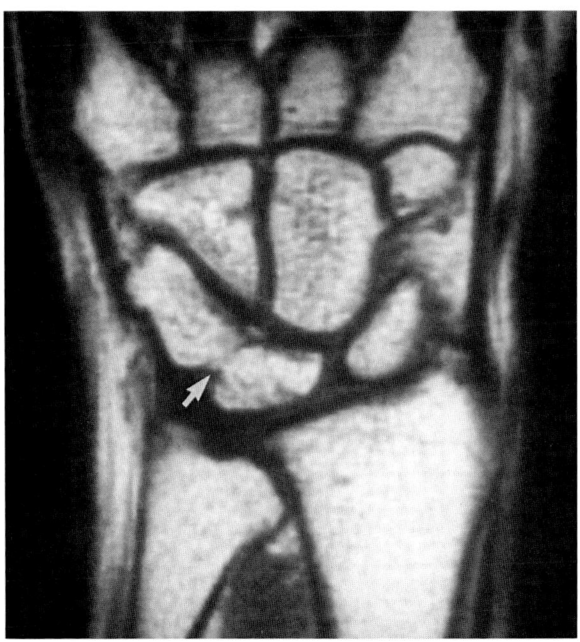

FIG. 11-22. Coronal SE 500/20 image of the wrist, demonstrating anomalous lunotriquetral (*arrow*) fusion.

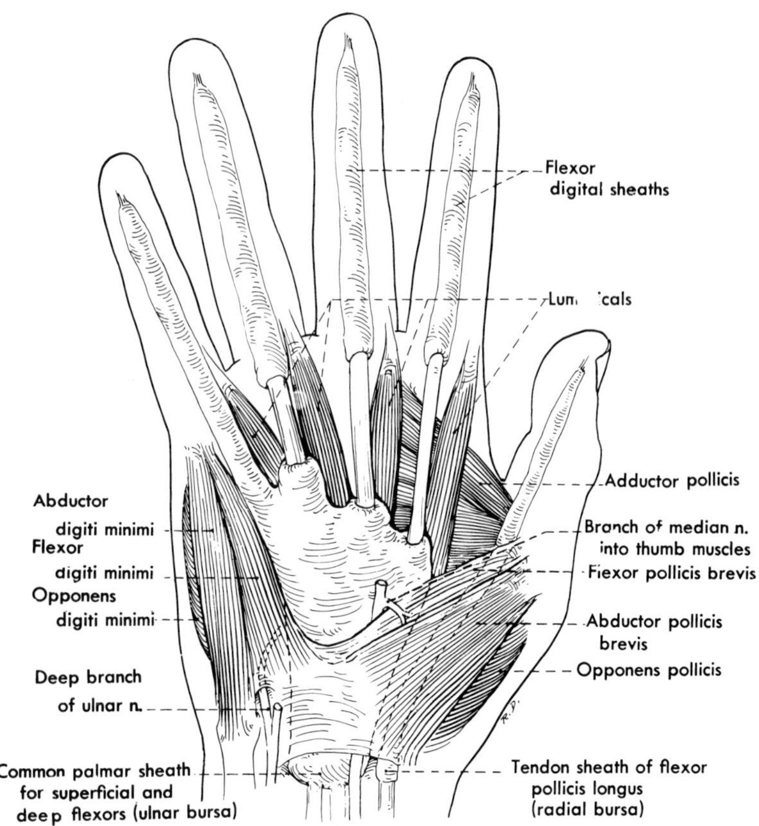

FIG. 11-23. Illustration of the flexor tendon sheaths. (From ref. 24, with permission.)

flexor tendon sheath ends in the midpalm (71.4°). The digital sheath of the fifth finger is contiguous in 80% of patients. The second to fourth flexor sheaths in the fingers do not usually communicate with the common flexor tendon sheath (Fig. 11-23) (24,34).

Problems with image quality, patient motion, and flow artifacts can result in diagnostic errors. Flow artifacts obscure lesions but may also be useful. For example, small ganglion cysts can be confused with vessels. When flow artifact is present, the two can easily be differentiated. There is no flow artifact from cysts (Fig. 11-24).

CLINICAL APPLICATIONS

Clinical applications for MRI of the hand and wrist have expanded dramatically due to improved surface

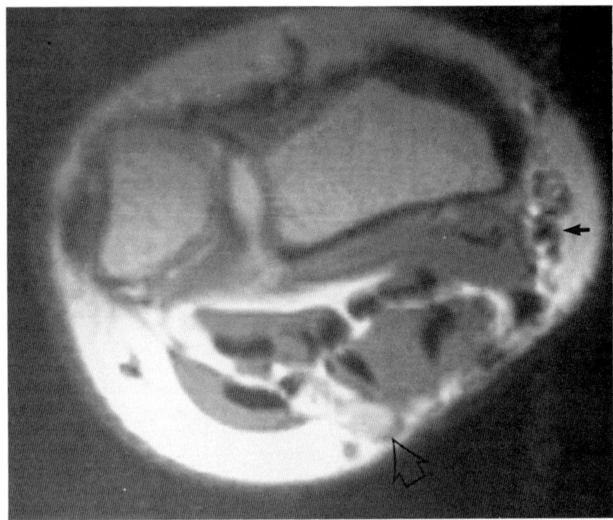
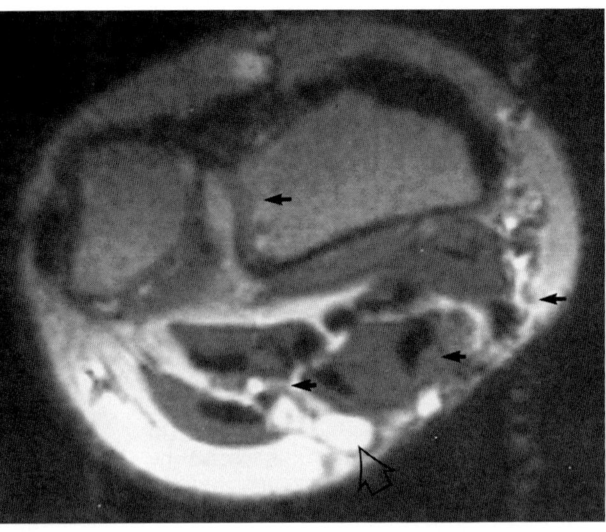

A,B

FIG. 11-24. SE 2,000/30 (**A**) and 2,000/60 (**B**) axial images of the wrist with multiple high-intensity spherical areas. The flow artifacts (*arrows*) differentiate vessels from the ganglion cyst (*open arrow*).

coil technology and new pulse sequences (25,49,51). Major applications for MRI in our practice include trauma, neoplasms, avascular necrosis, and infection. MRI may also be of value in imaging other conditions in the hand and wrist. However, experience is still evolving in these areas (56).

Trauma

Magnetic resonance imaging techniques can be useful in acute and chronic musculoskeletal injuries to the hand and wrist (10,22,28,56) (Table 11-3). Most acute skeletal injuries are adequately diagnosed with routine radiography. Conventional tomography or isotope studies are valuable supplemental radiographic techniques (9).

MRI is not frequently used for diagnosis of skeletal injuries in the hand and wrist. However, it is not unusual to detect subtle injuries that may not be evident with routine radiographs or tomography (Fig. 11-25) (10,27,33,53). Detection of stress fractures and osteochondral fractures with MRI has also been reported (19,27,53). Cortical bone appears black on MR images. Therefore, cortical fractures are most easily appreciated on T2 weighted images (SE 2,000/60–80). Edema and hemorrhage in marrow will also have higher signal intensity than normal marrow using these parameters (10,27,53). Fracture lines and adjacent reactive change have low signal intensity compared to normal marrow on T1 weighted (SE 500/20) sequences (Fig. 11-26). Compression injuries with trabecular condensation are seen as areas of low intensity on both T1 and T2 weighted sequences.

TABLE 11-3. *Hand and wrist trauma*

Anatomic region/indication	Imaging work-up
Osseous trauma	
Distal radius and ulna	Routine radiographs, tomography if needed
Carpal bones	Routine radiographs, radionuclide scans + tomography if indicated
Metacarpals and phalanges	Routine radiographs
Avascular necrosis ?	Routine radiograph, MRI if negative
Distal radioulnar joint (DRUJ) (subluxation–dislocation)	CT + arthrography or MRI using gradient-echo technique with cine (neutral, pronation, supination)
Ligament injuries	Arthrography
Capsules and ligaments MCP and IP joints	Arthrography
Muscle and tendon	MRI
Neural injury	MRI

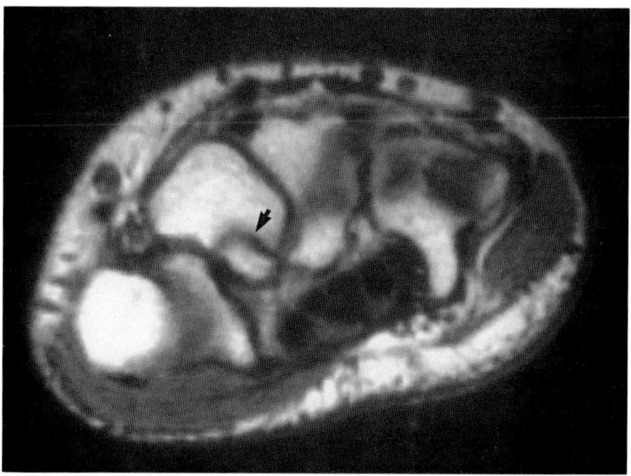

FIG. 11-25. SE 500/20 axial image of the wrist, demonstrating a fracture (*arrow*) along the palmar aspect of the trapezoid.

MRI is also useful for evaluating fracture healing, nonunion (Fig. 11-27), and early osteonecrosis (1,10, 26,37,41). Fibrous union has low signal intensity on both T1 and T2 weighted sequences. Increased signal intensity along the fracture line (due to fluid) is noted with T2 weighted sequences when nonunion occurs (10). Osteonecrosis following scaphoid fractures is easily detected with coronal MR images (Fig. 11-28). Initially, the signal intensity is diminished on T1 weighted images (1,37,41). As osteonecrosis progresses to sclerotic bone commonly seen on routine radiographs, the signal intensity is low on both T1 and T2 weighted sequences (10,26,37).

Articular or joint-related injuries of the hand and wrist are usually evaluated with arthrography, motion studies, stress views, and in certain cases postinjection CT or tomography (Table 11-3). Arthrography is still valuable for confirming suspected ligament injuries. In addition, diagnostic and therapeutic injections can be performed in conjunction with arthrography and tenography (10,52).

MRI is most useful for evaluating soft tissue trauma, specifically muscle and tendon injuries, neural compression syndromes, and capsule disruptions (10,28) (Table 11-3). Tears in the triangular fibrocartilage (TFC) can be detected, especially if they occur near the thicker ulnar margin (Fig. 11-29). Zlatkin et al. (56) and Golimbu et al. (22) reported accuracies of 95% for MR detection of TFC tears. A sensitivity of 100% and specificity of 92% were achieved with MRI compared to 89% and 90% for arthrography (56). However, near the apex (radial edge) the radiocarpal and distal radioulnar joint are separated by a thin segment. Therefore, injection of Gd-DTPA may be required to enhance detection accuracy in this region. Evaluation of the intercarpal ligaments and distal radioulnar joint is usually accomplished with arthrography and CT (52). However, MRI

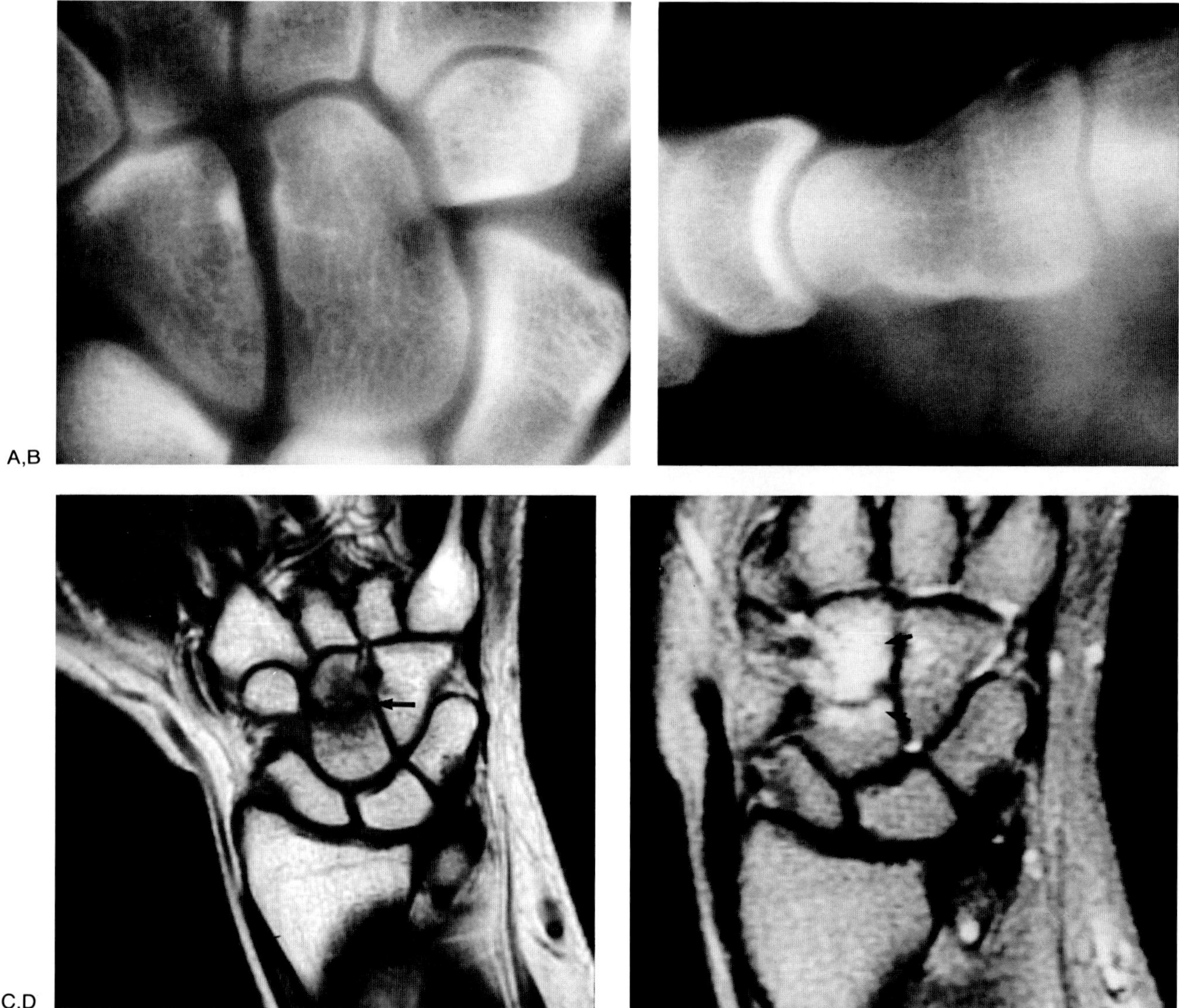

FIG. 11-26. Patient with wrist pain following trauma. The AP (**A**) and lateral (**B**) tomograms are normal. Coronal T1 (SE 500/20) (**C**) and T2 (SE 2,000/60) (**D**) images show a fracture through the midcapitate (*arrows*). (From ref. 10, with permission.)

has also demonstrated significant potential in these areas. Though experience is early, Zlatkin et al. (56) reported accuracy of 90% for the scapholunate ligament and slightly less accurate results (80%) for the lunotriquetral ligament.

Technique is very important. Dual coupled flat coils, a small field of view (8–12 cm), and T2 weighted sequences (SE 2,000/20,60) or gradient-echo sequences (TR 200–700; TE 12,31; flip angle 25°–30°) with T2* weighting are most useful. The coronal plane and thin (1–3 mm) slices are also best suited to evaluate the TFC and ligaments (10,56).

Muscle and tendon tears are also most easily demonstrated with T2 weighted sequences. To accurately define the extent of injury we usually use axial and either coronal or sagittal image planes. Subtle tendon abnormalities may be better demonstrated using gradient-echo motion studies (see Fig. 11-8) (10). Axial images in neutral, pronation, and supination are also best for evaluating the distal radioulnar joint.

Musculoskeletal Neoplasms

Bone tumors in the hand and wrist are uncommon compared to the lower extremities or axial skeleton. Benign tumors occur more frequently than malignant tumors (15,16,36). Generally, routine radiographs are most useful for determining the nature of the lesion, that is, whether a lesion is potentially benign or malignant.

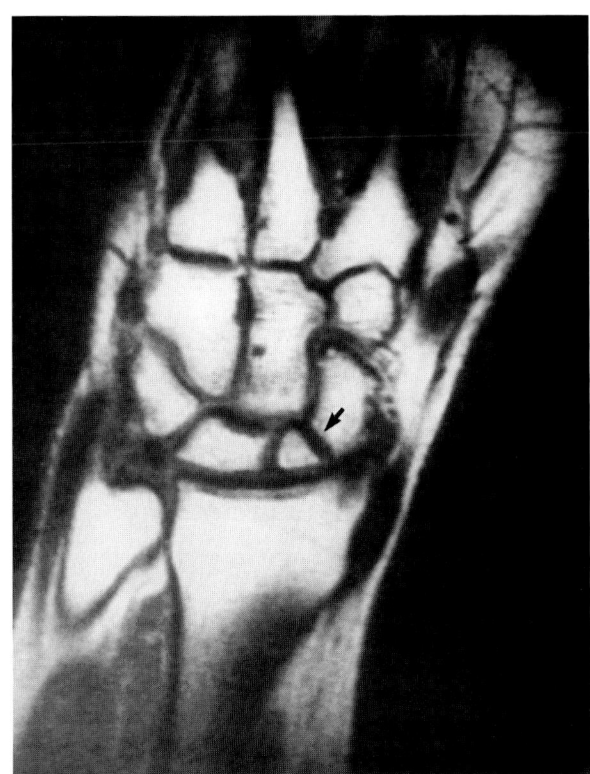

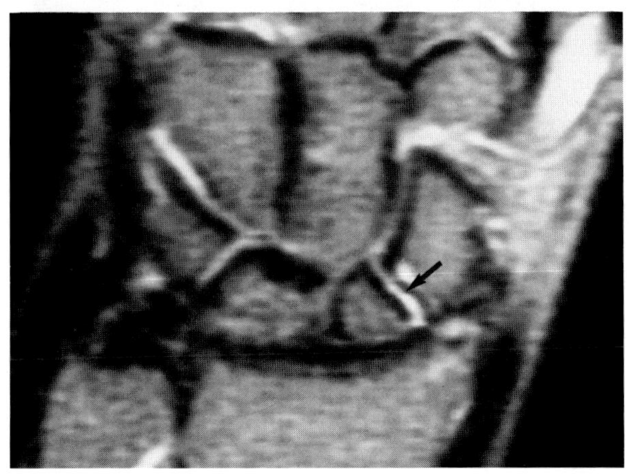

FIG. 11-27. Coronal MR images of the wrist following a scaphoid fracture. The T1 weighted image (**A**) shows a dark line (*arrow*) where the fracture had occurred. Fibrous tissue, sclerotic bone, or nonunion? The T2 weighted sequence (**B**) clearly shows fluid (*arrow*) passing through the fracture line and nonunion. Note that the signal intensity of the proximal fragment is normal, which excludes osteonecrosis.

Table 11-4 lists the most common benign and malignant bone neoplasms in the hand and wrist. The most common benign tumors in the hand and wrist as noted in Table 11-4 are, in order of decreasing frequency, endochondromas, osteochondromas, osteoid osteoma, giant cell tumor, and aneurysmal bone cysts. These lesions can usually be diagnosed accurately with routine radiographs and MRI is not indicated. In addition, certain of these lesions, such as osteoid osteoma, are more easily characterized with CT. To date, experience with MRI is limited; therefore, missed diagnosis could occur if MRI were performed instead of CT or unless plain films are available for comparison.

Malignant lesions of bone in the hand and wrist are even less common than benign lesions (see Table 11-4). As in other areas of the extremities, if a malignant lesions is suspected, MRI is superior to CT in demonstrating the extent of medullary bone, soft tissue, and neurovascular involvement. Most frequently, both T1 and T2 weighted sequences are needed to characterize lesions. T2 weighted sequences are best suited for soft tissue characterization and T1 weighted sequences for distinction between marrow and tumor (Fig. 11-30) (10,47).

The role of MRI in evaluation of soft tissue neoplasms differs significantly from osseous neoplasms (Fig. 11-30) (7,10,18,43,44). Routine radiographs are not usually able to identify soft tissue lesions. In addition, soft tissue contrast with MRI in the peripheral extremities is superior to CT. The ability to image in multiple planes with the variable pulse sequences and the superior soft tissue

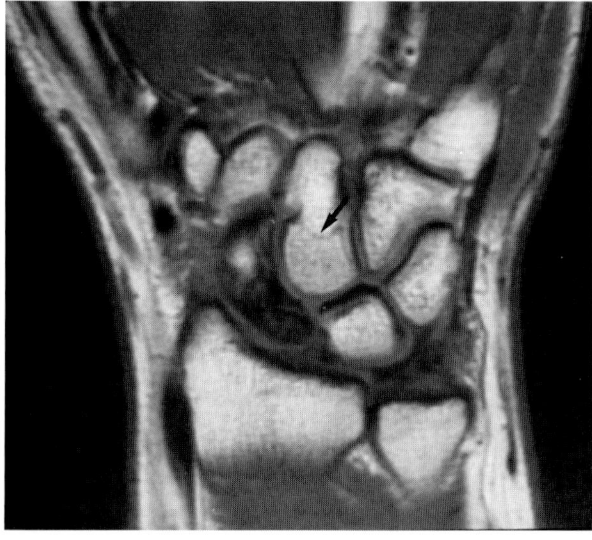

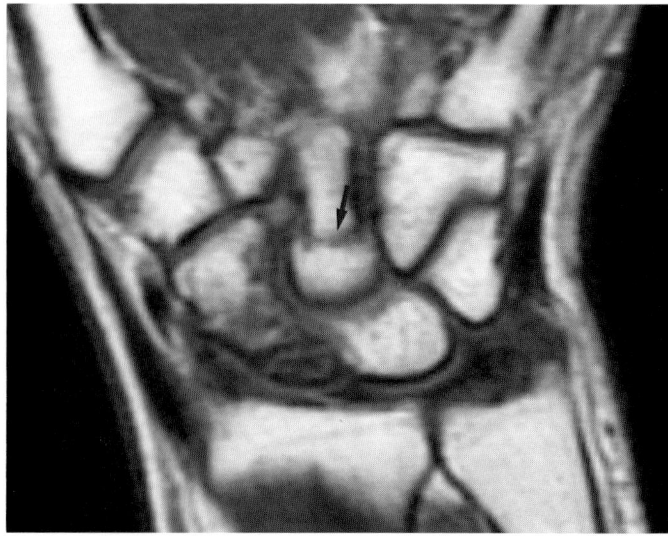

A,B

FIG. 11-28. Scaphoid fracture with osteonecrosis. **A:** T1 weighted coronal image shows loss of normal signal intensity in a large portion of the proximal scaphoid. There is no definite fracture. Note the questionable defect in the capitate (*arrow*). **B:** Two years later the fracture line and partially necrotic proximal scaphoid fragment are obvious. Note the capitate fracture is more obvious (*arrow*).

contrast of MRI make identification and characterization of soft tissues in the hand and wrist much easier compared with CT (10–12). Also, compared to skeletal lesions, differentiation of benign from malignant soft tissue neoplasms is more easily accomplished with MRI (10–12,48) (see Chapter 12). New angiographic software is also available that allows better definition of vascular lesions (Fig. 11-31).

Certain lesions peculiar to the hand and wrist deserve further discussion (15,36). Epidermoids, glomus tumors, ganglia, giant cell tumors of the tendon sheath, and mucoid cysts occur commonly in the hand and wrist (15,36).

Epidermoid tumors are most likely post-traumatic implants of epidermal tissue that form cysts. These lesions typically occur in the distal phalanx and vary in size from 1 to 20 mm. Pain over the lesion is common. A well-defined lucent lesion is usually noted radiographically. MRI is rarely indicated (36,38).

Glomus tumors arise in neuromyoarterial glomus, which is an end organ apparatus with an arteriovenous anastomosis without a capillary bed. The lesion occurs

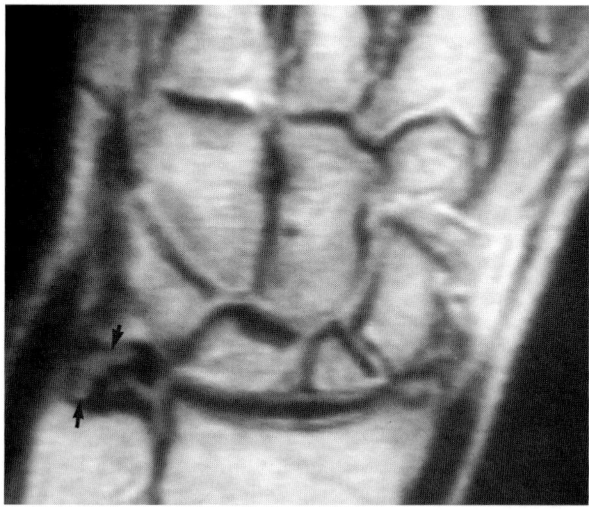

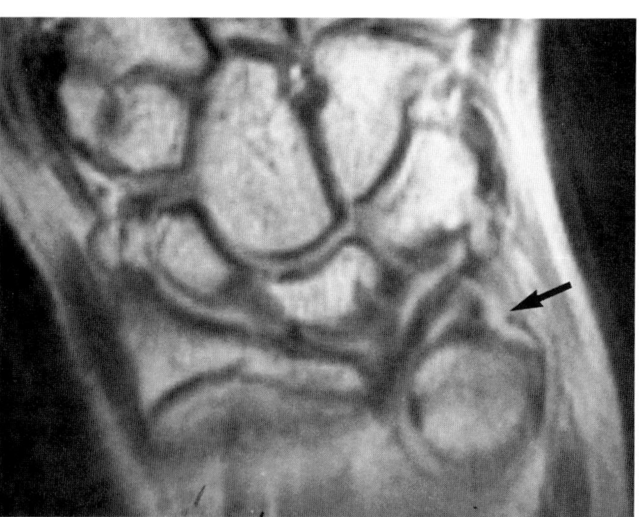

A,B

FIG. 11-29. Triangular fibrocartilage injuries. **A:** Coronal SE 2,000/30 image after wrist injury. There is a scaphoid fracture and increased signal in the TFC due to a tear in the ulnar aspect (*arrows*). **B:** Coronal SE 2,000/30 image with a tear in the TFC (*arrow*).

TABLE 11-4. *Bone tumors and tumorlike conditions of the hand and wrist (>8,000 tumors)* (16,36)

	Number of cases	Number (percentage) of tumors in hand and wrist
Benign		
Enchondromas	245	90 (37%)
Osteochondromas	727	28 (4%)
Giant cell tumors	425	63 (15%)
Osteoid osteoma	245	18 (7%)
Aneurysmal bone cysts	134	6 (4%)
Osteoblastoma	63	2 (3%)
Chondromyxoid fibroma	39	1 (2.5%)
Chondroblastoma	79	0 (0%)
Benign vascular tumors	80	0 (0%)
Neurolemmoma	10	0 (0%)
Fibrous defects	99	0 (0%)
Malignant		
Hemangioendothelioma	60	6 (10%)
Fibrosarcoma	207	1 (5%)
Metastasis	3,000	2 (4%)
Chondrosarcoma	634	14 (2.2%)
Parosteal osteosarcoma	56	1 (2%)
Malignant fibrous histiocytoma	52	1 (2%)
Osteosarcoma	1,274	13 (1%)
Ewing's sarcoma	402	5 (1%)
Lymphoma	469	4 (0.8%)
Myeloma	556	0 (0%)

most commonly in patients 30–50 years of age. Pain, often severe, is a common presenting complaint. These lesions are small (≤1 cm) and usually occur in the subungual or palmar aspect of the finger (15,36). These lesions usually have high signal intensity on T2 weighted sequences. However, MR findings are not specific.

Ganglion cysts are the most common soft tissue masses in the hand and wrist. Ganglion cysts are synovial outpouchings and are most common along the dorsal aspects of the hand and wrist (20,21). Ganglia are well marginated but vary in size. In some cases they appear as elongations of the tendon sheath. Most often they have high signal intensity on T2 weighted sequences and are near muscle intensity on T1 weighted sequences (Figs. 11-32 and 11-33). Slight shortening of T1 and T2 weighted relaxation times can occur with viscous or proteinaceous debris so that signal intensity is slightly reduced on T2 weighted and slightly increased on T1 weighted sequences (10).

Giant cell tumors of the tendon sheath are the second most common soft tissue mass in the hand (36). There are several features of this lesion that may assist in differentiation from a ganglion cyst. Giant cell tumors are most common along the dorsal tendons of the index, ring, and small fingers over the distal interphalangeal joints (36). Lesions occur less frequently in the wrist. Lesions are usually painless. Osteoarthritis and secondary bone erosion are commonly associated with tendon sheath giant cell tumors.

Paramagnetic effects of hemosiderin in giant cell tumors can be identified as areas of low signal intensity on T2 weighted images. This MR feature can assist in more clearly defining the nature of these lesions (Fig. 11-34) (10,12,13).

Mucoid cysts are cutaneous fluid-filled cysts that occur near the distal joints of the hand. These lesions are well defined, approximately 1 cm in size, and have a benign appearance on MR images. Differentiation from other benign lesions is not always possible based on image features alone (36).

Other soft tissue masses, specifically lipomas, hemangiomas, neurofibromas, and digital fibromas, also occur in the hand and wrist (15,36).

More detailed information regarding the utility and initial techniques for evaluation of musculoskeletal tumors is available in Chapter 12.

Infection

Routine radiographs including magnification views and tomography can be used as screening techniques for osteomyelitis (52). More sensitive and specific diagnosis may require the use of technetium bone scans and either indium-111 labeled white blood cells or gallium-67 radionuclide studies (8,17). A negative technetium-99m methyline diphosphonate scan is highly specific for excluding osteomyelitis or joint space infection (6,8). However, radionuclide studies are deficient in their ability to distinguish bone from soft tissue involvement (8,45,46). In these situations or in problem cases, MRI is very useful in demonstrating osteomyelitis. MRI may also be useful in demonstrating early erosive changes in the cartilage and effusions in joint space infections (5,8). To date, the appearance of the fluid has not been useful in differentiating infections, hemorrhage, and so on (Fig. 11-35) (5,8,40). Soft tissue abscesses can also be identified with MRI (4,6,8,35).

T2 weighted sequences are best for identification of synovial proliferation, joint effusions, and abscesses (5,6,8). T1 weighted or STIR sequences are optimal for identification of early changes in the marrow (10,47). A complete discussion of the role of MRI in evaluation of musculoskeletal infection is found in Chapter 13.

Arthritis

Routine radiographs have been valuable in staging and monitoring bone and joint changes in patients with inflammatory arthropathies (5,40). However, early soft tissue and cartilaginous changes are difficult to detect with these conventional techniques. High-field surface coil techniques are particularly useful for early detection

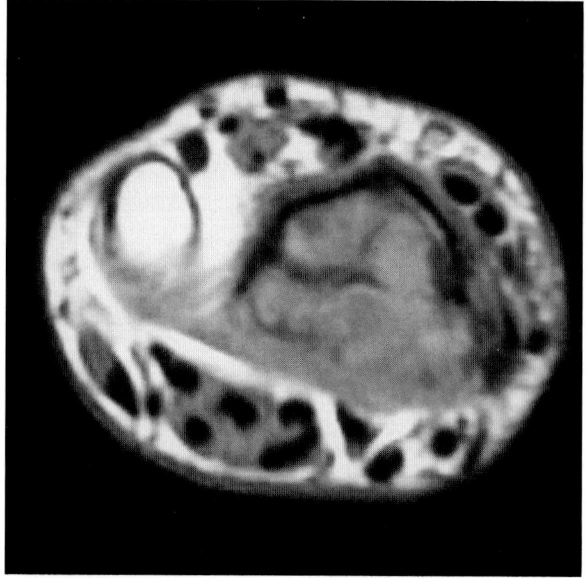

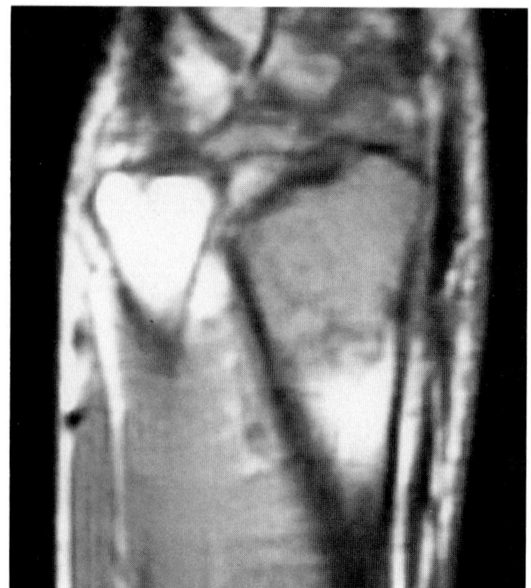

A,B

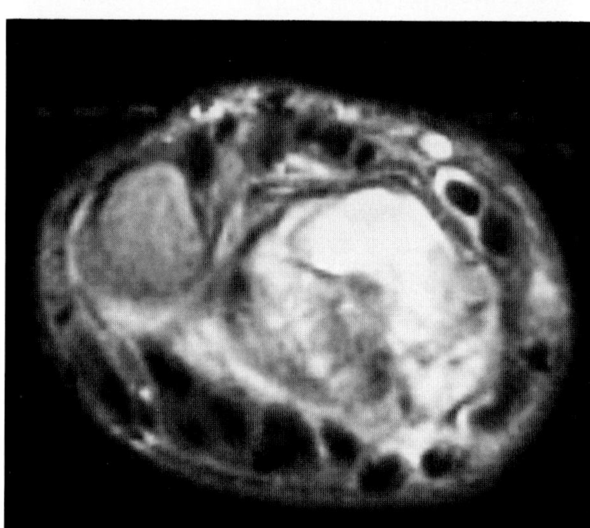

C

FIG. 11-30. Axial (**A**) and coronal (**B**) SE 500/20 and axial (**C**) SE 2,000/60 images of the wrist show a large destructive inhomogeneous lesion in the distal radius. This giant cell tumor would be difficult to diagnose based on MR images alone.

of subtle changes in the synovium, articular cartilage, and bone before they are evident radiographically (4,5,11,50,54). Synovial changes are most obvious on T2 weighted sequences (SE 2,000/60–80) (10). Inflamed synovium has high signal intensity and there is almost always an associated effusion. More chronic synovial proliferation (fronds) will appear as low signal intensity nodules or strands contrasted to the high signal intensity of fluid. Unfortunately, current MRI techniques have not been able to successfully differentiate changes (infection, blood, etc.) in joint fluid (5,40). Erosive changes are also nonspecific. However, early changes in unossified epiphyses are particularly easy to appreciate in early juvenile rheumatoid arthritis (39,54). Pigmented villonodular synovitis is an exception to the rule. In this con dition there is synovial inflammation that has high signal intensity on T2 weighted sequences. In addition, the hemosiderin deposition [at least 25% ferric (Fe^{3+})] causes shortening of T2 relaxation in the adjacent water molecules, leading to decreased signal intensity (shortening T2 relaxation time). This effect is even greater on high-field (1–1.5 T) units (42). Therefore, differentiation of PVNS from other arthropathies is possible with MRI.

Avascular Necrosis

MRI is a proven technique for detection of avascular necrosis (10,26,37). In the wrist, these changes are seen most commonly in the lunate and following scaphoid fractures (see Fig. 11-28). Carpal bones are smaller and, therefore, the MRI features of osteonecrosis may be more difficult to interpret. Uniform loss of signal intensity on short TE/TR sequences is the most reliable sign of avascular necrosis, specifically in the lunate (Fig.

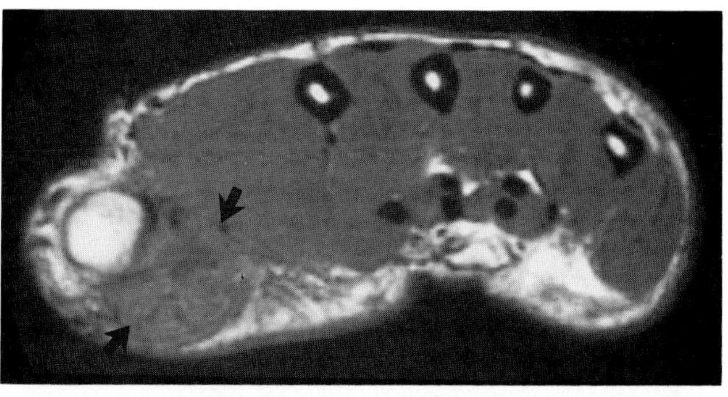

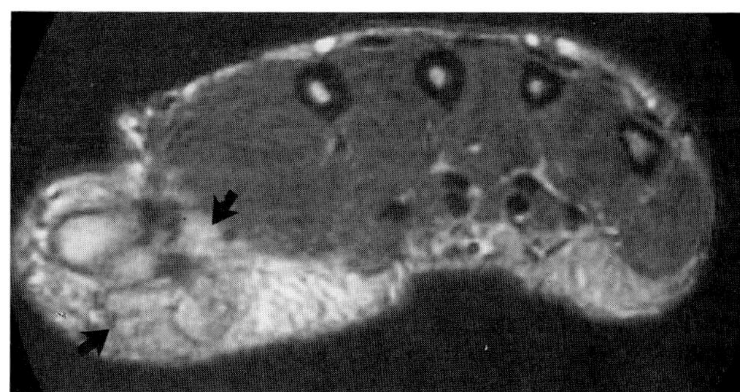

A,B

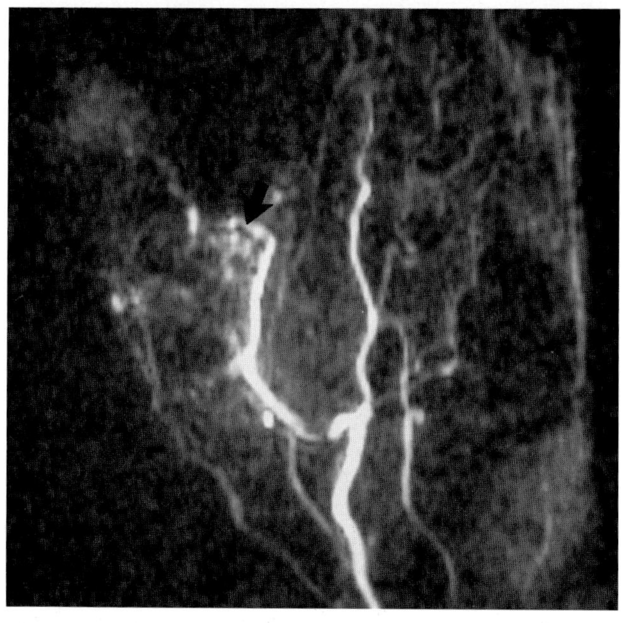

C

FIG. 11-31. Metastatic renal cell carcinoma. Axial SE 500/20 (**A**) and SE 2,000/60 (**B**) images show an inhomogeneous, irregular mass (*arrows*) in the thenar region. The coronal angiographic images (**C**) show the increased vascularity (*arrow*) of the lesion.

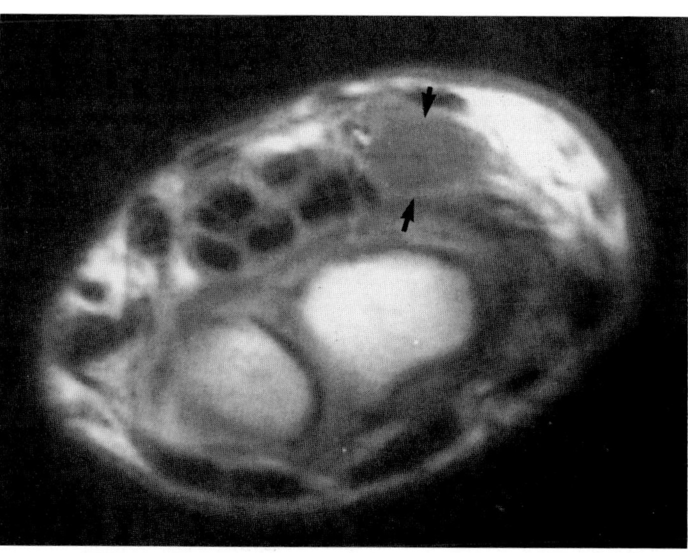

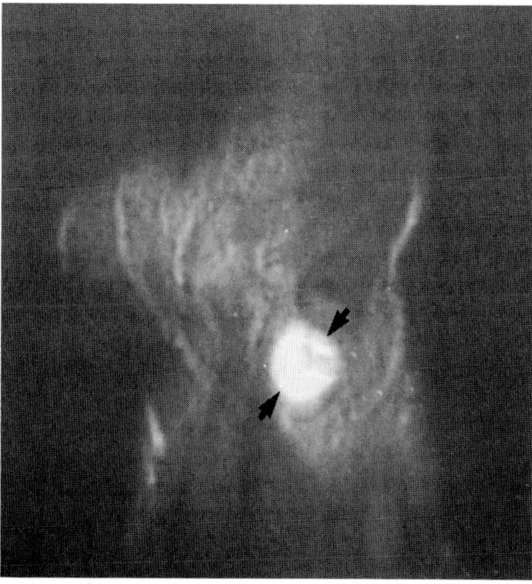

A,B

FIG. 11-32. Patient with ulnar neuropathy and wrist pain. **A:** Axial SE 500/20 image shows a well-defined muscle density mass (*arrows*) near the flexor tendons and ulnar nerve. **B:** Coronal SE 2,000/60 image shows the lesion to be well defined, homogeneous, and of high intensity (*arrows*). Diagnosis is ganglion cyst in Guyon's canal.

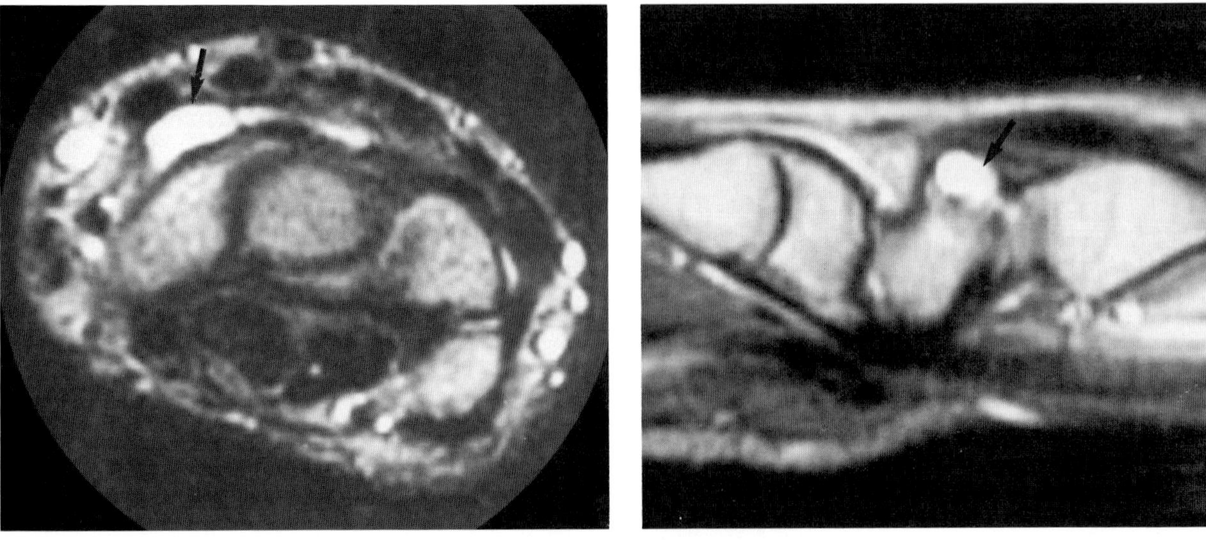

A,B

FIG. 11-33. Axial (**A**) and sagittal (**B**) SE 2,000/60 images demonstrating a ganglion cyst (*arrows*) dorsal to the scaphoid.

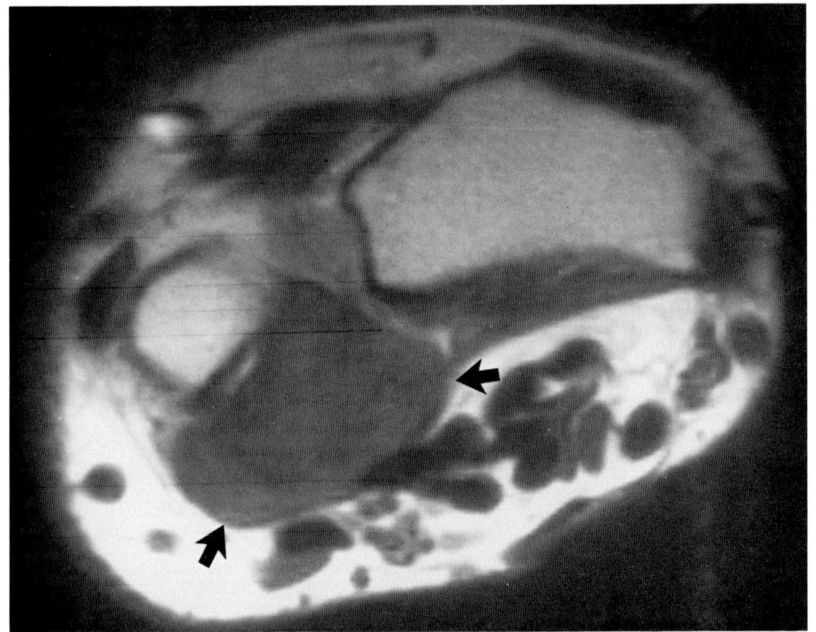

A

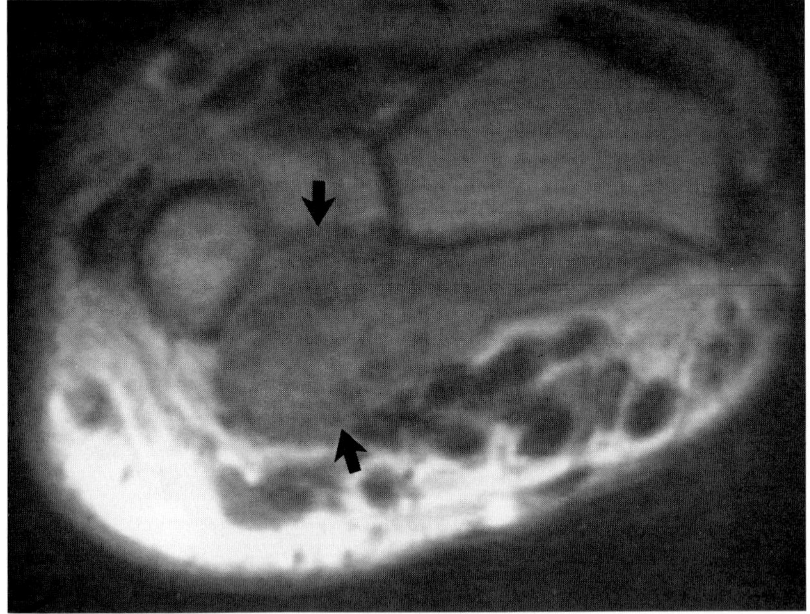

B

FIG. 11-34. Giant cell tumor of the tendon. Axial (**A**) SE 500/20 and (**B**) 2,000/60 images show a low-intensity lesion (*arrows*). The lack of signal intensity (most tumors are high intensity on T2 weighted sequences) on the T2 weighted sequence (**B**) suggests the possibility of giant cell tumor.

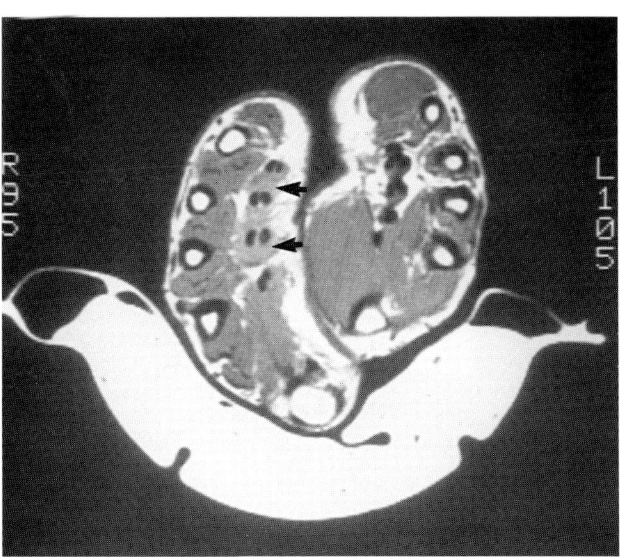

FIG. 11-35. Axial SE 800/25 images of the wrist, demonstrating normal flexor tendons on the left and thickening of the synovium on the right (*arrows*) due to tuberculous synovitis.

11-36) (12,37,41). Similar changes also can occur in the other carpal bones but are less common (Fig. 11-37). Patchy or focal signal intensity changes have also been noted (41). When small focal areas of reduced signal intensity are noted in the carpal bones on a T1 weighted sequence, the diagnosis may be more difficult (Fig. 11-38). Comparison with T2 weighted images is somewhat useful. In the early stages the signal intensity will be increased. Later, when bone sclerosis occurs, the signal intensity will be reduced on both T1 and T2 weighted sequences (37). In either setting comparison with routine radiographs is important. Well-marginated lucent areas are usually degenerative and should not be confused with osteonecrosis. This appearance can also be seen with conditions such as ulnolunate abutment syndrome (52).

MRI has been useful in the detection and monitoring of the response of avascular necrosis to conservative therapy. In several cases, the signal intensity in an otherwise low signal intensity lunate has returned to normal with conservative therapy (Fig. 11-36). This finding was correlated with improvement in the patient's symptoms. Although isotope studies can also be used for identification of avascular necrosis, the MR findings are more informative and the anatomy more clearly demonstrated (11,26,37,41).

Carpal Tunnel Syndrome

Patients with carpal tunnel syndrome present with chronic discomfort and tingling of the fingers in the median nerve distribution (thumb through radial side of the ring finger) (2,29–31). Thenar muscle atrophy may also be present. Most often patients are 30–60 years of age and females outnumber males by up to 5:1. The condition may be bilateral in up to 50% of cases (30). The condition is generally thought to be due to compression of the median nerve. Clinical features and nerve conduction studies have been the most common methods of diagnosis.

The superior soft tissue contrast obtained with MRI makes the technique ideal for identification of the nerves, vessels, and tendons in the carpal tunnel (Fig. 11-4D,E) (10,29–31,55). The median nerve typically lies just deep to the transverse carpal ligament and superficial to the flexor tendons (Fig. 11-39). On axial images

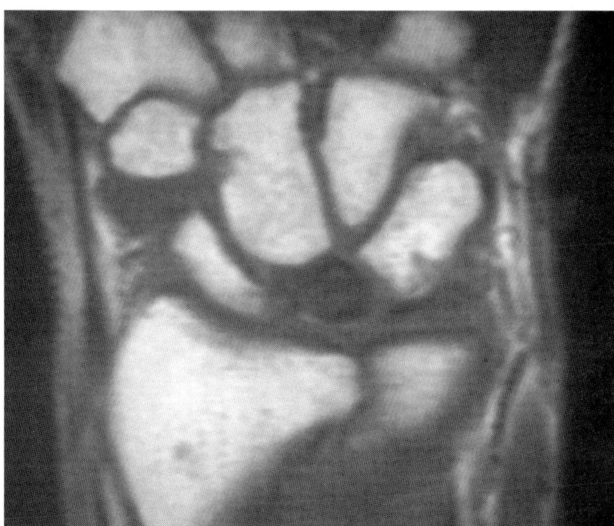

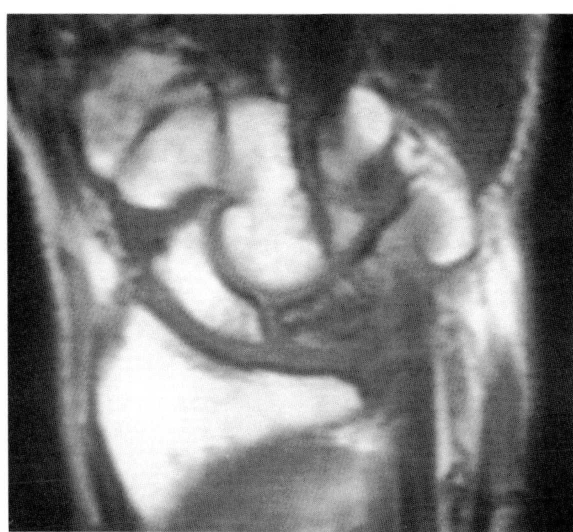

A,B

FIG. 11-36. AVN of the lunate. **A:** SE 500/20 image shows complete loss of signal intensity in the lunate. **B:** Follow-up examination after 6 months shows returning signal intensity, indicating revascularization.

A,B

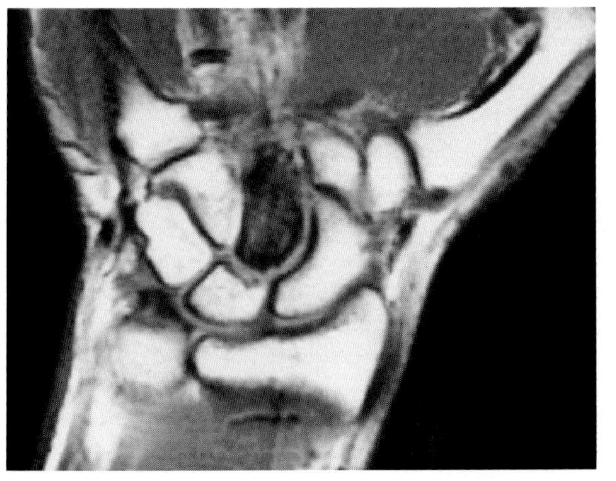

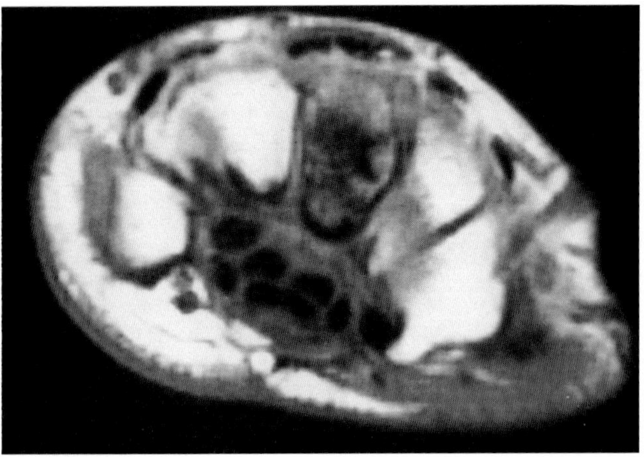

FIG. 11-37. Coronal (**A**) and axial (**B**) SE 500/20 images of the wrist show loss of normal marrow signal intensity in the capitate due to AVN.

A,B

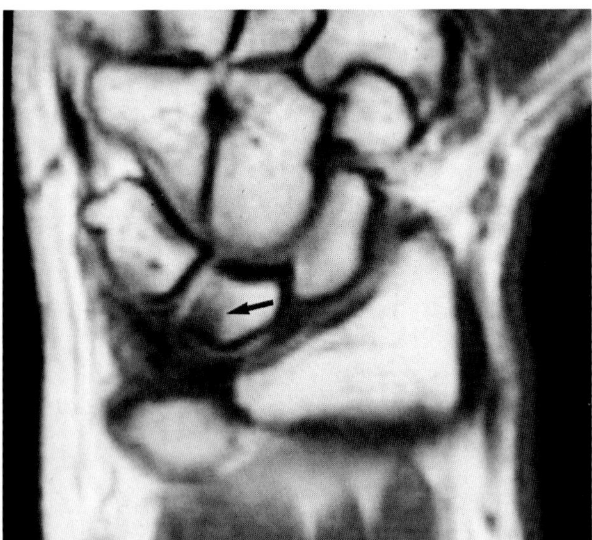

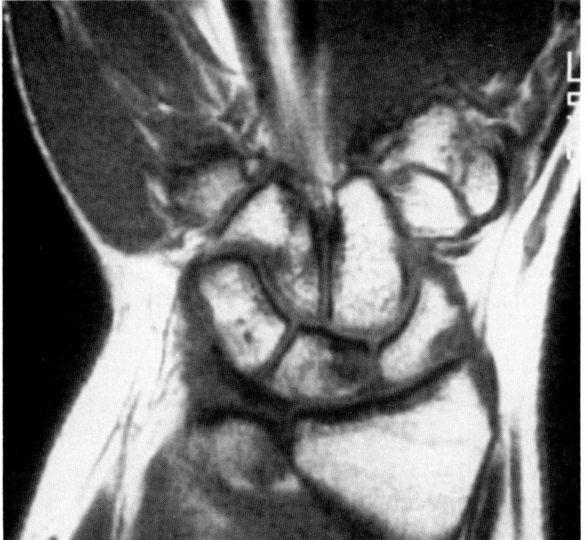

FIG. 11-38. Coronal SE 500/20 images of the wrist in two patients with wrist pain not related to AVN. **A:** Focal area of decreased signal intensity (*arrow*) in the ulnar aspect of the lunate due to ulnolunate abutment syndrome. **B:** Focal, well-marginated area of decreased signal intensity in the radial aspect of the lunate due to a degenerative cyst.

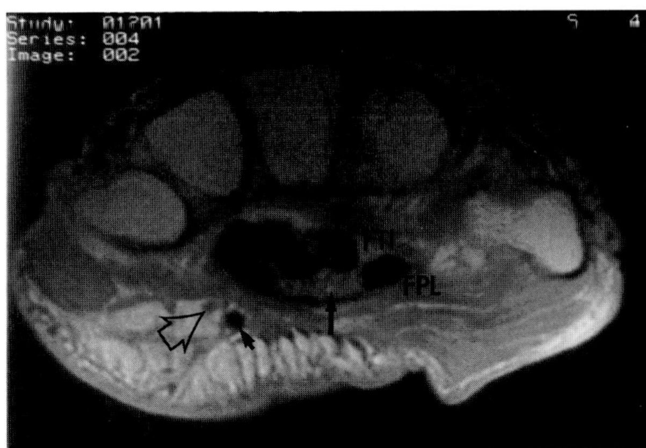

FIG. 11-39. Axial MR image of the wrist, demonstrating the normal shape of the median nerve (*large arrow*) and its relationship to the flexor tendon of the index finger (FTI) and flexor pollicis longus (FPL). Also note the position of the ulnar nerve (*open arrow*) and artery (*small arrow*).

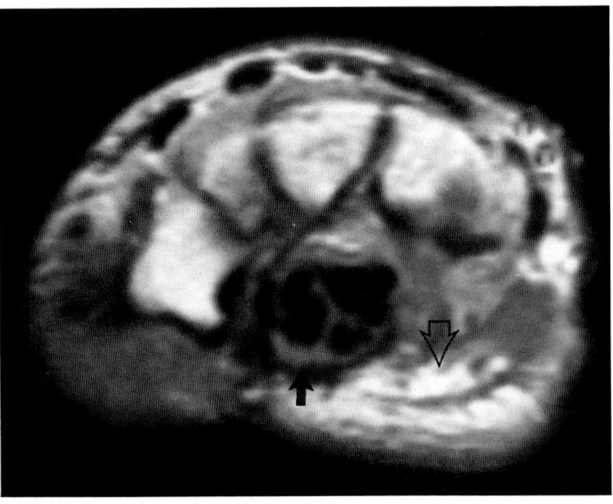

FIG. 11-40. Axial T2 weighted (SE 2,000/60) image of the wrist shows flattening of the median nerve (*arrow*) but no increase in signal intensity. There is superficial edema in the thenar region (*open arrow*).

the nerve is elliptical with signal intensity that is higher than the adjacent tendons (10,29–31,55).

The position and shape of the nerve may vary depending on the position of the wrist. Zeiss et al. (55) studied the position and configuration of the median nerve with the wrist in neutral, flexed, and extended positions. In the neutral position the median nerve is typically located either anterior to the superficial flexor tendon of the index finger or between this tendon and the flexor pollicis longus tendon. The nerve is more often between the flexor retinaculum and tendon to the index finger during extension. The nerve tends to flatten in the flexed position and again will most often lie anterior to the superficial flexor tendon to the index finger (55).

We prefer thin slice (3–5 mm) axial images with a small FOV (8–12 cm), 256 × 256 matrix, and surface coil technique to evaluate the carpal tunnel. Both T1 (SE 500/20) and T2 (SE 2,000/20,80) weighted sequences are obtained. It may be helpful to evaluate both wrists when symptoms are unilateral. This is especially useful when subtle MR changes are noted in the involved wrist. If the MRI of the wrist is normal, one must consider a lesion located more proximally such as the elbow, thoracic outlet, or cervical spine (30).

MRI can clearly define bone and soft tissue abnormalities that might cause compression of the median nerve. Early reviews have described swelling of the median nerve, flattening of the nerve (Fig. 11-40), bowing of the flexor retinaculum, and increased signal intensity of the nerve on T2 weighted sequences (Fig. 11-41). Other pathology such as synovitis in the tendon sheaths, muscle thickening, cysts, and soft tissue masses may also cause compression of the nerve (30,55). Since the pathology and therapy for carpal tunnel syndrome are controversial, we feel most comfortable, from an MRI standpoint, when a clearly defined lesion is identified as opposed to signal intensity changes or subtle changes in configuration of the nerve.

MRI can also be used to evaluate patients following surgical decompression (Fig. 11-42). Hematomas, hemorrhage, and other postoperative changes can affect the median and ulnar nerves.

Despite the uncertainties with diagnosis and therapy for carpal tunnel syndrome, we feel MRI is the imaging technique best suited to evaluate this region.

Ulnar Nerve Compression

Compression of the ulnar nerve can also occur at the wrist. Pain and tingling in the ulnar nerve distribution

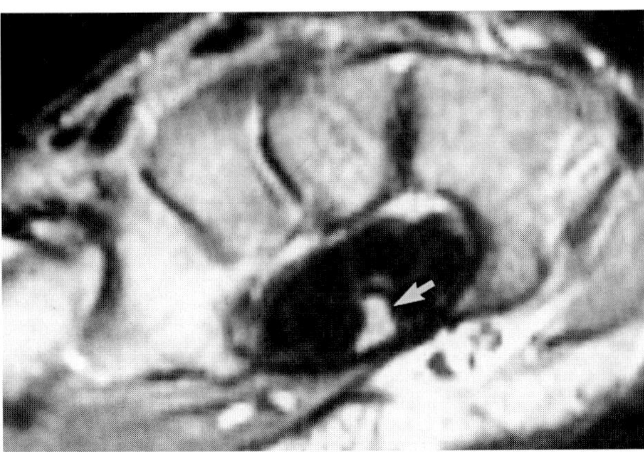

FIG. 11-41. Axial SE 2,000/60 image of the wrist, showing increased intensity and compression of the medial nerve (*arrow*).

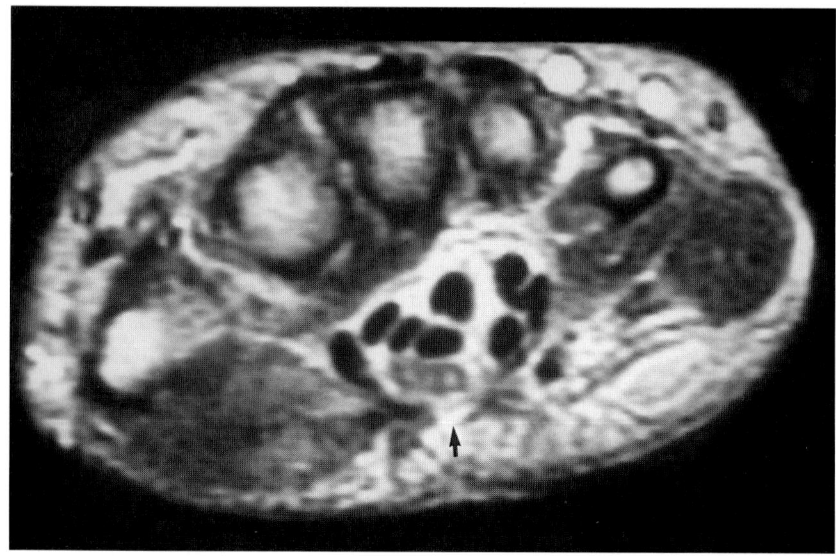

FIG. 11-42. Axial image (SE 2,000/60) of the wrist following carpal tunnel release. Note the defect in the ligament (*small arrow*) and the scattered areas of increased signal intensity in the median nerve. The patient was not symptomatic. The signal intensity in the nerve was similar preoperatively.

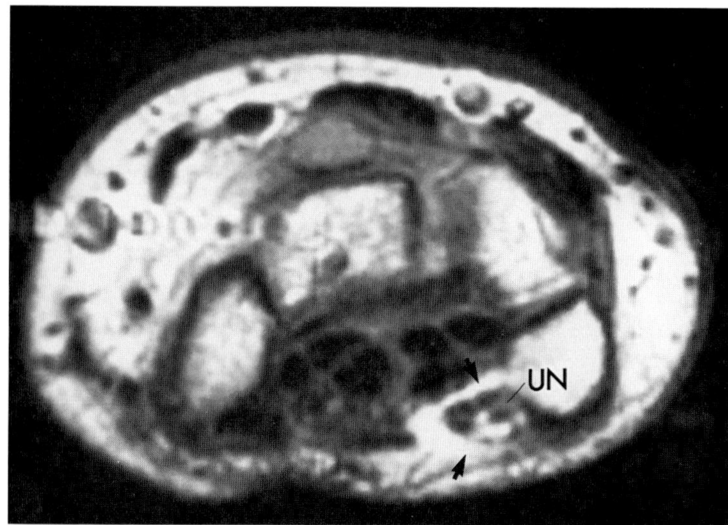

FIG. 11-43. Axial SE 2,000/60 image of the wrist, showing increased signal intensity along the margins and within Guyon's canal (*arrows*) due to post-traumatic inflammation. (UN, ulnar nerve.)

(hypothenar region and the ulnar side of the fourth and fifth fingers) may be the presenting complaints.

The MR technique and factors to evaluate are similar to those described with carpal tunnel syndrome. In our experience, ganglion cysts (Fig. 11-32) and/or inflammatory changes (Fig. 11-43) in Guyons canal have been the lesions most commonly associated with ulnar nerve symptoms (10,12,13).

Miscellaneous Conditions

There are numerous other abnormalities in the musculoskeletal system that may involve the hand and wrist. These include congenital abnormalities, metabolic diseases, and hematologic disorder. The exact role of MRI in these conditions is limited at this time (see Chapter 15).

REFERENCES

1. Amadio PC, Hanssen AD, Berquist TH. The genesis of Kienböck's disease: early diagnosis by magnetic resonance imaging. *J Hand Surg* 1987;12A:1044–1049.
2. Anderson JE. *Grant's atlas of anatomy,* 8th ed. Baltimore: Williams & Wilkins, 1983.
3. Baker LL, Hajek PC, Björkengren A, Galbraith R, Sartoris DJ, Gelberman RH, Resnick D. High-resolution magnetic resonance imaging of the wrist: normal anatomy. *Skeletal Radiol* 1987;16:128–132.
4. Beltran J, Caudill JL, Herman LA, Kantor SM, Hudson PN, Noto AM, Baran AS. Rheumatoid arthritis: MR imaging manifestations. *Radiology* 1987;165:153–157.
5. Beltran J, Noto AM, Herman LJ, Mosure JC, Burk JM, Christoforidis AJ. Joint effusions: MR imaging. *Radiology* 1986;158:133–137.
6. Beltran J, Noto AM, McGhee RB, Freedy RM, McCalla M. Infections of the musculoskeletal system: high-field-strength MR imaging. *Radiology* 1987;164:449–454.
7. Beltran J, Simon DC, Katz W, Weis LD. Increased MR signal intensity in skeletal muscle adjacent to malignant tumors: pathologic correlation and clinical relevance. *Radiology* 1987;162:251–255.
8. Berquist TH, Brown ML, Fitzgerald RH, May GR. Magnetic resonance imaging: application in musculoskeletal infection. *Magn Reson Imaging* 1985;3:219–230.
9. Berquist TH. *Imaging of orthopedic trauma and surgery.* Philadelphia: Saunders, 1986.
10. Berquist TH. Magnetic resonance imaging of the elbow and wrist. *Top Magn Reson Imaging* 1989;1(3):15–27.
11. Berquist TH, Ehman RL, Richardson ML. *Magnetic resonance of the musculoskeletal system.* New York: Raven Press, 1987.
12. Binkovitz LA, Ehman RL, Cahill DR, Berquist TH. Magnetic resonance imaging of the wrist: normal cross sectional imaging and selected abnormal cases. *Radiographics* 1988;8:1171–1202.
13. Binkovitz LA, Berquist TH, McLeod RA. Masses of the hand and wrist: detection and characterization using MR imaging. *AJR* 1990;154:323–326.
14. Brady TJ, Gebhardt MC, Pykett IL, et al. NMR imaging of forearms in healthy volunteers and patients with giant-cell tumor of bone. *Radiology* 1982;144:549–552.
15. Butler ED, Hamell JP, Seipel RS, deLorimier AA. Tumors of the hand. A 10 year survey and report of 437 cases. *Am J Surg* 1960;100:293–302.
16. Dahlin DC, Unni KK. *Bone tumors: general aspects and data on 8,542 cases,* 4th ed. Springfield, IL: CC Thomas, 1986.
17. Datz FL, Thorne DA. Effect of chronicity of infection on the sensitivity of the In-111 labeled leukocyte scan. *AJR* 1986; 147:809–812.
18. Dooms GC, Hricak H, Sollitto RA, Higgins CB. Lipomatous tumors and tumors with fatty component: MR imaging potential and comparison of MR and CT results. *Radiology* 1985;157:479–483.
19. Ehman RL, Berquist TH. Magnetic resonance imaging of musculoskeletal trauma. *Radiol Clin North Am* 1986;24:291–319.
20. Erickson SJ, Neeland JB, Middleton WD, Jesmanowicz A, Hiplo J, Lavson TL, Foley WD. MR imaging of the finger: correlation with normal anatomic sections. *AJR* 1989;152:1013–1019.
21. Feldman F, Singson RD, Staron RB. Magnetic resonance imaging of para-articular and ectopic ganglia. *Skeletal Radiol* 1989; 18:353–358.
22. Golimbu CN, Firoonia H, Melone CP, Rafii M, Weinreb J, Leber C. Tears of the triangular fibrocartilage of the wrist. MR imaging. *Radiology* 1989;173:731–733.
23. Hardy CJ, Katzberg RW, Frey RL, Szumowski J, Totterman S, Mueller OM. Switched surface coil system for bilateral MR imaging. *Radiology* 1988;167:835–838.
24. Hollinshead WP. *Anatomy for surgeons, Volume 3. The back and limbs.* New York: Harper & Rowe, 1982.
25. Koenig H, Lucas D, Meisser R. The wrist: a preliminary report on high-resolution MR imaging. *Radiology* 1986;160:463–467.
26. Lang P, Jergesen HE, Moseley ME, Block JE, Chafetz NI, Genant HK. Avascular necrosis of the femoral head: high-field-strength MR imaging with histologic correlation. *Radiology* 1988; 169:517–524.
27. Lee JK, Yao L. Stress fractures: MR imaging. *Radiology* 1988;169:217–220.
28. Louis DS, Buckwalter KA. Magnetic resonance imaging of the collateral ligaments of the thumb. *J Hand Surg* 1989;14A:739–741.
29. Mesgarzadeh M, Schneck CD, Bonakdapour A. Carpal tunnel: MR imaging. Part I: Normal anatomy. *Radiology* 1989;171:743–748.
30. Mesgarzadeh M, Schneck CD, Bonakdapour A, Mitra A, Conaway D. Carpal tunnel: MR imaging. Part II: Carpal tunnel syndrome. *Radiology* 1989;171:749–754.
31. Middleton WD, Kneeland JB, Kellman GM, et al. MR imaging of the carpal tunnel: normal anatomy and preliminary findings in the carpal tunnel syndrome. *AJR* 1987;148:307–316.
32. Middleton WD, Macrander S, Lawson TL, et al. High resolution surface coil magnetic resonance imaging of the joints: anatomic correlation. *Radiographics* 1987;7:645–683.
33. Mink JH, Deutsch AL. Occult cartilage and bone injuries of the knee: detection, classification and assessment with MR imaging. *Radiology* 1989;170:823–829.
34. O'Rahilly R. A survey of carpal and tarsal anomalies. *J Bone Joint Surg* 1953;35A:626–641.
35. Paajanen H, Grodd W, Revel D, Engelstad B, Brasch RC. Gadolinium-DTPA enhanced MR imaging of intramuscular abscesses. *Magn Reson Imaging* 1987;5:109–115.
36. Poznanski AK. *The hand in radiologic diagnosis.* Philadelphia: Saunders, 1984.
37. Reinus WR, Conway WF, Totty WG, et al. Carpal avascular necrosis: MR imaging. *Radiology* 1986;160:689–693.
38. Schajowics F, Aiello CL, Slullitel I. Cystic and pseudocystic lesions of the terminal phalanx with specific references to epidermoid cysts. *Clin Orthop* 1970;68:84–92.
39. Senac MO, Beutsch D, Bernstein BH, Stanley P, Crues JV III, Stoller DW, Mink J. MR imaging in juvenile rheumatoid arthritis. *AJR* 1988;150:873–878.
40. Sims RE, Genant HK. Magnetic resonance imaging of joint disease. *Radiol Clin North Am* 1986;24:179–188.
41. Sowa DT, Holder LE, Patt PG. Application of magnetic resonance imaging to ischemic necrosis of the lunate. *J Hand Surg* 1989;14A:1008–1016.
42. Spritzer CE, Dalinka MK, Kressel HY. Magnetic resonance imaging of pigmented villonodular synovitis: a report of two cases. *Skeletal Radiol* 1987;16:316–319.
43. Sundaram M, McGuire MH, Schajowic ZF. Soft tissue masses: histologic bases for decreased signal (short T2) on T2 weighted images. *AJR* 1987;148:1247–1250.

44. Sundaram M, McGuire MH, Herbold DR, Beshony S, Fletcher JW. High signal intensity soft tissue masses on T1 weighted pulsing sequences. *Skeletal Radiol* 1987;16:30–36.
45. Tang JS, Gold RH, Bassett LW, Seeger LL. Musculoskeletal infection of the extremities: evaluation with MR imaging. *Radiology* 1988;166:205–209.
46. Unger E, Moldofsky P, Gatenby R, Hartz W, Broder G. Diagnosis of osteomyelitis by MR imaging. *AJR* 1988;150:605–610.
47. Vogler JB III, Murphy WA. Bone marrow imaging. *Radiology* 1988;168:679–693.
48. Weekes RG, Berquist TH, McLeod RA, Zimmer WD. Magnetic resonance imaging of soft-tissue tumors: comparison with computed tomography. *Magn Reson Imaging* 1985;3:345–352.
49. Weiss KL, Beltran J, Shamam OM, Stilla RF, Levey M. High-field MR surface-coil imaging of the hand and wrist. Part I: Normal anatomy. *Radiology* 1986;160:143–146.
50. Weiss KL, Beltran J, Lubbers LM. High-field MR surface coil imaging of the hand and wrist. Part II: Pathologic correlations and clinical relevance. *Radiology* 1986;160:147–152.
51. Winkler ML, Ortendahl DA, Mills TC, Crooks LE, Sheldon PE, Kaufman L, Kramer DM. Characteristics of partial flip angle and gradient reversal MR imaging. *Radiology* 1988;166:17–26.
52. Wood MB, Berquist TH. The hand and wrist. In: Berquist, TH, ed. *Imaging of orthopedic trauma and surgery*. Philadelphia: Saunders, 1986:641–730.
53. Yao L, Lee JK. Occult intraosseous fracture: detection with MR imaging. *Radiology* 1988;167:749–751.
54. Yulish BS, Lieberman JM, Newman AJ, Bryan PJ, Mulopulos GP, Modic MT. Juvenile rheumatoid arthritis: assessment with MR imaging. *Radiology* 1987;165:149–152.
55. Zeiss J, Skie M, Ebraheim N, Jackson WT. Anatomic relations between the median nerve and flexor tendons in the carpal tunnel: MR evaluation in normal volunteers. *AJR* 1989;153:533–536.
56. Zlatkin MB, Chao PC, Osterman AL, Schnall MD, Dalinka MK, Kressel HY. Chronic wrist pain: evaluation with high-resolution MR imaging. *Radiology* 1989;173:723–729.

MRI of the Musculoskeletal System, 2nd Edition, edited by T. H. Berquist.
Raven Press, Ltd., New York © 1990.

CHAPTER 12

Musculoskeletal Neoplasms

Thomas H. Berquist

Techniques, 435
Positioning and Coil Selection, 435
Imaging Planes and Pulse Sequences, 436
Skeletal Neoplasms, 438
Benign Bone Neoplasms, 438
Malignant Bone Neoplasms, 441
Soft Tissue Neoplasms, 447
Benign Soft Tissue Neoplasms, 447
Malignant Soft Tissue Neoplasms, 455
Nonneoplastic Soft Tissue Masses, 458
Post-treatment Evaluation, 459
Metastases, 463
Specificity, 470
References, 470

Magnetic resonance imaging has become an accepted and valuable technique in the detection and staging of musculoskeletal neoplasms. Its superior soft tissue contrast and the ability to image in multiple planes provide significant advantages over other imaging techniques, including computed tomography (1,2,10,14,29,44 48,61,90).

New treatment techniques make it even more important to have as much information as possible regarding the nature and extent of bone and soft tissue neoplasms (5,75). This information allows more appropriate decisionmaking regarding the utility of limb salvage procedures, chemotherapy, radiation therapy, or combination therapy in managing musculoskeletal tumors. Imaging techniques provide valuable information for the surgeon or clinician treating patients with musculoskeletal neoplasms (75,106,107,116). Routine radiographs still play an important role in detection of characterization of skeletal lesions, especially benign bone tumors. Isotope scans can provide additional information, particularly in detection of skeletal metastasis. Both computed tomography (CT) and magnetic resonance imaging (MRI) have important roles in staging of skeletal neoplasms. Detection of soft tissue neoplasm requires the use of other imaging modalities. Ultrasound can differentiate solid from cystic lesions; however, until recently, CT was usually the technique of choice for detection and staging of soft tissue neoplasms. MRI has largely replaced CT, especially for evaluation of the extremities (14).

Certain aspects of musculoskeletal tumors have been discussed in previous chapters as they relate to specific anatomic regions. However, this chapter is designed to more fully discuss (a) techniques, (b) lesion detection and staging, (c) lesion characterization and specificity, (d) evaluation of metastasis, and (e) follow-up evaluation for differentiation of recurrent or residual tumor from postoperative or radiation changes.

TECHNIQUES

The basic principles of MRI and general techniques have been discussed in Chapters 1 and 3. However, certain aspects of MRI techniques for evaluating musculoskeletal neoplasm need to be reemphasized.

Positioning and Coil Selection

Positioning of patients and the choice of proper coils for studies of musculoskeletal neoplasms are essential to minimize motion artifacts and obtain optimal signal-to-noise ratios. Evaluation of the trunk and thighs is most efficacious using the body coil with the patient supine. If a gluteal soft tissue lesion is suspected, the prone position may be helpful to avoid distortion of the posterior soft tissues. The body coil also allows comparison of

T. H. Berquist: Mayo Medical School and Mayo Clinic, Rochester, Minnesota 55905.

both lower extremities and can provide more complete evaluation of the entire osseous or soft tissue region of interest (i.e., femur, tibia, etc.). In certain skeletal neoplasms, imaging the entire bone or region of interest is important to be certain that skip lesions are not overlooked (Fig. 12-1).

The peripheral lower extremities distal to the knee and the upper extremities are usually evaluated using flat surface coils or circumferential volume coils. These coils are important in achieving superior image quality and are selected on the basis of the body part and patient position needed for the examination. For example, a lesion in the shoulder might easily be evaluated using the $5\frac{1}{2}$ inch circular coil. A lesion in the humerus should be studied using a larger license plate shaped coil to include a larger area of the upper extremity (see Fig. 9-2). The circumferential volume extremity coil provides a more uniform signal, but it must be positioned in the center of the gantry with most imagers. Positioning is not difficult for evaluating the knee, calf, or foot and ankle, but evaluation of the forearm and wrist may require that the patient place his or her arm above the head (see Fig. 11-1). The latter position is uncomfortable and leads to motion artifacts, making it more difficult to obtain quality images.

New coils are now becoming available that allow superior image quality and more flexibility in the amount of area covered. These array coils will most likely be developed for the spine region first and will be very useful in evaluating large segments of the spine in patients with suspected lymphoma, myeloma, or metastatic disease (12).

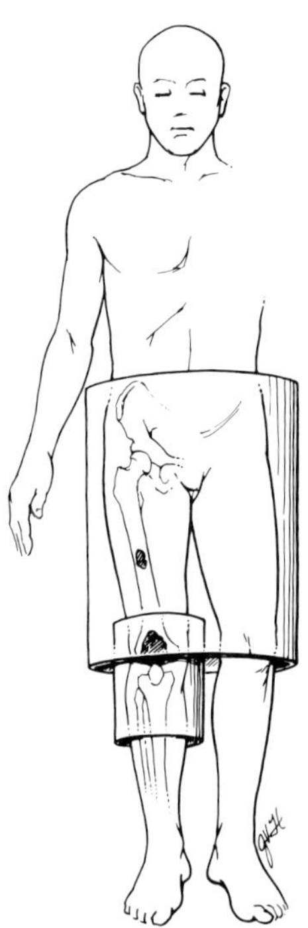

FIG. 12-1. Illustration of patient, demonstrating the body coil and an extremity coil. The body coil is preferred to avoid overlooking skip lesions. (From ref. 12, with permission.)

Imaging Planes and Pulse Sequences

In a given clinical setting there are numerous pulse sequences that could be used to evaluate the musculoskeletal system. These include the commonly utilized spin-echo sequences (short TE, TR; long TE, TR), inversion recovery sequences (IR), short TI inversion recovery sequences (STIR), gradient-echo sequences, and chemical shift sequences (6,12,41,53,98,105). For most patients with suspected bone or soft tissue neoplasms, spin-echo sequences are commonly employed. With these sequences, normal tissues have predictable signal intensity. Fat and bone marrow have high signal intensity and appear nearly white on MR images. Muscle has intermediate signal intensity, whereas cortical bone, ligaments, tendon, calcium, air, and fibrocartilage appear dark or black. Flowing blood usually gives no signal but this finding is inconsistent and varies with the flow rate and pulse sequences used. Nerves usually have slightly lower intensity than muscles (12).

Pathologic tissues generally have increased T1 and T2 relaxation times compared with normal tissues and therefore are seen as areas of low signal intensity or isointense with muscle on T1 weighted spin-echo sequences and high intensity on T2 weighted sequences (12). Because the location of the lesion may be equivocal, we generally use both T1 and T2 weighted sequences to evaluate musculoskeletal neoplasms. T1 weighted sequences (abnormal tissue is dark) provide the best contrast resolution in marrow and fat and T2 weighted sequences (abnormal tissue is white) are most useful in evaluating muscle and soft tissues such as ligaments and tendons, which normally appear dark. A double-echo T2 weighted sequence (TE 20–30, 60–80, and TR 2,000 msec) is generally used in the axial plane. Other parameters may vary depending on the size of the lesion expected. Smaller lesions should be studied with thin slices such as 3–5 mm with 1.5–2.5 mm interslice gaps, a 256×256 matrix and 1 excitation or a 192×256 matrix and either 1 or 2 excitations. The field of view should be varied with the extent of the lesion to be evaluated. In general, the smaller field of view is preferred if applicable. A typical T2 weighted sequence with a repetition time of 2,000 msec requires 8 min 56 sec to complete.

After the T2 weighted sequence is obtained and reviewed, a second T1 weighted sequence is normally performed. This short TE, TR (TE 20, TR 500–600) sequence can be performed in either the coronal or sagittal planes to evaluate the extent of lesions; in certain cases the axial plane is used so that the T1 and T2 weighted

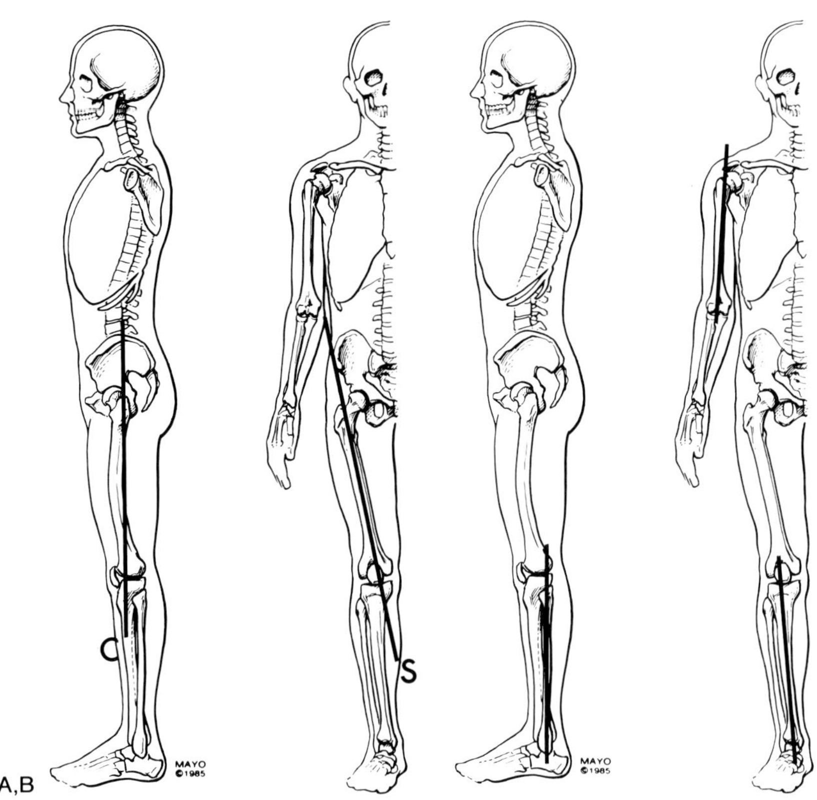

FIG. 12-2. Skeletal illustration demonstrating the oblique planes needed to accurately evaluate the long bones. **A:** The femur is most easily studied in the oblique sagittal plane (S) due to the normal bowing which would create more partial volume problems in the coronal plane (C). **B:** The oblique sagittal plane is also most useful for the upper extremity. Either the coronal or sagittal planes can be used for the tibia or fibula.

axial images can be more easily compared. In certain situations, oblique images are necessary to reduce the problems from partial volume effects (Fig. 12-2). Performing a second sequence in a plane that is 90° to the first sequence also more accurately demonstrates the extent of lesions.

If only two image sequences and two planes are required, a lesion can be identified and staged in 15–20 min. In some situations, where the lesion is more subtle, additional sequences may be required. For example, STIR sequences are very useful in evaluating subtle marrow abnormalities and are frequently added in addition to the conventional spin-echo sequences (Fig. 12-3). This technique (TI ~150, TE 30, TR 1,500) suppresses fat signal while providing an additive effect on T1 and T2 signal enhancement. The superior contrast achieved with this sequence can allow subtle lesions to be more easily identified (41,105). Some authors prefer short TE/TR spin-echo (SE 500/20) and STIR sequences to typical T1 and T2 weighted spin-echo sequences (53). STIR sequences can be performed more quickly (TR 1,500 compared to TR 2,000 for long TE/TR spin-echo sequence) than T2 weighted spin-echo sequences (10,53).

Recently, utilization of gadolinium-DTPA as a contrast medium has been suggested to improve characterization of musculoskeletal neoplasms. Some authors prefer T1 weighted sequences with and without gadolinium to the more conventional approach of using T1 and T2 weighted images (58,87). This would obviously reduce the examination time. Gadolinium-DTPA produces increased signal intensity in T1 weighted spin-echo images because of the reduction in T1 relaxation time (see Chapter 5). Therefore, zones in neoplasms that show marked increase signal intensity correlate with highly vascular regions, whereas zones that show low intensity or no intensity are thought to be due to necrosis. These data suggest that gadolinium may be valuable in identifying the areas of viable tumor within a mass, which is useful in determining whether residual tumor is still present. In addition, this information can be useful in biopsying lesions. One should try to avoid areas of necrosis and biopsy only those areas that would contain viable tumor (46,58,87). Early studies indicate that gadolinium-DTPA may also be useful in conjunction with gradient-echo sequences. However, this contrast medium is not currently used routinely in the musculoskeletal system.

Gradient-echo sequences are commonly used in the knee and for evaluating articular abnormalities. Recently, these techniques have also been used to perform two-dimensional and three-dimensional FT vascular studies (43,56). Motion has limited the effectiveness of MR angio in certain regions (abdomen, chest). However, new software techniques with gradient-echo sequences allow more effective vascular studies. Flow compensation, presaturation pulses, and breath-hold imaging can be performed using fast TE/TR gradient-

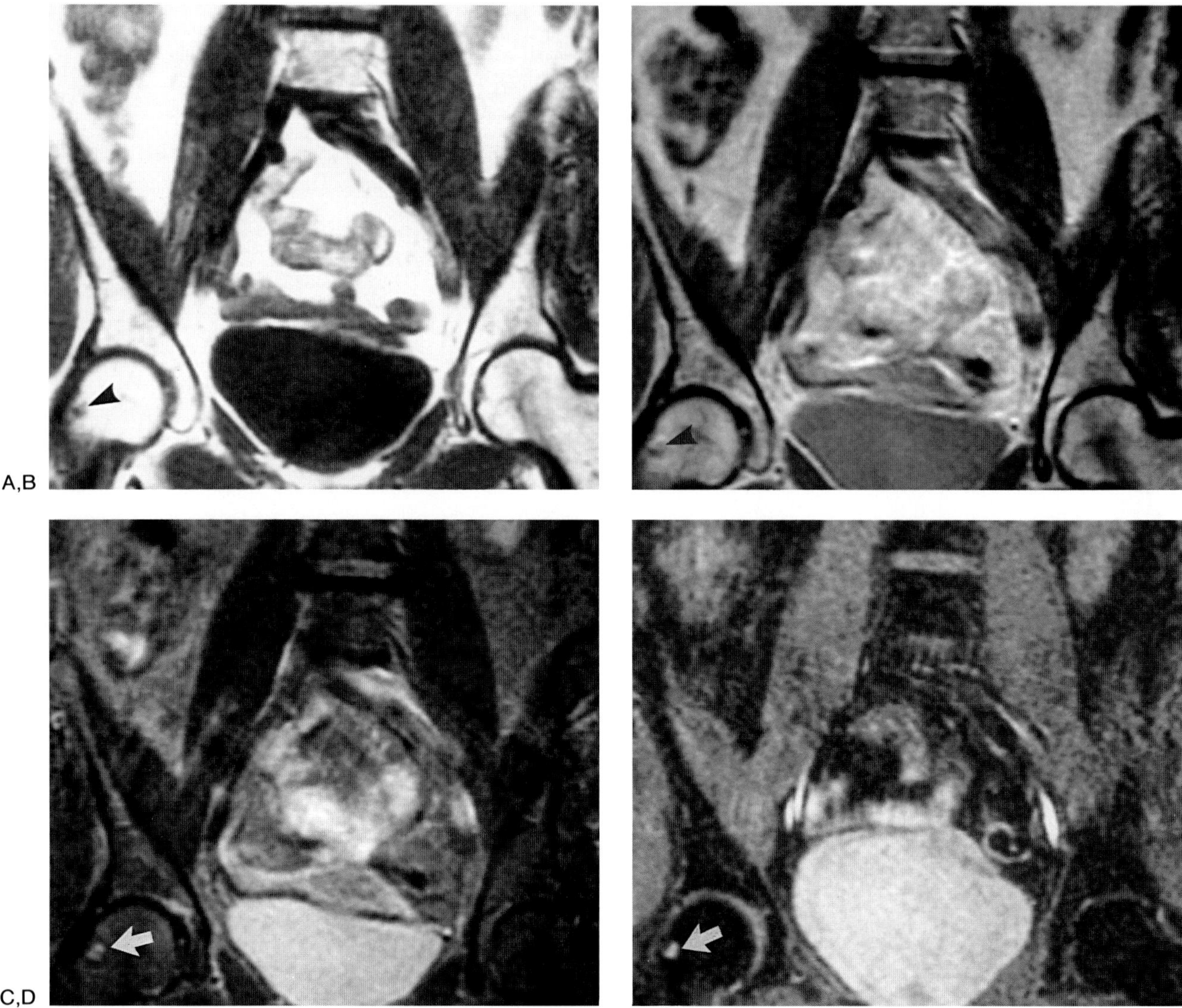

FIG. 12-3. Coronal images of the pelvis and hips using SE 500/20 (**A**), SE 2,000/30 (**B**), SE 2,000/60 (**C**), and STIR (**D**) images. The small cystic defect (*arrow*) in the right femoral neck is most obvious on the STIR sequence (**D**).

echo sequences. Edelman et al. (43) described a two-dimensional FT technique using TE 10, TR 30, flip angle of 20°–30°, and 5 mm thick slices. Presaturation pulses were used to suppress signal from incoming spins. These workers felt this method was superior to three-dimensional techniques in determining flow direction, differentiating arteries from veins, and defining normal and tumor vessels. Though many techniques are currently being evaluated, it is apparent that angiographic techniques will be valuable in MRI of neoplasms in the future.

SKELETAL NEOPLASMS

MRI can provide valuable information on primary benign and malignant bone lesions as well as skeletal metastasis (12,14,124). However, the proper categorization of lesions requires clinical data (patient's age, location of suspected lesion, onset of symptoms, etc.) and review of routine radiographs (Table 12-1). Routine radiographs are still extremely valuable in characterizing most skeletal neoplasms (12,112,130). In many cases, if a lesion has characteristic benign features, further imaging studies are not needed (12,31,130).

Benign Bone Neoplasms

Table 12-1 summarizes common benign bone neoplasms and lesions that may mimic neoplasms. Most benign lesions can be identified and characterized using routine radiography. However, when soft tissue and/or articular involvement is suspected or when the lesion is

TABLE 12-1. *Common benign skeletal neoplasms or neoplasm-like conditions (in order of decreasing frequency)* (34)

Lesion	Common locations	Age ranges
Osteochondroma	Femur, humerus, tibia, pelvis	10–40
Fibrous dysplasia	Skull, face, ribs, femur	10–30
Giant cell tumor	Femur, tibia, radius, sacrum	20–50 (after growth plate closure)
Osteoid osteoma	Femur, tibia, vertebrae	5–24
Aneurysmal bone cyst	Vertebrae, pelvis, tibia	10–20
Chondroma	Hand, femur, humerus, foot	10–40
Simple bone cyst	Humerus, femur, tibia	5–20
Fibrous defect	Femur, tibia	5–25
Hemangioma	Skull, vertebrae, femur	20–70
Chondroblastoma	Femur, humerus, tibia, pelvis	20–30
Osteoblastoma	Vertebrae, femur, tibia	20–40
Chondromyxoid fibroma	Tibia, femur, pelvis	20–30

not classically benign, MRI or CT may be useful before surgical resection is considered (12,112). Generally, MRI is most useful in detecting soft tissue extension. Soft tissue contrast is superior to that of CT and there is no beam hardening artifact using MR so the juxtacortical tissues can be identified more easily (Fig. 12-4) (12,80,137). The extent of neurovascular and medullary bone involvement is also more clearly demonstrated using multiplanar MRI. However, calcification and subtle cortical changes, especially in bones with little marrow such as the scapula and fibula or wing of the ilium, may be evaluated more easily with computed tomography (Fig. 12-5) (12,76,112). In addition, MRI or CT should also be considered when patients with benign lesions have symptoms that are suggestive of malignant degeneration (78). This can occur with osteochondromas, bone infarcts, and Paget's disease (12,34,70,96).

Although MRI is not commonly used to evaluate typically benign lesions, there have been several articles in the literature that describe characteristic MRI features of osteochondromas, chondromas, aneurysmal bone cysts, and fibrous defects (70,95,96,127,129).

Grossly, aneurysmal bone cysts contain cavernous anastomosing spaces filled with unclotted blood. It is not unusual to have fibrous or granular zones intermixed with the blood in these spaces (34). These histologic changes account for the variety of MRI appearances described in the literature.

Aneurysmal bone cysts are surrounded by a bony shell of variable thickness, which is seen as a well-marginated low-intensity rim on T1 and T2 weighted MR images (Fig. 12-6). The signal intensity of the lesion is usually increased on T2 weighted sequences and slightly greater than muscle intensity on T1 weighted sequences

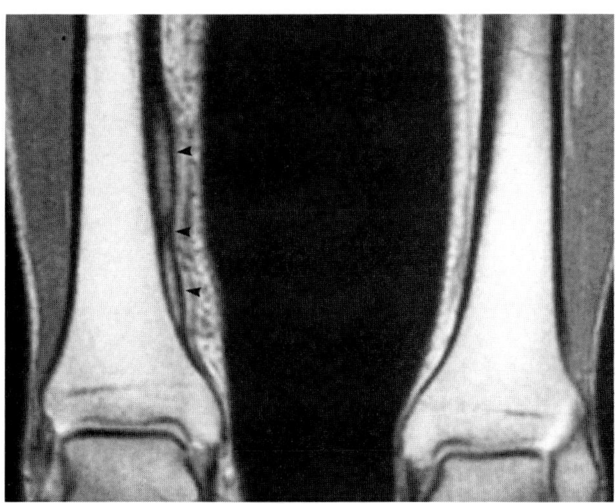

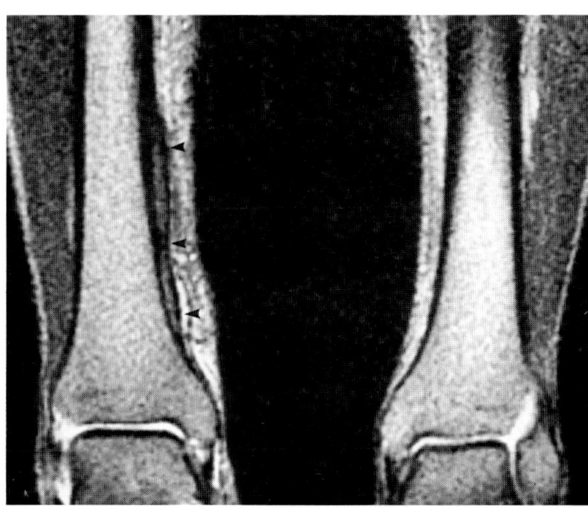

A,B

FIG. 12-4. Patient with leg pain and periosteal changes radiographically. Coronal SE 500/20 (**A**) and SE 2,000/60 (**B**) images demonstrate benign periosteal thickening (*arrowheads*) with no marrow or soft tissue mass.

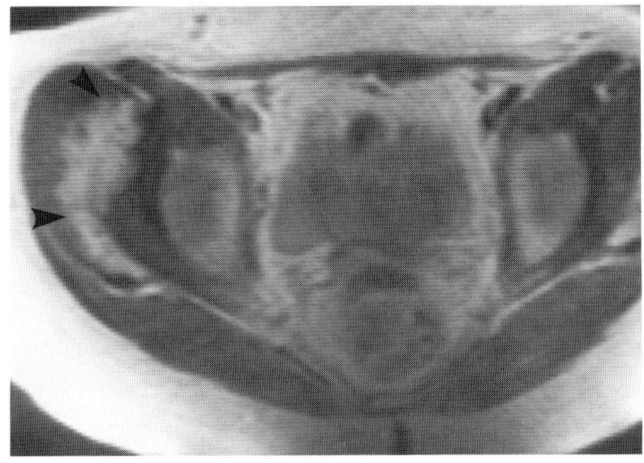

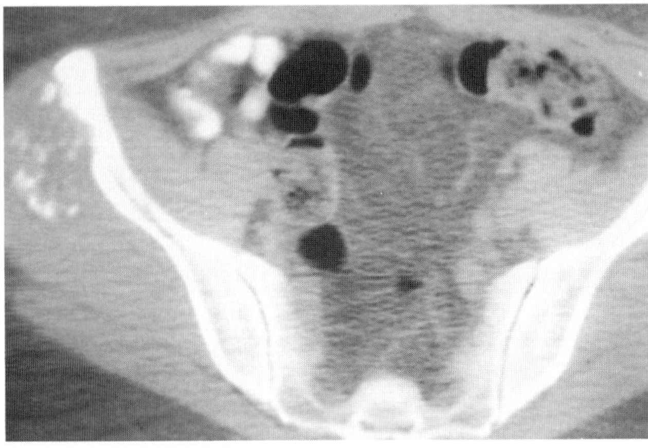

A,B

FIG. 12-5. Chondrosarcoma of the ilium. The MR image (SE 2,000/30) (**A**) clearly demonstrates the mass (*arrowheads*). However, CT image (**B**) demonstrates the soft tissue calcification, permitting more accurate tissue characterization. (From ref. 12, with permission.)

due to blood (138). Areas of solid tissue have intermediate intensity and can give the lesion an inhomogeneous appearance similar to malignancy (Fig. 12-7). Fluid-fluid levels have also been described (8,62,63). However, these changes are not specific and have been described with giant cell tumors, chondroblastomas, and telangiectatic osteosarcomas (65).

Fibrous defects and fibrous dysplasia are commonly encountered during interpretation of radiographs (Fig. 12-8). Similarly, these lesions may be identified with MRI. Although MRI features have been described, the variability in appearance can cause confusion if radiographs are not available for comparison (12).

Fibrous lesions are usually composed of dense fibrous tissue, which gives the lesion a muscle density on T1 weighted images and intermediate signal intensity or low intensity on T2 weighted images (95,127). Cystic areas are not uncommon (34). This can create an inhomogeneous lesion. Cystic areas are bright on T2 weighted sequences and low intensity on T1 weighted sequences. The margins of fibrous lesion tend to enhance after gadolinium-DTPA injection (95).

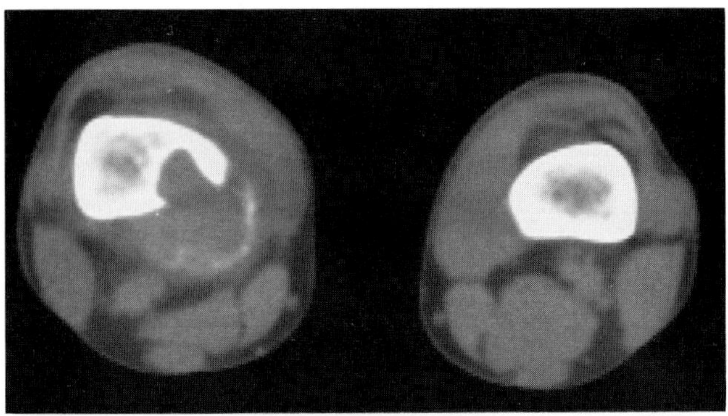

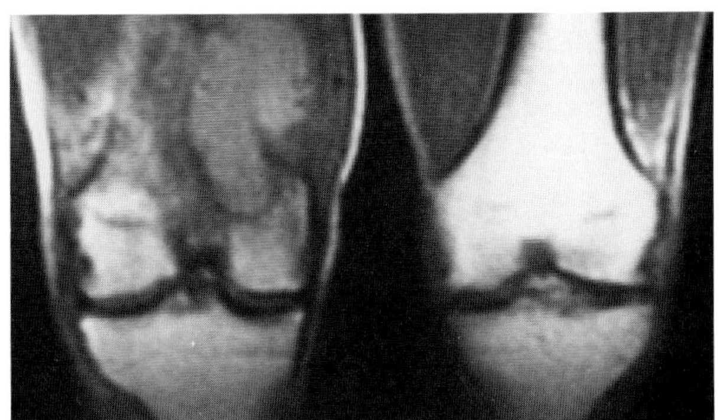

A,B

C

FIG. 12-6. Aneurysmal bone cyst. Axial CT image (**A**) shows a well-marginated defect in the femur with a rim of calcification at the periphery of the soft tissue component. Coronal SE 500/20 (**B**) image and axial SE 2,000/60 (**C**) image show a well-defined margin with signal intensity slightly greater than muscle on the T1 weighted image (**B**) and high intensity (>fat) on the T2 weighted image (**C**). Calcification is more easily appreciated with CT. (From ref. 138, with permission.)

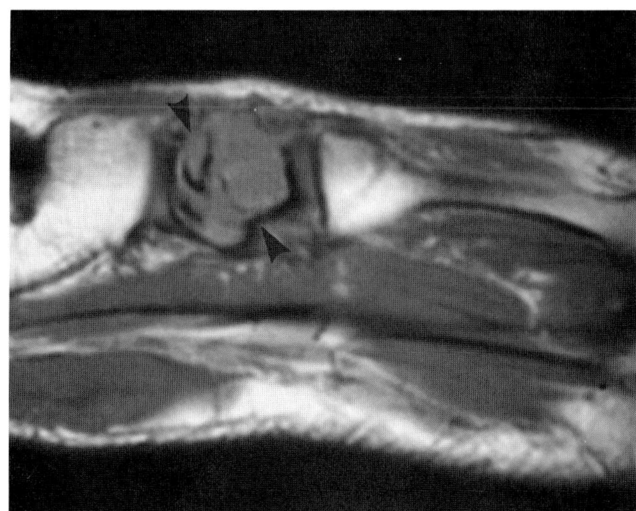

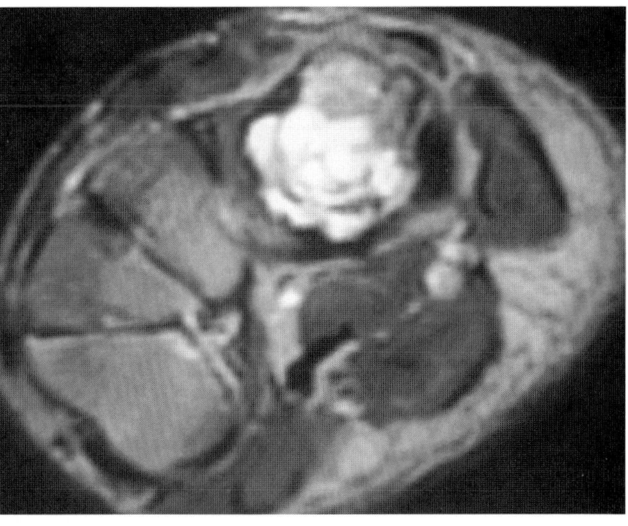

A,B

FIG. 12-7. Tarsal aneurysmal bone cyst. Sagittal SE 500/20 image (**A**) shows an irregular mass (*arrowheads*) in the bone with signal intensity slightly greater than muscle. Axial SE 2,000/60 image (**B**) shows an inhomogeneous high signal intensity lesion. The diagnosis of ABC could not be made based on these MR image features alone.

Osteochondromas are the most frequent benign bone tumors, comprising 35.8% of benign lesions in the Dahlin–Unni series (34). The lesions are usually asymptomatic but can cause neurovascular compression and rarely (1% solitary, 5+% multiple) become malignant (34,70). Routine radiographs and CT have a typical appearance so MRI is rarely indicated (Fig. 12-9). However, symptomatic lesions can effectively be evaluated with MRI. MRI can clearly demonstrate the signal intensity and thickness of the cartilaginous cap and perichondrium.

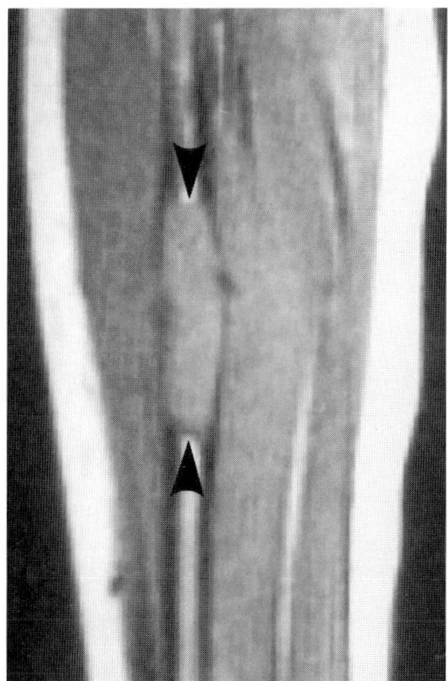

FIG. 12-8. Coronal SE 2,000/30 image of a fibular fibrous defect (*arrowheads*). The lesion is well marginated and similar in signal intensity to muscle.

The value of increased signal intensity in the cartilaginous cap in differentiating benign lesions from low-grade malignancy is controversial (Fig. 12-10). Also, neurovascular involvement is clearly defined using MRI (12,70). Although the thickness of the cap is controversial, some authors feel a cap measuring greater than 3 cm suggests chondrosarcoma (70). Incomplete resection of these structures can result in recurrence.

Chondromas (Fig. 12-11) or enchondromas have typical radiographic features. Therefore, MRI is rarely indicated except in patients with Maffucci's syndrome, where hemangiomas are associated and the incidence of malignant degeneration of the chondroma can exceed 50% (125).

Osteoid osteomas can be difficult to diagnose. Tomography, radionuclide scans, and CT have been most useful. MRI can also detect these lesions. However, if one is not familiar with their appearance, the lesion can easily be overlooked or misdiagnosed (12,134). The reactive change (sclerosis on radiographs) is demonstrated as low intensity on both T1 and T2 weighted sequences (Fig. 12-12). The nidus may be invisible on T1 weighted images but usually is demonstrated as a focal area of high signal intensity on T2 weighted spin-echo or T2* gradient-echo sequences. Comparison of MRI images with radiographs is essential with osteoid osteomas and other bone neoplasms (10).

Malignant Bone Neoplasms

Most malignant bone tumors are inhomogeneous on both T1 and T2 weighted sequences (12,17,18,50,52). The degree of inhomogeneity and signal intensity varies

Text continues on p. 446

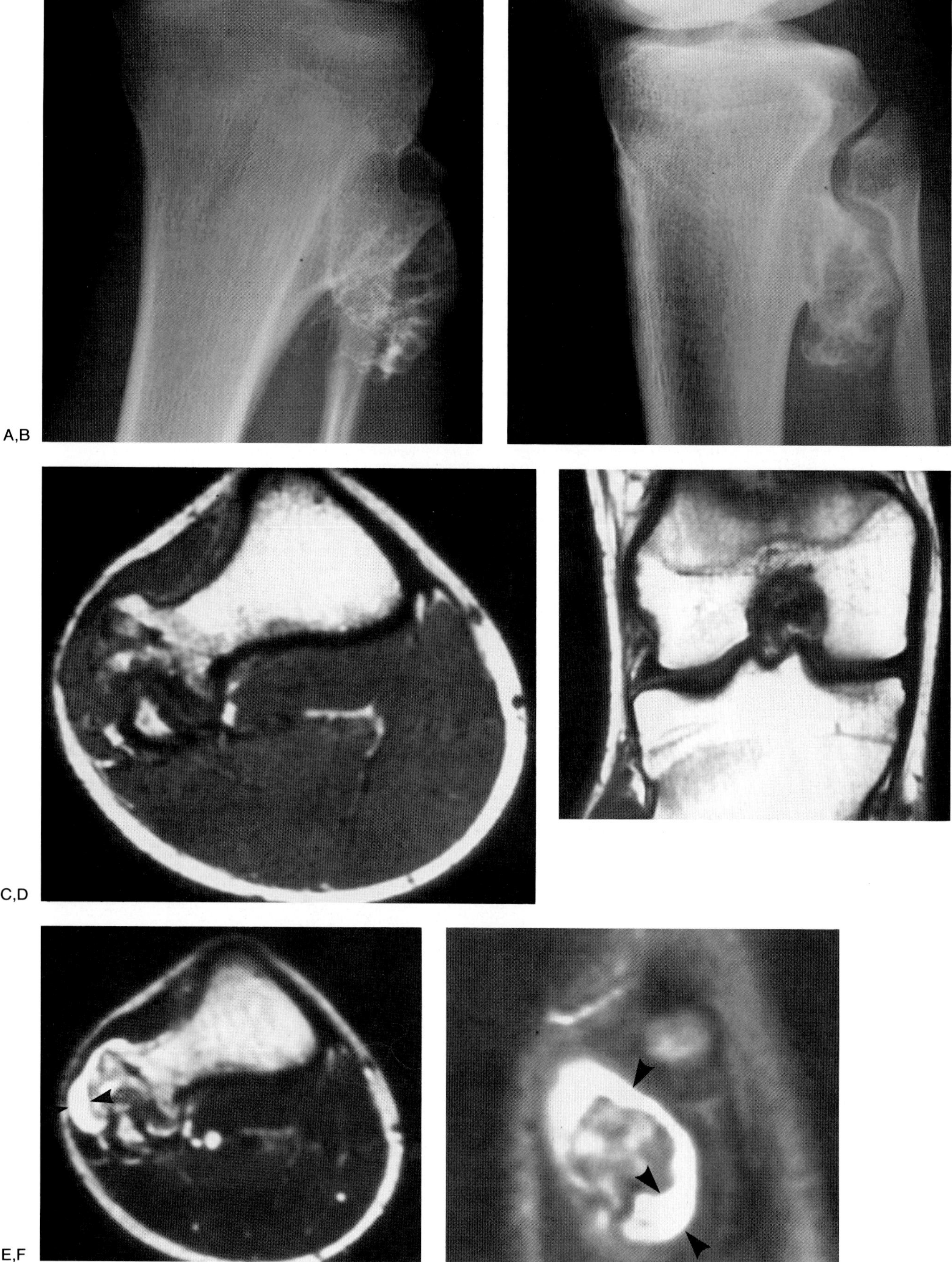

FIG. 12-9. Osteochondroma. AP (**A**) and oblique (**B**) radiographs of a classical osteochondroma. The patient was experiencing pain with a palpable mass. Axial (**C**) and coronal (**D**) SE 500/20 images demonstrate the osseous portion of the lesion but the cap is difficult to define. Axial (**E**) and sagittal (**F**) SE 2,000/60 images more clearly demonstrate the cap (*arrowheads*). Pain was due to peroneal nerve compression.

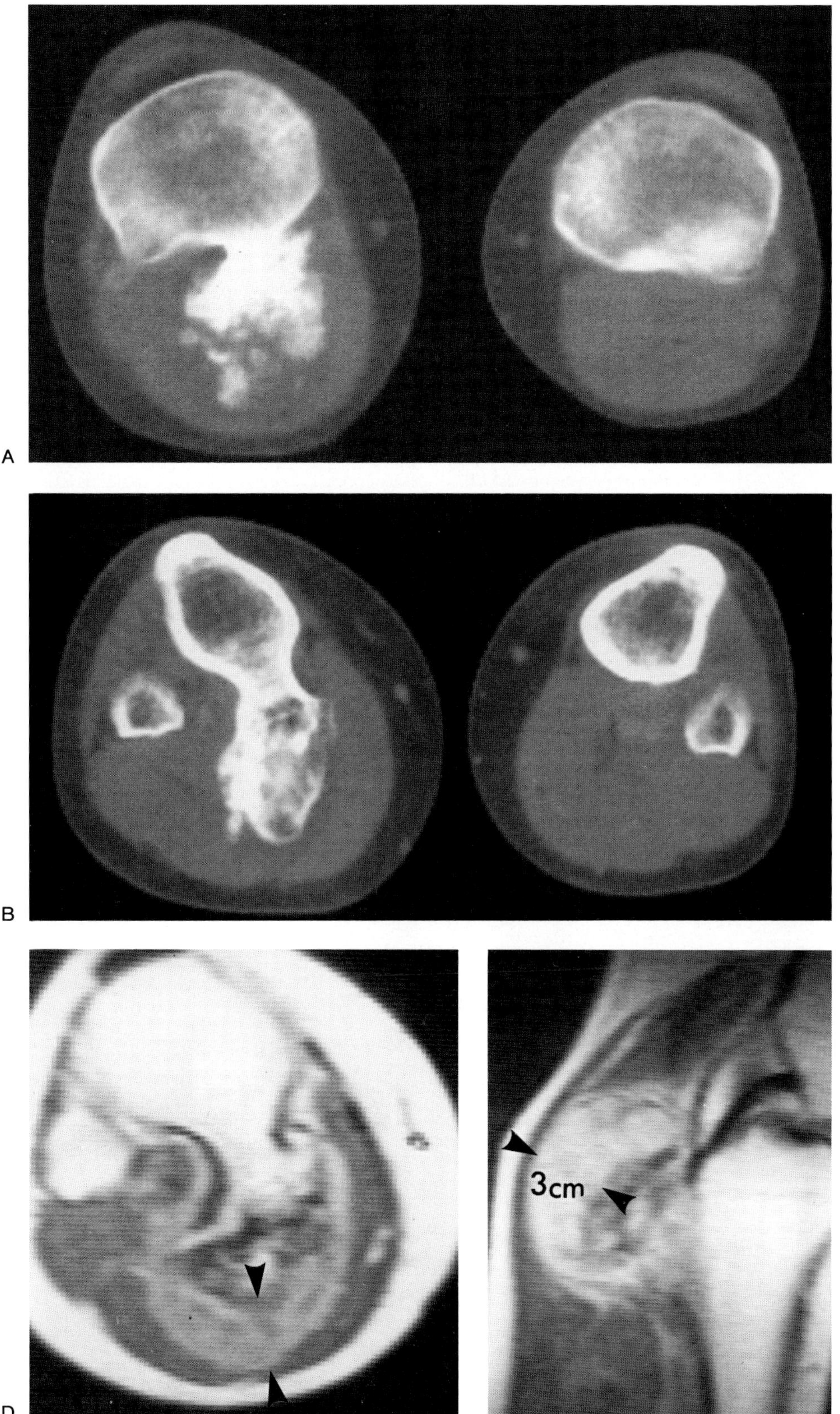

FIG. 12-10. CT images (**A,B**) of a right upper tibial osteochondroma. Axial (**C**) and sagittal (**D**) MR images show a thick cap (3 cm) (*arrowheads*) with signal intensity lower than demonstrated in Fig. 12-9. Histologically this patient had a grade 1 chondrosarcoma.

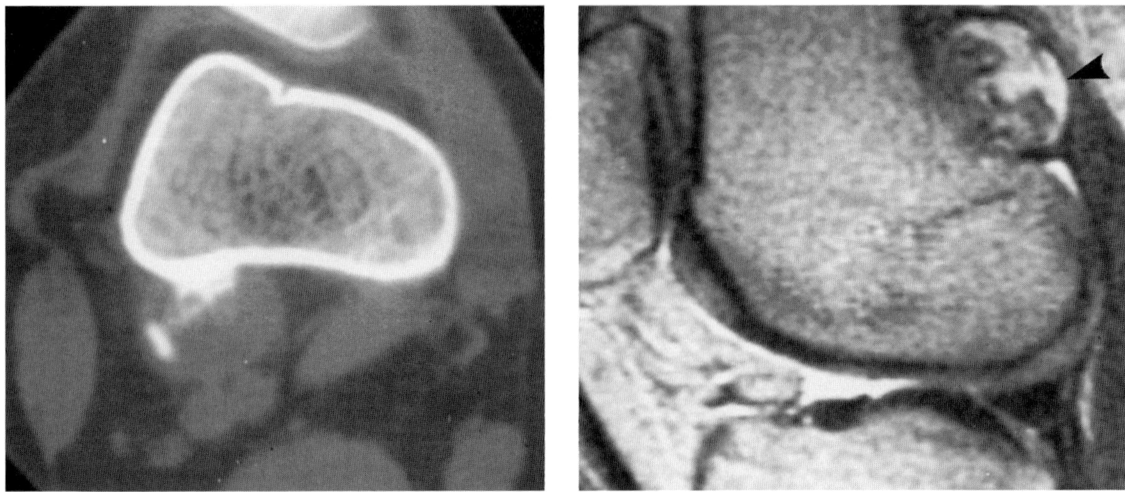

A,B

FIG. 12-11. Periosteal chondroma. CT scan (**A**) demonstrates a partially ossified soft tissue mass arising from the posterior femoral cortex. Sagittal SE 200/60 MR image (**B**) shows that the lesion is contiguous with bone and has a cartilaginous cap (*arrowhead*) similar to an osteochondroma.

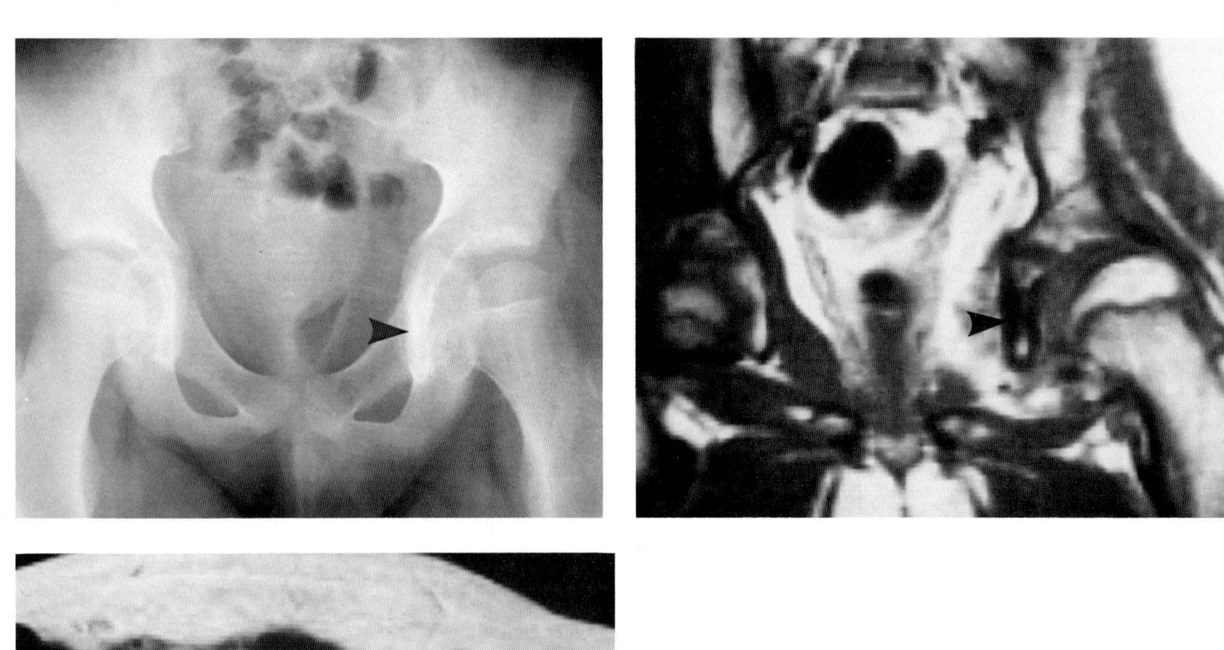

A,B

C

FIG. 12-12. Osteoid osteoma. AP radiograph of the pelvis (**A**) shows joint space widening and sclerosis of the medial acetabulum (*arrowhead*). SE 500/20 coronal (**B**) and axial (**C**) images show a low-intensity nidus medially (*arrowhead*) with synovial hypertrophy (*small arrowheads*).

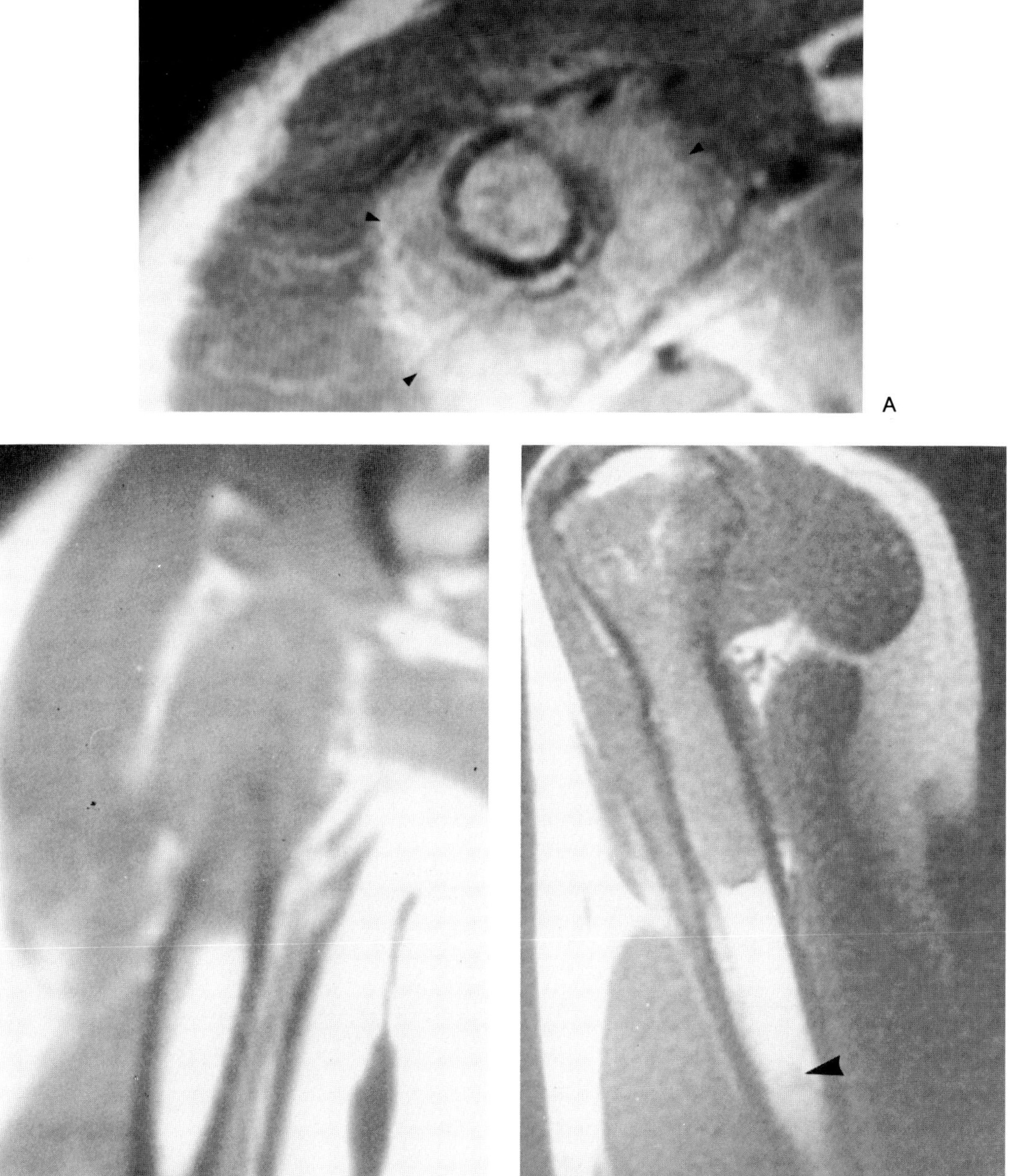

FIG. 12-13. Ewing's sarcoma of the humerus. Axial image (**A**) (SE 2,000/30) shows the soft tissue mass (*arrowheads*) and marrow change. Coronal SE 500/20 image (**B**) does not clearly demonstrate the extent of marrow involvement. Oblique sagittal SE 500/20 image (**C**) shows the extent of marrow involvement plus a distal skip lesion (*arrowhead*). (From ref. 12, with permission.)

TABLE 12-2. *Common 1° malignant skeletal lesions* (34)

Lesion	Location	Age	Gross pathologic histology	Image features
Osteosarcoma	Tibia, femur, humerus	15–35	Cortical destruction may encircle bone	Signal ↑T2WI[a]
			Periosteal evaluation	Signal ↓T2WI at margin, signal ↓T1WI[b]
			Marrow involvement with skip lesions in some cases	
			Osteosclerotic zones	Signals ↓T1WI and ↓T2WI
				Signals ↓T2WI and ↓T1WI
			Necrosis	
Ewing's sarcoma	Pelvis, femur, tibia	5–25	Long areas of marrow involvement	Signals ↑T2WI and ↓T1WI
			Necrosis and cyst formation	Signals ↑T2WI and ↓T1WI
			Hemorrhage	Signals ↑T2WI and ↑T1WI
Chondrosarcoma	Trunk, shoulder, humerus, femur	>40	Lobulated central marrow or peripheral and lobulated margin	Signals ↑T2WI and ↓T1WI
			Irregular calcification	Signals ↓T1WI and ↓T2WI
				T2WI, mucoid > hyaline
			Hyaline to mucoid matrix	
Fibrosarcoma	Tibia, femur Pelvis	20s–60s	Firm fibrous tissue	Intermediate signal T2WI
				T2WI and T1WI
			Necrosis and hemorrhage	Signal ↑T2W1 and ↓T1W1

[a] Signal T2WI, T2 weighted image.
[b] Signal T1WI, T1 weighted image.

with the type of tumor matrix (chondroid, osteoid, or fibrous) and the presence of hemorrhage and/or necrosis. Table 12-2 summarizes several of the more common malignant bone neoplasms and their histologic and therefore MRI features. It is evident from this small summary of four of the primary bone neoplasms that the histologic appearance, although it correlates to some degree with MRI findings, is not a useful feature for differentiating the various types of skeletal neoplasm. Characterizing lesions is much more easily accomplished with soft tissue masses. Therefore, the main value of MRI for primary skeletal bone tumors is to evaluate the extent of marrow and soft tissue involvement (12,17,50,52,112,137). Neurovascular displacement or encasement can also be evaluated easily with MRI (12,137).

In most cases, T1 weighted sequences are best for determining the extent of marrow involvement. Keep in mind it is important to include the entire osseous structure (such as the humerus or tibia) as well as the adjacent joints in the field of view (Fig. 12-13). This is important in staging the lesion so that the entire extent of marrow involvement and soft tissue involvement can be identified along with any potential skip lesions. Because of the improved contrast, T2 weighted sequences are more useful in evaluating cortical bone and juxtacortical soft tissue involvement (Fig. 12-14). MRI is also useful for evaluating periosteal changes and involvement of unossified epiphyseal bone (50,80). Lamellar periosteal reaction has low signal intensity on both T1 and T2 weighted sequences. More aggressive periosteal changes will have areas of increased signal intensity on T2 weighted sequences. This finding can be useful in characterizing the lesion (80).

Although calcification or areas of ossification within

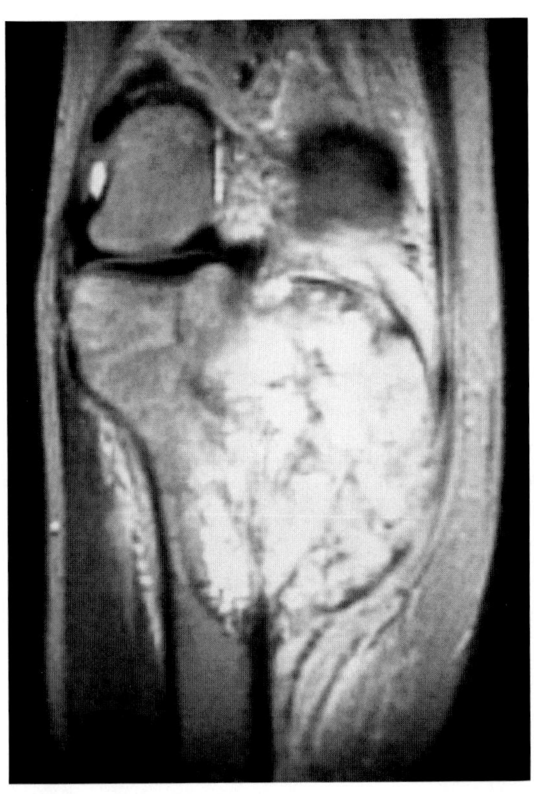

FIG. 12-14. Osteosarcoma. SE 2,000/60 image of the tibia, demonstrating an inhomogeneous high signal intensity tumor extending into the soft tissues.

neoplasms can be seen with MRI (low signal on both T1 and T2 weighted sequences), most imagers are more comfortable with identification of calcification and ossification on CT (112,119). Therefore, when these changes are evident on a routine radiograph, especially when a flat bone such as the ilium, fibula, or scapula is in question, CT might be preferred to MRI (12,119). In either case, it is important to compare radiographic findings with MRI findings to more thoroughly evaluate and characterize these neoplasms.

SOFT TISSUE NEOPLASMS

MRI has become the technique of choice for evaluation and characterization of soft tissue masses (12,15,16,23,35,81,114,123,131). Unlike skeletal neoplasms, in many cases the nature of the lesion can clearly be predicted by the morphologic features noted on MR examinations (15).

Benign Soft Tissue Neoplasms

Benign soft tissue masses are usually well marginated, have homogeneous signal intensity, and do not encase neurovascular structures or invade bone (12,115). T1 and T2 relaxation times of benign lesions overlap considerably with those of malignant lesions and thus have not been found to be useful in characterizing or predicting the histologic nature of these tumors (91). The identification of edema around lesions is controversial in differentiating benign from malignant masses. Beltran et al. (9) described edema around 13/25 malignant lesions compared to 9/25 benign masses. Others have reported edema more frequently with abscesses, hematomas, and vascular occlusion (58). However, the above imaging criteria (homogeneous signal intensity, well marginated, no neurovascular or osseous invasion) and rapidly expanding experience with MRI have allowed us to clearly define the nature of lesions, especially benign lesions, with significant frequency. In a recent blinded study (50 benign, 45 malignant lesions), we noted that observers correctly identified the histologic nature of benign lesions from 50 to 70% of the time. Lesions included benign neoplasms, hematomas, and abscesses. The accuracy for three observers (two relatively inexperienced, one experienced) was 87–95% in classifying the lesion as benign. The specificity among the three observers averaged 92% (15).

As experience has increased, we have gained considerable experience in the MRI appearance of several specific benign lesions (12,113,120). Lipomas are common benign soft tissue lesions that maintain a homogeneous high signal intensity (the same as subcutaneous fat) on both T1 and T2 weighted sequences (Fig. 12-15). These lesions are well marginated but may contain clearly defined fibrae septae (Fig. 12-16) (39,89). Occasionally, a small area of irregularity is noted as the tumor is distorted by adjacent muscle bundles. Liposarcoma should be considered when there are areas of inhomogeneity or significant irregularity of the margin is noted (12,72). Atypical lipomas in the extremities may cause confusion and are difficult to differentiate from low-grade liposarcomas (Fig. 12-17). Histologically, these lesions contain fat cells, multinucleated giant cells, and collagen bundles. Thus, the histology is not unlike a liposarcoma; however, atypical lipomas do not metastasize (20). From an imaging standpoint we should still describe such a lesion as potentially malignant since the image features, although different from a typical lipoma, do not allow us to differentiate low-grade liposarcoma and atypical lipomas (Figs. 12-18 to 12-20).

Benign cysts have high signal intensity on T2 weighted sequences and homogeneous low intensity on T1 weighted images (Fig. 12-21). These lesions are very distinct and well marginated, even when complicated by hemorrhage or infection (Fig. 12-22). When hemorrhage or infection has occurred, signal intensity of these

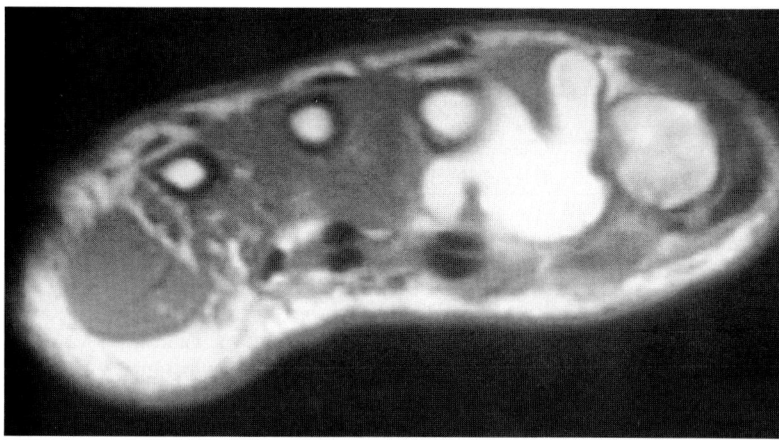

FIG. 12-15. Axial SE 500/20 image of the hand demonstrates a homogeneous lobulated lipoma between the first and second metacarpals.

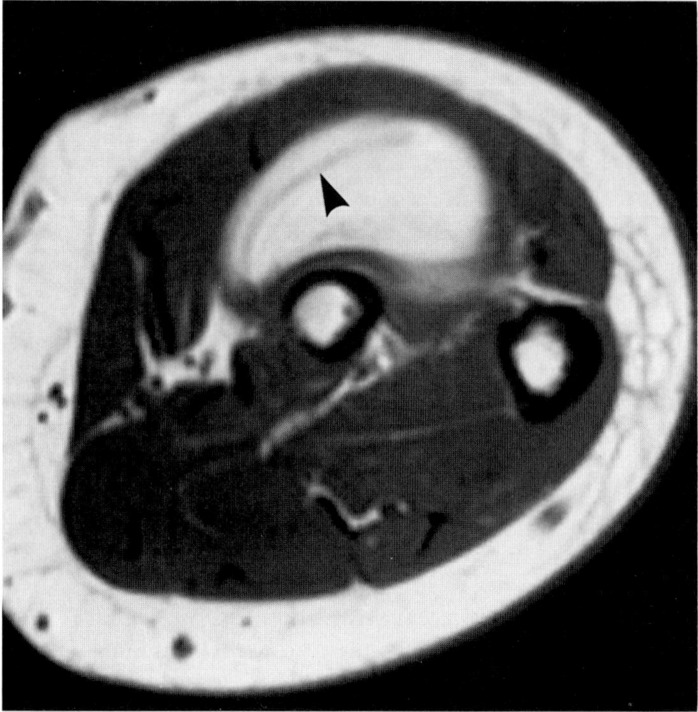
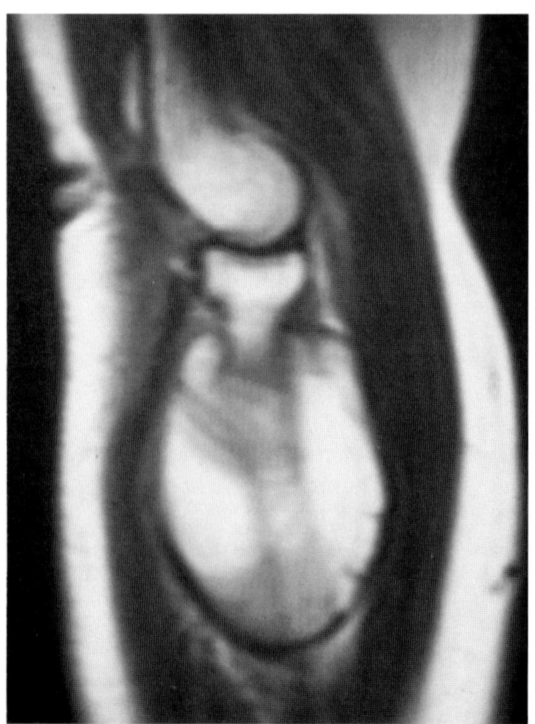

A,B

FIG. 12-16. Axial (**A**) and sagittal (**B**) SE 500/20 images demonstrating a typical lipoma with clearly defined (*arrowhead*) fibrous septae.

complicated cysts may be somewhat lower on T2 weighted sequences and slightly higher on T1 weighted sequences. In addition, cysts are typically associated with joints, which is an additional useful feature. The signal intensity of communicating articular cysts and ganglia does not differ significantly (19,47). Ganglia may be intraosseous, subperiosteal, or juxta-articular (47). Soft tissue ganglion cysts tend to occur in periarticular locations or along tendon sheaths. Most are smaller (1–4 cm) than popliteal cysts. Histologically, they are surrounded by a fibrous capsule with a fibroblastic lining, which simulates synovium. Fluid may be necrotic (high signal intensity on T2 weighted sequences) or mucoid and thick. In the latter case, the signal intensity may be somewhat decreased compared to synovial fluid. Location and image appearance generally permit a confident diagnosis of benign cyst or ganglion (12,47). A more complete discussion of cysts can be found in Chapters 7 and 11.

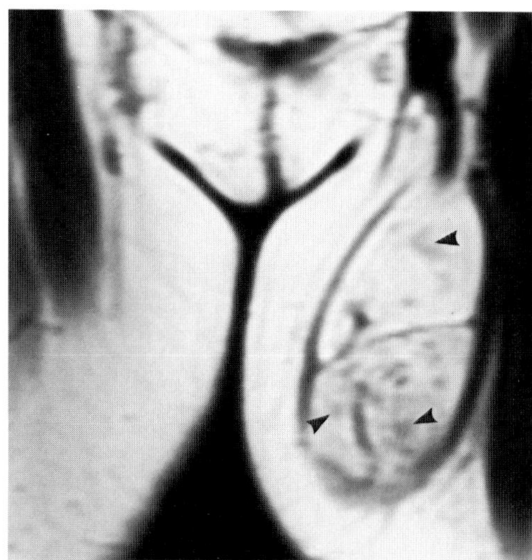

FIG. 12-17. Atypical lipoma of the thigh. Coronal SE 500/20 image shows a well-defined fat intensity mass with multiple low-intensity areas (*arrowheads*). Compare to Figs. 12-18 to 12-20.

Benign myxomas are uncommon, comprising only about 1% of all soft tissue tumors (45). These masses occur most frequently in older patients (40–70 years) and usually are slow growing and painless. The lesions occur most frequently in the shoulder, upper arm, buttock, and thighs. Histologically, myxomas are mucoid, largely avascular, and encapsulated (45). The MRI features are typically benign but also allow differentiation from other benign lesions such as lipomas. Myxomas are uniform intensity on both T1 and T2 weighted sequences (Fig. 12-23). Signal intensity is equal to or lower than muscle on T1 weighted and increased (>fat) on T2 weighted sequences (12,69).

Giant cell tumors of the tendon sheath also have MRI features that, along with location, can allow the diagnosis to be established (12,103). These lesions occur

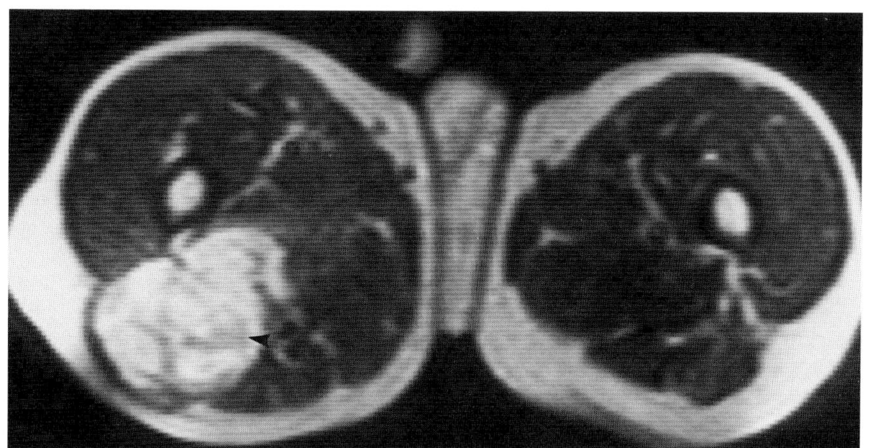
A

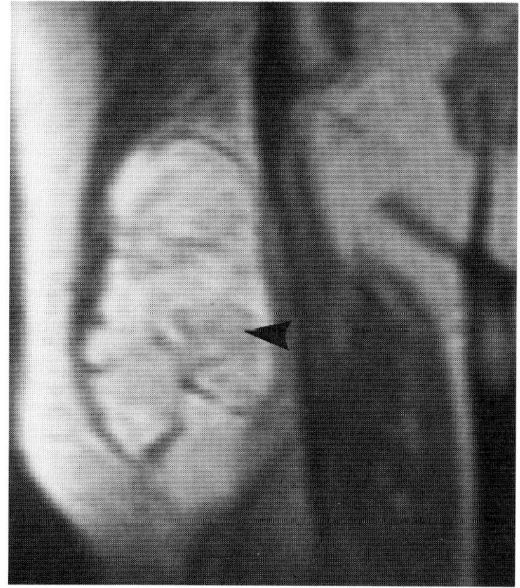
B

FIG. 12-18. Liposarcoma. Axial (**A**) and coronal (**B**) images demonstrate an inhomogeneous fatty tumor (*arrowheads*).

A

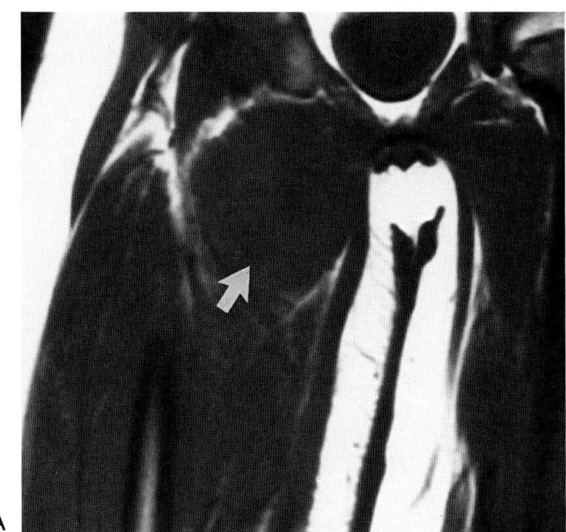

B

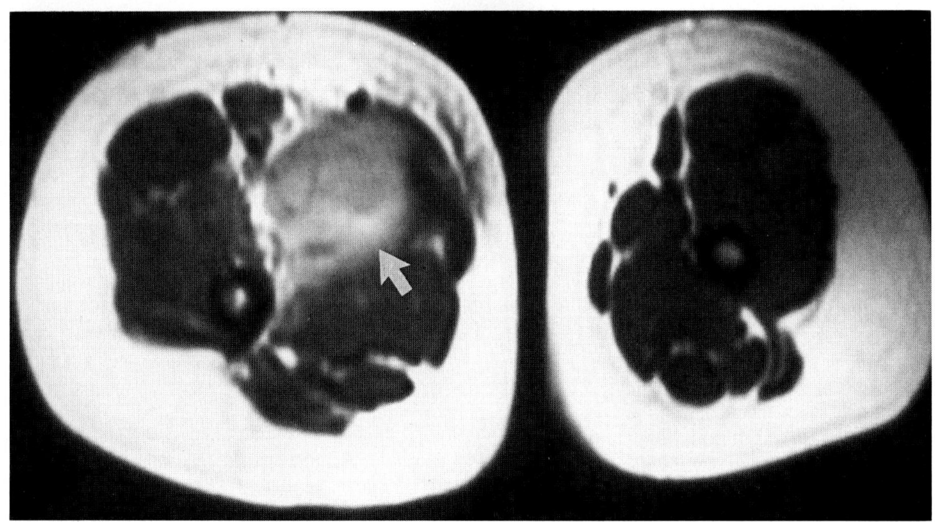

FIG. 12-19. Liposarcoma. Coronal SE 500/20 image (**A**) shows a large muscle intensity mass. Axial SE 2,000/30 image (**B**) shows an inhomogeneous mass with lower intensity than fat. There is very little fatty tissue in this mass.

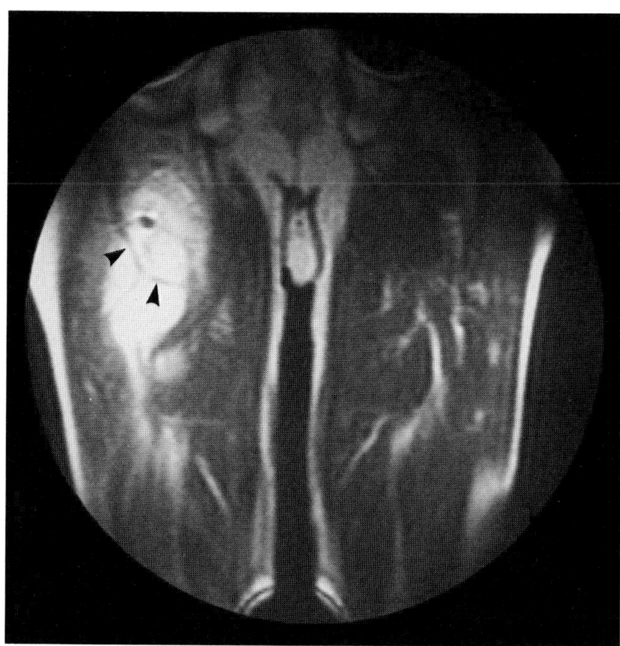

FIG. 12-20. Liposarcoma. Coronal SE 500/20 image shows a poorly marginated fatty mass encasing vascular structures (*arrowheads*).

along tendon sheaths and are composed of proliferating histocytes, giant cells, fibrous stroma, hemosiderin deposition, and foam-laden macrophages (45,103). The lesions are well marginated and signal intensity is decreased on T2 weighted sequences either diffusely or in scattered areas depending on the size of the lesion and hemosiderin deposition (Fig. 12-24) (103).

Most other benign lesions excluding lipomas are also well marginated and homogeneous with high signal intensity on T2 weighted sequences and low signal intensity on T1 weighted sequences (Fig. 12-25).

There are two notable exceptions to this rule concerning the morphologic appearance of benign lesions. Hemangiomas and other vascular malformations are often irregular, have mixed signal intensity, and may be extensive. Numerous vessels are usually obvious and when the MRI data are combined with the clinical data, the diagnosis is usually obvious (Fig. 12-26) (12,15, 26,28). Hemangiomas are typically divided into capillary and cavernous categories (45). The former have numerous small capillary-like vessels, whereas the cavernous variety contain large sinusoids filled with blood. Lesions are most common in the skin and subcutaneous tissues. However, hemangiomas are also common in the muscles of the peripheral extremities (12,26,45). Mixed vascular lesions such as angiolipoma can be somewhat confusing (Fig. 12-27). However, again the appearance of numerous serpiginous vessels usually allows diagnosis to be made with confidence. High signal intensity (blood) on both T1 and T2 weighted sequences is common (115,135). Local muscle atrophy has also been described (135). Differentiation of veins, arteries, and dilated lymphatic vessels is not always possible. However, newer GRASS imaging techniques and angiographic software packages allow the vascular nature of these lesions to be defined more clearly (Fig. 12-28). In some cases, selective angiography may still be necessary to identify feeding arteries and draining veins in arteriovenous malformations (12,15).

Desmoid tumors are aggressive, often hypocellular fibrous lesions (12,97,117). The margins are frequently irregular and the signal intensity is generally inhomogeneous. These lesions have a typically malignant appearance and are very aggressive clinically, resulting in extensive surgery for removal and frequent recurrence (Fig. 12-29). Sixty-eight percent recur after initial therapy. Recurrence is most common in females, in patients over 30 years of age, when lesions are noted in the foot or calf, and when marginal excisions were performed (97). A useful feature in identifying desmoid tumor is the significant amount of hypocellular or fibrous tissue that is evident within these lesions. This tissue has low or no signal intensity on both T1 and T2 weighted sequences (12,117). Demonstration of an irregular, inho-

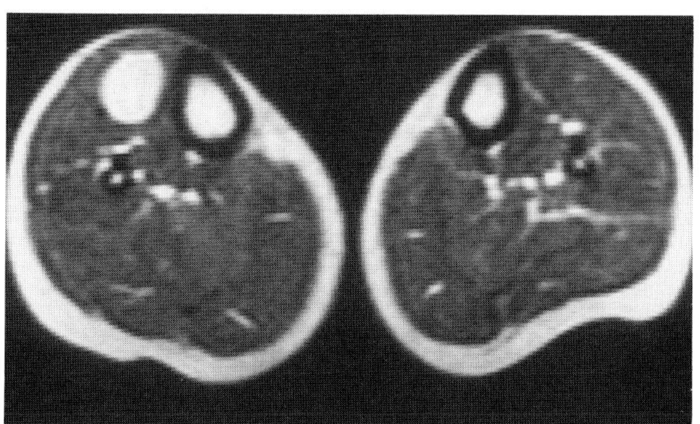

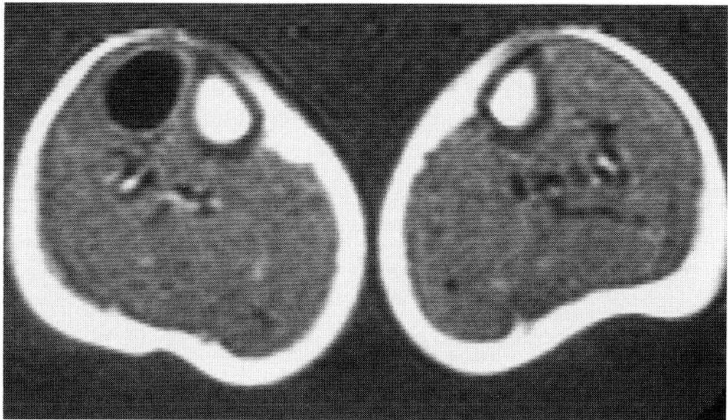

A,B

FIG. 12-21. Benign cyst. Axial T2 (**A**) and T1 (inversion recovery) (**B**) images of the leg show homogeneous high signal intensity on the T2 weighted image and low intensity on the T1 weighted image.

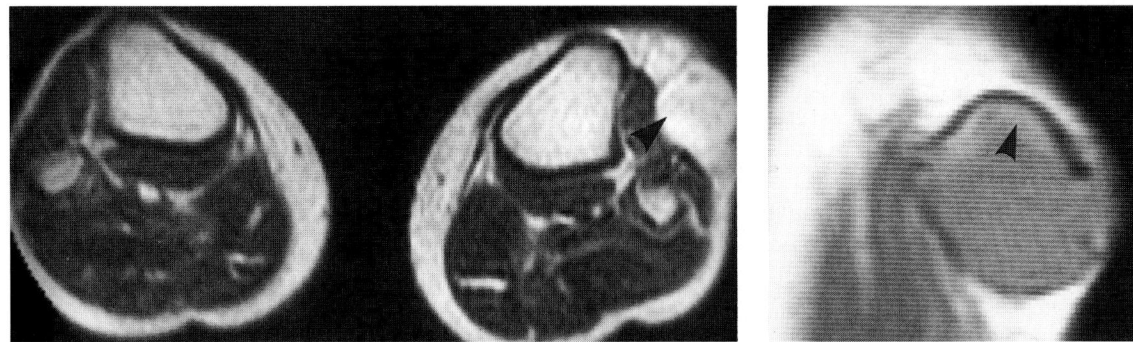

FIG. 12-22. Cyst with hemorrhage. Axial SE 2,000/60 image (**A**) shows a mass of intermediate intensity (*arrowhead*). Sagittal SE 500/20 image (**B**) shows a muscle intensity lesion with hemorrhage (*arrowhead*) near the margin.

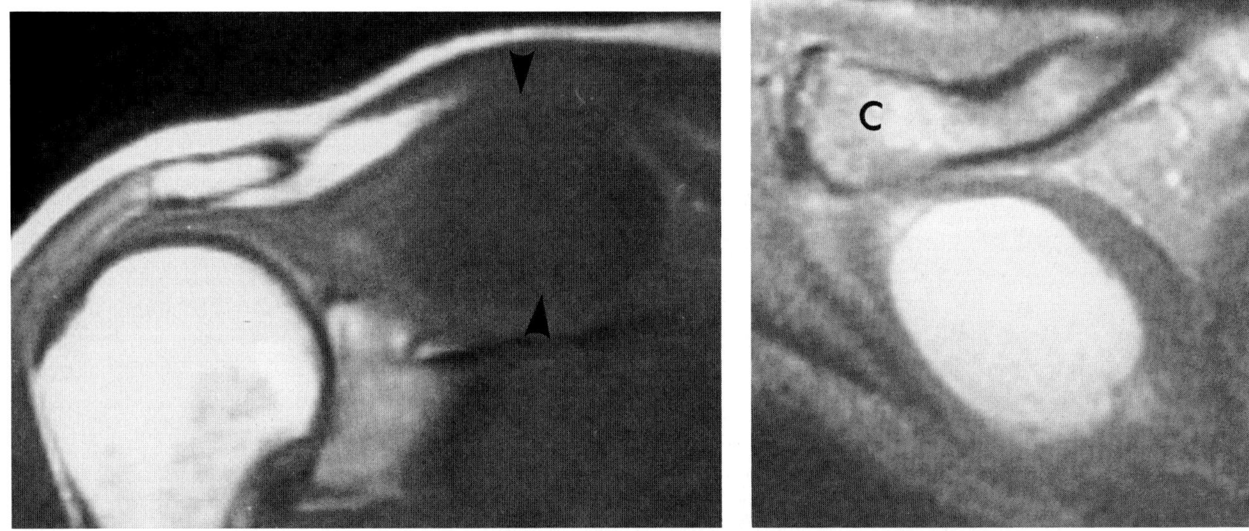

FIG. 12-23. Myxoma. Coronal SE 500/20 image (**A**) shows a homogeneous low-intensity (<muscle) mass (*arrowheads*) in the supraspinatus. Axial SE 2,000/60 image (**B**) shows the lesion to be homogeneous and high signal intensity (C, clavicle). (From ref. 12, with permission.)

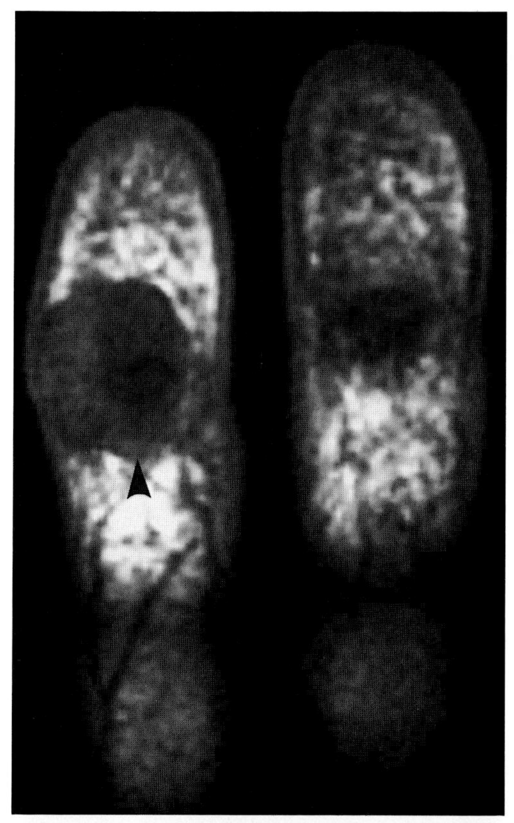

A

FIG. 12-24. Giant cell tumor of the tendon sheath. Coronal (**A**) and sagittal (**B**) SE 500/20 images show a low-intensity lesion (*arrowheads*) beginning along the flexor tendon and extending dorsally. Axial SE 2,000/60 image (**C**) shows the lesion (*arrows*) to be low intensity due to hemosiderin deposition.

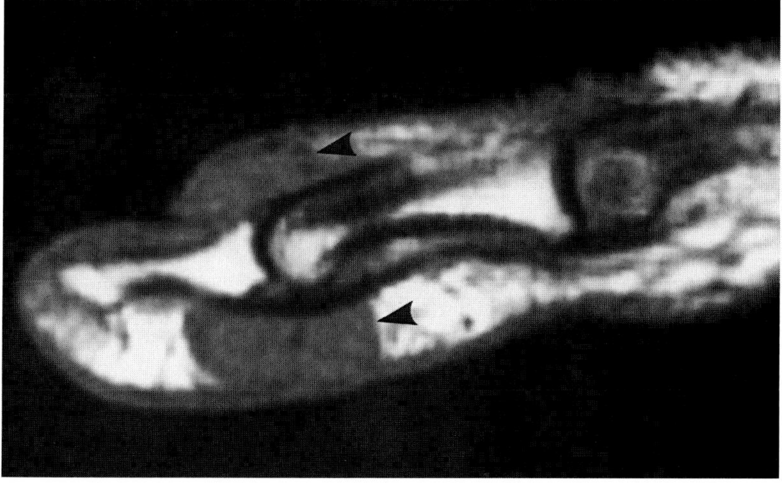

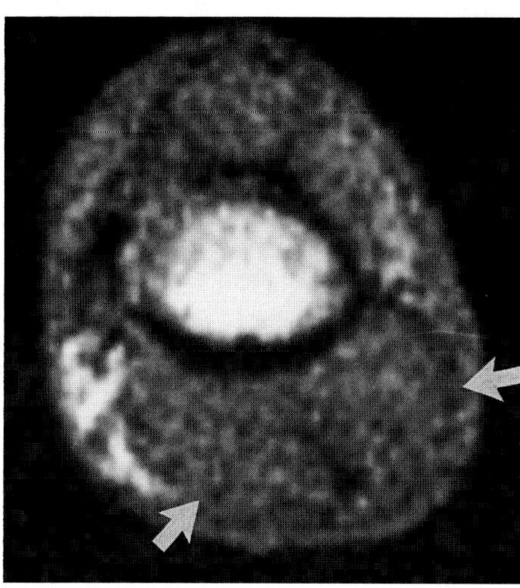

B,C

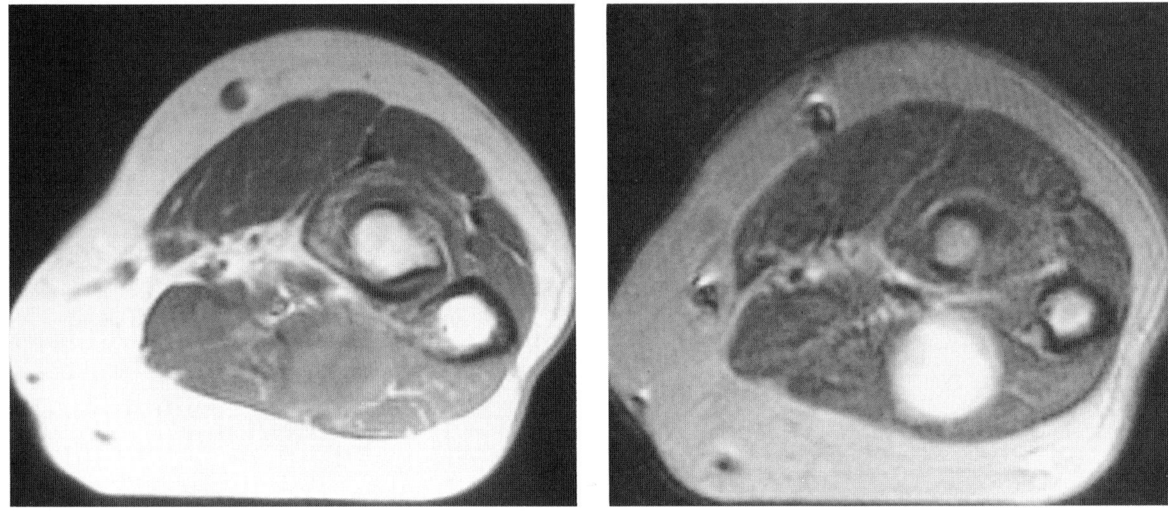

FIG. 12-25. Benign neuroma. SE 500/20 (**A**) and SE 2,000/30 (**B**) axial images show the typical appearance of a benign neuroma: well-marginated, high-intensity lesion on T2 and muscle intensity on T1 weighted sequences.

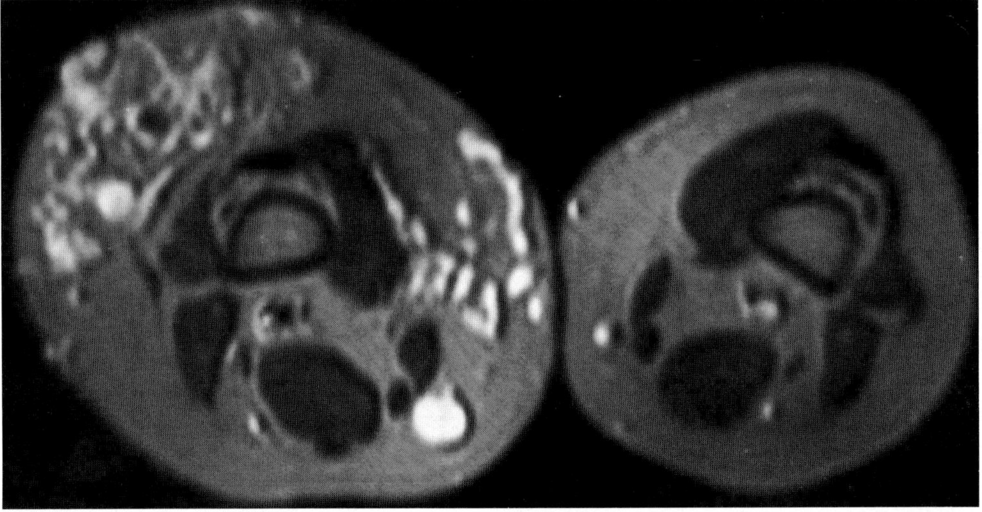

FIG. 12-26. Axial SE 2,000/60 image of the thighs, demonstrating an extensive hemangioma in the right thigh.

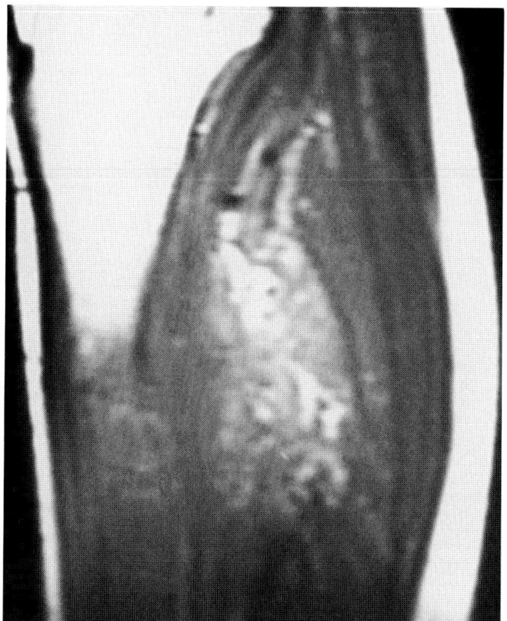

FIG. 12-27. Sagittal image of the calf, demonstrating a hemangioma with fatty tissue within and at the periphery of the lesion.

mogeneous lesion with significant scar tissue is typical in primary and recurrent desmoid tumors (Fig. 12-30). MRI is a useful technique for following these patients. Lesions can clearly be identified and size and other morphologic features monitored. Most surgeons will not reoperate if the lesion is not increasing in size (97).

Malignant Soft Tissue Neoplasms

Most malignant soft tissue tumors are irregular at least along a portion of their margin (Fig. 12-31) (12,15). Eighty-five percent of malignant lesions in our series demonstrated irregularity of a portion of the tumor margin (15). Irregular margins may also be due to local inflammation rather than malignant extension. Beltran et al. (9) described increased signal intensity surrounding masses on T2 weighted sequences. This finding was more common with malignant lesions but was also seen in some patients with infection and hemorrhage. This feature was not evident in any of seven benign neoplasms. Sensitivity of this finding in predicting malignancy was 80% and specificity 50% and the accuracy 54%.

Inhomogeneous signal intensity, however, is noted in most malignancies (95%) and may be a more useful sign in differentiating benign and malignant conditions. Generally, the signal intensity is inhomogeneous on both T1 and T2 weighted sequences. However, the inhomogeneity is usually most easily appreciated on the T2 weighted sequences (Fig. 12-32). Neurovascular encasement and bone involvement are also more common with malignant lesions (Figs. 12-20 and 12-33) (12,15,73,74).

There have been numerous articles that emphasize the inability of MRI to differentiate benign from malignant soft tissue masses (53,68,114). However, by using the above criteria, malignant lesions were accurately

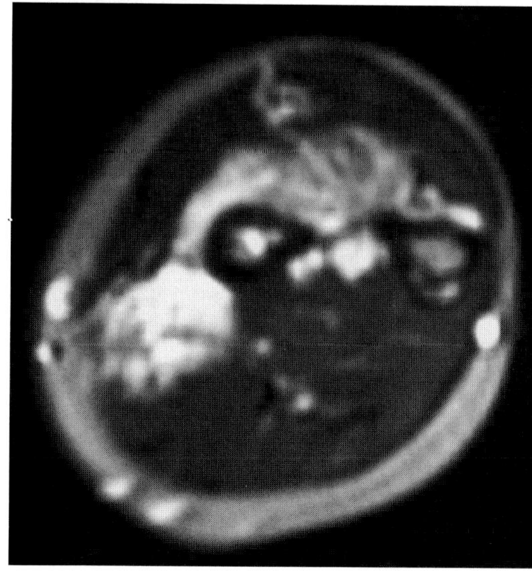

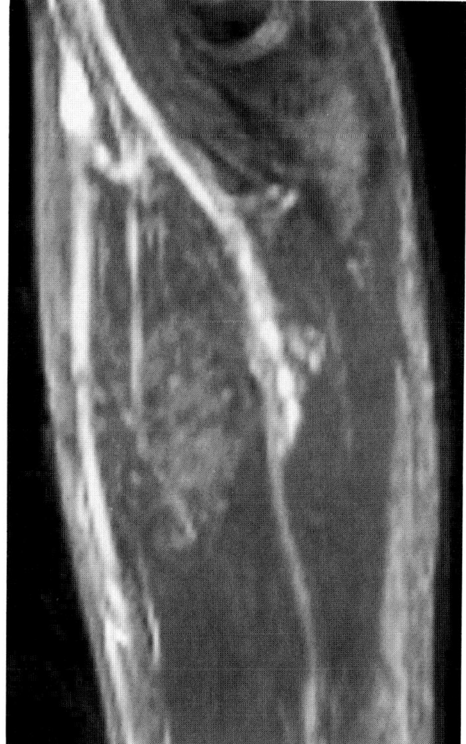

A,B

FIG. 12-28. Hemangioma. Axial SE 2,000/60 image (**A**) and sagittal GRASS image (**B**) demonstrate the hemangioma and vascular anatomy.

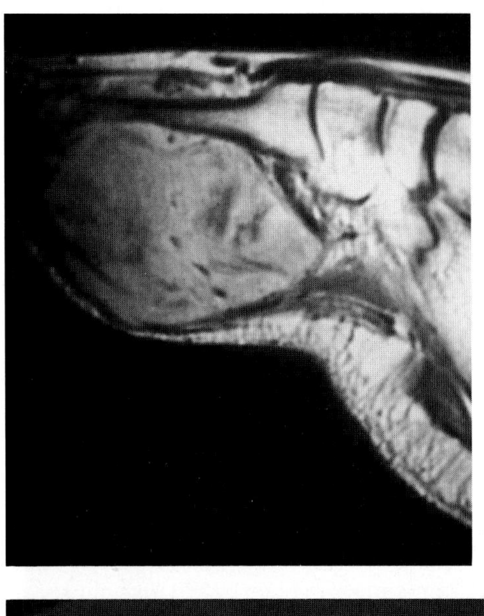
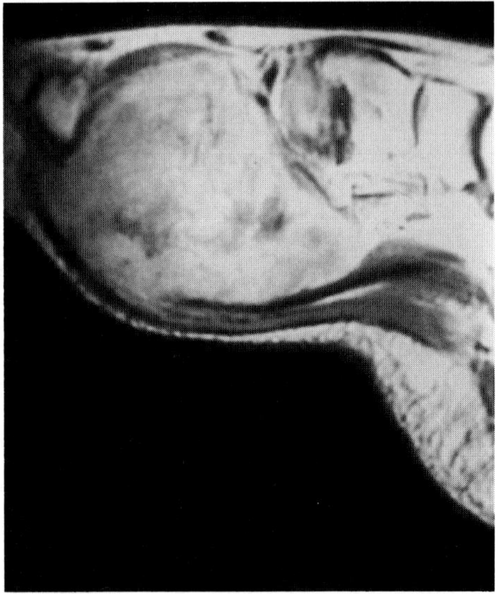

A

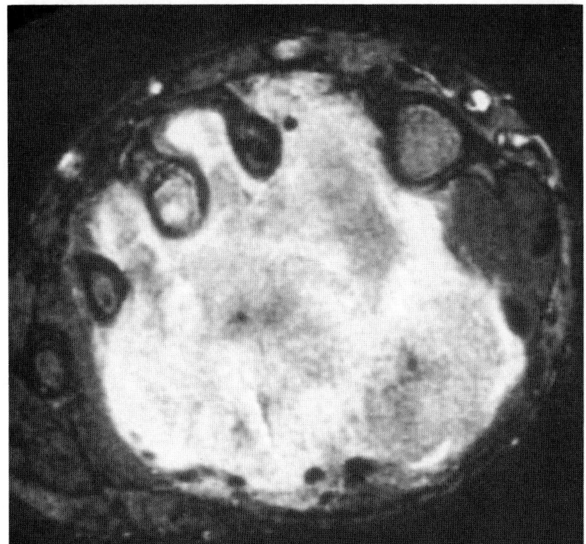

B

FIG. 12-29. Desmoid tumor of the foot. Sagittal SE 2,000/20 image (**A**) and axial SE 2,000/60 image (**B**) shows a large inhomogeneous plantar mass that encases the metatarsals.

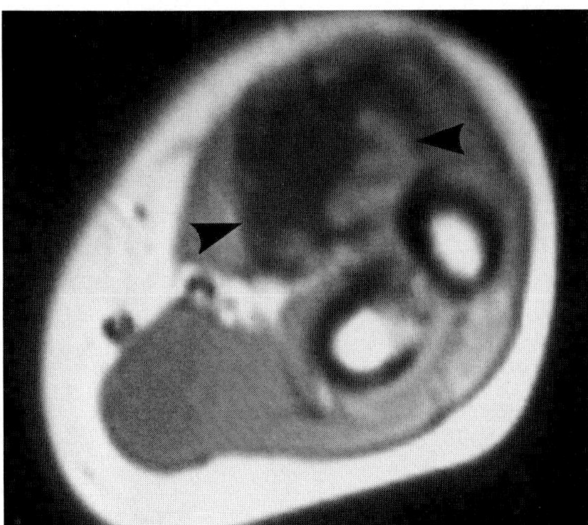

FIG. 12-30. Desmoid of the forearm. Axial image shows an irregular, low-intensity mass (*arrowheads*) due to fibrous tissue.

identified 91% of the time. More importantly, a negative predictive value of 94.5% for malignancy was demonstrated (15). These rates improve on the 80–88% accuracies reported with CT (60,132).

Despite the accuracy in determining the nature of the lesion (benign versus malignant) it is more difficult to predict the histology of malignant lesions (12,15,113). However, we have noted several lesions that can be confused with benign processes. Synovial sarcomas can be well marginated and cystic, mimicking a benign lesion (Fig. 12-34). These features were also noted in one soft tissue chondrosarcoma and hemangiopericytoma (Fig. 12-35) (15,25).

Patients who have had recent surgery or diagnostic needle biopsy are more difficult to evaluate with MRI. Inflammatory changes and/or hemorrhage or hematoma from the biopsy or surgery can create distortion of the mass and inhomogeneity in signal intensity which

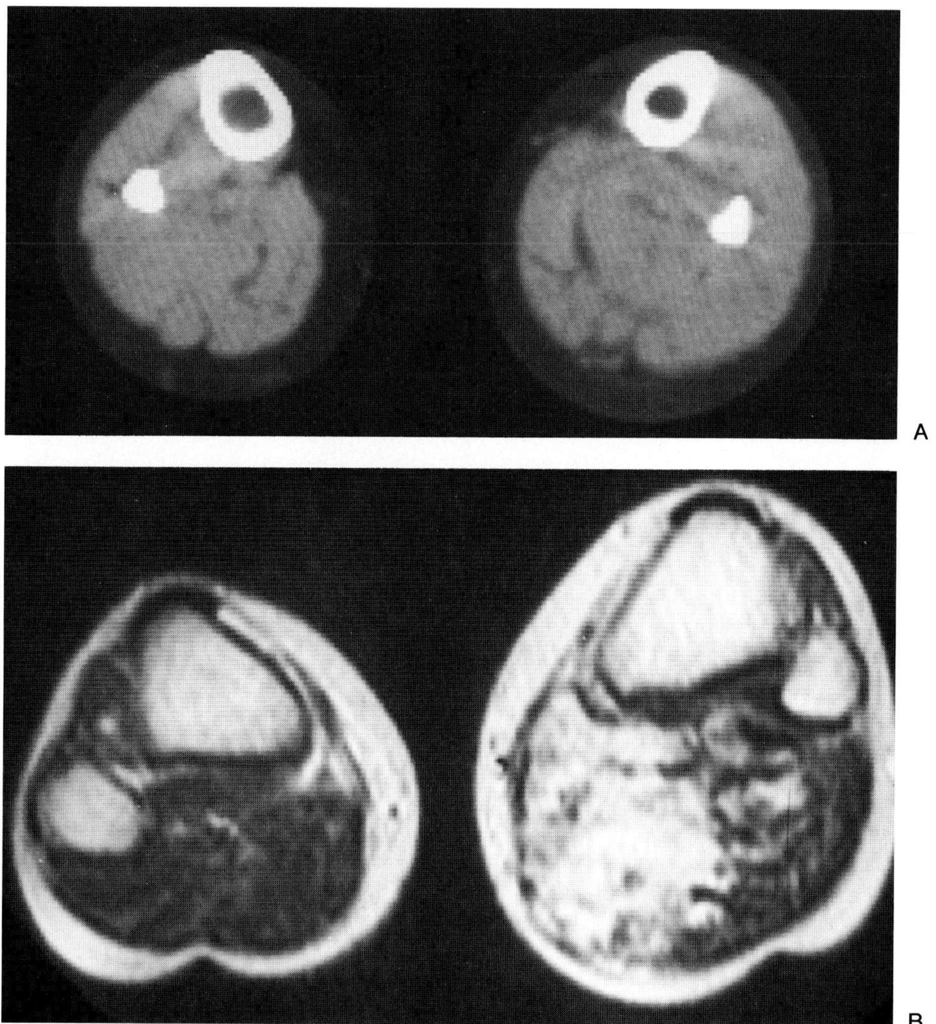

FIG. 12-31. Malignant fibrous histiocytoma. Axial CT image (**A**) shows a mass in the posterior compartment on the left. Axial SE 2,000/30 image (**B**) shows an inhomogeneous, markedly irregular lesion typical of malignancy. (From ref. 12, with permission.)

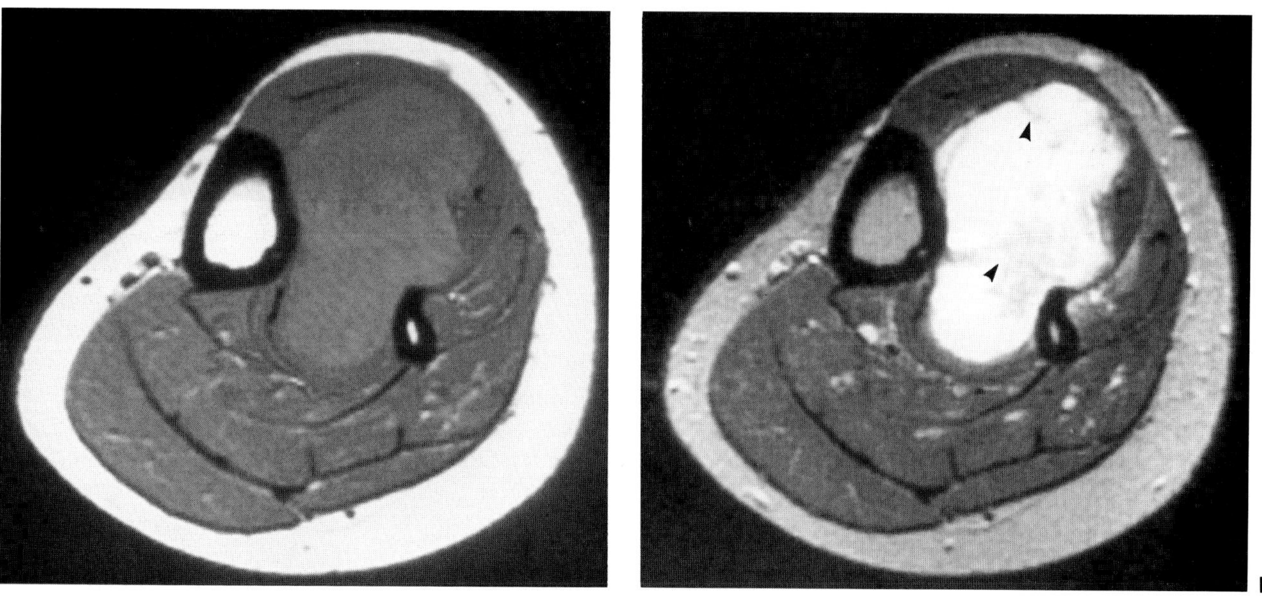

FIG. 12-32. Leiomyosarcoma of the calf. Axial SE 500/20 image (**A**) and SE 2,000/60 image (**B**). The lesion and subtle inhomogeneity (*arrowheads*) are most easily appreciated on the T2 weighted image (**B**).

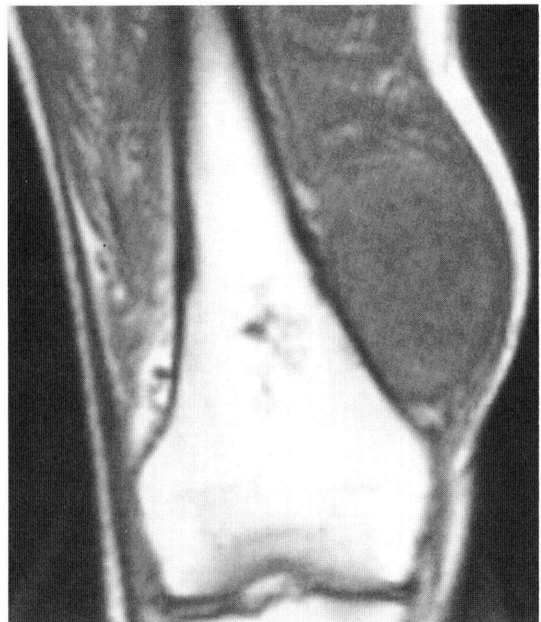

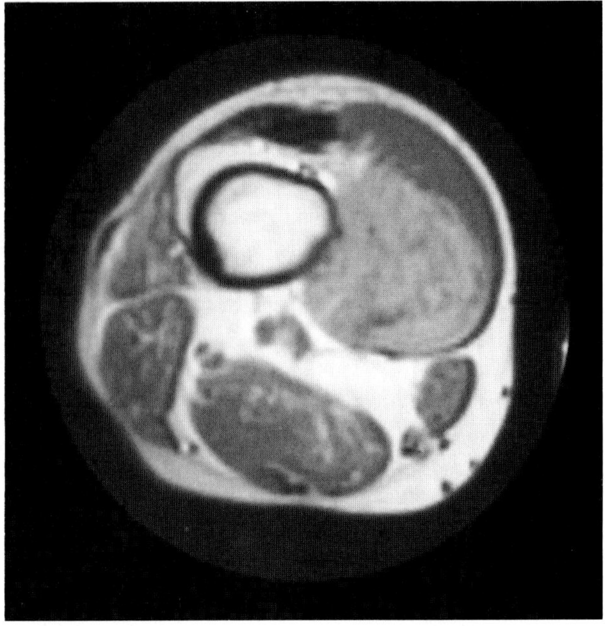

A,B

FIG. 12-33. Malignant fibrous histiocytoma. Coronal SE 500/20 image (**A**) and axial SE 2,000/30 image (**B**) show an inhomogeneous mass eroding the distal femur.

makes classification of these lesions more difficult (12,15).

Nonneoplastic Soft Tissue Masses

There are other soft tissue masses that can mimic neoplasms and occasionally cause confusion on MR images. Hematomas and abscesses (see Chapter 13) are the most common examples. When images are studied without knowledge of clinical history, these conditions can potentially be confused with neoplasms.

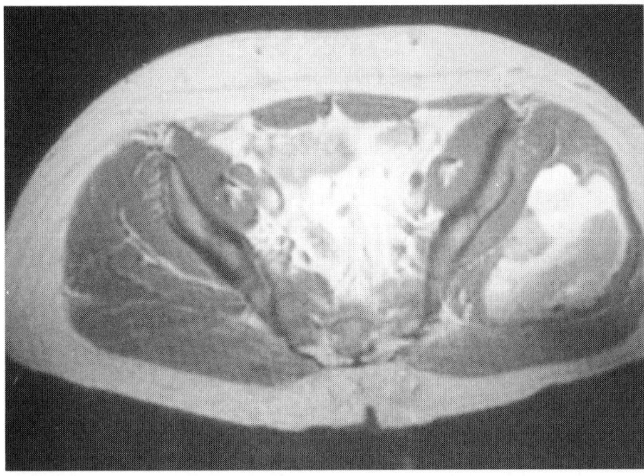

FIG. 12-34. Well-marginated cystic lesion with low intensity centrally which mimics a hematoma on this SE 2,000/30 image. Synovial sarcoma.

Abscesses generally have low inhomogeneous signal intensity on T1 weighted sequences and high slightly inhomogeneous signal intensity on T2 weighted sequences (see Figs. 13-11 and 13-12). The homogeneity of the signal intensity depends on the amount of necrotic tissue and protein within the lesion (12,27). Occasionally, signal intensity is more homogeneous and it can be difficult to differentiate an abscess from a cyst. However, generally there is more reactive edema around an abscess and a thick wall capsule is not unusual. Early studies with gadolinium-DTPA demonstrate enhanced signal intensity of the abscess wall and surrounding soft tissue. The clinical history is usually very useful in this setting. MRI experience in evaluation of abscess is less extensive than other soft tissue masses because clinical history is usually obvious and patients are more often referred for CT to detect and drain abscesses in the same setting.

Hematomas and hemorrhage can cause confusion; however, the MRI knowledge of these two lesions has increased and the understanding of these lesions is more clearly defined (30,81,118). In our blinded study, even the less experienced examiners correctly identified hematomas and differentiated them from neoplasms in 78% of patients.

Acute hematomas have high signal intensity on T2 weighted images and are near muscle density and can be overlooked on T1 weighted sequences (30,118). More data are available on the MRI features of subacute or chronic hematomas. In this setting, areas of increased signal intensity can be demonstrated on both T1 and T2 weighted sequences (Fig. 12-36) (115,126). On T1

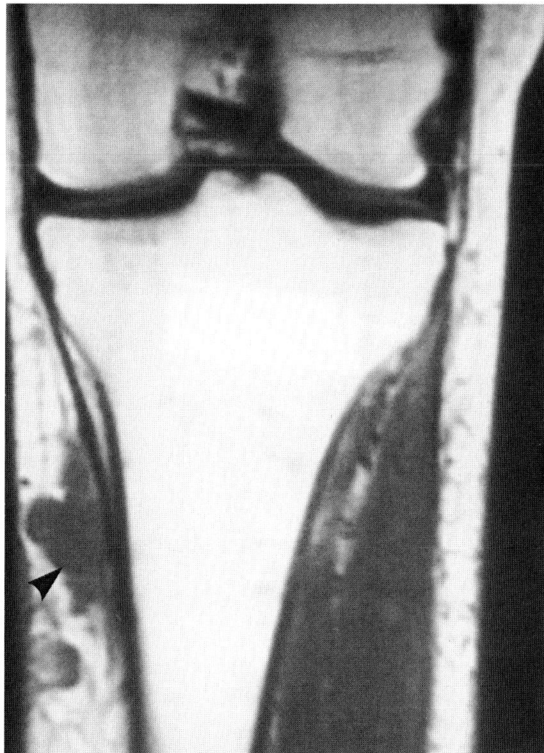

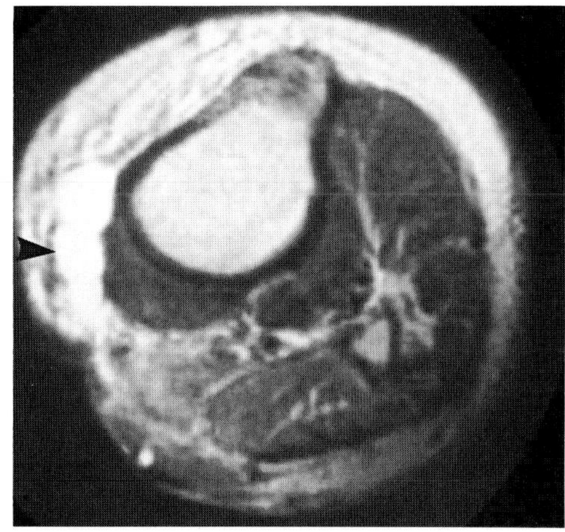

A,B

FIG. 12-35. Hemangiopericytoma. Coronal SE 500/20 image (**A**) shows a multilobulated low-intensity cystic lesion (*arrowhead*). The axial SE 2,000/60 image (**B**) demonstrates a lobulated homogeneous high signal intensity.

weighted sequences the central portion is low intensity with a high-intensity peripheral margin and dark outer rim. The area of high intensity is due to paramagnetic effects of hemoglobin breakdown products (14,44,126). On T2 weighted sequences the central portion of the hematoma is high intensity with a low-intensity rim (Fig. 12-37) (57). Hemophilic pseudotumors are rare (1–2% of patients with factor VIII or IX deficiency) but can have a similar appearance. The pelvis, thighs, and calves are the most common locations (133).

Post-treatment Evaluation

After radiation, surgery, or chemotherapy, it is difficult to determine the response to therapy and whether residual or recurrent tumor is present (12,24,77,88,101).

Differentiation of postoperative change for recurrent tumor is particularly difficult during the early postoperative period (Fig. 12-38). Reviews of CT findings in patients with suspected tumor occurrence have revealed that it is difficult to differentiate hematoma from recur-

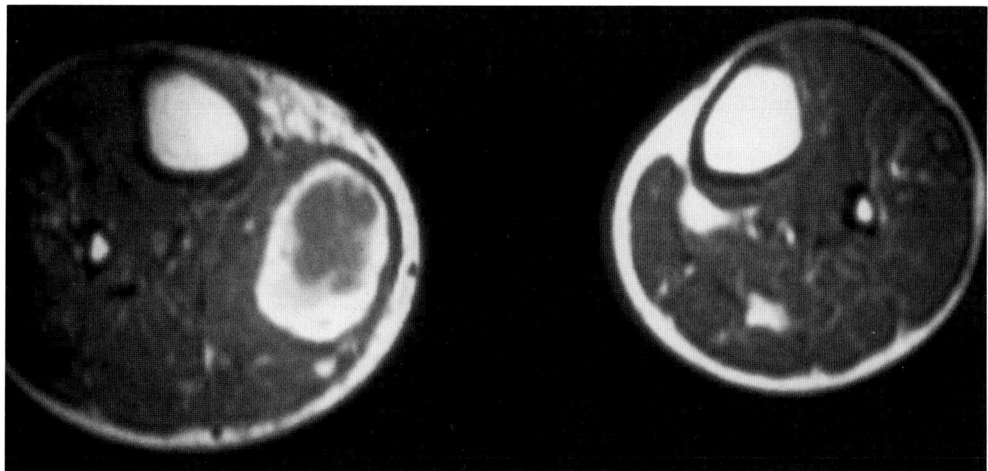

FIG. 12-36. Axial SE 2,000/30 image shows a high-intensity lesion with low signal intensity centrally due to paramagnetic effects. Subacute hematoma.

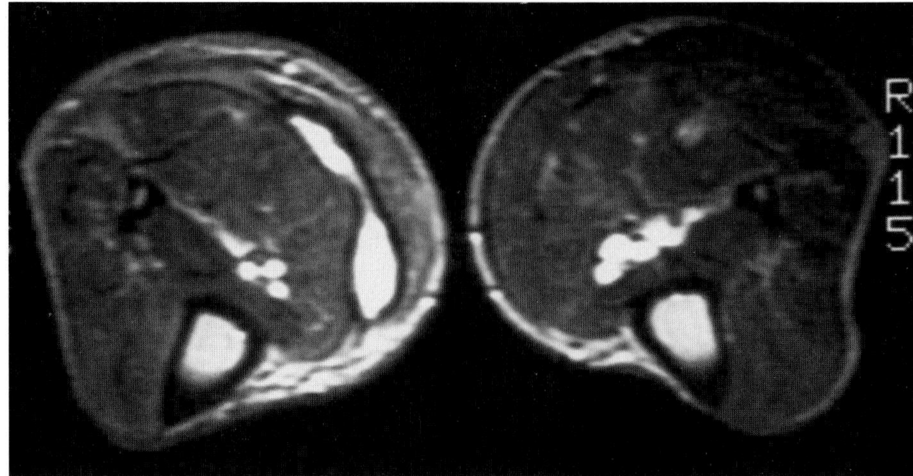

FIG. 12-37. Axial SE 2,000/60 image shows a high-intensity lesion with a dark rim in the left calf. Chronic hematoma.

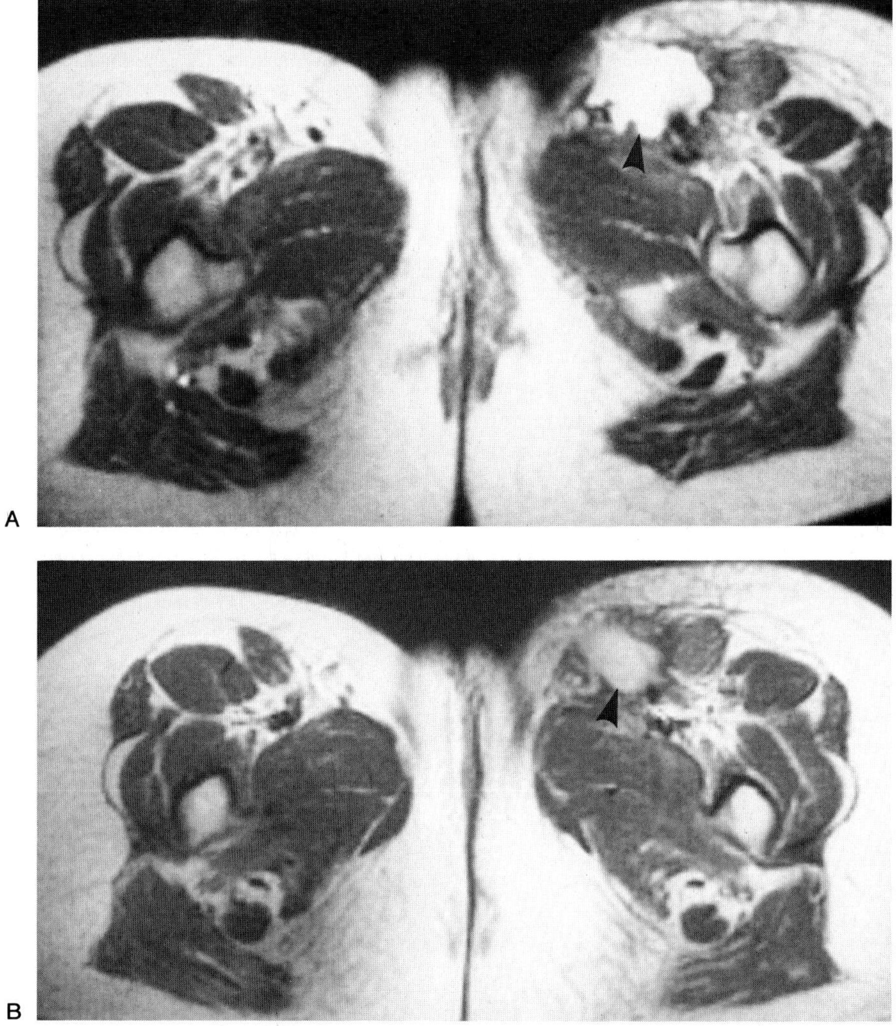

FIG. 12-38. Recurrent desmoid tumor? **A:** Immediate postoperative SE 2,000/30 image shows a large hematoma at the operative site (*arrowhead*). **B:** Follow-up image at 4 weeks shows the lesion is smaller, confirming a resolving hematoma.

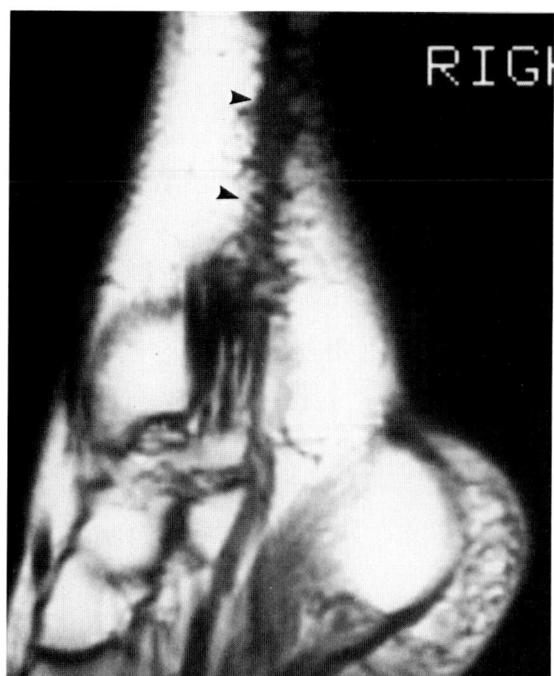

FIG. 12-39. Sagittal image of the ankle 1 year after surgery shows a typical irregular low-intensity scar (*arrowheads*) deep to the previous incision.

rence. Similar problems occur with MRI prior to the organization of scar tissue (12,24,51,66). Several techniques have been used to differentiate soft tissue and osseous neoplasms and postoperative, chemotherapeutic, and radiation changes. Evaluation of T1 and T2 weighted sequences alone is useful if scar tissue is fully organized (may require 6 months to 1 year, depending on the extent of treatment) (42,51,128). Scar tissue appears dark, similar to tendons on both T1 and T2 weighted sequences (Fig. 12-39 to 12-41). When low signal intensity was noted on T2 weighted sequences, Vanel et al. (128) reported a sensitivity of 96% in excluding recurrent tumor. Active processes (infection, hemorrhage, inflammation, and tumor) may have low signal intensity on T1 weighted sequences but will have high intensity on T2 weighted sequences (Fig. 12-41) (12,42,101).

During the early postoperative period the residual inflammation, blood, and other postoperative changes can easily obscure residual tumor (12,101). However, if a baseline examination is obtained at this time the progress of healing and detection of tumor can be accomplished more easily on follow-up examinations (Fig. 12-38).

Detection of residual tumor in marrow can be even more difficult (12,50). Following radiation therapy, fatty replacement of marrow is typical (Fig. 12-42). This can occur as soon as 10 days after therapy of 3,000 rads or more (92,94,104). Residual tumor can be seen as an area of low intensity on T1 weighted images and increased intensity on T2 weighted images (94).

Gadolinium-DTPA has also been used to differentiate scar from tumor. Enhancing lesions represent tumor or organizing scar or granulation tissue. However, well-organized scar tissue should not enhance on T1 weighted sequences after Gd-DTPA injection (66).

Limb salvage procedures are performed frequently using metal or ceramic implants. Both CT and MRI are degraded to some degree by metal artifact; however, if the metal is nonferromagnetic, the artifact may be much less significant with MRI, especially at lower field strengths (Fig. 12-43). Therefore, MRI should not be excluded and may be preferred for following patients in this setting (7,10,14).

Although spectroscopy has not yet achieved wide clinical usage, recent studies have demonstrated significant changes in inorganic phosphate, adenosine triphosphate, and other chemicals in patients who have been treated with chemotherapy (99,139). Ross et al. (99) studied 15 patients using MRI and ^{31}P spectroscopy. Tumors were noted to have increased adenosine tri-

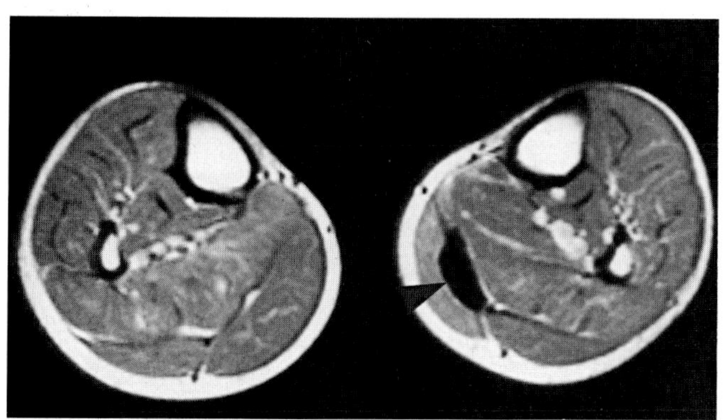

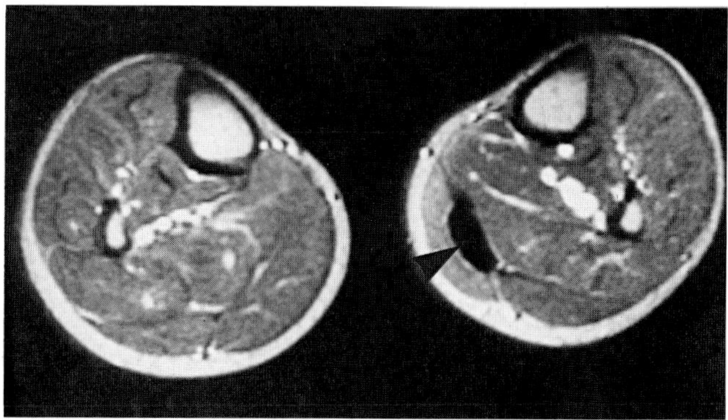

A,B

FIG. 12-40. Axial SE 500/20 (**A**) and SE 2,000/60 (**B**) images of the calves, demonstrating low signal intensity organized scar (*arrowhead*) on the left.

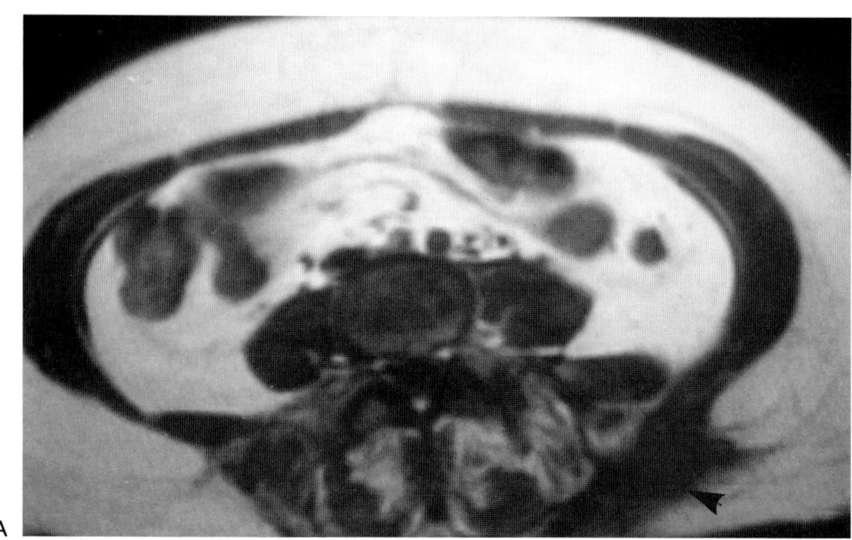

A

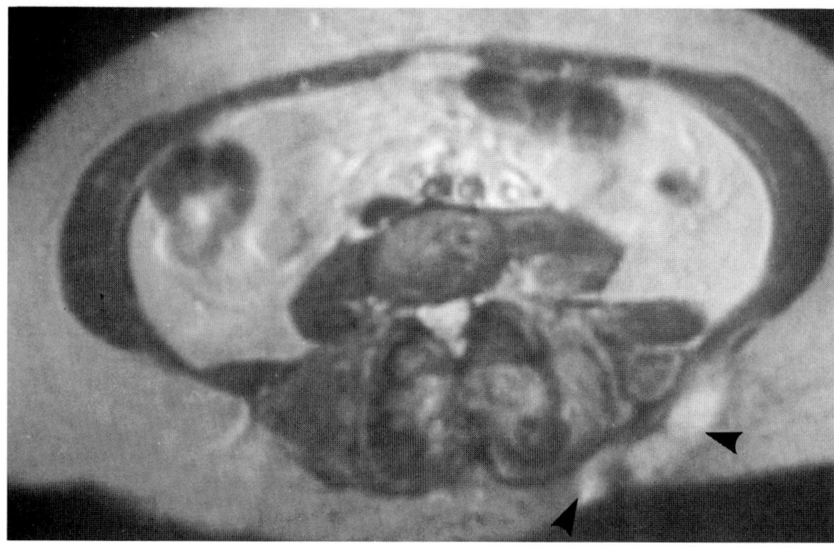

B

FIG. 12-41. Axial SE 500/20 (**A**) and SE 2,000/60 (**B**) images. Recurrence? There is an irregular area of low intensity (*arrowhead*) on (**A**). The lesion is high intensity on (**B**) (*arrowheads*), indicating an active process. (From ref. 12, with permission.)

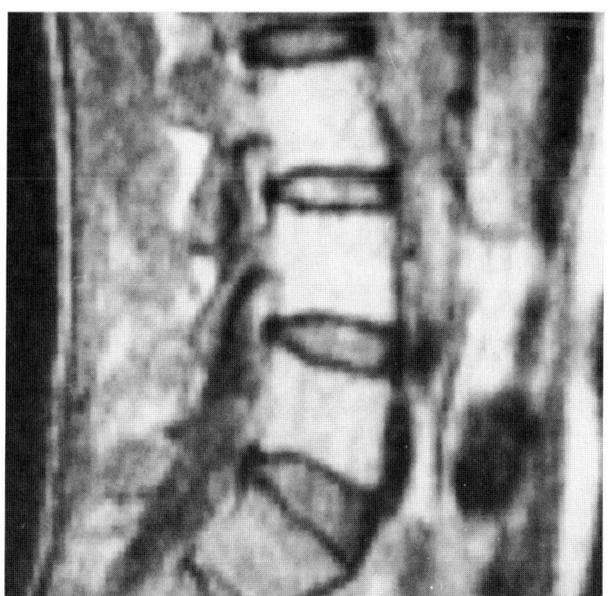

FIG. 12-42. Low-field sagittal image of the spine (SE 600/30) shows high signal intensity in L3–L5 due to fatty replacement following radiation.

phosphate and inorganic phosphate content. In addition, there was an abnormal phosphomonoester peak, indicating increased glycolysis. The abnormalities regressed during chemotherapy and returned in patients who had recurrent disease. Although these results are preliminary, spectroscopy seems to be more specific in following the response of neoplasms to therapy. There is also significant difference in these levels when comparing tumor and scar tissue (24).

METASTASES

Routine radiographs and radionuclide scans are most commonly used for screening and detection of skeletal metastases (12,13,14,64). In many situations these techniques are still most cost effective. However, isotope studies are not accurate in patients with multiple myeloma. In addition, patients with osteopenia (Fig. 12-44) or degenerative change or both may be difficult to evaluate using these techniques (12,14).

Recently, MRI has proved to be useful in early detection of marrow involvement by subtle metastases (Fig. 12-45), lymphoma (Fig. 12-46), leukemia, and multiple myeloma (Fig. 12-47) (3–5,11,32,33,54,109,121,122). Daffner et al. (33) studied 30 patients with multiple myeloma. Isotope scans were normal in all patients. MRI was positive in all 30 with no false positive or false negative examinations. Although lesions can be detected in many osseous structures, MRI is currently too time consuming to study the entire skeleton. However, the spine, pelvis, and upper femurs can be evaluated quickly using short TE, TR spin-echo sequences (SE 500/20). The T1 weighted sequence is ideal because tumor has

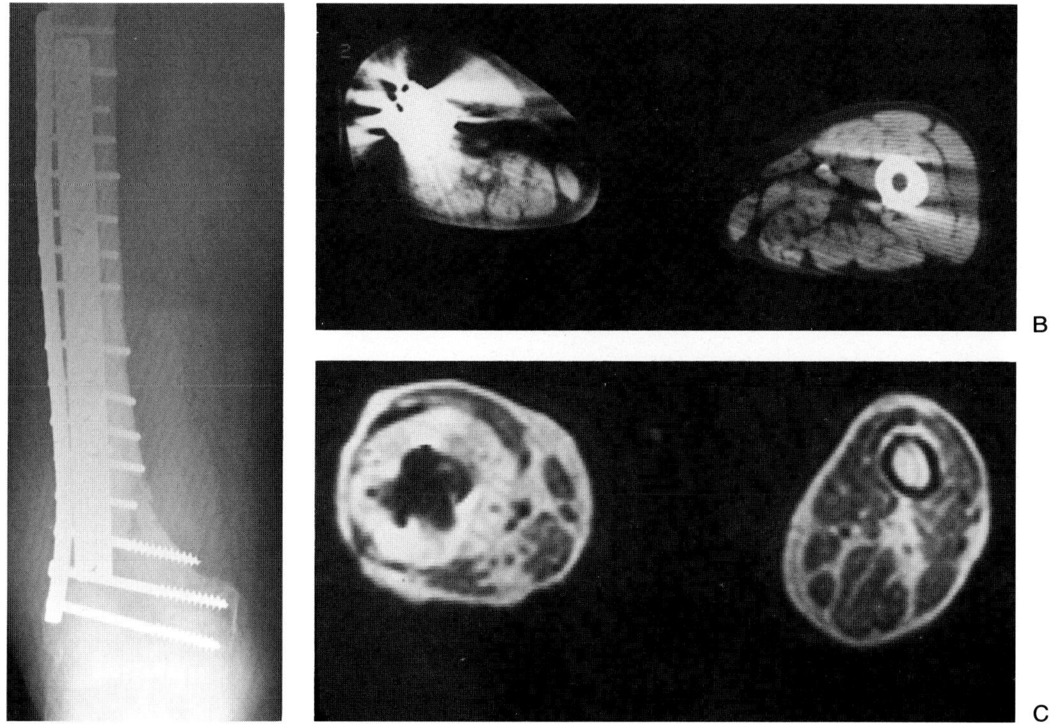

FIG. 12-43. A: Routine radiograph of the femur after limb salvage with plate and screw fixation. **B:** CT scan is badly degraded by metal artifact. **C:** MR image (SE 2,000/30) shows the soft tissue recurrence clearly.

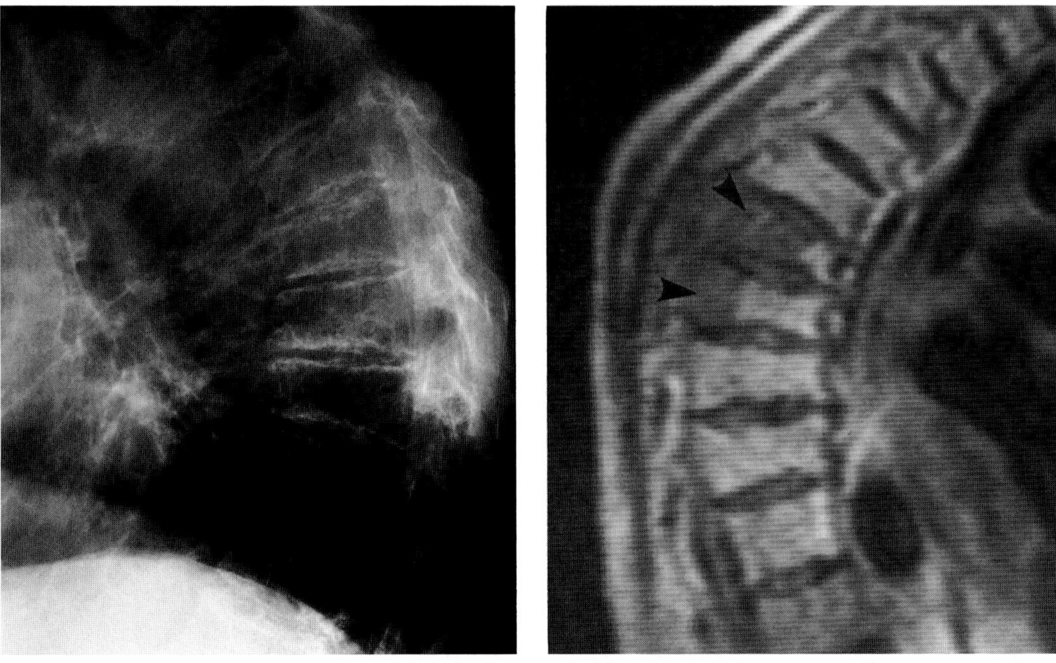

A,B

FIG. 12-44. A: Lateral radiograph of the thoracic spine, demonstrating osteopenia with wedging of multiple vertebrae. **B:** Low-field (0.15 T) sagittal SE 500/30 image shows metastasis (*arrowheads*) in two adjacent vertebrae.

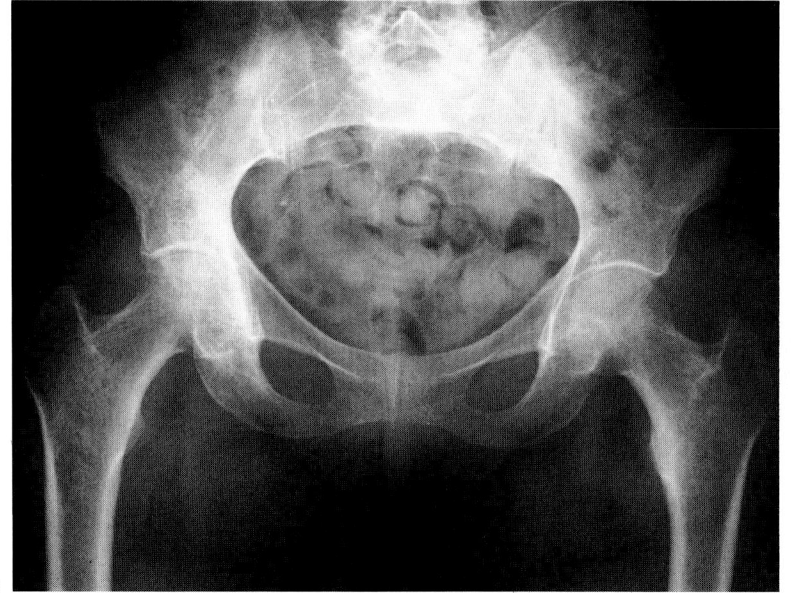

A,B

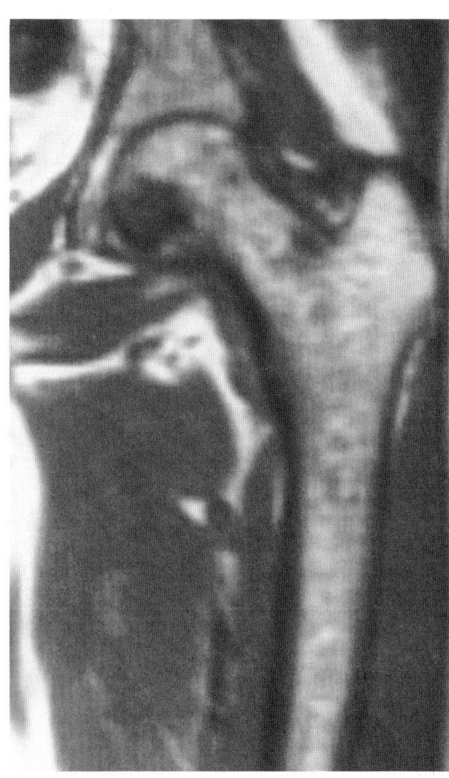

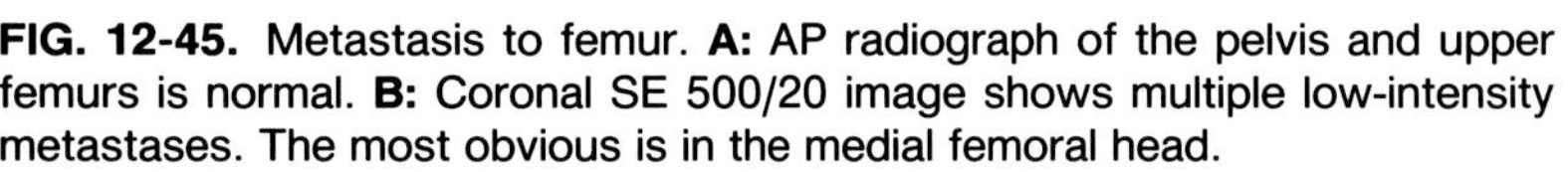

FIG. 12-45. Metastasis to femur. **A:** AP radiograph of the pelvis and upper femurs is normal. **B:** Coronal SE 500/20 image shows multiple low-intensity metastases. The most obvious is in the medial femoral head.

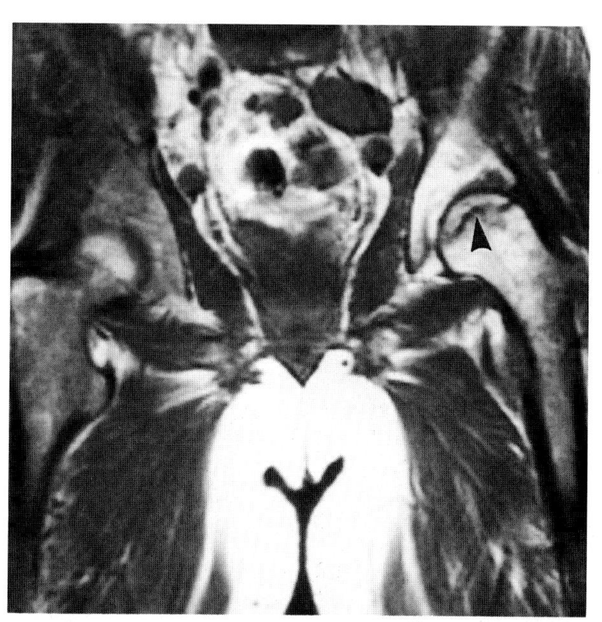

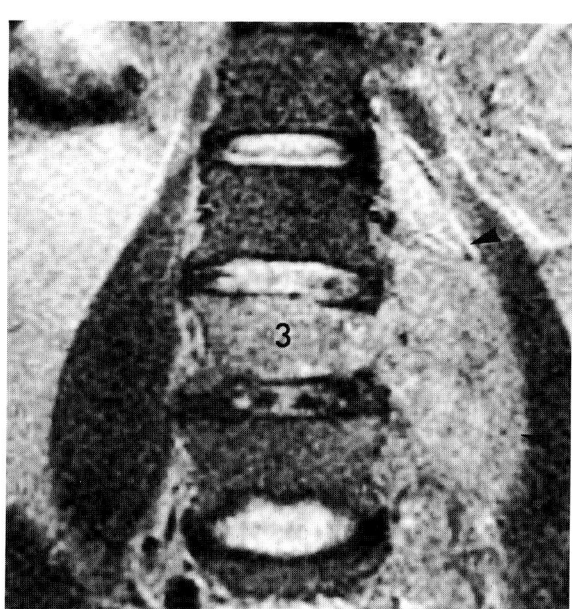

A,B

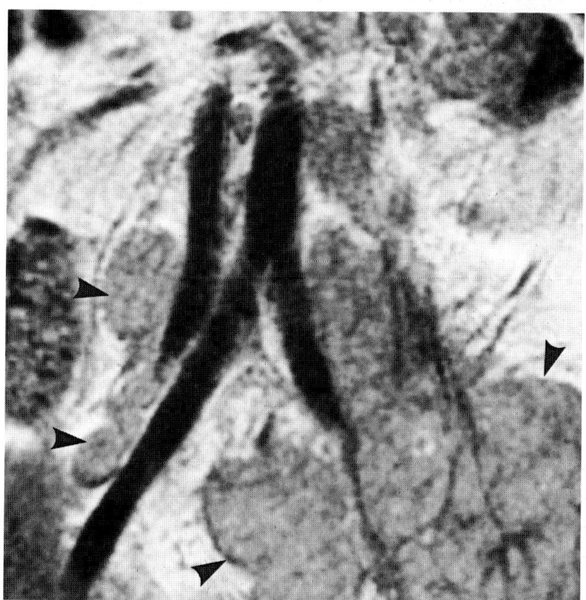

C

FIG. 12-46. Lymphoma. **A:** Coronal SE 500/20 image shows reduced signal intensity in the right femur and innominate bone due to lymphoma. Note the AVN in the left femoral head. **B:** Coronal SE 2,000/60 image of the lumbar region shows involvement of L3 and the left paraspinal soft tissues (*arrowheads*). **C:** Coronal SE 2,000/30 image of the aortoiliac region shows extensive adenopathy (*arrowheads*).

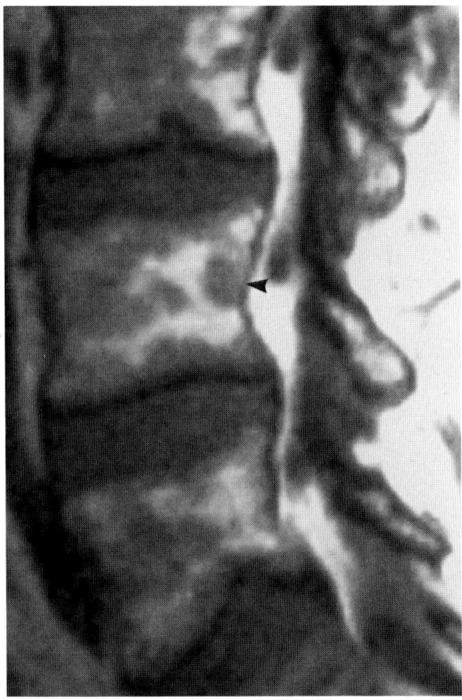

FIG. 12-47. Sagittal SE 500/20 image demonstrates focal (type 1) (*small arrowhead*) and diffuse marrow involvement due to multiple myeloma.

low intensity, providing excellent contrast with the high signal intensity of normal marrow. T1 weighted images of the spine are obtained in the sagittal plane. The pelvis and hips are examined in the coronal plane. In some cases additional image planes and pulse sequences may be needed to clarify suspicious areas. For example, T2 weighted or gradient echo T2* sequences may be needed to define the extent of cord involvement (Fig. 12-48). Patterns of marrow involvement have been described using T1 and T2 weighted sequences (4).

Type 1 lesions are focal and have low signal intensity on T1 and high signal intensity (>marrow fat) on T2 weighted sequences (Fig. 12-49). This image feature is seen with local lytic or destructive metastases or myeloma. Type 2, the second pattern, occurs with sclerotic or blastic lesions so that focal areas of low signal intensity are seen on both T1 and T2 weighted sequences (Fig. 12-50). These changes could also be identified with osteosclerotic myeloma and benign bone islands. Comparison with routine radiographs is essential with all patterns, especially type 2. The third pattern (4), type 3, is a diffuse inhomogeneous signal involving the vertebral body (Fig. 12-47). The final pattern, type 4, is diffuse homogeneous decreased signal intensity on T1 weighted images, and homogeneous increased intensity on T2 weighted sequences (4,12,121,122). Similar patterns can be identified with lymphoma, leukemia, and other infiltrative marrow diseases. A more complete discussion of these processes is included in Chapter 14.

In certain situations, additional pulse sequences or image planes may be required to improve lesion characterization and to clearly identify subtle lesions (3,12). Short T1 inversion recovery sequences (STIR) are very useful for identification of subtle bone and soft tissue involvement. Image time (TR 1,500, TI 150, TE 30) is shorter than a conventional T2 weighted spin-echo sequence (SE 2,000/60–80). Therefore, some authors prefer T1 weighted (SE 500/20) spin-echo and STIR

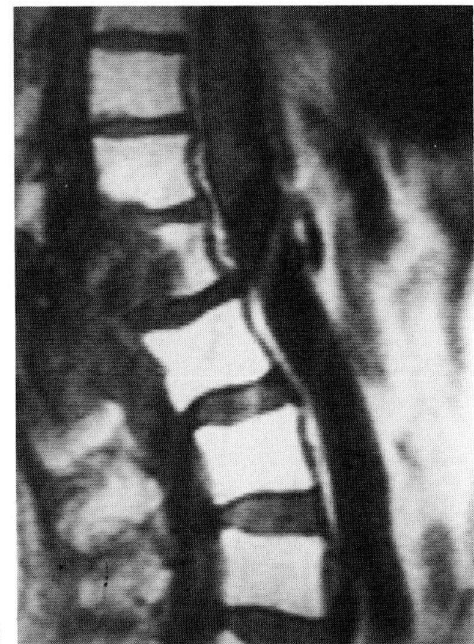

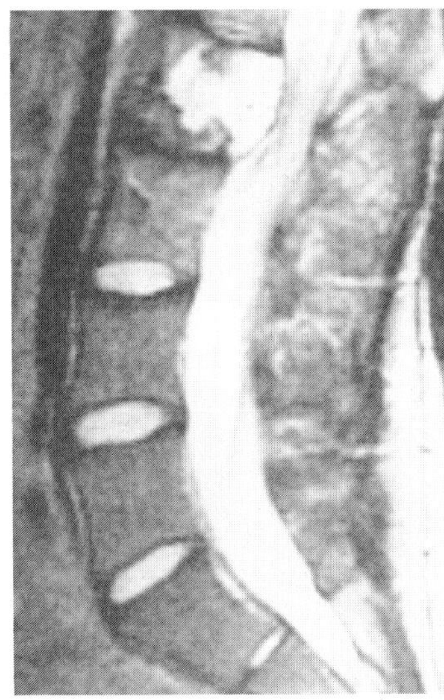

A,B

FIG. 12-48. Metastasis to the lumbar spine. **A:** SE 500/20 image clearly demonstrates the lesion in L1. **B:** The T2 weighted image in a different patient more clearly demonstrates the vertebral lesion and compression of the spinal canal.

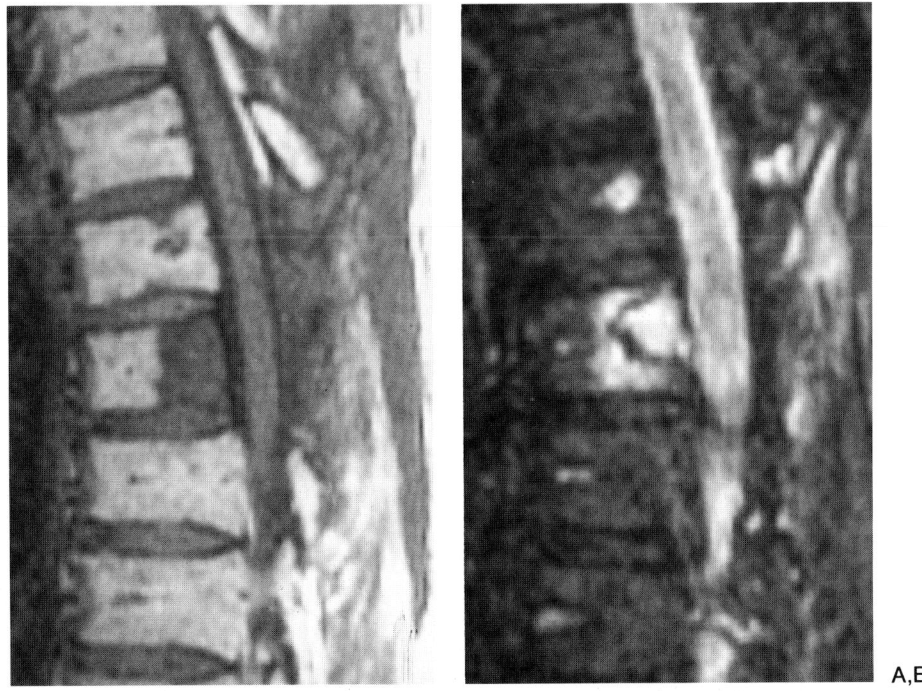

A,B

FIG. 12-49. Metastasis. Sagittal SE 500/20 (**A**) and gradient-echo (**B**) images show well-defined metastasis with low intensity on T1 (**A**) and high intensity on T2* (**B**) weighted images.

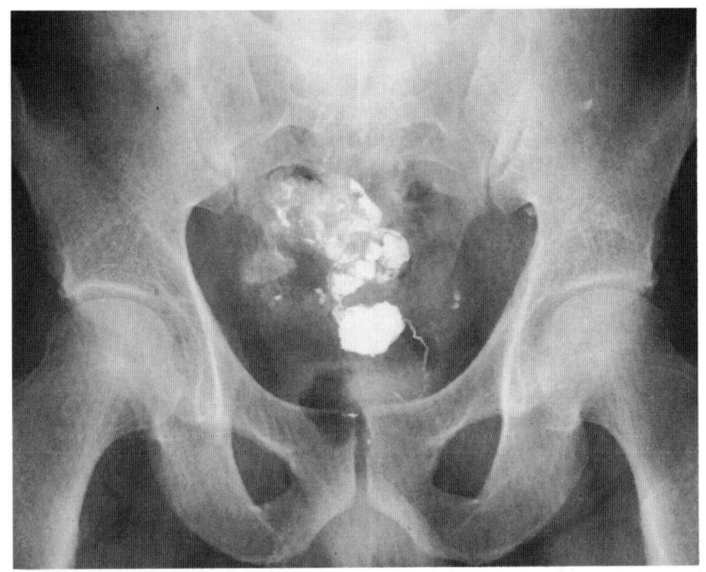

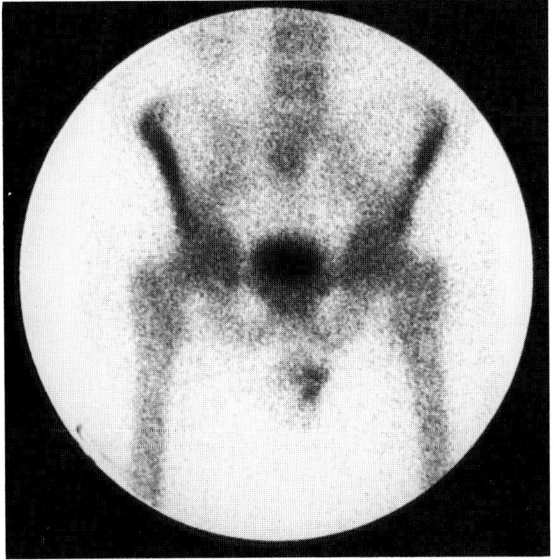

A,B

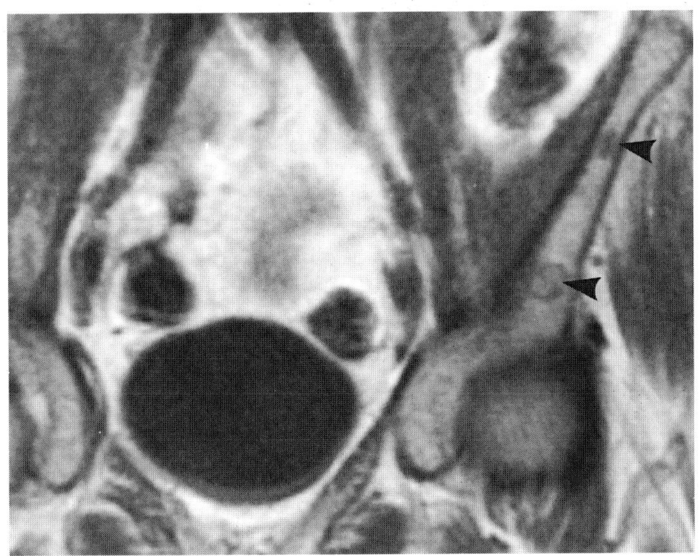

C

FIG. 12-50. Type 2 lesions of osteosclerotic myeloma. Routine radiograph (**A**) and technetium bone scan (**B**) are normal. Coronal SE 500/20 image (**C**) of the pelvis demonstrates two low-intensity lesions (*arrowheads*) due to osteosclerotic myeloma. Comparison with radiographs is essential.

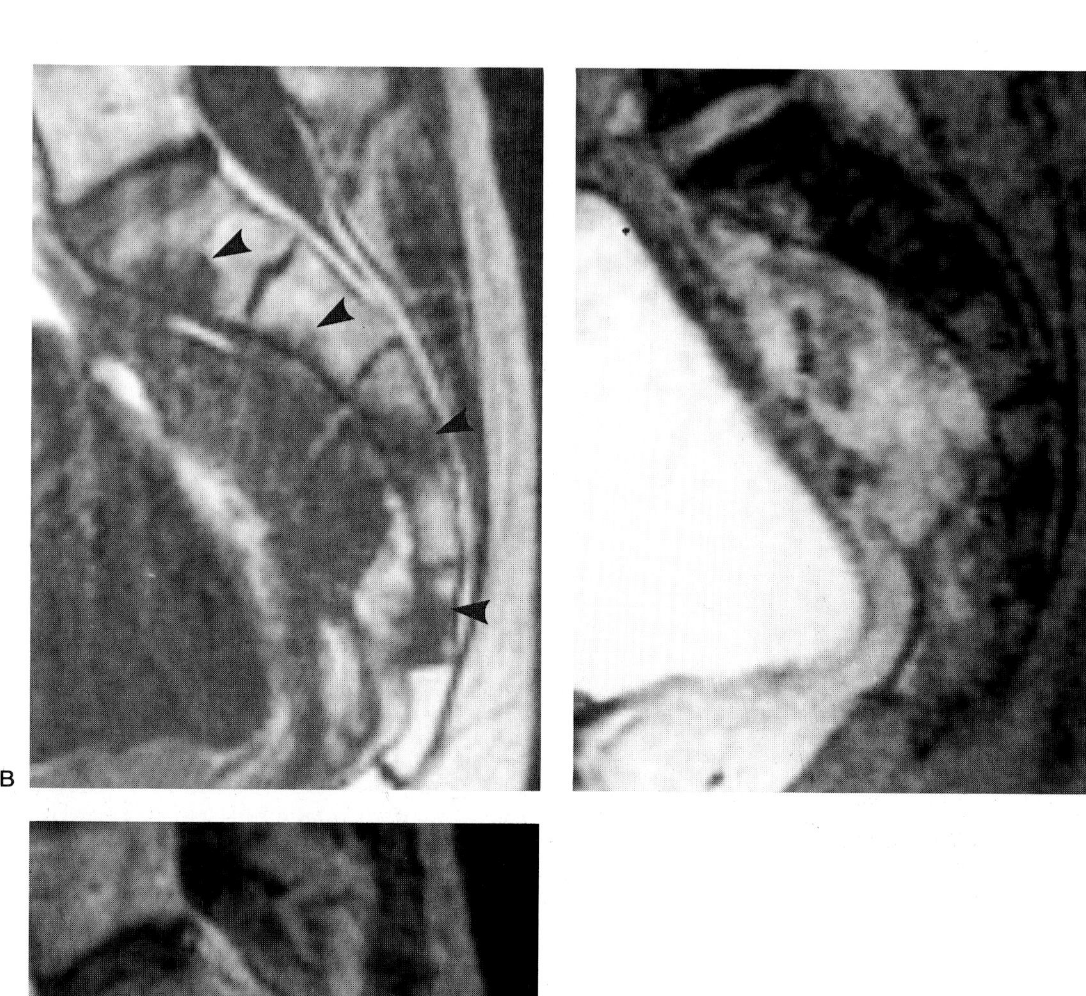

A,B

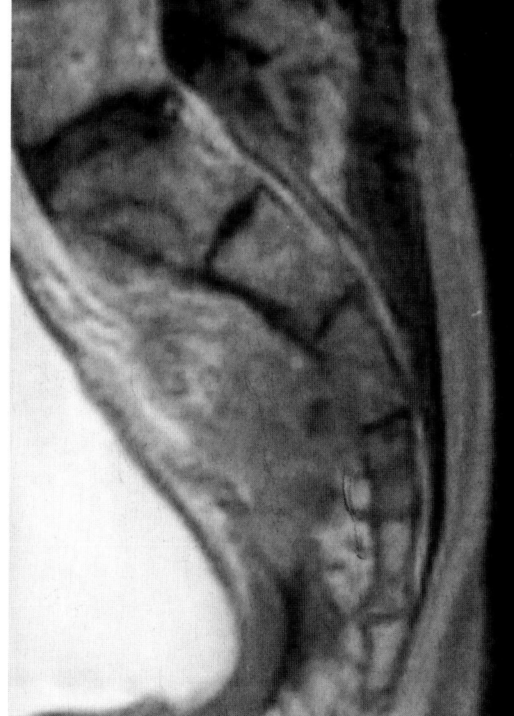

C

FIG. 12-51. Presacral rectal carcinoma recurrence and sacral metastasis. **A:** SE 500/20 image shows a presacral muscle density mass with multiple (*arrowheads*) vertebral metastases. **B:** Gradient-echo sequence shows the lesions are high intensity compared to the suppressed signal intensity of the normal marrow. **C:** Gd-DTPA enhanced SE 500/20 image shows the presacral mass has increased in signal intensity compared to the unenhanced scan (**A**). The sacral metastases are nearly isointense with marrow and more difficult to identify.

TABLE 12-3. *Vertebral lesions that can mimic metastasis (36,59,79,82,100,136)*

Diagnosis	MR features	Radiographic features
Degenerative disk disease (see Chapter 5)		
Type I	Vertebral end-plates ↓T1, ↑T2	Degenerative disk disease
Type II	Vertebral end-plates ↑T1, slight increase T2	Degenerative disk disease
Type III	Vertebral end-plates ↓T1, ↓T2	End-plate sclerosis or fibrosis
Schmorl's node	Disk enters end-plate	End-plate deformed
Infection	Disk ↑T2; end-plates ↑T2, ↓T1	Normal early, may have disk space narrowing or end-plate erosion
Hemangioma	Mottled ↑T2, ↑T1 focal ↑T2, ↑T1	Normal to prominent trabeculae
Fatty infiltrates	Focal ↑T1, intermediate T2	Normal
Compression fracture	Vertebral compression; normal signal intensity T1, T2 or linear area of ↑T2, ↓T1	Anterior or lateral wedging, no destruction

sequences to evaluate patients with suspected metastasis (14,21,110). Gadolinium-DTPA is useful for intradural metastasis (see Chapter 5) but STIR sequences are usually preferred for marrow and extradural disease (Fig. 12-51) (110). Relaxation times (T1 and T2) may be of some value but are currently not commonly employed in a clinical setting (111).

Differentiating metastatic or other malignant marrow processes from benign conditions and traumatic compression fractures is a common problem (38,40). Table 12-3 summarizes the nonmalignant conditions in the spine that can be confused with neoplastic involvement (59,82,100,136). Degenerative disk disease and marrow disorders are discussed in Chapters 5 and 14. We concentrate our discussion on traumatic versus neoplastic vertebral abnormalities. Clinical history and radiographic changes (see Table 12-3) are important. For example, are there multiple areas of involvement (Fig. 12-52)? Is there evidence of bone destruction or soft tissue mass? Most important is the history of trauma or a known primary malignancy. Location of the lesion is also important because compression in the upper thoracic region is more likely to be malignant than post-traumatic (59,136). Uniform compression of the end-plates is usually more often due to osteopenia or trauma (36). Irregularity of the end-plates is more common with metastasis. Multiple vertebral, soft tissue masses, and pedicle destruction indicate metastasis. However, soft tissue mass effect can also be seen with trauma (13).

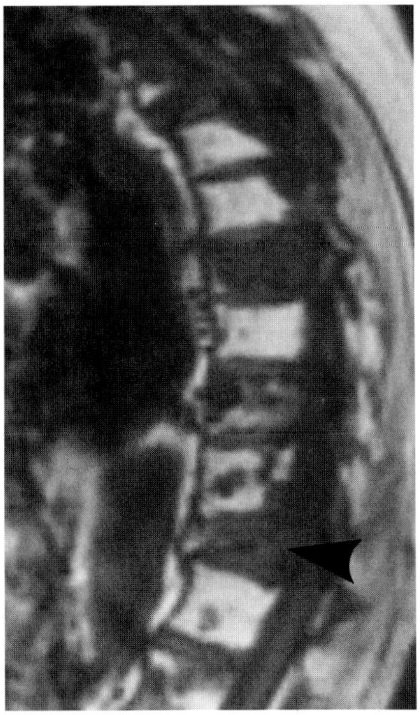

FIG. 12-52. Breast metastasis. SE 500/20 sagittal image shows multiple focal (type 1) metastases with diffuse involvement in several vertebrae. The compressed vertebra (*arrowhead*) has total replacement of normal marrow signal (*arrowhead*).

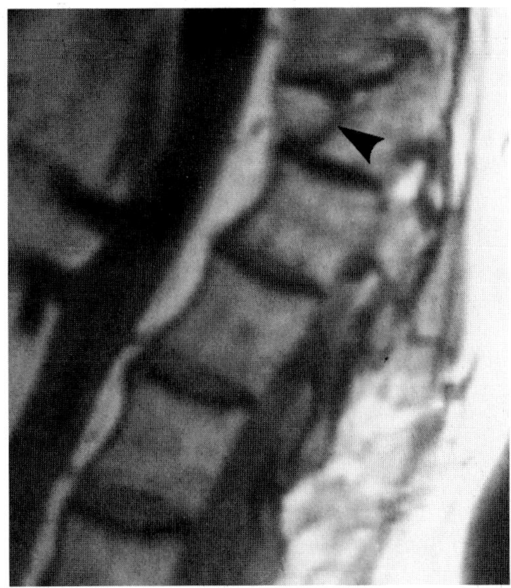

FIG. 12-53. Sagittal SE 500/20 image shows compression with a linear fracture (*arrowhead*) and normal signal intensity due to trauma.

MRI features of benign vertebral compression vary depending on the age of the injury. In the acute setting the vertebra may have uniform loss of signal intensity on T1 weighted sequences and increased intensity on T2, T2*, and STIR sequences (6,13,59,136). A linear fracture line (low signal intensity on T1), high signal or low signal (compressed trabeculae) intensity on T2 weighted sequences may also be evident early (Fig. 12-53 and Table 12-3). Absence of focal defects and soft tissue mass confirm the diagnosis of benign fracture (6,136). When marrow signal intensity remains normal in the presence of vertebral compression, the accuracy of calling the lesion benign is 94% (136).

When localized lesions are identified, it is necessary to obtain tissue to confirm tumor histology before planning therapy. Nonferromagnetic needles are available for MRI guided biopsy. Currently, however, fluoroscopic or CT guidance is much more efficient when needle biopsy is indicated.

SPECIFICITY

Progress continues to improve lesion characterization (benign, malignant, histologic specificity) and response to therapy. Morphologic data using common pulse sequences are useful, especially for soft tissue masses (115). However, additional sequences, use of gadolinium-DTPA, and spectroscopy are evolving and may be useful in this regard (139). Early studies with gadolinium have demonstrated a sharper, more rapid peak in enhancement for malignant lesions compared to benign masses (46).

Although relaxation times have not been useful (91,116), spectroscopy using ^{1}H and ^{31}P has begun to demonstrate potential in evaluating tumors and their response to therapy (22,37,49,55,67,83,85,86,129). Changes in the phosphomonoester (PME), phosphodiester (PDE), and inorganic phosphate (Pi) peaks have been used to evaluate tumor response to therapy. These peaks are elevated compared to normal tissue when active tumor is present. Creatine phosphate and nucleoside triphosphate (NTP) peaks are lower than normal (93,102). Ratios may also be useful in differentiating benign from malignant lesions. Malignant lesions have higher PME:NTP and PDE:NTP ratios and lower Pi:NTP ratios (84). The utility of these techniques for routine clinical practice is not yet established.

REFERENCES

1. Agartz I, Sääf J, Wahlund L, Wetterberg L. Magnetic resonance imaging at 0.02 T in clinical practice and research. *Magn Reson Imaging* 1987;5:179.
2. Aisen AM, Martel W, Braunstein EM, McMillin KI, Phillips WA, King TF. MRI and CT evaluation of primary bone and soft-tissue tumors. *AJR* 1986;146:749.
3. Albert S, Leeds NE. Fast proton density imaging of multiple myeloma in the vertebral column. Presented at the Society of Magnetic Resonance in Medicine, Amsterdam, The Netherlands, 1989.
4. Algra P, Bloem JL, Arndt JW, Verboom LJ, Falke THM, Tissing H. Sensitivity for MRI of vertebral metastasis: a comparison between MRI and bone scintigraphy. Presented at the Society of Magnetic Resonance in Medicine, Amsterdam, The Netherlands, 1989.
5. Avrahami E, Tadmor R, Dally O, Hadar H. Early MR demonstration of spinal metastases in patients with normal radiographs and CT and radionuclide bone scans. *J Comput Assist Tomogr* 1989;13:598–602.
6. Baker LL, Goodman SB, Perkash I, Lane B, Enzmann DR. Benign vs. pathologic compression fractures of vertebral bodies: assessment with conventional spin-echo, chemical-shift, and STIR MR imaging. *Radiology* 1990;174:495–502.
7. Bellon EM, Haacke EM, Coleman PE, Sacco DC, Steiger DA, Gangarosa RE. MR artifacts: a review. *AJR* 1986;147:1271.
8. Beltran J, Simon DC, Levy M, Herman L, Weis L, Mueller CF. Aneurysmal bone cysts: MR imaging at 1.5 T. *Radiology* 1986;158:689.
9. Beltran J, Simon DC, Katz W, Weis LD. Increased MR signal intensity in skeletal muscle adjacent to malignant tumors: pathologic correlation and clinical relevance. *Radiology* 1987;162:251.
10. Berquist TH. Magnetic resonance imaging: preliminary experience in orthopedic radiology. *Magn Reson Imaging* 1984;2:41.
11. Berquist TH. Magnetic resonance imaging in radiologic evaluation. In: Sim FH, ed. *Diagnosis and management of metastatic bone disease.* New York: Raven Press, 1987;43–49.
12. Berquist TH. Magnetic resonance imaging of musculoskeletal neoplasms. *Clin Orthop* 1989;244:101–118.
13. Berquist TH, Deutsch AL. Musculoskeletal neoplasms. In: Mink J, ed. *MRI of the musculoskeletal system: a teaching file.* New York: Raven Press, 1990.
14. Berquist TH, Ehman RL, Richardson ML. *Magnetic resonance of the musculoskeletal system.* New York: Raven Press, 1987.
15. Berquist TH, Ehman RL, King BF, Hodgman GA, Ilstrup DA. Differentiation of benign and malignant soft tissue masses with MRI: a blinded study. *Radiology* 1990;Aug.–Sept.
16. Bland KI, McCoy DM, Kinard RE, Copeland EM III. Application of magnetic resonance imaging and computerized tomography as an adjunct to the surgical management of soft tissue sarcomas. *Ann Surg* 1987;205:473–481.
17. Bloem JL, Taminiau AHM, Eulderink F, Hermans J, Pauwels EKJ. Radiologic staging of primary bone sarcoma: MR imaging, scintigraphy, angiography, and CT correlated with pathologic examination. *Radiology* 1988;169:805–810.
18. Boyko OB, Cory DA, Cohen MD, Provisor A, Mirkin D, DeRosa GP. MR imaging of osteogenic and Ewing's sarcoma. *AJR* 1987;148:317.
19. Burk LD, Dalinka MK, Kanal E, et al. Meniscal and ganglion cysts of the knee: MR evaluation. *AJR* 1988;150:331–336.
20. Bush CH, Spanier SS, Gillespy T. Imaging of atypical lipomas of the extremities: report of three cases. *Skeletal Radiol* 1988;17:472–475.
21. Carmody RF, Yang PJ, Seeley GW, Seeger JF, Unger EC, Johnson JE. Spinal cord compression due to metastatic disease: diagnosis with MR imaging versus myelography. *Radiology* 1989;173:225–229.
22. Chan L. The current status of magnetic resonance spectroscopy —basic and clinical aspects. *West J Med* 1985;143:773.
23. Chang AE, Matory YL, Dwyer AJ, et al. Magnetic resonance imaging versus computed tomography in the evaluation of soft tissue tumors of the extremities. *Ann Surg* 1987;205:340–348.
24. Charles HC, Baker ME, Hathorn JW, Sostman D. Differentiation of radiation fibrosis from recurrent neoplasia: a role for ^{31}P MR spectroscopy. *AJR* 1990;154:67–68.
25. Cohen EK, Kressel HY, Frank TS, Fallon M, Burk DL Jr, Dalinka MK, Schiebler ML. Hyaline cartilage-origin bone and soft-tissue neoplasms: MR appearance and histologic correlation. *Radiology* 1988;167:477.
26. Cohen EK, Kressel HY, Perosio T, Burk DL Jr, Dalinka MK, Schiebler ML, Fallon MD. MR imaging of soft-tissue hemangi-

omas: correlation with pathologic findings. *AJR* 1988;15:1079–1081.

27. Cohen JM, Weinreb JC, Maravilla KR. Fluid collections in the intraperitoneal and extraperitoneal spaces: comparison of MR and CT. *Radiology* 1985;155:705–708.
28. Cohen JM, Weinreb JC, Redman HC. Arteriovenous malformations of the extremities: MR imaging. *Radiology* 1986;158:475.
29. Cohen MD, Klatte EC, Baehner R, et al. Magnetic resonance imaging of bone marrow disease in children. *Radiology* 1984;151:715.
30. Cohen MD, McGuire W, Cory DA, Smith JA. MR appearance of blood and blood products: an *in vitro* study. *AJR* 1986;146:1293.
31. Cohen MD, Weetman RM, Provisor AJ, et al. Efficacy of magnetic resonance imaging in 139 children with tumors. *Arch Surg* 1986;121:522.
32. Colman LK, Porter BA, Redmond J III, Olson DO, Stimac GK, Dunning DM, Friedl KE. Early diagnosis of spinal metastases by CT and MR studies. *J Comput Assist Tomogr* 1988;12:423–426.
33. Daffner RH, Lupetin AR, Dash N, Deeb ZL, Sefczek RJ, Shapiro RL. MRI in the detection of malignant infiltration of bone marrow. *AJR* 1986;146:353.
34. Dahlin DC, Unni KK. *Bone tumors: general aspects and data on 8,542 cases.* Springfield, IL: CC Thomas, 1986.
35. Demas BE, Heelan RT, Lane J, Marcove R, Hajdu S, Brennan MF. Soft-tissue sarcomas of the extremities: comparison of MR and CT in determining the extent of disease. *AJR* 1988;150:615.
36. de Roose A, Kressel H, Spritzer C, Dalinka MK. MR imaging of changes at the endplate in degenerative lumbar disk disease. *AJR* 1987;149:531–534.
37. Dixon RM, Angus PW, Rajogopalan B, Radda GK. ^{31}P magnetic resonance studies of patients with lymphoma. Presented at the Society of Magnetic Resonance in Medicine, Amsterdam, The Netherlands, 1989.
38. Dooms GC, Fisher MR, Hricak H, Richardson M, Crooks LE, Genant HK. Bone marrow imaging: magnetic resonance studies related to age and sex. *Radiology* 1985;155:429.
39. Dooms GC, Hricak H, Sollitto RA, Higgins CB. Lipomatous tumors and tumors with fatty component: MR imaging potential and comparison of MR and CT results. *Radiology* 1985;157:479.
40. Dooms G, Mathurin P, Cornelis G, Malghem J, Maldague B. MR differential diagnosis between benign and malignant vertebral collapse. Presented at the Society of Magnetic Resonance in Medicine, Amsterdam, The Netherlands, 1989.
41. Duyer AJ, Frank JA, Sank VJ, Reinig JW, Hickey AM, Doppman JL. Short TI inversion-recovery pulse sequence: analysis and initial experience in cancer imaging. *Radiology* 1988;168:827–836.
42. Ebner F, Kressel HY, Mintz MC, et al. Tumor recurrence versus fibrosis in the female pelvis: differentiation with MR imaging at 1.5 T. *Radiology* 1988;166:333–340.
43. Edelman RR, Wentz KU, Mattle H, Zhao B, Liu C, Kim D, Laub G. Projection arteriography and venography: initial clinical results with MRI. *Radiology* 1989;172:351–357.
44. Ehman RL, Berquist TH, McLeod RA. MR imaging of musculoskeletal system: a 5-year appraisal. *Radiology* 1988;166:313.
45. Enzinger FM, Weiss SW. *Soft tissue tumors.* St. Louis, MO: CV Mosby, 1983.
46. Erlemann R, Reiser MF, Peters PE, et al. Musculoskeletal neoplasms: static and dynamic Gd-DTPA-enhanced MR imaging. *Radiology* 1989;171:767–773.
47. Feldman F, Singson RD, Staron RB. Magnetic resonance imaging of para-articular and ectopic ganglia. *Skeletal Radiol* 1989;18:353–358.
48. Fitzgerald RH, Berquist TH. Magnetic resonance imaging (editorial). *J Bone Joint Surg* 1986;68:799.
49. Francis IR, Chenevert TL, Collomb LG, Gubin B, Glazer DM. Clinical P-31 MR spectroscopy of malignant hepatic tumors using 1D SCI technique. Presented at the Society of Magnetic Resonance in Medicine, Amsterdam, The Netherlands, 1989.
50. Frouge C, Vanel D, Coffre C, Couanet D, Contesso G, Sarrazin D. The role of magnetic resonance imaging in the evaluation of Ewing sarcoma. *Skeletal Radiol* 1988;17:387–392.
51. Glazer HS, Lee JKT, Levitt RG, et al. Radiation fibrosis: differentiation from recurrent tumor by MR imaging. *Radiology* 1985;156:721.
52. Gillespy T, Manfrini M, Ruggieri P, Spanier SS, Pettersson H, Springfield DS. Staging of intraosseous extent of osteosarcoma: correlation of preoperative CT and MR imaging with pathologic macroslides. *Radiology* 1988;167:765–767.
53. Graif M, Pennock JM, Pringle J, Sweetnam DR, Jelliffe AJ, Bydder GM, Young IR. Magnetic resonance imaging: comparison of four pulse sequences in assessing primary bone tumors. *Skeletal Radiol* 1989;18:439–444.
54. Greco A, Jelliffe AM, Maher EJ, Leung AWL. MR imaging of lymphomas: impact on therapy. *J Comput Assist Tomogr* 1988;12:785–791.
55. Grossman RI, Hecht-Leavitt CM, Evans SM, et al. Experimental radiation injury: combined MR imaging and spectroscopy. *Radiology* 1988;169:305–309.
56. Haake EM, Masoruk TJ. The salient features of MR angiography. *Radiology* 1989;173:611–612.
57. Hahn PF, Saini S, Stark DD, Papanicolaou N, Ferrucci JT. Intraabdominal hematoma: the concentric ring sign in MR imaging. *AJR* 1987;148:115–119.
58. Harkens KL, Yuh WTC, Kathol MH, Moore TE, McGuire CW, Hawes DP, El-Khoury GY. Differentiating musculoskeletal neoplasm from nonneoplastic process: value of MR and Gd-DTPA. Presented at the Society of Magnetic Resonance in Medicine, Amsterdam, The Netherlands, 1989.
59. Hayes CW, Jensen ME, Conway WF. Non-neoplastic lesions of vertebral bodies. Findings in magnetic resonance imaging. *Radiographics* 1989;9:883–901.
60. Heiken JP, Lee JKT, Smathers RL, Totty WG, Murphy WA. CT of benign soft-tissue masses of the extremities. *AJR* 1984;142:575.
61. Hudson TM, Hamlin DJ, Enneking WF, Pettersson H. Magnetic resonance imaging of bone and soft tissue tumors: early experience in 31 patients compared with computed tomography. *Skeletal Radiol* 1985;13:134.
62. Hudson TM. Fluid-fluid levels in aneurysmal bone cyst: a CT feature. *AJR* 1984;141:1001.
63. Hudson TM, Hanlin DJ, Fitzsimmons JR. Magnetic resonance of fluid levels in aneurysmal bone cyst and in anticoagulated human blood. *Skeletal Radiol* 1985;13:267.
64. Jacobson AF, Stomper PC, Cronin EB, Kaplan WD. Bone scans with one or two new abnormalities in cancer patients with no metastasis: reliability of interpretation of initial correlative radiographs. *Radiology* 1990;174:503–507.
65. Kaplan PA, Murphey M, Greenway G, Resnick D, Sartoris DJ, Harms S. Fluid-fluid levels in giant cell tumors of bone: report of two cases. *J Comput Assist Tomogr* 1987;11:151–155.
66. Kim EE, Abello R, Holbert JM, et al. Differentiation of therapeutic changes from residual or recurrent musculoskeletal sarcomas using Gd-DTPA enhanced MRI. Presented at the Society of Magnetic Resonance in Medicine, Amsterdam, The Netherlands, 1989.
67. Koutcher JA, Ballon D, Graham M, Healey J, Casper ES. ^{31}P NMR spectral changes in sarcomas and squamous cell carcinomas with anti-neoplastic therapy. Presented at the Society of Magnetic Resonance in Medicine, Amsterdam, The Netherlands, 1989.
68. Kransdorf MJ, Jelinek JS, Moser RP Jr, Utz JA, Brower AC, Hudson TM, Berrey BH. Soft-tissue masses: diagnosis using MR imaging. *AJR* 1989;153:541–547.
69. Kransdorf MJ, Moser RP Jr, Jelinek JS, Weiss SW, Buetow PC, Berrey BH. Intramuscular myxoma: MR features. *J Comput Assist Tomogr* 1989;13:836–839.
70. Lee JK, Yao L, Wirth CR. MR imaging of solitary osteochondromas: report of eight cases. *AJR* 1987;149:557.
71. Linden A, Zankovick R, Theissen P, Diehl V, Schicha H. Malignant lymphoma: bone marrow imaging versus biopsy. *Radiology* 1989;173:335–339.
72. London J, Kim EE, Wallace S, Shirkhoda A, Coan J, Evans H. MR imaging of liposarcomas: correlation of MR features and histology. *J Comput Assist Tomogr* 1989;13:832–835.
73. Mahajan H, Kim EE, Wallace S, Abello R, Benjamin R, Evans

HL. Magnetic resonance imaging of malignant fibrous histiocytoma. *Magn Reson Imaging* 1989;7:283–288.
74. Mahajan H, Lorigan JG, Shirkhoda A. Synovial sarcoma: MR imaging. *Magn Reson Imaging* 1989;7:211–216.
75. Mankin HJ, Gebhardt MC. Advances in management of bone tumors. *Clin Orthop* 1985;200:73.
76. Martinez S, Vogler JA, Harrelson JM, Lyles KW. Imaging of tumoral calcinosis. New observations. *Radiology* 1990;174:215–222.
77. McKinstry CS, Steiner RE, Young AT, Jones L, Swirsky D, Aber V. Bone marrow in leukemia and aplastic anemia: MR imaging before, during and after treatment. *Radiology* 1987;162:701.
78. Mirra JM, Bullough PG, Marove RC, Jacobs B, Huros AG. Malignant fibrous histiocytoma and osteosarcoma in association with bone infarcts. *J Bone Joint Surg* 1979;56A:932–940.
79. Modic MT, Steinberg PM, Ross JS, Masary KTJ, Carter JR. Degenerative disk disease: assessment of changes in vertebral marrow with MR imaging. *Radiology* 1986;166:193–199.
80. Moore SG, Sebag GH, Dawson KL. MR evaluation of cortical bone and periosteal reaction in bone lesions: pathologic and radiographic correlation. Presented at the Society of Magnetic Resonance in Medicine, Amsterdam, The Netherlands, 1989.
81. Murphy WA, Totty WG, Carroll JE. MRI of normal and pathologic skeletal muscle. *AJR* 1986;146:565–574.
82. Naul LG, Peet GJ, Maupin WB. Avascular necrosis of the vertebral body: MR imaging. *Radiology* 1989;172:219–222.
83. Nederveen D, Jeneson JAL, Bakker CJG, Erich WBM. MR imaging of skeletal muscle of the forearm after handgrip exercise: a method to differentiate between trained and untrained muscles. Presented at the Society of Magnetic Resonance in Medicine, Amsterdam, The Netherlands, 1989.
84. Negendank WG, Crowley MG, Ryan JR, Keller NA, Evelhoch JL. Bone and soft-tissue lesions: diagnosis with combined H-1 MR imaging and P-31 MR spectroscopy. *Radiology* 1989; 173:181–188.
85. Ng TC, Majors AW, Vijayakumar S, et al. Response of human neoplasms to therapy: a study by ^{31}P-MRS. Presented at the Society of Magnetic Resonance in Medicine, Amsterdam, The Netherlands, 1989.
86. Nidecker AC, Müller S, Aue WP, Seelig J, Fridrich R, Remagen W, Hartweg H, Benz UF. Extremity bone tumors: evaluation by P-31 MR spectroscopy. *Radiology* 1985;157:167.
87. Paajanen H, Grodd W, Revel D, Engelstad B, Brasch RC. Gadolinium-DTPA enhanced MR imaging of intramuscular abscesses. *Magn Reson Imaging* 1987;5:109–115.
88. Pan G, Raymond AK, Carrasco CH, et al. Osteosarcoma: MR imaging after preoperative chemotherapy. *Radiology* 1990; 174:517–526.
89. Petasnick JP, Turner DA, Charters JR, Gitelis S, Zacharias CE. Soft-tissue masses of the locomotor system: comparison of MR imaging with CT. *Radiology* 1986;160:125.
90. Pettersson H, Gillespy T, Hamlin DJ, et al. Primary musculoskeletal tumors: examination with MR imaging compared with conventional modalities. *Radiology* 1987;164:237.
91. Pettersson H, Slone RM, Spanier S, Gillespy T III, Fitzsimmons JR, Scott KN. Musculoskeletal tumors: T1 and T2 relaxation times. *Radiology* 1988;167:783–785.
92. Ramsey RG, Zacharias CE. MR imaging of the spine after radiation therapy: easily recognizable effects. *AJR* 1985;144:1131.
93. Redmond OM, Stack JP, Dervan PA, Hurson BJ, Carney DN, Ennis JT. Osteosarcoma: use of MR imaging and MR spectroscopy in clinical decision making. *Radiology* 1989;172:811–815.
94. Remedios PA, Colletti PM, Raval JK, Benson RC, Chak LY, Boswell WD Jr, Halls JM. Magnetic resonance imaging of bone after radiation. *Magn Reson Imaging* 1988;6:301–304.
95. Ritschl P, Hajek PC, Pechmann U. Fibrous metaphyseal defects. *Skeletal Radiol* 1989;18:253–259.
96. Roberts MC, Kressel HY, Fallon MD, Zlatkin MB, Dalinka MK. Paget disease: MR imaging findings. *Radiology* 1989;173:341–345.
97. Rock MG, Pritchard DJ, Reiman HM, Soule EH, Brewster RC. Extra-abdominal desmoid tumors. *J Bone Joint Surg* 1984;66A:1369–1374.
98. Rosen BR, Fleming DM, Kushner DC, et al. Hematologic bone marrow disorders: quantitative chemical shift MR imaging. *Radiology* 1988;169:799–804.
99. Ross B, Helsper JT, Cox J, Young IR, Kempf R, Makepeace A, Pennock J. Osteosarcoma and other neoplasms of bone. Magnetic resonance spectroscopy to monitor therapy. *Arch Surg* 1987;122:1464.
100. Ross JS, Masaryk TJ, Modic MT, Carter JR, Mapstone T, Dengel FH. Vertebral hemangiomas: MR imaging. *Radiology* 1987;165:165.
101. Sanchez RB, Quinn SF, Walling A, Estrada J, Greenberg H. Musculoskeletal neoplasms after intraarterial chemotherapy: correlation with MR images with pathologic specimens. *Radiology* 1990;174:237–240.
102. Semmler W, Gademann G, Bachert-Baumann P, Zabel H, Lorenz WJ, van Kaick G. Monitoring human tumor response to therapy by means of P-31 spectroscopy. *Radiology* 1988;166:533.
103. Sherry CS, Harms SE. MR evaluation of giant cell tumors of the tendon sheath. *Magn Reson Imaging* 1989;7:195–201.
104. Shuman WP, Griffin BR, Haynor DR, Johnson JS, Jones DC, Cromwell LD, Moss AA. MR imaging in radiation therapy planning. *Radiology* 1985;156:143.
105. Shuman WP, Baron RL, Peters MJ, Tazioli PK. Comparison of STIR and spin echo MR imaging at 1.5T in 90 lesions of the chest, liver, and pelvis. *AJR* 1989;152:833–859.
106. Simon MA, Aschliman MA, Thomas N, Mankin HJ. Limb-salvage treatment versus amputation for osteosarcoma of the distal end of the femur. *J Bone Joint Surg* 1986;68A:1331–1337.
107. Simon MA, Nachman J. Current concepts review. The clinical utility of preoperative therapy for sarcomas. *J Bone Joint Surg* 1986;68A:1458–1464.
108. Sims RE, Genant HK. Magnetic resonance imaging of joint disease. *Radiol Clin North Am* 1986;24:179.
109. Smoker WRK, Godersky JC, Knutzon RK, Keyes WD, Norman D, Bergman W. The role of MR imaging in evaluating metastatic spinal disease. *AJR* 1987;149:1241–1248.
110. Stimac GK, Porter BA, Olson DO, Gerlock R, Genton M. Gadolinium-DTPA enhanced MR imaging of spinal neoplasms: preliminary investigation and comparison with unenhanced spin-echo and STIR sequence. *AJR* 1988;151:1185–1192.
111. Sugimura K, Yamasaki K, Kitagaki H, Tanaka Y, Kono M. Bone marrow diseases of the spine: differentiation with T1 and T2 relaxation times in MR imaging. *Radiology* 1987;165:541.
112. Sundaram M, McGuire MH. Computed tomography or magnetic resonance for evaluating the solitary tumor or tumor-like lesion of bone? *Skeletal Radiol* 1988;17:393–401.
113. Sundaram M, McGuire MH, Fletcher J, Wolverson MK, Heiberg E, Shields JB. Magnetic resonance imaging of lesions of synovial origin. *Skeletal Radiol* 1986;15:110.
114. Sundaram M, McGuire MH, Herbold DR. Magnetic resonance imaging of soft tissue masses: an evaluation of fifty-three histologically proven tumors. *Magn Reson Imaging* 1988;6:237–248.
115. Sundaram M, McGuire MH, Herbold DR, Beshony S, Fletcher JW. High signal intensity soft tissue masses on T1 weighted pulsing sequences. *Skeletal Radiol* 1987;16:30.
116. Sundaram M, McGuire MH, Herbold DR, Wolverson MK, Heiberg E. Magnetic resonance imaging in planning limb salvage surgery for primary malignant tumors of bone. *J Bone Joint Surg* 1986;68:809.
117. Sundaram M, McGuire MH, Schajowic ZF. Soft tissue masses: histologic bases for decreased signal (short T2) on T2 weighted images. *AJR* 1987;148:1247.
118. Swensen SJ, Keller PL, Berquist TH, McLeod RA, Stephens DH. Magnetic resonance imaging of hemorrhage. *AJR* 1985;145:921.
119. Tehranzadeh J, Mnaymneh W, Ghavam C, Morillo G, Murphy BJ. Comparison of CT and MR imaging in musculoskeletal neoplasms. *J Comput Assist Tomogr* 1989;13:466–472.
120. Tess JDT, Balzarini L, Ceglia E, Petrillo R, Musumeci R. MRI of lipomatous, fibrous and muscular tissue tumors. Presented at the Society of Magnetic Resonance in Medicine, Amsterdam, The Netherlands, 1989.
121. Tess JDT, Santoro A, Balzarini L, Ceglia E, Petrillo R, Bonadonna G, Musumeci R. Magnetic resonance staging of Hodgkin disease and non-Hodgkin lymphoma. Presented at the Society of

Magnetic Resonance in Medicine, Amsterdam, The Netherlands, 1989.
122. Thomsen C, Sorensen PG, Karle H, Christoffersen P, Henriksen O. Prolonged bone marrow T1-relaxation in acute leukaemia. *In vivo* tissue characterization by magnetic resonance imaging. *Magn Reson Imaging* 1987;5:251–257.
123. Totty WG, Murphy WA, Lee JKT. Soft-tissue tumors: MR imaging. *Radiology* 1986;160:135.
124. Turner DA. Nuclear magnetic resonance in oncology. *Semin Nucl Med* 1985;15:210.
125. Unger EC, Kessler HB, Kowalyshyn MJ, Lockman RD, Morea CT. MR imaging of Maffucci syndrome. *AJR* 1988;150:351–353.
126. Unger EC, Glazer HS, Lee JKT, Ling D. MRI of extracranial hematomas: preliminary observations. *AJR* 1986;146:403.
127. Utz JA, Kransdorf MJ, Jelinek JS, Moser RP Jr, Berrey BH. MR appearance of fibrous dysplasia. *J Comput Assist Tomogr* 1989;13:845–851.
128. Vanel D, Lacombe M, Covanet D, Kalifa C, Spielman M, Genin J. Musculoskeletal tumors: follow-up MR imaging after treatment with surgery and radiation therapy. *Radiology* 1987; 164:243.
129. van Vaals JJ, Bergman AH, van den Boogert HJ, van Gerwen PHJ, Heerschap A. ACE ^{1}H spectroscopic imaging over a localized volume of *in vivo* normal and pathologic rat brain. Presented at the Society of Magnetic Resonance in Medicine, Amsterdam, The Netherlands, 1989.
130. Watt I. Radiology in the diagnosis and management of bone tumors. *J Bone Joint Surg* 1985;67:520.
131. Weekes RG, Berquist TH, McLeod RA, Zimmer WD. Magnetic resonance imaging of soft-tissue tumors: comparison with computed tomography. *Magn Reson Imaging* 1985;3:345.
132. Weekes RG, McLeod RA, Reiman HM, Pritchard DJ. CT of soft-tissue neoplasms. *AJR* 1985;144:355–360.
133. Wilson DA, Prince JR. MR imaging of hemophilic pseudotumors. *AJR* 1988;150:349.
134. Yeager BA, Schiebler ML, Wertheim SB, Schmidt RG, Torg JS, Perosio PM, Dalinka MK. MR imaging of osteoid osteoma of the talus. *J Comput Assist Tomogr* 1987;11:916–917.
135. Yuh WTC, Kathol MH, Seim MA. Hemangiomas of skeletal muscle: MR findings in five patients. *AJR* 1986;149:765–768.
136. Yuh WTC, Zachar CK, Barloon TJ, Sato Y, Sichilo WJ, Hawes DR. Vertebral compression fractures: distinction between benign and malignant causes with MR imaging. *Radiology* 1989;172:215–218.
137. Zimmer WD, Berquist TH, McLeod RA, et al. Bone tumors: magnetic resonance imaging versus computed tomography. *Radiology* 1985;155:709.
138. Zimmer WD, Berquist TH, Sim FH, Wold LE, Pritchard DJ, Shives TC, McLeod RA. Magnetic resonance imaging of aneurysmal bone cyst. *Mayo Clin Proc* 1984;59:633–636.
139. Zlatkin MB, Lenkinski RE, Shinkwin M, et al. Combined MR imaging and spectroscopy of bone and soft tissue tumors. *J Comput Assist Tomogr* 1990;14:1–10.

MRI of the Musculoskeletal System, 2nd Edition, edited by T. H. Berquist.
Raven Press, Ltd., New York © 1990.

CHAPTER 13

Musculoskeletal Infection

Thomas H. Berquist

Infection in Nonviolated Tissue, 475
Joint Space Infection, 480
Septic Spondylitis, 482
Soft Tissue Infection, 483
Infection in Violated Tissue, 484
Surgical Reconstruction, 486
References, 489

Musculoskeletal infections may present with an acute, rapidly progressing course or in a more insidious fashion. The latter often follow trauma or surgery, such as after placement of orthopedic appliances (11). Early treatment, particularly in children with articular infections, is essential to prevent growth defects or joint ankylosis (17). Determination of the extent of involvement is important in planning proper medical or surgical management. Routine radiographs and computed tomography are useful for this purpose. Radioisotope studies are particularly sensitive in the early stages of infection (5,8,11,17,25).

Skeletal infections typically begin in medullary bone. The resulting hyperemia and inflammation cause alterations in signal intensity of medullary bone on MR images (7,17,23). The excellent tissue contrast and multiplanar imaging provided by MRI may allow earlier and more accurate assessment than current imaging techniques (3–7,24,30). Therefore, acute osteomyelitis may be evident on MR images when radiographs and CT are negative (7,17).

Discussion of the utility of MRI is facilitated by categorizing patients in the following manner: (a) infection in nonviolated tissue, (b) infection in violated tissue (previous trauma or surgery), and (c) evaluation of surgical techniques for treatment. The latter category includes patients treated with muscle or omental flaps and vascularized fibular grafts.

T. H. Berquist: Mayo Medical School and Mayo Clinic, Rochester, Minnesota 55905.

INFECTION IN NONVIOLATED TISSUE

Osteomyelitis presents a diagnostic and therapeutic challenge regardless of the age group. Early diagnosis and management are essential to avoid irreversible bone and soft tissue damage. Hematogenous osteomyelitis, which occurs more commonly in children than adults, may be acute, subacute, or chronic and most commonly involves the long bones of the lower extremities. In neonates and adults, the epiphysis is not protected: vascular channels cross the growth plate, allowing infection to involve both the metaphysis and epiphysis with a high incidence of joint space involvement (8,11,34). In patients 1–16 years of age, the growth plate prevents spread of infection to the epiphyses and joint space involvement is less common unless the metaphysis is intracapsular (8).

Infections typically involve the metaphyseal portion of long bones or areas near the physis in flat bones, such as the ilium. Radiologic changes are nonspecific in the early stages of infection. Localized swelling and distortion of the tissue planes may be the only early findings. Bone destruction is usually not appreciated until 35–40% of the involved region is destroyed and thus is generally not evident for 10–14 days (8,11,34). In addition, the degree of involvement is often underestimated on routine radiographs. In this situation, conventional or computed tomography may be useful to more clearly define the extent of involvement. Computed tomography has been especially useful in determining the extent of disease prior to planning operative therapy (29).

Radioisotope studies provide a sensitive tool for early detection of osteomyelitis. Technetium, gallium-67, and

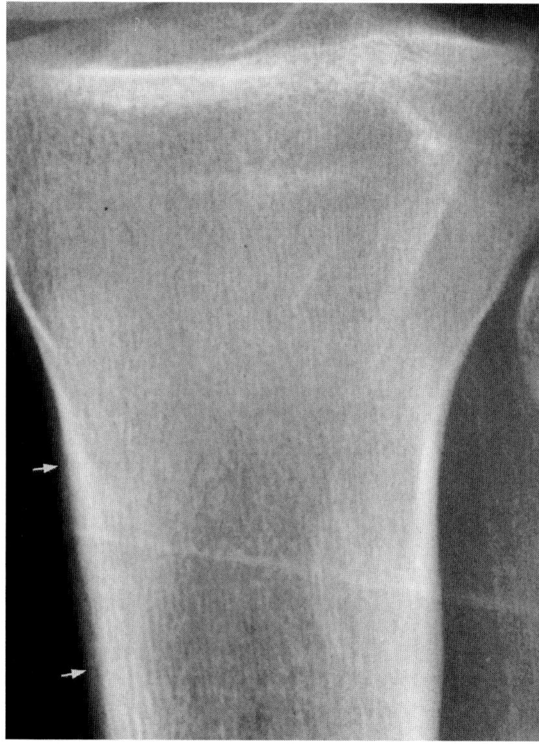

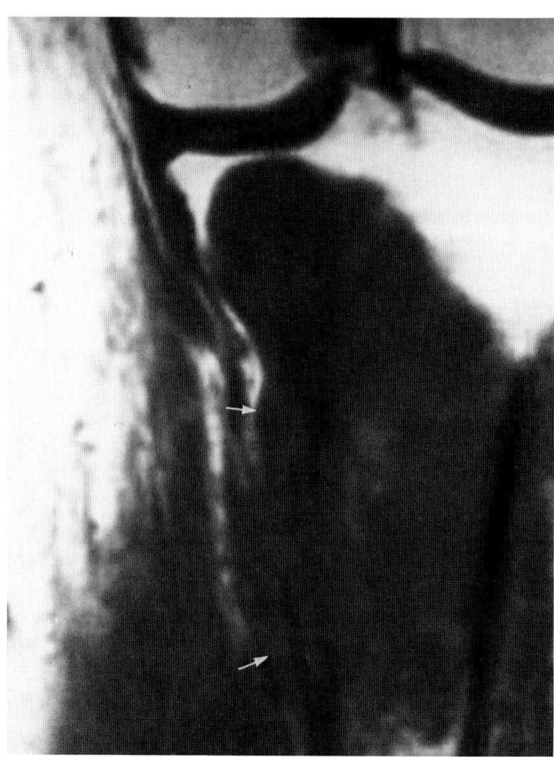

A,B

FIG. 13-1. A: Oblique view of the upper tibia shows subtle periosteal reaction (*arrows*). **B:** Coronal SE 500/20 image shows a large area of reduced signal intensity with involvement of the cortex and periosteum (*arrows*). It is difficult to separate the soft tissue changes on this sequence.

indium-111 labeled leukocytes provide sensitive and fairly specific methods for diagnosis of infection (7,8,11,18,21). However, the anatomic extent may be inaccurate, especially in the articular regions, and differentiation of soft tissue from bone involvement is not always possible (7).

Motion artifact is generally not a problem in the lower extremities. Therefore, MRI is particularly suited to evaluate osteomyelitis in these areas. Anatomic detail is

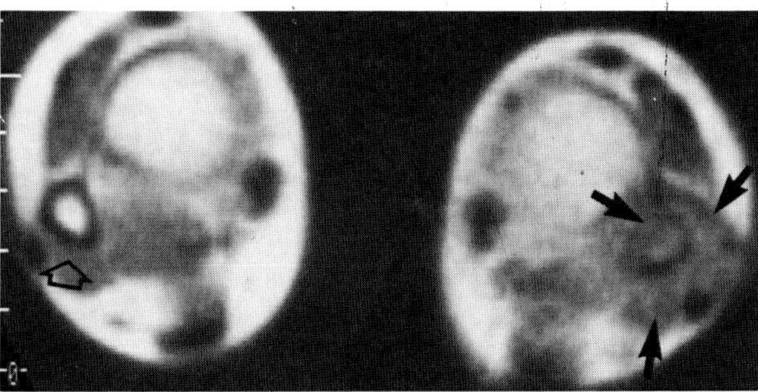

FIG. 13-2. Osteomyelitis of the distal left fibula. Spin-echo (SE 500/20) sequence demonstrates decreased signal intensity in the medullary bone with similar changes in the periosteum and soft tissues (*black arrows*). Note the normal right fibula (*open arrow*) and similar density of the muscle and soft tissue infection using this sequence. (From ref. 7, with permission.)

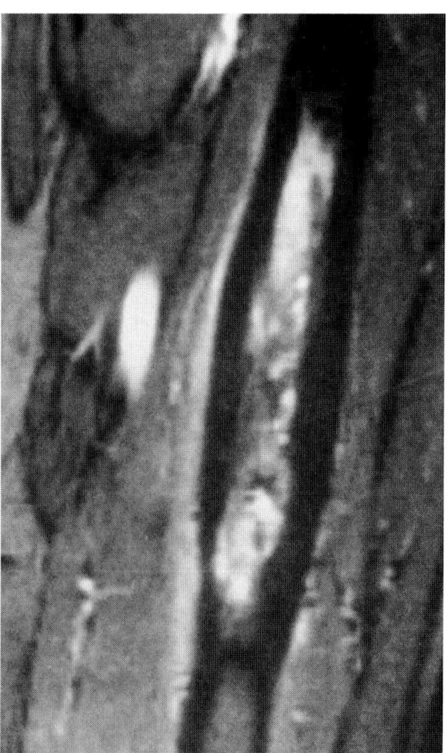

FIG. 13-3. Chronic osteomyelitis of the left femur. Coronal (SE 2,000/80) sequence shows thickening of the cortex with increased signal intensity in the marrow, thickened cortex, and soft tissue inflammation medially.

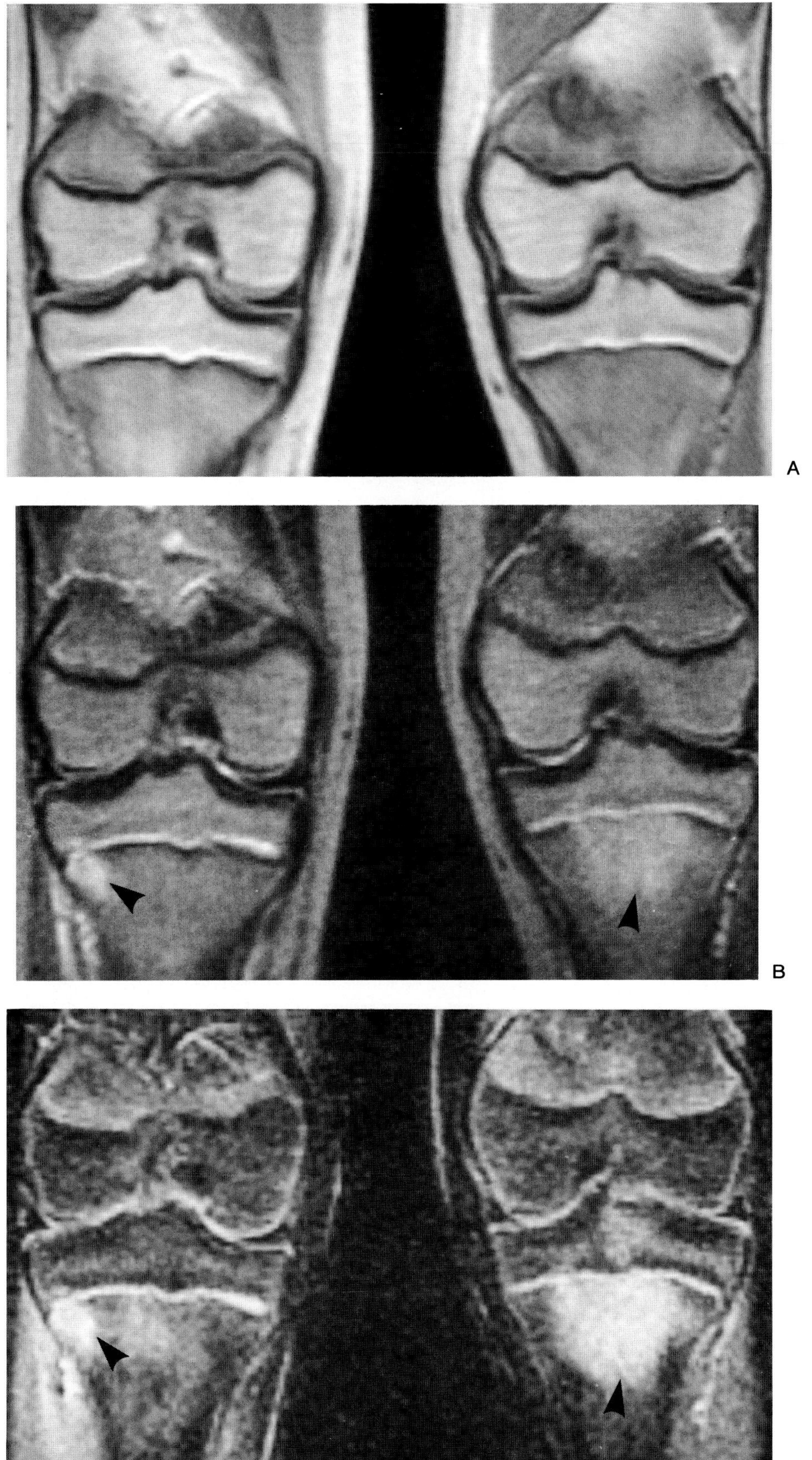

FIG. 13-4. Bilateral tibial osteomyelitis. **A:** SE 2,000/20 images show excellent anatomic detail. However, the areas of infection are not clearly demonstrated. **B:** SE 2,000/60 images show increased intensity in the metaphyses bilaterally (*arrowheads*). **C:** STIR sequence results in improved contrast between marrow and infection (*arrowheads*).

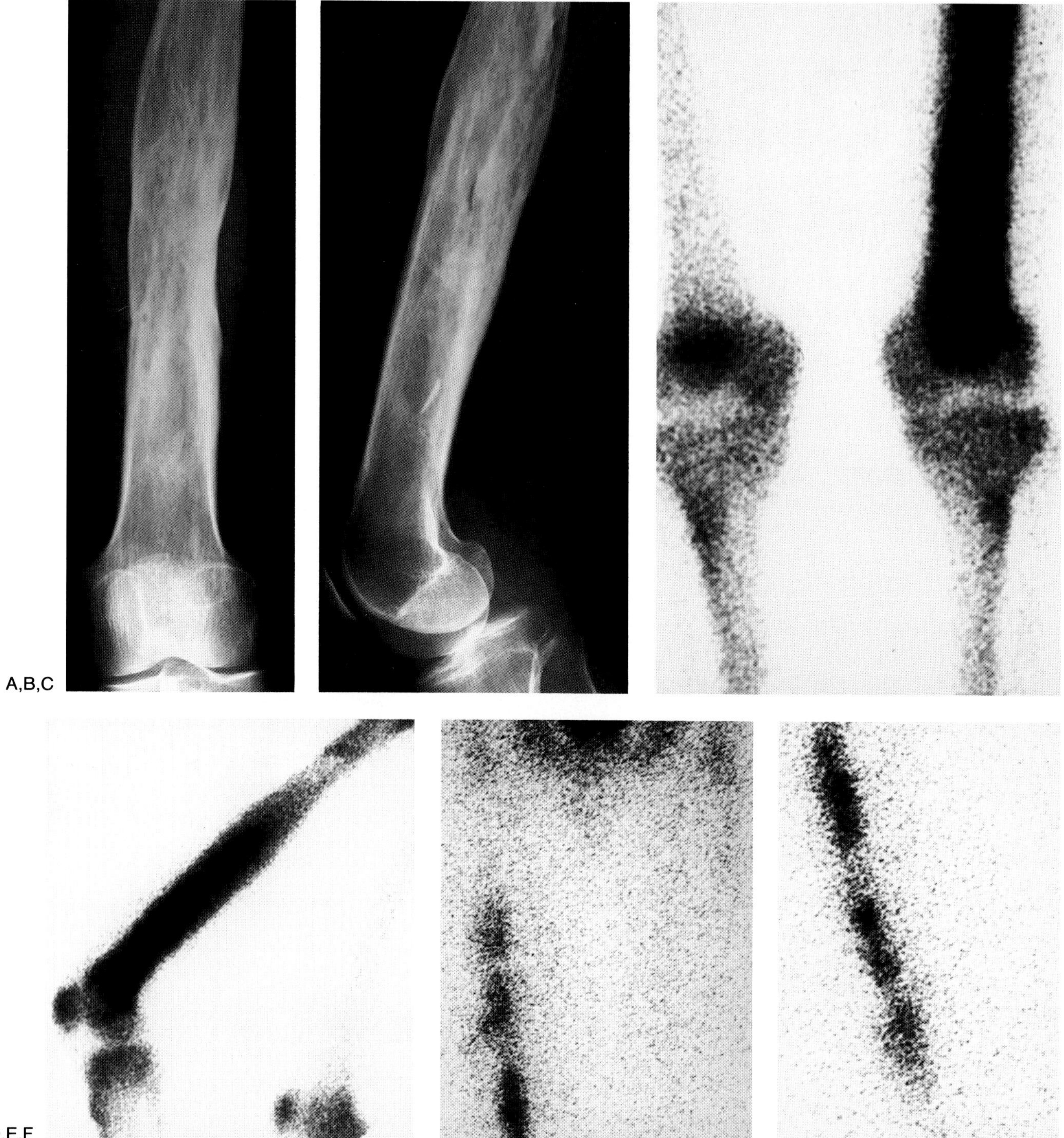

FIG. 13-5. AP (**A**) and lateral (**B**) radiographs of the femur in a patient with suspected osteomyelitis. Technetium-99m scans (**C,D**) show marked increased uptake in the distal femur. Indium-111 labeled white blood cell images in the AP (**E**) and lateral (**F**) projections show scattered areas of uptake in the femur. Soft tissue involvement? Coronal SE 500/20 image (**G**) demonstrates decreased signal intensity in the femur. Note the metal artifact (*arrowheads*). Axial T2 weighted image (**H**) shows increased signal intensity in the marrow with a localized (*arrowhead*) juxtacortical abscess.

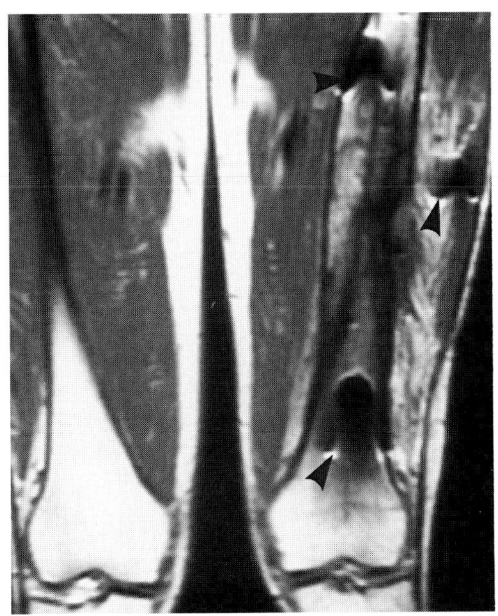

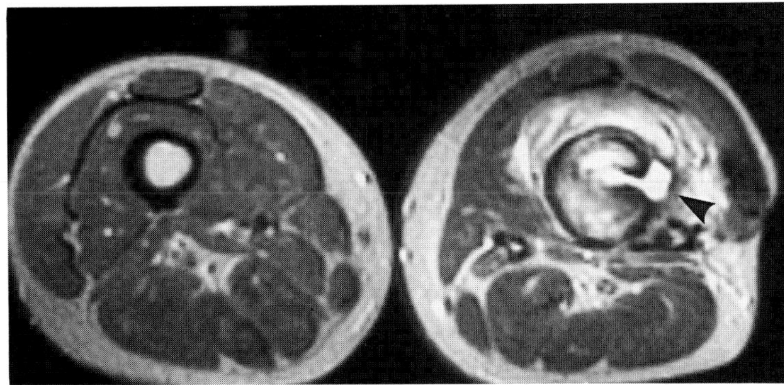

G,H

FIG. 13-5. *Continued.*

superior to that provided by isotope studies, and subtle bone and soft tissue changes are more easily appreciated than on radiographs or CT examinations (2,6,7, 13,17,36). In determining the effectiveness of MRI in evaluating infection, the following questions must be answered: (a) Can MRI detect infection as early as or earlier than isotope studies? (b) Which pulse sequences and MR techniques are most specific? (c) Can healing and treatment be effectively monitored?

As with other musculoskeletal pathology, examination of patients with infection requires at least T1 (SE 500/20 or inversion recovery) and T2 (spin-echo with long TE [≥60] and TR [>2,000]) weighted sequences (7,26,32,40,43). These sequences are needed to provide the necessary contrast between normal and abnormal tissue and to detect and characterize subtle abnormalities. T1 weighted spin-echo sequences (SE 500/20) can be performed quickly and provide high spatial resolution (7,17,23). Infection is demonstrated as an area of decreased signal intensity compared to the high signal intensity of normal marrow (Fig. 13-1). Changes in cortical bone, periosteum, and muscle are often less obvious (Fig. 13-2). Inversion recovery sequences may detect more subtle changes but images are "noisier" and scans require more time (TR usually ≥2,000). T2 weighted sequences (SE 2,000/60) demonstrate infection as areas of high signal intensity. The second echo (2,000/60) is ideal for distinguishing abnormal areas in cortical bone and soft tissues. Fat signal is reduced so areas of marrow inflammation are increased in intensity compared to marrow (Fig. 13-3). In certain situations, more than two sequences may be required to improve tissue characterization. For example, short TI inversion recovery (STIR) sequences (Fig. 13-4) or chemical shift imaging may provide valuable information about fat, water (cellular elements), or inflammatory changes in bone marrow (39).

The anatomic extent of osteomyelitis can clearly be demonstrated by MRI (7,24). The extent of disease, including detection of skip areas, is easily established using transaxial images in combination with either the sagittal or coronal images (see Figs. 13-1 to 13-4). This information is particularly valuable in planning surgical debridement.

Animal studies have demonstrated excellent correlation between gross histology and image features (12,25). There have also been several studies comparing isotope studies, CT, and MRI in detection of early osteomyelitis. Chandnani et al. (12) compared CT and MRI. MRI

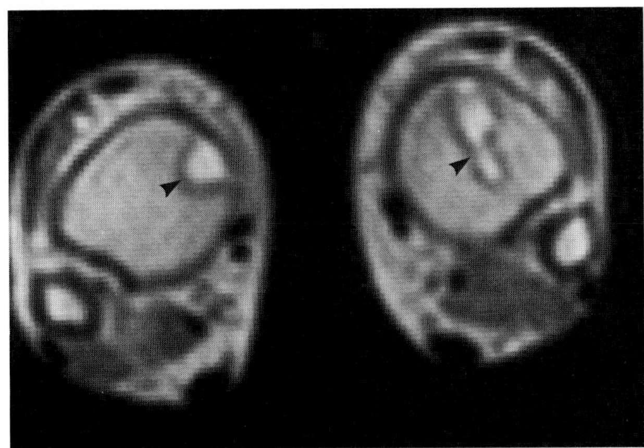

FIG. 13-6. Osteomyelitis in the tibias. High signal intensity areas in the marrow are surrounded by a thin fibrous margin (*arrowheads*).

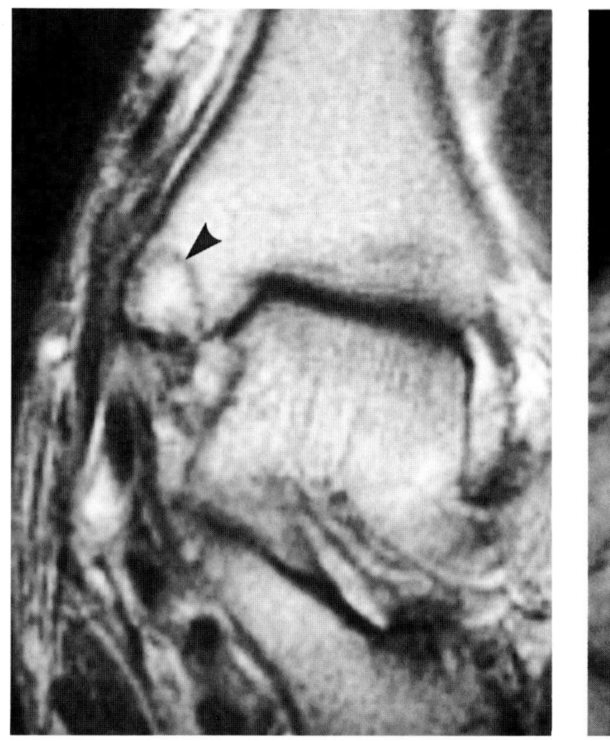

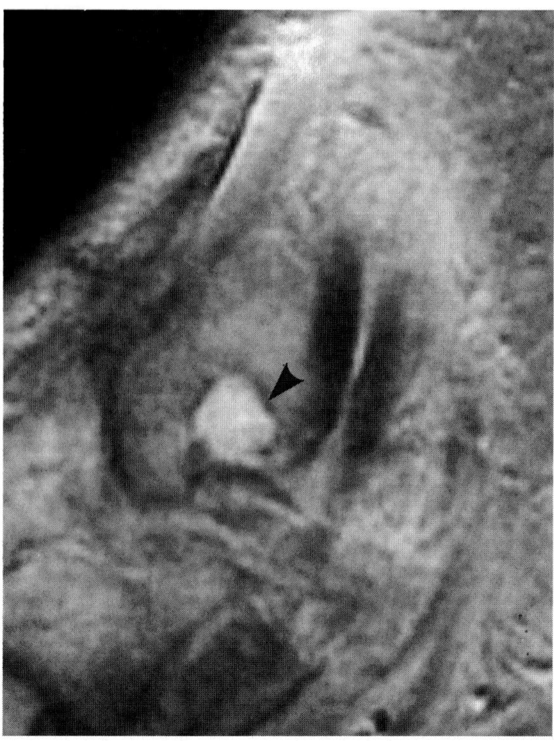

A,B

FIG. 13-7. Osteomyelitis of the medial malleolus. SE 2,000/20 coronal (**A**) and SE 2,000/60 sagittal (**B**) images show a focal area of osteomyelitis with a well-defined margin.

demonstrated a 94% sensitivity compared to 66% for CT. Both techniques were equally specific in excluding osteomyelitis. Unger et al. (40) reported an overall accuracy of 94% for MRI compared to 71% for technetium bone scans. MRI was particularly useful in separating bone and soft tissue processes compared to isotope scintigraphy. Gallium-67 and indium-111 labeled white blood cells are more specific for infection than technetium scans (5,21). Beltran et al. (5) compared technetium-99m MDP, gallium-67, and MRI in evaluating musculoskeletal infection. All techniques were equally effective in detecting osseous infection. However, MRI was more sensitive (100% to 69% for isotope scans) in identifying abscesses and distinguishing abscesses from cellulitis (Fig. 13-5).

The specificity of MRI in diagnosing osteomyelitis needs to be more clearly defined. Increased signal intensity in marrow, cortical bone, periosteum, and soft tissue is noted on T2 weighted, STIR, and gradient-echo (T2*) sequences (Fig. 13-5). Decreased signal intensity is evident when T1 weighted sequences are used (Fig. 13-1) (5,7,32,40). Similar findings, however, have also been noted with neoplasms. The only reliable image feature noted to date has been increased signal in medullary bone with a well-defined lucent margin (Figs. 13-6 and 13-7) (7). This observation has been noted with both infection and benign tumors (43). Infection must be present for several weeks to allow the reactive region in the medullary bone, which is responsible for this finding, to develop. Calculated T1 and T2 values overlap with other types of pathology. In addition, early studies show that these data do not accurately predict when the infection has been completely eradicated (25).

Despite the sensitivity of MRI, certain questions regarding osteomyelitis in nonviolated bone remain unanswered. To date, we have noted that MR images demonstrate changes earlier than radiographs, as well as provide better anatomic definition (7,17,30,43). However, it is not certain if MRI can detect abnormalities earlier than radioisotopes. By the time that the majority of patients present for evaluation, infections are already well established and the earliest phase of this process has passed. It is thus difficult to assess the relative usefulness of isotopes and MRI. Gallium-67 and indium-111 labeled WBCs may be more specific; however, anatomic detail is less than that provided by MRI (Fig. 13-5) (7).

JOINT SPACE INFECTION

Infectious arthritis is generally monoarticular and, like osteomyelitis, commonly involves the lower extremities (8,11,20). Joint space changes and soft tissue swelling may be noted on radiographs, but early bone changes are not appreciated for 1–2 weeks in a pyogenic infection and may take months to develop with tuber-

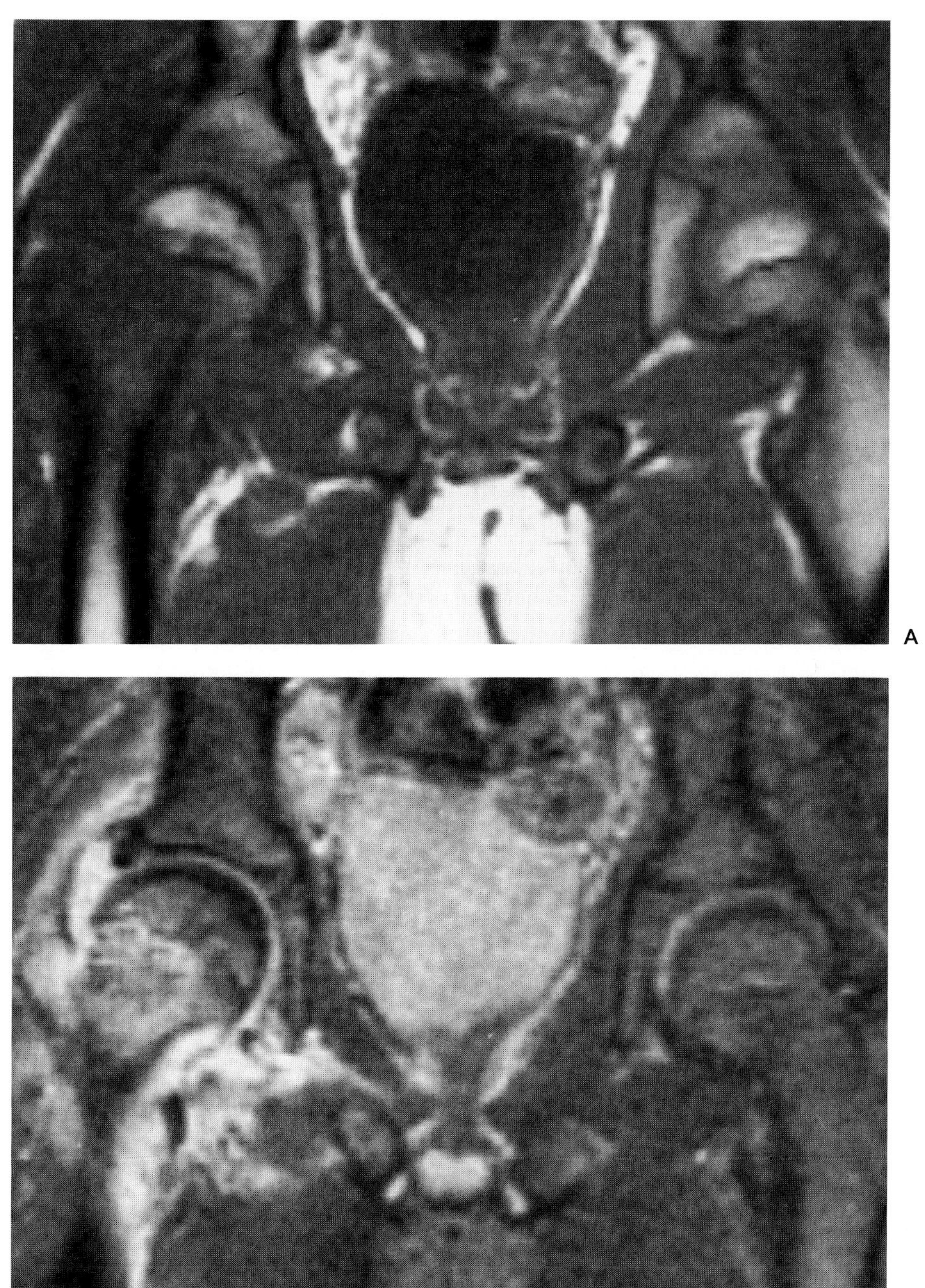

FIG. 13-8. Coronal SE 500/20 (**A**) and SE 2,000/60 (**B**) images of the hips in a child with joint space infection and osteomyelitis of the femoral neck.

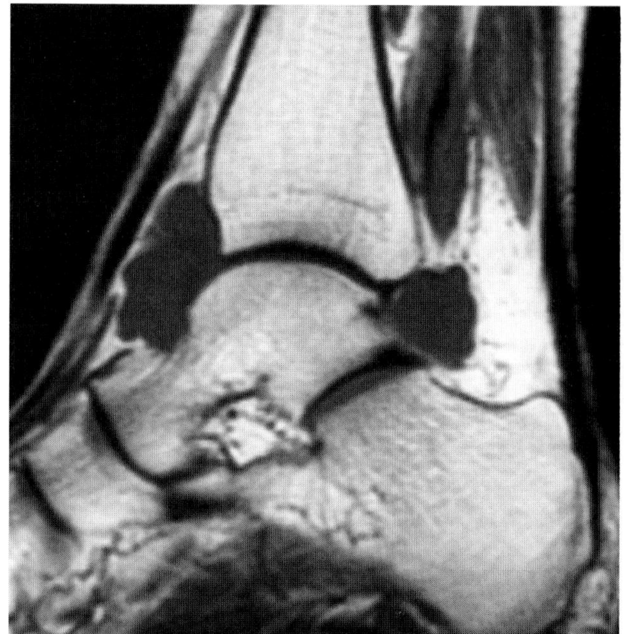
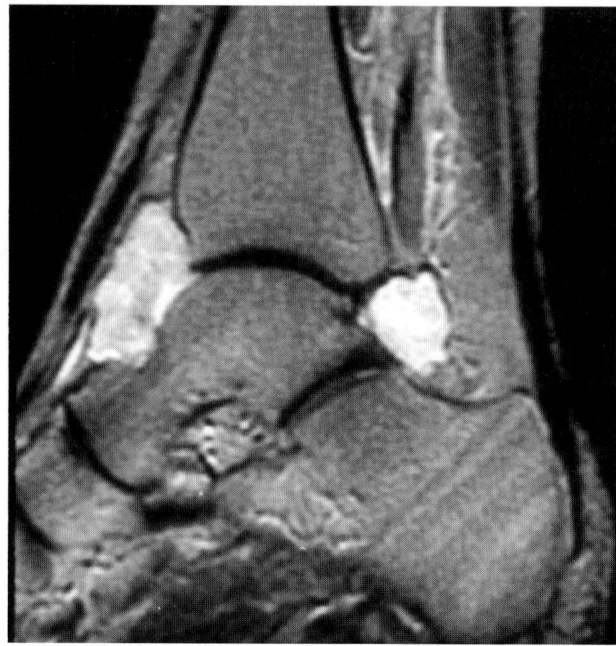

A,B

FIG. 13-9. SE 500/20 (**A**) and SE 2,000/60 (**B**) sagittal images demonstrating a large effusion. No infection. Compare the signal intensity of this case to the infection in Fig. 13-7. There is no detectable difference in signal intensity.

culous arthritis (8,20). Isotope scans using ^{99m}Tc are sensitive in detecting early changes, but nonspecific. Gallium-67 and indium-111 labeled WBC scans are more specific in this regard (8,18,21).

The role of MRI in joint space infection is unclear. Early bone and soft tissue changes and effusions are easily detected (Fig. 13-8). However, the early erosive changes are not specific and could be noted with many other arthritides. Characterization of the type of fluid present in the joint would be useful (4). Generally, the T1 and T2 relaxation times of transudates are longer than exudates (10,14,35). Infected fluid and blood in the joint tend to have more intermediate signal intensity and may be inhomogeneous on T2 weighted images (10). Normal synovial fluid has a uniformly high signal intensity using this sequence (Figs. 13-8 and 13-9) (4). This information is obviously not sufficient to avoid joint aspiration to identify the offending organism.

SEPTIC SPONDYLITIS

Various terms have been applied to inflammatory changes in the disk space or vertebrae. Disk space narrowing with an elevated sedimentation rate has been termed "diskitis," "infectious diskitis," and "intervertebral disk space inflammation" (9,11). In adults, the disk is relatively avascular, and infection usually spreads to the disk via the vertebral body rather than the hematogenous route—pyogenic vertebral osteomyelitis (8,9,11). Septic spondylitis is a general term that includes the spectrum of childhood diskitis and adult vertebral osteomyelitis (11).

Diagnosis of septic spondylitis can be difficult with routine imaging techniques. The first radiographic changes, disk space narrowing with adjacent swelling, may not be evident for several weeks (8). Thus, serial spine films are especially helpful in differentiating septic spondylitis from other causes of disk space narrowing (degenerative, traumatic, etc.). Lucent zones in the adjacent vertebrae follow disk narrowing by several weeks, and if left unchecked, progressive collapse and kyphotic deformity can occur (8,11).

Technetium scans may be difficult to interpret, especially in adults with degenerative disease, previous laminectomy, or fusion. Increased accuracy is achieved using gallium-67 and indium-111 labeled white blood cells (11).

CT has played a valuable role in evaluating the disk, vertebra, and surrounding soft tissues. CT guided aspiration is also useful in defining the infecting organism so that the appropriate antibiotics can be used (29). MRI, however, can demonstrate changes earlier and more clearly than either CT or routine radiographs (15,22). This is largely due to the improved soft tissue contrast and the ability to perform direct coronal and sagittal imaging (Fig. 13-10). In patients with suspected vertebral osteomyelitis, MRI was found to be both accurate and sensitive. T1 weighted sequences (SE 500/20) demonstrate decreased signal in the vertebral bodies and in-

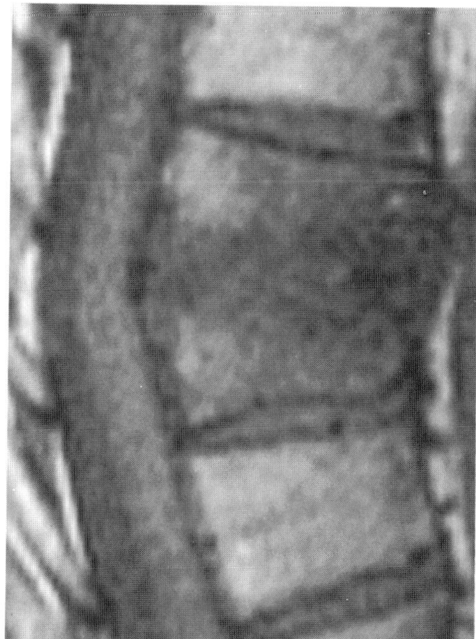

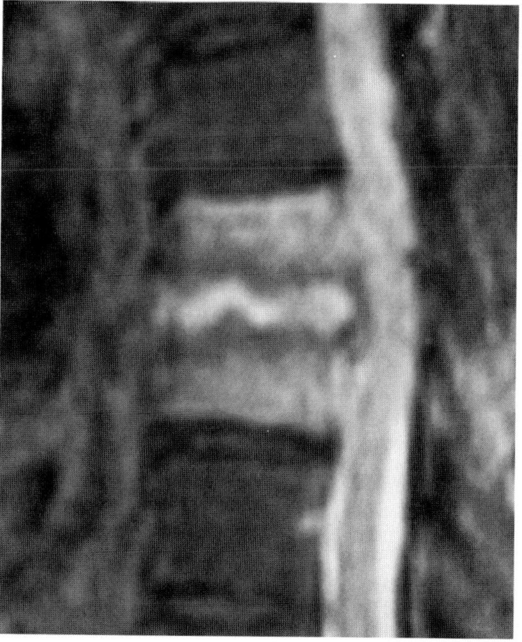

A,B

FIG. 13-10. Sagittal SE 500/20 (**A**) and SE 2,000/60 (**B**) images of the spine, demonstrating low signal intensity in the vertebra and disk on the T1 weighted image (**A**) and marked increased intensity on the T2 weighted sequence (**B**).

volved disk. T2 weighted spin-echo sequences (SE 2,000/60) reveal higher signal intensity than normal disks or marrow in the involved areas. In addition, sagittal MR images provide a noninvasive means for evaluating kyphotic angulation and the extent of spinal canal involvement (22). See Chapter 5 for a more complete discussion on vertebral infection.

SOFT TISSUE INFECTION

The superior soft tissue contrast of MRI is ideally suited for identification of soft tissue inflammation and abscesses (Fig. 13-5) (36). Localization of the infected area, specifically the relationship to bone and neurovascular structures, is easily accomplished without injec-

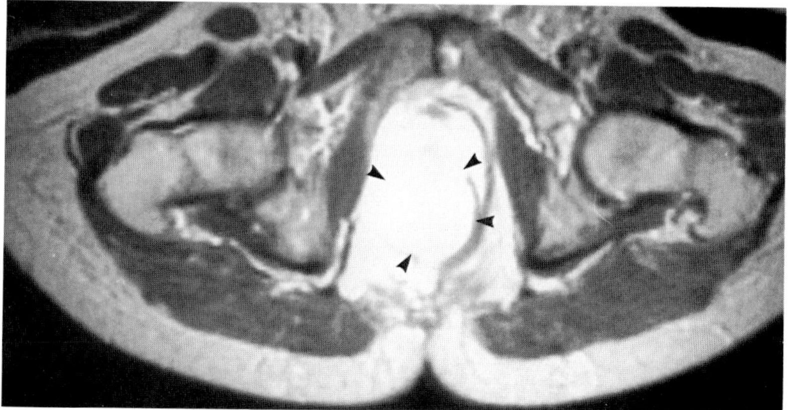

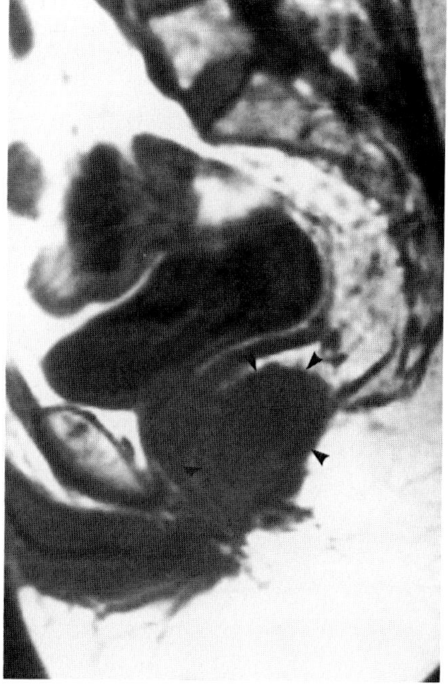

A,B

FIG. 13-11. Axial SE 2,000/60 (**A**) and sagittal SE 500/20 (**B**) images show a well-defined homogeneous lesion. This abscess fluid has uniformly high intensity on T2 (**A**) and low intensity on T1 (**B**) weighted sequences.

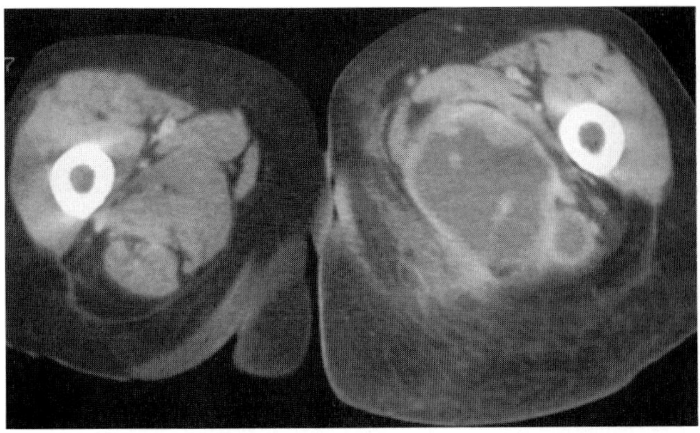

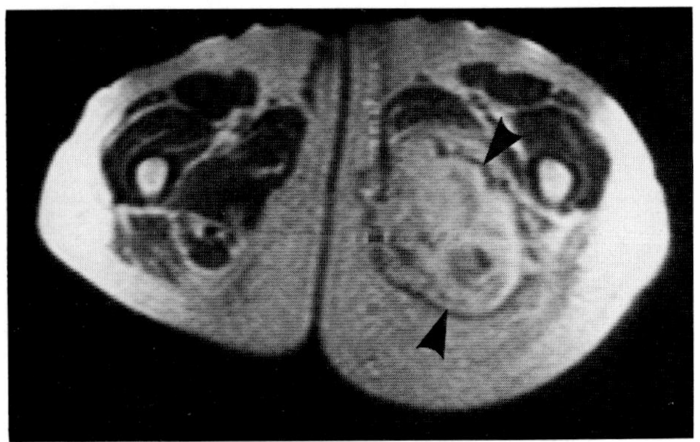

A,B

FIG. 13-12. Thigh abscess. **A:** CT scan shows a large fluid-filled abscess with a thick irregular capsule. The capsule enhances on this contrast examination. **B:** T2 weighted MR image shows the abscess (*arrowheads*) has intermediate intensity and is inhomogeneous.

tion of contrast medium (7,23). Both T1 and T2 weighted images are used to assist in defining the nature of the lesion and to define its extent. The signal intensity of abscess fluid may be inhomogeneous and have high to intermediate signal intensity on T2 weighted and STIR sequences (Fig. 13-11). Signal intensity varies slightly depending on the protein content and necrotic debris in the abscess (Fig. 13-12) (14,35). Abscesses are typically similar to or slightly lower in intensity than muscle on T1 weighted sequences (3,7,12). Gadolinium has been used to enhance the hyperemic margins or capsules of chronic abscesses. This technique may assist in improving the diagnostic specificity.

Reports suggest that MRI is more sensitive than CT for detection of abscesses (5,12). The choice of technique should be varied with the clinical setting. In patients with recent surgery or strong clinical indication of abscess formation, CT may be more useful. This is especially true if abdominal or pelvic abscesses (Fig. 13-11) are suspected and percutaneous drainage is considered. The examination and intervention can be accomplished at the same time. Patients with subtle clinical findings and when extremity involvement is suspected are more appropriately evaluated with MRI.

INFECTION IN VIOLATED TISSUE

Detection of infection in patients with violated bone and soft tissue presents a difficult diagnostic challenge. This includes patients with previous fracture or surgical intervention, either for fracture reduction or joint replacement (11,27,28,42). Radiographs and tomograms may be difficult to interpret in the early phases of infection due to the changes of fracture healing (Fig. 13-5A,B). Subtle changes adjacent to metal fixation devices and joint replacements are also not seen for weeks. The usually reliable ^{99m}Tc scan can remain positive for more than 10 months following fracture or surgery, but ^{111}In-labeled leukocytes and gallium-67 scans have been more successful in these patients (21). The anatomic detail and combination of joint aspiration and anesthetic injection have made subtraction arthrography a very useful exam for patients with joint replacement and suspected infection (11).

In a review of the MRI studies in over 50 patients with infection in violated bone and soft tissues, we observed abnormalities in all examinations. However, in many cases it was difficult to differentiate areas of osteomyelitis from zones of fracture healing. Fracture healing re-

TABLE 13-1. *MRI features of infection*

	Marrow		Cortical bone		
	Normal	Infection	Normal	Infection	Soft tissues
SE 500/20 (T1WI)	Fat density	Dark	Black	Dark (may be slightly gray)	May be difficult to evaluate (Figs. 13-1 and 13-2)
Inversion recovery	Fat density	Dark	Black	Dark (may be slightly gray)	Signal decreased relative to muscle, nerve, fat
SE 2,000/60 (T2WI)	Low intensity	High intensity	Black	High intensity	Signal increased relative to muscle and fat
Short TI inversion recovery (STIR)	Low intensity	High intensity	Low intensity	High intensity	Signal intensity of infection > muscle > fat

T1WI, T1 weighted image.
T2WI, T2 weighted image.

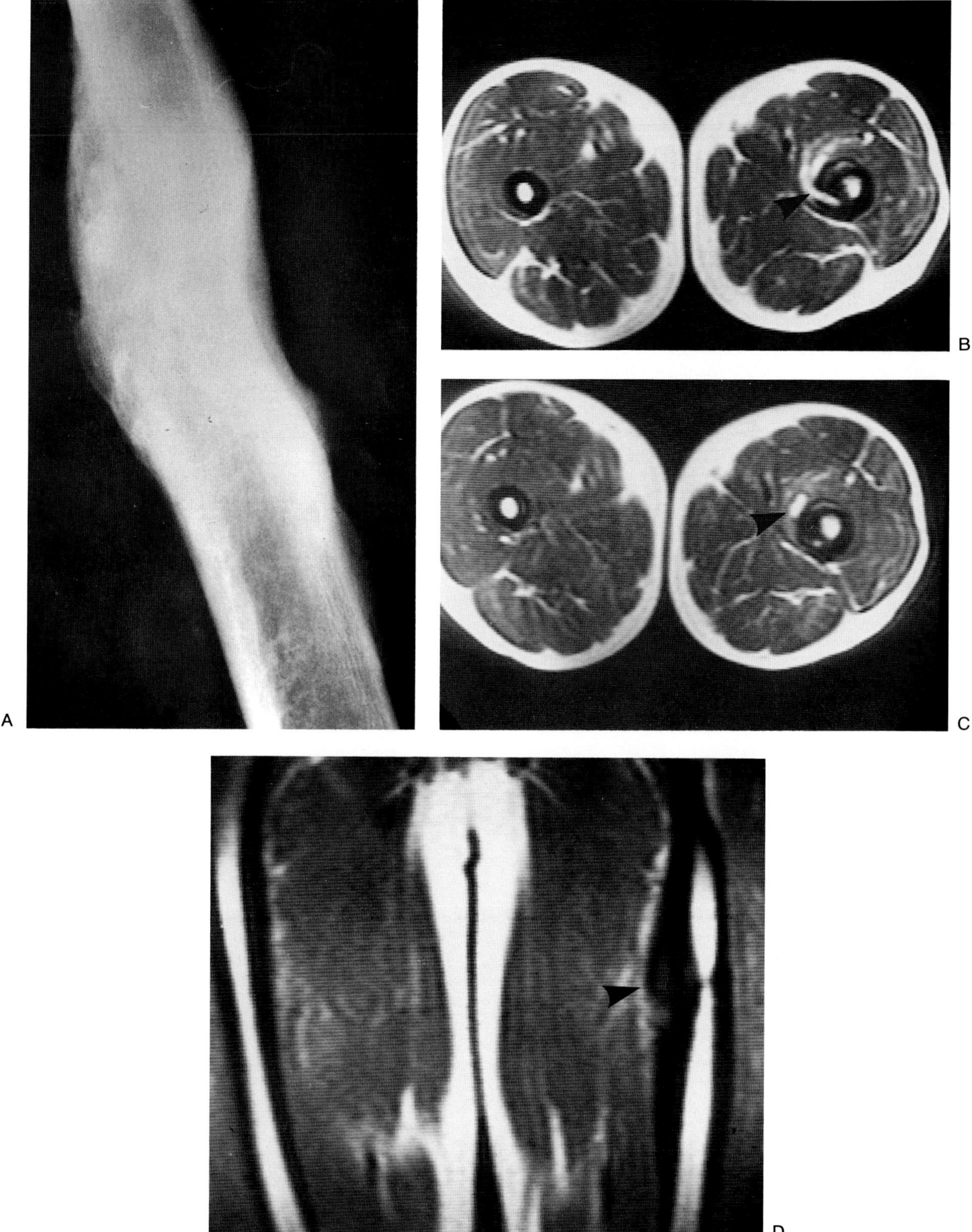

FIG. 13-13. Femoral osteomyelitis following fracture. **A:** Radiograph demonstrating old fracture deformity with sclerosis and cortical thickening. **B,C:** Axial MR images (SE 2,000/30) show cortical irregularity on the left with increased signal intensity in the cortex and soft tissues (*arrowheads*), indicating infection. **D:** Coronal T1 weighted image shows cortical changes medially (*arrowhead*).

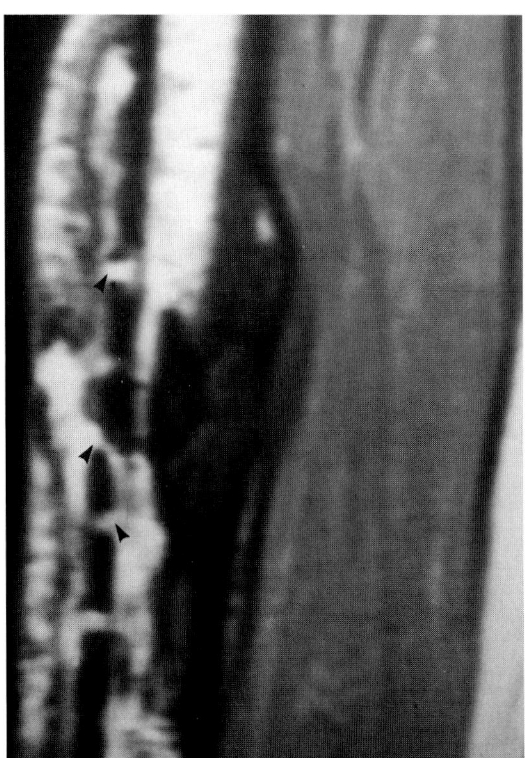

FIG. 13-14. Sagittal SE 2,000/30 image of the tibia in a patient with previous fixation of a fracture. There is a large low signal intensity sequestrum (*large arrowhead*). Fluid exits the screw tracts (*small arrowheads*) into juxtacortical abscess cavities.

sults in cortical thickening with granulation tissue and fibrocartilage in the region of the fracture. T2 weighted images are most useful because they provide the best contrast between cortical bone and granulation tissue or fibrocartilage. Subtle changes in medullary bone can be seen with STIR sequences (see Table 13-1). Areas of inflammation or active infection have longer T2 relaxation times due to increased free water content compared to the areas of healing (Fig. 13-13). Hemorrhage also has a long T2, but at low and medium field strengths, the T2 shortens over a 10–17 day period, which may assist in differentiating hemorrhage or hematoma from untreated areas of infection (31).

Routine radiographs, tomography, and CT are clearly very useful for identifying sequestra, which appear as areas of decreased signal on MR images (Fig. 13-14). The artifact created by metal implants (on MR images), though often minimal, may prohibit evaluation of subtle bone changes immediately adjacent to the metal (Fig. 13-15). However, we have found that periosteal changes and soft tissue abnormalities can easily be detected even in the region of the hip, where the amount and configuration of the metal tends to cause more artifact (6,7).

SURGICAL RECONSTRUCTION

A high percentage of adult patients with chronic osteomyelitis require surgical therapy for excision of ne-

A,B

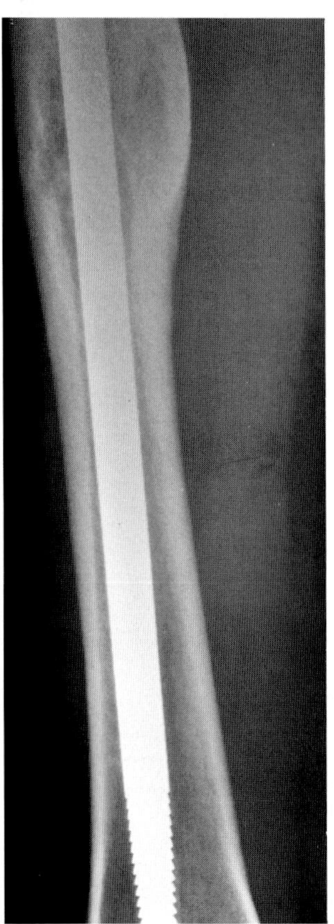

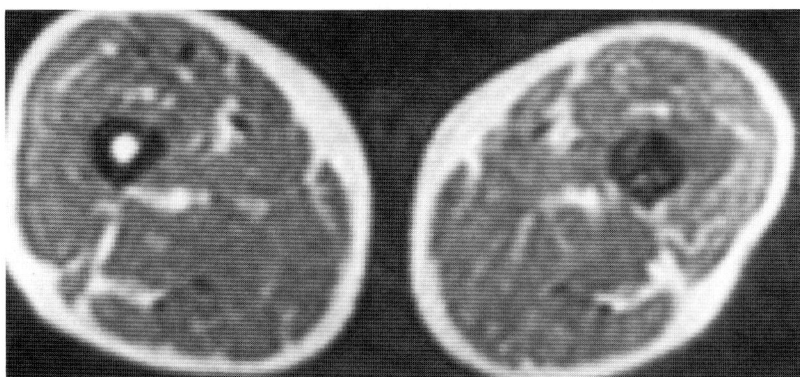

FIG. 13-15. Old femoral fracture with medullary wall for fixation. There was pain in the midfemur with abundant callus on the radiograph (**A**). MR image (0.15 T, SE 2,000/30) (**B**) shows no significant artifact and no evidence of infection.

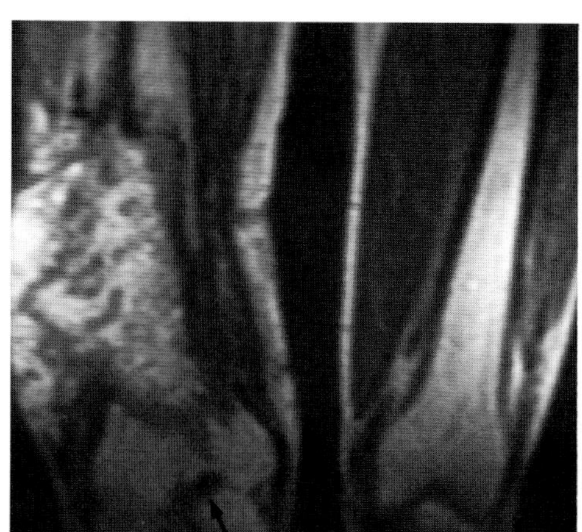

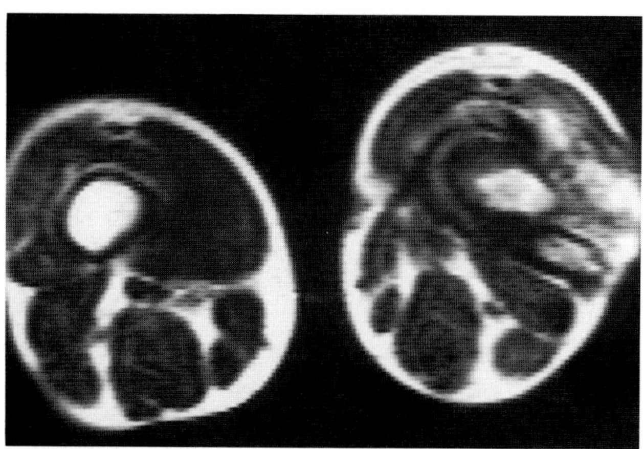

A,B

FIG. 13-16. Chronic osteomyelitis of the distal femur with vascularized omental graft. The coronal (**A**) and axial (**B**) (TE 30, TR 500) MR images show that the graft fills the dead space. The omental fat has high signal intensity and appears viable. There is an area of decreased intensity in the distal femur (*arrow*), representing a separate area of infection.

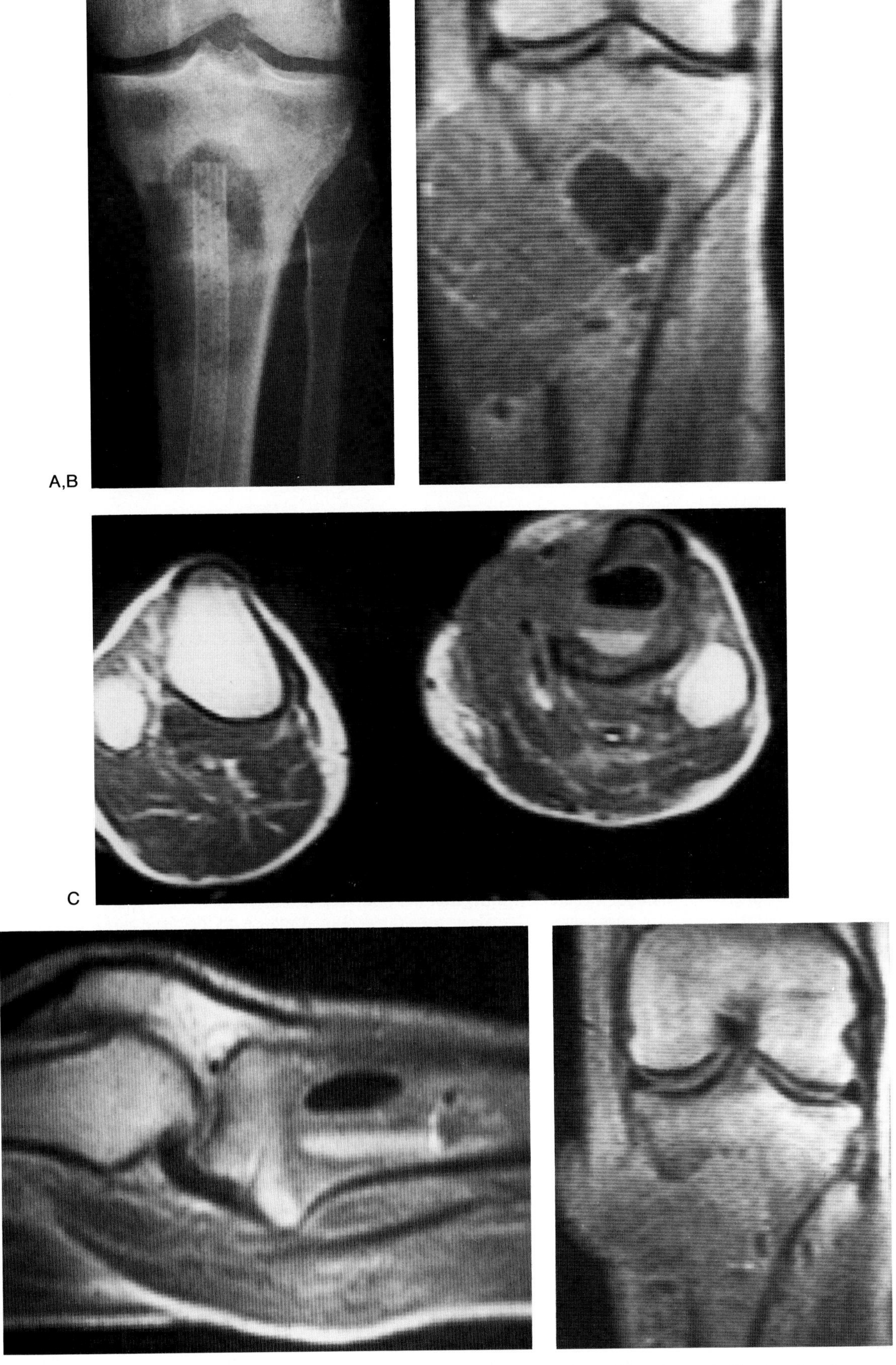

FIG. 13-17. Osteomyelitis of the proximal tibia treated with muscle flap. AP radiograph (**A**) showing the bone defect in the upper tibia. Coronal (**B**), axial (**C**), and sagittal (**D**) MR images using partial saturation techniques show a large residual dead space with air, blood, and fluid in the dead space. This is an ideal medium for recurrent infection. The patient was returned to surgery and the dead space (**E**) filled by repositioning the flap.

crotic or infected tissue. The use of free vascularized muscle, omental, and bone grafts is increasing in the treatment of patients with chronic osteomyelitis (1,16,19,37,38,41). Reconstructive procedures may be needed depending on the vascularity of adjacent tissue and the size and type of defect (38). There are several basic goals regardless of the tissue or technique used. These include (a) wound coverage, (b) obliteration of dead space (which may permit survival of existing organisms or provide a medium for recurrent infection), and (c) provision of optimal vascular supply to the described area (37,38,41).

Preoperative assessment should include review of the necessary information and planning of the surgical approach; postoperative assessment should determine whether or not the surgical goals have been achieved. Preoperatively, MRI is an ideal way to assess the extent of bone and soft tissue involvement, as well as to detect skip areas. Preoperative images also serve as a valuable baseline to later determine whether the surgical goals are achieved (Fig. 13-16).

MRI is well suited to evaluate defect coverage or dead space, residual infection, and hematomas or fluid collections that may serve as media for recurrent infection (Fig. 13-17). MRI is particularly useful in the evaluation of omental (Fig. 13-16) and muscle flaps (Fig. 13-17). Vascularized fibular grafts can be evaluated but the small amount of marrow presents certain problems, since there is little fibular marrow to image in the axial plane. This can be improved by using coronal and sagittal views, which increase the marrow volume imaged and allow the position as well as the proximal and distal attachments of the grafts to be more easily evaluated.

Recently, Gd-DTPA has been used to confirm viability of vascularized grafts. Varnell et al. (33) demonstrated that viable grafts enhanced while those with early vascular occlusion did not enhance.

Further studies and follow-up of these patients will be needed to determine the effectiveness of MRI in evaluating viability and flow factors in the grafts. Spectroscopy may also play a role in graft evaluation, especially early ischemic changes.

REFERENCES

1. Arnold PG, Irons GB. Lower extremity muscle flaps. *Orthop Clin North Am* 1984;15:441–449.
2. Baker HL Jr, Berquist TH, Kispert DB, et al. Magnetic resonance imaging in a routine clinical setting. *Mayo Clin Proc* 1985;60:75–90.
3. Beltran J, Noto AM, McGhee RB, Freedy RM, McCalla MS. Infections of the musculoskeletal system: high-field-strength MR imaging. *Radiology* 1987;164:449–454.
4. Beltran J, Noto AM, Herman LJ, Mosure JC, Burk JM, Christoforidis AJ. Joint effusions: MR imaging. *Radiology* 1986; 158:133–137.
5. Beltran J, McGhee RB, Shaffer PB, et al. Experimental infections of the musculoskeletal system: evaluation with MR imaging and Tc-99m MDP and Ga-67 scintigraphy. *Radiology* 1988;167:167–172.
6. Berquist TH. Magnetic resonance imaging: preliminary experience in orthopedic radiology. *Magn Reson Imaging* 1984;2:41–52.
7. Berquist TH, Brown ML, Fitzgerald RH Jr, May GR. Magnetic resonance imaging: application in musculoskeletal infection. *Magn Reson Imaging* 1985;3(3):219–230.
8. Bonakdapour A, Gaines VD. The radiology of osteomyelitis. *Orthop Clin North Am* 1983;14:21–37.
9. Boston HC, Bianco AJ Jr, Rhodes KH. Disk space infections in children. *Orthop Clin North Am* 1975;6:953–964.
10. Brown JJ, vanSonnenberg E, Gerber KH, Strich G, Wittich GR, Slatsky RA. Magnetic resonance relaxation times of percutaneously obtained normal and abnormal body fluids. *Radiology* 1985;154:727–731.
11. Brown ML, Kamida CB, Berquist TH, Fitzgerald RH Jr. An imaging approach to musculoskeletal infections. In: Berquist TH, ed. *Imaging of orthopedic trauma and surgery.* Philadelphia: Saunders, 1986;731–753.
12. Chandnani VP, Beltran J, Morris CS, et al. Acute experimental osteomyelitis and abscesses: detection with MR imaging versus CT. *Radiology* 1990;174:223–226.
13. Cohen MD, Klatte EC, Baehner R, et al. Magnetic resonance imaging of bone marrow disease in children. *Radiology* 1984;151:715–718.
14. Cohen JM, Weinreb JC, Maravilla KR. Fluid collections in the intraperitoneal and extraperitoneal spaces: comparison of MR and CT. *Radiology* 1985;155:705–708.
15. deRoos A, vanMeerten ELVP, Bloem JL, Bluemm RG. MRI of tuberculous spondylitis. *AJR* 1986;146:79–82.
16. Fitzgerald RH, Ruttle PE, Arnold PG, Kelly PJ, Irons GB. Local muscle flaps in the treatment of chronic osteomyelitis. *J Bone Joint Surg* 1985;67A:175–185.
17. Fletcher BD, Scoles PV, Nelson AD. Osteomyelitis in children: detection by magnetic resonance. *Radiology* 1984;150:57–60.
18. Howie DW, Savage JP, Wilson TG. The technetium phosphate bone scan in the diagnosis of osteomyelitis in children. *J Bone Joint Surg* 1983;65A:431–437.
19. Irons GB, Fisher J, Schmitt EH. Vascularized muscular and musculocutaneous flaps for management of osteomyelitis. *Orthop Clin North Am* 1984;15:473–480.
20. Kelly PJ, Martin WJ, Coventry MB. Bacterial arthritis in the adult. *J Bone Joint Surg* 1970;52A:1595–1602.
21. Merkel KD, Brown ML, Dewanjee MK, Fitzgerald RH Jr. Comparison of indium-labeled leukocyte imaging with sequential technetium–gallium scanning in diagnosis of low-grade musculoskeletal sepsis: a prospective study. *J Bone Joint Surg* 1985;67A:465–476.
22. Modic MT, Feiglin DH, Piraino DW, Boumphrey F, Weinstein MA, Duchesneau PM, Rehm S. Vertebral osteomyelitis: assessment using MR. *Radiology* 1985;157:157–166.
23. Modic MT, Pflanze W, Feiglin DHI, Belhobeck G. Magnetic resonance imaging of musculoskeletal infections. *Radiol Clin North Am* 1986;24:247–258.
24. Moon KL Jr, Genant HG, Helms CA, Chafetz NI, Crooks LE, Kaufman L. Musculoskeletal applications of nuclear magnetic resonance. *Radiology* 1983;147:161–171.
25. Petersen SA. Alterations of blood flow by a local muscle flap in treatment of chronic osteomyelitis in a canine model. Thesis, Mayo Graduate School of Medicine, Rochester, MN, 1989.
26. Quinn SF, Murray W, Clark RA, Cochran C. MR imaging of chronic osteomyelitis. *J Comput Assist Tomogr* 1988;12:113–117.
27. Santoro JP, Cachia VV, Sartoris DJ, Resnick D. Nonspecific inflammation in the foot demonstrated by magnetic resonance imaging. *J Foot Surg* 1988;27:478–483.
28. Seabold JE, Nepola JV, Conrad GR, Marsh JL, Montgomery WJ, Bricker JA, Kirchner RT. Detection of osteomyelitis at fracture non-union sites: comparison of two scintigraphic methods. *AJR* 1989;152:1021–1027.
29. Seltzer SE. Value of computed tomography in planning medical and surgical treatment of chronic osteomyelitis. *J Comput Assist Tomogr* 1984;8:482–487.
30. Scott JA, Rosenthal DI, Brady TJ. The evaluation of musculoskel-

etal disease with magnetic resonance imaging. *Radiol Clin North Am* 1984;22:917–924.
31. Swensen SJ, Keller PL, Berquist TH, McLeod RA, Stephens DH. Magnetic resonance of hemorrhage. *Am J Roentgenol* 1985;145:921–927.
32. Tang JSH, Gold RH, Bassett LW, Seeger LL. Musculoskeletal infection of the extremities: evaluation with MR imaging. *Radiology* 1988;166:205–209.
33. Varnell RM, Flint DW, Dalley RW, Moravilla KR, Cummings CW, Shuman WP. Myocutaneous flap failure: early detection with Gd-DTPA-enhanced MR imaging. *Radiology* 1989;173:755–758.
34. Waldvogel FA, Medoff G, Sehwartz MN. Osteomyelitis: a review of clinical features, therapeutic considerations, and unusual aspects. *N Engl J Med* 1970;282:198–206.
35. Wall SD, Fisher MR, Amparo EG, Hricak H, Higgins CB. Magnetic resonance imaging in the evaluation of abscesses. *Am J Roentgenol* 1985;144:1217–1221.
36. Weekes RG, Berquist TH, McLeod RA, Zimmer WD. Magnetic resonance imaging of soft tissue tumors: comparison with computed tomography. *Magn Reson Imaging* 1985;3:345–352.
37. Weiland AJ, Moore JR, David RK. The efficacy of free tissue transfer in treatment of osteomyelitis. *J Bone Joint Surg* 1984;66A:181–193.
38. Weiland AJ. Symposium: the use of muscle flaps in the treatment of osteomyelitis in the lower extremity. *Contemp Orthop* 1985;10:127–159.
39. Wismer GL, Rosen BR, Buxton R, Start DD, Brady TJ. Chemical shift imaging of bone marrow: preliminary experience. *Am J Roentgenol* 1985;145:1031–1037.
40. Unger E, Moldofsky P, Gatenby R, Hartz W, Broder G. Diagnosis of osteomyelitis by MR imaging. *AJR* 1988;150:605–610.
41. Wood MB, Cooney WP III. Vascularized bone segment transfers for management of chronic osteomyelitis. *Orthop Clin North Am* 1984;15:401–472.
42. Yuh WTC, Corson JD, Baraniewski HM, et al. Osteomyelitis of the foot in diabetic patients: evaluation with plain film, ^{99m}Tc-MDP bone scintigraphy, and MR imaging. *AJR* 1989;152:795–800.
43. Zimmer WD, Berquist TH, McLeod RA, et al. Bone tumors: MRI vs CT. *Radiology* 1985;155:709–718.

MRI of the Musculoskeletal System, 2nd Edition, edited by T. H. Berquist.
Raven Press, Ltd., New York © 1990.

CHAPTER 14

Diffuse Marrow Diseases

James B. Vogler III and William A. Murphy, Jr.

Normal Bone Marrow, 491
Anatomy and Physiology, 491
MRI Features, 493
Technical Considerations, 499
Diffuse Marrow Disorders, 502
Reconversion, 502
Myeloid Depletion, 503
Bone Marrow Ischemia, 505
Marrow Infiltration or Replacement, 508
Bone Marrow Edema, 511
Pitfalls, 515
References, 515

As one of the larger and more important organs in the human body, bone marrow plays important physiologic roles in both health and disease. In healthy individuals its function is to provide a continual supply of red cells, platelets, and white cells to meet the body's demands for oxygenation, coagulation, and immunity. As such, bone marrow frequently becomes a target, either directly or indirectly, of many varied disease processes. The way in which marrow responds can, at times, be dramatic.

Until recently, *in vivo* imaging of certain physiologic functions and anatomic features of bone marrow has been limited. Historically, many methods have been used and still remain useful, despite shortcomings. Plain film radiography provides an excellent anatomic overview but is limited in detecting even considerable amounts (30–50%) of trabecular bone loss that might result from an intramedullary process. More importantly, it does not detect the cellular changes in marrow. Scintigraphy affords a physiologic survey of either marrow elements themselves or the surrounding osseous elements. Physiologic processes such as hematopoiesis and phagocytosis can be evaluated (15). Lack of anatomic detail and low specificity, however, are recognized shortcomings. Computed tomography (CT) provides transaxial images with excellent in-plane spatial resolution (on the order of 0.35 mm) and contrast resolution (on the order of 0.5%) (25). These capabilities allow excellent definition of cortical bone, trabecular bone, and, to a lesser degree, the intramedullary space. The nature of CT is such that extended anatomic regions cannot be evaluated without sacrificing resolution or substantially increasing radiation exposure.

Combining multiplanar images, excellent spatial resolution, superior contrast discrimination, and high sensitivity, magnetic resonance imaging (MRI) has greatly improved the ability for *in vivo* assessment of normal and abnormal bone marrow. With this instrument, the continuous change of normal bone marrow patterns throughout life and the varied responses of marrow cell populations to disease can be monitored.

NORMAL BONE MARROW

Anatomy and Physiology

The basic microstructure of bone marrow consists of a trabecular framework housing fat cells and hematopoietic cells both supported by a system of reticulum cells, nerves, and vascular sinusoids (59). The trabecular or cancellous bone is composed of primary and bridging secondary trabeculae. This tissue provides both architectural support and a mineral depot. Cellular constituents of marrow include all stages of erythrocytic and leukocytic development, as well as fat cells and reticulum cells

J. B. Vogler III: Department of Radiology, Mayo Clinic, Jacksonville, Florida 32224.
W. A. Murphy, Jr.: Mallinckrodt Institute of Radiology, Washington University School of Medicine, St. Louis, Missouri 63110.

(52). Erythroid, granulocytic, and megakaryocytic cell lines replenish the body's supply of red cells, white cells, and platelets. The role of fat cells in marrow function is unclear. Speculation exists that they provide surface and nutritional support and possibly growth factors for hematopoiesis (59). Reticulum cells consist of phagocytic cells (macrophages), which play a role in immunity, and undifferentiated nonphagocytic cells (5), whose role remains unclear.

The various components of normal marrow (fat cells, hematopoietic cells, reticulum cells, trabeculae, vessels, and nerves) may be simplified into a unifying concept —that of red and yellow marrow. That fraction of bone marrow actively involved in the production of blood cells is termed hematopoietic or "red marrow." The remaining fraction, the fat cell population, which is hematopoietically inactive, is termed "yellow marrow." Important anatomic and compositional differences exist between these two types of marrow (52). On average, red marrow contains approximately 40% water, 40% fat, and 20% protein and has a rich, arborized vascular network. Yellow marrow contains approximately 15% water, 80% fat, and 5% protein and has a sparse vascular network.

At birth, virtually the entire marrow space contains red marrow. During growth and development, conversion of red to yellow marrow occurs and has a predictable and orderly pattern. This conversion begins in the immediate postnatal period and is first evident in the terminal phalanges of the hands and feet (21). The process then progresses from peripheral (appendicular) toward central (axial) with respect to the skeleton as a whole and from diaphyseal to metaphyseal in individual long bones (Fig. 14-1). The rate and extent of conversion are not uniform but vary according to site in a particular bone as well as among bones (Fig. 14-2).

Epiphyses and apophyses must be considered independently. These structures lack marrow until they begin to ossify. What remains unclear is how much red marrow appears at these sites and how long it remains. Undoubtedly, any red marrow contained in these structures undergoes rapid conversion to yellow marrow. Thus, as a general rule, epiphyseal and apophyseal ossification centers can be thought of as containing yellow marrow from very early and then throughout life.

Usually by 25 years of age the process of primary marrow conversion is complete and a balanced distribution of red and yellow marrow has been achieved (27,40,43,47). This balance will vary from person to person as it is influenced by age, gender, and health. Similarly, the balance achieved in individual bone varies by location. Red marrow is predominantly concentrated in the axial skeleton (skull, vertebrae, ribs, sternum, and pelvis) and the proximal appendicular skeleton (proximal femora and humeri) (Fig. 14-3). Yellow marrow occupies the remaining portion of the appendicular skeleton and can be scattered throughout the axial skeleton.

The boundaries of red and yellow marrow are not absolute and variations in this generally accepted adult pattern do exist (Fig. 14-3). Islands of hematopoietic tissue may be found in areas dominated by fatty marrow and vice versa. Likewise, it is not at all unusual to find red marrow occupying up to two-thirds of the femoral and humeral shafts (27,28,52). The red/yellow marrow distribution continues to change slowly with advancing age as the red marrow fraction in individual bones declines (19). Factors modulating this conversion of red to yellow marrow are largely unknown; however, temperature (30), vascularity (47), and low oxygen tension (58) have been implicated.

The process of red to yellow marrow conversion is, at times, halted or reversed as alterations in the body's

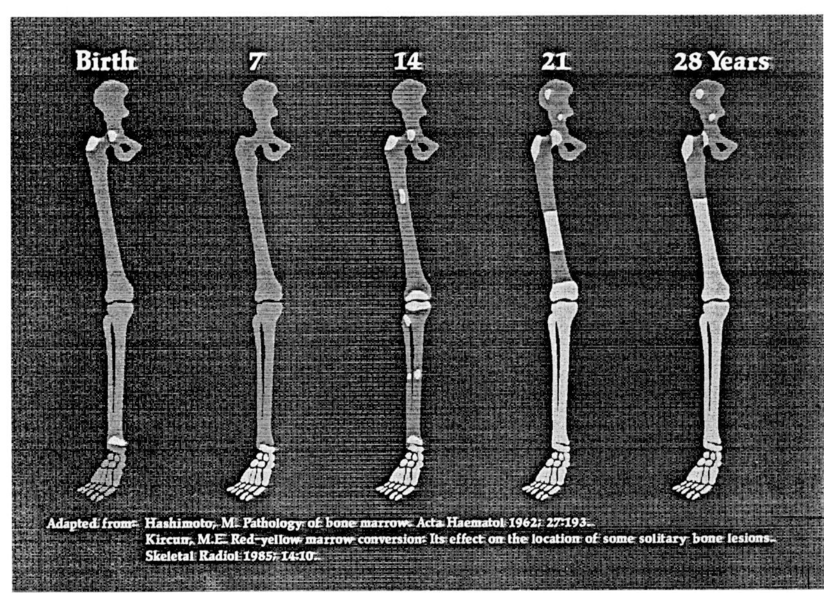

FIG. 14-1. Age-related changes in red/yellow marrow distribution. The natural conversion of red to yellow marrow is illustrated by drawings of the right lower extremity at 7 year increments. At birth, virtually the entire ossified skeleton contains red marrow. Conversion of red to yellow marrow begins shortly after birth and is first evident in the distal appendicular skeleton (hands and feet). Through the ensuing years, the process gradually progresses from distal to proximal with respect to the skeleton as a whole and from diaphyseal to epiphyseal in individual long bones. (Adapted from refs. 28 and 34.)

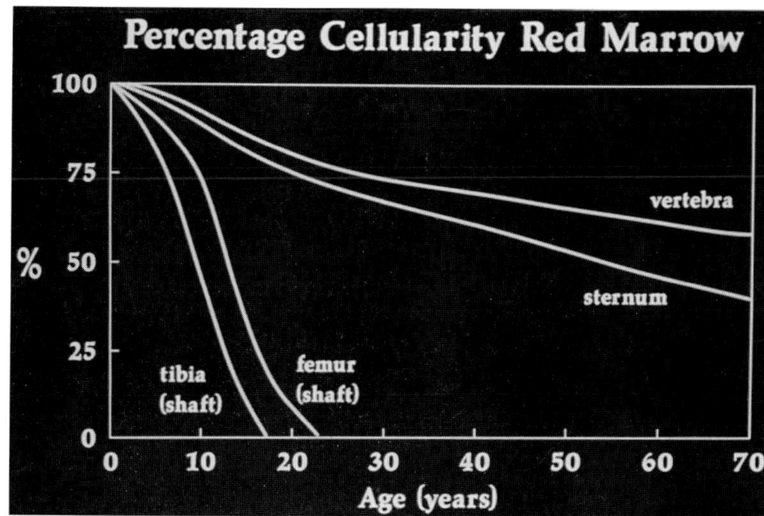

FIG. 14-2. Conversion of red to yellow marrow. Changes in the red marrow fraction (percentage cellularity red marrow) at specific anatomic sites are illustrated on this graph. The rate and extent of conversion differ between axial (vertebra and sternum) and appendicular (tibia and femur) sites. The axial skeleton demonstrates a more gradual decline in the red marrow fraction with substantial amounts of red marrow persisting throughout life. The rate of red to yellow marrow conversion in the appendicular skeleton is more rapid with little red marrow persisting in the tibial and femoral shafts beyond 25 years of age. (Adapted from ref. 13.)

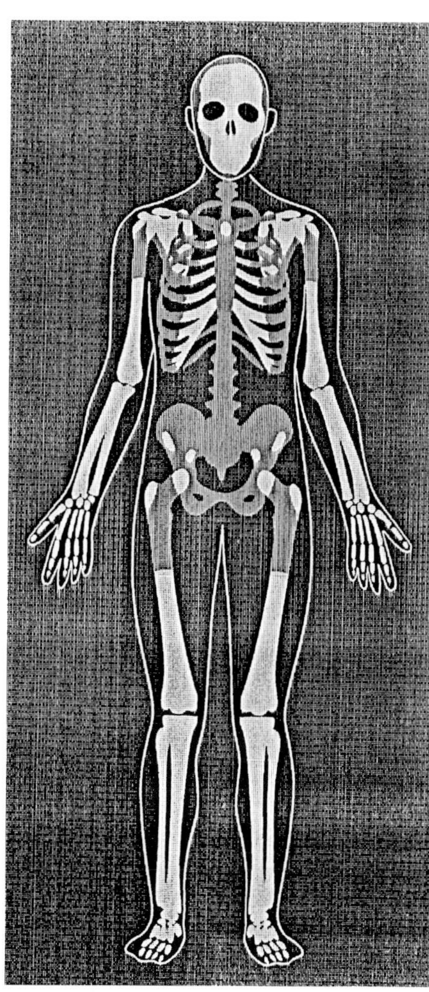

FIG. 14-3. Adult pattern of red/yellow marrow. Usually by 25 years of age the primary conversion of red to yellow marrow has been accomplished and the adult distribution of red/yellow marrow established. Red marrow is concentrated in the axial and proximal appendicular skeleton while yellow marrow occupies the remainder of the appendicular skeleton. (Adapted from refs. 28 and 34.)

demand for hematopoiesis provoke a "reconversion" of yellow marrow to red marrow. During this reconversion, yellow marrow is transformed to red marrow throughout the skeleton in the reverse sequence of the primary red to yellow marrow conversion described previously. Thus, the process occurs first in the axial skeleton followed by the appendicular skeleton in a proximal to distal sequence (12,13,43,47) (Fig. 14-4). Temperature (30), oxygen tension (58), and elevated erythropoietin (31) are again implicated in initiating and modulating this process, although the actual mechanisms and controlling factors remain largely unknown.

MRI Features

Fat, water, protein, and mineral are the basic constituents of bone marrow that contribute to the formation of its MR image. As relative amounts of these constituents change, the signal intensity of marrow is altered accordingly. Fat cells are responsible for the greatest fraction of marrow signal on T1 weighted images. Most protons in fat are contained in hydrophobic CH_2 groups and demonstrate very efficient spin–lattice relaxation, resulting in a particularly short T1 relaxation time and thus high signal intensity on T1 weighted spin-echo images (63). Spin–spin relaxation of fat is less efficient, resulting in some prolongation of its T2 relaxation time and thus moderate signal intensity on T2 weighted spin-echo images.

Water in tissue is thought to exist in different forms. Tissues rich in free water (extracellular water) show longer T1 and T2 relaxation times, while those having greater amounts of bound (intracellular) water demonstrate a shortening of T1 and T2 relaxation values (38). The relative contribution of each type of water to overall

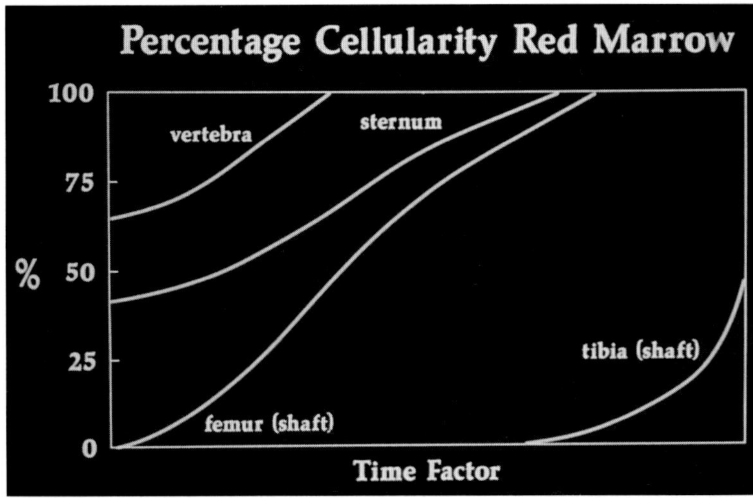

FIG. 14-4. Reconversion of yellow to red marrow. Yellow marrow is reconverted to red marrow in response to the body's demand for increased hematopoietic capacity. This reconversion process is first evident in the axial skeleton (vertebra and sternum), where the rate and extent of the process usually exceed that of the appendicular skeleton (femur and tibia). The extent of axial and appendicular involvement is influenced by the severity and duration of the inciting stimulus. (Adapted from ref. 13.)

marrow signal is not clearly defined. Nevertheless, as the amount of marrow water increases, it is logical to expect lower signal intensity on T1 weighted images and higher signal intensity on T2 weighted images.

The contribution of protein to marrow signal intensity is poorly understood. Protein in general has a long T1 relaxation time due to the large size of the molecules (38). Yet, protein in solution will result in a shortening of the T1 relaxation time of that solution. The individual contribution of these competing signal patterns to overall marrow signal intensity remains unclear.

Mineral contributes in a negative fashion to bone marrow signal intensity through two different mechanisms. First, due to a lack of mobile protons, the mineral matrix produces little or no signal. Second, inhomogeneous susceptibility where mineral matrix interfaces with water or fat results in local field gradients and signal loss. The mineral matrix of bone marrow is contained in trabecular bone. Since metaphyses and epiphyses contain greater amounts of trabecular bone, signal intensity at these sites is altered accordingly.

Signal characteristics of red and yellow marrow will vary among the different pulse sequences. The vast majority of clinical studies and most of the basic knowledge of MR marrow patterns to date have been based on routine spin-echo pulse sequences with T1 and T2 weighted images. Thus, spin-echo pulse sequences will be used to describe typical signal patterns of yellow and red marrow (40,49,62,66).

Yellow marrow, owing to its high fat composition (80%), displays signal intensity comparable to that of subcutaneous fat on T1 and T2 weighted images (Fig. 14-5). For comparison purposes, it is higher in signal intensity than muscle on both pulse sequences. Having larger fractions of water (40%) and protein (40%) with a smaller fraction of fat (20%), red marrow displays signal intensity lower than that of yellow marrow on T1 weighted images. As a reference, its signal intensity is generally slightly greater than normal muscle. On T2 weighted images, the signal intensity of red marrow increases (probably as a result of its water fraction) and approaches that of yellow marrow. With STIR imaging or heavy T2 weighting (TR values exceeding 3,000 msec and TE values greater than 90 msec), red marrow signal intensity may even exceed that of yellow marrow (Fig. 14-6). Thus, on T1 weighted pulse sequences in normal individuals, yellow marrow will be higher in signal intensity than red marrow, which in turn is higher in signal intensity than muscle. With increasing repetition times and echo delays, the signal intensity of red marrow approaches that of yellow marrow and both remain higher in signal than muscle, but lower in signal than fluid.

The T1 weighted MRI appearance of marrow in any particular bone will be determined by the relative fractions of red marrow, yellow marrow, and trabecular bone. At locations where the red marrow fraction is high, overall marrow signal intensity will be lower than at sites where little red marrow is found (Fig. 14-5). Thus, overall marrow signal intensity in vertebral bodies (sites where the red marrow fraction remains relatively high throughout life) will be lower than marrow signal intensity in the distal appendicular skeleton, where little red marrow persists in adulthood. In the normal individual, the red/yellow marrow and trabecular bone fractions change continuously but slowly throughout life. This is reflected in the changing marrow appearance seen on MRI of patients at various ages. For example, measured T1 relaxation times of vertebral bodies decline with age (18), probably reflecting a decreasing fractional volume of hematopoietic marrow with concomitant increase in fatty marrow. This decrease in T1 values is most pronounced in the first four decades of life, when normal conversion of red to yellow marrow is

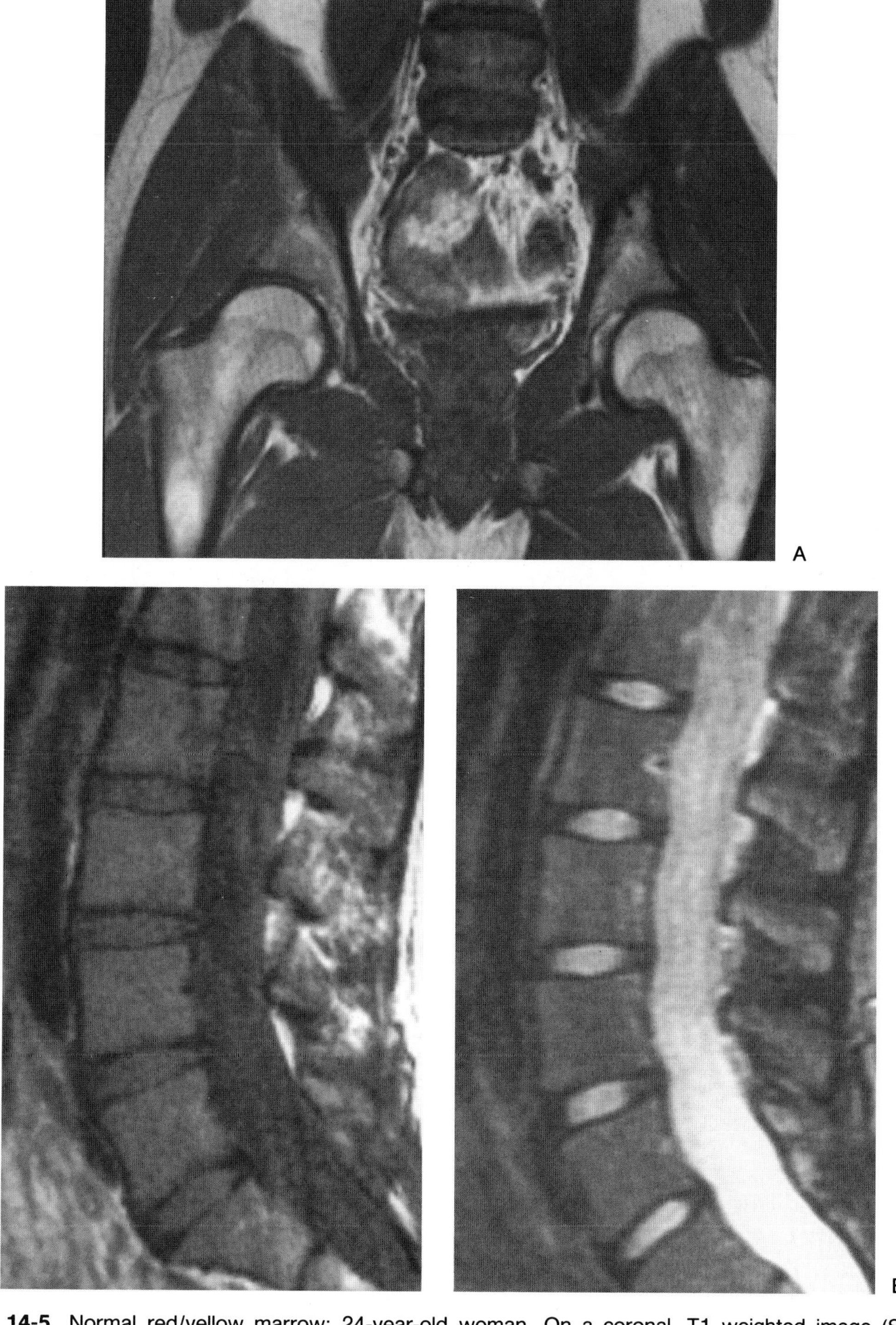

FIG. 14-5. Normal red/yellow marrow: 24-year-old woman. On a coronal, T1 weighted image (SE 600/20) of the pelvis (**A**), signal characteristics of red and yellow marrow are apparent. Yellow marrow (seen in the proximal femoral shafts and femoral epiphyses) is roughly isointense to subcutaneous fat. Red marrow (present in the femoral metaphyses, pelvis, and lumbar vertebrae) is lower in signal intensity than yellow marrow but slightly higher in signal intensity than muscle. Note that regions containing higher fractions of red marrow (lumbar vertebra) demonstrate lower signal intensity than areas where the red marrow fraction is less (femora). Sagittal T1 (SE 500/20) (**B**) and T2 weighted (SE 2,000/80) (**C**) images of the lumbar spine show red marrow as having slightly higher signal intensity than fluid (CSF) on T1 weighted images and lower signal intensity than fluid on T2 weighted images. Note also that the signal intensity of red marrow is approaching that of subcutaneous fat on the T2 weighted image.

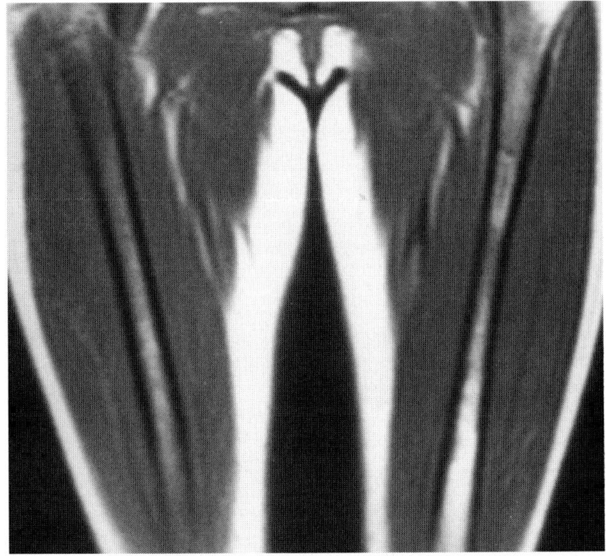

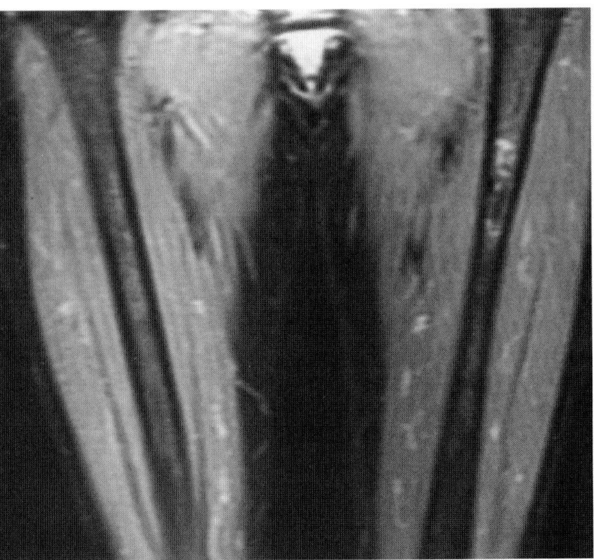

A,B

FIG. 14-6. Normal marrow: 30-year-old woman. **A:** On a coronal, T1 weighted image (SE 500/20) of the thighs, marrow can be seen occupying the mid and proximal femoral shafts. Yellow marrow is evident in the distal femoral shafts and left greater trochanter (right greater trochanter not included on this section). **B:** A coronal STIR image at approximately the same level demonstrates the red marrow to have signal intensity exceeding that of the nulled yellow marrow. (The focal area of increased signal intensity in the proximal left femur is believed to represent an enchondroma.)

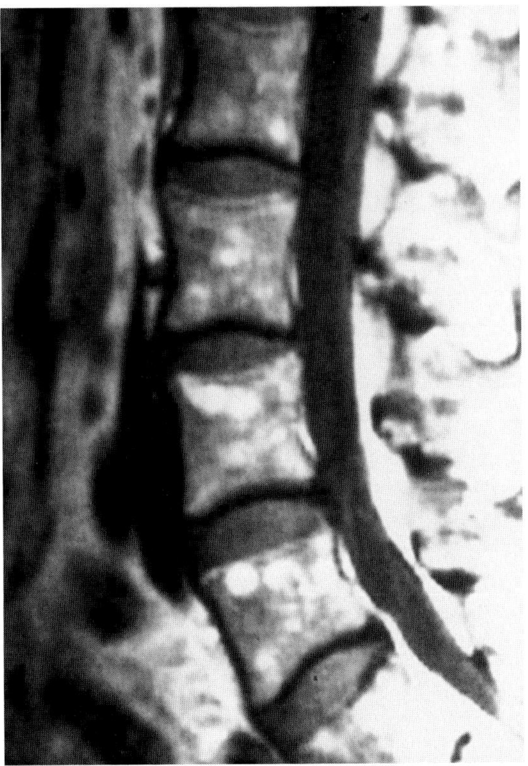

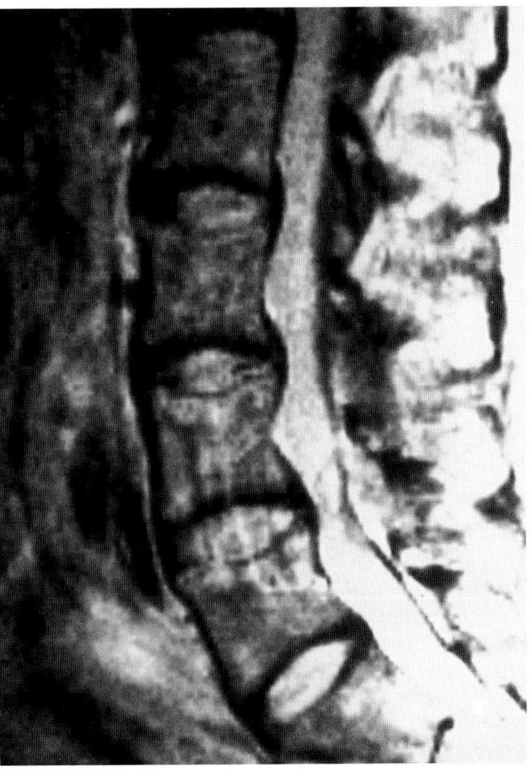

A,B

FIG. 14-7. Focal fatty conversion: 56-year-old man. **A:** A sagittal T1 weighted image (SE 500/20) of the lumbar spine demonstrates focal areas of increased signal intensity (comparable to subcutaneous fat) subjacent to the superior end-plates of L4 and L5 and centrally in the L3 vertebral body. **B:** These areas show some loss of signal intensity on a T2 weighted image (SE 2,000/60) and are representative of focal fatty conversion of vertebral red marrow.

occurring. Beyond the fourth decade, loss of trabecular bone mass and the resulting reduction of vertebral mineral content (by approximately 40% in men and 55% in women by age 75) (24) contributes to the decline in T1 values. T2 relaxation times show a similar decline with age. Loss of trabecular bone with replacement by fat cells as occurs in osteoporosis may help explain differences in the range of T1 and T2 values for men and women, which is similar under the age of 40 years but slightly higher in women after 50 years of age (18).

Other factors can influence the MRI appearance of vertebral marrow through mechanisms that are, at present, incompletely understood. As the normal age-related conversion of red to yellow marrow occurs in the spine, the process may assume a more focal (rather than diffuse) pattern (26). This focal conversion to fatty marrow is more evident in the posterior elements, about the central venous channels, and at the periphery of vertebral bodies, particularly the end-plates (Fig. 14-7). Marrow involved in this process assumes a spotty appearance (particularly on T1 weighted images) as the bright foci of fat intermix with the lower signal intensity red marrow. The process is more prevalent with increasing age and may be present in up to 60% of patients. Among the hypotheses put forward to explain this phenomenon is that of chronic stress and biomechanical stimuli causing diminished vascularity at involved sites, prompting the conversion of red to yellow marrow.

Certain common disease-related alterations in the MRI appearance of vertebral marrow may also occur. Adjacent to degenerating intervertebral disks, marrow can assume a bandlike configuration of variable signal intensity (16). Bands of decreased signal on short and long TR/TE images are occasionally observed and probably reflect sclerosis and/or fibrosis adjacent to the end-plate. A more common pattern is bands of increased signal intensity (similar to fat) on short TR/TE and long TR/TE images likely representing focal conversion of hematopoietic to fatty marrow possibly as a result of ischemia associated with degenerative disk disease (Fig. 14-8). Rarely, a pattern of decreased signal intensity on short TR/TE images and increased signal intensity on long TR/TE images will be observed (Fig. 14-9). This pattern may indicate an increase in local marrow water content possibly as a result of focal inflammation or ischemia.

In the appendicular skeleton and in individual long bones, common local MR marrow patterns also exist. Distal to the humeri and femora in the adult appendicular skeleton, the MRI appearance is that of fatty marrow with homogeneous signal intensity on short and long TR/TE sequences. Known anatomic features that alter this pattern include local variations in trabecular bone content and remnants of the growth plate (physeal scar). At sites where trabecular bone is in abundance, the marrow will generally demonstrate slightly lower signal

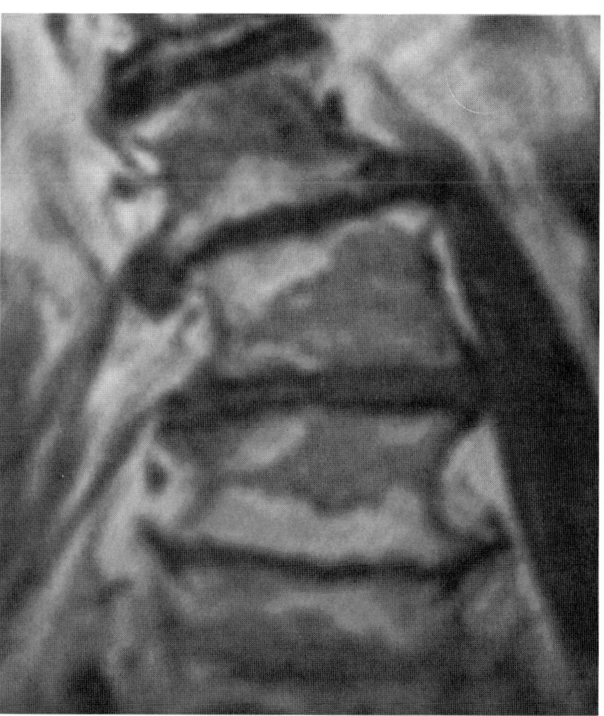

FIG. 14-8. Vertebral marrow alterations associated with degenerative disk disease: 79-year-old woman. On a coronal T1 weighted image (SE 600/20) of the lumbar spine, bands of high signal intensity (comparable to fat) are noted subjacent to the vertebral end-plates. These bands indicate areas of focal conversion of red to yellow marrow seen in association with degenerative disc disease. Note the residual areas of red marrow located in the central portions of the vertebral bodies.

intensity on both long and short TR/TE sequences. This is most commonly encountered in the metaphyseal/epiphyseal regions of long bones. Likewise, trabeculae that are oriented and reinforced along skeletal stress lines produce bands of lower signal intensity in the marrow. Compressive and tensile trabeculae coursing through the femoral head and neck are good examples of this. The physeal scar appears as a thin, transverse band of low signal intensity on T1 and T2 weighted images. It is a constant finding at expected locations in the appendicular skeleton. Bone reinforcement lines, if thick enough, would be expected to produce a similar appearance.

The femora and humeri warrant special attention because they are the long bones that consistently contain the greatest concentration of hematopoietic marrow in adults and, in essence, are the sites of transition between the "fatty" appendicular marrow and the "hematopoietic" axial marrow. In these bones, red marrow is commonly found in the proximal two-thirds (Fig. 14-10) with the greatest fraction usually in the proximal one-third. Less commonly, foci of red marrow may be evident in the distal one-third of these bones. This finding, by itself, should not be considered abnormal.

At sites where red marrow is present, a variety of

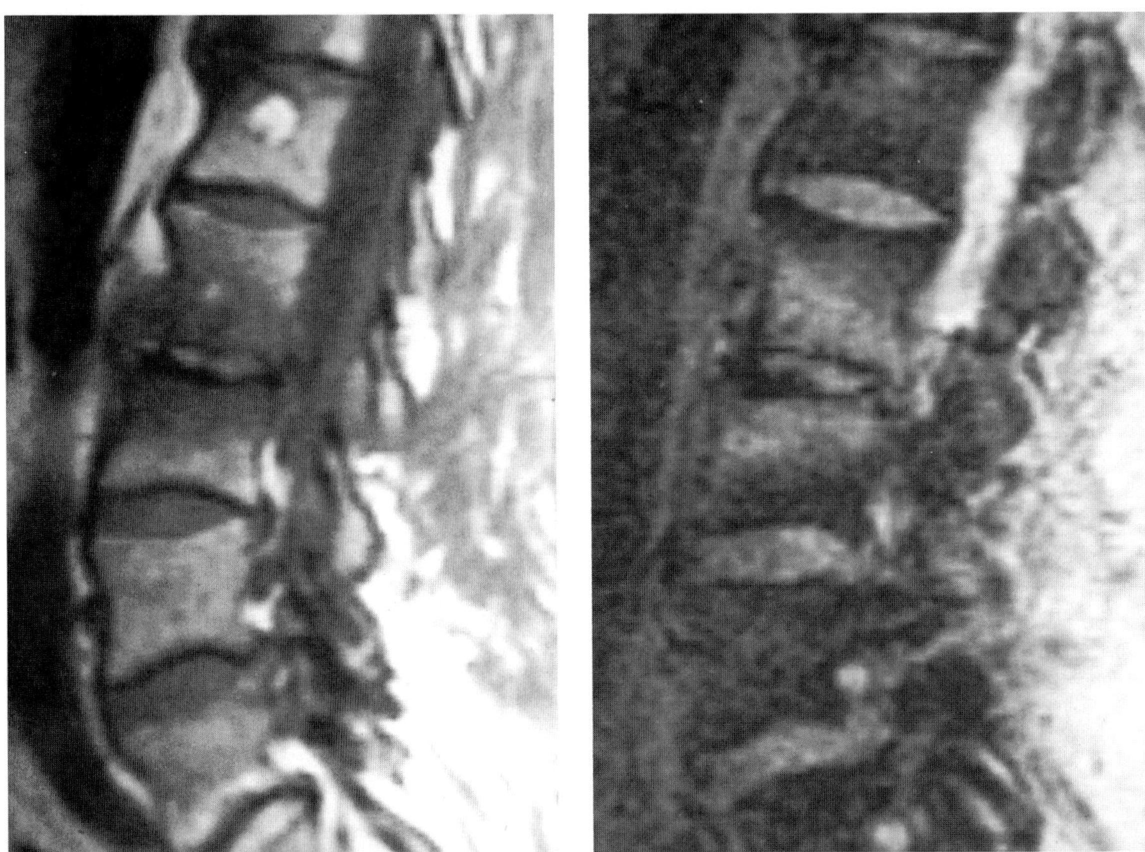

FIG. 14-9. Vertebral marrow alterations associated with degenerative disk disease: 68-year-old man. Bands of low signal intensity are noted subjacent to the end-plates at the L2–L3 interspace on a sagittal T1 weighted image (SE 600/20) (**A**). These bands show increased signal intensity on a T2 weighted image (SE 2,000/80) (**B**), presumably reflecting increased local marrow water in response to degenerative disk disease.

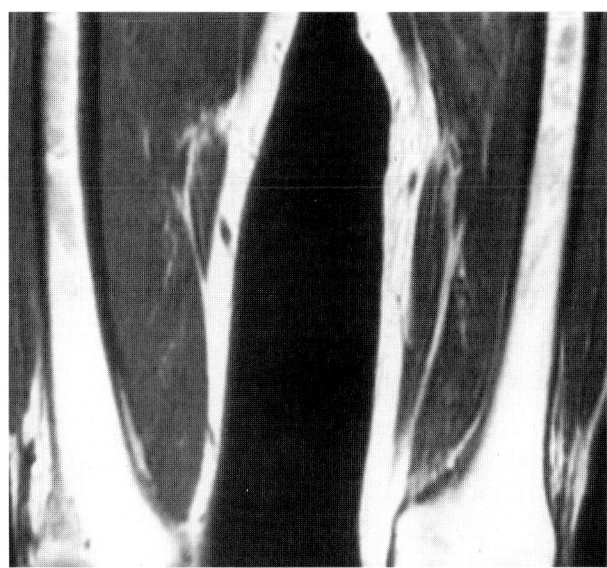

FIG. 14-10. Normal marrow distribution: 48-year-old man. Islands of red marrow (identified as foci of decreased signal intensity in the bright fatty marrow) can be seen to extend to the junction of the middle and distal thirds of the femora. This finding is not unusual and should not by itself be considered abnormal (SE 500/20).

signal patterns may be observed reflecting relative red/yellow fractions and distribution. A common pattern observed is islands of red marrow scattered throughout a background of fatty marrow (Fig. 14-10). The islands may have a variety of configurations ranging from small and circular to large and geographic. Less commonly in the long bones, foci of yellow marrow are evident in a background of red marrow, resembling the phenomenon of focal fat conversion in the vertebral bodies.

The amount and distribution of red marrow in these bones may not be perfectly uniform or symmetric. At the extremes, some individuals demonstrate virtually no red marrow in the femora or humeri while others display large amounts. Most individuals fall somewhere between. Minor differences in the amount and distribution of red marrow from side to side are expected. However, marked asymmetry is unusual and warrants explanation. Likewise, the signal intensity of red marrow, although variable among individuals, is roughly symmetric in the same individual.

TECHNICAL CONSIDERATIONS

In the MR evaluation of bone marrow and bone marrow disorders, the major technical considerations to be addressed are pulse sequences, slice parameters, imaging planes, contrast agents, and types of coil to be used.

The MRI appearance of bone marrow varies greatly between pulse sequences. Numerous pulse sequences have been and continue to be developed, each with its own nuances aimed at improving some aspect of MRI. What role, if any, many of these will play in bone marrow evaluation is unclear. Spin-echo pulse sequences with T1 and T2 weighted images have traditionally been the method used in MRI of marrow and, as such, much of the current knowledge about normal and abnormal bone marrow is based on this type of imaging.

Evaluating bone marrow with spin-echo pulse sequences usually requires both T1 and T2 weighted images. Repetition times used in obtaining these images need not be absolute but can vary depending on the anatomic region to be covered. Larger anatomic areas require longer repetition times. As a general guideline, however, the TR for a T1 weighted sequence should be kept below 700 msec and the TR for a T2 weighted sequence should exceed 2,000 msec. Accepted echo delays for T1 weighted images are less variable, generally being less than 30 msec and preferably at 20 msec or shorter. To achieve adequate T2 weighting, TE values of 80 msec or greater are necessary. Thus, by using these guidelines, a routine MR evaluation of bone marrow would include T1 weighted images using a TR of 500 msec and TE of 20 msec in addition to T2 weighted images obtained with a TR of 2,000 msec and a TE of 80 msec.

Studies obtained in this manner take advantage of many inherent marrow properties. On the T1 weighted images, contrast is predominantly a function of T1 relaxation time. Due to the short T1 of lipid, the signal from fatty marrow is optimized (Fig. 14-11). Tissues containing lesser amounts of fat or having longer T1 relaxation times become conspicuous against the background of high-signal fatty marrow. Thus, bone, red marrow, muscle, and most pathologic processes can readily be identified. T1 weighted images also provide excellent anatomic detail.

On T2 weighted images, contrast predominantly reflects differences in T2 relaxation times (Fig. 14-11). With progressive T2 weighting, the signal intensity of red marrow slowly increases while that of yellow marrow slowly declines, making it more difficult to discriminate between the two. Since many pathologic processes have very long T2 relaxation times (greatly exceeding those of red and yellow marrow), they are conspicuous in the marrow. Difficulty arises, however, when an insufficiently T2 weighted pulse sequence is used, in essence narrowing the T2 contrast difference between a pathologic process and normal marrow, thus resulting in the pathologic process becoming less conspicuous.

Addition of other pulse sequences to routine spin-echo evaluation may prove beneficial in certain instances. Chemical shift imaging may improve lesion detection and red/yellow marrow discrimination on T1 weighted sequences. This form of imaging is based on the differing precession rates or resonant frequencies of fat and water protons in biologic tissue—about 3.5 ppm

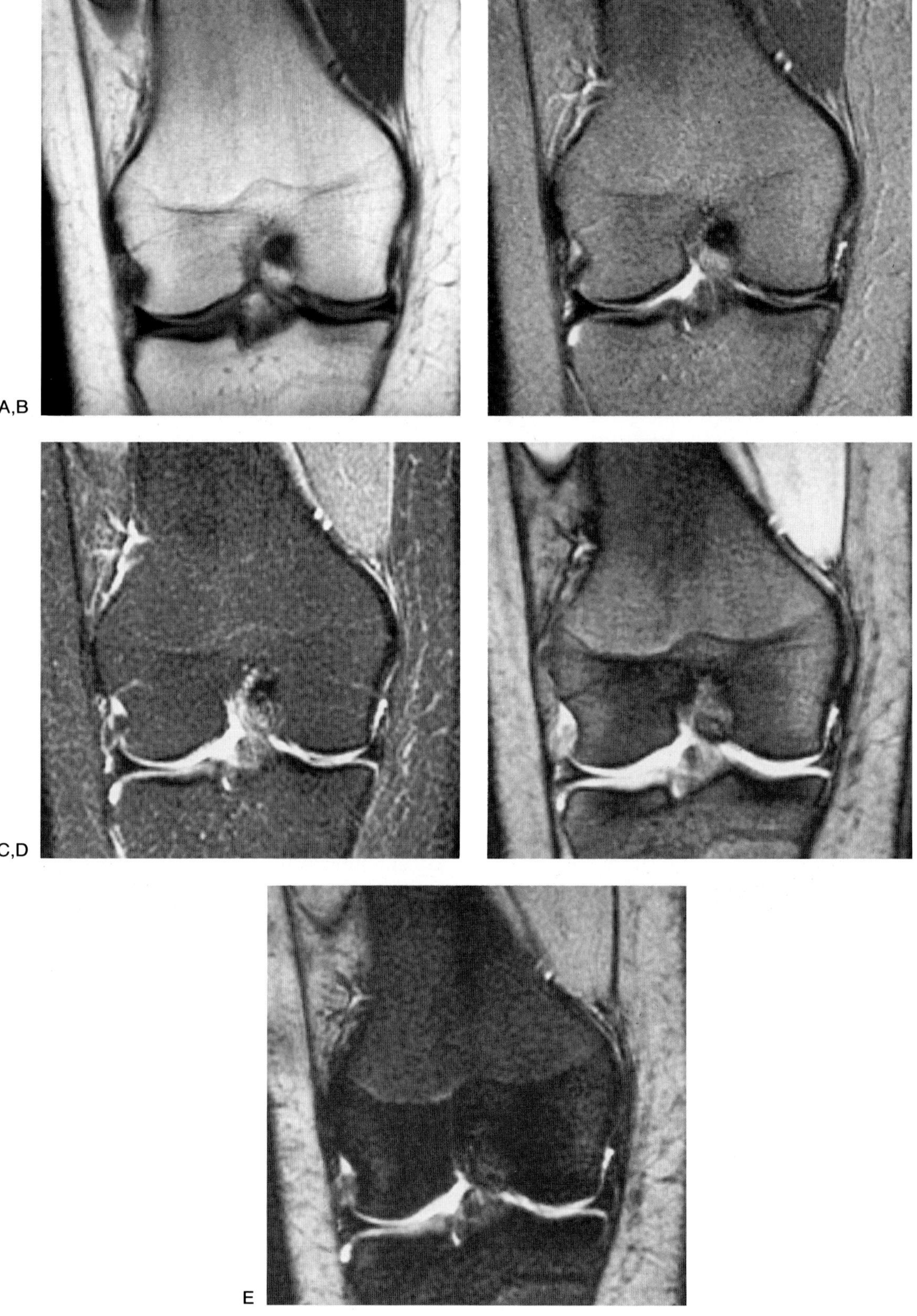

FIG. 14-11. Appearance of bone marrow on different pulse sequences. Coronal images of the right knee are obtained by using different pulse sequences to demonstrate the variable appearance of bone marrow with changing scanning parameters. (All images obtained at a field strength of 1.5 T.) **A:** Spin-echo, T1 weighted image (TR = 500, TE = 20). Bone marrow in the distal femur and proximal tibia is roughly isointense with subcutaneous fat. This is the expected appearance of fatty marrow on T1 weighted images. **B:** Spin-echo, T2 weighted image (TR = 2,000, TE = 60). With increasing repetition times and echo delays, the signal intensity of fatty marrow declines as does that of subcutaneous fat. **C:** STIR (TR = 1,500, TE = 30, TI = 140). Since the signal of fat is nulled on STIR images, fatty marrow will appear

or 75–150 Hz for scanners operating in the range of 0.5–1 T (65). By using chemical shift techniques like the one described by Dixon (17), fat and water molecules present in the same voxel will cancel, producing no net signal in the respective pixel. Thus, when tissues containing excess water (most pathologic processes) occur in fatty marrow, a dark interface appears along the perimeter, making that tissue more conspicuous. Red marrow, due to its higher water content, is also more conspicuous. Some chemical shift sequences allow for selective fat or water images.

A particular form of inversion recovery, STIR, can also improve lesion detection. In this pulse sequence, the signal from fat is nulled, making it appear dark on the images (Fig. 14-11). Tissues having T1 or T2 relaxation values that differ from fat will have greater signal intensity than fat. In fact, due to the nature of inversion recovery sequences, T1 and T2 values become additive, making STIR imaging perhaps the most sensitive of all pulse sequences for detecting marrow abnormalities. Limitations of this sequence include lesser anatomic definition than T1 weighted spin-echo images secondary to loss of the fat signal, restrictions in the size of the anatomic region that can be covered, and long scan times.

Gradient-echo pulse sequences provide an alternative to STIR and T2 weighted images, yet at much shorter scan times (Fig. 14-11). Numerous gradient-echo sequences exist (GRASS, FLASH, FISP, etc.). All are based on the generation of a gradient echo rather than the classic 180° refocusing pulse used in spin-echo pulse sequences. The flip angle (theta, θ) can be varied on gradient-echo scans, enabling substantial reduction in imaging time. Contrast in these pulse sequences is a function of many different factors including T1, T2, T2*, TR, TE, and theta (29,65). These sequences are very sensitive to field inhomogeneities and chemical shift and susceptibility effects. By varying TR, TE, and theta, the contrast between marrow and most pathologic processes can be increased. Gradient-echo sequences do not suffer the same restrictions in anatomic detail and amount of anatomic coverage as STIR imaging.

To date, the role of MR contrast agents (e.g., gadolinium) in evaluation of diffuse marrow disease has not been defined. These agents appear to hold promise for demonstrating the extent of marrow involvement by neoplastic processes in certain settings and may improve the specificity of MR for separating benign from malignant disorders. At present though, routine use of these agents for evaluating diffuse marrow disorders cannot be recommended.

Size of the anatomic region to be evaluated influences many of the MR scanning parameters including surface coil selection, slice thickness, and interslice gap. Smaller anatomic regions may better be imaged with surface coils, whereas larger regions require body coils. Comparison with the contralateral extremity is generally desirable, necessitating use of a body coil. Slice thicknesses on the order of 5 mm with no interslice gap usually provide the resolution necessary in small anatomic areas. However, 1 cm slices with 1–3 mm gaps are often needed to cover larger regions. Signal-to-noise considerations also influence slice thickness and interslice gap in addition to matrix size and number of excitations (Nex). Generally, matrices on the order of 128 × 256 with two excitations provide adequate signal-to-noise for evaluating large anatomic regions.

Clinical settings that account for the majority of MR examinations for diffuse marrow disease include: (a) a follow-study to further define abnormalities encountered on other radiologic procedures; (b) a "screen" of the marrow for possible involvement by processes not readily imaged with other modalities (e.g., myeloma); (c) a method of assessing response to therapy; and (d) a procedure to localize potential sites for biopsy.

The sensitivity of MRI for detecting marrow abnormalities may indicate a future role for this modality in the initial staging of certain tumors likely to metastasize to bone (breast, prostate, lung). MR examination will need to be tailored in each of these situations. It is not possible to image the entirety of an individual's bone marrow. Thus, any screening protocol should be directed at evaluating skeletal sites where the likelihood of involvement is highest. In adults, this would mean evaluating the axial skeleton since most diffuse marrow disorders tend to follow the distribution of red marrow. Imaging of marrow in the ribs and skull is limited due to the size and shape of these bones. Time limitations usually prohibit evaluating all at-risk sites. As a reasonable compromise, one could consider evaluating the pelvis (including proximal femora) and the lumbar spine (including portions of the lower thoracic spine). Reasonable parameters for such an evaluation might include those listed in Table 14-1.

←

dark. **D:** GRASS (TR = 700, TE = 12, flip angle = 25°). Gradient-echo sequences at low flip angles (theta) tend to accentuate T2 characteristics of tissues and fluids. Note that the fatty marrow is not as bright as on the T1 weighted image (**A**) and the synovial fluid displays increased signal intensity. **E:** GRASS (TR = 700, TE = 31, flip angle = 25°). Many factors contribute to signal intensity on gradient-echo sequences. Susceptibility effects and field inhomogeneities may in part account for the marked decrease in fatty marrow signal on this image.

TABLE 14-1. *Marrow screening protocol*[a]

	Plane	TR	TE	FOV	Slice thickness	Gap	Matrix	Nex
Pelvis	Coronal	700	20	32	5 mm	1 mm	256 × 192	2
L spine	Sagittal	500	20	24	4 mm	1 mm	256 × 192	2

[a] Obtain STIR or T2 weighted images of either pelvis or L spine.

DIFFUSE MARROW DISORDERS

Bone marrow responds to insult and disease through a select number of mechanisms. These pathophysiologic responses can be identified and categorized on MR images. The concept provides a useful means of grouping the various disorders that affect marrow and for understanding associated marrow signal patterns. Five pathophysiological mechanisms are to be considered. First, reconversion, where the normal pathophysiologic process of converting red marrow to yellow marrow is reversed such that yellow marrow is "reconverted" to red marrow. Persistent red marrow hyperplasia should be considered a subcategory of this mechanism. Second, myeloid depletion, in which all marrow cells other than fat are destroyed or disappear. Third, ischemia, where all marrow elements are lost. Fourth, infiltration, where normal marrow is invaded by abnormal elements. And, finally, the process of marrow edema, where excess water appears in the marrow tissue. This conceptualized categorization is neither distinct nor all inclusive, but it does provide a useful framework for discussion (62).

Reconversion

When the body's demand for hematopoiesis exceeds the ability of existing red marrow to meet that demand, a process is initiated whereby yellow marrow is "reconverted" to red marrow. This reconversion follows the reverse sequence of normal red to yellow marrow conversion. It is first evident in the axial skeleton and then progresses toward the distal appendicular skeleton in a proximal to distal pattern. Thus, in a given case, if reconversion is suspected in the appendicular skeleton, then it should be evident, often to a greater degree, in the axial skeleton. Pathologically, the process is heralded by capillary proliferation and sinusoid formation in the subendosteal portions of the fatty marrow (51).

The process of reconversion will generally be symmetric throughout the skeleton, although not necessarily uniform in any particular bone. The extent of reconversion depends on the severity and duration of the stimulus. Mild cases may show only hyperplasia of axial marrow, while in extreme cases involvement may be evident in distal appendicular regions.

Causes of reconversion vary and span a spectrum of diverse disorders. Hematopoietic processes such as chronic anemias (sickle cell, thalassemia, etc.), marrow replacement disorders (metastatic disease, etc.), and myeloproliferative conditions (myeloma, leukemia) are among some of the processes that may incite this phenomenon. In hematopoietic conditions, the severity and chronicity of the anemia will determine the extent of reconversion and/or the degree of persistent red marrow hyperplasia. In patients with sickle cell disorders, the amount of marrow lost due to osteonecrosis also influences the degree of reconversion. In a similar fashion, metastases and myeloproliferative disorders cause distal reconversion through loss of hematopoietic capacity in proximal replaced marrow. Since these types of disorder generally follow the distribution of red marrow (involving the axial skeleton before appendicular sites), identifying reconversion in the extremities of one of these patients is an ominous sign suggesting extensive replacement of axial marrow. Situations such as this are not common, however, and care must be taken when trying to diagnose reconversion on the basis of MRI. To date, there is no reliable means of differentiating reconverted marrow from other marrow infiltrative disorders. In most cases, bone marrow biopsy will be necessary to make that determination.

The MRI appearance of reconversion and diagnostic criteria for this process are not well established and, as such, recognition of reconversion is probably low. MR images of patients in whom this phenomenon is operative display expected findings of an expanded red marrow fraction (49). Signal intensity of the hyperplastic marrow at any particular location will vary, depending on the red marrow fraction present and the degree of hyperplasia (cellularity). On short TR/TE sequences, involved sites display decreased marrow signal intensity (Fig. 14-12), while on longer TR/TE images the signal intensity increases relative to that of fatty marrow. Actual signal intensity observed is influenced by the degree of cellularity, the amount of red marrow water, and the scanning parameters used. When severe red marrow hyperplasia is present, its signal intensity on T1 weighted images may be equal to or slightly lower than that of muscle (Fig. 14-13). On T2 weighted images, signal intensity of hyperplastic marrow may slightly exceed the signal intensity of fatty marrow.

The process of reconversion may involve individual bones to varying degrees, producing a spectrum of MRI appearances. In early or mild cases, islands of regenerat-

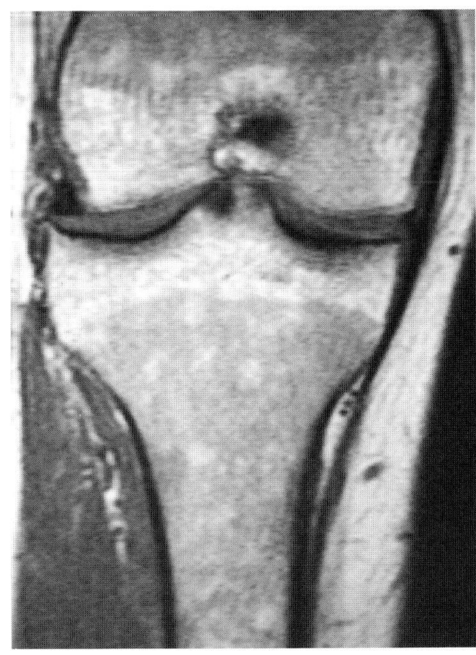

FIG. 14-12. Reconversion/persistent red marrow hyperplasia in anemia: 20-year-old man. A coronal, T1 weighted image (SE 600/17) of the right knee illustrates many features of the reconversion process in a patient with anemia (believed to be alpha thalassemia minor). The fatty marrow that is typically present in the distal femur and proximal tibia of a patient this age has largely been reconverted to (or persists from childhood as) hematopoietic marrow. The large fraction of red marrow present in the distal femur and proximal tibia is evidenced by decreased overall marrow signal intensity at these sites (compare to the normal pattern in Fig. 14-10). Note that there has even been some reconversion of yellow marrow to red marrow in the epiphyses.

ing red marrow are scattered throughout the marrow space, producing a "spotty" or geographic appearance, while in severe cases there may be diffuse involvement of the entire marrow compartment.

The MR signal pattern and distribution of the reconversion phenomenon is by no means specific. Differentiation of this process from normal variation in red marrow distribution may be difficult at times. More concerning, however, is that some neoplastic processes (metastases, myeloma, leukemia) may display T1 and T2 signal characteristics similar to normal red marrow. This problem is magnified when dealing with hyperplastic or reconverted marrow because red marrow cellularity and water fraction are increased in this setting, hypothetically resulting in greater overlap with neoplastic conditions.

Myeloid Depletion

With depletion of the myeloid (hematopoietic) fraction of bone marrow, the marrow space becomes filled with fatty marrow. MR images reflect this change as the marrow assumes signal characteristics of yellow marrow on both T1 and T2 weighted sequences. The degree to which this occurs will be influenced by the severity and duration of the incitive process. Conditions that result in myeloid depletion include aplastic anemia, radiation therapy, and chemotherapy.

In patients with aplastic anemia, the marrow becomes hypocellular or, in extreme cases, acellular. In hypocellular cases, residual amounts of red marrow will be evident as small areas of decreased signal intensity against a background of bright fatty marrow on T1 weighted se-

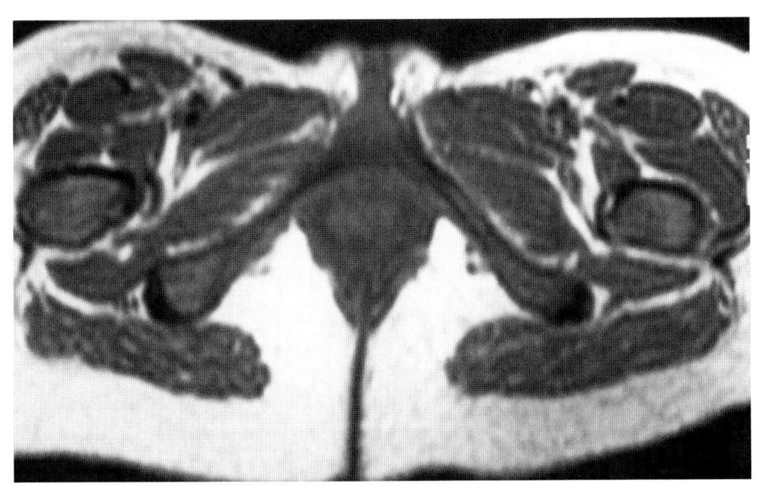

FIG. 14-13. Reconversion in anemia: 29-year-old woman. This patient has chronic anemia due to blood loss from untreated cervical carcinoma. An axial, T1 weighted image (SE 500/20) below the level of the lessor trochanters demonstrates the femoral bone marrow to have decreased signal intensity, comparable to that of muscle. This appearance has resulted from a combination of reconversion of yellow to red marrow and red marrow hyperplasia. The degree of hyperplasia has caused the marked lowering of the marrow signal intensity.

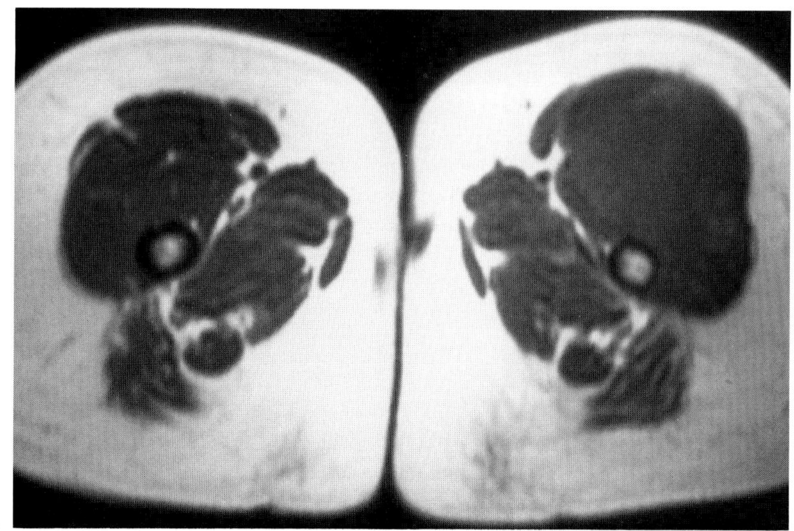

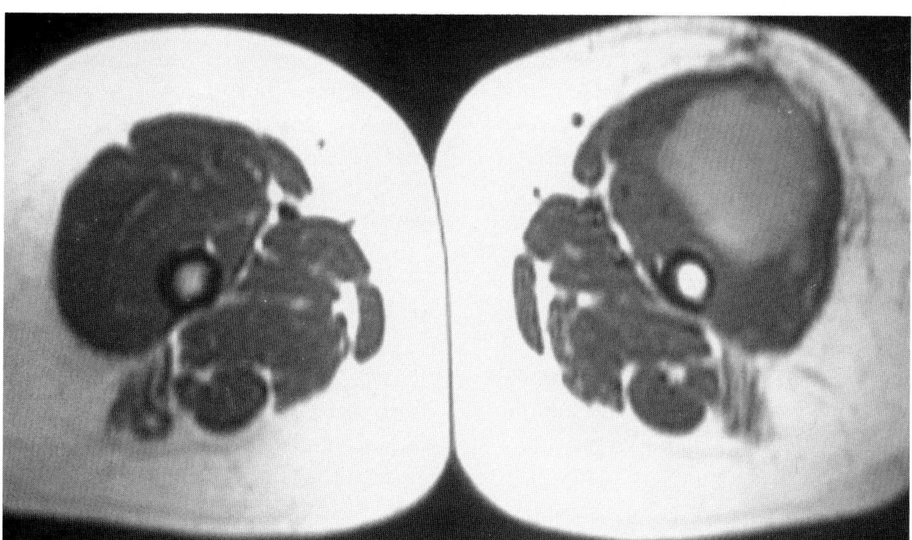

FIG. 14-14. Myeloid depletion from radiation therapy: 28-year-old woman. **A:** An axial, T1 weighted image (SE 500/20) of the proximal thighs in this patient with a malignant fibrous histiocytoma (anterior compartment of the left thigh) demonstrates normal red/yellow marrow signal intensity in both femoral shafts. Note the symmetrical intermediate signal intensity of both medullary spaces. **B:** Following radiation therapy to the left thigh, there has been a significant change in the signal intensity of the left femoral marrow. An axial, T1 weighted image (SE 500/20) obtained at the same level as (**A**) demonstrates marked increase in the signal intensity of the left femoral marrow such that it is now isointense with subcutaneous fat. This change reflects loss of red marrow or myeloid depletion due to radiation therapy. Only fatty marrow is evident on the left following the therapy. Note also how the soft tissue tumor has become necrotic.

quences (33); while in acellular cases, the marrow demonstrates diffuse high signal, reflecting a preponderance of fatty marrow (11,32,45). With treatment, islands of regenerating hematopoietic tissue begin to reappear in the fatty marrow (33) and, at some point in time, will become evident as spotty foci of decreased signal intensity on T1 weighted images. With time, these areas of low signal intensity may increase in size, coalesce, and become diffuse in patients responding to therapy. This response may be regionally limited at any particular time. Axial response is expected to precede appendicular response. The exact sequence of response throughout the skeleton, however, is not known.

Irradiation of marrow and systemic or regional chemotherapy exert toxic effects on red marrow. Early pathologic findings following these insults may include marrow congestion and edema (37). These acute changes then subside and hematopoietic tissue gradually disappears, leaving the marrow predominantly fatty in nature. MR findings at the earliest stages of involvement are not well established. Preliminary reports focusing on vertebral irradiation (54) describe either no change or slight change in the MR pattern within the first week following radiation therapy. The slight change consists of decrease in marrow signal intensity on T1 weighted images and increase in signal intensity on T2 weighted and STIR images, presumably due to edema. At 4 weeks postirradiation, the marrow becomes either mottled and heterogeneous or displays central fatty marrow. With time, older patients tend to show diffuse fatty marrow throughout involved vertebral bodies, while young patients show diffuse fatty marrow centrally and what is presumed to be red marrow around the periphery of the vertebral body. This pattern observed in younger patients may represent regenerating red marrow from end-plate sinusoids.

MR findings at later stages of marrow ablation are as expected. Involved marrow follows the signal pattern of fatty marrow on both T1 and T2 weighted sequences. These changes may be evident diffusely throughout the skeleton in the setting of systemic chemotherapy, while they are more likely to be regionally limited in radiation therapy (Fig. 14-14) or local chemotherapy (e.g., intra-arterial chemotherapy).

Bone Marrow Ischemia

Although usually focal in nature, bone marrow ischemia may be present at multiple sites throughout the

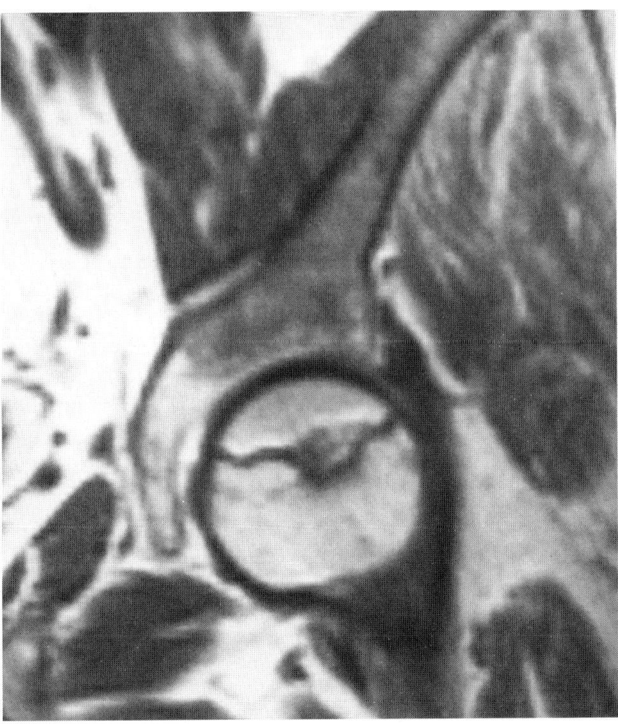

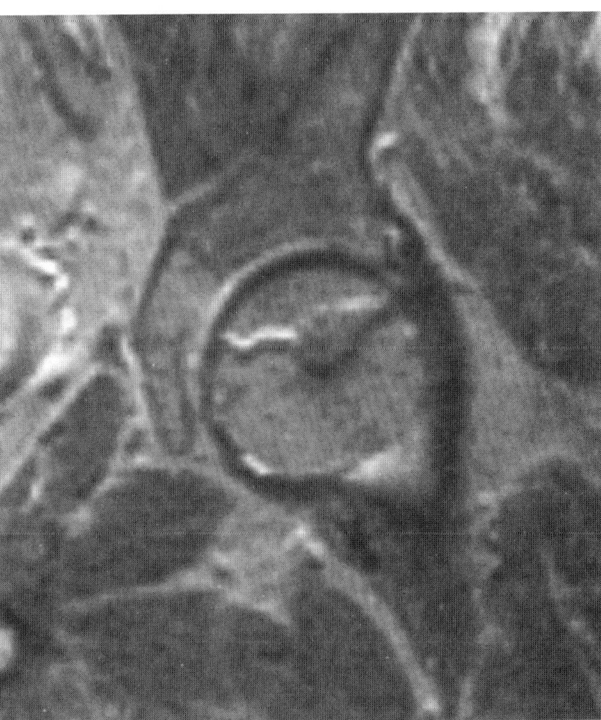

A,B

FIG. 14-15. Marrow ischemia from avascular necrosis: 59-year-old man. **A:** A coronal, T1 weighted image (SE/600/20) of the left hip demonstrates many features of ischemic marrow disease. A serpiginous line of decreased signal intensity defines the ischemic area in the superior portion of the femoral head. The marrow signal intensity within the ischemic region is comparable to the signal intensity of fatty marrow in the remainder of the femoral head. This pattern is associated with a less advanced stage of avascular necrosis. **B:** On a coronal T2 weighted image (SE 2,000/80) at the same location, the "double-line sign" of avascular necrosis becomes evident as a band of high signal intensity is seen to accompany the serpiginous dark line.

skeleton in select individuals. Settings that predispose to this occurrence include collagen vascular diseases (systemic lupus erythematosus), exogenous steroid administration, marrow packing diseases (Gaucher's), sickle cell anemia, pancreatitis, and radiation therapy among others. In the absence of disease-specific findings, the distribution and appearance of osteonecrosis in these diverse disorders may be identical and thus differentiation of the disorders on the basis of MR findings may not be possible. Two basic types of marrow ischemia are to be considered: avascular necrosis and bone infarction. Details of the basic pathophysiology of marrow ischemia have been discussed elsewhere in this text and only portions will be reemphasized in this chapter.

Avascular necrosis is most frequently encountered in the subarticular regions of long bones. Anatomic sites particularly prone to this process include femoral heads, humeral heads, and femoral condyles. The appendicular skeleton is more often involved than the axial skeleton, probably reflecting the propensity of osteonecrosis for fatty marrow over hematopoietic marrow. This propensity presumably reflects the differing vascular systems of red and yellow marrow (being rich in red marrow and sparse in yellow marrow). This concept has been supported by identification of an increased prevalence of fatty marrow in the proximal femora of patients with nontraumatic avascular necrosis (40); however, the concept is yet to be substantiated on subsequent studies.

Bone infarction occurs most frequently in the shafts of long bones. Favored anatomic sites include femora, humeri, and tibiae. Although flat bones are by no means immune, occurrence at these sites is less frequently detected. As with avascular necrosis, the appendicular skeleton is more often involved than the axial skeleton.

Regardless of the cause or site of involvement, histopathologic changes occurring in ischemic marrow are similar, therefore producing similar MRI appearances. Although the cause is ischemia, manifestations of the process represent a balance of progressive cell death and host response through repair.

Controversy exists as to just how early in osteonecrosis MRI will be able to detect signal alterations in ischemic marrow. Since fat cells form the basis of the high signal intensity of normal marrow, speculation exists that marrow signal changes may begin with the death of fat cells (approximately 2–5 days following the insult) (57). However, there is cause to believe that the death of fat cells may not immediately alter signal intensity since signal derived from depot lipid may persist for an extended time span after cell death (20). That being the case, signal changes will not become apparent until later in the process when depot lipid is altered. To date, this issue has not been resolved.

A variety of shapes and signal patterns are produced in the setting of avascular necrosis of the femoral head. Morphologic configurations include oval, ring, geometric, and band patterns (57). In commonly encountered signal patterns, the involved marrow signal may be homogeneous or inhomogeneous; however, some component of diminished signal intensity on T1 weighted images is usually present. This reflects replacement of fatty marrow by some balance of edema, amorphous cellular debris, granulation tissue, and fibrosis. Variable signal changes are evident on T2 weighted images, ranging from low to high signal intensity when compared to normal fatty marrow. Uncommonly, avascular necrosis has been shown to present as diffuse signal abnormality in the femoral head and neck with extension into the intertrochanteric region (60). The abnormal areas demonstrate low signal intensity on short TR/TE images—a pattern associated with bone marrow edema and similar to that seen in patients with reflex sympathetic dystrophy. Also, there probably are cases in which MRI will be negative yet the patient goes on to develop avascular necrosis. As with other marrow disorders, biopsy may be necessary to establish a diagnosis when MRI is equivocal. Despite recognized limitations, there is general agreement that MRI remains the most sensitive imaging method for detecting avascular necrosis.

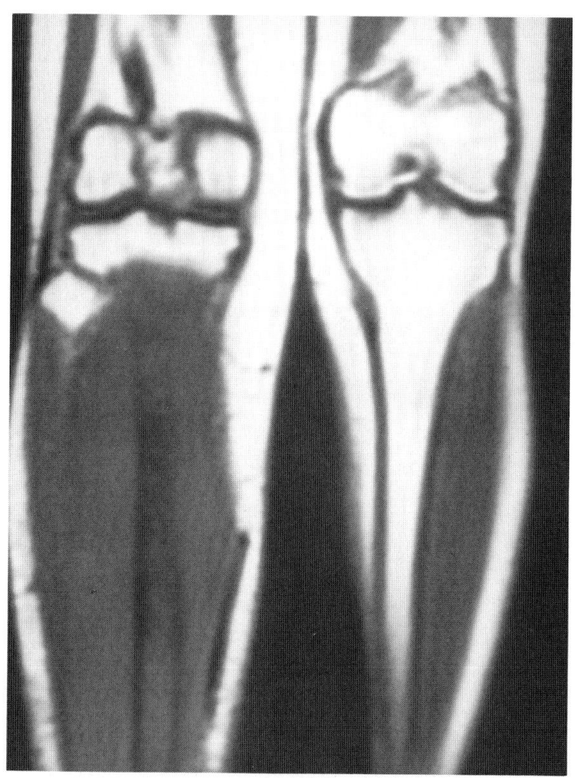

FIG. 14-16. Marrow infiltration in lymphoma: 38-year-old man. On a coronal, T1 weighted image (SE 500/20) of the legs, lymphomatous marrow infiltration is apparent in the right tibia. Involved marrow demonstrates decreased signal intensity on the T1 weighted image. The tumor extent can readily be identified in the high-signal fatty marrow. Compare to the normal left side.

A,B
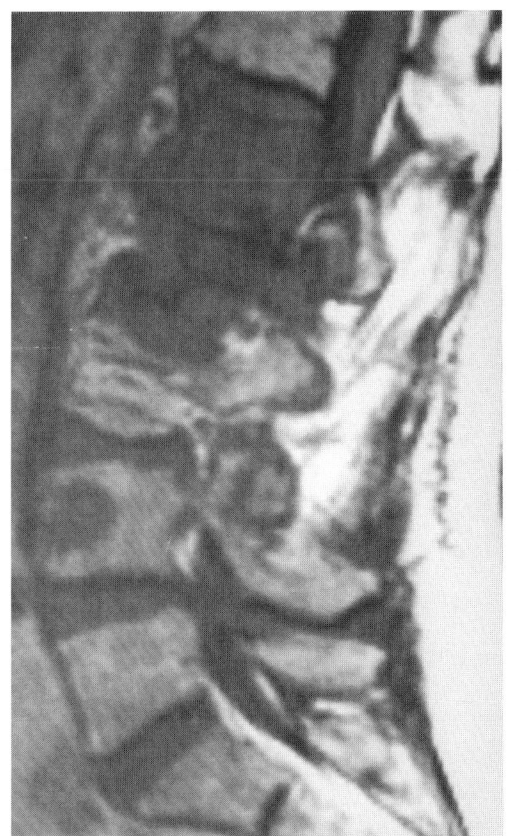
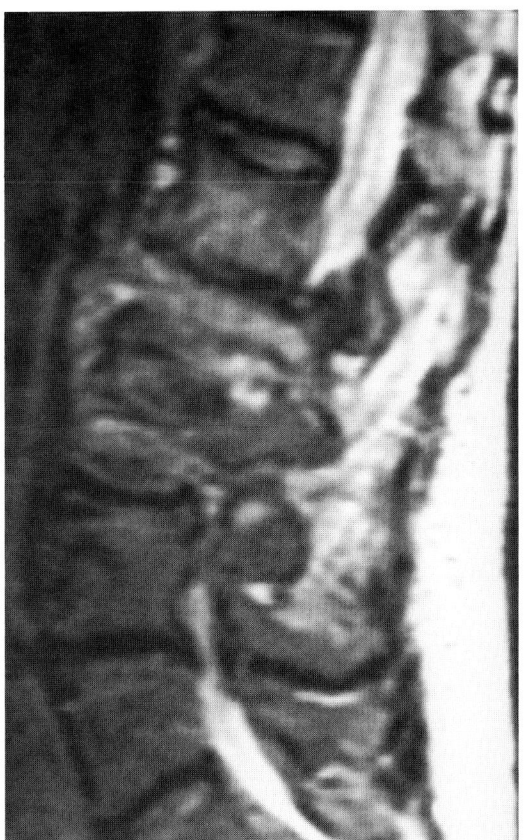

C
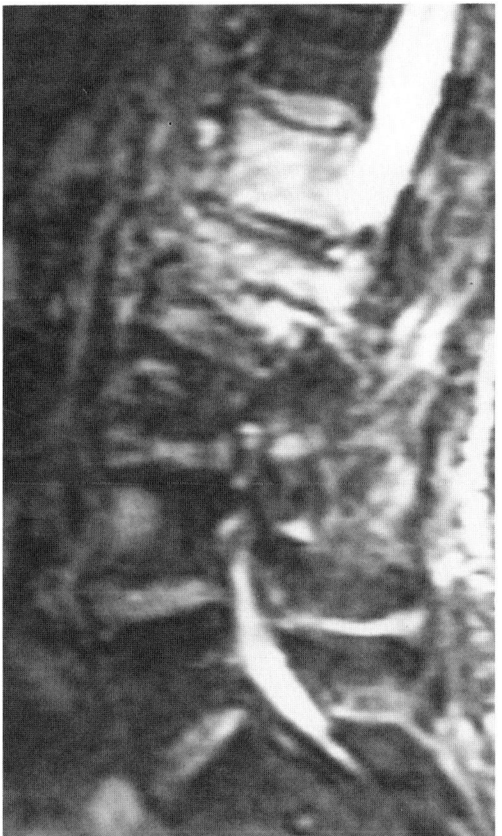

FIG. 14-17. Marrow infiltration in metastatic disease: 76-year-old woman. **A:** The expected appearance of metastatic disease is evident on this T1 weighted sagittal image (SE 600/20) of the lumbar spine. Involved areas of the L1, L2, and L4 vertebral bodies demonstrate decreased signal intensity. (Compression deformities of the L2 and L3 vertebral bodies are present.) **B:** On a T2 weighted sagittal image (SE 2,000/80), the metastatic deposits demonstrate varying degrees of increase in signal intensity. The lesion in L4 is roughly isointense with surrounding marrow while the lesions in L1 and L2 are higher in signal intensity than normal marrow. **C:** These same lesions become hyperintense and are much more conspicuous on a sagittal STIR image (1,500/43/160).

The different morphologic and signal patterns probably reflect chronologic stages of the ischemic process. Signal patterns identifying fat and/or edema in the involved area suggest an earlier stage, while patterns associated with fibrosis imply a more advanced process. When a reactive interface forms histologically between viable and necrotic tissue, the MR image may demonstrate a "double-line sign" (a band of low signal intensity on T1 weighted images that is partially hyperintense on T2 weighted images) (Fig. 14-15). Presumably, the high-signal component of this double line represents vascularized fibroblastic repair tissue that contains increased amounts of water. Widening and geographic change of this interface within the boundaries of the involved area could indicate progressive repair. Likewise, subchondral fractures (indicating a more advanced stage of disease) may produce signal changes in the ischemic area (39).

Occasionally, other marrow abnormalities will be present (such as hyperplastic marrow and hemosiderosis in a patient with sickle cell anemia) that will identify a specific disorder as the etiology of ischemic marrow disease. Often, however, no such markers can be found and the differential diagnosis must rely on the patients' clinical setting.

Marrow Infiltration or Replacement

A wide variety of disorders alter marrow by infiltrating or replacing normal components. Included in this group are neoplastic processes, inflammatory conditions, myeloproliferative disorders, lipidoses, and histiocytoses. The effect of these different processes on marrow signal patterns depends largely on the type of cells/tissue infiltrating the marrow, the degree of cellularity, associated water content or edema, and other complicating factors such as hemorrhage, necrosis, fibrosis, and inflammatory debris. Substantial overlap between the disorders exists, making histologic determination based on MR findings alone unreliable, thus necessitating bone marrow biopsy to make that determination if necessary.

Neoplastic processes, whether primary or metastatic, alter marrow by infiltration. With rare exception, the tumor cells have long T1 values and variable T2 values (48). Measured T1 and T2 relaxation times for a spectrum of infiltrative processes (9,10,67) demonstrate no reliable means of identifying specific histologic types or even differentiating benign from malignant tumors. In certain settings (e.g., leukemia) when the diagnosis is established, however, T1 relaxation values may be helpful in documenting new disease, remission, and relapse (41).

MR signal characteristics of infiltrative lesions vary. With the exception of melanoma, however, all demonstrate some decreased signal intensity on T1 weighted images (8,11,14,55), making them conspicuous in the higher signal intensity of surrounding fatty marrow (Fig. 14-16). Melanoma, on the other hand, may demonstrate increased signal on T1 weighted images, presumably resulting from the paramagnetic effect of melanin.

A,B
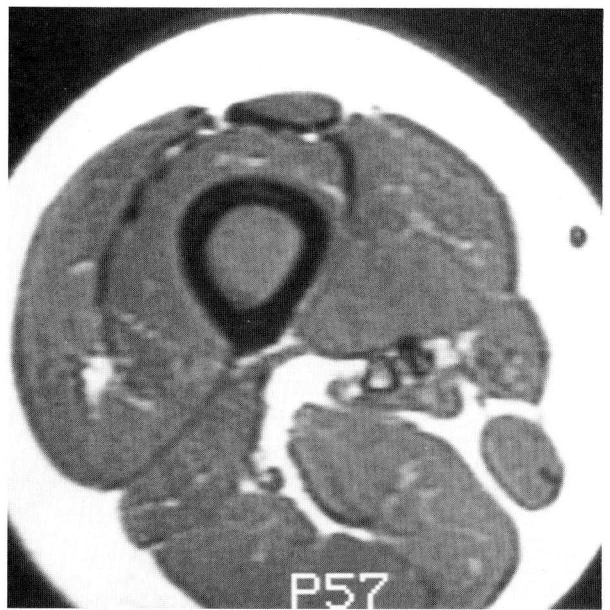

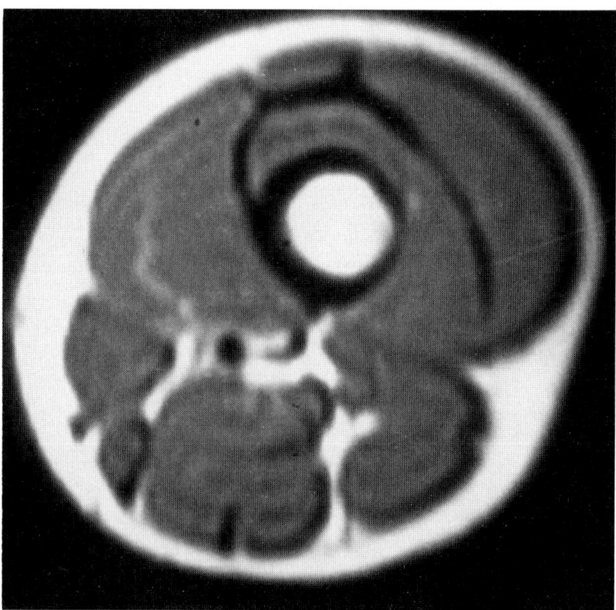

FIG. 14-18. Marrow infiltration in leukemia: 26-year-old woman. An axial, T1 weighted image (SE 500/20) of the right thigh (**A**) demonstrates diffuse lowering of marrow signal intensity due to the prolonged T1 values of leukemic marrow. The marrow signal intensity is roughly comparable to that of muscle. Compare with normal marrow signal intensity at the same anatomic site in a similar age patient (**B**) (SE 500/20).

T2 signal intensities of infiltrative processes are much more variable. Although most of the disorders will demonstrate some prolongation of T2 relaxation times, causing them to appear higher in signal intensity than surrounding marrow (Fig. 14-17), many will not. This variability results not only from tumor cell type but also from cellularity, water content, and complicating or associated factors (fibrosis, necrosis, hemorrhage, inflammatory debris) (23). On occasion, the cellularity and water fraction of an infiltrative process may approach that of hyperplastic or even normal red marrow. In these instances, T1 and T2 signal characteristics of the normal and abnormal marrow may appear similar. At times, other pulse sequences (e.g., STIR) may demonstrate subtle T1 and T2 relaxation differences not apparent on spin-echo images. However, due to substantial overlap in signal characteristics, reliable differentiation of neoplastic and nonneoplastic marrow is not always possible without biopsy.

The skeletal distribution of neoplastic disorders tends to follow the pattern of red marrow distribution (34). This occurs predominantly for two reasons. First, many primary neoplasms (myeloma, leukemia, histiocytic lymphoma, Ewing's sarcoma) are thought to originate in red marrow. Second, other disorders, such as metastases, spread hematogenously, thus favoring the rich vascularity of red marrow to the sparse vascularity of yellow marrow. These tendencies may be of diagnostic and prognostic importance. Finding a metastatic lesion in the distal appendicular skeleton (where red marrow is generally sparse) may indicate extensive axial involvement with reconversion of appendicular fatty marrow to red marrow and subsequent involvement with metastatic disease.

Despite limitations in tissue characterization, most evidence would suggest that the local extent of marrow involvement by primary and metastatic tumors can be reliably determined (1,7,8,46,55,68). Similarly, "skip" lesions are readily identified. This information is valuable not only for staging purposes but as a means of identifying potential biopsy sites and for assessing therapy or disease progression.

MRI features of a number of infiltrative disorders have been described. Studies of leukemic patients (32,33,37,41,45) have identified marrow alterations before, during, and after treatment. Involvement may be diffuse or spotty depending on the extent of disease. The most common pattern observed in leukemic marrow is prolongation of T1 relaxation values (41,44,45,56), resulting in an overall lowering of marrow signal intensity on T1 weighted images (Fig. 14-18). Ongoing studies (42) indicate a significant difference between T1 values in patients with newly diagnosed and relapse leukemia as compared with patients in remission and normal age-matched controls (Fig. 14-19). A T1 value less than 600 msec correlates with a disease-free state, while a T1 value greater than 750 msec correlates with disease (newly diagnosed or relapse). Changes in T2 relaxation times are more variable. Although there may be some prolongation of these times, measured values show no statistically significant difference from those of age-matched controls. Of the various types of leukemia, patients with chronic myelogenous leukemia (particularly during blast phases) (Fig. 14-20) and acute lymphocytic leukemia (pretreatment or in relapse) demonstrate the most profound MR findings.

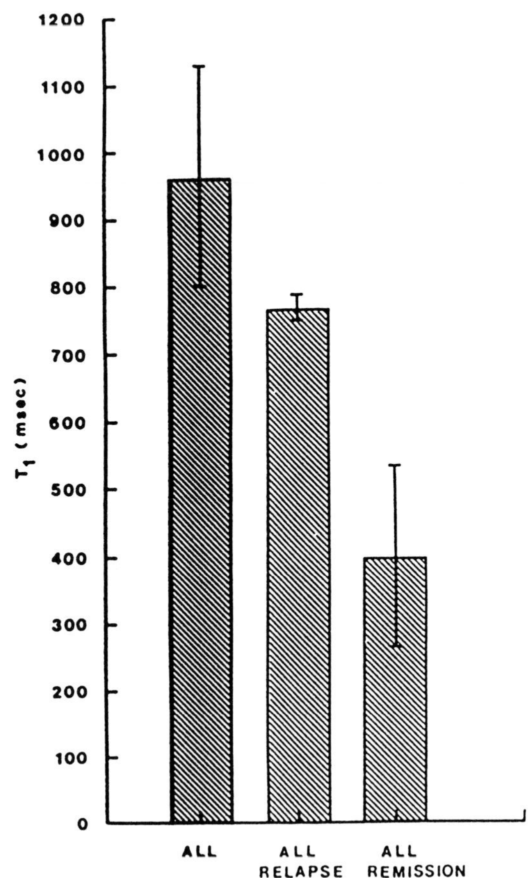

FIG. 14-19. T1 relaxation times of vertebral bone marrow in patients with acute lymphocytic leukemia (ALL). Mean T1 relaxation times (± standard deviation) of patients with newly diagnosed ALL, ALL in relapse, and ALL in remission are illustrated. Note that there is a significant difference between patients with disease and patients in a disease-free state. (Adapted from ref. 41.)

Leukemic marrow often demonstrates changing MR patterns following chemotherapy or radiation therapy for ablation of leukemia. Acutely, these changes are consistent with edema and congestion of the marrow (37). After the acute alterations have resolved, MR findings reflect normocellular or hypocellular marrow with corresponding T1 values and signal intensity. Quantitative MRI is a potential means for monitoring marrow changes in these patients.

Myelomatous involvement of bone marrow has no

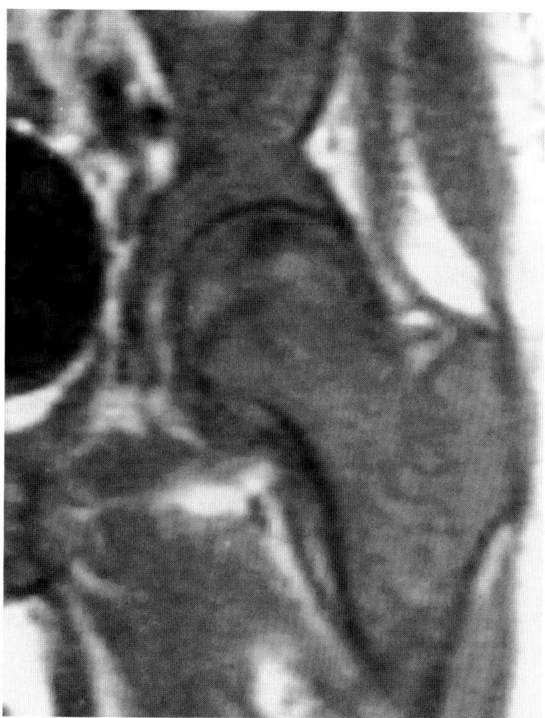

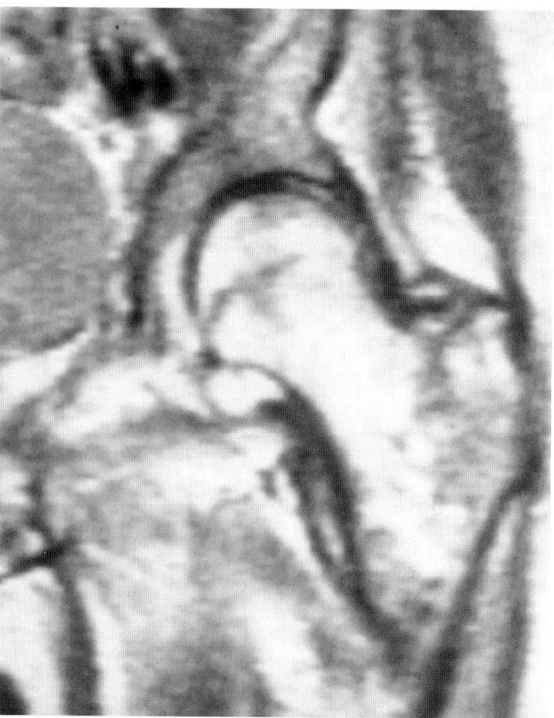

A,B

FIG. 14-20. Marrow infiltration in chronic myelogenous leukemia (blast crisis): 66-year-old man. **A:** Diffuse lowering of marrow signal intensity is evident on this coronal, T1 weighted image (SE 525/32) of the left hip. **B:** The involved marrow demonstrates a marked increase in signal intensity on a T2 weighted image (SE 2,000/60). The marked increase in T2 signal intensity of leukemic marrow in this case may not be encountered in all forms of leukemia or even in different stages of the disease. (Courtesy of M. B. Desai, M.D., New York.)

characteristic that distinguishes it from other infiltrating processes on MR images (14,44). The usual appearance is a nonspecific decrease in signal intensity of involved areas on T1 weighted images (Fig. 14-21). Affected sites may demonstrate diffuse or spotty involvement depending on the severity of the process. On T2 weighted images, untreated lesions demonstrate increased signal intensity, while foci that have responded to therapy remain low in signal intensity (Fig. 14-22) (23). Without a substantial increase in signal intensity of neoplastic marrow on T2 weighted images, differentiation between myeloma and normal red marrow may be difficult. Despite this limitation, MRI is currently the most sensitive imaging modality available for detecting myelomatous marrow involvement. MR evaluation of patients with myeloma has demonstrated disease despite negative radionuclide bone scans and plain films.

Other myeloproliferative disorders (myelofibrosis, polycythemia vera, mastocytosis) have not been extensively studied to date. In myelofibrosis (35), the marrow is replaced to varying degrees by fibrosis. The fibrosis, along with hypercellularity, results in a lowering of marrow signal intensity on T1 weighted images (Fig. 14-23). Due to the nature of replacement tissue (fibrous), marrow signal intensity is likewise diminished on T2 weighted images. In more advanced cases, where a larger amount of fibrous tissue is present, marrow signal intensity may be substantially lower than that of muscle on longer TR/TE images.

Lipidoses (Gaucher's disease, Niemann–Pick disease) have likewise received little attention. The most extensively studied among these has been Gaucher's disease (36,50). In this condition, glucocerebroside-laden cells (Gaucher's cells) accumulate in various tissues throughout the body—particularly the liver, spleen, lymph nodes, and bone marrow. Involvement of marrow generally occurs in the axial and proximal appendicular skeleton before peripheral sites are affected—probably reflecting the predilection of this disease for red marrow. As a result, epiphyses and apophyses are usually spared until late in the disease. Involved sites demonstrate decreased signal intensity (Fig. 14-24) on both T1 and T2 weighted images (36). In affected marrow, marked shortening of T2 relaxation time appears to be the principal cause of diminished signal on both T1 and T2 weighted images. Presumably this T2 shortening relates to the presence of fast-exchanging protons in the glucocerebroside. Both homogeneous and inhomogeneous patterns of involvement may be observed. Intramedullary osteonecrosis is a recognized complication of

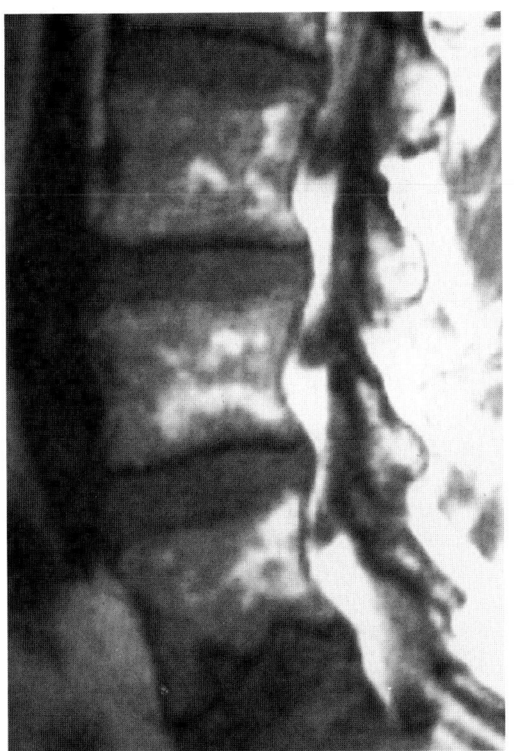

FIG. 14-21. Marrow infiltration in myeloma: 53-year-old man. A sagittal, T1 weighted image (SE 500/20) of the lumbar spine demonstrates patchy areas of decreased signal intensity throughout the visualized vertebral marrow. This appearance is not specific for myeloma as it could occur in several other conditions. Nevertheless, the extent of marrow involvement is readily appreciated.

Gaucher's disease and, when present, will produce expected alterations in the described MR marrow patterns of these patients. Marrow infarction and other osseous complications in patients with Gaucher's disease appear to correlate with the extent of marrow involvement as defined by MRI (50).

Inflammatory processes result in replacement or infiltration of normal marrow by inflammatory tissue. In the case of osteomyelitis, proliferating bacteria evoke this inflammatory response, which results in increased fluid accumulation in the marrow. Intramedullary pressure may increase and be accompanied by marrow infarction. Increased water content and cellularity result in decreased marrow signal intensity on T1 weighted images and increased signal intensity on T2 weighted images (3,22). MR patterns may vary somewhat depending on the stage of osteomyelitis (3,4,22,61). Adjacent soft tissue changes and poorly marginated areas of involvement appear to be features of acute, subacute, and recurrent osteomyelitis. Margins of involved sites are generally better defined in chronic osteomyelitis. Although more commonly confined to one location, osteomyelitis can, on occasion, be multifocal in nature (Fig. 14-25).

Bone Marrow Edema

Most processes that produce an MR pattern of bone marrow edema (trauma, skeletal stress, reflex sympa-

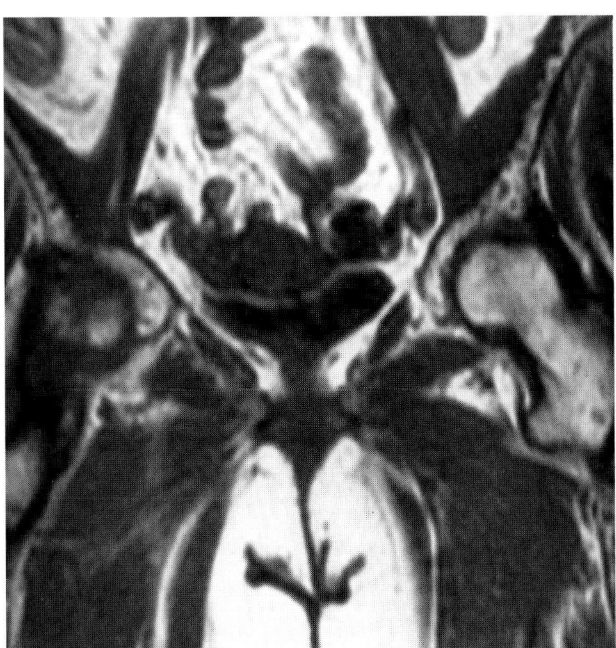

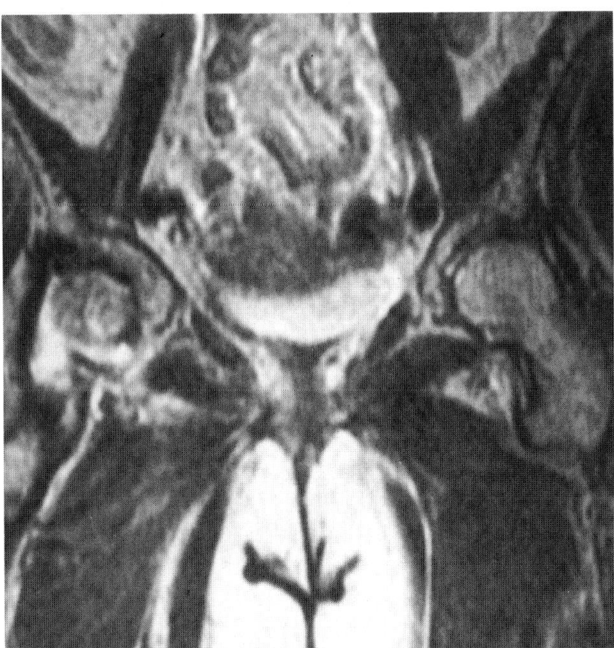

A,B

FIG. 14-22. Marrow infiltration in myeloma: 68-year-old man. Coronal images of the pelvis demonstrate the expected appearance of myeloma that has responded to therapy. Spotty areas of decreased signal intensity scattered throughout the marrow on a T1 weighted (SE 600/20) image (A) remain low in signal intensity on long TR/TE sequences (SE 2,000/80) (B).

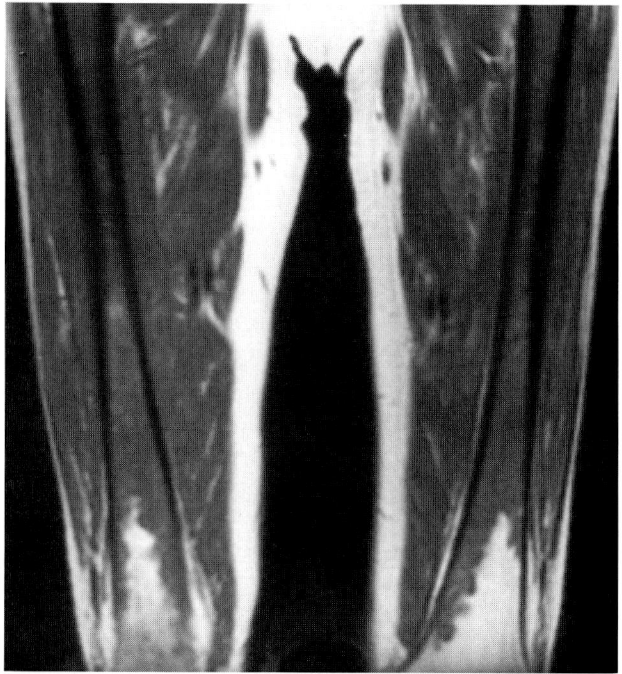

FIG. 14-23. Marrow infiltration in myelofibrosis: 66-year-old man. A coronal, T1 weighted image (SE 500/20) of the thighs demonstrates infiltration/replacement of marrow in the femoral shafts by tissue that is low in signal intensity. This low signal intensity tissue indicates fibrotic marrow. The extent of involvement can readily be determined in this condition.

thetic dystrophy) are regionally limited—often affecting only one anatomic site. In this setting, these processes can be readily distinguished from other diffuse marrow disorders. Confusion may arise, however, when one of the marrow edema processes affects multiple sites. Such can be the case in patients with insufficiency fractures of the pelvis. In these individuals, it is not uncommon to have concurrent insufficiency fractures in both sacral alae, the parasymphyseal regions, and the supra-acetabular areas. The multiplicity of involvement may raise concern for metastatic disease; however, when involvement is restricted to any or all of these sites, the possibility of insufficiency fractures should be considered. In many cases, computed tomography of the sacrum will resolve the issue by defining the fractures.

MRI features of marrow edema processes include decreased marrow signal intensity on T1 weighted images and increased marrow signal intensity on T2 weighted images. These findings are consistent with expected marrow alterations from increased extracellular (interstitial) water. It appears that the amount of extra water controls the degree of signal intensity alteration—ranging from barely perceptible to quite conspicuous. Initiating and controlling factors of this edema are not clear; however, the process is thought to be modulated through control of hypervascularity or hyperperfusion (64).

A,B

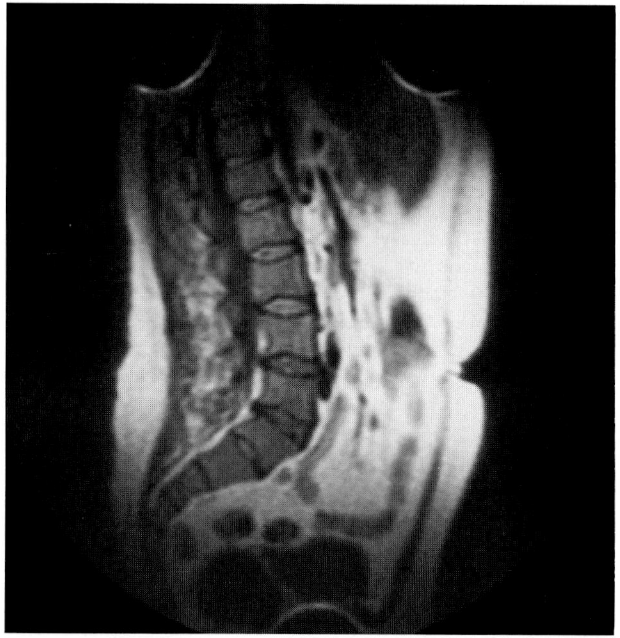

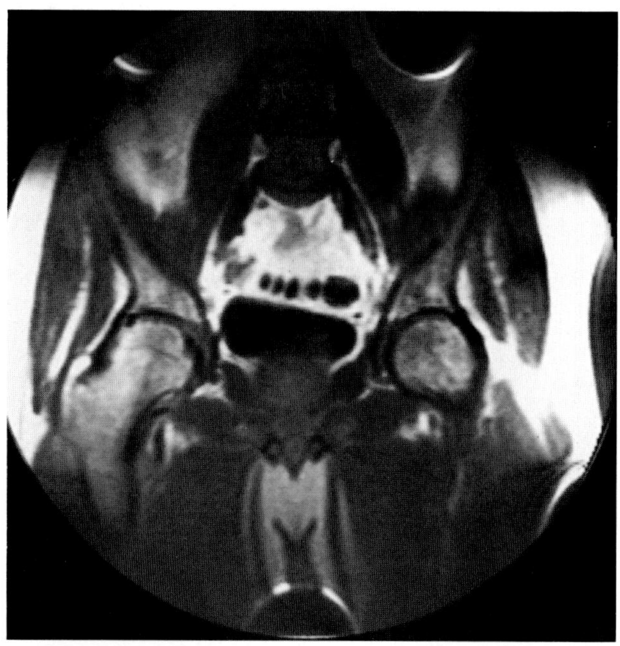

FIG. 14-24. Marrow infiltration in Gaucher's disease: 45-year-old man. Sagittal lumbar (**A**) and coronal pelvis (**B**) T1 weighted images (0.35 T, SE 500/30) demonstrate marrow involvement in Gaucher's disease. There is diffuse, decreased marrow signal intensity in the lumbar spine and spotty decreased signal intensity in proximal femoral and pelvic marrow. The decreased signal intensity probably reflects a combination of Gaucher's cells and residual hematopoietic elements.

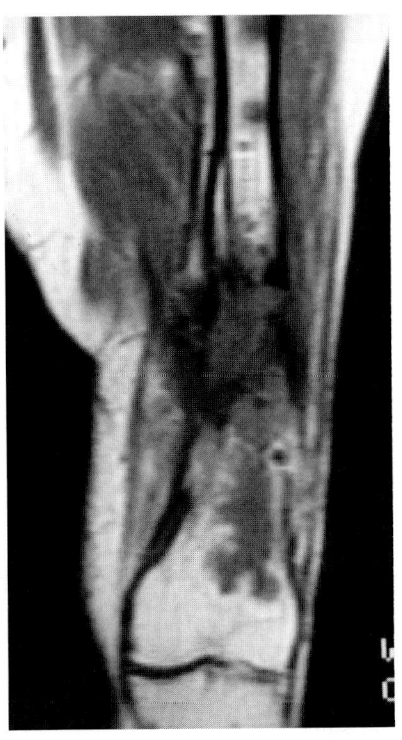

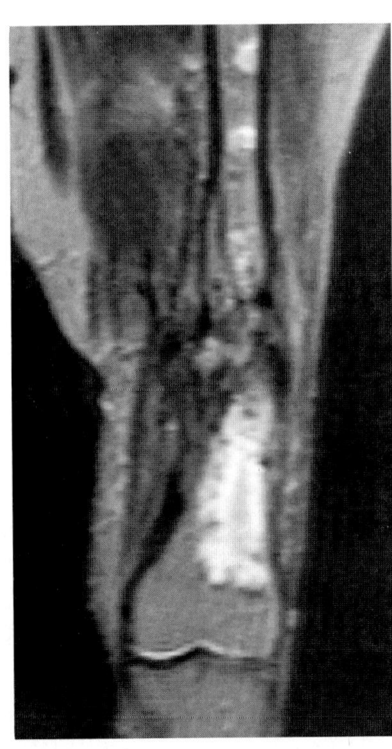

A,B

FIG. 14-25. Marrow infiltration in infection: 50-year-old man. Coronal T1 (SE 700/17) (**A**) and T2 weighted (SE 3,000/90) (**B**) images of the left femur demonstrate multiple foci of osteomyelitis throughout the medullary space. The foci demonstrate typical signal alterations encountered in osteomyelitis being low in signal intensity on T1 weighted images and high in signal intensity on T2 weighted images.

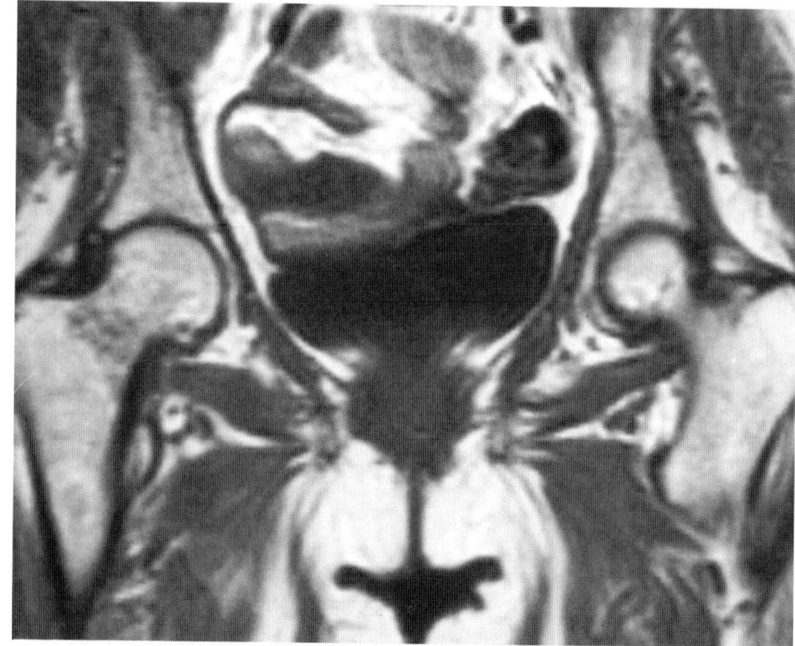

A

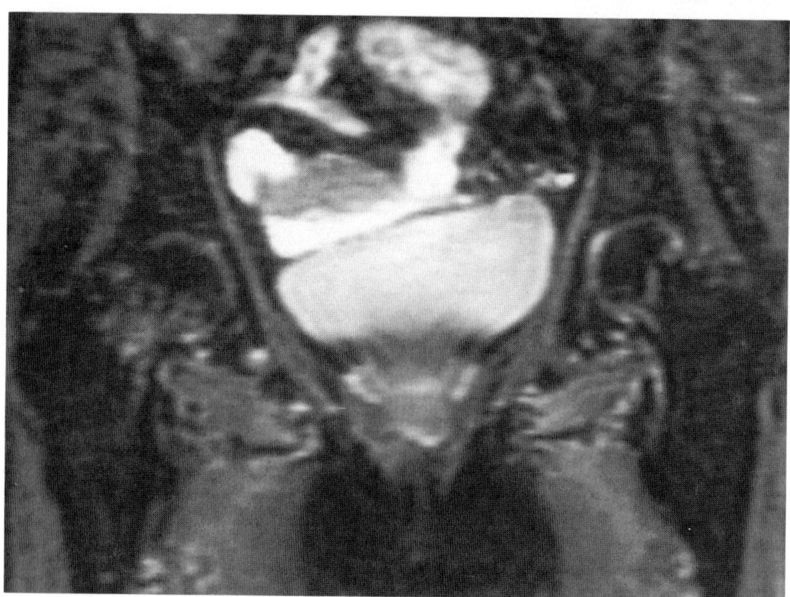

B

FIG. 14-26. Marrow edema from stress fracture: 69-year-old woman. **A:** An irregular band of decreased signal intensity is identified in the right femoral neck on this T1 weighted image (SE 600/20). **B:** The involved area demonstrates increased signal intensity on a STIR image (2,000/43/165). This pattern presumably reflects marrow edema associated with a stress fracture of the femoral neck.

Direct trauma with or without fracture, insufficiency fractures, and stress fractures can produce signal changes in bone marrow (53,67). These changes consist of irregular areas of low signal intensity on T1 weighted images which increase in signal intensity (greater than fat) on T2 weighted or STIR images (Fig. 14-26). The degree of T1 and T2 signal intensity alteration varies from subtle to profound, presumably reflecting the amount of edema present. Similarly, the extent of trauma-related marrow involvement can range from discrete areas intimately associated with the site of injury to diffuse regional marrow involvement. Although the MR signal patterns described above are consistent with increased tissue water, some contribution from hemorrhage may be present depending on the degree and time course of the injury. This contribution remains unclear at present because MRI features of intraosseous hemorrhage have not been described experimentally or clinically and time-related changes observed in hemorrhage at other extracranial locations are yet to be observed in bone marrow injuries. In bone contusion, trabecular fractures, presumably present in most instances, may not be apparent on MRI studies, conventional films, or tomograms.

Reflex sympathetic dystrophy and related disorders such as transient or migratory osteoporosis (6,64) produce bone marrow changes through complex and poorly understood mechanisms—the net result of which appears to be accumulation of increased marrow water or edema. Factors associated with the edema such as mild inflammation, hyperemia, and increased bone turnover are evident on radionuclide studies and/or histologically. Increased tissue water produces expected MR signal patterns at involved sites. Regions of low signal intensity are evident on T1 weighted images and are correspondingly bright on T2 weighted images. The extent of marrow involvement is variable. In transient osteoporosis of the hip, the femoral head and neck may be diffusely involved while the acetabulum may or may not be affected. MR signal patterns of involved marrow appear to return to normal with resolution of the syndrome (6).

PITFALLS

Most of the pitfalls encountered in interpreting MRI studies for diffuse marrow disorders probably relate to distinguishing between normal hematopoietic marrow and pathologic processes. This distinction becomes extremely difficult when the pathologic tissue demonstrates signal intensity similar to that of normal red marrow on both T1 and T2 weighted images. Disease processes most likely to present in this fashion include metastases, myeloma, and leukemia. At present, there is no reliable means of distinguishing such disorders from red marrow through the use of MRI. MR spectroscopy and MR contrast agents have hypothetical potential in this regard but are, to date, unproven. In unclear cases, bone marrow aspiration or biopsy will be necessary to establish a diagnosis.

Focal marrow processes are much more common but less likely to be confused with diffuse marrow disease. Included among these processes are focal fat replacement and degenerative changes occurring about joints. Focal fat replacement demonstrates signal patterns of normal marrow fat on T1 and T2 weighted images. Also, this fat replacement is typically found at certain locations in vertebral bodies (end-plates, periphery, and about the central venous plexus). Vertebral marrow changes that occur in the setting of degenerative disc disease are generally characteristic and have been discussed earlier in this chapter. Degenerative changes occurring at synovial articulations can also result in changes in the MRI appearance of subjacent bone marrow. Subchondral sclerosis may appear as regions of decreased signal intensity on T1 and T2 weighted images. Subchondral cyst formation usually appears as a circular area of decreased signal intensity on T1 weighted images that becomes bright on T2 weighted images (following the signal pattern of synovial fluid). Usually, the MR findings associated with degenerative disease can be explained with plain films of the region.

With MRI, *in vivo* evaluation of normal and abnormal marrow is now possible to an extent never before realized. Valuable information about the appearance and distribution of normal red and yellow marrow is being acquired. With this comes the potential for better understanding disease processes and their effects on bone marrow. This information impacts the manner in which marrow diseases are diagnosed and monitored.

Limitations and pitfalls in MRI of marrow diseases are also being recognized. Although these recognized limitations may dampen somewhat the initial enthusiasm about the capabilities of MRI, the potential of this modality in bone marrow evaluation remains great.

REFERENCES

1. Aisen AM, Martel W, Braunstein EM, McMillin KI, Phillips WA, Klink TF. MRI and CT evaluation of primary bone and soft tissue tumors. *AJR* 1986;146:749–756.
2. Beltran J, Herman LJ, Burk JM, et al. Femoral head avascular necrosis: MR imaging with clinical-pathologic and radionuclide correlation. *Radiology* 1988;166:215–220.
3. Beltran J, Noto AM, McGhee RB, Freedy RM, McCalla MS. Infections of the musculoskeletal system: high-field-strength MR imaging. *Radiology* 1987;164:449–454.
4. Berquist TH, Brown ML, Fitzgerald RH Jr, May GR. Magnetic resonance imaging: application in musculoskeletal infection. *Magn Reson Imaging* 1985;3:219–230.
5. Biermann A, Von Keyserlingk DG. Ultrastructure of reticulum cells in the bone marrow. *Acta Anat* 1978;100:34–43.
6. Bloem JL. Transient osteoporosis of the hip: MR imaging. *Radiology* 1988;167:753–755.
7. Bohndorf K, Reiser M, Lochner B, de Lacroix WF, Steinbrich W. Magnetic resonance imaging of primary tumours and tumour-like lesions of bone. *Skeletal Radiol* 1986;15:511–517.
8. Boyko OB, Cory DA, Cohen MD, Provisor A, Mirkin D, DeRosa GP. MR imaging of osteogenic and Ewing's sarcoma. *AJR* 1987;148:317–322.
9. Brady TJ, Gebhardt MC, Pykett IL, et al. NMR imaging of forearms in healthy volunteers and patients with giant-cell tumor of bone. *Radiology* 1982;144:549–552.
10. Cherryman GR, Smith FW. NMR scanning for skeletal tumours. *Lancet* 1984;1:1403–1404.
11. Cohen MD, Klatte EC, Baehner R, et al. Magnetic resonance imaging of bone marrow disease in children. *Radiology* 1984;151:715–718.
12. Custer RP. Studies on the structure and function of bone marrow. I. Variability of the hemopoietic pattern and consideration of method for examination. *J Lab Clin Med* 1932;17:951–959.
13. Custer RP, Ahlfeldt FE. Studies on the structure and function of bone marrow. II. Variations in cellularity in various bones with advancing years of life and their relative response to stimuli. *J Lab Clin Med* 1932;17:960–962.
14. Daffner RJ, Lupetin AR, Dash N, Deeb ZL, Sefczek RJ, Schapiro RL. MRI in the detection of malignant infiltration of bone marrow. *AJR* 1986;146:353–358.
15. Datz FL, Taylor A Jr. The clinical use of radionuclide bone marrow imaging. *Semin Nucl Med* 1985;15:239–259.
16. de Roos A, Kressel HY, Spritzer C, Dalinka M. MR imaging of marrow changes adjacent to end plates in degenerative lumbar disk disease. *AJR* 1987;149:531–534.
17. Dixon WT. Simple proton spectroscopic imaging. *Radiology* 1984;153:189–194.
18. Dooms GC, Fisher MR, Hricak H, Richardson M, Crooks LE, Genant HK. Bone marrow imaging: magnetic resonance studies related to age and sex. *Radiology* 1985;155:429–432.
19. Dunnill MS, Anderson JA, Whitehead R. Quantitative histological studies on age changes in bone. *J Pathol Bacteriol* 1967;94:275–291.

20. Ehman RL, Berquist TH, McLeod RA. MR imaging of the musculoskeletal system: a 5-year appraisal. *Radiology* 1988;166:313–320.
21. Emery JL, Follett GF. Regression of bone-marrow haemopoiesis from the terminal digits in the foetus and infant. *Br J Haematol* 1964;10:485–489.
22. Fletcher BD, Scoles PV, Nelson AD. Osteomyelitis in children: detection by magnetic resonance. Work in progress. *Radiology* 1984;150:57–60.
23. Fruehwald FXJ, Tscholakoff D, Schwaighofer B, et al. Magnetic resonance imaging of the lower vertebral column in patients with multiple myeloma. *Invest Radiol* 1988;23:193–199.
24. Genant HK, Cann CE. Quantitative computed tomography for assessing vertebral bone mineral. In: Genant HK, Chafetz H, Helms CA, eds. *Computed tomography of the lumbar spine.* San Francisco: University of California, 1982:289–314.
25. Genant HK, Wilson JS, Bovill EG, et al. Computed tomography of the musculoskeletal system. *J Bone Joint Surg* [*Am*] 1980;62:1088–1101.
26. Hajek PC, Baker LL, Goobar HE, et al. Focal fat deposition in axial bone marrow: MR characteristics. *Radiology* 1987;162:245–249.
27. Hashimoto M. The distribution of active marrow in the bones of normal adults. *Kyushu J Med Soc* 1960;11:103–111.
28. Hashimoto M. Pathology of bone marrow. *Acta Haematol* 1962;27:193–216.
29. Hendrick RE, Kneeland JB, Stark DD. Maximizing signal-to-noise and contrast-to-noise ratios in FLASH imaging. *Magn Reson Imaging* 1987;5:117–127.
30. Huggins C, Blocksom BH Jr. Changes in outlying bone marrow accompanying a local increase of temperature within physiological limits. *J Exp Med* 1936;64:253–274.
31. Jacobsen EM, Davis AK, Alpen EL. Relative effectiveness of phenylhydrazine treatment and hemorrhage in the production of an erythropoietic factor. *Blood* 1956;11:937–945.
32. Kangarloo H, Dietrich RB, Taira RT, et al. MR imaging of bone marrow in children. *J Comput Assist Tomogr* 1986;10:205–209.
33. Kaplan PA, Asleson RJ, Klassen LW, Duggan MJ. Bone marrow patterns in aplastic anemia: observations with 1.5 T MR imaging. *Radiology* 1987;164:441–444.
34. Kricun ME. Red–yellow marrow conversion: its effect on the location of some solitary bone lesions. *Skeletal Radiol* 1985;14:10–19.
35. Lanir A, Aghai E, Simon JS, Lee RGL, Clouse ME. MR imaging in myelofibrosis. *J Comput Assist Tomogr* 1986;10:634–636.
36. Lanir A, Hadar H, Cohen I, et al. Gaucher disease: assessment with MR imaging. *Radiology* 1986;161:239–244.
37. McKinstry CS, Steiner RE, Young AT, Jones L, Swirsky D, Aber V. Bone marrow in leukemia and aplastic anemia: MR imaging before, during, and after treatment. *Radiology* 1987;161:239–244.
38. Mitchell DG, Burk DL Jr, Vinitski S, Rifkin MD. The biophysical basis of tissue contrast in extracranial MR imaging. *AJR* 1987;149:831–837.
39. Mitchell DG, Kressel HY, Arger PH, Dalinka M, Spritzer CE, Steinberg ME. Avascular necrosis of the femoral head: morphologic assessment by MR imaging, with CT correlation. *Radiology* 1986;161:739–742.
40. Mitchell DG, Rao VM, Dalinka M, et al. Hematopoietic and fatty bone marrow distribution in the normal and ischemic hip: new observations with 1.5 T MR imaging. *Radiology* 1986;161:199–202.
41. Moore SG, Gooding CA, Brasch RC, et al. Bone marrow in children with acute lymphocytic leukemia: MR relaxation times. *Radiology* 1986;160:237–240.
42. Moore SG, Sebag GH. Prolongation of T1 relaxation time in leukemia. *Radiology* 1990 (In Press).
43. Neumann E. Das gesetz der verbreitung des gelben und roten, markes in den extremitatenknochen. *Centralblatt Med Wiss* 1882;20:321–323.
44. Nyman R, Rehn S, Glimelius B, et al. Magnetic resonance imaging in diffuse malignant bone marrow diseases. *Acta Radiol (Diagn)* 1987;28:199–205.
45. Olson DL, Shields AF, Scheurich CJ, Porter BA, Moss AA. Magnetic resonance imaging of the bone marrow in patients with leukemia, aplastic anemia, and lymphoma. *Invest Radiol* 1986;21:540–546.
46. Pettersson H, Gillespy R III, Hamlin DJ, et al. Primary musculoskeletal tumors: examination with MR imaging compared with conventional modalities. *Radiology* 1987;164:237–241.
47. Piney A. The anatomy of the bone marrow. *Br Med J* 1922;2:792–795.
48. Ranade SE, Shah S, Advani SH, Kasturi SR. Pulsed nuclear magnetic resonance studies of human bone marrow. *Physiol Chem Phys* 1977;9:297–299.
49. Rao VM, Fishman M, Mitchell DG, et al. Painful sickle cell crisis: bone marrow patterns observed with MR imaging. *Radiology* 1986;161:211–215.
50. Rosenthal DI, Scott JA, Barranger J, et al. Evaluation of Gaucher disease using magnetic resonance imaging. *J Bone Joint Surg* [*Am*] 1986;68:802–808.
51. Sabin FR. Bone marrow. *Physiol Rev* 1928;8:191–244.
52. Snyder WS, Cook MH, Nasset ES, Karhausen LR, Howells GP, Tipton IH. *Report of the task group on reference man.* Oxford: Pergamon, 1974:79–98.
53. Stafford SA, Rosenthal DI, Gebhardt MD, Brady TJ, Scott JA. MRI in stress fracture. *AJR* 1986;147:553–556.
54. Stevens SK, Moore SG, Kaplan ID. Early and late bone marrow changes following radiation: magnetic resonance evaluation. *AJR* 1990;154:745–790.
55. Sundaram J, McGuire MH, Herbold DR. Magnetic resonance imaging of osteosarcoma. *Skeletal Radiol* 1987;16:23–29.
56. Thomsen C, Sorensen PG, Karle H, Christoffersen P, Henriksen O. Prolonged bone marrow T1-relaxation in acute leukemia: *in vivo* tissue characterization by magnetic resonance imaging. *Magn Reson Imaging* 1987;5:251–257.
57. Totty WG, Murphy WA, Ganz WI, Kumar B, Daum WJ, Siegel BA. Magnetic resonance imaging of the normal and ischemia femoral head. *AJR* 1984;143:1273–1280.
58. Tribukait B. Experimental studies on the regulation of erythropoiesis with special reference to the importance of oxygen. *Acta Physiol Scand* 1963;58(suppl 208):1–48.
59. Trubowitz S, Davis S. The bone marrow matrix. In: *The human bone marrow: anatomy, physiology, and pathophysiology.* Boca Raton, FL: CRC, 1982:43–75.
60. Turner DA, Templeton AC, Selzer PM, Rosenberg AG, Petasnick JP. Femoral capital osteonecrosis: MR finding of diffuse marrow abnormalities without focal lesions. *Radiology* 1989;171:135–140.
61. Unger E, Moldofsky P, Gatenby R, Hartz W, Broder G. Diagnosis of osteomyelitis by MR imaging. *AJR* 1988;150:605–610.
62. Vogler III JB, Murphy WA. Bone marrow imaging. Radiology 1988;168:679–693.
63. Wehrli FW, MacFall JR, Shutts D, Breger R, Herfkens RJ. Mechanisms of contrast in NMR imaging. *J Comput Assist Tomogr* 1984;8:369–380.
64. Wilson AJ, Murphy WA, Hardy DC, Totty WG. Transient osteoporosis: transient bone marrow edema? *Radiology* 1988;167:757–760.
65. Winkler ML, Ortendahl DA, Mille TC, et al. Characteristics of partial flip angle and gradient reversal imaging. *Radiology* 1988;166:17–26.
66. Wismer GL, Rosen BR, Buxton R, Stark DD, Brady TJ. Chemical shift imaging of bone marrow: preliminary experience. *AJR* 1985;145:1031–1037.
67. Yao L, Lee JK. Occult intraosseous fracture: detection with MR imaging. *Radiology* 1988;167:749–751.
68. Zimmer WD, Berquist TH, McLeod RA, et al. Bone tumors: magnetic resonance imaging versus computed tomography. *Radiology* 1985;155:709–718.

MRI of the Musculoskeletal System, 2nd Edition, edited by T. H. Berquist.
Raven Press, Ltd., New York © 1990.

CHAPTER 15

Miscellaneous Conditions

Thomas H. Berquist

Myopathies, 517
Arthropathies, 518
Pediatric and Congenital Disorders, 523
Miscellaneous Bone Disorders, 526
References, 526

As the techniques in magnetic resonance imaging (MRI) have improved, the applications have continued to expand (17). Most of these applications have been discussed in the previous pathologic and anatomic chapters. However, certain evolving applications deserve more mention here.

MYOPATHIES

The MR applications and characteristics of soft tissue infection, trauma, and neoplasms have been discussed in previous chapters. Early experience suggests MRI may also play a significant role in evaluation of other primary muscle and neuromuscular disorders. Both imaging and spectroscopy will be of value in this regard (3,7,9,14–16,18,19,23,25,32,34,37,41,46,56,58,60).

There are numerous inflammatory and metabolic myopathies, neural myopathies, and forms of muscular dystrophy that could potentially be studied with imaging techniques and/or magnetic resonance spectroscopy. To date, none of these techniques has provided specific information for the exact histologic type of process or specific myopathy. Conventional imaging techniques provide limited information about nonneoplastic muscle diseases. Routine radiographic techniques are of little value even when low kV or xerox techniques are used. Several authors have studied computed tomographic features of myopathy (20,38,46). O'Doherty et al. (38) described patterns of muscle replacement using computed tomography (CT). Both localized and diffuse low-density areas were noted in patients with pseudohypertrophic muscular dystrophy. Changes in selected muscle groups have been reported in Duchenne's muscular dystrophy. Hawley et al. (20) demonstrated that CT scans of patients with neuromuscular diseases initially showed atrophy of muscles followed by decreased muscle density. Primary myopathies revealed similar changes but in reverse order with decreased density preceding muscle atrophy. The low-density areas in muscles seen on CT are likely due to fat and/or connective tissue replacement.

MRI has superior soft tissue contrast compared to CT. Therefore, detection of early muscle changes can be more easily accomplished. From an imaging standpoint, the findings seen on MRI may be no more specific than

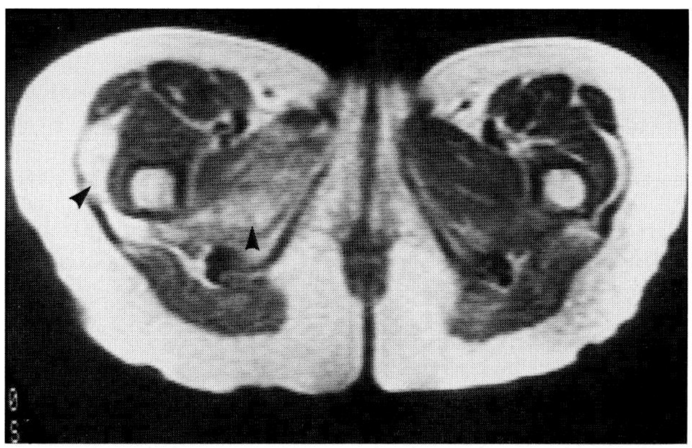

FIG. 15-1. Axial SE 2,000/30 image of the upper thighs, demonstrating an infiltrative process in the adductor muscles on the right and inflammation of the tensor fascia lata (*arrowheads*) due to nodular polymyositis.

T. H. Berquist: Mayo Medical School and Mayo Clinic, Rochester, Minnesota 55905.

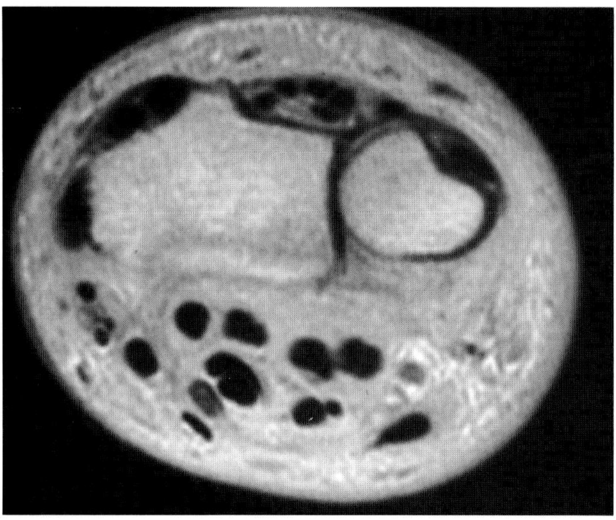

FIG. 15-2. Axial SE 2,000/60 image of the wrist, demonstrating complete fatty replacement of the muscles due to a chronic neuropathy.

CT. However, certain important changes can be noted with MRI. The muscle groups can easily be distinguished and the extent of involvement determined by using multiple image planes. Using both T1 and T2 weighted sequences makes it possible to distinguish early edema or inflammation (high signal intensity on T2 and low intensity on T1 weighted images) from fatty infiltration or replacement, which is seen as intermediate signal intensity on both T1 and T2 weighted sequences. Other changes such as increase or decrease in muscle volume and fibrous replacement can also be identified (Figs. 15-1 and 15-2).

Borghi et al. (9) also studied T1 relaxation times. They noted that T1 relaxation times were considerably reduced in patients with myopathy (normal 450–800 msec, myopathy $\leq$ 500 msec). This is undoubtedly due to replacement of muscle with fat and fibrous tissue. Although further studies are needed, these data may be useful in differentiating myopathy from other pathology such as neoplasms where T1 values are elevated.

The potential imaging role of MRI in evaluating myopathies include the following: (a) clearly defining the muscle groups involved, (b) differentiating atrophy and fatty replacement for more acute inflammatory changes, (c) following treatment phases and progression of disease, and (d) localizing optimal sites for biopsy. The current use of imaging parameters alone does not obviate the need for clinical and histochemical studies to completely define the pathologic process.

Significant progress has been made in evaluating the utilization of spectroscopy for defining muscular and neuromuscular inflammatory diseases (Fig. 15-3). With higher magnetic field strengths, imaging and spectroscopic studies with nuclei such as ^{31}P, ^{21}Na, and ^{13}C may be possible. Conditions such as inflammatory myopathies, metabolic myopathies, muscular dystrophies, and neuropathic muscular changes have been studied that demonstrate changes in organic phosphate and phosphocreatine ratios as well as other phosphate metabolites. These studies are not only useful in more specifically identifying the pathologic process but also show potential in monitoring the response of patients to drug therapy (14,34,46,58,60). Further data are necessary before the role of spectroscopy in evaluating myopathies and neuromuscular disorders is completely understood.

ARTHROPATHIES

The role of MRI in evaluating specific arthropathies has been discussed briefly in each of the preceding anatomic chapters, specifically as they might apply to a given articular region. This section is intended to discuss in more detail the imaging and spectroscopic applications of magnetic resonance in evaluating inflammatory

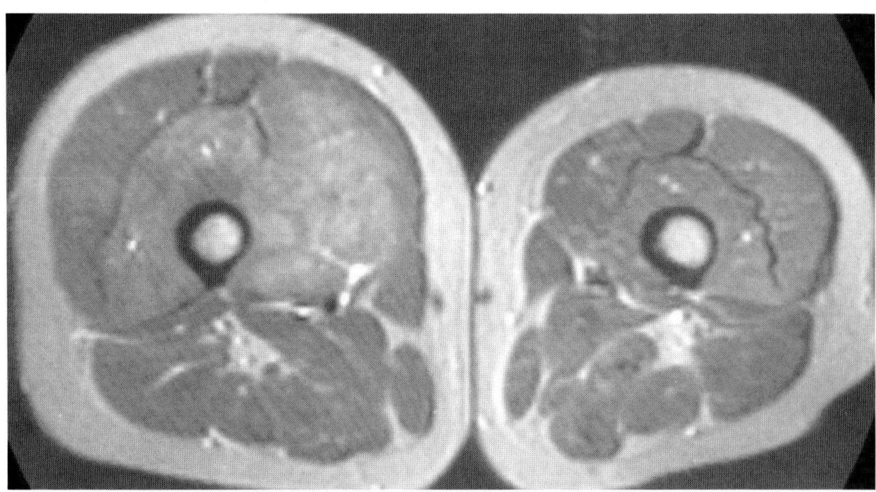

FIG. 15-3. Axial SE 2,000/30 images of the thighs, showing generalized hypertrophy on the right with increased signal intensity in the anterior musculature. Eosinophilic myositis.

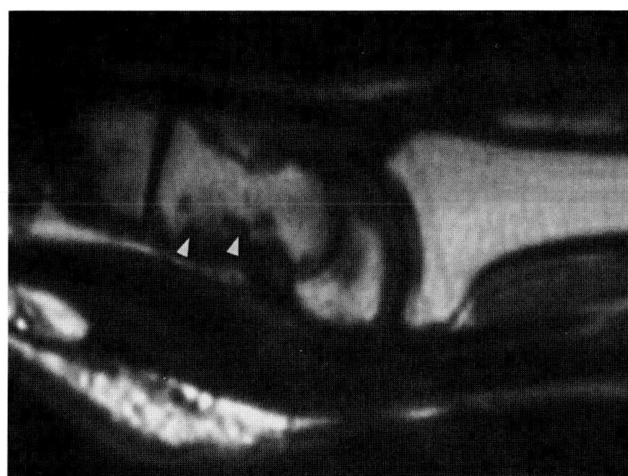

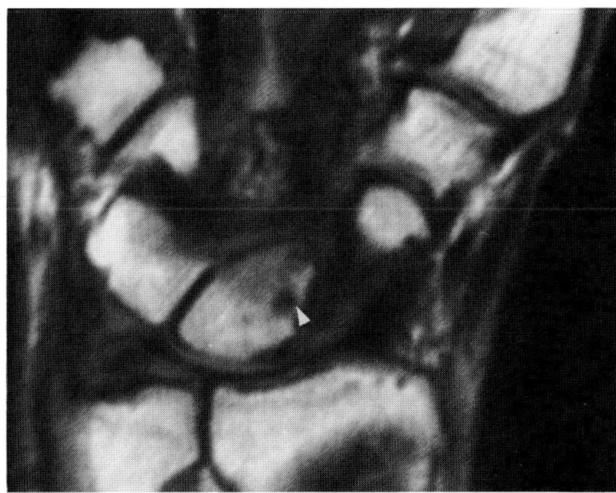

A,B

FIG. 15-4. SE 500/20 sagittal (**A**) and coronal (**B**) images of the wrist demonstrate early erosive changes (*arrowheads*) due to rheumatoid arthritis.

arthropathies. Infection was discussed in Chapter 13; therefore, joint space infection will not be completely reevaluated here.

Currently, diagnosis of rheumatoid and other types of arthritis is based on laboratory studies, clinical data, and radiographic techniques (radiographs, xerograms, and magnification techniques) (30,35,40,42,48,52,64). Soft tissue changes occur prior to bony erosion and articular destruction. The superior soft tissue contrast of MRI and the ability to differentiate cortical bone, articular cartilage, and the soft tissues of the joints should provide improved early detection of inflammatory arthropathies. Although specificity of MRI is still being evaluated, new pulse sequences, utilization of gadolinium, and spectroscopy show promise in increasing the accuracy of MRI in diagnosis of arthritis (2,5,10,13,21,26,45).

There have been several articles in the recent literature describing the utility of MRI in evaluating rheumatoid arthritis and juvenile rheumatoid arthritis (1,4,62). As with other articular disorders, synovial proliferation and inflammatory soft tissue changes precede cartilage and bone changes by months to years. Clinical, laboratory, and later radiographic findings have been used to monitor patients with both rheumatoid and juvenile rhcumatoid arthritis. Clinical fcaturcs of rhcumatoid arthritis with peripheral extremity involvement, usually symmetrical, are useful. The problems are somewhat different with juvenile rheumatoid arthritis in that 80% of patients become symptomatic by age 7 and, therefore, bone changes may be difficult to evaluate with routine radiographs. Epiphyses may be incompletely ossified, making evaluation more difficult with routine radiographs (1,51,62).

MRI has demonstrated the capability for evaluating early soft tissue changes in patients with rheumatoid and juvenile rheumatoid arthritis. Initially, both T1 and T2 weighted sequences were employed to detect early bone (Fig. 15-4) and soft tissue changes. Subtle synovial changes are usually more easily appreciated with T2 weighted spin-echo sequences (SE 2,000/20,60) or gradient-echo sequences. More recently, gadolinium-DTPA has been evaluated in an attempt to identify early synovial changes. Reiser et al. (45) studied 34 joints pre- and post-gadolinium injection and found significant rapid enhancement of the proliferating inflamed synovium compared to the very minimal changes noted in bone and the adjacent soft tissues. This finding, though useful in early identification of inflammation, is not spe-

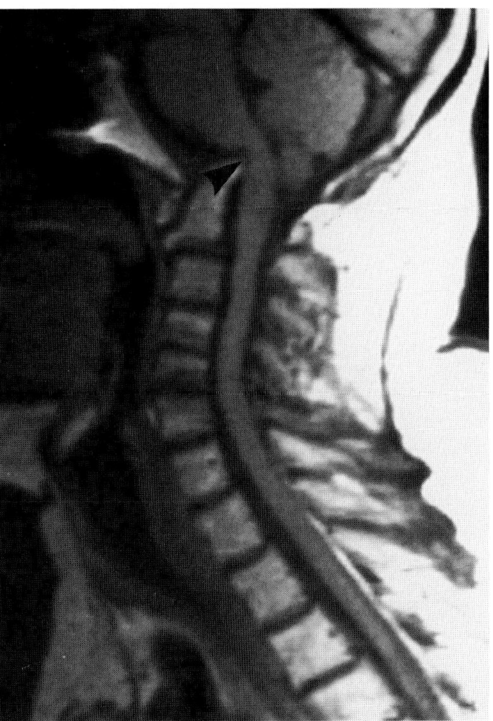

FIG. 15-5. Sagittal SE 500/20 image of the cervical spine in a patient with rheumatoid arthritis. Note the position of the odontoid and brain stem compression (*arrowhead*).

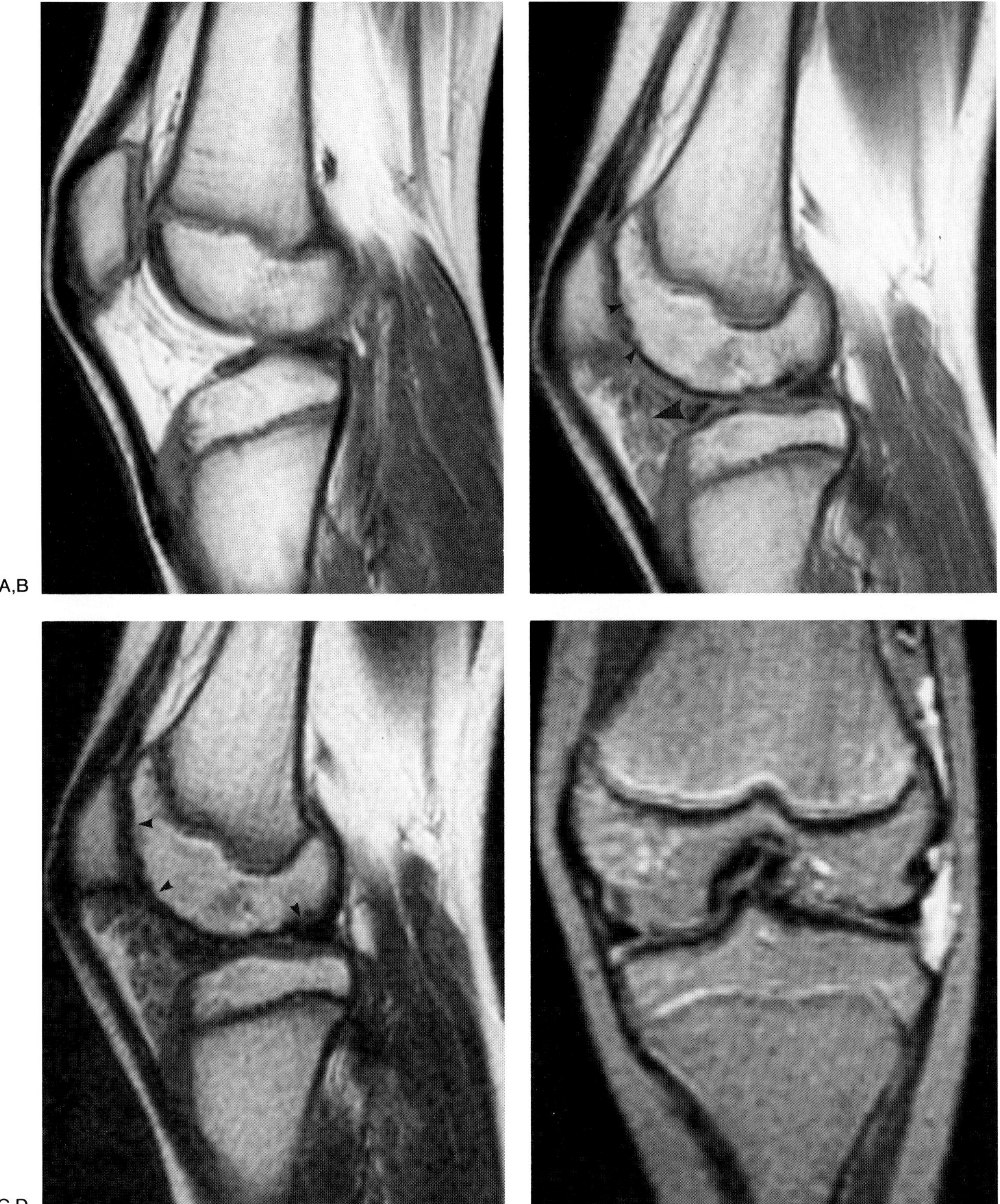

FIG. 15-6. Juvenile rheumatoid arthritis. Sagittal SE 500/20 (**A**) image of the normal knee. SE 500/20 (**B**) and SE 2,000/60 (**C**) images of the involved knee. There is irregularity of the epiphysis (*small arrowheads*) and decreased signal intensity in the infrapatellar fat on both sequences (*large arrowhead*) due to chronic synovial proliferation. Coronal SE 2,000/60 (**D**) image shows soft tissue inflammation and increased signal intensity in the femoral epiphysis due to hyperemia.

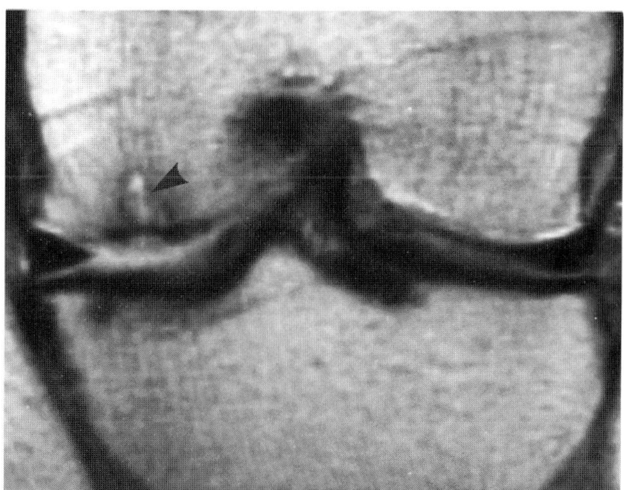

FIG. 15-7. SE 2,000/60 coronal image of the knee, demonstrating medial compartment osteoarthritis with a small cartilage defect and subchondral cyst formation (*arrowhead*).

cific. Spectroscopy may also play a role in identification of early and subtle soft tissue changes (6,57). To date, MRI is most often used to evaluate patients with indeterminate arthritides, early erosive and soft tissue changes, and changes in the cervical spine region often associated with rheumatoid arthritis (Fig. 15-5). MRI may be particularly useful in children, where unossified cartilage and the monoarticular involvement, not uncommonly seen with juvenile rheumatoid arthritis, may make clinical evaluation more difficult (Fig. 15-6) (51,55).

Degenerative or osteoarthritis has also been typically evaluated with routine radiographs. However, use of surface coils has allowed early detection of subtle cartilaginous and joint space changes in this type of arthropathy as well (8,31). Grading systems for osteoarthritis, specifically for the hips (see Chapter 6), have been developed (53,61). When compared with radiographic grading systems, it is apparent that MRI is most useful in evaluating subtle changes. Once radiographic and clinical symptoms become more advanced, there is little to be gained from using MRI to evaluate these patients (Figs. 15-7 and 15-8) (12,30,31,53,61).

Pigmented villonodular synovitis is a relatively uncommon disorder characterized by synovial proliferation with hemosiderin deposition in the involved synovial tissues. Pigmented villonodular synovitis occurs most commonly in the second through fifth decades with an age range of 10–90 years, although most patients are in their early 20s. The disease is usually monoarticular, which assists in diagnosis. Clinically, the involved joint is usually painful and palpable soft tissue masses may be evident. Synovial involvement may be localized, although a more diffuse form of synovial involvement is evident in up to 75% of cases. The knee is the most commonly involved joint and is reportedly involved in up to 80% of cases (22,33,54).

Radiographically changes occur in approximately 80% of cases. The most common abnormality seen is soft tissue swelling and effusion. Increased density may be evident due to hemosiderin deposition. Cystic erosions occur in bone in up to 50% of patients (54). MR features of pigmented villonodular synovitis are fairly typical, allowing diagnosis of the condition in many cases, especially when coupled with the clinical findings. Both T1 and T2 weighted sequences are important in order to accurately characterize the synovial changes

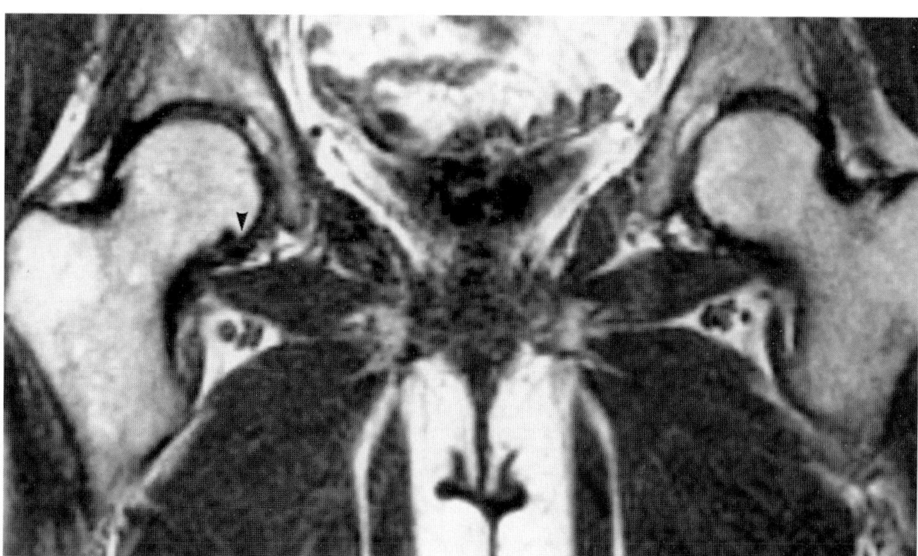

FIG. 15-8. Osteoarthritis of the right hip. There is joint space narrowing with marrow extending into the small osteophytes (*arrowheads*).

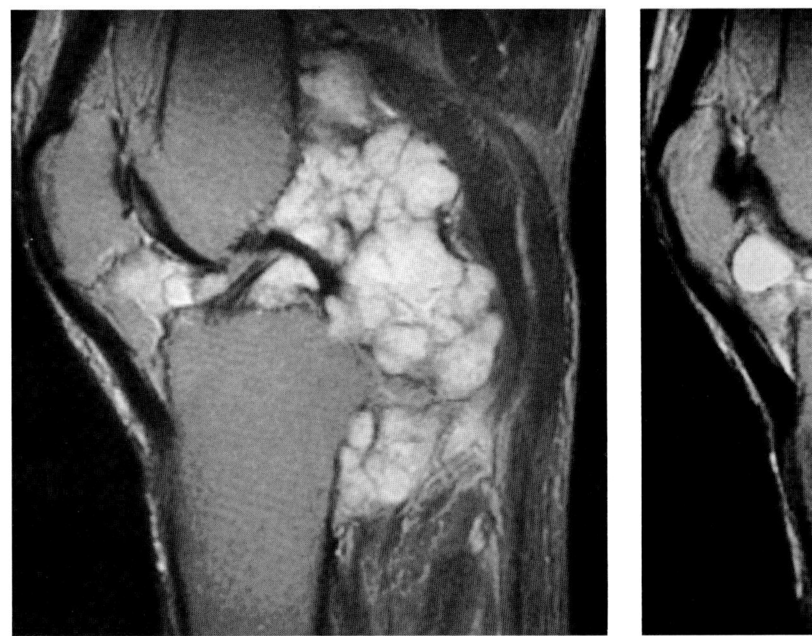
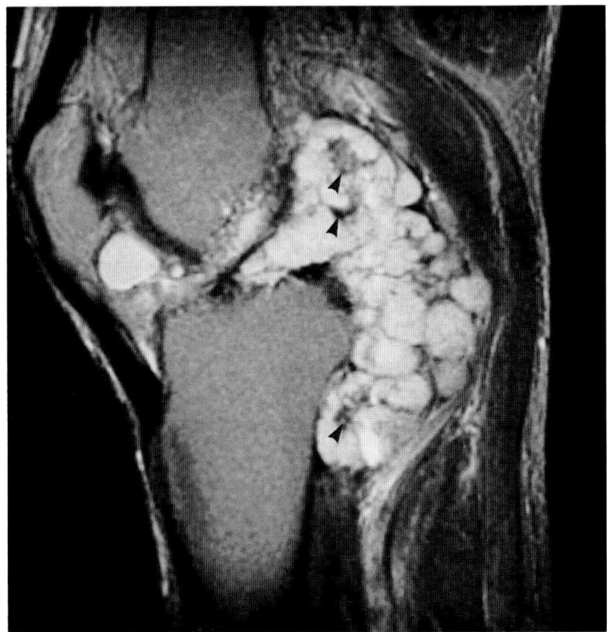

A,B

FIG. 15-9. Synovial chondromatosis. SE 2,000/60 images (**A**) and (**B**) show extensive synovial inflammation with cyst formation. There is a palpable soft tissue mass in the popliteal space. Note the small chondromatous areas (*arrowheads*). Compare to Fig. 7-69—PVNS.

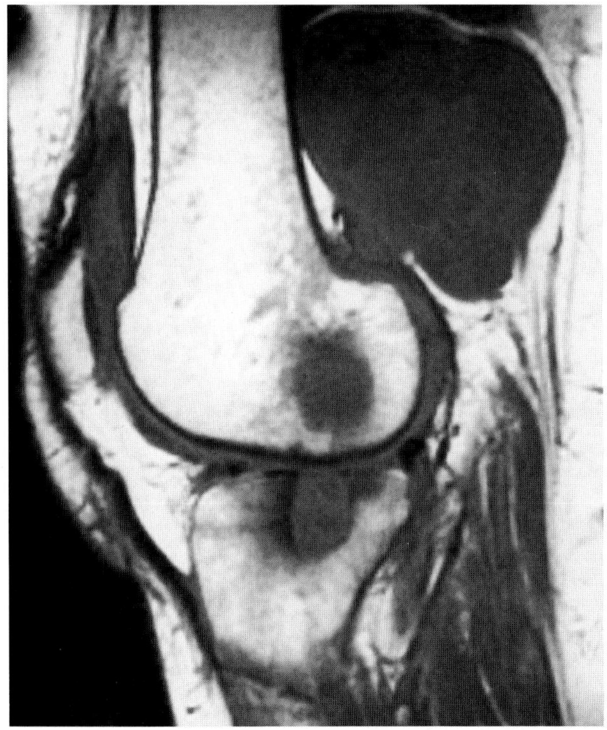
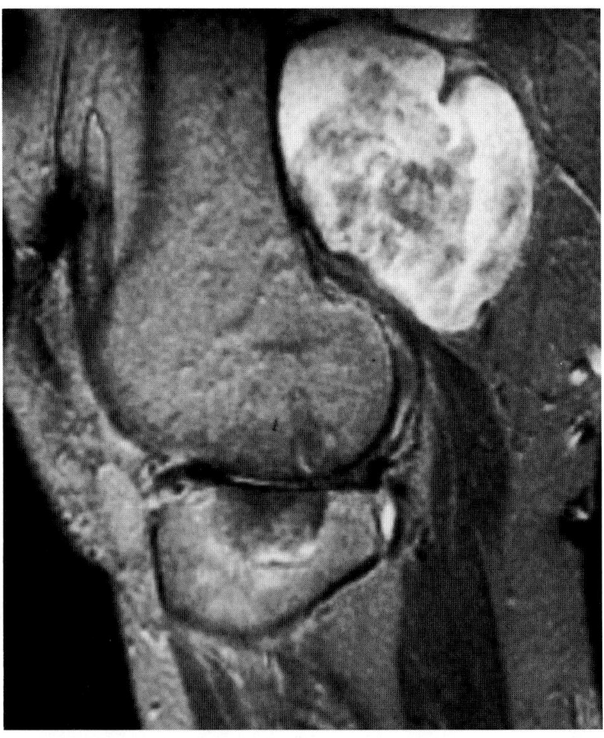

A,B

FIG. 15-10. Tuberculous arthritis. SE 500/20 (**A**) and SE 2,000/60 (**B**) images show a large mass with multiple low-intensity regions on the T2 weighted sequence (**B**) due to chronic fibrotic synovial proliferation. There are also cystic changes in the bone which can also occur with PVNS (see Fig. 7-69).

and hemosiderin deposition (see Fig. 7-69). The synovial nodules or areas of proliferation containing hemosiderin are demonstrated as large globular areas of low signal intensity on both T1 and T2 weighted sequences (22,54). Although these findings are fairly specific in early cases when only subtle synovial changes are present or in certain other conditions where there is advanced synovial proliferation, the diagnosis can be more difficult. Patients with conditions such as synovial chondromatosis (Fig. 15-9) and chronic long-standing infection (Fig. 15-10) may be difficult to differentiate from PVNS (see Fig. 7-69) in certain cases.

The literature has also discussed the MRI applications for evaluation of patients with hemophilic arthropathy. Again, synovial changes, changes in articular cartilage and bone, and hemorrhagic changes seen with this condition can be identified more easily than with routine radiographs (27,43,63).

New pulse sequences that may be more effective in evaluating articular cartilage changes, such as the gradient-echo sequences, use of gadolinium, and fluid analysis with conventional imaging techniques, have been unsuccessful in specifically identifying the type of arthritis with the exception of pigmented villonodular synovitis (2,5,10,30,35,40,42,48,52,64). Early work with spectroscopy may enhance the specificity of MRI in this regard (6,57).

PEDIATRIC AND CONGENITAL DISORDERS

Routine radiographs continue to play a major role in identification of major congenital disorders. MRI offers several potential advantages for the study of congenital disorders, specifically as they relate to the growth plate and unossified epiphyses. There is no ionizing radiation with MRI and images of the extremities can be obtained in the axial plane as well as coronal, sagittal, and off-axis planes to better define osseous and cartilaginous development (Fig. 15-11).

Other pediatric conditions have evolved more rapidly. In fact, many of the conditions described in the previous chapters such as trauma, infection, osteonecrosis and osteochondroses, pediatric hip disorders (Chapter 6), and tarsal coalition (Chapter 8) are common applications in pediatric practice. These applications will not be reemphasized here (24,29,47,49,59).

Growth plate deformities, specifically those related to trauma, are a common problem in pediatric orthopedic practice. Partial physeal arrest is particularly apt to

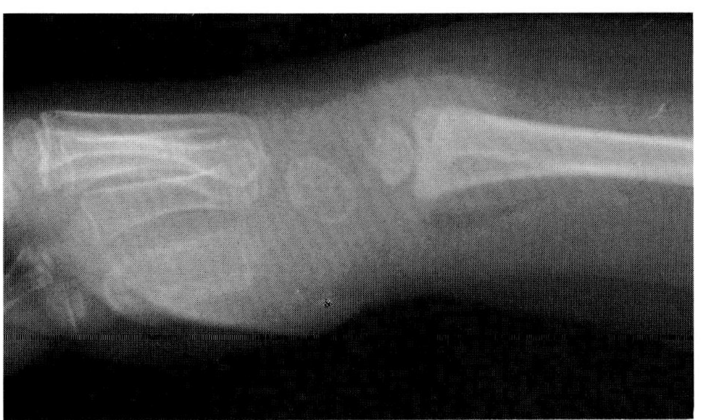

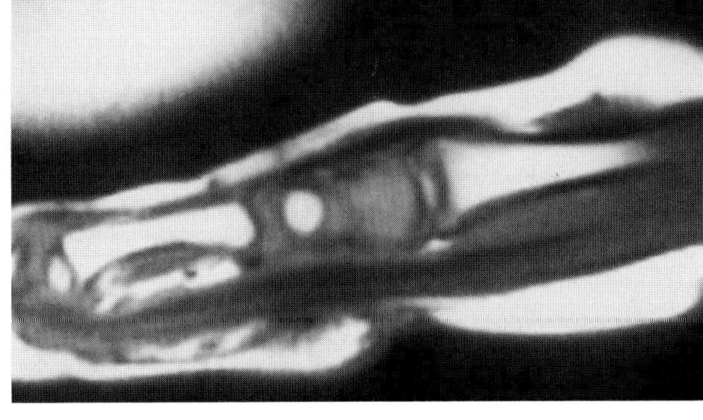

A,B

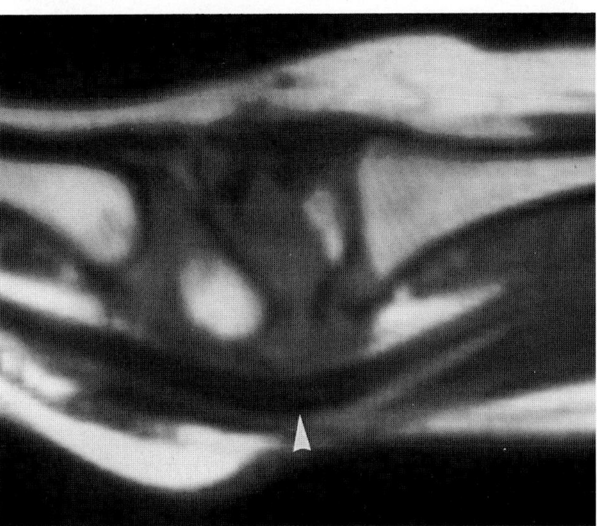

C

FIG. 15-11. Three-year-old with pain and function loss in the wrist. **A:** Lateral radiograph shows incomplete ossification of the carpal bones. **B:** Sagittal SE 500/20 image of the normal wrist. **C:** Sagittal image of the involved wrist shows carpal collapse with shortening of the involved wrist. Note the volar displacement (*arrowhead*) of the flexor tendon.

cause problems. This is due to progressive angular deformity that occurs due to segmental growth of a portion of the growth plate while the injured portion is arrested. Although these changes are most often due to trauma, physeal arrest can also occur with infection, tumors, therapeutic radiation, burns, electrical injuries, and metabolic and hematologic abnormalities (39).

Generally, imaging of growth plate abnormalities has been accomplished with conventional or computed tomography. This is usually adequate to assess the percentage of growth plate arrest or closure prior to consideration of surgical therapy. Recently, MRI has provided valuable information in evaluating patients with growth plate deformities. This is true in both preoperative (Fig. 15-12) and postoperative (Fig. 15-13) situations. MRI is particularly suited to situations where growth plate deformity is significant and tomographic or CT planes are difficult to obtain. Both T1 and T2 weighted sequences are useful to evaluate activity in the growth plate. Increased signal intensity is seen along growth plates with growth potential. Scar tissue has low signal intensity on both T1 and T2 weighted sequences. Bony bridges are seen as areas of sclerotic bone or have signal intensity similar to marrow (Fig. 15-13).

A,B

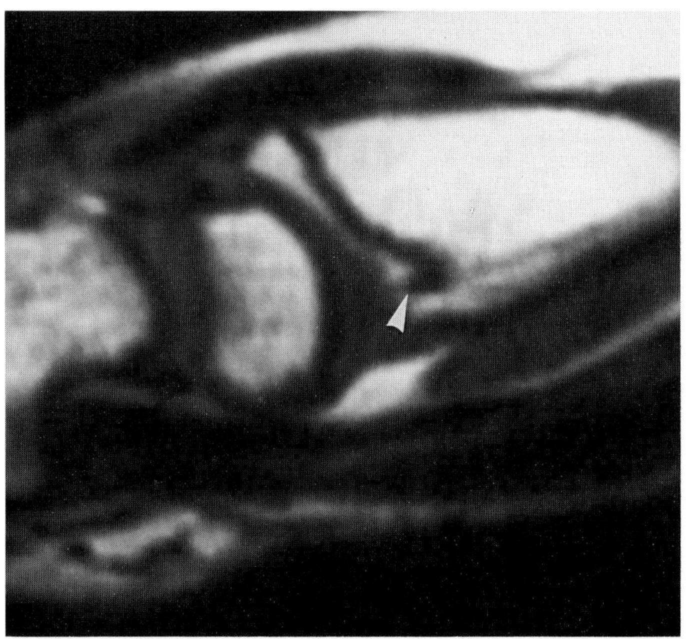

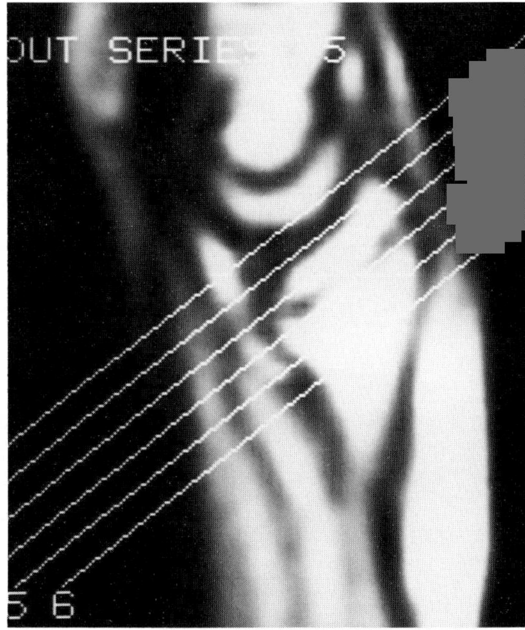

C

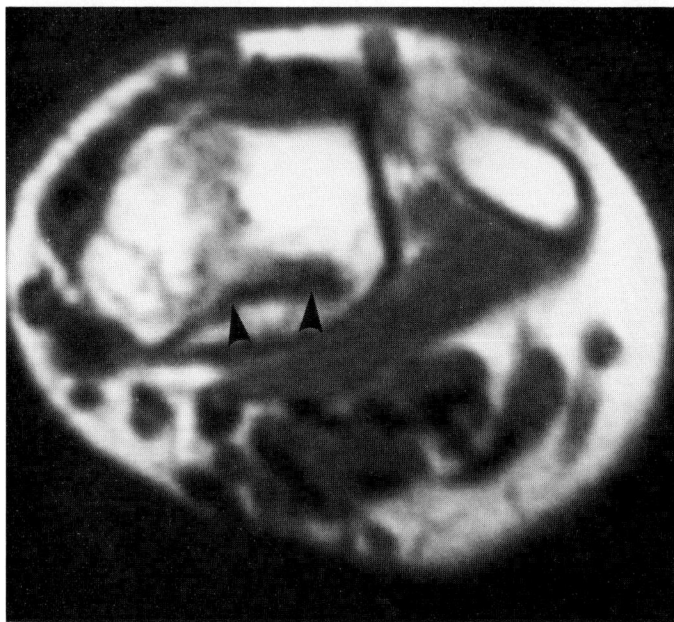

FIG. 15-12. Old wrist fracture with dorsal overgrowth. **A:** Sagittal SE 500/20 image shows volar closure of the growth plate (*arrowhead*). **B:** Sagittal scout with axial selection planes. **C:** The axial image shows the area of involvement (*arrowheads*).

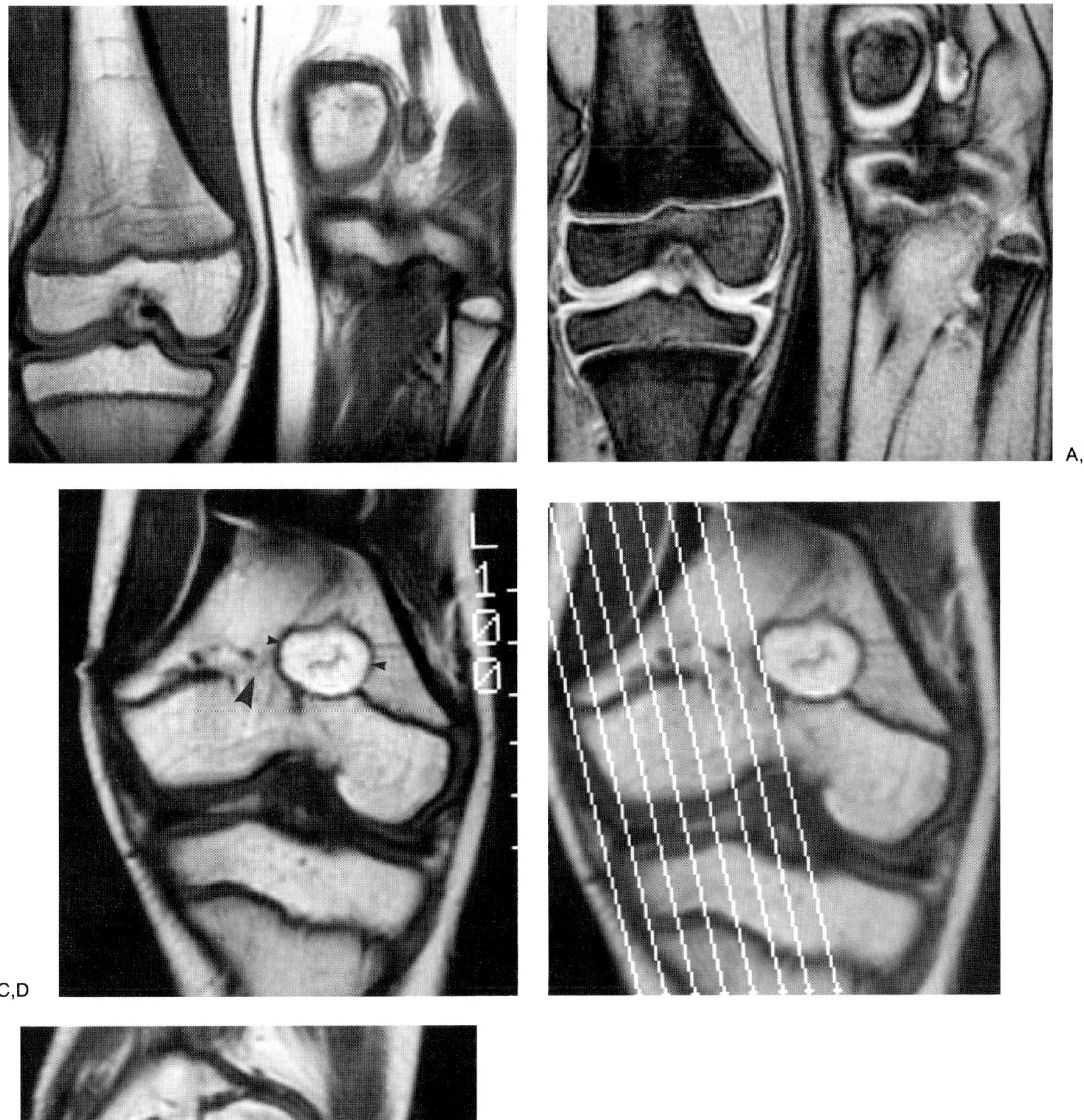

A,B

C,D

E

FIG. 15-13. Old distal femoral injury with leg length discrepancy on the left. A bony bar has been resected and filled with a fat plug. SE 500/20 (**A**) and gradient-echo (MPGR—FA 25°, TE 31, TR 700) (**B**) images show a normal right leg with increased signal in the normal growth plates on the right. The left leg is short. Coronal SE 500/20 (**C**) image demonstrates the fat plug (*small arrowheads*) and a small bony bar (*large arrowhead*). Oblique sagittal images were selected (**D**) which allow a true sagittal view of the growth plate (**E**), which confirms only a small (<10%) bar (*arrowhead*).

MISCELLANEOUS BONE DISORDERS

Many of the bone disorders have been described in previous chapters, specifically Chapter 14 on diffuse marrow disorders. Certain marrow conditions—specifically, metabolic disease, hemoglobinopathies, and infiltrative disorders—are still typically evaluated with more conventional imaging techniques (11,17,28,44,50,53). Although imaging abnormalities are frequently nonspecific, new data using spectroscopy may be beneficial in certain metabolic conditions involving bone minerals (36).

The applications of MRI have evolved rapidly in the past several years, largely due to significant improvements in higher field magnets, surface coil technology, and pulse sequences. The addition of gadolinium-DTPA as a contrast agent will no doubt further enhance the sensitivity and specificity of this technique. The role of spectroscopy continues to evolve but to date it is not commonly used in clinical practice for magnetic resonance studies.

REFERENCES

1. Aisen AM, Marte W, Ellis JH, McCune WJ. Cervical spine involvement in rheumatoid arthritis: MR imaging. *Radiology* 1987;165:159–163.
2. Baker DG, Schumacher HR Jr, Wolf GL. Nuclear magnetic resonance evaluation of synovial fluid and articular tissues. *J Rheumatol* 1985;12:1062–1065.
3. Barfuss H, Fischer H, Hentschel D, Ladebeck R, Vetter J. Whole-body MR imaging and spectroscopy with a 4-T system. *Radiology* 1988;169:811–816.
4. Beltran J, Caudill JL, Herman LA, Kantor SM, Hudson PN, Noto AM, Baran AS. Rheumatoid arthritis: MR imaging manifestations. *Radiology* 1987;165:153–157.
5. Berquist TH. The elbow and wrist. *Top Magn Reson Imaging* 1989;1(3):15–27.
6. Blatter DD. Phosphorus-31 magnetic resonance spectroscopy of experimentally induced arthritis in rats. *Skeletal Radiol* 1987;16:183–189.
7. Boeve WJ, Kamman RL, Mooyaart EL, Hoekstra HJ, Thijn CJP, Koops HS. *In vivo* phosphorus magnetic resonance spectroscopy of bone and soft tissue tumors. Presented at the Society of Magnetic Resonance in Medicine, Amsterdam, The Netherlands, 1989.
8. Bongartz G, Bock E, Horbach T, Requardt H. Degenerative cartilage lesions of the hip—magnetic resonance evaluation. *Magn Reson Imaging* 1989;7:179–186.
9. Borghi L, Savoldi F, Scelsi R, Villa M. Nuclear magnetic resonance response of protons in normal and pathologic muscles. *Exp Neurol* 1983;81:89–96.
10. Brasch RC, Bennett HF. Consideration in the choice of contrast media for MR imaging. *Radiology* 1988;166:897–899.
11. Brasch RC, Wesbey GE, Gooding CA, Koerper MA. Magnetic resonance imaging of transfusional hemosiderosis complicating thalassemia major. *Radiology* 1984;150:767–771.
12. Chao PW, Zlatkin MB, Dalinka M, Kressel HY. High resolution MRI of the hip at 1.5 T using a surface coil pair and small fields of view for evaluation of the cartilaginous surface of the hip. Presented at the Society of Magnetic Resonance in Medicine, Amsterdam, The Netherlands, 1989.
13. Deutsch AL, Mink JH. Articular disorders of the knee. *Top Magn Reson Imaging* 1989;1(3):43–56.
14. Dunn JF, Frostick S, Radda GK. Changes in high energy phosphate compounds associated with the primary defect in Duchenne's muscular dystrophy: a study of the MDX mouse. Presented at the Society of Magnetic Resonance in Medicine, Amsterdam, The Netherlands, 1989.
15. Edwards RHT, Dawson MJ, Griffith JR, Gorton R, Wilk C. Nuclear magnetic resonance spectroscopy in research and clinical diagnosis. *Eur J Clin Invest* 1983;13:429–431.
16. Edwards RHT, Dawson MJ, Wilkie RE, Shaw D. Clinical use of nuclear magnetic resonance in investigation of myopathy. *Lancet* 1982;1:725–731.
17. Ehman RL, Berquist TH, McLeod RA. MR imaging of the musculoskeletal system: a 5-year appraisal. *Radiology* 1988;166:313–320.
18. Fotedar LK, Narayana PA, Slopis JM, Pivarnik JM, Fenstermacher MJ, Butler IJ. Proton MRS of exercise-induced changes in human gastrocnemius muscle. Presented at the Society of Magnetic Resonance in Medicine, Amsterdam, The Netherlands, 1989.
19. Hands LJ, Bore PJ, Galloway G, Morris PJ, Radda GK. Muscle metabolism in patients with peripheral vascular disease investigated by ^{31}P nuclear magnetic resonance spectroscopy. *Clin Sci* 1986;71:283–290.
20. Hawley RJ, Schellinger D, O'Doherty DS. Computed tomographic patterns of muscle in neuromuscular diseases. *Arch Neurol* 1984;41:383–387.
21. Heuck AF, Steiger P, Stoller DW, Glüer CC, Genant HK. Quantification of knee joint fluid volume by MR imaging and CT using three-dimensional data processing. *J Comput Assist Tomogr* 1989;13:287–293.
22. Jelinek JS, Kransdorf MJ, Utz JA, Berrey BH Jr, Thomson JD, Heekin RD, Radowich MS. Imaging of pigmented villonodular synovitis with emphasis on MR imaging. *AJR* 1989;152:337–342.
23. Jeneson JAL, Nederveen D, Bakker CJG. Dynamic exercise of the human forearm muscles: a combined ^{1}H MRI and ^{31}P MRS study. Presented at the Society of Magnetic Resonance in Medicine, Amsterdam, The Netherlands, 1989.
24. Johnson ND, Wood BP, Noh KS, Jackman KV, Westesson P, Katzberg RW. MR imaging anatomy of the infant hip. *AJR* 1989;153:127–133.
25. Keller U, Oberhänsli R, Huber P, et al. Phosphocreatine content and intracellular pH of calf muscle measured by phosphorus NMR spectroscopy in occlusive arterial disease of the legs. *Eur J Clin Invest* 1985;15:382–388.
26. Kneeland JB, Erickson SJ, Jesmanowicz A, Hyde JS. High resolution MR imaging of the hand. Presented at the Society of Magnetic Resonance in Medicine, Amsterdam, The Netherlands, 1989.
27. Kulkarni MV, Drolshagen LF, Kaye JJ, Green NE, Burks DD, Janco RL, Nance EP Jr. MR imaging of hemophiliac arthropathy. *J Comput Assist Tomogr* 1986;10:445–449.
28. Lanir A, Hadar H, Cohen I, Tal Y, Benmair J, Schreiber R, Clouse ME. Gaucher disease: assessment with MR imaging. *Radiology* 1986;161:239–244.
29. Lee MS, Harcke HT, Kumar SJ, Bassett GS. Subtalar joint coalition in children: new observations. *Radiology* 1989;172:635–639.
30. Lehner KB, Rechl HP. Normal morphology and degeneration of hyaline articular cartilage in MR—imaging: an *in vitro* study in bovine patellae and human arthritic femoral heads. Presented at the Society of Magnetic Resonance in Medicine, Amsterdam, The Netherlands, 1989.
31. Li KC, Higgs J, Aisen AM, Buckwalter KA, Martel W, McCune WJ. MRI in osteoarthritis of the hip: gradations of severity. *Magn Reson Imaging* 1988;6:229–236.
32. Mancini DM, Ferraro N, Tuchler M, Chance B, Wilson JR. Detection of abnormal calf muscle metabolism in patients with heart failure using phosphorus-31 nuclear magnetic resonance. *Am J Cardiol* 1988;62:1234–1240.
33. Mandelbaum BR, Grant TT, Hartzman S, et al. The use of MRI to assist in diagnosis of pigmented villonodular synovitis of the knee joint. *Clin Orthop* 1988:231:135–139.
34. Matthews PM, Allaire C, Shoubridge E, Karpati G, Arnold DL. Phosphorus MRS in the clinical assessment of myopathies. Presented at the Society of Magnetic Resonance in Medicine, Amsterdam, The Netherlands, 1989.
35. Mitchell MJ, Sartoris DS, Resnick D. The foot and ankle. *Top Magn Reson Imaging* 1989;1(3):75–84.
36. Moore JR, Ackerman JL. Phosphorus-31 imaging of bone and

synthetic bone minerals. Presented at the Society of Magnetic Resonance in Medicine, Amsterdam, The Netherlands, 1989.

37. Murphy WA, Totty WG, Carroll JE. MRI of normal and pathologic skeletal muscle. *AJR* 1986;146:565–574.
38. O'Doherty DS, Schellinger D, Raptopoulos V. Computed tomographic patterns of pseudohypertrophic muscular dystrophy: preliminary result. *J Comput Assist Tomogr* 1977;14:482–486.
39. Ogden JA. Current concepts review. The evaluation and treatment of partial physeal arrest. *J Bone Joint Surg* 1987;69A:1297–1302.
40. Oloff-Solomon J, Solomon MA. Special radiographic techniques in the evaluation of arthritic disease. *Clin Podiatr Med Surg* 1988;5:25–36.
41. Park JH, Brown RL, Park CR, Cohn M, Chance B. Evaluation of muscle fiber heterogeneity by ^{31}P magnetic resonance spectroscopy. Presented at the Society of Magnetic Resonance in Medicine, Amsterdam, The Netherlands, 1989.
42. Paul PK, Mezrich R, Wang JZ. Soft tissue quantification by MRI to study the progress of joint inflammation. Presented at the Society of Magnetic Resonance in Medicine, Amsterdam, The Netherlands, 1989.
43. Pettersson H, Gillespy T, Kitchens C, Kentro T, Scott KN. Magnetic resonance imaging in hemophilic arthropathy of the knee. *Acta Radiol* 1987;28:621–625.
44. Rao VM, Fishman M, Mitchell DG, et al. Painful sickle cell crisis: bone marrow patterns observed with MR imaging. *Radiology* 1986:161:211–215.
45. Reiser MF, Bongartz GP, Erlemann R, Schneider M, Pauly T, Sittek H, Peters PE. Gadolinium-DTPA in rheumatoid arthritis and related disease: first results with dynamic magnetic resonance imaging. *Skeletal Radiol* 1989;18:591–597.
46. Rott HD, Breimesser FH, Rödl W. Imaging technics in muscular dystrophies. *J Genet Hum* 1985;33:397–403.
47. Rush BH, Bramson RT, Ogden JA. Legg–Calvé–Perthes disease: detection of cartilaginous and synovial changes with MR imaging. *Radiology* 1988;167:473–476.
48. Sanchez RB, Quinn SF. MRI of inflammatory synovial processes. *Magn Reson Imaging* 1989;7:529–540.
49. Scoles PV, Yoon YS, Makley JT, Kalamchi A. Nuclear magnetic resonance imaging in Legg–Calvé–Perthes disease. *J Bone Joint Surg* 1984;66:1357–1363.
50. Sebes JI. Diagnostic imaging of bone and joint abnormalities associated with sickle cell hemoglobinopathies. *AJR* 1989;152:1153–1159.
51. Senac MO Jr, Deutsch D, Bernstein BH, Stanley P, Crues JV III, Stoller DW, Mink J. MR imaging in juvenile rheumatoid arthritis. *AJR* 1988;150:873–878.
52. Sims RE, Genant HK. Magnetic resonance imaging of joint disease. *Radiol Clin North Am* 1986;24:179–188.
53. Smith DK, Totty WG. Articular disorders of the hip. *Top Magn Reson Imaging* 1989;1(3):29–41.
54. Spritzer CE, Dalinka MK, Kressel HY. Magnetic resonance imaging of pigmented villonodular synovitis: a report of two cases. *Skeletal Radiol* 1987;16:316–319.
55. Stack JP, Redmond O, Kirby B, Ryan M, Coghlan R, Ennis J. Rheumatoid disease of the wrist: evaluation by MRI. Presented at the Society of Magnetic Resonance in Medicine, Amsterdam, The Netherlands, 1989.
56. Strear CM, Bolinger L, Leigh JS. Nuclear Overhauser studies *in vivo* ^{31}P muscle spectra. Presented at the Society of Magnetic Resonance in Medicine, Amsterdam, The Netherlands, 1989.
57. Terrier F, Hricak H, Revel D, Alpers CE, Reinhold CE, Levine J, Genant HK. Magnetic resonance imaging and spectroscopy of periarticular inflammatory soft tissue changes in experimental arthritis of the rat. *Invest Radiol* 1985;20:813–823.
58. Thomsen C, Jensen KE, Henriksen O. *In vivo* measurements of T2 relaxation times of ^{31}P metabolites in human gastrocnemius muscle. Presented at the Society of Magnetic Resonance in Medicine, Amsterdam, The Netherlands, 1989.
59. Toby EB, Koman LA, Bechtold RE. Magnetic resonance imaging of pediatric hip disease. *J Pediatr Orthop* 1985;5:665–671.
60. van Echteld CJA, Kirkel HJ, Dekker T, Vermeulen JWAH, Luyten PR. A ^{31}P NMR saturation transfer study of creatine kinase activity in human calf muscle employing a progressive saturation sequence with adiabatic pulses. Presented at the Society of Magnetic Resonance in Medicine, Amsterdam, The Netherlands, 1989.
61. Wradzilo W, Schneider S, Richter G, Kauffmann G, Hiltbrand E, Gottschlich K. Magnetic resonance imaging of the hyaline joint cartilage of the hip. Presented at the Society of Magnetic Resonance in Medicine, Amsterdam, The Netherlands, 1989.
62. Yulish BS, Lieberman JM, Newman AJ, Bryan PJ, Mulopulos GP, Modic MT. Juvenile rheumatoid arthritis: assessment with MR imaging. *Radiology* 1987;165:149–152.
63. Yulish BS, Lieberman JM, Strandjord SE, Bryan PJ, Mulopulos GP, Modic MT. Hemophilic arthropathy: assessment with MR imaging. *Radiology* 1987;164:759–762.
64. Zlatkin MB, Dalinkia MK. The glenohumeral joint. *Top Magn Reson Imaging* 1989;1(3):1–13.

Subject Index

A
Abdominal aorta, 170
Abductor digiti minimi
  action, 280–282, 413
  blood supply, 280–282
  innervation, 280–282, 413
  insertion, 280–282, 413
  origin, 280–282, 413
Abductor hallucis
  action, 280–282
  blood supply, 280–282
  innervation, 280–282
  insertion, 280–282
  origin, 280–282
Abductor pollicis brevis
  action, 413
  innervation, 413
  insertion, 413
  origin, 413
Abductor pollicis longus
  action, 375
  innervation, 375
  insertion, 375
  origin, 375
Abscess, 457, 482
  epidural, 127, 132
    postcontrast, 132
  foot, 305, 306
  paraspinal, 127, 132
    postcontrast, 132
  tibia, 484
Accessory soleus muscle, 285
Ace-Fischer external fixation device, 62
Acetabular labral tear, 185
Acetabular labrum, 163
Acetabulum, 163
  hip, 160
  pelvis, 160
  thigh, 160
Achilles tendon
  plantar flexion, 297
  tear, 290, 291–293
    healed, 293
  trauma, 290–291
Acromioclavicular joint, 317, 320, 324, 334
Acromioclavicular ligament, 334, 335
Acromion, 322, 324
Acromioplasty, 349–350
Acute lymphocytic leukemia, bone marrow, 509
Adductor brevis, 164, 166, 168
  function, 165
  innervation, 165
  insertion, 165
  origin, 165
Adductor hallucis
  action, 280–282
  blood supply, 280–282
  innervation, 280–282
  insertion, 280–282
  origin, 280–282
Adductor longus, 164, 166, 168
  function, 165
  innervation, 165
  insertion, 165
  origin, 165
Adductor magnus, 164, 166, 169–170
  function, 165
  innervation, 165
  insertion, 165
  origin, 165
Adductor origin tear, 185
Adductor pollicis
  action, 413
  innervation, 413
  insertion, 413
  origin, 413
Adenocarcinoma metastasis, 131
Age
  annulus fibrosus, 95
  degenerative disc disease, 105
  end-plate change, 105
  nucleus pulposus, 95
  vertebral body, 105
Alar ligament, 101
Aliasing, 22
Anconeus
  action, 374
  blood supply, 374
  innervation, 374
  insertion, 374
  origin, 374
Anemia, reconversion, 505
Aneurysm, magnetic field, 54
Aneurysmal bone cyst, 438–439
  hand, 423
  tarsus, 440
  wrist, 423
Angiography, dural arteriovenous fistula, 140, 142
Ankle
  anterolateral musculature, 278–279
  arthritis, 302–305
  articular anatomy, 273–275
  avascular necrosis, 305–308
  axial images, 256
  bone neoplasm, 297–302
  compartment syndrome, 296
  coronal image, 263
  effusion, 305
  infection, 302–305
  interosseous ligament, 273–274
  ischemic necrosis, 308–309
  joint capsule, 273–274
  lateral ligament, 273–274
  medial ligament, 273–274
  MRI, 253–309
    acquisitions, 255
    applications, 285–309
    coil selection, 253–254
    field of view, 255
    image time, 255
    matrix, 255
    normal variants, 284–285
    patient positioning, 253–254
    pitfalls, 284
    slice thickness, 255
    techniques, 253–254
  muscle origin, 275
  muscles, 276
  neurovascular structures, 294
  osteonecrosis, 305–308
  plantar fasciitis, 296
  post-traumatic, 305
  posterior musculature, 275–278
  skeletal anatomy, 273–275
  soft tissue anatomy, 275
  soft tissue disease, 308–309
  soft tissue tumor, 302
  steroid, 352
  tendons, 294
  trauma, 285–297
    soft tissue, 285–297
  upper, 258
Annulus fibrosus, 95
  age, 95
Antecubital fossa, 381
Anterior tibial tendon
  partial tear, 296
  trauma, 295–296
Apical ligament, 101
Apophyses, 492
Arachnoid, 102
Arachnoiditis
  postoperative evaluation, 111
  T1 weighting, 111
Arcuate ligament, 210
Arm
  capsular abnormalities, 349–351
  MRI
    applications, 343–354
    excitations, 314
    field of view, 314
    image time, 314
    matrix, 314
    postoperative changes, 348
    pulse sequence, 314
    slice thickness/gap, 314
    technique, 316
  muscular anatomy, 337–341
  osseous anatomy, 334–337
  osteonecrosis, 351–353
  upper, 328
Arnold-Chiari malformation, 137–138
  type I, 138
  type II, 138
  type III, 138

Artery of Adamkiewicz, 102
  medullary arteriovenous malformation, 140
Arthritis
  ankle, 302–305
  calf, 302–305
  foot, 302–305
  hand, 425–426
  infectious, 478–480
  knee, 247–248
  rheumatoid. *See* Rheumatoid arthritis
  tuberculous, 522
  wrist, 425–426
Arthrography, knee injury, 232, 233
Arthropathy, 518–523
  hip, 189–190, 191
    cartilage change, 190
    synovial change, 190
  inflammatory
    elbow, 390
    forearm, 390
Articular cartilage, defects, 383
Artifact, 13, 15–16, 22
  cast, 62–63
  cerebrospinal fluid, 88–89
  cochlear implant, 56
  dental appliance, 56
  dressing, 62–63
  external fixation devices, 59–62, 63
  foreign body, 56–57
  frequency effects, 20
  genitourinary prosthesis, 56
  hip prosthesis, 57, 58, 59
  image fold over, 21
  linear, 68
  metallic, 21
  methyl methacrylate, 59, 62
  motion, 88
  orthopedic appliance, 57–62
  patient motion, 21
  phase effects, 20
  radiofrequency, 21
  sources, 15–16
  truncation, 88–90
  vascular appliance, 56
Astrocytoma, spine, 123, 128
  postcontrast T1 weighting sequences, 123
Atlanto-occipital membrane
  anterior, 101
  posterior, 101
Atlas, 95
Attenuation, 23
Avascular necrosis, 174–180
  ankle, 305–308
  bone marrow ischemia, 505–506
  capitate, 430
  elbow, 388–389
  etiology, 174
  femoral condyle, 243
  femoral head, 177
    focal lesion, 182
    patterns, 180
    signal intensity, 180
  foot, 305–308
  forearm, 388–389
  hand, 426–429
  hip, 149, 162
    computed tomography, 176
    core decompression, 174
    coronal T1 weighting, 176
    diagnosis, 174–180
    differential diagnosis, 176–178
    focal area, 178
    histologic phases, 178, 180
    isotope study, 176
    linear subchondral defects, 177
    low-intensity margin, 178
    sagittal images, 176, 177
    signal intensity, 178, 180
    staging, 176
    surface coil, 176
    T2 weighting, 176
    therapy, 174–180
    vascular anatomy, 174, 175
  lunate, 429
  pelvis, 149
  steroid, 243, 352
  talus, 306, 307, 308
  wrist, 426–429
Axilla, 328
Axillary region
  neural anatomy, 342
  vascular anatomy, 342
Axis, 95

B

B_0, 23
B_1, 23
Back pain
  postoperative evaluation, 111
  recurrent, 111, 115
Baker's cyst, knee, 244
Bandwidth, 23
Basivertebral vein, 102
Biceps brachii
  action, 374
  blood supply, 374
  innervation, 374
  insertion, 374
  origin, 374
Biceps femoris, 169–170, 214
  function, 165
  innervation, 165, 215
  insertion, 165, 215
  origin, 165, 215
Biceps tendon, 320
  GRASS (gradient recalled acquisition in steady state), 383–384
Biceps tendon rupture, 383
Blood
  signal intensity, 45
    even echo rephasing, 47
    flow-related enhancement, 45–47
    laminar flow, 47, 48
    plug flow, 47, 48
    saturation effects, 45
    spin dephasing effect, 47
    washout effect, 48, 49
  T1 relaxation time, 46
Blood supply, spinal cord, 102
Blount's disease, 245
Body coil
  pelvis, 149–162
  sacroiliac joint, 149–162
  spine, 87
Bone bruise, 240
Bone infarct, 174–180
  etiology, 174
  femur, 180
  pelvis, 180
Bone island, benign, 189
Bone marrow
  acute lymphocytic leukemia, 509
  age-related changes, 492
  anatomy, 491–493
  components, 492
  degenerative disc disease, 498
  fat, 493
  femur, 497
  FISP (fast imaging with steady-state precession), 501
  FLASH (fast low angle shot), 501
  focal fatty conversion, 496
  gradient-echo, 501
  GRASS (gradient recalled acquisition in steady state), 501
  humerus, 497
  hyperplastic, 508
  infiltration, 508–511
  mineral, 494
  MRI, 493–499
    pitfalls, 515
    spin-echo pulse sequences, 499
    T1 weighting, 499–501
    T2 weighting, 499–501
    technical considerations, 499–501
  myelomatous involvement, 509–510
  normal, 491–499
  physiology, 491–493
  protein, 493
  red to yellow marrow conversion, 492–493
  replacement, 508–511
  screening protocol, 502
  short T1 inversion recovery sequence, 501
  water, 493–494
Bone marrow ischemia, 505–508
  avascular necrosis, 505–506
Bone necrosis, 174–180. *See also* Avascular necrosis etiology, 174
Bone neoplasm. *See also* specific type
  ankle, 297–302
  benign, 438–440
  elbow, 384–388
  foot, 297–302
  forearm, 384–388
  malignant, 440–446
Bone sclerosis, 180
  osteoid osteoma, 190
BOSS (bimodal out of slice saturation), 14
Brachial artery, 380, 381
Brachial plexus, 325, 326, 330
  branches, 341
  lesions, 354–355
  metastasis, 354
  MRI
    excitations, 314
    field of view, 314
    image time, 314
    matrix, 314
    pulse sequence, 314
    slice thickness/gap, 314
    technique, 316, 334
  neurovascular anatomy, 341–342
Brachialis, 381
  action, 374
  blood supply, 374
  innervation, 374
  insertion, 374
  origin, 374
Brachioradialis
  action, 375
  innervation, 375
  insertion, 375
  origin, 375
Breast carcinoma metastasis, marrow fat signal, 115, 120
  contrast administration, 115, 120
Bursa
  elbow, 371–373
  knee, 210, 212
  shoulder, 339, 341

Bursitis, 185
  foot, 296

C

Calcaneal fracture, complex, 287
Calcaneofibular ligament, 273, 274
Calcaneus, 260, 261, 263
  infarct, 308
  plantar flexion, 297
Calcification, 180
Calf
  anterolateral musculature, 278–279
  arthritis, 302–305
  articular anatomy, 273–275
  compartment syndrome, 300
  infection, 302–305
  leiomyosarcoma, 456
  lower, axial image, 257
  middle, axial image, 256
  MRI, 253–309
    acquisitions, 255
    applications, 285–309
    coil selection, 253–254
    field of view, 255
    image time, 255
    imaging parameters, 254–255
    matrix, 255
    normal variants, 284–285
    patient positioning, 253–254
    pitfalls, 284
    pulse sequences, 254–255
    slice thickness, 255
    techniques, 253–255
  muscles, 277
  neoplasm, 297–302
  neurovascular anatomy, 278
  posterior musculature, 275–278
  skeletal anatomy, 273–275
  soft tissue anatomy, 275
  soft tissue disease, 308–309
  superficial muscles, 275
  trauma, 285–297
    compartment syndrome, 297
    hematomas, 297, 299
    soft tissue, 285–297
    venous abnormalities, 297, 298
  upper, 256
Capitate, 419
  avascular necrosis, 430
Capitate fracture, 424
Capitellum, 361, 370
  osteonecrosis, 389
Cardiac gating, motion, 88
Cardiac motion, spine, sagittal thoracic, 88
Carotid artery, 330
Carpal bone, 405, 406, 411
  incomplete ossification, 523
Carpal row, distal, 400
Carpal tunnel, 415
Carpal tunnel release, 432
Carpal tunnel syndrome, 429–431
Carr-Purcell-Meiboom-Gill sequence, 23
Carr-Purcell sequence, 23
Cast, artifact, 62–63
Cauda equina
  beading, 125
  intradural nodule, 124
Caudal regression syndrome, 137
Cavernous hemangioma
  gradient-echo, 112, 119
  T1 weighting, 112, 119
  T2 weighting, 112, 119
Cerebrospinal fluid
  artifact, 88–89
  flow compensation gradient, 90
  frequency gradient direction, 90
  gradient-echo, 93, 102
  motion, 88
  phase gradient direction, 90
  presaturation pulse, 90
  T1 weighting, 102
  T2 weighting, 102
Cervical decompressive laminectomy, 109
Cervical interspace, gradient-echo, 93
Cervical nerve, 101–102
Cervical nerve root, 101
Cervical spinal canal
  gradient-echo, 91
  T1 weighting, 91
Cervical spine, rheumatoid arthritis, 519
Cervical vertebra, 90, 95
Chemical shift imaging, 15, 18, 19, 20, 23
  elbow, 370
  forearm, 370
  pulse sequence, 18
Chemical shift spatial offset, 23
Chest, lateral, 332
Chiari malformation, 137–138
Child
  disorders of, 190–192, 523–254
  hip disorder, 190–192
Chondroblastoma, knee, 244
Chondroma, 440
  periosteal, 443
Chondromalacia patella, 236
  arthroscopic classification of, 236
  MRI classification of, 236
Chondrosarcoma
  age, 445
  gross pathologic histology, 445
  ilium, 439
  image features, 445
  location, 445
Chordoma, 119
Circumflex artery, 170
Claustrophobia, 53
Clavicle, 334
Coccygeal vertebra, 90
Cochlear implant, artifact, 56
Coherence, 23
Coil. *See also* specific type
  selection, 63–65
  spine, 102
Collateral ligament, 210, 213, 370
  fibular, 233
  lateral, injury, 233
  medial, injury, 233
  trauma, 227–233
    MRI vs. arthrography, 232, 233
    repair evaluation, 232–233
  variations, 217–218
Collateral ligament tear, medial, 227–233, 235
Compartment syndrome
  ankle, 296
  calf, 300
  foot, 296
Computed tomography, fundamental principles, 1–2
Computed tomography myelography
  disc herniation, 110
  epidural abscess, 127
  paraspinal abscess, 127
Condylar head, 76
Congenital disorder, 523–524
Contrast
  gradient-echo, 37–39
  pulse sequence, 35–36
  relaxation time, 35–36
Contrast agent, spine, 102
Conus, 101, 134, 136
  abnormal vessels, 143
  cystic mass, 129
  enhancing mural nodule, 129
  gradient-echo, 96–97
Coracoacromial ligament, 334, 335
Coracohumeral ligament, 335, 337
Coracoid, 318, 320, 323
Cord edema, 131
Coronary ligament, 210, 213
Correlation time
  T1, 30
  T2, 30
    protons, 30
Corticosteroid
  ankle, 352
  avascular necrosis, 243, 352
  elbow, 352
  femoral condyle, 243
  femoral head, 174
  hip, 352
  knee, 243, 352
  shoulder, 352
  tibia infarct, 243
Cranial chordoma, 119
Cranial vertebral junction, T1 weighting, high-resolution, 92
Craniovertebral junction, 138
Cruciate ligament, 210, 211
  anterior, 204, 210, 213
    normal, 228, 229
  extended, 214
  flexed, 214
  posterior, 204, 207, 210, 218
    normal, 229
  scout image, 227
  trauma, 227–233
    MRI vs. arthrography, 232, 233
    repair evaluation, 232–233
  variations, 217–218
Cruciate ligament tear
  anterior, 227–233
  posterior, 227–233
Cruciform ligament, 101
Cuboid, 274
  giant cell tumor, 301
Cuneiform, 266, 274
  intermediate, 272
Cyst. *See also* specific type
  benign, 446–447, 450
  elbow, 386
  forearm, 386
  hemorrhage, 451

D

Decompressive laminectomy, 111, 115, 133
Degenerative disc disease, 105–108
  age, 105
  bone marrow, 498
Deltoid, 337
  action, 339
  innervation, 339
  insertion, 339
  origin, 339
Deltoid ligament, 273
Demyelinating plaque, 135
Dental appliance, artifact, 56
Descending aorta, 333

Desmoid tumor, 187, 304, 353, 450–454, 455
  elbow, 386
  foot, 455
  forearm, 386, 388, 455
  recurrent, 459
Diabetes, 304, 306
Diastematomyelia, 134, 137
Diffuse marrow disorder, 502–515
  reconversion, 502–503
Diplomyelia, 137
Disc
  intervertebral
    field of view, 98
    gradient-echo, 93, 95
    normal anatomy, 95
    T1 weighting, 95
    T2 weighting, 95
    water content, 95
  normal anatomy, 95
Disc disease, 105–111
  degenerative, 105–108
  nonsurgical lesions, 105–108
  surgical lesions, 108
Disc extrusion, 108, 114
  gadolinium, 110, 113
Disc fragment
  lateral, 110, 113
  recurrent, 111, 117
Disc herniation, 108–111
  anterior, 108
  asymptomatic, 110
  central, 108, 111
  lateral, 108, 110, 113
  lumbar, 110
    myelography, 110
  midline, 108, 110–111, 114
    calcified, 114
  posterior, 108
  recurrent, 111, 116
    postcontrast MRI, 111, 115
  thoracic region, 110–111, 114
Disc protrusion, 108
  recurrent, 111, 115, 116, 117
Disc space, pyogenic, 126–127, 131
Discitis, pyogenic, 126–127
Discoid meniscus, 226–227
  clinical features, 227
  types, 226
Diskitis, 480
Distal carpal row, 400
Dorsal dermal sinus, 134
Dorsal ligament, 412
Dorsal root ganglion, T1 weighting, 98–99
Dressing, artifact, 62–63
Dual switchable coil, 63
Duchenne's muscular dystrophy, 417
Dura, 102
Dural arteriovenous fistula
  angiography, 140, 142
  myelogram, 140, 142
  T2 weighting, 140, 142
Dural sac, T1 weighting, 98–99
Dural scarring, 111, 116
  postcontrast MRI, 111, 115
  postoperative evaluation, 111

E

Echo planar imaging, 23
Edema
  bone marrow, 511–515
  transient, 181
    differential diagnosis, 181
Elbow
  anatomy, 370–382
  anterior, 367
  articular capsule, 370
  articular structures, 370–371
  avascular necrosis, 388–389
  axial image, 359, 360
  bone neoplasm, 384–388
  bursa, 371–373
  chemical shift, 370
  cyst, 386
  desmoid tumor, 386
  extensors, 376, 377–380
    deep, 379–380
  FLASH (fast low angle shot), 370
  flow artifact, 382
  gradient-echo, 370
  GRASS (gradient recalled acquisition in steady state), 370, 372
  GRIL (gradient recalled acquisition in steady state interleaved), 370
  infection, 390
  inflammatory arthropathy, 390
  inversion recovery, 370
  ligaments, 371
  lipoma, 386
  major arterial anatomy, 381
  middle, 366
  MRI, 357–393
    coil selection, 357–358
    excitations, 359
    field of view, 359
    image time, 359
    matrix, 359
    patient positioning, 357–358
    pitfalls, 382
    slice thickness, 359
    techniques, 357–370
  muscular anatomy, 371–377
  neoplasm, 384–388
  nerve compression syndrome, etiology, 392
  nerve entrapment syndrome, 390–393
  neurovascular anatomy, 380–382
  osteoid osteoma, 385
  osteonecrosis, 388–389
  posterior, 366
  sclerosis, 385
  short T1 inversion recovery sequence, 370
  skeletal neoplasm, 385
  soft tissue neoplasm, 384–388
  steroid, 352
  superficial flexor muscles, 376
  T1 weighting, 370
  trauma, 382–384
Enchondroma, 440
  metatarsal, 301
End-plate change
  age, 105
  T1 weighting, 105, 106
  T2 weighting, 105, 106
  type 1, 105, 106
  type II, 105, 106
  type III, 105, 107
Endochondroma
  hand, 423
  wrist, 423
Enhancement, flow-related, 23
Eosinophilic myositis, 518
Ependymoma
  filum terminale, vs. intradural neurilemoma, 123, 126
  postcontrast image, 126
  spinal cord cyst, 123
  spine, 123, 126, 127
    filum terminale, 123, 126
  syrinx, 126
  vs. hemangioblastoma, 127
Epidermoid tumor
  hand, 424
  wrist, 424
Epidural abscess, 127, 132
  postcontrast, 132
Epidural scar, 111, 116, 117
Epidural soft tissue mass, contrast, 111, 117
Epidural vein, anterior longitudinal, 102
Epiphyses, 492
Ewing's sarcoma
  age, 445
  gross pathologic histology, 445
  humerus, 444
  image features, 445
  knee, 244
  location, 445
  pelvis, 244
Extensor carpi radialis brevis
  action, 375
  innervation, 375
  insertion, 375
  origin, 375
Extensor carpi radialis longus
  action, 375
  innervation, 375
  insertion, 375
  origin, 375
Extensor carpi ulnaris
  action, 375
  innervation, 375
  insertion, 375
  origin, 375
Extensor digiti minimi
  action, 375
  innervation, 375
  insertion, 375
  origin, 375
Extensor digitorum
  action, 375
  innervation, 375
  insertion, 375
  origin, 375
Extensor digitorum brevis
  action, 282
  blood supply, 282
  innervation, 282
  insertion, 282
  origin, 280–282
Extensor digitorum longus, 279
  action, 276
  blood supply, 276
  innervation, 276
  insertion, 276
  origin, 276
Extensor digitorum longus tendon, trauma, 295–296
Extensor hallucis longus, 279
  action, 276
  blood supply, 276
  innervation, 276
  insertion, 276
  origin, 276
Extensor hallucis longus tendon
  ganglion cyst, 303
  trauma, 295–296
Extensor indicis
  action, 375

innervation, 375
insertion, 375
origin, 375
Extensor pollicis brevis
action, 375
innervation, 375
insertion, 375
origin, 375
Extensor pollicis longus
action, 375
innervation, 375
insertion, 375
origin, 375
External fixation device, 59–62, 63
Extradural lesion, spine, 112–115
contrast studies, 115
MRI vs. myelopathy, 112–115

F

Facet joint, 101
field of view, 98
hypertrophy, 109
Failed back syndrome, postoperative evaluation, 111
FAST (flow artifact suppression technique), 14
Fast scanning technique, 14–15, 17
BOSS (bimodal out of slice saturation), 17
FAST (flow artifact suppression technique), 17
FFE (fast field echo), 17
FISP (fast imaging with steady-state precession), 17
FLASH (fast low angle shot), 17
GMR (gradient moment refocusing), 17
GRASS (gradient recalled acquisition in steady state), 17
GRIL (gradient recalled acquisition in steady state interleaved), 17
MAST (motion artifact suppression technique), 17
ROPE (respiratory ordered phase encoding), 17
SAT (saturation), 17
Fat
bone marrow, 493
knee capsule, 218
lateral collateral ligament, 218
medial collateral ligament, 218
precession, 15, 18
selective images, 44, 45
suppression, short T1 inversion recovery sequence, 15, 19, 20
T1, 40–41
T2, 40–41
Fatty infiltration, relaxation time, 33
Femoral artery, 174, 175, 214
common, 170
deep, 171
superficial, 171
Femoral circumflex artery
lateral, 174, 175
medial, 174, 175
Femoral condyle, 206, 209
avascular necrosis, 243
lower, 201
margin, 205
osteonecrosis, spontaneous, 244
steroid, 243
upper, 200
Femoral fracture, 183
post-traumatic neuroma, 183
Femoral head, 153
avascular necrosis, 177
focal lesion, 182
patterns, 180
signal intensity, 180
corticosteroid, 174
hip, 160
pelvis, 160
thigh, 160
upper, 152
Femoral neck, 153, 182
herniation pit, 173
osteomyelitis, 479
Femoral neck fracture, 182
Femoral nerve, 172, 214
Femoral triangle
muscular boundaries, 170
neurovascular structures, 170
Femoral vein, thrombosis, 46
Femur, 189
bone infarct, 180
bone marrow, 497
hip, 161
infection, 484
leg length discrepancy, 525
marrow pattern variation, 173
metastasis, 463
musculoskeletal neoplasm, 437
osteomyelitis, 474, 476, 477
after fracture, 483
vascularized omental graft, 485
pelvis, 161
screws, 60
thigh, 161
upper, 154
FFE (fast field echo), 14
Fibrocartilage complex, 411
Fibrocartilaginous meniscus, 207, 209, 213
Fibromatosis, 304
Fibrosarcoma
age, 445
gross pathologic histology, 445
image features, 445
location, 445
Fibrosis, relaxation time, 33
Fibrous defect, fibula, 439–440
Fibrous dysplasia, 439
Fibrous histiocytoma, malignant, 456, 457
Fibrous lesion, 439
Fibula, 273
fibrous defect, 439–440
metal screws, 59
musculoskeletal neoplasm, 437
osteomyelitis, 474
upper, 202
Fibular head, 202
lateral margin, 203
Field echo, 14
Field of view
facet joint, 98
intervertebral disc, 98
intervertebral foramen, 98
L4 interspace, 98
L5 interspace, 98
nerve root, 98
neural foramen, 98
pelvis, 149–162
respiratory compensation technique, 149, 150
selection, 72
Field strength, spine, 87
Filter, 23
Filum terminale
ependymoma, vs. intradural neurilemoma, 123, 126
thickened, 134
FISP (fast imaging with steady-state precession), 14, 37–38, 68
bone marrow, 501
FLASH (fast low angle shot), 14, 37–38, 68
bone marrow, 501
elbow, 370
forearm, 370
vs. GRASS (gradient recalled acquisition in steady state), 38
Flat coil, 63, 64
Flexor carpi radialis
action, 375
innervation, 375
insertion, 375
origin, 375
Flexor carpi ulnaris, 418
action, 375
innervation, 375
origin, 375
Flexor digiti minimi brevis
action, 280–282, 413
blood supply, 280–282
innervation, 280–282, 413
insertion, 280–282, 413
origin, 280–282, 413
Flexor digitorum, 419
Flexor digitorum brevis
action, 280–282
blood supply, 280–282
innervation, 280–282
insertion, 280–282
origin, 280–282
Flexor digitorum longus
action, 276
blood supply, 276
innervation, 276
insertion, 276
origin, 276
Flexor digitorum longus tendon, incomplete tear, 295
Flexor digitorum profundus
action, 375
innervation, 375
insertion, 375
origin, 375
Flexor digitorum superficialis
action, 375
innervation, 375
insertion, 375
origin, 375
Flexor hallucis brevis
action, 280–282
blood supply, 280–282
innervation, 280–282
insertion, 280–282
origin, 280–282
Flexor hallucis longus
action, 276
blood supply, 276
innervation, 276
insertion, 276
origin, 276
Flexor hallucis longus tendon, trauma, 291–295
Flexor pollicis brevis
action, 413
innervation, 413
insertion, 413
origin, 413

Flexor pollicis longus, 431
action, 413
innervation, 413
insertion, 413
origin, 413
Flexor retinaculum, 418
Flexor tendon, 406
tuberculous synovitis, 429
volar displacement, 523
Flexor tendon sheath, 420
variations, 419–420
Flip angle, 23
Flip angle radiofrequency stimulation, 16
Flow artifact, 13–14
elbow, 382
ganglion cyst, 420
ulnar nerve, 382
wrist, 69
Flow compensation, 13–14
gradient moment nulling, 15
spatial presaturation, 15
Flow compensation gradient
cerebrospinal fluid, 90
motion, 88
Flow-related enhancement, 23, 45–47
Foot
abscess, 305, 306
anterolateral musculature, 278–279
arthritis, 302–305
articular anatomy, 273–275
avascular necrosis, 305–308
bone neoplasm, 297–302
bursitis, 296
compartment syndrome, 296
coronal image, 263
desmoid tumor, 455
dorsal neurovascular anatomy, 283
fourth muscle layer, 283
infection, 302–305
ischemic necrosis, 305–308
MRI, 253–309
acquisitions, 255
applications, 285–309
coil selection, 253–254
field of view, 255
image time, 255
matrix, 255
normal variants, 284–285
patient positioning, 253–254
pitfalls, 284
slice thickness, 255
techniques, 253–254
muscle layers, 280, 281
muscle origin, 275
musculature, 270, 280–282
neuroma, 302
neurovascular supply, 284
osteonecrosis, 305–308
plantar fasciitis, 296
plantar neurovascular anatomy, 284
posterior musculature, 275–278
second muscle layer, 283
skeletal anatomy, 273–275
soft tissue anatomy, 275
soft tissue disease, 308–309
soft tissue tumor, 302
superficial muscle layers, 280, 281
sustentacular level, 268
third muscle layer, 283
trauma, 285–297
soft tissue, 285–297
Forearm
anatomy, 370–382
anterior, 367
avascular necrosis, 388–389
axial image, 359, 360
bone neoplasm, 384–388
chemical shift, 370
cyst, 386
deep flexors, 379
desmoid tumor, 386, 388, 455
distal, 397
FLASH (fast low angle shot), 370
gradient-echo, 370
GRASS (gradient recalled acquisition in steady state), 370
GRIL (gradient recalled acquisition in steady state interleaved), 370
infection, 390
inflammatory arthropathy, 390
intermediate flexor compartment, 378
inversion recovery, 370
lipoma, 386
major arterial anatomy, 381
middle, 366
MRI, 357–393
applications, 382–393
coil selection, 357–358
excitations, 359
field of view, 359
image planes, 358–370
image time, 359
matrix, 359
patient positioning, 357–358
patient rotation, 359
pitfalls, 382
pulse sequences, 358–370
slice thickness, 359
techniques, 357–370
muscular anatomy, 371–377
neoplasm, 384–388
nerve compression syndrome, etiology, 392
nerve entrapment syndrome, 390–393
neuroma, 391
neurovascular anatomy, 380–382
posterior, 366
pronators, 377
proximal, 364, 365
sarcoma, 388
short T1 inversion recovery sequence, 370
skeletal neoplasm, 385
soft tissue neoplasm, 384–388
superficial extensor muscle, 378
superficial flexor muscle, 378
supinators, 377
T1 weighting, 370
trauma, 382–384
Forefoot, 273
Foreign body, artifact, 56–57
Fourier transform, two-dimensional, 5
Fourier transform imaging, 23
Fracture healing, 482–484
Free induction decay, 3–4, 23
Freiberg's disease, 307
Frequency encoding, 7, 9, 23
Frequency gradient direction, cerebrospinal fluid, 90
Frequency gradient direction reversal, motion, 88
Fusiform intramedullary widening, spinal cord, 126

G

Gadolinium, disc extrusion, 110, 113
Ganglion cyst, 447
extensor hallucis longus tendon, 303
flow artifact, 420
Guyon's canal, 427
hand, 425
knee, 244–246, 247
meniscal cyst, 224–226
scaphoid, 428
wrist, 425
Gastrocnemius, 214
action, 276
blood supply, 276
hematoma, 299
innervation, 276
insertion, 276
medial head tear, 298
origin, 276
tear, 300
Gaucher's disease, 510, 512
Gauss, 23
Gemellus
inferior, 167
function, 165
innervation, 165
insertion, 165
origin, 165
superior, 167
function, 165
innervation, 165
insertion, 165
origin, 165
Genicular artery, 214
Geniculate vessel, inferior, 217, 218
Genitourinary prosthesis, artifact, 56
Giant cell tumor, 428
cuboid, 301
hand, 423, 425, 426
knee, 244
tendon sheath, 246–247, 447–450, 452
wrist, 423, 425, 426
Gibb's phenomenon, 88–90
Glenohumeral articulation, 335
Glenohumeral joint, 321, 334
infection, 351
inflammatory disease, 351
MRI, techniques, 314–316
Glenoid, 318, 323
lower, 319
posterior, 321
upper, 318
Glenoid fossa, 76
Glenoid labrum, normal, 351
Glial mesenchymal tumor, intradural metastatic deposits, 124
Glomus tumor
hand, 424
wrist, 424
Gluteal nerve, superior, 171–172
Gluteal region, neurovascular anatomy, 171
Gluteus maximus, 164
function, 165
innervation, 165
insertion, 165
origin, 165
Gluteus medius, 164, 166, 167
function, 165
innervation, 165
insertion, 165
origin, 165
Gluteus minimus, 164, 166
function, 165
innervation, 165
insertion, 165
origin, 165

GMR (gradient moment refocusing), 14
Gracilis, 164, 166, 169, 214
  function, 165
  innervation, 165, 215
  insertion, 165, 215
  origin, 165, 215
Gradient activation, 5, 6
Gradient-echo, 23, 68
  bone marrow, 501
  cavernous hemangioma, 112, 119
  cerebrospinal fluid, 93, 102
  cervical interspace, 93
  cervical spinal canal, 91
  contrast, 37–39
  conus, 96–97
  elbow, 370
  forearm, 370
  intervertebral disc, 93, 95
  ligamentum flavum, 101
  meniscal cyst, 226
  meniscal tear, 220
  motion, 88
  phase interference effects, 38
  spinal canal, diaphragm motion, 104
  spinal cord, 93, 102
    diaphragm motion, 104
    distal, 96–97
    lumbar, 97
    thoracic, 97
  spinal nerve root, 93
  spoiled, 37–38
  steady-state, 37–38
  T1 weighting, 101
  T2 weighting, 101
  vertebral body, 93, 95
Gradient magnetic field, 24
Gradient moment nulling, 13–14
  flow compensation, 15
Gradient moment ruling, pulse sequence, 14
Gradient recalled echo, 14, 17
Gradient recalled echo production, pulse sequence, 16
Gradient reversal, 14, 17
Gradient sequence, 5–7
Granuloma, noncaseating, 133
Granulomatous infection, radial nerve, 393
GRASS (gradient recalled acquisition in steady state), 14, 37–38, 68
  biceps tendon, 383–384
  bone marrow, 501
  elbow, 370, 372
  forearm, 370
  hand, 71
  hemangioma, 387
  vs. FLASH (fast low angle shot), 38
GRIL (gradient recalled acquisition in steady state interleaved), 14
  elbow, 370
  forearm, 370
  knee, 70
  meniscus, 70
GRIL-GRASS (gradient recalled acquisition in steady state interleaved), 68
Growth plate deformity, 523
Growth plate fracture, 240
Guyon's canal, 399, 418
  ganglion cyst, 427
  post-traumatic inflammation, 432
Gyromagnetic ratio, 24

H

Hamate, hook, 400, 419
Hamstring muscle, 164, 166, 169–170, 214
Hamstring tear, 184
Hand
  arthritis, 425–426
  articular anatomy, 411–413
  avascular necrosis, 426–429
  distal, 397
  dorsal carpal bones, 405
  dorsal image, 404
  endochondroma, 423
  epidermoid tumor, 424
  ganglion cyst, 425
  giant cell tumor, 423, 425, 426
  glomus tumor, 424
  GRASS (gradient recalled acquisition in steady state), 71
  infection, 425
  ligamentous anatomy, 411–413
  MRI, 395–433
    anatomic variants, 419
    anatomy, 410–410
    clinical applications, 420–433
    coil selection, 395–396
    field of view, 395, 396
    image planes, 407
    osteology, 411
    pitfalls, 419–420
    positioning, 395–396
    pulse sequences, 407
    techniques, 345, 407, 410
  mucoid cyst, 425
  muscular anatomy, 413–418
  musculoskeletal neoplasm, 422–425
  neurovascular anatomy, 418–419
    volar aspect, 416
  osteochondroma, 423
  osteoid osteoma, 423
  trauma, 421–422
Head coil, 63, 64
Heart valve, magnetic field, 54–55
Heel, stress fracture, 286
Helium gas, 21, 22
Hemangioblastoma
  spine, 123–125, 128–130
    vs. intramedullary arteriovenous malformation, 125, 130
  von Hippel-Lindau disease, 123–125, 128
Hemangioma, 450, 453, 454
  GRASS (gradient recalled acquisition in steady state), 387
  thigh, 187
Hemangiopericytoma, 458
Hematoma, 41–44, 184, 185, 457–458
  chronic, 459
  gastrocnemius, 299
  high field, 42
  low field, 42
  medium field, 42
  relaxation time, 33–35
  resolving, 459
  subacute, 458
  T1 weighting, 43
Hemophilic arthropathy, 523
Hemorrhage, 457–458
  cyst, 451
  medial gastrocnemius, 299
Hemosiderosis, 45, 508
Hemostasis clip, magnetic field, 54
Hepatocellular carcinoma, marrow fat, 112, 118
Herniation pit
  femoral neck, 173
  hip, 179
  pelvis, 173
Hindfoot, 273
Hip
  acetabulum, 160
  acquisitions, 162
  anatomy, 162–172
  anterior aspect, 156
  arthropathy, 189–190, 191
    cartilage change, 190
    synovial change, 190
  avascular necrosis, 149, 162
    computed tomography, 176
    core decompression, 174
    coronal T1 weighting, 176
    diagnosis, 174–180
    differential diagnosis, 176–178
    focal area, 178
    histologic phases, 178, 180
    isotope study, 176
    linear subchondral defects, 177
    low-intensity margin, 178
    sagittal images, 176, 177
    signal intensity, 178, 180
    staging, 176
    surface coil, 176
    T2 weighting, 176
    therapy, 174–180
    vascular anatomy, 174, 175
  coronal images, pubic symphysis, 156
  femoral head, 160
  femur, 161
  fibrous capsule, 163
  field of view, 162
  greater trochanteric level, 157
  herniation pit, 179
  hyaline cartilage, 163
  iliopectineal eminence, 159
  image time, 162
  inflamed bursae, 172
  joint space infection, 479
  lymphoma, 189, 190
  marrow pattern variation, 173
  matrix, 162
  middle, 157
  MRI pitfalls, 172–174
  muscles, 165
  muscular anatomy, 163–170
  neoplasm, 186–189
  neurovascular anatomy, 170–172
  osseous anatomy, 162–163
  osteoarthritis, 189–190, 191, 521
    cartilage change, 190
    synovial change, 190
  osteomyelitis, 190
    short T1 inversion recovery sequence, 190
  pulse sequence, 162
  sciatic notch, 159
  slice thickness, 162
  soft tissue variants, 172
  steroid, 352
  supporting ligaments, 163, 164
  synovial membrane, 163
  T1 weighting, 162
  T2 weighting, 162
  trauma, 181–186
    compartment syndromes, 185
    muscle, 182–185
    nerve injuries, 185

Hip (*contd.*)
soft tissue, 182–185
two-plane T2 weighting, 185
vascular anatomy, 174, 175
Hip arthroplasty, orthopedic appliance, 58, 59, 61
Hip disease, congenital, 192
Hip fracture, 182
Hip prosthesis, artifact, 57, 58, 59
Histiocytoma
partial saturation, 40
T2 weighting, 40
Houlder, vascular anatomy, 343
Humeral head, 318, 320, 324
lateral, 325
lower, 319
upper, 327
Humerus, 334, 340, 370
bone marrow, 497
Ewing's sarcoma, 444
upper, 329
Hyperplastic marrow, 508

I

Iliac artery, 170
Iliac spine
anterior inferior, 152
avulsion stress injury, 183
anterior superior
hip, 161
pelvis, 161
thigh, 161
Iliac vessel
external, 170
internal, 170
Iliacus
function, 165
innervation, 165
insertion, 165
origin, 165
Iliofemoral ligament, 163, 164
Iliopectineal eminence
hip, 159
pelvis, 159
thigh, 159
Iliopsoas, 164, 167, 169
function, 165
inflammation after trauma, 186
innervation, 165
insertion, 165
origin, 165
Iliopsoas bursa, neoplasm, differential diagnosis, 187, 188
Iliopsoas inflammation, 185
Ilium, 163
chondrosarcoma, 439
Image acquisition time, 24
Image pixel, object voxel, 35
Index finger, 407
flexor tendon, 431
Infection
ankle, 302–305
calf, 302–305
elbow, 390
femur, 484
foot, 302–305
forearm, 390
glenohumeral joint, 351
hand, 425
marrow infiltration, 513
MRI, 473–487
cortical bone, 482
joint space, 478–480
marrow, 482
nonviolated tissue, 473–478
soft tissue, 481–482
violated tissue, 482–484
shoulder, 351
wrist, 425
Infectious arthritis, 478–480
Inflammation, relaxation time, 32
Inflammatory arthropathy
elbow, 390
forearm, 390
Inflammatory disease
glenohumeral joint, 351
shoulder, 351
Infrapatellar plica, 236, 237
Infraspinatus, 337
action, 339
innervation, 339
insertion, 339
origin, 339
Inguinal region, lymphoma, 189, 190
Innominate bone, 162
Intercondylar eminence, 209
loose fragment, 239
Intercondylar spine region, osteoarthritis, 243, 245
Interosseous
action, 413
innervation, 413
insertion, 413
origin, 413
Interosseous dorsal
action, 280–282
blood supply, 280–282
innervation, 280–282
insertion, 280–282
origin, 280–282
Interpulse time, 24
Interspinous ligament, 101
Intervertebral disc
field of view, 98
gradient-echo, 93, 95
normal anatomy, 95
T1 weighting, 95
T2 weighting, 95
water content, 95
Intervertebral disc space inflammation, 480
Intervertebral foramen, 330
field of view, 98
lateral parasagittal section, 94
Intradural extramedullary lesion, spine, 115–123
contrast, 121
Intradural metastasis, spine, 123, 124, 125
enhancing nodules, 123, 124
noncontrast MRI, 123, 124
Intradural nodule
cauda equina, 124
melanoma, 124
Intramedullary expansion, 144
Intramedullary lesion, spine, 123–125
Intraparenchymal cord hematoma, 141, 144
Intrapatellar fat pad, 210, 211
Intrapatellar synovial fold, 210, 211
Intraspinal fat, T1 weighting, 98–99
Intrasynovial space, 210
Inversion recovery, 24
elbow, 370
forearm, 370
Inversion recovery pulse sequence, 7, 10, 11
Ischemic necrosis
ankle, 305–308
calf, 305–308
dural, 111, 115, 116
foot, 305–308
Ischiofemoral ligament, 163, 164
Ischium, 158, 163
Isochromat
phase angle
laminar flow, 48
plug flow, 47, 48
spin-echo signal, 47

J

Joint space infection, 191, 478–480
hip, 479
Jugular vein, external region, 331
Juvenile rheumatoid arthritis, 519–524

K

Knee
anatomy, 197, 198–214
anterior joint, 207
arthritis, 247–248
articular anatomy, 198–212
Baker's cyst, 244
bone anatomy, 198–212
bursa, 210, 212
capsular attachments, 211
chondroblastoma, 244
coronal capsule, 212
Ewing's sarcoma, 244
extended, 214
flexed, 214
flexion, 239
flexors, 214, 215
ganglion cyst, 244–246, 247
giant cell tumor, 244
GRIL (gradient recalled acquisition in steady state interleaved), 70
joint space, 220
ligament anatomy, 220
ligament trauma, 227–233
MRI vs. arthrography, 232, 233
repair evaluation, 232–233
ligaments, 212, 213
loose bodies, 238, 239, 240
medial soft tissues, 205
meniscus, 213
midjoint, 207
MRI, 195–248
acquisitions, 196
anatomic variants, 217
applications, 219–248
contrast, 195
cross artifact, 216
extremity coil, 195, 196
field of view, 196
flow artifact, 214–216
flow artifacts, vs. articular defect, 216
gradient-echo, 196–197
image geometry, 195
image time, 196
interpretation errors, 216–219
long TR, multiecho spin-echo sequences, 196
marrow artifact, 216, 217
matrix, 196
multiplanar GRASS (gradient recalled acquisition in steady state), 206, 216
peroneal nerve, 214
pitfalls, 214–219
pulsatile motion artifact, 216

pulse sequence, 195, 196
radial imaging, 197, 198
sagittal plane flow artifact, 214–216
slice thickness, 196
spin-echo, 196
supine position, 195, 196
techniques, 195–198
three-dimensional FT acquisition, 197–198
vs. arthrography, 195
muscles, 212–214
muscular anatomy, 220
musculoskeletal neoplasms, 244–247
neurovascular supply, 214, 215
osteochondrosis, 242–243
osteomyelitis, 69
osteonecrosis, 242–243
MRI features, 243–244
radiographic features, 243–244
spontaneous, 243–244
osteosarcoma, 244
periarticular ligaments, 210
popliteal cyst, 244
posterior soft tissue, 206
primary skeletal neoplasms, 244, 245
radial GRIL (gradient recalled acquisition in steady state interleaved), 208–209
sagittal capsule, 212
short T1 inversion recovery sequence, 69
soft tissue masses, 244–247
soft tissue tumors, 245
steroid, 243, 352
synovial disease, 247–248
synovial lining, 211, 212
synovial plica, 233–236
transverse ligament, 212
Knee capsule, 210
fat, 218
synovial membrane, 209
Knee coil, 63
Knee fracture, 238–240
Kohler's disease, 307

L

L4 interspace, field of view, 98
L5 interspace, field of view, 98
Labrum, normal, 318
Lacertus fibrosis, 392
Larmor frequency, 2
Lateral collateral ligament, fat, 218
Lateral epicondyle, 360, 368
Lateral malleolus, 264, 270
Lateral meniscus, 207, 213
anatomy, 219
complex degenerative tear, 223
discoid, 218, 219
tangential sections, 219
Lateral parasagittal section, intervertebral foramen, 94
Lateral talus, 270
Lateral tibial condyle, 209
Latissimus dorsi, 340
action, 339
innervation, 339
insertion, 339
origin, 339
Leg
anterior compartment, muscles, 279
lateral muscle group, 279
muscles, 276
Legg-Calve-Perthes disease, 191, 192
Leiomyosarcoma, calf, 456
Leptomeningeal enhancement, 132, 133
Leptomeningeal tumor, 123, 125
Leukemia, marrow infiltration, 508, 509
Levator scapulae, 340
action, 339
innervation, 339
insertion, 339
origin, 339
Ligament of Testut, 412
Ligament of Wrisberg, 218
Ligamentum flavum, 101
gradient-echo, 101
hypertrophy, 109
thickening, 109
Ligamentum mucosum, 210, 211
Ligamentum teres, 163
Linear artifact, 68
Lipidosis, 510, 512
Lipoma, 446
elbow, 386
forearm, 386
spine, 121, 123
Liposarcoma, 446, 448, 449, 450
Longitudinal ligament
anterior, 95–101
posterior, 101
Longitudinal magnetization, 24
Longitudinal relaxation, 3–5, 24
Lumbar spine
coronal images, 100
metastasis, 465
MRI, scout view, 104
Lumbar vertebra, 90
Lumbosacral plexus, 171
Lumbrical
action, 280–282, 413
blood supply, 280–282
innervation, 280–282, 413
insertion, 280–282, 413
origin, 280–282, 413
Lunate, 411
avascular necrosis, 429
ulnolunate abutment syndrome, 340
Lunocapitate region, 408
Lymphoma, 464
hip, 189, 190
inguinal region, 189, 190
marrow infiltration, 506

M

Macroscopic magnetization vector, 3, 4, 24
Magnetic field, 5
aneurysm, 54
heart valve, 54–55
hemostasis clip, 54
surgical clip, 54–55
Magnetic field gradient, 24
Magnetic resonance, 24
Magnetic shielding, 18–21
Magnetic susceptibility, 24
Malleolus, 260
Mandibular condyle, 75
Marrow fat
breast carcinoma metastasis, 115, 120
hepatocellular carcinoma, 112, 118
metastasis, 112, 118
multiple myeloma, 112, 118
prostate carcinoma, 112, 118
Marrow fat signal, breast carcinoma metastasis, contrast administration, 115, 120
MAST (motion artifact suppression technique), 14
Matrix, 72
Medial collateral ligament, fat, 218
Medial collateral ligament tear, 217
Medial compartment, 205
Medial cuneiform, 271
Medial epicondyle, 360
Medial femoral condyle, 209
Medial gastrocnemius, hemorrhage, 299
Medial malleolus, 265, 268, 273
osteomyelitis, 478
Medial meniscus
anatomy, 219
normal, 224
normal anterior horn, 212, 214
posterior, 217
tangential sections, 219
Medial talus, 269
Medial tendon, trauma, 294–295
Medial tibial condyle, 209
Median nerve, 380, 381, 392, 419, 429–430
branches, 417
Mediopatellar plica, 236, 237
Medullary arteriovenous malformation, 140–141, 144
anterior spinal artery, 140
artery of Adamkiewicz, 140
Medullary artery, great anterior, 102
Melanoma, intradural nodule, 124
Meningioma
calcification, 115
postcontrast, 115, 121
spine, 115, 121
contrast, 115, 121
Meningocele, 134, 136
Meningomyelocele, 134
Meniscal cyst, 222, 224–226
etiology, 226
ganglion cyst, 224–226
gradient-echo, 226
popliteal cyst, 224–226
presentations, 224
T2 weighting, 226
Meniscal tear, 214, 219–224
bucket handle, 221–223, 224
causes, 219
examination techniques, 219–220
grade 1, 220, 222, 224
grade 2, 221, 222
grade 3, 221, 222
grade 4, 221, 222, 223
gradient-echo, 220
grading system, 220
MRI accuracy, 224
MRI sensitivity, 224, 225
MRI specificity, 224
MRI vs. arthrography, 224
radial, 221, 223, 224
stable peripheral, 225
T2 weighted spin-echo, 220
T1 weighting, 220
three-dimensional gradient-echo, 220
types, 221
vertical, 221
Meniscosynovial junction, concave, 217
Meniscus
attachments, 220
GRIL (gradient recalled acquisition in steady state interleaved), 70
ligament anatomy, 220
osteoarthritis, 243, 245

Meniscus (*contd.*)
  radial GRIL (gradient recalled acquisition in steady state interleaved), 208–209
  tendon anatomy, 220
Metacarpal, 411
  third, 409
Metacarpal head
  first, 401
  second to fifth, 402
  third, 402
Metacarpal joint, first, 401
Metacarpophalangeal joint, ligaments, 412
Metartarsal region, middle, 267
Metastatic disease, marrow infiltration, 112, 118, 507
Metatarsal, 274
  enchondroma, 301
  fifth, 272
  first, 271
  proximal, 266
  second, 271
Metatarsal head, 307
Methyl methacrylate
  artifact, 59, 62
  tibia, 62
Midcapitate fracture, 422
Midcarpal articulation, 411
Midfoot, 273, 274
Mineral, bone marrow, 494
Motion
  artifact, 88
  cardiac gating, 88
  cerebrospinal fluid, 88
  flow compensation gradient, 88
  frequency gradient direction reversal, 88
  gradient-echo, 88
  phase gradient direction reversal, 88
  presaturation pulse sequence, 88
  respiratory gating, 88
  spine
    patient, 88
    physiologic, 88
  T1 weighting, 88
  T2 weighting sequence, 88
Motion compensation technique, 13–14
MRI
  acronym, 12, 14
  ankle, 253–309
    acquisitions, 255
    applications, 285–309
    coil selection, 253–254
    field of view, 255
    image time, 255
    matrix, 255
    normal variants, 284–285
    patient positioning, 253–254
    pitfalls, 284
    slice thickness, 255
    techniques, 253–254
  arm
    applications, 343–354
    excitations, 314
    field of view, 314
    image time, 314
    matrix, 314
    postoperative changes, 348
    pulse sequence, 314
    slice thickness/gap, 314
    technique, 316
  arteries, 45–50
  biological effects, 16–18
  bone marrow, 493–499
    pitfalls, 515
    spin-echo pulse sequences, 499
    T1 weighting, 499–501
    T2 weighting, 499–501
    technical considerations, 499–501
  brachial plexus
    excitations, 314
    field of view, 314
    image time, 314
    matrix, 314
    pulse sequence, 314
    slice thickness/gap, 314
    technique, 316, 334
  calf, 253–309
    acquisitions, 255
    applications, 285–309
    coil selection, 253–254
    field of view, 255
    image time, 255
    imaging parameters, 254–255
    matrix, 255
    normal variants, 284–285
    patient positioning, 253–254
    pitfalls, 284
    pulse sequences, 254–255
    slice thickness, 255
    techniques, 253–255
  coordinate system, 3, 4
  elbow, 357–393
    coil selection, 357–358
    excitations, 359
    field of view, 359
    image time, 359
    matrix, 359
    patient positioning, 357–358
    pitfalls, 382
    slice thickness, 359
    techniques, 357–370
  emergency procedures, 22
  FDA guidelines, 18, 21
  foot, 253–309
    acquisitions, 255
    applications, 285–309
    coil selection, 253–254
    field of view, 255
    image time, 255
    matrix, 255
    normal variants, 284–285
    patient positioning, 253–254
    pitfalls, 284
    slice thickness, 255
    techniques, 253–254
  forearm, 357–393
    applications, 382–393
    coil selection, 357–358
    excitations, 359
    field of view, 359
    image planes, 358–370
    image time, 359
    matrix, 359
    patient positioning, 357–358
    patient rotation, 359
    pitfalls, 382
    pulse sequences, 358–370
    slice thickness, 359
    techniques, 357–370
  fundamental principles, 1–2
  glenohumeral joint, techniques, 314–316
  gradient fields, 16–18
  hand, 395–433
    anatomic variants, 419
    anatomy, 410–410
    clinical applications, 420–433
    coil selection, 395–396
    field of view, 395, 396
    image planes, 407
    osteology, 411
    pitfalls, 419–420
    positioning, 395–396
    pulse sequences, 407
    techniques, 345, 407, 410
  high static magnetic fields, 16
  historical development, 1
  infection, 473–487
    cortical bone, 482
    joint space, 478–480
    marrow, 482
    nonviolated tissue, 473–478
    soft tissue, 481–482
    violated tissue, 482–484
  knee, 195–248
    acquisitions, 196
    anatomic variants, 217
    applications, 219–248
    contrast, 195
    cross artifact, 216
    extremity coil, 195, 196
    field of view, 196
    flow artifact, 214–216
    flow artifacts, vs. articular defect, 216
    gradient-echo, 196–197
    image geometry, 195
    image time, 196
    interpretation errors, 216–219
    long TR, multiecho spin-echo sequences, 196
    marrow artifact, 216, 217
    matrix, 196
    multiplanar GRASS (gradient recalled acquisition in steady state), 206, 216
    peroneal nerve, 214
    pitfalls, 214–219
    pulsatile motion artifact, 216
    pulse sequence, 195, 196
    radial imaging, 197, 198
    sagittal plane flow artifact, 214–216
    slice thickness, 196
    spin-echo, 196
    supine position, 195, 196
    techniques, 195–198
    three-dimensional FT acquisition, 197–198
    vs. arthrography, 195
  lumbar spine, scout view, 104
  musculoskeletal neoplasm, 435–469
    coil selection, 435–436
    imaging planes, 436–438
    metastases, 462–469
    patient positioning, 435–436
    recurrence, 461, 462
    specificity, 469
    techniques, 435–438
  operational, 21–22
  patient selection, 53–63
    claustrophobia, 53
    clinical status, 53–54
    electrical device, 54
    metal implant, 54
    weight, 53
  quench, 21, 22
  radiofrequency radiation, 18
  relative temporal placement, 12
  safety issues, 22

security issues, 22
shoulder
applications, 343–354
excitations, 314
field of view, 314
matrix, 314
postoperative changes, 348
pulse sequence, 314
slice thickness/gap, 314
trauma, 343–348
vs. arthrography, 348
site considerations, 18–21
spine
circular coil, 102
contrast agents, 105
examination technique, 102–105
gadolinium diethylenetriaminepentaacetic acid, 105
gradient-echo sagittal sequence, 102–103
license plate coil, 102
multispecialty expertise, 87
pathologic conditions, 105–145
protocol, 104, 105
surface coil, 102–105
T1 weighting sagittal sequence, 102–103
T2 weighting sagittal sequence, 102–103
technical considerations, 87–90
technique selection, 39–45
temporomandibular joint, 75–84
degenerative joint disease, 80–83
disc dessication, 80, 83
fast gradient-echo images, 78–79
fractured implant, 83, 84
grade 1 joint, 81
grade 2 joint, 82
grading system, 81
GRASS (gradient recalled acquisition in steady state), 81
GRIL (gradient recalled acquisition in steady state interleaved), 78
normal silastic implant, 83, 84
postoperative evaluation, 84
sagittal plane T1 weighted images, 77–79
surface coil, 78
T1, 81
technique, 77–79
three-dimensional volume acquisition, 79
vs. computed tomography, 84
time-varying magnetic fields, 16–18
timing variation, 12
trauma
accuracy, 347–348
diagnostic criteria, 347
vs. arthrography, 348
vascular structure appearance, 45–50
veins, 45–50
wrist, 395–433
anatomic variants, 419
anatomy, 410
field of view, 395, 396
osteology, 411
pitfalls, 419–420
pulse sequences, 407
techniques, 345, 407, 410
MRI system, diagram, 4
Mucoid cyst
hand, 425
wrist, 425
Multiple coil array, 63
Multiple myeloma, 465
marrow fat, 112, 118
Multiple sclerosis, 133, 135
plaques, 133, 135
postcontrast, 133–134
Musculoskeletal neoplasm. *See also* Neoplasm; Specific type
femur, 437
fibula, 437
hand, 422–425
MRI, 435–469
coil selection, 435–436
imaging planes, 436–438
metastases, 462–469
patient positioning, 435–436
recurrence, 461, 462
specificity, 469
techniques, 435–438
tibia, 437
wrist, 422–425
Musculoskeletal tissue
relaxation time, 31–32
effects of pathology, 32–35
signal intensity, 66–68
Myelocele, 134
Myelocystocele, 134
Myelofibrosis, marrow infiltration, 512
Myelogram
disc herniation, 110
dural arteriovenous fistula, 140, 142
spinal canal stenosis, 108
Myeloid depletion, 503–505
radiation therapy, 504
Myeloma, marrow infiltration, 511
Myelomalacia, 108, 109
Myelomeningocele, 136
Myelopathy
high cervical, 135
progressive thoracic, 132, 141
Myeloproliferative disorder, 510
Myopathy, 417
Myositis, eosinophilic, 518
Myxoma, 451
benign, 447

N

Navicular, 265, 274
spontaneous osteonecrosis, 307
Neck, 326, 333
lateral, 331
Neoplasm. *See also* specific type
calf, 297–302
elbow, 384–388
forearm, 384–388
fourth ventricular, 125
hip, 186–189
iliopsoas bursa, differential diagnosis, 187, 188
partial saturation, 41
pelvis, 186–189
relaxation time, 32–33
shoulder, 353–354
soft tissue, 39
spine, 111–131
T2 weighting, 41
thigh, 186–189
vs. adipose tissue, 40–41
Nerve compression syndrome
elbow, etiology, 392
forearm, etiology, 392
ulnar nerve, 392
Nerve entrapment syndrome
elbow, 390–393
forearm, 390–393
Nerve root
field of view, 98
T1 weighting, 98–99
Nerve sheath tumor, spine, 121
Neural foramen
field of view, 98
T1 weighting, 98–99
Neurilemoma, 121, 122
Neurofibroma
necrotic, 187
spine, 121
Neurogenic tumor, spine, 115–121, 122
Neuroma, 304
benign, 453
foot, 302
forearm, 391
Neuropathy, wrist, 518
Niemann-Pick disease, 510, 512
Nodular polymyositis, 417
Nuclear magnetic resonance
experiment, 2
signal, 3–4
Nucleus pulposus, 95
age, 95
herniated, 108–111
anterior, 108
asymptomatic, 110
central, 108, 111
lateral, 108
midline, 108
posterior, 108

O

Object voxel, image pixel, 35
Oblique popliteal ligament, 210
Obturator artery, 170
Obturator externus, 169
function, 165
innervation, 165
insertion, 165
origin, 165
Obturator internus, 167
function, 165
innervation, 165
insertion, 165
origin, 165
Obturator nerve, 172, 214
Odontoid process, 95
Off-resonance, 2
Olecranon bursa, 372
Opponens digiti minimi
action, 413
innervation, 413
insertion, 413
origin, 413
Opponens pollicis
action, 413
innervation, 413
insertion, 413
origin, 413
Orthopedic appliance
artifact, 57–62
hip arthroplasty, 58, 59, 61
Osgood-Schlatter disease, 245
Osteoarthritis, 521
hip, 189–190, 191, 521
cartilage change, 190
synovial change, 190

Osteoarthritis (*contd.*)
  intercondylar spine region, 243, 245
  medial compartment, 521
  meniscus, 243, 245
  MRI stages, 191
  radiographic stages, 191
Osteochondral fracture, 240
Osteochondritis dissecans, 240–242
Ostcochondroma, 440, 441
  hand, 423
  tibia, 442
  wrist, 423
Osteochondrosis, knee, 242–243
Osteoid osteoma, 187, 189, 443
  bone sclerosis, 190
  elbow, 385
  hand, 423
  synovial hypertrophy, 190
  wrist, 423
Osteomyelitis, 191, 473–478
  femoral neck, 479
  femur, 474, 476, 477
    after fracture, 483
    vascularized omental graft, 485
  fibula, 474
  hip, 190
    short T1 inversion recovery sequence, 190
  knee, 69
  medial malleolus, 478
  pelvis, 190
    short T1 inversion recovery sequence, 190
  short T1 inversion recovery sequence, 69
  surgical reconstruction, 484–487
  thigh, 190
    short T1 inversion recovery sequence, 190
  tibia, 477
    bilateral, 475
    muscle flap, 486
Osteonecrosis, 174–180, 307, 423
  ankle, 305–308
  arm, 351–353
  capitellum, 389
  elbow, 388–389
  etiology, 174
  femoral condyle, spontaneous, 244
  foot, 305–308
  knee, 242–243
    MRI features, 243–244
    radiographic features, 243–244
    spontaneous, 243–244
  scaphoid fracture, 424
  shoulder, 351–353
Osteopenia
  thoracic spine, 463
  vertebra, 463
Osteoporosis
  migratory, 181
  transient, differential diagnosis, 181
Osteosarcoma
  age, 445
  gross pathologic histology, 445
  image features, 445
  knee, 244
  location, 445
Osteosclerotic myeloma, 466

P

Paget's disease, 182, 189
Palm
  central compartments, 419
  hypothenar compartments, 419
  thenar compartments, 419
Palmar arch, deep, 417
Palmar ligament, 412
Palmaris brevis
  action, 413
  innervation, 413
  insertion, 413
  origin, 413
Palmaris longus
  action, 375
  innervation, 375
  insertion, 375
  origin, 375
Paraplegia, 144
Paraspinal abscess, 127, 132
  postcontrast, 132
Paraspinal fat, T1 weighting, 98–99
Partial saturation, 24
  histiocytoma, 40
  neoplasm, 41
  Schwannoma, 40
Partial saturation pulse sequence, 7, 9, 10
Partial volume coil, 63–65
Patella
  axial image, 199
  lower, 200
  upper, axial image, 199, 200
  Wiberg types, 209
Patellar cartilage, 236
Patellar disorder, 236–238
Patellar ligament, 168, 210
  sagittal images, 233, 236
Patellar retinaculum, 209, 210
Patellofemoral instability, 236–238
Patellofemoral pain syndrome, 236
Patient positioning
  body part, 63
  expected examination time, 63
  lower extremity, 63
  size, 63
  upper extremity, 63–65
Pectineus, 168, 169
  function, 165
  innervation, 165
  insertion, 165
  origin, 165
Pectoralis major, 340–341
  action, 339
  innervation, 339
  insertion, 339
  origin, 339
Pectoralis minor, 340–341
  action, 339
  innervation, 339
  insertion, 339
  origin, 339
Pediatric disorder, 523–524
  hip, 190–192
Pelvic fracture, 182
Pelvis
  acetabulum, 160
  acquisitions, 162
  anatomy, 162–172
  articulations, 163
  avascular necrosis, 149
  body coil, 149–162
  bone infarct, 180
  coronal images, pubic symphysis, 156
  Ewing's sarcoma, 244
  femoral head, 160
  femur, 161
  field of view, 149–162
  herniation pit, 173
  iliopectineal eminence, 159
  image time, 162
  inflamed bursae, 172
  marrow pattern variation, 173
  matrix, 162
  MRI pitfalls, 172–174
  muscles, 165
  muscular anatomy, 163–170
  neoplasm, 186–189
  neurovascular anatomy, 170–172
  osseous anatomy, 162–163
  osteomyelitis, 190
    short T1 inversion recovery sequence, 190
  pulse sequence, 162
  sciatic notch, 159
  slice thickness, 162
  soft tissue variants, 172
  T1 weighting, 149–162
  T2 weighting, 149–162
  technique, 149–162
  trauma, 181–186
    compartment syndromes, 185
    muscle, 182–185
    nerve injuries, 185
    soft tissue, 182–185
    two-plane T2 weighting, 185
Perimedullary arteriovenous fistula, 141, 145
Peroneal artery, 284
Peroneal groove, 263
Peroneal nerve
  common, 280
  deep, 280, 284
Peroneal tendon, 273, 274
  ruptures, 289, 290
  subluxing, 288
  trauma, 288–290
Peroneus brevis, 278
  action, 276
  blood supply, 276
  innervation, 276
  insertion, 276
  origin, 276
Peroneus brevis tendon, incomplete tear, 290
Peroneus longus, 278
  action, 276
  blood supply, 276
  innervation, 276
  insertion, 276
  origin, 276
Peroneus longus rupture, complete, 289
Peroneus tertius, 279
  action, 276
  blood supply, 276
  innervation, 276
  insertion, 276
  origin, 276
Pes anserine bursitis, 245
Phalangeal base, proximal, 402
Phalanx, 274, 411
  middle, 411
  proximal, 411
  second to fourth, 403
Phase, 24
Phase angle, isochromat
  laminar flow, 48
  plug flow, 47, 48
Phase encoding, 7–9, 24
Phase gradient direction, cerebrospinal fluid, 90
Phase gradient direction reversal, motion, 88
Pia mater, 102

Pial vein, 102
Pigmented villonodular synovitis, 248, 391, 521–523
Piriformis, 166–167, 168
  function, 165
  innervation, 165
  insertion, 165
  origin, 165
Pisiform, 411
Pisotriquetral articulation, 399
Pixel, 35
Pixel size reduction, 72
Plantar artery, medial, 284
Plantar fasciitis
  ankle, 296
  foot, 296
Plantar fibromatosis, 304
Plantaris
  action, 276, 280–282
  blood supply, 276, 280–282
  innervation, 276, 280–282
  insertion, 276, 280–282
  origin, 276, 280–282
Plateau fracture, 240, 242
Plica, 233–236
  infrapatellar, 236, 237
  mediopatellar, 236, 237
  suprapatellar, 236
  T1 weighting, 236
  T2 weighting, 236
Polyradiculopathy, 125
Popliteal artery, 214, 278
Popliteal cyst
  knee, 244
  meniscal cyst, 224–226
Popliteal vein, lumen, 46
Popliteus, 214
  action, 276
  blood supply, 276
  innervation, 276
  insertion, 276
  origin, 276
Popliteus tendon, 217
Posterior band, 75
Posterior tibial tendon
  complete tear, 295
  tendon sheath fluid, 295
Precession, 2, 24
  fat, 15, 18
  water, 15, 18
Presaturation pulse
  cerebrospinal fluid, 90
  motion, 88
Progressive thoracic myelopathy, 132, 141
Pronator quadratus
  action, 375
  innervation, 375
  insertion, 375
  origin, 375
Pronator teres, 392
  action, 374, 375
  blood supply, 374
  innervation, 374, 375
  insertion, 374, 375
  origin, 374, 375
Prostate carcinoma, marrow fat, 112, 118
Protein, bone marrow, 493
Psoas major
  function, 165
  innervation, 165
  insertion, 165
  origin, 165
Psoas minor
  function, 165
  innervation, 165
  insertion, 165
  origin, 165
Pubis, 163
Pubofemoral ligament, 163, 164
Pulse sequence, 7–12, 13, 25
  chemical shift imaging, 18
  contrast, 35–36
  gradient moment ruling, 14
  gradient recalled echo production, 16
  inversion recovery, 7, 10, 11
  partial saturation, 7, 9, 10
  spatial presaturation, 15
  spin-echo, 7–12, 13
Pulse sequence selection, 65–69
Pyogenic discitis, 126–127
  vertebral body, 127, 131

Q

Quadratus femoris, 167
  function, 165
  innervation, 165
  insertion, 165
  origin, 165
Quadratus plantae
  action, 280–282
  blood supply, 280–282
  innervation, 280–282
  insertion, 280–282
  origin, 280–282
Quadriceps femoris, 168, 169
  function, 165
  innervation, 165
  insertion, 165
  origin, 165
Quadriceps tendon, 168
  sagittal images, 233, 236
  tear, 236
Quadriplegia, 144

R

Radial acquisition technique, 197
  knee, 197, 198
Radial artery, 381
Radial GRIL (gradient recalled acquisition in steady state interleaved)
  knee, 208–209
  meniscus, 208–209
Radial head, 361, 370
Radial ligament, 370
Radial neck, 361
Radial nerve, 380, 381
  granulomatous infection, 393
Radial tuberosity, 361
Radicular vein, 102
Radiculomedullary artery, 102
Radiocapitate ligament, 412
Radiocapitellar joint
  lateral, 368
  ulnar aspect, 369
Radiocarpal joint, 411
Radiofrequency shielding, 18–21
Radiolunotriquetral ligament, 412
Radioscapholunate ligament, 412
Radioulnar joint, 398
  distal, 411
Radioulnar region, 409
Rectal carcinoma
  recurrence, 467
  sacral metastasis, 467
Rectus femoris, 168
  function, 165
  innervation, 165, 215
  insertion, 165, 215
  origin, 165, 215
Red marrow, 492
  normal, 495
  signal characteristics, 494
Reflex sympathetic dystrophy, 181, 514
Relaxation time, 28–29
  contrast, 35–36
  fibrosis, 33
  hematoma, 33–35
  inflammation, 32
  musculoskeletal tissue, 31–32
    effects of pathology, 32–35
  neoplasm, 32–33
  significance, 29–31
Rephasing gradient, 25
Resonance, 2, 25
Respiratory compensation technique, field of view, 149, 150
Respiratory gating, motion, 88
Rhabdomyolysis, 185
Rheumatoid arthritis, 519–524
  cervical spine, 519
  wrist, 519
Rhomboid, 340
Rhomboideus major
  action, 339
  innervation, 339
  insertion, 339
  origin, 339
Rhomboideus minor
  action, 339
  innervation, 339
  insertion, 339
  origin, 339
ROPE (respiratory ordered phase encoding), 14
Rotator cuff muscle, 337
Rotator cuff syndrome, 343–347
Rotator cuff tear, 343–347
  chronic, 346–347
  incomplete, 346–347

S

Sacral vertebra, 90
Sacroiliac joint, 151
  body coil, 149–162
  technique, 149–162
Sacrum, 150, 162
  blastic metastasis, 188
  mixed blastic and lytic lesion, 188
Sarcoid myelitis, 128, 133
Sarcoma, forearm, 388
Sartorius, 168, 214
  function, 165
  innervation, 165, 215
  insertion, 165, 215
  origin, 165, 215
SAT (saturation), 14
Saturation recovery, 25
Scaphoid, 398, 411, 419
Scaphoid fracture
  non-union, 423
  osteonecrosis, 424
Scaphotrapezial articulation, 408
Scapula, 334, 340
  lateral, 332
Scapular spine, 323
Scar, 460
  epidural, 111, 116, 117

Schmorl's nodule, 108, 111
Schwannoma
  partial saturation, 40
  T2 weighting, 40
Sciatic nerve, 171–172, 214
Sciatic notch, 151
  hip, 159
  pelvis, 159
  thigh, 159
Sclerosis, elbow, 385
Scoliosis, 103
  congenital, 137
    coronal plane, 137
  T1 weighting, 103
Semimembranosus, 169–170, 214
  function, 165
  innervation, 165, 215
  insertion, 165, 215
  origin, 165, 215
Semitendinosus, 169–170, 214
  function, 165
  innervation, 165, 215
  insertion, 165, 215
  origin, 165, 215
Septic spondylitis, 480–481
Serratus anterior, 340
  action, 339
  innervation, 339
  insertion, 339
  origin, 339
Sharpey's fiber, 95
Shimming, 20
  active, 20
  passive, 20
  shim coil, 20
Short T1 inversion recovery sequence
  bone marrow, 501
  elbow, 370
  fat suppression, 15, 19, 20
  forearm, 370
  knee, 69
  osteomyelitis, 69
Shoulder, 317, 320, 333
  anterior capsular attachments, 337
  bursa, 339, 341
  capsular abnormalities, 349–351
  capsular attachments, 335–337
  extrinsic muscles, 339, 340
  infection, 351
  inflammatory disease, 351
  ligaments, 334–335
  MRI
    applications, 343–354
    excitations, 314
    field of view, 314
    matrix, 314
    postoperative changes, 348
    pulse sequence, 314
    slice thickness/gap, 314
    trauma, 343–348
    vs. arthrography, 348
  muscular anatomy, 337–341
  neoplasm, 353–354
  osseous anatomy, 334–337
  osteonecrosis, 351–353
  post-traumatic pain, 344
  skeletal neoplasms, 353
  steroid, 352
  vascular supply, 342, 343
Shoulder fracture, 344
Signal decay, 3, 4
Signal intensity
  blood, 45
    even echo rephasing, 47
    flow-related enhancement, 45–48
    laminar flow, 47, 48
    plug flow, 47, 48
    saturation effects, 45
    spin dephasing effect, 47
    washout effect, 48, 49
  musculoskeletal tissue, 66–68
  vertebral body, 95
    increased marrow fat signal, 95, 101
    radiation therapy, 95, 101
Skeletal neoplasm, 438–440. *See also* specific type
Slice selection, 69–72
Soft tissue disease
  ankle, 308–309
  calf, 308–309
  foot, 308–309
Soft tissue infection, 481–482
Soft tissue mass, nonneoplastic, 457–458
Soft tissue neoplasm, 446–469. *See also* specific type
  ankle, 302
  benign, 446–457
  elbow, 384–388
  foot, 302
  forearm, 384–388
  malignant, 454–457
  nonneoplastic, 457–458
Soleus
  action, 276
  blood supply, 276
  edema, 298
  innervation, 276
  insertion, 276
  origin, 276
Space of Poirier, 412
Spatial encoding, 5, 6
Spatial presaturation, 13–14
  flow compensation, 15
  pulse sequence, 15
Spatial resolution, 72
Spin, 2, 25
Spin density, 3–4, 29
  calculated maps, 44
  supplementary images, 44
Spin echo, 25
Spin-echo formation, 11–12
Spin-echo imaging, 25
Spin-echo pulse sequence, 7–12, 13
Spin-echo signal, isochromat, 47
Spin-lattice relaxation, 4, 5
Spin-lattice relaxation time. *See* T1
Spin-spin relaxation, 3, 5
Spin-spin relaxation time. *See* T2
Spina bidifa aperta, 134
Spina bifida, 134
Spinal artery
  anterior, 102
  posterior, 102
Spinal bifida occulta, 134
Spinal canal
  gradient-echo, diaphragm motion, 104
  narrowing, 114
  stenosis, 108, 109
    myelogram, 108
  T1 weighting, thoracic, 94
  T2 weighting
    midline sagittal thoracic, 94
    progressive weighting, 94
Spinal column, normal anatomy, 90–95
Spinal cord
  atrophy, 109
  blood supply, 102
  cystic mass, 129
  disc fragment, calcified, 114
  dural covering, 102
  enhancing mural nodule, 129
  fusiform intramedullary widening, 126
  gradient-echo, 93, 102
    diaphragm motion, 104
    distal, 96–97
    lumbar, 97
    thoracic, 97
  infection, 127
  inflammation, 127
  intramedullary expansion, 132, 133, 134
  normal anatomy, 101–102
  size, 101
  T1 weighting, 102
    lumbar, 97
    thoracic, 97
  T2 weighting, white vs. gray matter, 102
  thoracic, 89
    sagittal, 88
  transverse myelitis, 128–133, 134
Spinal cord cyst, 138–140
Spinal cord infarct, 144, 145
Spinal cord parenchyma, 127, 132
Spinal dysraphism, 134–137
  occult, 134, 136
Spinal ligament, normal anatomy, 95–101
Spinal lipoma, 134
Spinal nerve
  neural foramina, 90–95
  normal anatomy, 101–102
Spinal nerve root
  dural covering, 102
  gradient-echo, 93
Spine, 87–145. *See also* specific type
  astrocytoma, 123, 128
    postcontrast T1 weighting sequences, 123
  body coil, 87
  body habitus, 90
  cardiac motion, sagittal thoracic, 88
  congenital abnormalities, 134–138
  demyelinating disease, 133–134
  ependymoma, 123, 126, 127
    filum terminale, 123, 126
  extradural lesion, 112–115
    contrast studies, 115
    MRI vs. myelopathy, 112–115
  field strength, 87
  hemangioblastoma, 123–125, 128–130
    vs. intramedullary arteriovenous malformation, 125, 130
  inflammatory conditions, 126–133
  intradural extramedullary lesion, 115–123
    contrast, 121
  intradural metastasis, 123, 124, 125
    enhancing nodules, 123, 124
    noncontrast MRI, 123, 124
  intramedullary lesion, 123–125
  intramedullary metastases, 125, 131
  intraspinal component size, 90
  lipoma, 121, 123
  meningioma, 115, 121
    contrast, 115, 121
  motion
    patient, 88
    physiologic, 88
  MR1, computed tomography myelography, 108
  MRI
    circular coil, 102

contrast agents, 105
examination technique, 102–105
gadolinium diethylenetriaminepentaacetic acid, 105
gradient-echo sagittal sequence, 102–103
license plate coil, 102
multispecialty expertise, 87
pathologic conditions, 105–145
protocol, 104, 105
surface coil, 102–105
T1 weighting sagittal sequence, 102–103
T2 weighting sagittal sequence, 102–103
technical considerations, 87–90
neoplasm, 111–131
nerve sheath tumor, 121
neurofibroma, 121
neurogenic tumor, 115–121, 122
normal anatomy, 90–102
postcontrast studies, 125, 131
spinal curvature, 90
surface coil, 87–88
multiple, 87–88
trauma, 138–139
ascending myelopathy, 140
intramedullary expansion, 139, 140
midthoracic vertebral bodies, 140
post-traumatic cyst, 139, 140
retropulsed fracture fragment, 139
T8 paraplegia, 139
vascular malformation, 139–145
view field, 87
Spondylitis, septic, 480–481
Spondylosis, 108, 109
Steroid
ankle, 352
avascular necrosis, 243, 352
elbow, 352
femoral condyle, 243
femoral head, 174
hip, 352
knee, 243, 352
shoulder, 352
tibia infarct, 243
Stress fracture, 181–182, 240, 241
heel, 286
marrow edema, 514
Subarachnoid space, narrowing, 109
Subchondral cyst, 521
Subclavius, 340–341
action, 330
innervation, 330
insertion, 330
origin, 330
Subscapular bursa, 335–337
Subscapularis, 337
action, 339
innervation, 339
insertion, 339
origin, 339
Subtalar joint, posterior, 261
Supinator
action, 374
blood supply, 374
innervation, 374
insertion, 374
origin, 374
Suprapatellar bursa, 210
Suprapatellar plica, 236, 237
Supraspinatus, 317, 337
action, 339
innervation, 339
insertion, 339
origin, 339
Supraspinous ligament, 101
Surface coil, 63
spine, 87–88
multiple, 87–88
Surgical clip, magnetic field, 54–55
Sustentacular region, 262
Sustentaculum tali, 295
Symphysis, 163
Syndesmosis
lower, 259
upper, 258
Syndesmotic recess, 273
Synovial chondromatosis, 240, 522
Synovial disease, knee, 247–248
Synovial herniation, 174
Synovial hypertrophy, osteoid osteoma, 190
Synovial sarcoma, 187, 457
Synovitis, 391
Syrinx, ependymoma, 126
Syrinx cavity, 128
Systemic lupus, 144

T

T1, 25, 28
calculated maps, 44
correlation time, 30
defined, 3
fat, 40–41
water, 28, 30–31
T2, 25, 28–29
calculated maps, 44
correlation time, 30
protons, 30
defined, 3
diagrammatic representation, 3
fat, 40–41
supplementary images, 44
water, 30–31
T2* ("T-two-star"), 25
T1 relaxation time, blood, 46
T2 weighted spin-echo, meniscal tear, 220
T1 weighting, 36–37
arachnoiditis, 111
cavernous hemangioma, 112, 119
cerebrospinal fluid, 102
cervical spinal canal, 91
cranial vertebral junction, high-resolution, 92
dorsal root ganglion, 98–99
dural sac, 98–99
elbow, 370
end-plate change, 105, 106
evaluation, 37
forearm, 370
gradient-echo, 101
hematoma, 43
hip, 162
intervertebral disc, 95
intraspinal fat, 98–99
meniscal tear, 220
motion, 88
nerve root, 98–99
neural foramen, 98–99
paraspinal fat, 98–99
pelvis, 149–162
plica, 236
scoliosis, 103
selection, 36, 65–72
spinal canal, thoracic, 94
spinal cord, 102
lumbar, 97
thoracic, 97
thigh, 162
tibia, 66
uses, 36
vertebral body, 95
T2 weighting, 36–37
cavernous hemangioma, 112, 119
cerebrospinal fluid, 102
dural arteriovenous fistula, 140, 142
end-plate change, 105, 106
evaluation, 37
gradient-echo, 101
hip, 162
histiocytoma, 40
intervertebral disc, 95
meniscal cyst, 226
motion, 88
neoplasm, 41
pelvis, 149–162
plica, 236
Schwannoma, 40
selection, 36, 65–72
spinal canal
midline sagittal thoracic, 94
progressive weighting, 94
spinal cord, white vs. gray matter, 102
thigh, 162
uses, 36
vertebral body, 95
Talar dome fracture, 286
Talofibular ligament
anterior, 273, 274
posterior, 273, 274
Talus, 273
avascular necrosis, 306, 307, 308
lateral, 270
medial, 269
middle, 269
Tarsal condition, 309
Tarso-metatarsal joint, 274
Tarsus, aneurysmal bone cyst, 440
TE, 25
Temporal bone, eminence, 75, 76
Temporomandibular joint
anatomy, 75–77
closed lock presentation, 76
disc, 75
internal derangement, 76–77, 80–84
lower joint, 75
meniscus, 76–77, 80–84
MRI, 75–84
degenerative joint disease, 80–83
disc dessication, 80, 83
fast gradient-echo images, 78–79
fractured implant, 83, 84
grade 1 joint, 81
grade 2 joint, 82
grading system, 81
GRASS (gradient recalled acquisition in steady state), 81
GRIL (gradient recalled acquisition in steady state interleaved), 78
normal silastic implant, 83, 84
postoperative evaluation, 84
saggital plane T1 weighted images, 77–79
surface coil, 78
T1, 81
technique, 77–79
three-dimensional volume acquisition, 79
vs. computed tomography, 84
upper joint, 75
Tendon sheath, 217
giant cell tumor, 246–247, 447–450, 452

Tensor fasciae latae, 164, 166, 168
  function, 165
  innervation, 165
  insertion, 165
  origin, 165
Teres major, 340
  action, 339
  innervation, 339
  insertion, 339
  origin, 339
Teres minor, 337
  action, 339
  innervation, 339
  insertion, 339
  origin, 339
Tesla, 25
Tethered cord, 134
Thenar eminence, 414–416
  metastatic renal cell carcinoma, 427
Thenar muscle, 405
Thenar region, 400
Thigh
  abductors, 168
  acetabulum, 160
  acquisitions, 162
  adductors, 164, 166
  anatomy, 162–172
  anterior muscles, 169
  anteromedial neurovascular supply, 172
  coronal images, pubic symphysis, 156
  extensors, 164
  femoral head, 160
  femur, 161
  field of view, 162
  flexors, 164, 166
  hemangioma, 187
  iliopectineal eminence, 159
  image time, 162
  inflamed bursae, 172
  matrix, 162
  MRI pitfalls, 172–174
  muscular anatomy, 163–170
  neoplasm, 186–189
  neurovascular anatomy, 170–172
  osseous anatomy, 162–163
  osteomyelitis, 190
    short T1 inversion recovery sequence, 190
  pulse sequence, 162
  rotators, 164, 167
  sciatic notch, 159
  slice thickness, 162
  soft tissue variants, 172
  T1 weighting, 162
  T2 weighting, 162
  trauma, 181–186
    compartment syndromes, 185
    muscle, 182–185
    nerve injuries, 185
    soft tissue, 182–185
  upper, 155
Thoracic myelopathy, 119
Thoracic spine, 333
  osteopenia, 463
Thoracic vertebra, 90
Three-dimensional gradient-echo, meniscal tear, 220
Thrombosis, femoral vein, 46
TI, 25
Tibia, 202, 240, 241, 273
  abscess, 484
  infarct, 308
  metal screws, 59
  methyl methacrylate, 62
  musculoskeletal neoplasm, 437
  osteochondroma, 442
  osteomyelitis, 477
    bilateral, 475
    muscle flap, 486
  periosteal reaction, 474
  posterior, 206
  T1 weighting, 66
  upper, 201, 202
Tibia infarct, steroid, 243
Tibial artery
  anterior, 280, 283, 284
  posterior, 284
Tibial condyle, 209
Tibial nerve, 278
Tibialis anterior, 279
  action, 276
  blood supply, 276
  innervation, 276
  insertion, 276
  origin, 276
Tibialis posterior
  action, 276
  blood supply, 276
  innervation, 276
  insertion, 276
  origin, 276
Tibiofibular articulation, 198–209, 203
Tibiotalar joint, posterior, 264
Tissue characterization, 27–29
TR, 25
Transverse ligament, 214
Transverse myelitis, spinal cord, 128–133, 134
Transverse relaxation, 3, 5
Trapezius, 340
  action, 339
  innervation, 339
  insertion, 339
  origin, 339
Trapezoid fracture, 421
Trauma
  Achilles tendon, 290–291
  ankle, 285–297
    soft tissue, 285–297
  anterior tibial tendon, 295–296
  calf, 285–297
    compartment syndrome, 297
    hematomas, 297, 299
    soft tissue, 285–297
    venous abnormalities, 297, 298
  collateral ligament, 227–233
    MRI vs. arthrography, 232, 233
    repair evaluation, 232–233
  cruciate ligament, 227–233
    MRI vs. arthrography, 232, 233
    repair evaluation, 232–233
  elbow, 382–384
  extensor digitorum longus tendon, 295–296
  extensor hallucis longus tendon, 295–296
  flexor hallucis longus tendon, 291–295
  foot, 285–297
    soft tissue, 285–297
  forearm, 382–384
  hand, 421–422
  hip, 181–186
    compartment syndromes, 185
    muscle, 182–185
    nerve injuries, 185
    soft tissue, 182–185
    two-plane T2 weighting, 185
  medial tendon, 294–295
  MRI
    accuracy, 347–348
    diagnostic criteria, 347
    vs. arthrography, 348
  pelvis, 181–186
    compartment syndromes, 185
    muscle, 182–185
    nerve injuries, 185
    soft tissue, 182–185
    two-plane T2 weighting, 185
  peroneal tendon, 288–290
  posterior tibial, flexor digitorum longus tendon, 291–295
  spine, 138–139
    ascending myelopathy, 140
    intramedullary expansion, 139, 140
    midthoracic vertebral bodies, 140
    post-traumatic cyst, 139, 140
    retropulsed fracture fragment, 139
    T8 paraplegia, 139
  thigh, 181–186
    compartment syndromes, 185
    muscle, 182–185
    nerve injuries, 185
    soft tissue, 182–185
  wrist, 421–422
    soft tissue trauma, 421–422
Triangular fibrocartilage complex, 411
Triangular fibrocartilage tear, 421, 424
Triceps brachii
  action, 374
  blood supply, 374
  innervation, 374
  insertion, 374
  origin, 374
Triceps tendon rupture, 383
  snapping, 383
Triquetrum, 411
Trochanter
  greater, 153
    hip, 161
    pelvis, 161
    thigh, 161
  lesser, 154
Trochlea, 370
Truncation artifact, 88–90
Tuberculous arthritis, 522
Tuberculous spondylitis, 127
Tuberculous synovitis, flexor tendon, 429
Tumor, malignant soft tissue, 29
Two-dimensional Fourier transform, 5

U

Ulna, 370, 411
Ulnar artery, 381, 418, 431
Ulnar nerve, 380, 418, 431
  deep branch, 417
  flow artifact, 382
  nerve compression syndrome, 392
Ulnar nerve compression, 431–433
Ulnar-trochlear articulation, 369
Ulnar vein, 418
Ulno-triquetral ligament, 412
Ulnolunate abutment syndrome, lunate, 340

V

Vascular appliance, artifact, 56
Vascular tumor nodule, 129
Vastus intermedius
  function, 165

innervation, 165, 215
insertion, 165, 215
origin, 165, 215
Vastus lateralis, 168, 169
function, 165
innervation, 165, 215
insertion, 165, 215
origin, 165, 215
Vastus medialis
function, 165
innervation, 165
insertion, 165
muscle tear, 184
origin, 165
Vertebra, 90. *See also* specific type
breast metastasis, 468
lesions mimicking metastasis, 468
osteopenia, 463
Vertebral body
age, 105
gradient-echo, 93, 95
pyogenic discitis, 127, 131
signal intensity, 95
increased marrow fat signal, 95, 101
radiation therapy, 95, 101
T1 weighting, 95
T2 weighting, 95
Vertebral column, 101
View field, spine, 87
Volar carpal ligament, 418
Von Hippel-Lindau disease, hemangioblastoma, 123–125, 128
Voxel, 35, 47

W

Water
bone marrow, 493–494
cytoplasm two-state model for organization, 31
precession, 15, 18
selective images, 44, 45
T1, 28, 30–31
T2, 30–31
Whole volume coil, 63–65
Wrist, 71
aneurysmal bone cyst, 423
anomalous lunotriquetral fusion, 419
arthritis, 425–426
articular anatomy, 411–413
avascular necrosis, 426–429
compartments, 412–413
distal, 397
dorsal image, 404
endochondroma, 423
epidermoid tumor, 424
extensor muscles, 414
flexor muscles, 414
flow artifact, 69
ganglion cyst, 425
giant cell tumor, 423, 425, 426
glomus tumor, 424
infection, 425
ligamentous anatomy, 411–413
MRI, 395–433
anatomic variants, 419
anatomy, 410–410
field of view, 395, 396
osteology, 411
pitfalls, 419–420
pulse sequences, 407
techniques, 345, 407, 410
mucoid cyst, 425
muscular anatomy, 413–418
musculoskeletal neoplasm, 422–425
neurovascular anatomy, 418–419
volar aspect, 416
osteochondroma, 423
osteoid osteoma, 423
radial deviation, 415
rheumatoid arthritis, 519
trauma, 421–422
soft tissue trauma, 421–422
ulnar deviation, 415
volar aspect, 406
Wrist fracture, 524

Y

Yellow marrow, 492
normal, 495
signal characteristics, 494